3RD EDITION

BATES' NURSING GUIDE TO PHYSICAL EXAMINATION AND HISTORY TAKING

Beth Hogan-Quigley, DNP, MSN, RN, CRNP
Biobehavioral Health Sciences Department
University of Pennsylvania School of Nursing
Philadelphia, Pennsylvania

Mary Louise Palm, MS, RN
Associate Clinical Professor Emerita
University of Rhode Island College of Nursing
Kingston, Rhode Island

Wolters Kluwer

Philadelphia • Baltimore • New York • London
Buenos Aires • Hong Kong • Sydney • Tokyo

Not authorised for sale in United States, Canada, Australia, New Zealand, Puerto Rico, and U.S. Virgin Islands.

Vice President and Publisher: Julie K. Stegman
Manager, Nursing Education and Practice Content: Jamie Blum
Senior Acquisitions Editor: Jonathan Joyce
Supervisory Development Editor: Staci Wolfson
Senior Editorial Coordinator: Emily Buccieri
Editorial Assistant: Molly Kennedy
Marketing Manager: Brittany Riney
Senior Production Project Manager: Sadie Buckallew
Manager, Graphic Arts & Design: Stephen Druding
Art Director, Illustration: Jennifer Clements
Manufacturing Coordinator: Margie Orzech
Prepress Vendor: Aptara, Inc.

3rd edition

9 8 7 6 5 4 3 2 1

Printed in China

Library of Congress Cataloging-in-Publication Data
Names: Hogan-Quigley, Beth, author. | Palm, Mary Louise, author.
Title: Bates' nursing guide to physical examination and history taking / Beth Hogan-Quigley, Mary Louise Palm.
Other titles: Nursing guide to physical examination and history taking
Description: Third edition. | Philadelphia, PA : Wolters Kluwer, [2022] | Includes bibliographical references and index.
Identifiers: LCCN 2021025722 | ISBN 9781975161095 (hardback)
Subjects: MESH: Nursing Assessment | Physical Examination | Medical History Taking | BISAC: MEDICAL / Nursing / Assessment & Diagnosis
Classification: LCC RT48.6 | NLM WY 100.4 | DDC 616.07/5–dc23
LC record available at https://lccn.loc.gov/2021025722

shop.lww.com

CCS0821

My heartfelt appreciation and unwavering love for my family:
Peter, for climbing every mountain with me,
Megan, Colleen, Joe, and Rae for making my heart smile,
My parents, Jim and Betty for believing in me,
and Kristin, who will always SHINE on all of us.
I have had the pleasure to work with amazing people
throughout my nursing career.
I am grateful for these opportunities.
BETH HOGAN-QUIGLEY

With much appreciation and thanks to my family:
My husband, William J. Palm, for his support and
love during this project.
My children, Aileene, Bill, and Andy, with love.
Special thanks to my colleagues and students, who encouraged and
supported me throughout my teaching career.
MARY LOUISE PALM

REVIEWERS

Donna Driscoll, DNP, RN, CEN
Faculty
Plymouth State University
Plymouth, New Hampshire

Joan Dugas, PhD(c), RN, CNE
Clinical Associate Professor
University of Rhode Island
Kingston, Rhode Island

Teresa Phillips, EdD, MSN, RN, CCRN, RCIS
Professor
Mount Vernon Nazarene University
Mount Vernon, Ohio

Megan Ray, MSN, RN
Nursing Instructor
College of Saint Mary
Omaha, Nebraska

Lisa L. Sitler, PhD, MSN-Ed, PHNA-BC, SANE
Director of School of Nursing
William Woods University
Fulton, Missouri

Karen Wajda, MSN, RN
Assistant Professor of Nursing
Walsh University
North Canton, Ohio

Ashley York, DNP, AGNP-C, WHNP-BC, NCMP, COI
Assistant Professor
Samford University
Birmingham, Alabama

PREFACE

Bates' Nursing Guide to Physical Examination and History Taking is relevant to the diverse health care arena. Nurses are at the front lines, coordinating and providing holistic care for patients in a multitude of health care delivery systems. The ever-changing world paired with complex patient needs present nursing the opportunity to lead the coordination and provision of holistic care for patients in many venues. Assessment is a key nursing responsibility that ensures the patient receives optimal care. The text provides assessment tools to assist the student with obtaining a thorough history and performing a comprehensive physical examination of each patient. The student will learn how to utilize communication techniques, ask the pertinent subjective questions, and recognize verbal and nonverbal cues while eliciting information related to patient concerns in each body system. The student will utilize subjective findings and critical thinking skills to prioritize and guide the physical examination. The history taking paired with objective findings obtained during the assessment will provide the basis for the analysis and development of the plan of care. Salient points related to health promotion and disease prevention are highlighted for nurses for educating patients, families, and communities.

Bates' Nursing Guide builds on student's knowledge of human anatomy and physiology relevant to the acquisition of patient assessment skills. Throughout the book, the focus and emphasis are the "healthy" patient with common findings or diseases rather than the rare or obscure disorder. Occasionally, physical signs of rare disorders are included if they hold a solid niche in classic physical examination or represent a disorder that is critical to the life of the patient. Each chapter reflects current information, listing key citations that closely align content with new evidence from the health care literature. Coordinating colors help readers find chapter sections and tables more easily and highlight insets of key material and special tips for challenging aspects of examination such as the cranial nerves or assessing lung fields.

BATES' NURSING GUIDE: HIGHLIGHTS

The book is divided into three units: *Foundations, Body Systems,* and *Special Lifespan Considerations.*

Unit 1, Foundations

- *Chapter 1, Introduction to Health Assessment and Social Determinants of Health,* presents the role of the nurse in assessment, including the concept of health and what defines a "healthy" individual. The indicators and purpose of Healthy People 2030 are identified, as are the components of a health assessment in relation to where a person lives and how this intertwines with health risks and outcomes.

- *Chapter 2, Critical Thinking and Clinical Judgment in Health Assessment* focuses on how to think "like a nurse," utilizing a case study approach to implement the nursing process.

- *Chapter 3, Interviewing and Communication,* leads the nursing student through therapeutic communication techniques, shares mnemonics for assessment questions, and identifies strategies for handling difficult patients.

- *Chapter 4, The Health History,* describes the different types of health histories, the purpose for each, and the components of a comprehensive health history.

- *Chapter 5, Cultural and Spiritual Assessment,* explains why culture and spirituality are important in the health assessment and case studies demonstrate cultural humility.

- *Chapter 6, Physical Examination: Getting Started,* introduces a logical sequence of the physical examination with an explanation of the techniques and visualization of the equipment.

- *Chapter 7, General Survey Including Vital Signs and Pain,* and *Chapter 8, Nutrition and Hydration* continue the process of data collection and expand the process of clinical reasoning for nurses.

Unit 2, Body Systems

Chapters 9 through 21 are devoted to the techniques of the regional examination of each of the body systems. These chapters are arranged in a "head-to-toe" sequence, just as the patient examination should flow. Each chapter contains:

- A review of relevant anatomy and physiology
- Key questions for a relevant nursing health history
- Updated information for health promotion and counseling
- Well-described and well-illustrated techniques of examination
- Extensive citations from the clinical literature
- Tables to assist nursing students in recognizing and comparing normal and abnormal findings

The unit concludes with *Chapter 22, Putting the Physical Examination All Together*, which assists the student nurse in performing a "head-to-toe" examination following a systems integration sequence. Students frequently need this step-by-step guidance as they learn new skills and process how the objective data are collected in a systematic manner.

Unit 3, Special Lifespan

Chapter 23, Assessing Children: Infancy through Adolescence, and *Chapter 24, Assessing Older Adults* relate to special ages in the life cycle and how the assessment techniques and physical examination findings may differ.

This textbook is written for the undergraduate nursing student and geared to the generalist nurse. The focus of the book is **nursing** physical examination and history taking. The health history and the physical examination are both essential for patient assessment and care.

Students are advised to return to chapters, especially in the *Foundations* unit, as they gain additional experience with patients. Each patient brings a unique background and set of abilities, ideas, issues, coping mechanisms, and family and community dynamics to the health care setting. These attributes mixed with a disease process can be confounding to even the seasoned nurse.

Students may study or review the "Anatomy and Physiology" sections according to their individual needs. They can study the "Physical Examination" sections to learn how to perform the relevant examination, practice it under faculty guidance, and review the section again afterward to consolidate their learning.

Students and faculty will benefit from identifying common abnormal findings, which appear in two places. The red marginal text of the "Physical Examination" sections presents possible abnormal findings. Tables in each chapter will deepen students' understanding of important clinical conditions, what they should be looking for, and why they are asking certain questions. However, students should not try to memorize all the detail that is presented. As students work to master the skills of assessment, they should return to the related signs and remember ideal findings.

As students progress through each body system, they should study the documentation for the sample patient, Mrs. N, found in Chapter 2, *Critical Thinking and Clinical Judgment in Health Assessment*. Students should make frequent references to the sections in each of the body systems chapters titled "Recording Your Findings" that display samples of a patient record. This cross-checking will help students learn how to describe and organize information from the interview and physical examination into an understandable documentation format. Furthermore, studying Chapter 22, *Putting the Physical Examination All Together*, will help students integrate the body systems examinations into a coordinated head-to-toe physical examination.

STUDENT AND INSTRUCTOR RESOURCES

Student Resources

Student resources to accompany this text are available online at thePoint®.

Resources include journal articles, NCLEX-style review questions, a Spanish-English audio glossary, Watch and Learn video clips, and Concepts in Action animations.

Instructor Resources

Instructor resources are also available on thePoint® and include the following:

- Test Generator containing over 400 multiple choice questions
- PowerPoint presentations
- Image Bank featuring all of the figures from each chapter
- Guided Lecture Notes for presenting key information to your students
- Assignments and Prelecture Quizzes for gauging student understanding
- Discussion Topics to encourage critical thinking
- Case Studies providing real-life application of concepts

A FULLY INTEGRATED COURSE EXPERIENCE

We offer an expanded suite of digital solutions to support instructors and students using *Bates' Nursing Guide to Physical Examination and History Taking,* 3rd edition, that elevate the learning experience. To learn more about any of these solutions, please contact your local Wolters Kluwer representative.

Lippincott CoursePoint and CoursePoint+: An Adaptive Learning Experience

Lippincott® CoursePoint is an integrated, digital curriculum solution for nursing education that provides a completely interactive experience geared to help students understand, retain and apply their course knowledge and be prepared for practice. The time-tested, easy-to-use and trusted solution includes engaging learning tools, evidence-based practice, case studies, and in-depth reporting to meet students where they are in their learning, combined with the most trusted nursing education content on the market to help prepare students for practice. This easy-to-use digital learning solution of *Lippincott® CoursePoint+,* combined with unmatched support, gives instructors and students everything they need for course and curriculum success!

Lippincott® CoursePoint+ includes:

- Leading content provides a variety of learning tools to engage students of all learning styles.
- A personalized learning approach gives students the content and tools they need, giving them data for focused remediation and a boost to their confidence and competence.
- Powerful tools, including varying levels of case studies, interactive learning activities, and adaptive learning powered by PrepU, help students learn the critical thinking and clinical judgment skills to help them become practice-ready nurses.
- Preparation for Practice improves student competence, confidence, and success in transitioning to practice.
  - vSim® for Nursing: Co-developed by Laerdal Medical and Wolters Kluwer, vSim® for Nursing simulates real nursing scenarios and allows students to interact with virtual patients in a safe, online environment.
  - Lippincott® Advisor for Education: With over 8,500 entries covering the latest evidence-based content and drug information, Lippincott® Advisor for Education provides students with the most up-to-date information possible, while giving them valuable experience with the same point-of-care content they will encounter in practice.
- Unparalleled reporting provides in-depth dashboards with several data points to track student progress and help identify strengths and weaknesses.
- Unmatched support includes training coaches, product trainers, and nursing education consultants to help educators and students implement CoursePoint with ease.

ACKNOWLEDGMENTS

We appreciate the many professionals at Wolters Kluwer who provided guidance throughout the writing of the third edition of *Bates' Nursing Guide to Physical Examination and History Taking*. We had the good fortune to work with many outstanding professionals who took the lead at varying stages of the project. We also are thankful for the numerous individuals working diligently behind the scenes to bring this latest edition to fruition.

Individual acknowledgments and appreciation are warranted for those we worked most closely:

Jonathan Joyce, Senior Acquisitions Editor, laid the groundwork for the third edition.

Staci Wolfson, Supervisory Development Editor, Nursing Content Publishing, was our go-to person. She communicated with us frequently and was available at a moment's notice.

Emily Buccieri, Senior Editorial Coordinator, had a keen eye for details and offered her expertise.

Karan Rana, project manager at Aptara, orchestrated the page proofs.

Our colleagues provided expertise and support for our endeavor and helped make this text a reality.

Connie Scanga, PhD, provided additional clarification on various aspects of anatomy and physiology.

Colleen Quigley assisted with photography.

Megan Quigley developed computer graphics at a moment's notice.

To our students, past and present, who inspire us to write and educate the nurses of the future.

CONTENTS

UNIT 1

Foundations

1 INTRODUCTION TO HEALTH ASSESSMENT AND SOCIAL DETERMINANTS OF HEALTH

KEY TERMS		
health	nursing health assessment	social determinants of health (SDOH)

Learning Objectives

The student will:

1. Define and identify social determinants of health.
2. Define health and health assessment.
3. Explain the components of the health assessment.
4. Identify the health indicators and purpose of *Healthy People 2030*.
5. Define the nurse's role in assessment.

Health assessment is an integral part of nursing practice. There are over 3.8 million registered nurses nationwide working in a variety of capacities (Smiley et al., 2018). Nurses are visible in both inpatient and outpatient facilities, homes, work sites, and in various community settings. Every nurse, no matter where the practice is situated, is assessing health (American Association of Colleges of Nursing, 2008).

Social determinants of health (SDOH) are proven to affect a person's health and are the effects of where people work, live, play, and learn (Centers for Disease Control and Prevention, 2020). SDOH are associated with health risks and outcomes. If a person lives at the poverty level, it limits its accessibility to safe neighborhoods, nutritious foods, and education, all factors in better health outcomes (Hahn et al., 2018). Addressing SDOH positively impacts the health of people and their communities and takes a step forward in achieving health equity.

In nursing, regardless of which career path you take, assessment techniques are essential. Astute attention to details, use of appropriate questions, and a keen awareness of what a person says and does shape the plan of care to optimize each individual's health status throughout the lifespan.

HEALTH

There are eight dimensions to health. **Health** is a relative state in which a person strives to meet their potential and includes the areas of wellness with the ultimate goal of improving health. The eight dimensions are: physical, emotional, social, spiritual, environmental, intellectual, financial, and occupational (U.S. Department of Health and Human Services Substance Abuse and Mental Health Services Administration [SAMHSA], 2016). Health is the sum of these and is not solely defined as the absence of disease or eating right, but rather by the contributions of all dimensions. The health care team must take into account all of these domains (Fig. 1-1).

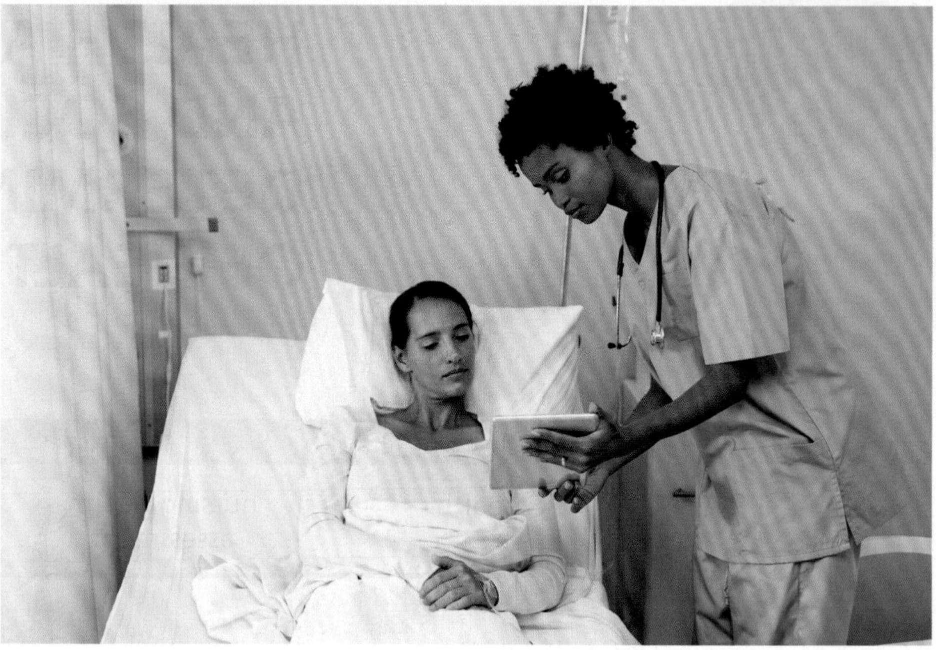

FIGURE 1-1 Collaboration to determine the best assessment strategies (wavebreakmedia/Shutterstock).

Health is influenced by all eight dimensions (Fig. 1-2, Box 1-1). A person's ability to adapt while not compromising the different components is important for health maintenance. Health is not a constant and cannot be taken for granted. The ability to juggle and align the eight dimensions in a harmonious network leads to a healthy state for an individual.

In all aspects, it is best to work with the patient to enable partnering in choices. This allows the patient to make decisions regarding health care. The more a patient participates in these decisions, the better the outcomes are for a long-term healthier lifestyle. Reminding ourselves of the social determinants of health and how they may affect each person individually is important in determining the plan of care.

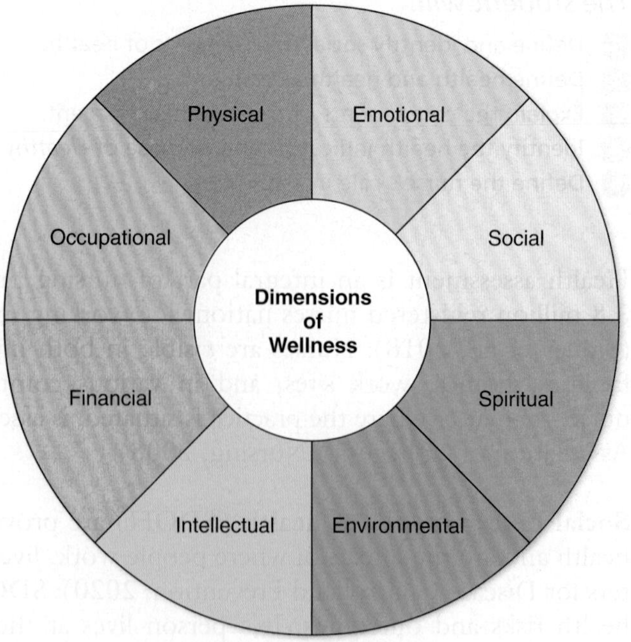

FIGURE 1-2 Eight dimensions of wellness.

BOX 1-1 EIGHT DIMENSIONS OF HEALTH AND WELLNESS

Physical wellness takes into consideration multiple areas including activity level and exercise, proper nutrition, and sleep. It also looks at promoting healthy coping behaviors and identifying nonhealthy behaviors such as smoking, excess caffeine intake, or substance abuse.

Emotional health is the ability to handle life and its challenges that may arise. The ability to be resilient and use coping mechanisms effectively, including strong relationships with others, are recognized.

Social wellness is a sense of inclusiveness and connection. If a patient feels isolated, figuring out family dynamics and a potential support system are important. Providing information about self-help groups, health resources, and local organizations can promote additional avenues for socialization.

Spiritual health involves a person's sense of values and beliefs. A patient may wish to speak with a spiritual advisor or may utilize meditation or some other form of self-care. Often, it is best to broach this topic and let the patient take the lead on how to handle spiritual care, as this dimension is individual.

Environmental wellness encompasses the patient's surroundings, which may be in the home or outside and can affect health. Neighborhood safety related to violence or inside the home related to physical or sexual abuse are examples of factors to assess. Overall disorganization may negatively influence how one feels and affect health.

Intellectual wellness is the ability to advance knowledge and is different for each person. A patient may need guidance in areas to enhance this component and suggestions might be to read, engage in a new hobby, tutor others, or learn a new language.

Financial aspects of health are often stressful. Finances for the basics such as shelter, food, and health care may be lacking. Insurance may not cover all facets of care or specific providers. Illness often leads to decreased income with increased costs for care and medication.

Occupational wellness involves the work milieu, including the type of job, relationships with coworkers, and management of stress levels. This is important in conjunction with a healthy work–life balance.

HEALTH ASSESSMENT

The **nursing health assessment** entails both a comprehensive health history and a complete physical examination, which are used to evaluate the health status of a person. The ability to solicit information, understand the findings, and apply knowledge can initially be daunting to the new nurse. The nursing health assessment involves a systematic data collection that provides information to facilitate a plan to deliver the best care for the patient.

The first part of the health assessment is the health history, which also incorporates the eight dimensions. The nurse asks pertinent questions to gather data from the patient and/or family. Past medical records may also be used to collect additional information. Learning about the patient's physical, emotional, social, financial, occupational, environmental, intellectual, and spiritual beliefs and issues contributes to a well-rounded history.

The second component of the health assessment is the physical examination. The nurse uses a structured head-to-toe examination to identify changes in the patient's body systems. An unusual or abnormal finding may support the history data or trigger additional questions.

Concept Mastery Alert

Types of Health Assessments

When determining the type of health assessment to complete, the nurse needs to consider the patient's current situation and condition. A focused assessment is completed on a patient who has already had a comprehensive examination and is being seen for a follow-up visit. A patient who presents with a new problem of a serious or critical nature would require an emergency assessment to determine the patient's current status. However, if this patient is now stable and the acute condition has subsided, the nurse needs to complete a comprehensive health assessment to evaluate all body systems to better decide which system is contributing to the patient's current problem.

The purpose of the nursing health assessment is to determine a patient's health status, risk factors, and need for education as a basis for developing a nursing plan of care. The ability of the nurse to extrapolate the findings, prioritize them, and finally formulate and implement the plan of care is the overall goal. This is called the nursing process. The information obtained throughout the health assessment should be documented in a clear, concise manner. This information is collated in the patient's medical records.

The health assessment is similar to a puzzle. When the nurse meets a patient, it is like opening the puzzle box and dumping out the pieces. Each piece of the history and examination data represents a different aspect of the patient's life, which form a picture of who the patient is. The review of systems in the health history is like the corner and edge pieces of a puzzle that form the frame, in this case, the basis for the assessment and how to proceed with the physical examination. Once the frame is in place it is easier to complete the puzzle. Listening and understanding a patient is key to having the pieces fit (Fig. 1-3). The health assessment assists the nurse with discovering a patient's needs. As a rapport with the patient develops, more details are acquired. As the information is collated, actual health risks emerge, and eventually those last hard-to-fit puzzle pieces are found, which represent the potential health risks. This intricate puzzle is a person's life, and the pieces need to fit correctly for the person to maintain health and quality of life. As the puzzle takes shape, a picture is formed. Likewise, the nurse is able to see the patient as an individual more clearly and is able to create a specific nursing plan of care.

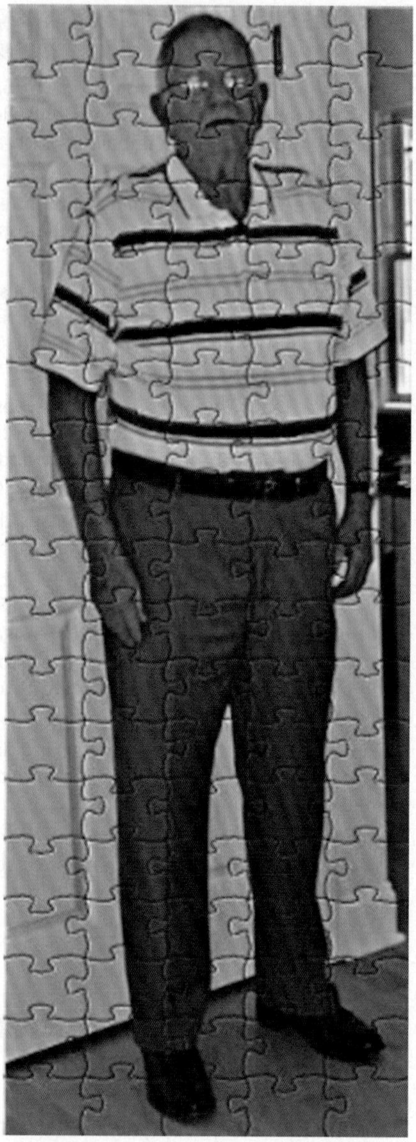
FIGURE 1-3 Individual health assessments explore the pieces of each unique puzzle.

The assessment is typically performed on the patient's arrival to a health care facility. The extent of the health assessment is determined by the acuity of the patient's condition and the site of the care. For example:

- The patient in critical condition brought into a busy emergency department would be asked basic questions revolving around the event that precipitated the admission and whether the patient is on medications, has any allergies, or has any adverse reactions. The thorough health history would be completed when the patient was stable and able to answer questions.

- The patient who has a professional relationship with the nurse and had a thorough health assessment at the initial meeting does not need to have a health history repeated on each visit. Updates based on new events would be added as necessary.

- The nursing home admission of a patient with dementia may require the health assessment information to be supplemented with information from the family, past health care providers, and/or medical records, based on the ability of the patient to remember information.

Each person needs a complete health assessment. Ideally this is done on admission, but extenuating circumstances may prohibit its completion in detail at this time. The sooner the health assessment is completed fully, the better the nurse knows the patient, and more holistic care can be provided to ensure health promotion and quality of life.

Nursing and medical professionals both perform health assessments, and although the assessment techniques may be similar, the use is different. A medical diagnosis refers to the disease process and illness. This diagnosis is at the discretion of the physician. In contrast, the focus of the nursing analysis is on the patient's response to the medical condition or disease. An example is the medical diagnosis of hypertension; the physician focuses on figuring out the etiology of the disease and how to treat the high blood pressure using medical or surgical interventions. The nurse focuses on how to treat the patient's potential responses, such as fear of the diagnosis, risk of falling related to the potential for fainting, lack of knowledge regarding new medications, and the need for education about lifestyle changes involving diet and exercise. The nursing assessment identifies many contributing factors to the individual's health and wellness, including the eight dimensions. The health assessment facilitates data collection specific to the patient. As the nurse spends time with the patient, identification of concerns or changes are uncovered. Any deviation is noted, as are the coping mechanisms and resources the patient has available. This information is used to determine health problems or other potential problems. In the hypertension example, the patient may be a smoker or have had a family member who had a stroke related to high blood pressure. Concerns over the financial implications, inability to lift items, or dealing with stress at work might be shared. Taking all dimensions into account when developing the nursing care plan and working with the individual patient are paramount in health promotion and nursing care.

Once the plan is in place, evaluation continually occurs, and reconfiguring the plan may be necessary. The health care team meets to collaborate on plans for patients and decides the best overall care. This occurs throughout the lifespan, from the inception of life until death. The collaboration of the health care team is invaluable and may include nurses, physicians, nutritionists, social workers, physical therapists, occupational therapists, speech therapists, dentists, and more. These professionals all work together on the same team for the benefit of the patient. The partnership and coordination with all members of the team, with input from the patient as a key stakeholder and team member, is crucial to the success of the plan.

Through the health assessment, nurses detect areas of concern, requiring immediate attention, as well as health maintenance or improvement needs. Nurses have taken the lead in health promotion and disease prevention and assist patients with changing behaviors and lifestyles to obtain optimal health. Such changes enable individuals to increase control of and improve their overall health. Selecting the level of care and teaching is governed by the nurse as care is rendered. During the overall assessment of the patient, the nurse uses the findings to decide the areas that take precedence.

Concept Mastery Alert

Addressing Health Concerns

When the assessment uncovers possible additional health issues, the nurse should extend the allotted time to sufficiently gather additional information critical to creating an effective plan of care. The most effective time to gather such information is during the assessment that is currently being performed.

Health promotion and disease prevention are essential areas of patient education. Maintaining health is a balancing act influenced by behaviors and choices. Health education is a vital component of nursing practice. The nurse assists people in making connections between a healthy lifestyle and disease prevention. Additional components that contribute to health include the individual's personality and attitude, resilience, family dynamics, access to health care and resources, nutrition, exercise, culture, and beliefs.

Healthy People 2030 is a campaign that uses a framework for improved health based on the National Health Promotion and Disease Prevention objectives set forth by the Secretary of Health and Human Services advisory committee (Hahn et al., 2018). The U.S. Department of Health and Human Services provides the data online and invites health care leaders and individuals in the community to voice their opinions regarding the focus for the next decade (Hahn et al., 2018). The national health objectives in *Healthy People 2030* are broad and take into consideration the results of the *Healthy People 2020* outcomes. These are based on current data, new developments, and challenges that are prevalent or emerging in the United States related to American risk factors, health issues, and diseases of concern (*Healthy People 2030,* 2020). The goals and objectives serve to improve the health of individuals and communities, targeting 10-year increments. The overall goal is to increase quality of life by creating guidelines for a healthy lifestyle as well as educating people and cultivating an awareness that will assist in the elimination of national health disparities. *Healthy People 2030* promotes health and disease prevention as it improves the quality and length of a person's life (*Healthy People 2030,* 2020). *Healthy People* initiatives include the SDOH and address physical and social environments to promote health for everyone as a main goal (Hahn et al., 2018).

The *Healthy People 2030* indicators pertinent to individuals are determined as the nurse completes the health assessment on each patient. Using the website healthypeople.gov, the nurse can identify health indicators, appropriate interventions, and resources (*Healthy People 2030,* 2020).

Role of the Nurse in Assessment

Nurses deliver care across the lifespan in a variety of practice arenas. A small sample of the groups served are pediatrics, geriatrics, medical, surgical, mental health, maternity, and community health. Nurses assess patient needs, develop interventions, and educate and counsel individuals, families, groups, and communities toward higher levels of health and wellness. Nurses view health as the focus with the patient, the environment, and the nurse all influencing the health status of the patient. It is crucial to use all eight dimensions that affect the patient's health, as this guides the nursing plan of care. Also important is the patient's view and definition of health. One person may view health as being free of disease. Another may indicate health as good control of blood pressure. One person has a chronic disease and the other does not, but they may both see themselves as healthy. When meeting with the patient, ask what their goals and views are:

"What would you like to accomplish during this visit?"
"Tell me how you see yourself with regard to health."
"Tell me why you are here today."

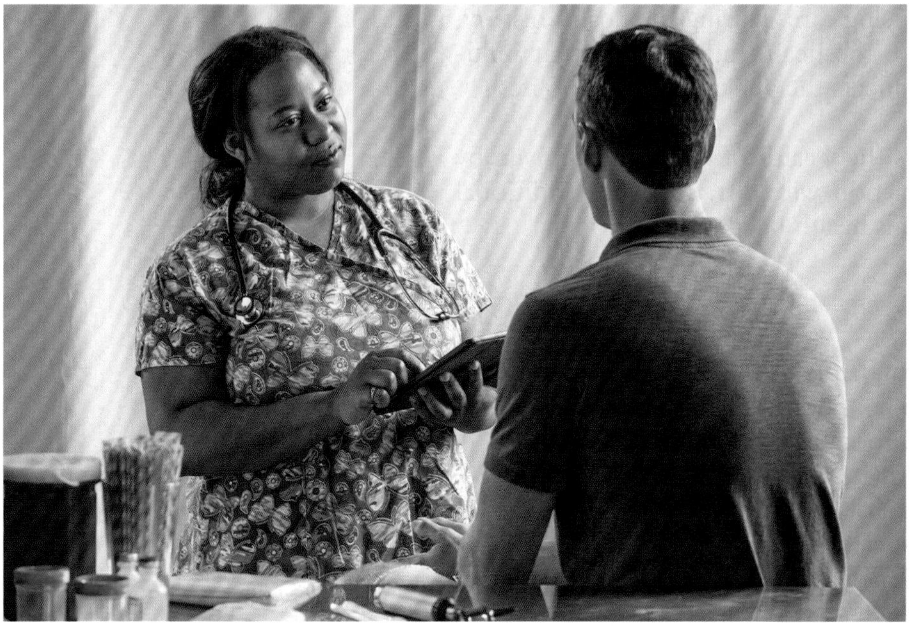

FIGURE 1-4 Nurse taking a health history (Burlingham/Shutterstock).

Focusing on the answers (verbal) and the actions (nonverbal) of the patient, the nurse is constantly assessing and formulating a plan of care so that the patient can achieve the best possible health (Fig. 1-4).

Health goes beyond the individual patient. It also encompasses the community. Nurses are involved in shaping public policy and in social, economic, and workplace decisions. For the nurse to assist a patient with health, a healthy environment must be nurtured. The community and the environment need to be defined and realistic goals set for possible change, such as access to healthy foods. In the context of environment, what does this mean? Accessibility to healthy school lunch programs and proximity to grocery stores with affordable, fresh produce. This sets a path for prevention of illness and maintenance of health and wellness. Nurses assess the individual, family, and the community; however, the focus of this text will be the assessment of the individual.

Nurses are instrumental in the care of patients. They oversee the holistic care of each patient. The nurse's initial role in health assessment is to collect data. Constant observation and attention to details and nuances are critical. Each person comes with a vast array of information and is influenced by the surroundings, including the physical, emotional, intellectual, and spiritual environments. This extensive body of knowledge and the responsibility that each patient encounter requires can seem overwhelming to the new nurse. As the nurse becomes more proficient and comfortable in the role, the knowledge base and expertise increase and foster confidence.

As a nurse, it is vital to sift through all the patient information and make decisions about what information will impact patient safety and quality of care. The ability to identify what is important on a daily basis for each individual patient is paramount for nursing care. During the health history, the nurse asks questions to determine the health information that influences the day-to-day care and how it affects the person's quality of life.

The following brief encounter depicts the wealth of information given by one patient. During this short interaction with Mr. P., what additional questions are you forming related to his health needs?

CASE STUDY

Mr. P. arrives at the clinic with complaints of blurred vision. During the health history, the patient also confides to the nurse that he has not been able to make it to the bathroom in time and has been incontinent frequently. He verbalizes that he is upset that he is unable to see well which has slowed down his mobility. The decrease in mobility and incontinence have limited his social life with friends and he is becoming more irritable and feeling lonely. He admits to feeling like he wants to sleep all the time.

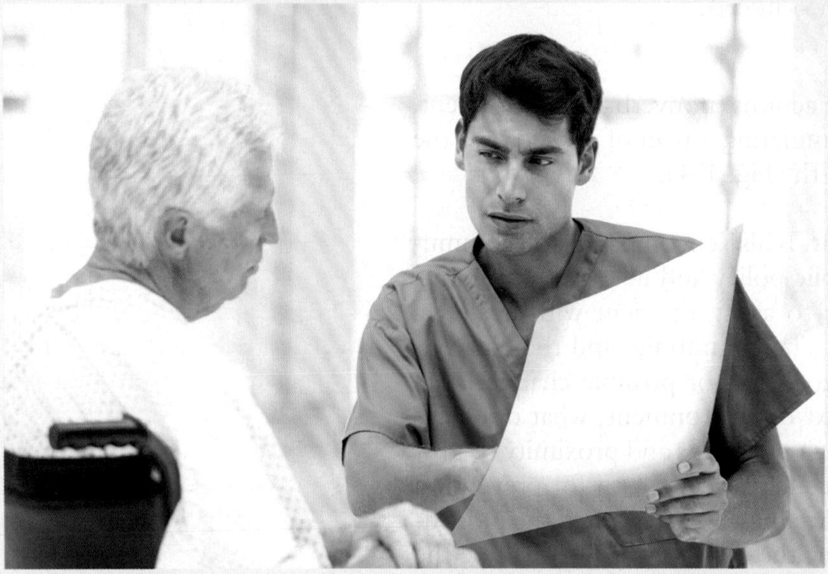

Monkey Business Images/Shutterstock.

The nurse is already formulating additional questions to correlate with the standard health history based on what the patient has disclosed. As you read through this book, you will learn more questions to ask, those that are system-specific as well as those regarding overlapping systems. How you interpret this nurse–patient interaction will be much different after you learn how to do a health assessment.

As a student nurse, you might take the encounter at face value and attribute Mr. P.'s downward spiral to his initial report of blurred vision. However, after a thorough assessment, you may uncover additional issues and determine that his vision problem is not the root of his irritability and fatigue.

There is too little information available in this scenario to determine what is going on with this patient. It is important to allot a sufficient amount of time to do a detailed health assessment. Once more details are uncovered, more possibilities arise. Mr. P. could potentially have multiple issues, such as diabetes, a brain tumor, depression, blurred vision, or benign prostatic hypertrophy. However, these discoveries will not be unearthed without more information.

Accurate health history taking and physical assessment are the foundation of nursing practice. Nurses rely heavily on these skills in all aspects of nursing. The puzzle will be pieced together during the nursing history and assessment. For example, the patient recovering from an illness or surgery needs to be carefully assessed each shift, with changes noted that may indicate potentially dire consequences.

Assessing the patient by using the eight dimensions is at the forefront of the nurse's responsibilities. Physically, the nurse may discover a change in vital signs, nausea, difficulty swallowing, or incontinence. Mentally, the patient may be experiencing changes in the level of consciousness and not know where they are or even who they are. Emotionally, is the patient more subdued, angry, or crying after a visit from a family member? The nurse will pursue the reasons behind a mood change in the patient. Could there be abuse, money concerns, or a fear of abandonment? The nurse has developed a rapport with the patient and is now able to delve into territory that may have been previously off limits. Once these issues are acknowledged, the patient can develop a healthier life with appropriate interventions and options. Developmentally, a patient may need guidance in areas such as problem solving or moral understanding. Socially, the patient may be isolated from their support system in the hospital and need additional outlets. Providing information about self-help groups or health resources can provide additional avenues for people socially. Spiritually, it is best to let the patient take the lead on how to handle spiritual care, as this dimension is personal. If the patient wishes, connecting them with clergy of the same denomination while in the hospital may be welcome, or assisting with transportation to worship services when at home may be reasonable. In all aspects, it is best to work with the patient to enable partnering in choices, addressing access and how social determinants of health may impact these choices. This allows the patient to make decisions regarding their own health care. The more a patient participates in these decisions, the better the outcomes are in the long term toward a healthier lifestyle.

Teaching opportunities for the patient and family present themselves during health assessments. The nurse uses information detected in the assessment to work with the patient to enhance quality of life. For example, the person who is overweight and has an increased body mass index might need assistance with meal planning or an exercise regimen. A plan that includes the family may be the best solution for one individual, but another may do better with an outside support group. A mutually agreed upon plan will assist the patient in maintaining autonomy to achieve the highest possible level of wellness.

The nurse's ability to detect a change in a patient's physical, emotional, environmental, intellectual, financial, occupational, social, or spiritual self, whether slight or significant, is instrumental in providing the best care. Just as a detective asks questions, the nurse finds clues and follows up on information in order to solve patient problems. Knowing how to facilitate the nursing health assessment by asking appropriate questions to obtain more information helps solve the mystery and create a nursing care plan. The care plan is evaluated periodically, and changes are made to update the plan. The nurse, like a detective, is always reassessing the patient and their case for changes in order to achieve the best results. Each relies on both the science and art of their respective profession.

The nursing process will be explained in detail in Chapter 2, "Critical Thinking and Clinical Judgment in Health Assessment."

REFERENCES

American Association of Colleges of Nursing. (2008). *The Nursing Fact Sheet.* American Association of Colleges of Nursing. Retrieved June 8, 2020, from https://www.aacnnursing.org/News-Information/Fact-Sheets/Nursing-Fact-Sheet

Centers for Disease Control and Prevention. (2020). Social determinants of health: Know what affects health. Retrieved June 8, 2020, from https://www.cdc.gov/socialdeterminants/index.htm

Hahn, R. A., Truman, B. I., & Williams, D. R. (2018). Civil rights as determinants of public health and racial and ethnic health equity: Health care, education, employment, and housing in the United States. *Population Health, 4,* 17–24. https://doi.org/10.1016/j.ssmph.2017.10.006

Healthy People 2030. Retrieved May 1, 2020, from http://www.healthypeople.gov.

Smiley, R. A., Lauer, P., Bienemy, C., Berg, J. G., Shireman, E., Reneau, K. A., & Alexander, M. (2018). The 2017 National Nursing Workforce Survey. *Journal of Nursing Regulation, 9*(3), supplement (S1–S54).

U.S. Department of Health and Human Services Substance Abuse and Mental Health Services Administration (SAMHSA). (2016). The eight dimensions of wellness. http://www.samhsa.gov/wellness-initiative/eight-dimensions-wellness

2 CRITICAL THINKING AND CLINICAL JUDGMENT IN HEALTH ASSESSMENT

KEY TERMS

assessment	objective data	subjective data

Learning Objectives

The student will:

1. Define subjective and objective data.
2. Identify appropriate subjective questions for the health history.
3. Explain the nursing process.
4. Explain the clinical reasoning process and its relationship to the nursing process.
5. Identify a patient's problems prioritized by severity.
6. Create a nursing care plan for a patient.
7. Analyze a written patient history and physical examination findings to identify patient problems and develop a nursing care plan.
8. Evaluate and revise a care plan based on a simulation of a patient.

The goal of health assessment by the nurse is the development of an individualized plan of care for each patient. The nursing process is *a problem-solving process* the nurse uses to identify patient problems; set goals and develop an action plan; implement the plan; and evaluate the outcome by determining if the interventions resolved or improved the patient's problem or if the plan needs to be revised.

There are five steps in the nursing process, and they include assessment, diagnosis, planning, implementation, and evaluation.

During the **assessment** phase, the nurse gathers patient data via the health history and examination of the patient. A *clinical reasoning* process is then used to analyze the patient data and develop hypotheses about the patient's problem or problems. Once the problems are defined, the nurse develops the plan of care and implements and evaluates it. During the process, the nurse records the patient assessment findings and the plan of care in the patient record to communicate the patient's story and the nurse's clinical reasoning and plan to the other health care team members. This chapter will discuss types of patient data, the clinical reasoning process, and the nursing process.

Critical thinking is ongoing, as is assessment of the patient. The two are intricately intertwined, and neither exists in isolation. The health assessment is the discovery and collation of facts from both the health history and physical examination. The comprehensive health history and physical assessment build the foundation of the clinical assessment (Fig. 2-1).

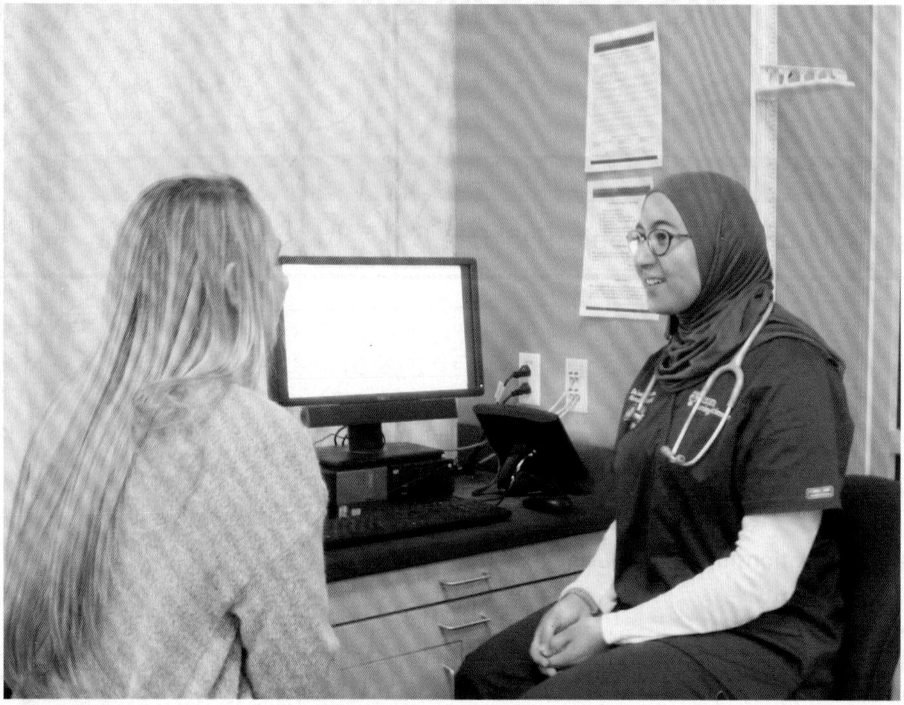

FIGURE 2-1 The clinical assessment comprises the comprehensive health history and physical assessment.

TYPES OF PATIENT DATA

Through skilled interviewing, the nurse will gather the history from the patient or the family; this is the **subjective data**, which are also known as *symptoms*. After the interview and collection of subjective data, the nurse will perform either a head-to-toe physical examination or a systems-specific examination based on the patient's information. The **objective data** are the information gathered from the physical examination and the laboratory tests. These are primarily factual and descriptive and are also known as *signs*. Table 2-1 outlines the differences between subjective and objective data.

TABLE 2-1 Differences between Subjective and Objective Data

Subjective Data: Symptoms	Objective Data: Signs
What the patient describes or tells you	What you detect during the examination
The history, from chief complaint through review of systems	All physical examination findings and laboratory results; measurable data
Example: Mrs. G is a 54-year-old veteran who reports pressure over her left chest "like an elephant sitting there," which radiates to her left neck and arm.	*Example:* Mrs. G is an older, overweight female, who is pleasant and cooperative. Height 5 ft 4 in, weight 150 lb, BMI 26, BP 160/80 right arm, sitting, HR 96 and regular, respiratory rate 24 and regular, temperature 97.5°F oral

As you learn the techniques of history taking and physical examination, remember the important differences between *subjective information* and *objective information*. These distinctions are equally important for organizing written and oral presentations about patients into a logical and understandable format.

Obtaining Subjective Data

During the history, a rapport develops between the nurse and the patient, and a mutual trust begins. As the fact-finding mission of the health history proceeds and data are collected, the nurse is putting pieces of the patient's puzzle together. By asking questions, the nurse clarifies the patient's problems and teaching needs. Each time the patient has a positive response to a question, the topic should be addressed further. As a new nurse, the questions you need to ask may seem endless, and the use of the mnemonic "OLD CART" is instrumental in assisting you with formulating the questions. Remember to ask one question at a time to ensure a thorough understanding on both the patient's and nurse's parts. The patient needs to understand each specific question, and questions should be asked one at a time. Once the question is answered clearly, moving to the next question is appropriate. An organized and deliberate interaction by the nurse enables an understanding of which answers pertain to the specific question.

OLD CART
Onset
Location
Duration
Characteristic symptoms
Associated manifestations
Relieving factors
Treatment

CLINICAL TIP
Remember to open the chief complaint (CC) interview with a broad, open-ended question; for example, "Tell me about your headache from when it began until now." Then use the OLD CART mnemonic to identify missing data.

Mr. C. is a 57-year-old male who presents to the clinic with complaints of a headache. During questioning, you refer to "OLD CART:"

Onset: When the sign or symptom began
When did the headache begin?
Location: Where the sign or symptom is located
Where exactly is the headache? Can you point to it? Does it radiate?
Duration: How long the sign or symptom has been present
Does the headache come and go? Is it continuous? What time of day is it most severe?
Characteristic symptoms: What the symptom feels like, how it is described, and the severity
How does the headache feel? Is it throbbing? Sharp? Stabbing? Describe it. Rate it on a scale of 1 to 10, with 10 being the worst pain you have ever felt in your life.
Associated manifestations: What else is going on when the patient experiences the sign(s) or symptom(s)
Does anything else happen when you get the headaches? Blurred vision? Nausea? Vomiting? Seizures?
Relieving factors: Anything the patient has tried to relieve the headache
What have you tried to make your headache subside? Cool compresses? Rest in a dark room? Did it work?
Treatments: Any interventions the patient has previously tried
Has the patient seen a health care provider? Tried any remedies like medications (prescription, over-the-counter, or herbal) or acupuncture to make the headache go away? Does it work?

NURSING PROCESS

The nurse collects patient information to synthesize (assessment), decide what is most important (nursing analysis), develop a plan (goals/plan), implement the plan (interventions), and determine whether it is working for the patient (evaluation). This occurs in a multitude of sites and settings with all types of people. Examples are numerous:

- At the community clinic, while assessing length and weight, you note that a 2-month-old has not gained any weight in the past month.
- At the senior center, you note that the blood pressure reading of one of the members is 192/104 mm Hg, R arm, sitting.
- Postoperatively, you assess your patient and find him crying uncontrollably.

These scenarios can have different outcomes based on how the nurse and patient handle the situation. As a student nurse, you may find yourself in a quandary, uncertain of how to handle a situation or what to tackle first. Developing your knowledge base and diagnostic reasoning skills will assist with the problem-solving process. The nursing process facilitates logical and efficient structuring of the patient's care.

The nursing process is the broad systematic framework that provides a methodical base for the practice of nursing. This problem-solving approach addresses the human responses and needs of each patient, family, and community. The nursing process is also the scaffold that the American Nurses Association uses to develop the Standards of Nursing Practice.

The patient is the focus in the nursing process, with the nurse assisting the patient in achieving optimal health using individualized interventions. This is a mutually agreed upon plan of care which contributes to the patient's involvement and increased success.

The five steps of the nursing process are assessment, analysis, planning, implementation, and evaluation. These five steps are all incorporated into the patient's plan of care and revised as the patient's health status changes (Table 2-2).

A nursing analysis is designed in response to an issue a person, family, or community is having in response to a health condition or vulnerable situation. The nursing analysis guides the plan of care and selection of individualized nursing interventions to attain positive outcomes (Benner, 2001).

TABLE 2-2 Assessment, Analysis, Planning, Implementation, Evaluation

Assessment	• *Assessment is the subjective and objective data gathered during the initial health history and physical examination and collected on each patient encounter.* • This data is instrumental in devising a plan of care for the patient. • Therapeutic communication is essential to elicit pertinent information about the patient, the family, and the community in order to provide the best care for the patient. • As you document your findings, cluster key points and relevant pieces of information together. • This will help you formulate the preliminary problem list. • The assessment phase continues throughout the entire patient encounter, which provides the potential for updates in the plan of care based on new assessments and data.
Analysis	• *Analysis in the nursing process has a nursing focus and is based on real or potential health problems or human responses to health problems.* • The nurse uses clinical reasoning to formulate analyses based on the assessment data and the patient's problem list. • The analysis sets the stage for the remainder of the care plan.
Planning	• *Planning is devising the best course of action to address the patient's analyses.* • During planning, the nurse and patient select goals for each analysis in order to alleviate, decrease, or prevent the problems addressed in the nursing analysis. • There should be a short-term goal (STG) and a long-term goal (LTG) with realistic time frames incorporated. • Developing a successful plan requires good interpersonal skills and sensitivity to the patient's goals, economic means, competing responsibilities, and family structure and dynamics. • Interventions are then developed for each goal.
Implementation	• *Implementation of the interventions can be completed by the patient, the family, or members of the health care team.* • The interventions should clearly relate to the nursing analysis and the planned goals. • The interventions are individualized for each patient and will be modified as the patient's status or environment changes to support positive outcomes.
Evaluation	• *Evaluation is a continuing process to determine if the goals have been attained.* • The nursing care plan is revised based on the patient's condition and whether the goals are realistic or appropriate for the patient. • The intervention and evaluation process is ongoing and confirms that the nursing care is relevant.

ASSESSMENT AND ANALYSIS: THE PROCESS OF CLINICAL REASONING

The process of clinical reasoning may seem mysterious to beginning students. Assessment appears to take place in the experienced nurse's mind. These expert nurses often think quickly, with little overt or conscious effort. They differ widely in personal style, communication skills, clinical training, experience, and interests. Some nurses find it difficult to explain the logic behind their clinical thinking. As an active learner, it is expected that you will ask teachers and clinicians to elaborate on the fine points of their clinical reasoning and decision making (Benner et al., 2009; Choi & Choi, 2016; Den Hertog & Niessen, 2019). Using the nursing process and care planning as a student is instrumental in learning to think like a nurse. This framework is concrete and organized. Using the step-by-step approach facilitates the learning process (Fig. 2-2).

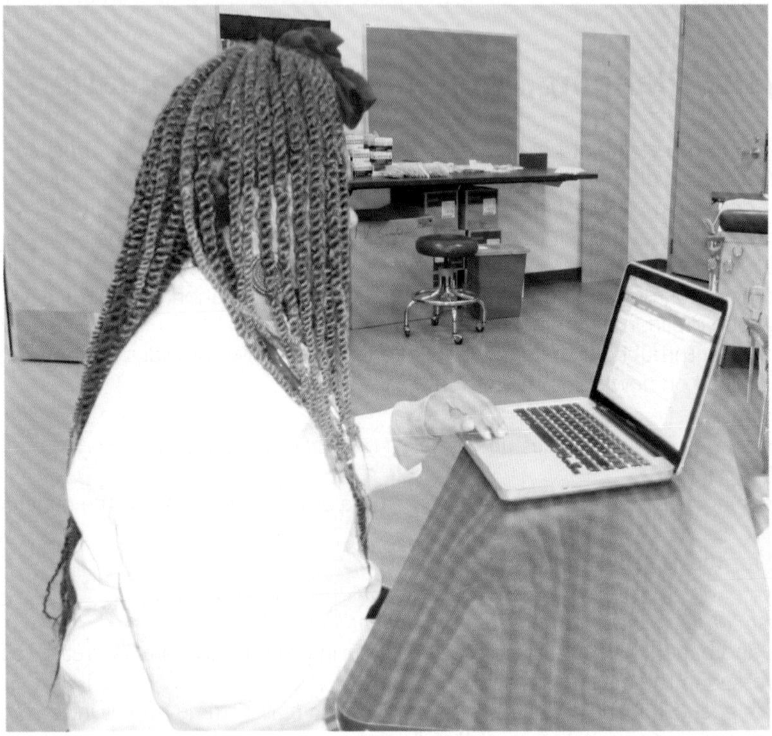

FIGURE 2-2 Using the nursing process and care planning as a student helps in learning to think like a nurse.

Cognitive psychologists have shown that clinicians use three types of reasoning for clinical problem solving: pattern recognition, development of schemas, and application of relevant basic and clinical science (Geist et al., 2019; Herdman & Kamitsuru, 2018). As you gain experience, your clinical reasoning will begin at the outset of the patient encounter, not at the end. The novice nurse needs to see all the pieces and the plan of care in a systematic fashion where they are able to evaluate the situation, while the experienced nurse may appear to figure out the plan from the onset. Ultimately, as students gain experience over the first few years in practice, this acumen will be acquired, too (Kim et al., 2020; Koharchik et al., 2015; Melin-Johansson et al., 2017).

Identifying Problems and Making Nursing Analyses: Steps in Clinical Reasoning

The process of using clinical reasoning to make a nursing analysis generally follows a set of ordered steps.

- *Identify abnormal or positive findings.* Make a list of the patient's *symptoms,* the *signs* you observed during the physical examination, and any laboratory reports available to you. Also identify positive responses during the health history. For example, the patients living in a community with a high crime level is important when organizing the issue/problem list and in development of the plan.

- *Cluster the findings.* This step may be easy. The symptom of a scratchy throat and the sign of an erythematous inflamed pharynx, for example, clearly localize the problem to the pharynx. A complaint of headache leads you quickly to the structures of the skull and brain. However, do not forget to include information on the patient's stress level due to being laid off work and lack of income. Other symptoms may present greater difficulty. Chest pain, for example, can originate in the coronary arteries, the stomach and esophagus, or the muscles and bones of the chest. If the pain is exertional and relieved by rest, either the heart or the musculoskeletal components of the chest wall may be involved. If the patient notes pain only when carrying groceries with the left arm, the musculoskeletal system becomes the likely culprit.

  When localizing findings, be as specific as your data allow, but bear in mind that you may have to settle for a body region, such as the chest, or a body system, such as the musculoskeletal system. On the other hand, you may be able to define the exact structure involved, such as the left pectoral muscle. Some symptoms and signs cannot be localized, such as fatigue or fever but are still useful in the next set of steps. In addition, obtaining more information regarding psychosocial issues may add more depth when trying to pinpoint the underlying problem.

- *Interpret findings in terms of probable process.* Patient problems stem from different causes, including changes like disease processes, relationships, nutritional, immunologic, infectious, congenital, traumatic, toxic, economic, and cultural causes, and many more. Analyze the data to evaluate the patient's health status (Fig. 2-3). It is important to differentiate a problem that should be treated by a nurse versus one that should be referred to another health care professional.

- *Make hypotheses about the nature of the patient's problem.* Draw on all the knowledge and experience you can muster; it is in this step that reading is most useful for learning about patterns

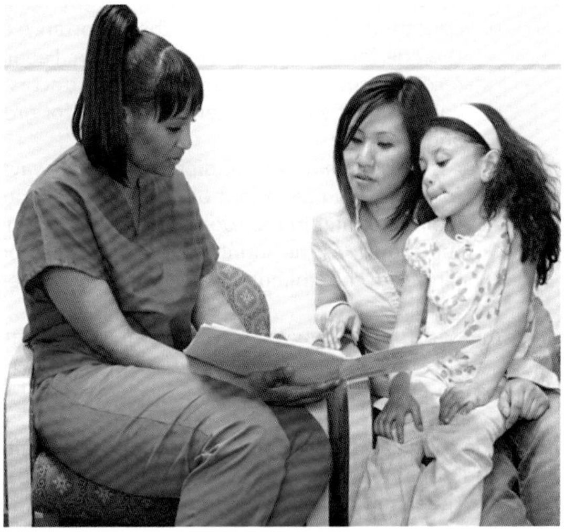

FIGURE 2-3 Sifting through data. (Reprinted with permission from Stephen, T. C., & Skillen, D. L. (2021). *Canadian nursing health assessment: A best practice approach* (2nd ed.). Wolters Kluwer Health.)

of abnormalities, diseases, and issues that help cluster your patient's findings. You may need to gather more data to rule in or out your hypotheses (Box 2-1).

BOX 2-1 **CLINICAL REASONING: DEVELOPING HYPOTHESES ABOUT PATIENT PROBLEMS**

The Nursing Process

1. Assessment
   Select the most specific and critical findings to support your problem list. At the community clinic while assessing length and weight of infants, you note that a 2-month-old has gained 7 lb in the past month. The mother reports that the child does not sleep through the night and the family of seven is living in a hotel room. The baby's crying is waking everyone up, so she has started feeding him more, hoping he will sleep when he is full. On further questioning, you find out that the 2-month-old baby is also eating rice cereal six to seven times a day. This information is critical in building a thorough assessment.
2. Analysis
   Use your inferences as multiple options for this child and family. The top nursing analysis could be:
   Altered infant feeding patterns related to excess food intake
   or
   Overweight
   Other possible nursing analyses that may not be the best or top priority include:
   Knowledge deficiency
   Deficient fluid volume risk
   Disturbance in sleep patterns: Sleep deprivation risk
   Constipation risk
3. Planning/Outcomes
   Develop goals for the nursing analysis that are realistic and timely.
   Nursing analysis: Altered infant feeding patterns related to excess food intake
   The goals for this child might be:
   STG: The infant will receive adequate nutrition for growth appropriate to age within 1 day.
   LTG: The infant will maintain current weight over the next month.
4. Implementation/interventions:
   The nursing interventions should help achieve the goals stated.
   a. Record daily weights and weekly length in a journal.
   b. Educate the family regarding the importance of formula and/or breast milk only at this age for development and nutrition. Feeding the baby cereal at this age is not recommended as the baby's digestive tract is not ready to digest the cereal. The baby will get all the nutrients necessary for growth and development from formula and/or breast milk.
   c. Assist the family with finding alternative ways to calm the baby rather than using food. An example might be to take a walk outside as this will relax the baby and maintain quiet in the room. Another solution is to go into the bathroom and run the shower as the sound of the water may be calming to the child and separate him from the siblings so they are able to sleep; this will limit distractions to both groups.
   d. Record the sleep/wake cycle and include when and what the baby is eating. Once this is recorded, develop a schedule that will support healthy patterns for the family.
5. Evaluation
   The child and family should continue to be monitored to determine if adjustments or additional teaching is necessary. Assess the child's length and weight every week and ask the family if they are obtaining more sleep. See the "Evaluating Clinical Findings" section.

- By consulting the clinical literature, you embark on the lifelong goal of *evidence-based decision making* (Melnyk et al., 2014; Morris, 2016; My Family Health Portrait, 2020).

Until you gain broader knowledge and experience, you may not be able to develop highly specific hypotheses, but you should still proceed as far as you can with the data and knowledge you have. The following steps should help:

- Test the hypothesis and establish a working nursing analysis. Nursing analyses are based primarily on changes in a person's life, altered processes, and specific causes. You will frequently see patients whose complaints do not fall neatly into these categories. Some symptoms defy analysis and are medically unexplained. You may never be able to move beyond simple descriptive categories such as "fatigue" or "anorexia." Other problems relate to stressful events in the patient's life. Events such as losing a job or loved one may increase the risk for subsequent illness. Identifying these events and helping the patient develop coping strategies are as important as managing a headache or a duodenal ulcer.

- Another increasingly prominent category on problem lists is *health maintenance*. Routinely listing health maintenance helps track several important health concerns more effectively: immunizations, screening measures (e.g., mammograms, prostate examinations), instructions regarding nutrition and self-examinations, recommendations about exercise or use of seat belts, and responses to important life events.

- Develop a plan agreeable to the patient. Develop and record a *plan* for each patient problem. Your *plan* flows logically from the problems or diagnoses you have identified. Specify which steps are needed next. These steps range from monitoring daily weights to consultation to timing of dressings or medication administration, to arranging a family meeting. You will find that you will follow many of the same nursing analyses over time, but the plan is often more fluid, encompassing changes and modifications that emerge from each patient encounter. The *plan* should reference the analysis, therapy, and patient education for each individual. The nursing analysis may be the same, but the remainder of the care plan can be much different.

- Before finalizing your plan, it is important to share your assessment and clinical thinking with the patient and seek out their opinions, concerns, and willingness to proceed with the interventions. Remember that patients may need to hear the same information multiple times and ways before they comprehend it. The patient should always be an active participant in the plan of care.

Concept Mastery Alert

Nursing Analysis

Diagnostic reasoning involves a step-by-step process. In the first step, the nurse gathers data to identify what is and is not normal for the patient. In the second step, the nurse uses this information to look for cues that suggest or indicate whether the findings from the first step are related, thus clustering the data. From there, the nurse analyzes the data and applies knowledge and experience to make hypotheses about the patient's problem.

Concept Mastery Alert

Identifying Abnormal Data

If a nurse recognizes that a patient is at risk for cardiovascular disease, this is an example of identifying abnormal data. Although it may seem like this critical thinking step is interpreting the nurse's findings, interpretation happens after data are clustered.

RECORDING YOUR FINDINGS: THE CASE OF MRS. N

Now turn to the case of Mrs. N and scrutinize the history, physical examination, assessment, and plan.

CASE STUDY

The Case of Mrs. N

1/12/21 11:00 a.m.
Mrs. N is a pleasant, 54-year-old widowed salesperson residing in Amarillo, Texas.

Referral. None.

Source and Reliability. Self seems reliable.

Chief Complaint: "My head hurts."

Present Illness: Mrs. N reports increasing problems with frontal headaches over the past 3 months. These are usually bifrontal, throbbing, and mild to moderately severe. She has missed work on several occasions because of associated nausea and vomiting. Headaches average once a week related to stress and last 4 to 6 hours. Relieved by sleep and putting a damp towel on forehead. Little relief from aspirin. No associated visual changes, motor-sensory deficits, or paresthesias.

"Sick headaches" with nausea and vomiting began at age 15, recurred through her mid-20s, decreased to one every 2 or 3 months, and almost disappeared.

Patient reports increased pressure at work from a new and demanding boss and worried about daughter (see *Personal and Social History*). Thinks headaches similar to headaches had in the past. Wants to be sure because mother died of a stroke. Concerned they interfere with work, make her irritable with family. Eats three meals a day, drinks three cups of coffee per day; cola at night.

Medications. Aspirin, one to two tablets every 4 to 6 hours as needed. "Water pill" in the past for ankle swelling, none recently.

Allergies. Ampicillin causes rash.

Tobacco. About one pack of cigarettes per day since age 18 (36 pack-years).

Alcohol/drugs. Wine rarely. No illicit drugs.

Past History

Childhood Illnesses. Measles, chickenpox. No scarlet fever or rheumatic fever.

Adult Illnesses. Medical: Pyelonephritis, 2012, with fever and right flank pain; treated with ampicillin; developed generalized rash with itching several days later. Reports kidney x-rays normal; no recurrence of infection. *Surgical:* Tonsillectomy, age 6; appendectomy, age 13. Sutures for laceration, 2015, after stepping on glass. *Ob/Gyn:* G3

Gravida (G) is the number of times the patient has been pregnant including any current pregnancy.

Para (P) is broken down into:
- T: term births
- P: preterm births
- A: abortions
- L: living children

or TPAL

P3–0–0–3, normal vaginal deliveries. Menarche age 12. Last menses 6 months ago. Little interest in sex, not sexually active. No concerns about HIV infection. *Psychiatric:* None.

Health Maintenance. Immunizations: Oral polio vaccine, year uncertain; Tdap, 2015; flu vaccine, 2020, no reaction. *Screening tests:* Last Pap smear, 2018, normal. No mammograms to date.

Family History

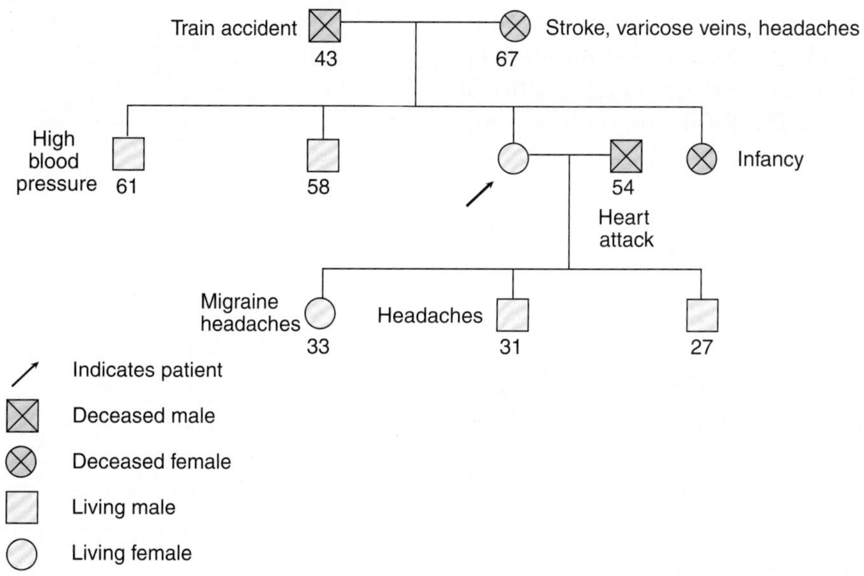

OR

Father died at age 43 in train accident. Mother died at age 67 from stroke; had varicose veins, headaches.

Brother, 61, hypertension; brother, 58, mild arthritis; sister, died in infancy of unknown cause.

Husband died, 54 of heart attack.

Daughter, 33, with migraine headaches; son, 31, headaches; son, 27, well.

Denies family history of diabetes, tuberculosis, heart or kidney disease, cancer, anemia, epilepsy, or mental illness.

CLINICAL TIP

The *family history* can be recorded as a diagram or a narrative. The diagram is more helpful than the narrative for tracing genetic disorders. The negatives from the family history should follow either format.

The U.S. Surgeon General Initiative and National Human Genome Research Institute website has a tool to construct a family tree as both a chart and a drawing that can be printed to share with health care providers at https://www.genome.gov/For-Patients-and-Families/Family-Health-History (Stec, 2015).

Personal and Social History

Born and raised in Lake City, finished high school, married at age 19. Worked as sales clerk for 2 years, moved with husband to Amarillo, had three children. Returned to work 15 years ago because of financial pressures. Children all married. Four years ago, Mr. N died suddenly of a heart attack, leaving little savings. Mrs. N has moved to a small apartment near daughter, Dorothy. Dorothy's husband, Arthur, misuses alcohol. Mrs. N's apartment is a haven for Dorothy and her two children, Kevin, 6 years, and Kyra, 3 years. Mrs. N feels responsible for helping them; feels tense and nervous but denies depression. She has friends but rarely discusses family problems: "I'd rather keep them to myself. I don't like gossip." No church or other organizational support. She is typically up at 7:00 a.m., works 9:00 a.m. to 5:30 p.m., eats dinner alone.

Exercise and Diet

Gets little exercise. Diet high in carbohydrates.

Safety Measures

Seat belt regularly. Sunblock SPF 15. Medications in unlocked medicine cabinet. Cleaning solutions in unlocked cabinet below sink. Shotgun and box of shells in unlocked closet.

Review of Systems

General. Has gained about 10 lb in the past 4 years.
Skin. Denies rashes or other changes.

Head, Eyes, Ears, Nose, Throat (HEENT). See *Present Illness.* Denies history of head injury. *Eyes:* Reading glasses for 5 years, last checked 1 year ago. Denies diplopia, blurring, halos, tearing, pain. *Ears:* Able to hear. Denies tinnitus, vertigo, infections. *Nose, sinuses:* Occasional mild cold. Denies hay fever, sinus trouble. *Throat (or mouth and pharynx):* Some bleeding of gums recently. Last dental visit 2 years ago. Occasional canker sore.

Neck. Denies lumps, goiter, pain. No swollen glands.

Breasts. Denies lumps, pain, discharge. Does breast self-examination sporadically.

Respiratory. Denies cough, wheezing, shortness of breath. Sleeps with one pillow. Last chest x-ray, 2000, St. Mary's Hospital; unremarkable.

Cardiovascular. Denies heart disease or high blood pressure; last blood pressure taken in 2016. Denies dyspnea, orthopnea, chest pain, palpitations, electrocardiogram (ECG).

Gastrointestinal. Appetite "good;" denies nausea, vomiting, indigestion. Bowel movement about once daily, hard stools when tense; denies diarrhea, bleeding, pain, jaundice, gallbladder, or liver problems.

Urinary. Denies frequency, dysuria, hematuria, or recent flank pain; nocturia × 1, large volume. Occasionally loses some urine when coughs hard.

Genital. Denies vaginal, or pelvic infections or dyspareunia. Last Pap smear 2018, negative results.

Peripheral Vascular. Varicose veins appeared in both legs during first pregnancy. For 10 years, has had swollen ankles after prolonged standing; wears light elastic pantyhose; tried "water pill" 5 months ago but didn't help; denies history of phlebitis or leg pain.

Musculoskeletal. Mild, aching, low back pain, often after a long day of work; no radiation down the legs; back exercises in past, none currently. No other joint pain.

Psychiatric. Denies history of depression or treatment for psychiatric disorders. See also *Present Illness* and *Personal and Social History.*

Neurologic. Denies fainting, seizures, motor or sensory loss. Memory intact.

Hematologic. Except for bleeding gums, denies easy bleeding, anemia.

Endocrine. Denies thyroid trouble, temperature intolerance, symptoms or history of diabetes. Minimal sweating.

Physical Examination

Mrs. N is a short, overweight, middle-aged woman. Animated and responds quickly to questions. Somewhat tense with moist, cold hands. Hair fixed neatly, clothes immaculate, color is tan, and lies supine without discomfort.

Vital Signs. Ht (without shoes) 157 cm (5 ft 2 in). Wt (dressed) 65 kg (143 lb). Body mass index (BMI) 26. Blood pressure (BP) 164/98 right arm, supine; 160/96 left arm, supine. Heart rate (HR) 88 and regular. Respiratory rate (RR) 18. Temperature (oral) 98.6°F.

Skin. Cool, moist, tan. Scattered cherry angiomas over upper trunk. Nails without clubbing, cyanosis.

Head, Eyes, Ears, Nose, Throat (HEENT). Head: Hair coarse, full, brown. Scalp without lesions, normocephalic/atraumatic. *Eyes:* Distant vision 20/30 in each eye. Visual fields full by confrontation. Conjunctiva pink; sclera white. PERRLA. EOMs intact. Disc margins sharp without hemorrhages, exudates. No arteriolar narrowing. *Ears:* Soft, light brown cerumen partially obscures right TM; left canal clear, TM with cone of light. Acuity hears whispered voice at 1 ft BL. Weber midline. 2AC> BC. *Nose:* Mucosa pink, septum midline. No sinus tenderness or polyps. *Mouth:* Oral mucosa pink. Several interdental papillae red, slightly swollen. Dentition intact. Tongue midline, with 3-mm × 4-mm shallow white ulcer on red base on undersurface near tip; tender but not indurated. Tonsils absent. Pharynx without exudates.

Neck. Neck supple. Trachea midline. Thyroid isthmus barely palpable, lobes not felt.

PERRLA
*P*upils
*E*qual
*R*ound
*R*eact to
*L*ight
*A*ccommodate

EOM
*E*xtra
*O*cular
*M*ovements

TM
*T*ympanic
*M*embrane

Lymph Nodes. Small (<1 cm), soft, nontender, and mobile tonsillar and posterior cervical nodes bilaterally. No axillary or epitrochlear nodes. Several 0.5-cm inguinal nodes bilaterally, soft, equal nontender, mobile.

Thorax and Lungs. Thorax symmetric with equal excursion. Lungs resonant. Breath sounds vesicular with no added sounds. Diaphragm descends 4 cm bilaterally.

Cardiovascular (CV). JVP 1 cm above the sternal angle at 30 degrees. Carotid upstrokes brisk without bruits. Apical impulse discrete and tapping, barely palpable in the fifth left interspace, 8 cm lateral to the midsternal line. S_1, S_2; no S_3 or S_4. A II/VI medium-pitched midsystolic murmur at the second right interspace; does not radiate to neck. No diastolic murmurs.

JVP
*J*ugular
*V*enous
*P*ressure

Breasts. Pendulous, left slightly larger than right. No dimpling, retractions, rashes, masses; nipples without discharge.

Abdomen. Protuberant. Well-healed 5-cm × 0.25-cm scar, right lower quadrant. Bowel sounds active. No tenderness or masses. Liver span 7 cm in right midclavicular line; edge smooth, palpable 1 cm below RCM. Spleen and kidneys not felt. No CVAT.

RCM
*R*ight
*C*ostal
*M*argin

CVAT
Angle between the 12th rib and the vertebral column
*C*osto
*V*ertebral
*A*ngle
*T*enderness

Genitalia. External genitalia without lesions. Internal examination deferred. Vaginal mucosa pink.

Rectal. Stool brown, negative for occult blood.

Extremities. Warm without edema. BL calves supple, nontender.

BL
Bilateral

Peripheral Vascular. Trace edema at both ankles. Moderate varicosities of saphenous veins, both in lower extremities. No stasis pigmentation or ulcers.

	Radial	Femoral	Popliteal	Dorsalis Pedis	Posterior Tibial
RT	2+	2+	2+	2+	2+
LT	2+	2+	2+	Absent	2+

Musculoskeletal. No joint deformities. FROM in hands, wrists, elbows, shoulders, spine, hips, knees, ankles.

FROM
*F*ull
*R*ange
*o*f
*M*otion

Neurologic. Mental Status: Tense but alert and cooperative. Thought coherent. AA&O × 4. *Cranial Nerves:* II to XII intact. *Motor:* Equal intact muscle bulk and tone. Strength 5/5 throughout. *Cerebellar:* RAMs, point-to-point movements intact. Gait stable, fluid. *Sensory:* Pinprick, light touch, position sense, vibration, and stereognosis intact. Romberg negative.

AA&O × 4
*A*wake
*A*lert
*O*riented (to person, place, time, situation)

RAM
*R*apid
*A*lternating
*M*ovements

Reflexes:

	Biceps	Triceps	Brachioradialis	Patellar	Achilles	Plantar
RT	2+	2+	2+	2+	1+	↓
LT	2+	2+	2+	2+	1+	↓

Recording reflexes uses a grading system.

Laboratory Data: None currently. See *Plan.*

Generating the Problem List

Now that you have completed your assessment and written record, you will find it helpful to generate a *problem list* that summarizes the patient's problems. *List the most active and serious problems first, and record their date of onset.* Some nurses make separate lists for active or inactive problems; others make one list in order of priority. On follow-up visits, the problem list helps you remember to check the status of problems the patient may not mention. The problem list also allows other members of the health care team to review the patient's health status at a glance.

A sample problem list for Mrs. N is provided. You may wish to give each problem a number and use the number when referring to specific problems in subsequent notes.

CASE STUDY

Problem List: The Case of Mrs. N from Assessment Data

Date Entered	Problem No.	Problem
1/12/21	1	Headaches
	2	Elevated blood pressure
	3	Overweight
	4	Family stress
	5	Tobacco use since age 18
	6	Low back pain
	7	Health maintenance
	8	Occasional incontinence
	9	History of right pyelonephritis, 2012
	10	Varicose veins
	11	Allergy to ampicillin

The list illustrated here includes problems that need attention now, such as Mrs. N's headaches, as well as problems that need future observation and attention, such as her blood pressure. Listing the allergy to ampicillin warns you not to distribute medications in the penicillin family. Some symptoms such as canker sores and hard stools do not appear on this list because they are minor concerns and do not require attention during this visit. Problem lists with too many relatively insignificant items diminish in value. If these symptoms increase in importance, they can always be added at a later visit.

The Challenges of Clinical Data

As you can see from the case of Mrs. N, organizing the patient's clinical data poses several challenges. The beginning student must decide whether to cluster the patient's symptoms and signs into one problem or into several problems. The amount of data may appear unmanageable. The quality of the data may be prone to error. However, there are some guidelines to help address these challenges.

- Consider whether to cluster data into single or multiple problems. One of the greatest difficulties facing students is how to cluster clinical data. Do select data fit into one problem or several problems? The patient's *age* may help—young people are more likely to have a single disease, while older people tend to have multiple diseases. The *timing* of symptoms is also often useful. For example, an episode of pharyngitis 6 weeks ago is probably unrelated to fever, chills, pleuritic chest pain, and cough that prompt a visit today. To use timing effectively, you need to know the natural history of various diseases and conditions. A yellow penile discharge followed 3 weeks later by a painless penile ulcer suggests two problems: gonorrhea and primary syphilis. In contrast, a penile ulcer followed in 6 weeks by a maculopapular skin rash and generalized lymphadenopathy suggests two stages of the same problem: primary and secondary syphilis.

- Involvement of *different body systems* may help to cluster the clinical data. If symptoms and signs occur in a single system, one disease may explain them. Problems in different, apparently unrelated systems often require more than one explanation. Again, knowledge of disease patterns is necessary. You might decide, for example, to group a patient's high blood glucose and blurred vision together and place them in the "head, eyes, ears, nose, and throat" system, and label the constellation "hyperglycemia." You would develop another explanation for the patient's mild fever, left lower quadrant tenderness, and diarrhea.

- Some diseases involve more than one body system. As you gain knowledge and experience, you will become increasingly adept at recognizing *multisystem conditions* and building plausible explanations that link together their seemingly unrelated manifestations. To explain cough, hemoptysis, and weight loss in a 60-year-old plumber who has smoked cigarettes for 40 years, you probably would rank lung cancer high in the problem list. You might support your list with your observation of the patient's cyanotic fingernails. With experience and continued reading, you will recognize that his other symptoms and signs can be linked to the same diagnosis. Dysphagia would reflect extension of the cancer to the esophagus, pupillary asymmetry would suggest pressure on the cervical sympathetic chain, and jaundice could result from metastases to the liver.

- Be prepared to sift through an extensive array of data. It is common to confront a relatively long list of symptoms and signs and an equally long list of potential explanations. One approach is to *tease out separate clusters of observations and analyze one cluster at a time*, as just described. You can also *ask a series of key questions* that may steer your thinking in one direction and allow you to temporarily ignore the others. For example, you may ask what produces and relieves the patient's chest pain. If the answer is exercise and rest, you can focus on the cardiovascular and musculoskeletal systems and set the gastrointestinal system aside. If the pain is substernal and burning and occurs only after meals, you can logically focus on the gastrointestinal tract. A series of discriminating questions helps you form a decision tree or algorithm that is helpful in collecting and analyzing clinical data and reaching logical conclusions and explanations (Storey et al., 2019).

- Assess the quality of the data. Almost all clinical information is subject to error. Patients forget to mention symptoms, confuse the events of their illness, avoid recounting embarrassing facts, and often slant their stories to what they think the nurse wants to hear. Nurses may misinterpret patient statements, overlook information, fail to ask "the one key question," jump prematurely to conclusions and analyses, or forget an important part of the examination, such as the funduscopic examination in a woman with a headache. You can avoid some of these errors by acquiring the habits of skilled nurses, summarized in Box 2-2 (Umberger et al., 2017).

BOX 2-2 TIPS FOR ENSURING THE QUALITY OF PATIENT DATA

- Ask open-ended questions and listen carefully and patiently to the patient's story.
- When a patient answers "yes" to a question, continue further using "OLD CART" for additional details.
- Craft a thorough and systematic sequence to history taking and physical examination.
- Keep an open mind toward both the patient and the data.
- Always include "the worst-case scenario" in your list of possible explanations of the patient's problem, and make sure it can be safely eliminated.
- Analyze any mistakes in data collection or interpretation.
- Confer with colleagues and review the pertinent literature to clarify uncertainties.
- Apply principles of data analysis to patient information and testing.

Compose the record as soon as possible after seeing the patient before your findings fade from memory. Record key points from each segment of the health history during the interview, leaving spaces for filling in details later. A sample progress note based on this patient's case follows.

Sample Progress Note

A month later, Mrs. N returns for a follow-up visit. The format of the office progress note is quite variable, but it should meet the same standards as the initial assessment. The note should be clear, sufficiently detailed, and easy to follow. It should reflect your clinical reasoning and delineate your assessment and plan. Be sure to learn the documentation standards for billing in your institution, because this can affect the detail and type of information needed in your progress notes.

The note below follows the "SOAP" format: *s*ubjective, *o*bjective, *a*ssessment, and *p*lan. You will see many other styles, some focused on the "patient-centered" record. The terms for SOAP are often not listed, but instead implied. Frequently, nurses record the history and physical examination, then document the plan with the listing of each problem and its assessment.

CASE STUDY

The Case of Mrs. N: Progress Note

2/12/21

Mrs. N returned to the clinic for follow-up for her migraine headaches. She stated that she has fewer headaches since avoiding caffeinated beverages. She is now drinking decaffeinated coffee and has stopped drinking colas. She has joined a support group and started exercising to reduce stress. She is still having one to two headaches a month with some nausea, but they are less severe and generally relieved with nonsteroidal antiinflammatory drugs (NSAIDs). She denies any fever, stiff neck, associated visual changes, motor-sensory deficits, or paresthesia.

She has been checking her blood pressure at home. It is running about 150/90 mm Hg. She is walking 30 minutes three times a week in her neighborhood and has reduced her total daily calorie intake. She has been unable to stop smoking. She has been doing the pelvic floor muscle exercises but still has some leakage with coughing or laughing.

Medications: Motrin 400 mg up to three times daily as needed for headache

Allergies: Ampicillin causes rash

Tobacco: One pack per day since age 18

Physical Examination: Pleasant, overweight, middle-aged woman, who is animated and somewhat tense. Ht 157 cm (5 ft 2 in). Wt 63 kg (140 lb). BMI 26. BP 150/90. HR 86 and regular. RR 16. Afebrile.

Skin: No suspicious nevi. *HEENT:* Normocephalic, atraumatic. Pharynx without exudates. *Neck:* Supple, without thyromegaly. *Lymph nodes:* No lymphadenopathy. *Lungs:* Resonant and clear. *CV:* JVP 6 cm above the right atrium; carotid upstrokes brisk, no bruits. S_1, S_2. No murmurs. No S_3, S_4. *Abdomen:* Active bowel sounds. Soft, nontender, no hepatosplenomegaly. *Extremities:* Without edema.

Labs: Basic metabolic panel and urinalysis from 1/25/21 unremarkable. Pap smear normal.

Impression and Plan

1. Migraine headaches—now down to one to two per month due to reductions in caffeinated beverages and stress. Headaches are responding to NSAIDs.
   a. Affirm need to stop smoking and to continue exercise program.
   b. Affirm patient's participation in support group to reduce stress.
2. Elevated blood pressure—BP remains elevated at 150/90.
   a. Educate on newly prescribed diuretic.

   b. Patient to take blood pressure three times a week and bring recordings to next office visit.
   c. Affirm need to exercise, lose weight, and stop smoking.
3. Cystocele with occasional stress incontinence—stress incontinence improved with pelvic floor muscle exercises but still with some urine leakage. Urinalysis from last visit—no infection.
   a. Educate on newly prescribed vaginal estrogen cream.
   b. Patient to continue pelvic floor muscle exercises.
4. Overweight—has lost ~3 lb.
   a. Patient to continue exercise.
   b. Review diet history; affirm weight reduction.
5. Family stress—patient handling this better. See *Plan*.
6. Occasional low back pain—no complaints today.
7. Tobacco use—see *Plan*.
8. Health maintenance—Pap smear sent last visit. Mammogram scheduled. Colonoscopy recommended.

The following case study details the nursing process in the case of Mrs. N. Included are the problem list, which has been developed from the assessment; the nursing analyses formulated from the problem list; the plan, including the STG and the LTG; the interventions/implementation; and the evaluation. Each nursing care plan would be individualized and updated for the specific patient.

CASE STUDY

The Nursing Process in the Case of Mrs. N

1. Headaches

Assessment: A 54-year-old woman with a history of migraine headaches since childhood with a throbbing vascular pattern and frequent nausea and vomiting. Headaches are associated with stress and relieved by sleep and cold compresses. There is no papilledema, and there are no motor or sensory deficits on the neurologic examination. The differential diagnosis includes tension headache, also associated with stress, but there is no relief with massage, and the pain is more throbbing than aching. There is no fever, stiff neck, or focal findings to suggest meningitis, and the lifelong recurrent pattern makes subarachnoid hemorrhage unlikely (usually described as "the worst headache of my life").

Nursing Analysis: Acute pain related to headaches

Plan:

STG: The patient will have decreased severity and frequency of headaches within 1 week as documented in journal/phone app entries.

LTG: The patient will have acceptable relief options as evidenced by her return to activities of daily living and work within 2 weeks.

Interventions:

- Log headaches—onset, location, duration, characteristic symptoms, associated manifestations, relieving factors, and treatment.
- Discuss biofeedback and stress management.
- Advise patient to avoid caffeine, including coffee, colas, and other carbonated beverages.
- Start NSAIDs for headache as needed and prescribed by nurse practitioner or physician.
- Follow-up appointment in 2 weeks and call physician/nurse practitioner sooner if signs/symptoms increase.

Evaluation[1]: Ideally, the patient will no longer have headaches; however, if they do persist, then the plan and goals need to be revised and/or the interventions adjusted.

[1]Evaluations will be completed for each nursing analysis based on the individual patient and will be updated accordingly.

2. Elevated Blood Pressure

Assessment: Systolic hypertension with wide cuff is present. May be related to obesity and/or to anxiety from the initial visit or white coat hypertension. No evidence of end-organ damage to retina or heart.

Nursing Analysis: Knowledge deficiency related to the relationship between increased blood pressure and increased weight and/or stress

Plan:

STG: The patient will verbalize understanding within 5 days of importance of decreasing blood pressure and how to begin the process of diet changes, exercise, and stress reduction to assist in lowering blood pressure.

LTG: The patient will have decreased blood pressure to below 140/90 within 1 month.

Interventions:

- Discuss standards for assessing blood pressure.
- Recheck blood pressure in 2 weeks using wide cuff.
- Check basic metabolic panel; review urinalysis.
- Introduce weight reduction, exercise, and stress reduction techniques.
- Reduce salt intake.

3. Overweight

Assessment: Patient 5 ft 2 in, weighs 143 lb, BMI is ~26

Nursing Analysis: Altered health maintenance related to increased food consumption in response to stressors and insufficient energy expenditure for intake

Plan:

STG: The patient will verbalize commitment to a weight loss program within 2 days.

LTG: The patient will decrease weight by 5 lb within 1 month (143 to 138 lb).

Interventions:

- Explore diet history; ask patient to keep food intake diary or use app for tracking food intake.
- Explore motivation to lose weight; set target for weight loss by next visit.
- Schedule visit with dietitian.
- Discuss exercise program, specifically, walking 30 minutes 5 to 6 days a week.

4. Family Stress

Assessment: Son-in-law with alcohol misuse; daughter and grandchildren seeking refuge in patient's apartment, leading to tension in these relationships. Patient also has financial constraints. Stress currently situational. No current evidence of major depression.

Nursing Analysis: Caregiver fatigue related to daughter/grandchildren situation

Plan:

STG: Mrs. N will verbalize a plan to decrease strain within 5 days.

LTG: Mrs. N will partake in the plan and have decreased signs/symptoms of stress within 1 month.

Interventions:

- Explore patient's views on strategies to cope with stress.
- Explore sources of support, including Al-Anon for daughter and financial counseling for patient.
- Continue to monitor for depression.

5. Tobacco Use

Assessment: One pack per day for 36 years.

Nursing Analysis: Altered health maintenance related to insufficient knowledge of effects of tobacco use and resources available to quit

Plan:

STG: The patient will verbalize plan to quit within 2 days.

LTG: The patient will decrease or quit smoking within 1 month.

Interventions:

- Educate patient on short- and long-term effects of smoking on self and grandchildren.
- Identify benefits of quitting smoking (e.g., money savings, health).
- Devise strategies to decrease/eliminate smoking.
- Offer referral to tobacco cessation program.

6. Occasional Musculoskeletal Low Back Pain

Assessment: Usually with prolonged standing. No history of trauma or motor vehicle accident. Pain does not radiate; no tenderness or motor-sensory deficits on examination.

Nursing Analysis: Impaired comfort related to back pain

Plan:
STG: The patient will demonstrate abdominal exercises that will strengthen back within 4 days.
LTG: Patient will rate back pain as 1 to 2 on pain scale within 1 month of using interventions.

Interventions:
- Rate pain on scale of 1 to 10.
- Use heating pad to decrease pain.
- Review benefits of weight loss and exercises to strengthen low back muscles.
- Continue daily exercises to strengthen abdominal muscles.
- Refer to exercise therapist for evaluation and additional exercises as needed.

7. Health Maintenance

Assessment: Last Pap smear 2018; has never had a mammogram.

Nursing Analysis: Altered health maintenance related to insufficient knowledge of screening and prevention

Plan:
STG: The patient will verbalize importance of health and prevention within 1 day.
LTG: The patient will have scheduled/completed all preventative screenings within 1 month.

Interventions:
- Teach Mrs. N breast self-awareness.
- Schedule mammogram.
- Send Pap smear today.
- Provide three stool guaiac cards; discuss screening colonoscopy at next visit.
- Update immunizations.
- Suggest dental care for mild gingivitis.
- Gun lock and store shells in a separate area.
- Advise patient to move medications and caustic cleaning agents to locked cabinet, if possible, above shoulder height.

8. Occasional Stress Incontinence

Assessment: Incontinence reported with coughing, suggesting alteration in bladder neck anatomy. No dysuria, fever, flank pain. Not taking any contributing medications. Usually involves small amounts of urine, no dribbling, doubt urge or overflow incontinence. Patient is perimenopausal.

Nursing Analysis: Functional urinary stress incontinence related to loss of muscle tone

Plan:
STG: Mrs. N will verbalize understanding of stress incontinence and exercises within 2 days.
LTG: Mrs. N will report decreased or elimination of stress incontinence within 2 months.

Interventions:

- Explain cause of stress incontinence.
- Review urinalysis.
- Teach pelvic floor muscle exercises.

The remaining problems on the list do not need a care plan; they are provided as points to be aware of, such as the allergy to ampicillin, or to observe and incorporate into the patient's plan of care if they come into the forefront as more of an issue.

9. History of Right Pyelonephritis, 2012

No pain.

10. Varicose Veins, Lower Extremities

No complaints currently.

11. Ampicillin Allergy

Developed rash but no other allergic reaction.

EVALUATING CLINICAL FINDINGS

Symptoms, physical findings, tests, and x-rays should help reduce uncertainty about whether a patient does or does not have a given condition. Clinical data, including laboratory work, however, are inherently imperfect. Learn to apply the principles of *reliability, validity, sensitivity,* and *specificity* to your clinical findings (Box 2-3).

LIFELONG LEARNING: INTEGRATING CLINICAL REASONING, ASSESSMENT, AND ANALYSIS OF CLINICAL EVIDENCE

As nursing students progress and become novice nurses and then develop into more experienced clinicians, it becomes easier to integrate assessment, reasoning, and analysis into patient care. The two major aspects of data collection that are used to formulate a plan of care are patient history as well as physical examination and laboratory reports.

Nurses make use of many assessment tools. These tools are used in areas of prevention such as falls, malnutrition, and skin breakdown. Screening tests for alcohol (AUDIT-C) or developmental delays (Denver II) are examples of additional tools. The concepts of sensitivity and specificity help in both the collection and the analysis of data. They even underlie some of the basic strategies of interviewing. Questions with high sensitivity, if answered in the affirmative, may be particularly useful for screening and for gathering evidence to support a hypothesis. For example, "Are you confined to bed?" is a highly sensitive question for detecting risk of skin breakdown. For patients who are immobile, there would be few false-negative responses. Thus, it is a good first screening question. However, because there are indicators other than activity and mobility that determine skin breakdown,

BOX 2-3 PRINCIPLES OF TEST SELECTION AND USE

Reliability

Indicates how well repeated measurements of the same relatively stable phenomenon will give the same result, also known as *precision*. Reliability may be measured for one observer or for more than one observer.

Example: If, on several occasions, one nurse consistently percusses the same span of a patient's liver dullness, *intra-observer reliability* is good. If, on the other hand, several observers find quite different spans of liver dullness on the same patient, *interobserver reliability* is poor.

Validity

Indicates how closely a given observation agrees with "the true state of affairs," or the best possible measure of reality.

Example: Noninvasive blood pressure measurements by sphygmomanometers are less valid than intra-arterial pressure tracings.

Sensitivity

Identifies the proportion of people who test positive in a group of people known to have the disease or condition, or the proportion of people who are *true positives* compared with the total number of people who actually have the disease. When the observation or test is negative in people with the disease, the result is termed *false negative. Good observations or tests have a sensitivity of more than 90% and help rule out disease because there are few false negatives. Such observations or tests are especially useful for screening.*

Example: The sensitivity of the Homans sign in the diagnosis of deep venous thrombosis (DVT) of the calf is 50%. In other words, compared with a group of patients with DVT confirmed by phlebogram, a much better test, only 50% will have a positive Homans sign, so this sign, if absent, is not helpful because 50% of patients may still have a DVT.

Specificity

Identifies the proportion of people who test negative in a group of people known to be *without* a given disease or condition, or the proportion of people who are *true negatives* compared with the total number of people without the disease. When the observation or test is positive in people without the disease, the result is termed *false positive.* Good observations or tests have a specificity of more than 90% and help "rule in" disease because the test is rarely positive when disease is absent, and there are few false positives.

Example: The specificity of serum amylase in patients with possible acute pancreatitis is 70%. In other words, of 100 patients without pancreatitis, 70% will have a normal serum amylase; in 30%, the serum amylase will be falsely elevated.

To help remember the meaning of sensitivity, experts state when the *se*n*s*itivity of a symptom or sign is high, a *n*egative response rules *out* the target disorder, and the acronym for this property is "*SnNout*" (Xiao et al., 2017).

Likewise, when the *sp*ecificity is high, a *p*ositive test result rules *in* the target disorder. The acronym is "*SpPin*" (Xiao et al., 2017).

it is not highly specific. Decreased sensory perception, friction, malnutrition, and increased moisture each is a reasonably sensitive attribute of skin breakdown and would add importantly to the growing evidence.

Data also come from the physical assessment and examination of the skin. Combining data from the history and physical examination allows screening of patients at risk for skin breakdown.

Skilled nurses use this kind of logic to generate tentative nursing analyses as soon as the patient describes the *chief complaint*, then build evidence for one or more of these analyses and discard others as they continue with the history and examination. The nurse searches explicitly for other possible manifestations of skin breakdown such as history of cerebrovascular accident or diminished lower extremity pulses of atherosclerotic peripheral

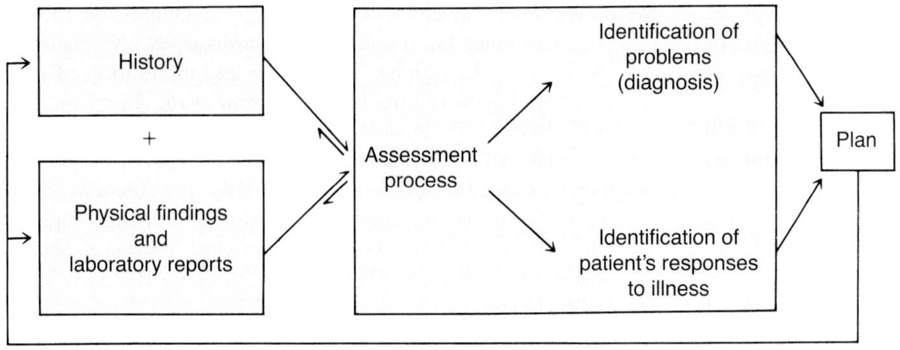

FIGURE 2-4 The process of clinical reasoning.

vascular disease. By generating diagnoses early and testing them sequentially, experienced nurses improve their efficiency and enhance the relevance and value of the data they collect. Once the analyses have been identified, the nurse develops appropriate nursing care plans.

This sequence of collecting data and testing hypotheses is diagrammed in Figure 2-4.

After the plan has been implemented, the process recycles. The nurse gathers more data, assesses the patient's progress, modifies the problem list if indicated, and adjusts the plan accordingly. As you gain experience, the interplay of assessment, data collection, and knowledge from the clinical literature will become increasingly familiar. You will come to value the challenges and rewards of clinical reasoning and assessment that make patient care so meaningful.

BIBLIOGRAPHY

CITATIONS

Benner, P. (2001). *From novice to expert: Excellence and power in clinical nursing practice*. Commemorative Edition. Prentice Hall.

Benner, P. E., Tanner, C. A., & Chesla, C. A. (2009). *Expertise in nursing practice: Caring, clinical judgment & ethics* (2nd ed.). Springer Pub.

Choi, J., & Choi J. E. (2016). Enhancing patient safety using clinical nursing data: a pilot study. *Studies in Health Technology Informatics*, *225*, 103–107.

Den Hertog, R., & Niessen, T. (2019). The role of patient preferences in nursing decision-making in evidence-based practice: Excellent nurses' communication tools. *Journal of Advanced Nursing*, *75*(9), 1987–1995. https://doi-org.proxy.library.upenn.edu/10.1111/jan.14083.

Geist, M. J., Sanders, R., Harris, K., Arce-Trigatti, A., & Hitchcock-Cass, C. (2019). Clinical Immersion: An Approach for Fostering Cross-disciplinary Communication and Innovation in Nursing and Engineering Students. *Nurse Educator*, *44*(2), 69–73. https://doi.org/10.1097/NNE.0000000000000547

Herdman, T. H., & Kamitsuru, S. H. (2018). *Nursing diagnoses: Definitions and classifications, 2018–2020* (11th ed.). Thieme.

Kim, J., Macieira, T. G. R., Meyer, S. L., Maggie, M. A., Raga, R. I. B., Smith, M. B., Citty, S. W., Schentrup, D. M., Nealis, R. M., & Keenan, G. M. (2020). Towards Implementing SNOMED CT in Nursing Practice: A Scoping Review. *International Journal of Medical Informatics*, *134*, 104035. https://doi.org/10.1016/j.ijmedinf.2019.104035.

Koharchik, L., Caputi, L., Robb, M., Culleiton, A. L. (2015). Fostering clinical reasoning in nursing students. *The American Journal of Nursing*, *115*(1), 58–61. https://doi.org/10.1097/01.naj.0000459638.68657.9b.

Melin-Johansson, C., Palmqvist, R., Rönnberg, L. (2017). Clinical Intuition in the nursing process and decision-making—A mixed-studies review. *Journal of Clinical Nursing*, *26*(23–24), 3936–3949. https://doi-org.proxy.library.upenn.edu/10.1111/jocn.13814.

Melnyk, B. M., Gallagher-Ford, L., Long, L. E., & Fineout-Overholt, E. (2014). The establishment of evidence-based practice competencies for practicing registered nurses and advanced practice nurses in real-world clinical settings: proficiencies to improve healthcare quality, reliability, patient outcomes, and costs. *Worldviews on Evidence-Based Nursing*, *11*(1), 5–15. https://doi.org/10.1111/wvn.12021.

Morris, J. (2016). The use of team-based learning in a second year undergraduate pre-registration nursing course on evidence-informed decision making. *Nurse Education in Practice, 21*, 23–28. https://doi.org/10.1016/j.nepr.2016.09.005.

My Family Health Portrait. Genome.gov. Retrieved June 1, 2020, from https://www.genome.gov/For-Patients-and-Families/Family-Health-History

Stec, M. W. (2015). Health as expanding consciousness. *Nursing Science Quarterly, 29*(1), 54–61. https://doi.org/10.1177/0894318415614901.

Storey, S., Wagnes, L., Lamothe, J., Pittman, J., Cohee, A., & Newhouse, R. (2019). Building evidence-based nursing practice capacity in a large statewide health system. *The Journal of Nursing Administration, 49*(4), 208–214. https://doi.org/10.1097/nna.0000000000000739.

Umberger, R. A., Hatfield, L. A., Speck, P. M. (2017). Understanding negative predictive value of diagnostic tests used in clinical practice. *Dimensions of Critical Care Nursing, 36*(1), 22–29. https://doi.org/10.1097/dcc.0000000000000219.

Xiao, S., Widger, K., Tourangeau, A., & Berta, W. (2017). Nursing process health care indicators. *Journal of Nursing Care Quality, 32*(1), 32–39. https://doi.org/10.1097/ncq.0000000000000207.

ADDITIONAL REFERENCES

Alfaro-LeFevre, R. (2013). *Critical thinking, clinical reasoning, and clinical judgment: A practical approach* (5th ed.). Saunders/Elsevier.

Black, A. T., Balneaves, L. G., Garossino, C., Puyat, J. H., & Qian, H. (2015). Promoting evidence-based practice through a research training program for point-of-care clinicians. *Journal of Nursing Administration, 45*(1), 14–20. https://doi.org/10.1097/NNA.0000000000000151

Carpenito-Moyet, L. J. (2012). *Nursing diagnosis: Application to clinical practice* (14th ed.). Lippincott Williams & Wilkins.

Cathcart, E. B., Greenspan, M. (2013). The role of practical wisdom in nurse manager practice: why experience matters. *Journal of Nursing Management, 21*(7), 964–970. https://doi.org/10.1111/jonm.12175.

Cherry, B., & Jacob, S. R. (2014). *Contemporary nursing: Issues, trends, & management* (6th ed.). Elsevier.

Gengo E Silva, R. C., Dos Santos Diogo, R. C., da Cruz, D. A. L. M., Ortiz, D., Ortiz, D., Peres, H. H. C., & Moorhead, S. (2018). Linkages of Nursing Diagnoses, Outcomes, and Interventions Performed by Nurses Caring for Medical and Surgical Patients Using a Decision Support System. *International Journal of Nursing Knowledge, 29*(4), 269–275. https://doi.org/10.1111/2047-3095.12185

Leoni-Scheiber, C., Mayer, H., & Müller-Staub, M. (2019). Relationships between the Advanced Nursing Process quality and nurses and patient characteristics: A cross-sectional study. *Nursing Open, 7*(1), 419–429. https://doi.org/10.1002/nop2.405.

LoBiondo-Wood, G., & Haber, J. (2014). *Nursing research: Methods and critical appraisal for evidence-based practice* (8th ed.). Elsevier.

Lockwood, C., & Lee, Y. M. (2015). Evidence-based nursing: A Singaporean perspective. *Singapore Nursing Journal, 42*(2), 8–12.

Matney, S. A., DaDamio, R., Couderc, C., Dlugos, M., Evans, J., Gianonne, G., Haskell, R., Hardiker, N., Coenen, A., & Saba, V. K. (2008). Translation and integration of CCC nursing diagnoses into ICNP. *Journal of the American Medical Informatics Association, 15*(6), 791–793. https://doi.org/10.1197/jamia.m2801.

Miguel, S., Caldeira, S., & Vieira, M. (2018). The Adequacy of the Q Methodology for Clinical Validation of Nursing Diagnoses Related to Subjective Foci. *International Journal of Nursing Knowledge, 29*(2), 97–103. https://doi.org/10.1111/2047-3095.12163

Müller-Staub, M., Needham, I., Odenbreit, M., Lavin, M. A., van Achterberg, T. (2008). Implementing nursing diagnostics effectively: cluster randomized trial. *Journal of Advanced Nursing, 63*(3), 291–301. https://doi.org/10.1111/j.1365-2648.2008.04700.x

Nettina, S. M. (2013). *Lippincott manual of nursing practice handbook* (10th ed.). Lippincott Williams & Wilkins.

Pinto, S. M., Caldeira Berenguer, S. M., & Martins, J. C. (2016). Is Impaired Comfort a Nursing Diagnosis? *International Journal of Nursing Knowledge, 27*(4), 205–209. https://doi.org/10.1111/2047-3095.12121

Polit, D. F., & Beck, C. T. (2010). Generalization in quantitative and qualitative research: Myths and strategies. *International Journal of Nursing Studies, 47*(11), 1451–1458. https://doi.org/10.1016/j.ijnurstu.2010.06.004

Renolen, Å., & Hjälmhult, E. (2015). Nurses experience of using scientific knowledge in clinical practice: a grounded theory study. *Scandinavian Journal of Caring Sciences, 29*(4), 633–641. https://doi.org/10.1111/scs.12191

Richards, D. A., & Borglin, G. (2011). Complex interventions and nursing: looking through a new lens at nursing research. *International Journal of Nursing Studies, 48*(5), 531–533. https://doi.org/10.1016/j.ijnurstu.2011.02.013

Scala, E., Price, C., & Day, J. (2016). An integrative review of engaging clinical nurses in nursing research. *Journal of Nursing Scholarship, 48*(4), 423–430. https://doi.org/10.1111/jnu.12223

Sieloff, C. L., & Raph, S. W. (2011). Nursing theory and management. *Journal of Nursing Management, 19*(8), 979–980. https://doi.org/10.1111/j.1365-2834.2011.01334.x

Stavor, D. C., Zedreck-Gonzalez, J., & Hoffmann, R. L. (2017). Improving the use of evidence-based practice and research utilization through the identification of barriers to implementation in a critical access hospital. *Journal of Nursing Administration, 47*(1), 56–61. https://doi.org/10.1097/NNA.0000000000000437

Tastan, S., Linch, G. C., Keenan, G. M., Stifter, J., McKinney, D., Fahey, L., Lopez, K. D., Yao, Y., & Wilkie, D. J. (2014). Evidence for the existing American Nurses Association-recognized standardized nursing terminologies: a systematic review. *International Journal of Nursing Studies, 51*(8), 1160–1170. https://doi.org/10.1016/j.ijnurstu.2013.12.004

Williams, B., Perillo, S., & Brown, T. (2015). What are the factors of organizational culture in health care settings that act as barriers to the implementation of evidence-based practice? A scoping review. *Nurse Education Today, 35*(2), e34–e41. https://doi.org/10.1016/j.nedt.2014.11.012

3 INTERVIEWING AND COMMUNICATION

KEY TERMS

active listening
confidentiality
disease
Health Insurance Portability and Accountability Act (HIPAA)
illness
motivational interviewing
open-ended questions
paralanguage

Learning Objectives

The student will:

1. Describe the phases of the nurse–patient interview.
2. Identify environmental elements that support successful interviewing.
3. Begin the interview with broad open-ended questions then move to focused questions to clarify topics.
4. Use therapeutic communication techniques during the patient interview.
5. Demonstrate increased comfort when interviewing patients on sensitive subjects.
6. Discuss strategies for handling patients with specific needs.
7. Utilize ethical principles when interviewing patients.

The health history interview is a conversation with a purpose. As you learn to elicit the patient's history, you will draw on many interpersonal skills that you use every day, but with important differences. Unlike social conversation, in which you can freely express your own needs and interests, the primary goal of the nurse–patient interview is to improve the well-being of the patient. At its most basic level, the purpose of conversation with a patient is threefold: to establish a trusting and supportive relationship, to gather information, and to offer information (Fig. 3-1).

Relating effectively with patients is among the most valued skills of nursing care. Using techniques that promote trust and convey respect allow the patient's story to unfold in its most full and detailed form. Establishing a

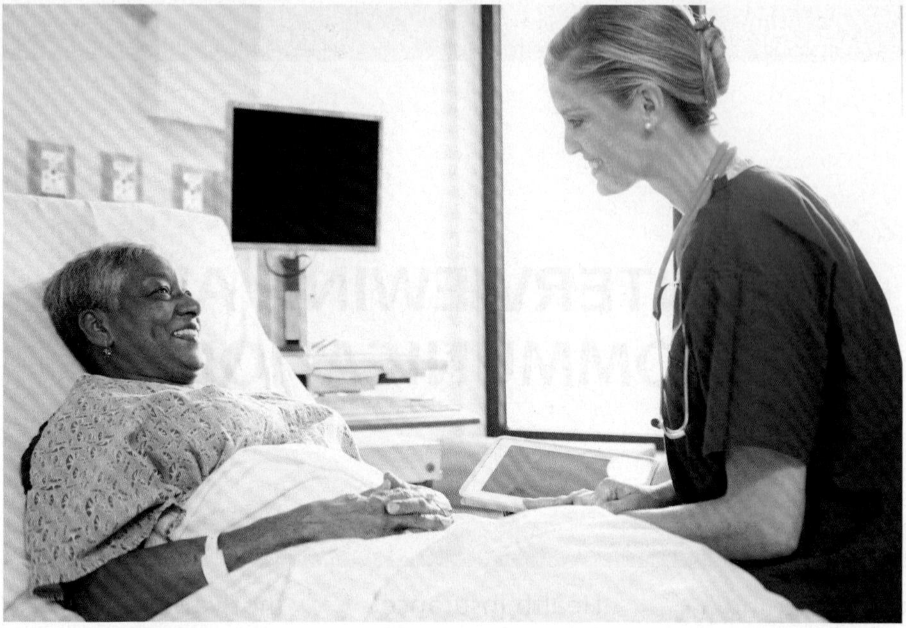

FIGURE 3-1 The health history interview helps establish a trusting and supportive relationship and allows the nurse to gather information and offer information.

supportive interaction helps the patient feel more at ease when sharing information and becomes the foundation for therapeutic nurse–patient relationships (Lein & Wills, 2007). Illness can make patients feel scared and isolated. A strong nurse–patient relationship can reduce feelings of isolation and fear.

This chapter introduces the essentials of interviewing. It emphasizes interviewing techniques but covers fundamental communication skills that will be continually used in conversations with patients. The chapter covers the phases of interviewing, important therapeutic communication techniques, and strategies for interviewing special patients.

The process of interviewing patients requires sensitivity to the patient's feelings and behavioral cues and is much more than just asking a series of questions. This process differs from the *format* of the health history as presented in Chapter 4, "The Health History." Both are necessary to care for patients but serve different purposes.

- The *health history format* is a structured framework for organizing patient information in *written, electronic, or verbal form* to communicate effectively with other health care providers. The patient's information is concisely organized into categories of present, past, and family health. The format identifies the specific information that must be obtained from the patient. As noted in Chapter 2, "Critical Thinking and Clinical Judgment in Health Assessment," the health history provides data for the nurse to generate an initial patient problem list.

- The *interviewing process* that actually generates the health information is much more fluid and demands effective communication and relational skills. It requires not only knowledge of the data needed but also the ability to elicit accurate information and the interpersonal skills that allow you as the nurse to respond to the patient's feelings and concerns.

Underlying these interviewing skills is a mindset that allows the nurse to collaborate with the patient and build a healing relationship. If the patient's greatest need is for support and empathy, encouraging the patient to discuss the *experience of illness* is therapeutic, as shown by the words below from a nurse working with a patient with long-standing and severe arthritis:

> *The patient had never talked about what the symptoms meant to her. She had never said: "This means that I can't go to the bathroom by myself, put my clothes on, even get out of bed without calling for help." When we finished the physical examination, I said something like, "Rheumatoid arthritis really has not been nice to you." She burst into tears, and her daughter did also, and I sat there, close to losing it myself. She said, "You know, no one has ever talked about it as a personal thing before. No one's ever talked to me as if this were a thing that mattered, a personal event." That was the significant moment in the encounter. I didn't really have much else to offer... but something really meaningful had happened between us, something that she valued and would carry away with her* (Hastings, 1989).

Motivational interviewing is an evidence-based method of therapeutic communication that enhances the nurse–patient relationship and the patient's understanding of their health needs. It helps patients identify, create, and implement changes in behaviors to improve or maintain health. To begin implementing motivational interviewing in your daily interaction with patients remember the acronym, "OARS" (Bershad, 2019; Carr, 2017):

- *O*pen-ended questions. Invite the patient to tell their story in their own words. Avoid "why" questions, which may seem judgmental to the patient. "Tell me about..." will sound nonjudgmental.

- *A*ffirmation. When the patient reveals a healthy habit or good decision, affirm this choice. For example, when a patient reports they taped a medication reminder to the bathroom mirror, affirm that is a good way not to forget to take medication.

- *R*eflective listening. To ensure you understand the correct meaning of a patient statement or the emotion the patient is feeling, you can reflect back the statement or feeling you hear. For example, "It sounds like you are feeling hopeless since your cancer returned."

- *S*ummarize and teach back. Summarize what the patient said, especially any strengths or plans the patient has told you regarding their problem. If you made a plan with the patient, ask them to repeat the information to reinforce it and make sure they understood the plan correctly.

PHASES OF INTERVIEWING

There are four general phases of each interview (Box 3-1).

BOX 3-1 PHASES OF THE INTERVIEW

1. Pre-interview: Setting the stage for a smooth interview
   - Self-reflection
   - Reviewing patient record
   - Setting interview goals
   - Reviewing own clinical behavior and appearance
2. Introduction: Putting the patient at ease and establishing trust
   - Greeting the patient and establishing rapport
   - Establishing the agenda for the interview
3. Working: Obtaining patient information
   - Inviting the patient's story
   - Identifying and responding to emotional cues
   - Expanding and clarifying the patient's story
   - Generating and testing diagnostic hypotheses
   - Negotiating a plan, including further evaluation, treatment, education and self-management support and prevention
4. Termination
   - Summarizing important points
   - Discussing plan of care

Phase 1: Pre-Interview

Interviewing patients requires planning. There are several preliminary steps that are crucial to success: taking time for self-reflection, reviewing the patient record, setting goals for the interview, reviewing your behavior and appearance, adjusting the environment, and being ready to take brief notes.

Take Time for Self-Reflection

As nurses, we encounter a wide variety of patients, each one unique. Establishing relationships with people from a broad spectrum of ages, social classes, races, ethnicities, and states of health or illness is an opportunity and privilege. Being consistently respectful and open to individual differences is one of the nurse's challenges. Because we bring our own values, assumptions, and biases to every encounter, we must look inward to clarify how our own expectations and reactions may affect what we hear and how we behave. Self-reflection is a continual part of professional development in nursing that enhances the care of our patients (Antai-Otong, 2007).

Review the Medical and Nursing Records

Before seeing the patient, review the medical and nursing records. This information helps identify areas to explore with the patient. Review identifying data such as age, gender, address, and health insurance, and peruse the problem list, medication list, and details such as documentation of allergies. The chart often provides valuable information about past diagnoses and treatments, but it is important to not let previous documentation bias your problem solving or prevent you from developing new approaches or ideas. Remember that information in the record comes from different observers and that standardized forms reflect different institutional norms. Details and nuances of patient information can be lost in electronic charting programs with drop-down menus. Data may be incomplete or even out of alignment with what you learn from the patient—understanding such discrepancies may prove helpful to the patient's care.

Set Goals for the Interview

Before talking with the patient, clarify the goals for the interview. Goals range from following up on health care issues, identifying new problems, and completing forms for health care institutions to obtaining a basis for developing a plan of care. *A nurse must balance these provider-centered goals with patient-centered goals.* There can be discrepancies between the needs of the nurse, the needs of the institution, and needs of the patient and family. If you take a few minutes to think through the goals ahead of time, the interview will be smoother.

Review Clinical Behavior and Appearance

Just as the nurse carefully observes the patient throughout the interview, the patient will be watching the nurse. Consciously or not, the nurse sends messages through both words and behavior. Posture, gestures, eye contact, and tone of voice all convey the extent of interest, attention, acceptance, and understanding. The skilled interviewer appears calm and unhurried, even if time is limited. Reactions that indicate disapproval, embarrassment, impatience, or boredom block communication, as do behaviors that condescend, stereotype, criticize, or belittle the patient or family. Professionalism requires the nurse maintain equanimity.

CLINICAL TIP
During the COVID-19 pandemic, nurses were concerned that wearing personal protection equipment (PPE), including the use of masks, inhibited the patient's ability to see their faces and prevented the patient seeing how much they cared. Wearing pictures of themselves without PPE helped contribute to bonding.

Personal appearance also affects the clinical relationship. Patients find cleanliness, neatness, conservative dress, and a name tag reassuring (Fig. 3-2). Remember to keep *the patient's perspective* in mind in order to build the patient's trust.

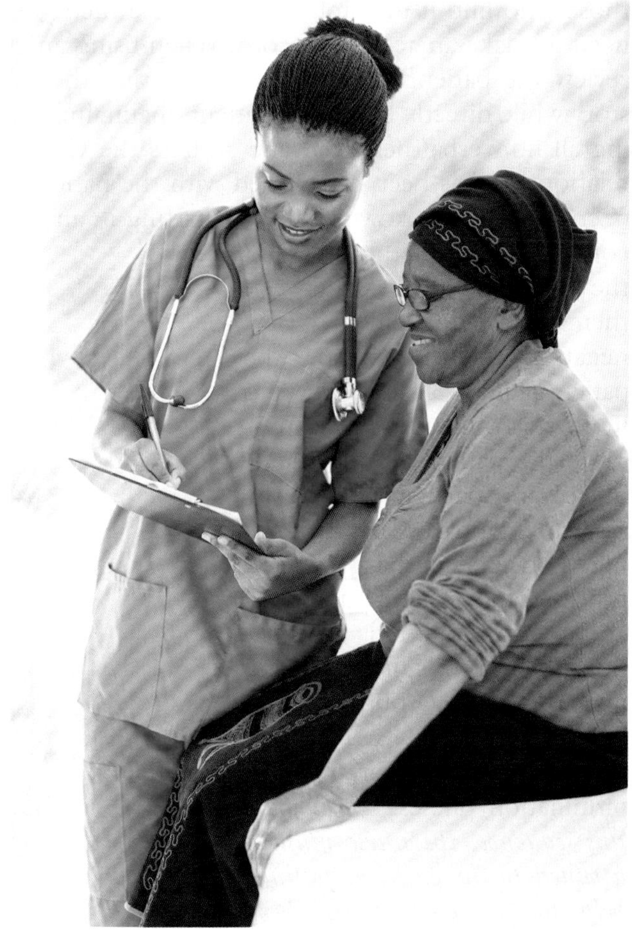

FIGURE 3-2 Personal appearance is critical in making a good first impression. (michaeljung/Shutterstock)

Adjust the Environment

Make the interview setting as private and comfortable as possible. A proper environment improves communication, though a hospitalized patient may need to be interviewed in a two-bed room or an emergency department. If there are privacy curtains, ask permission to pull them shut. Suggest moving to an empty room instead of talking in a waiting area. Adjust the room temperature for the patient's comfort when needed; for example, an older adult patient may appreciate a warmer room. *As the nurse, it is part of your job to make adjustments to the location and seating that make you and the patient more comfortable.* These efforts are always worth the time.

Concept Mastery Alert

Adjusting the Environment

To facilitate any patient interview and promote optimal communication, it is important that the nurse ensures that the environment for conducting the interview is comfortable and private. This may require interviewing the patient in an empty room, such as a conference room or exam room. This is done even before the nurse meets with the patient in phase 2.

Take Notes

No one can remember all the details of a comprehensive history. Write down short phrases, specific dates, or words, but do not let note taking or written or electronic forms distract you from the patient. Maintain eye contact and note when the patient points to a body part when describing a symptom. Whenever the patient is talking about sensitive or disturbing material, put down your pen or move away from the keyboard and focus solely on the patient. Most patients are accustomed to note taking, but for those who find it uncomfortable, explore their concerns and explain your need to make an accurate record. When using an electronic health record, review the patient's record before entering the room; elicit the patient's story while directly facing the patient, maintaining eye contact, and observing all nonverbal behavior; and address the viewing screen only after the relationship has been established with the patient included in the process (Cerrato, 2013; Stokowski, 2013). Charting in an electronic record with the computer between the nurse and the patient puts a barrier between them that the patient may view negatively. Sitting beside the patient (Fig. 3-3) while charting in an electronic record can promote the patient's understanding of and participation in the assessment process. By becoming "partners" in the assessment process and asking questions about the collected information, the patient's health literacy may improve (Drobny, 2017). The interview moves through the introduction, working, and termination phases. *Throughout this sequence, the nurse must be attuned to the patient's feelings, help the patient express them, respond to their content, and validate their significance.*

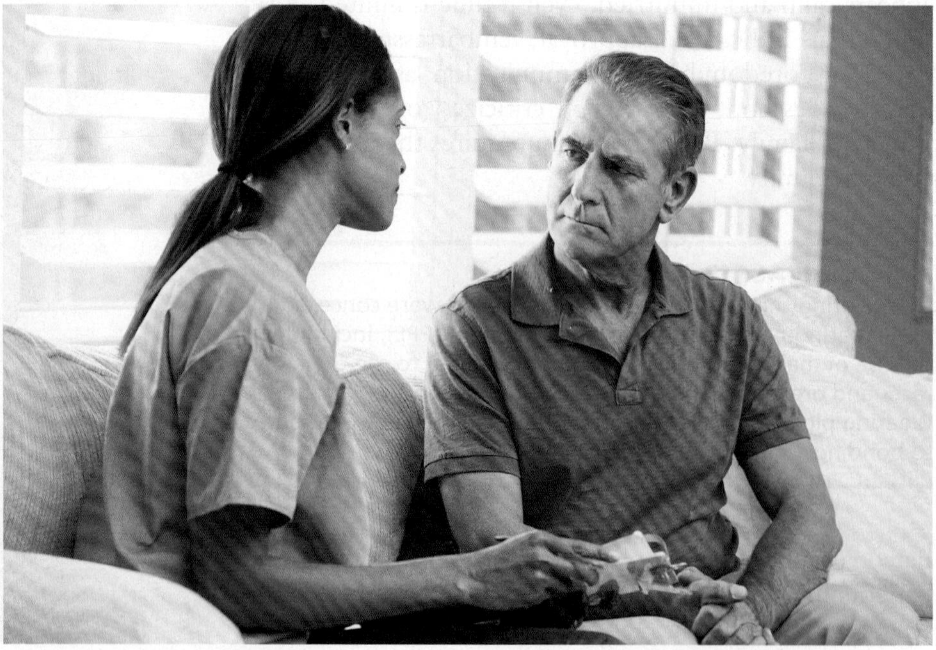

FIGURE 3-3 Sitting beside the patient can promote the patient's understanding of and participation in the assessment process. (Monkey Business Images/Shutterstock)

As a beginning student, concentrate primarily on gathering the patient's story and creating a shared understanding of the problem. As you become a practicing nurse, reaching agreement on a plan for further evaluation and treatment becomes more important. Whether the interview is comprehensive or focused, you should move through this sequence with close attention to the patient's feelings and affect, always working on strengthening the relationship.

Phase 2: Introduction

Greet the Patient and Establish Rapport

The initial moments of an encounter with the patient lay the foundation for an ongoing relationship. How you greet the patient and other visitors in the room, provide for the patient's comfort, and arrange the physical setting all shape the patient's first impressions.

As you begin, *greet the patient* by name and introduce yourself, giving your own name. If possible and culturally appropriate, shake hands with the patient. If this is the first contact, explain your role, including your status as a student and how you will be involved in the patient's care.

Using a formal title to address the patient—Mr. O'Neil or Ms. Washington, for example—is always best (Sheldon & Foust, 2014). If you are unsure how to pronounce the patient's name, do not be afraid to ask. You can say, "I am afraid of mispronouncing your name. Could you say it for me?" Then repeat it to make sure that you heard it correctly. Also ask the patient how they would like to be addressed and what pronouns they prefer to use. See the section, "The LBGTQIA Patient." Except with children or adolescents, avoid first names unless you have specific permission from the patient or family. Addressing an unfamiliar adult as "granny" or "dear" can be depersonalizing and demeaning, as well as unprofessional.

When visitors are in the room, be sure to acknowledge and greet each one in turn, inquiring about each person's name and relationship to the patient. Whenever visitors are present, *you are obligated to maintain the patient's confidentiality*. Let the patient decide if visitors or family members should remain in the room before conducting the interview. "Would you prefer if I spoke to you alone or with your sister present?"

Consider the best way to *arrange the room* and distance from the patient. Remember that cultural background and individual taste influence preferences about interpersonal space. Choose a distance that facilitates conversation and allows good eye contact, probably within a few feet of the patient, close enough to be intimate but not intrusive. Pull up a chair and if possible, sit at eye level with the patient. Move any physical barriers, such as desks or bedside tables, out of the way. Avoid arrangements that convey disrespect or inequality of power, such as interviewing a patient on a bedpan or commode. Such arrangements are unacceptable. Lighting also makes a difference. Sitting between a patient and a bright light or window may make the patient squint uncomfortably to see you.

Provide the patient with undivided attention. Spend enough time on small talk to put the patient at ease, and avoid looking down to take notes, read the chart, or scan a computer screen. In a first meeting, demonstrate interest in the patient as a person (Riley, 2020).

Establish the Agenda

Once rapport has been established, the nurse is ready to pursue the patient's reason for seeking health care. This reason is traditionally designated the *chief complaint*, but when there are three or four reasons for the visit, the phrase *presenting problems* may be preferable. Begin with **open-ended questions** that allow full freedom of response like, "What concerns bring you here today?" or "How can I help you?" Helpful open-ended questions include "Are there specific concerns that prompted you to schedule this appointment?" and "What made you decide to come in to see us today?" Note that these questions encourage the patient to express any possible concerns and do not restrict the patient to a problem per se. Sometimes patients do not give a specific problem; it is a well-person visit, and they ask for "just a check-up."

An important fact to remember is that the first problem the patient brings up is not necessarily the most important one. In fact, when the chief reason for coming is psychosocial, it is usually *not* the first reason the patient mentions. The order in which problems are presented is not always connected to their clinical importance.

Identifying all the concerns at the beginning of the interview allows the patient and the nurse to negotiate which concerns are most pressing for the visit and which can be postponed to a follow-up appointment. Questions such as "Is there anything else?" or "Have we got everything?" help elicit the patient's complete list of reasons for coming to the health care facility. The nurse may also have concerns such as blood pressure management or diabetic diet maintenance. Identifying the full agenda or even the "real reason" for the visit at the outset makes use of the time available more meaningful, facilitates time management, and reduces the short shrift given to late-emerging concerns. However, negotiating the agenda at the outset still does not always prevent the patient from mentioning a new problem while leaving.

Phase 3: Working Phase

Invite the Patient's Story

Once the agenda has been decided, invite the patient's story by asking about the patient's foremost concern, saying, "Tell me more about..." Encourage the patient to tell the story in their own words. Avoid biasing the patient's story. That is, *do not add new information* and *do not*

See the sections, "Guided Questioning: Options to Expand and Clarify the Patient's Story" and "Encouraging with Continuers."

interrupt. Instead, use active listening skills, such as leaning forward as you listen and using continuers such as nodding your head and offering phrases like "uh huh," "go on," or "I see." *Follow the patient's lead*. Asking specific questions prematurely or suggesting solutions before the patient's story is complete risks losing the information being sought. Once interrupted, patients rarely return to telling their stories. After the patient completes the initial description of each problem, use *focused questions to explore the patient's story in more depth*, for example, "How would you describe the pain?" "What happened next?" and "Did you notice this occurs at a certain time?" Using guided questioning allows the nurse to obtain a complete picture of the patient's concern (Riley, 2020).

Identify and Respond to the Patient's Emotional Cues

Emotional distress is frequently associated with illness. Patients may withhold their true concerns during health care visits but offer various clues that may be direct or indirect, verbal or nonverbal, and expressed as ideas or emotions. Acknowledging and responding to these clues help build rapport, expand the nurse's understanding of the illness, and improve patient satisfaction (Riley, 2020).

If the patient has not mentioned their perspective on illness during the open-ended portion of the interview, explore this perspective prior to the directive. Probe the personal context of the illness by asking, "How has this affected you?" "What do you make of this?" or "How did you feel about that?" or by stating, "Many people would be frustrated by something like this." In addition, explore the patient's ideas about the effect of the illness on their life. See Box 3-2 for the different ways clues about the patient's perspective on illness may be expressed.

BOX 3-2 CLUES TO THE PATIENT'S PERSPECTIVE ON ILLNESS

- Direct statement(s) by the patient of explanations, emotions, expectations, and effects of the illness
- Expression of feelings about the illness
- Attempts to explain or understand symptoms
- Speech clues (e.g., repetition, prolonged reflective pauses)
- Sharing a personal story
- Behavioral clues indicative of unidentified concerns, dissatisfaction, or unmet needs such as reluctance to accept recommendations, seeking a second opinion, or early return appointment

Respond immediately when you hear an emotional cue. Appropriate response techniques include reflection, synonyms, and feedback indicating support and partnership. A mnemonic for responding to emotional cues is *NURS*: *n*aming—"That sounds like a scary experience;" *u*nderstanding or legitimization—"It's understandable that you feel that way;" and *res*pecting—"You've done better than most people would with this."

NURS
N—Naming
U—Understanding
ReS—Respecting

Expand and Clarify the Patient's Story

After eliciting the patient's story as fully as possible in a nondirective manner and exploring the patient's lived experience of the illness, guide the patient in elaborating on the areas of the health history that seem most significant. Clarify the attributes of each symptom, including context, associations, and chronology. For pain and many other symptoms, understanding these essential characteristics, summarized as follows as the seven key attributes of a symptom, is critical.

To pursue the seven attributes, two mnemonics may help:

- OLD CART (Box 3-3), or *o*nset, *l*ocation, *d*uration, *c*haracteristic symptoms, *a*ssociated manifestations, *r*elieving/exacerbating factors, and *t*reatment
- OPQRST, or *o*nset, *p*alliating/*p*rovoking factors, *q*uality, *r*adiation, *s*ite, and *t*iming

BOX 3-3 THE SEVEN ATTRIBUTES OF A SYMPTOM (OLD CART)

1. *O*nset: When did (does) it start; setting in which it occurs, including environmental factors, personal activities, emotional reactions, or other circumstances that may have contributed.
2. *L*ocation: Where is it? Does it radiate?
3. *D*uration: How long does it last?
4. *C*haracteristic symptoms: What is it like? How severe is it? (For a subjective symptom like pain, ask the patient to rate it on a scale of 1 to 10.)
5. *A*ssociated manifestations: Have you noticed anything else that accompanies it?
6. *R*elieving/exacerbating factors: Is there anything that makes it better or worse?
7. *T*reatment: What have you done to treat this? Was it effective?

See Chapter 2, "Critical Thinking and Clinical Judgment in Health Assessment" for more symptom attribute questions using OLD CART.

Whenever possible, *use the patient's words,* making sure you clarify their meaning. Do not use medical terminology or medical jargon, because it confuses and frustrates patients. Define medical terminology for the patient in layman's terms. Be aware of how quickly jargon like "take a history" and "work you up" can creep into discussions. Choose instead plain English words such as "I'd like to learn more about your illness" or "Doing these examinations can help us understand what's causing your illness."

It is important to establish *the sequence and timing* of each patient symptom if you are to arrive at accurate assessments. Encourage a chronologic account by stating, "Please describe the *symptom* from when it began to now" or "Please start at the beginning, or the last time you felt well, and go step by step." You may also choose to ask such questions as "What then?" or "What happened next?" To fill in specific details, guide the patient's story by employing different types of questions and the techniques of skilled interviewing. Use focused questions to elicit information that the patient has not already offered. *In general, an interview moves back and*

See Box 3-5 "Techniques of Skilled Interviewing" and the section "Moving from Open-Ended to Focused Questions."

forth from open-ended questions to increasingly focused questions and then on to another open-ended question, returning the lead in the interview to the patient.

Generating and Testing Diagnostic Hypotheses

The skills of diagnostic reasoning are developed over time with practice. As the history is gathered, one develops and tests hypotheses about the patient problem or problems. Identifying the attributes and details of the patient's symptoms is fundamental to recognizing patterns of problems and generating nursing analyses.

Some students visualize the process of evoking a full description of the symptom as "the cone" (Fig. 3-4).

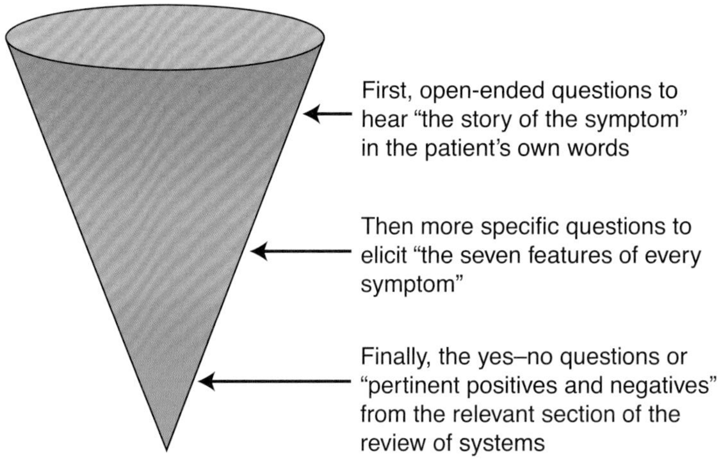

First, open-ended questions to hear "the story of the symptom" in the patient's own words
Then more specific questions to elicit "the seven features of every symptom"
Finally, the yes–no questions or "pertinent positives and negatives" from the relevant section of the review of systems

FIGURE 3-4 Each symptom has its own "cone."

For example, for a patient with a cough, these questions would come from the "Respiratory" section of the "Review of Systems." See Chapter 4, "The Health History."

Each symptom has its own "cone," which is documented in the "History of Present Illness" section of the written record.

Appropriate questions about symptoms are also suggested in each of the chapters on the regional physical examinations. This is one way to build evidence for and against various diagnostic possibilities. The challenge is not letting this kind of inquiry dominate the interview and displace learning about the patient's perspective, conveying concern for the patient's well-being, and building the relationship.

See also Chapter 2, "Critical Thinking and Clinical Judgment in Health Assessment."

Create a Shared Understanding of the Problem

The literature makes it clear that delivering effective health care requires exploring the deeper meanings patients attach to their symptoms. Although the "seven attributes of a symptom" add important details to the patient's history, the disease/illness distinction model helps health care practitioners understand the full impact on the patient (Kleinman et al., 1978). This model acknowledges the different yet complementary perspectives of the nurse and the patient. **Disease** is the explanation that the *nurse* uses to account for the symptoms. It is the way that the nurse organizes what is learned from the patient that leads to a nursing diagnosis. **Illness** can be defined as how the *patient* experiences the disease, including its effects on relationships, functioning, and sense of well-being. Many factors may shape this experience, including prior personal or family health, the effect of symptoms on everyday life, individual outlook and style of coping, and expectations about medical and nursing care. The melding of these perspectives forms the basis for identifying nursing analyses and creating a plan of care. *The interview needs to incorporate both these views.*

Even a chief complaint as straightforward as a sore throat can illustrate these divergent views. The patient may be most concerned about pain and difficulty swallowing, missing time from work, or a cousin who was hospitalized with tonsillitis. The nurse, however, may focus on specific points in the history that differentiate streptococcal pharyngitis from other causes or on a history of an allergy to penicillin. To understand the patient's expectations, the nurse needs to go beyond just the attributes of a symptom. Learning about the patient's perception of illness means asking patient-centered questions in the four domains of feelings. This information is crucial to patient satisfaction, effective health care, and patient follow-through.

A mnemonic for the patient's perspective on the illness is *FIFE*, *f*eelings, *i*deas, effect on *f*unction, and *e*xpectations (Box 3-4).

BOX 3-4 EXPLORE THE PATIENT'S PERSPECTIVE (FIFE)

- The patient's *f*eelings, including fears or concerns, about the problem
- The patient's *i*deas about the nature and the cause of the problem
- The effect of the problem on the patient's life and *f*unctioning
- The patient's expectations of the disease, of the clinician, or of health care, often based on prior personal or family experiences

To uncover the patient's feelings, the nurse might ask, "What concerns you most about the pain?" or "How has this been for you?" To explore the patient's thoughts about the cause of the problem, the nurse could say, "Why do you think you have this stomachache?" Because self-treatment suggests the patient's thinking, you may ask, "What have you tried?"

A patient may worry that the pain is a symptom of serious disease and want reassurance. Alternatively, the patient may be less concerned about the cause of the pain and just want relief. To determine the effect of the illness on the patient's lifestyle and function, particularly for patients with chronic illness, ask, "What can't you do now that you could do before?" or "How has your backache (for example) affected your ability to work? Your life at home? Your social activities? Your role as a parent?

Your function in intimate relationships? The way you feel about yourself as a person?"

You also need to find out what the patient expects from you, the nurse, or from health care in general by continuing the conversation in such a way as, "I am glad that the pain is almost gone. How specifically can I help you now?" Even if the stomach pain is almost gone, the patient may need a work excuse to take to an employer.

Negotiate a Plan

Learning about the effects of the illness gives the nurse and the patient the opportunity to create a complete and congruent picture of the problem. This multifaceted picture then forms the basis for planning further evaluation (e.g., physical examination, laboratory tests, consultations) and negotiating a nursing care plan. It also plays an important role in building rapport with the patient.

See also the Chapter 2 discussion of developing a plan that is agreeable to the patient.

Phase 4: Termination

Summarize Important Points and Discuss Plan

Let the patient know that the end of the interview is approaching to allow time for the patient to ask any final questions. Make sure the patient understands the mutual plans you have developed. For example, before gathering your papers or standing to leave the room, you can say, "We need to stop now. Do you have any questions about what we've covered?" As you close, summarizing the patient's problems and reviewing the plan of care and follow-up are helpful. "So, you will take the medicine as we discussed, check your blood glucose daily, and make a follow-up appointment for 4 weeks. Do you have any questions about this?" Address any related concerns or questions that the patient raises. At the end of the interview, use the "teach-back" method to ensure the patient remembers and understands the information and plan of care. Ask the patient to repeat the plan of care (Bershad, 2019).

The patient should have a chance to ask any final questions; however, the last few minutes are not the time to bring up new topics. If that happens and the concern is not life-threatening nor requires immediate attention, assure the patient of your interest and make plans to address the problem at a future time.

THERAPEUTIC COMMUNICATION TECHNIQUES

This section describes the skills that form the basic tools of interviewing. The nurse employs these interviewing skills to achieve the tasks described in the "Phases of Interviewing" section more effectively. Practice improves interviewing skills. Being observed and recorded during an interview allows for feedback from an experienced interviewer. The techniques of skilled interviewing are listed in Box 3-5.

BOX 3-5 THE TECHNIQUES OF SKILLED INTERVIEWING

- Active listening
- Guided questioning
- Nonverbal communication
- Empathic responses
- Validation
- Reassurance
- Summarizing
- Transitions
- Empowering the patient

Active Listening

Underlying all the techniques is the habit of *active listening*. **Active listening** is the process of paying close attention to what the patient is communicating, being aware of the patient's emotional state, and using verbal and nonverbal skills to encourage the speaker to continue and expand (Antai-Otong, 2007). This takes practice. It is easy to drift into thinking about the next question or the potential nursing analyses.

Guided Questioning: Options to Expand and Clarify the Patient's Story

There are several ways you can ask for more information from the patient without interfering with the flow of the patient's story. The goal is to facilitate the patient's fullest communication. Learning the techniques in Table 3-1 encourages patient disclosures while minimizing the risk for distorting the patient's ideas or missing significant details. This is how one avoids asking a series of specific questions, which takes more time and makes the patient feel more passive.

Nonverbal Communication

Communication that does not involve speech occurs continuously and provides important clues to feelings and emotions. Becoming sensitive to nonverbal messages allows the nurse to both "read the patient" more effectively and send messages. Pay close attention to eye contact, facial expression, posture, head position and movement such as shaking or nodding, interpersonal distance, and placement of the arms or legs—crossed, neutral, or open. Be aware that some nonverbal language is universal and some is culturally bound.

Matching your position to the patient's position can signify increased rapport, just as mirroring your position can signify the patient's increasing sense of connectedness. One can also mirror the patient's **paralanguage**, or qualities of speech, such as pacing, tone, and volume, to increase rapport. Moving closer or using physical contact like placing your hand on the patient's arm can convey empathy or help the patient gain control of difficult feelings. Sensitivity to the patient's culture must guide the use of nonverbal communication.

TABLE 3-1 Guided Questioning Techniques

Technique	Description	Reasoning	Examples
Moving from open-ended to focused questions	Start with general questions; follow up with more specific questions.	Helps patient describe the problem Avoids leading questions that might suggest the answer to the patient	"Tell me about your chest pain." "What else?" "Where did you feel it?" "Show me." "Anywhere else?" "To which arm?"
Graded response questions	Ask questions that require a graded response rather than a single answer.	Produces a more useful quantitative answer	Instead of "Do you get tired climbing steps?" ask "How many steps can you climb before you get short of breath?"
Asking questions one at a time	Rather than asking a series of questions that may confuse the patient, pause between each problem and make eye contact to allow the patient time to answer.	Reduces patient confusion	"Have you had any of the following problems? Tuberculosis (pause)? Pleurisy (pause)? Bronchitis (pause)?"
Offering multiple choices for answers	Provide multiple possible responses for a question you ask rather than leaving them entirely open-ended.	Minimizes bias or leading the patient erroneously Helps patients articulate their symptoms	"Which of the following words best describes your pain: aching, sharp, pressing, burning, shooting, or something else?"
Clarifying patient's meaning	Clearing up words that patients use that are ambiguous or have unclear associations	Prevents misunderstanding the meaning of the patient's responses	"Tell me exactly what you meant by 'the flu.'" "You said you were behaving just like your mother. What did you mean?"
Encouraging with continuers	Using posture, gestures, or words to encourage the patient to say more	Makes the patient feel comfortable sharing potentially intimate details	Leaning forward, making eye contact, and using phrases like "Mm-hmm," "go on," or "I'm listening" to maintain the flow of the patient's story
Reflection	A simple reflection or echoing back of the patient's words	Encourages the patient to express both factual details and feelings	Patient: "The pain got worse and began to spread." Response: "Spread?" Patient: "Yes, it went to my shoulder and down my left arm to the fingers. It was so bad that I thought I was going to die." Response: "You thought you were going to die." Patient: "Yes, it was just like the pain my father had when he had his heart attack, and I was afraid the same thing was happening to me."

Empathic Responses

Conveying empathy greatly strengthens patient rapport. As patients talk, they may express—with or without words—feelings they may or may not have consciously acknowledged. *To provide empathy, first identify the patient's feelings.* At first, this may seem unfamiliar or uncomfortable. When you sense important but unexpressed feelings from the patient's face, voice, words, or behavior, inquire about them rather than assuming that you know how the patient feels. You may simply ask, "How did you feel about that?" Patients may hold back their feelings, unsure of how they will be received. Unless you let patients know that you are interested in feelings as well as facts, you may miss important insights.

Once you have identified the feelings, respond with understanding and acceptance. Responses may be as simple as "I understand," "That sounds upsetting," or "You seem sad." Empathy may also be nonverbal—for example, offering a tissue to a crying patient or gently placing your hand on the patient's arm (Fig. 3-5). For a response to be empathic, it must reflect a precise understanding of what the patient is feeling. If your response acknowledges how upset a patient must have been at the death of a parent when in fact the death relieved the patient of a long-standing financial and emotional burden, you have misunderstood the situation. Instead of making assumptions, you can ask directly about the patient's emotional response. "I am sorry about the death of your father. What has that been like for you?"

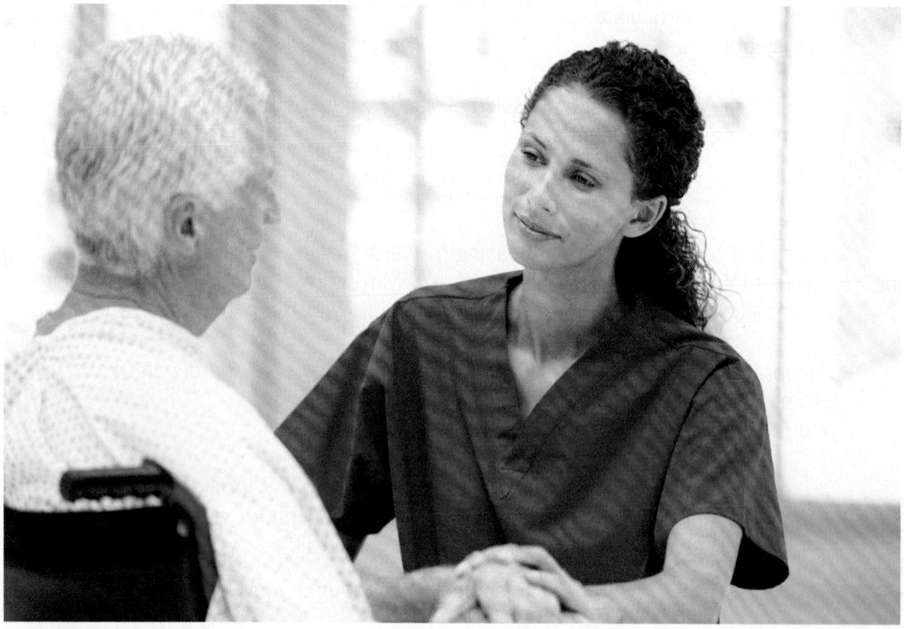

FIGURE 3-5 Empathy may be nonverbal.

Validation

Another important way to make a patient feel affirmed is to validate or acknowledge the legitimacy of the emotional experience. A patient who has been in a car accident but has no physical injury may still be experiencing significant distress. You can reassure the patient by stating something like, "Being in that accident must have been scary. Car accidents are always unsettling because they remind us of our vulnerability and mortality. That could explain why you still feel upset." It helps the patient feel that such emotions are legitimate and understandable.

Reassurance

When you are talking with patients who are anxious or upset, it is tempting to try to reassure them. Saying, "Don't worry. Everything is going to be alright" may reassure the patient about the wrong thing and provide false reassurance. Moreover, premature reassurance may block further disclosures, especially if the patient feels that the nurse is uncomfortable with the patient's anxiety or has not appreciated the extent of their distress.

The first step to effective reassurance is simply identifying and acknowledging the patient's feelings. This promotes a feeling of connection. The actual reassurance comes much later after the interview, the physical examination, and perhaps some diagnostic studies have been completed. At that point, you can interpret for the patient what you think is happening and deal openly with expressed concerns. True reassurance comes from conveying information in a competent manner, making the patient feel confident that problems have been fully understood and will be addressed.

Summarizing

Giving a capsule summary of the patient's story during the course of the interview serves several different functions. It communicates to the patient that you have been listening carefully. It identifies what you know and what you do not know. "Now, let me make sure that I have the full story. You said you've had a cough for 3 days, that it's especially bad at night, and that you have started to bring up yellow phlegm. You have not had a fever or felt short of breath, but you do feel congested with difficulty breathing through your nose." Following with an attentive pause or asking, "Is there anything else?" lets the patient add other information and correct any misunderstanding.

Summarizing can be used at different points in the interview to structure the visit, especially at times of transition (see the next section). This technique also allows you to organize your clinical reasoning and to convey it to the patient, making the relationship more collaborative. *It is also a useful technique for learners when they draw a blank on what to ask the patient next.*

Transitions

Patients have many reasons to feel vulnerable during a health care visit. To put them more at ease, tell them when you are changing directions during the interview. Just as clear signs along the highway give a sense of confidence, this "sign posting" gives patients a greater sense of control. As you move from one part of the history to the next and on to the physical examination, orient the patient with brief transitional phrases like, "Now I'd like to ask some questions about your past health." Make clear what the patient should expect or do next. "Before we move on to reviewing all your medications, was there anything else you want to discuss about past health problems?" "Now I would like to examine you. I will step out for a few minutes. Please undress and put on this gown." Specifying that the gown should close in the back protects the patient's modesty and can make examiners more comfortable.

Empowering the Patient

Patients have many reasons to feel vulnerable. They may be in pain or worried about a symptom. They may be unfamiliar or overwhelmed with accessing the health care system. Differences of gender, ethnicity, race, or class may also contribute to power differentials. However, ultimately, patients are responsible for their own care. Patients who are self-confident and understand the recommendations are most likely to adopt offered advice, make lifestyle changes, or take medications as prescribed.

Box 3-6 lists principles that help nurses share power with patients. Although many of them have been discussed in other sections of this chapter, the need to reinforce each patient's primary responsibility for their health is so fundamental that it is worth summarizing them here.

BOX 3-6 EMPOWERING THE PATIENT: PRINCIPLES OF SHARING POWER

- Evoke the patient's perspective.
- Convey interest in the person, not just the problem.
- Follow the patient's leads.
- Elicit and validate emotional content.
- Share information with the patient, especially at transition points during the visit.
- Make your clinical reasoning transparent to the patient.
- Reveal the limits of your knowledge.

ADAPTING THE INTERVIEW FOR SPECIFIC PATIENTS

Each patient is unique and has the potential to present the nurse with interviewing challenges. Your proficiency handling these situations will develop throughout your career. *Always remember the importance of listening to the patient and clarifying the patient's concerns.*

The Silent Patient

Novice interviewers are often uncomfortable with periods of silence and feel obligated to keep the conversation going. Silence has many meanings and many purposes. Patients frequently fall silent for short periods to collect thoughts, remember details, or decide whether you can be trusted with certain information. The period of silence usually feels much longer to the nurse than it does to the patient. The nurse should appear attentive and give brief encouragement to continue when appropriate. During periods of silence, watch the patient closely for nonverbal cues, such as difficulty controlling emotions (Fig. 3-6).

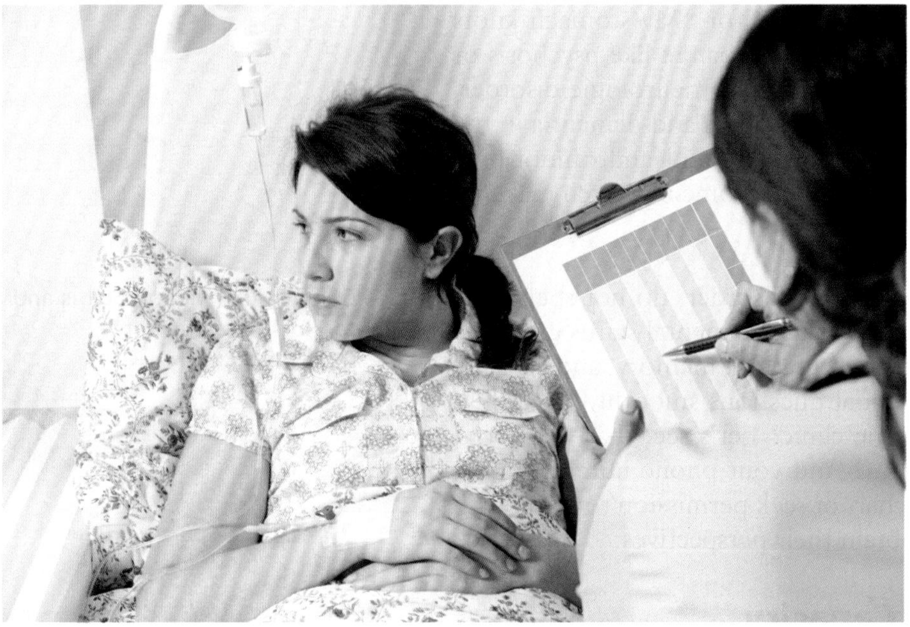

FIGURE 3-6 Patients may fall silent for short periods to collect thoughts, remember details, or decide whether you can be trusted with certain information.

Silence may be part of the patient's culture or be the patient's response to how you are asking questions. Are you asking too many short-answer questions in rapid succession? Have you offended the patient in any way by signs of disapproval or criticism? Have you failed to recognize an overwhelming symptom such as pain, nausea, or dyspnea? If so, you may need to ask the patient directly, "You seem very quiet. Have I done something to upset you?"

Patients with depression or dementia may lose their usual spontaneity of expression, give short answers to questions, and then fall silent. If you have already tried guiding them through recent events or a typical day, try shifting your inquiry to the symptoms of depression or begin an exploratory mental status examination.

See Chapter 19, "Mental Status and Mental Health Assessment."

The Confusing Patient

Some patients present a confusing array of *multiple symptoms*. They seem to have every symptom that you ask about. With these patients, focus on the meaning or function of the symptom, emphasizing the patient's perspective, and guide the interview into a psychosocial assessment. There is little profit to exploring each symptom in detail. Although the patient may have several illnesses, a psychological disorder may also be present.

At other times, you may feel baffled, frustrated, and confused because you cannot make sense out of the patient's story. The history is vague and

See Table 24-1, "Delirium and Dementia."

difficult to understand, ideas are poorly connected, and language is hard to follow. Even though you word your questions carefully, you cannot seem to get clear answers. The patient's manner of relating to you may also seem peculiar, distant, aloof, or inappropriate. Symptoms may be described in bizarre terms like "My fingernails feel too heavy" or "My stomach knots up like a snake." Perhaps there is a mental status change like psychosis or delirium, a mental illness such as schizophrenia, or a neurologic disorder. Consider delirium in acutely ill or intoxicated patients and dementia in the elderly. Such patients give histories that are inconsistent and cannot provide a clear chronology about what has happened. Some may even make up information to fill in the gaps in their memories.

When you suspect a psychiatric or neurologic disorder, do not spend too much time gathering a detailed history. Shift to the mental status examination, focusing on level of consciousness, orientation, memory, and capacity to understand. You can work in the initial questions smoothly by asking, "When was your last appointment at the clinic? Let's see, that was about how long ago?" "Your address now is…? And your phone number?" You can check these responses against the chart or seek permission to speak with family members or friends and then obtain their perspectives.

See Chapter 19, "Mental Status and Mental Health Assessment."

The Patient with Altered Capacity

Some patients cannot provide their own histories because of delirium from illness, dementia, or other health or mental health conditions. Others are unable to relate certain parts of their histories, such as events related to febrile illnesses or seizures. Under these circumstances, you need to determine whether the patient has *decision-making capacity* which is the ability to understand information related to health, to make health choices based on reason and a consistent set of values and to declare preferences about treatments. The term "capacity" is preferable to the term "competence," which is a legal term. You do not need to consult a colleague in psychiatry to assess capacity unless mental illness impairs decision making. For many patients with psychiatric conditions or even cognitive impairments, their ability to make decisions remains intact.

For patients with decision-making capacity, obtain their consent before talking about their health with others. Even if patients communicate only with facial expressions or gestures, you must maintain confidentiality and elicit their input. Assure patients that any shared history will be kept confidential, and clarify what you can discuss with others. Your knowledge about the patient can be quite comprehensive, yet others may offer surprising and important information. A spouse, for example, may report significant family strains, depressive symptoms, or drinking habits that the patient has denied. Consider dividing the interview into two segments—one with the patient and the other with both the patient and a second informant. Each interview has its own value. Information from other sources often gives you helpful ideas for planning the patient's care but remains confidential. Also learn the tenets of the **Health Insurance Portability and Accountability Act (HIPAA)** passed by Congress in 1996, which sets strict standards for disclosure for both institutions and providers when sharing patient information (Health Information Privacy—HIPPA for Professionals, 2020).

For patients with impaired capacity, you will often need to find a *surrogate informant* or *decision maker* to assist with the history. Check whether the patient has a *durable power of attorney for health care* or a *health care proxy*. If not, in many cases, the patient may have a spouse or family member who can represent the patient's wishes and fill this role.

Apply the basic principles of interviewing to your conversations with patients' relatives or friends. Find a private place to talk. Introduce yourself, state your purpose, inquire how they are feeling under the circumstances, and recognize and acknowledge their concerns. As you listen to their versions of the history, assess the quality of their relationships with the patient because it may color their credibility. Establish how they know the patient. For example, when a child is brought in for health care, a grandparent who provides daily day care while parents work may have the most inclusive knowledge of the child's course of illness. Always seek the best-informed source. Occasionally, a relative or friend insists on being with the patient during your evaluation. Try to find out why, and assess the patient's wishes.

The Talkative Patient

The garrulous, rambling patient may be difficult to interview, especially when faced with limited time and the need to "get the whole story." Several techniques are helpful. Give the patient free rein for the first 5 or 10 minutes, listening closely to the conversation. Perhaps the patient simply needs a good listener and is expressing pent-up concerns, or the patient's style is to tell stories. In some cultures, social conversation of various lengths before "getting down to business" is considered polite. Does the patient seem obsessively detailed? Is the patient unduly anxious or apprehensive? Is there flight of ideas or a disorganized thought process that suggests a cognitive disorder?

Focus on what seems most important to the patient. Show your interest by asking questions in those areas. Interrupt only if necessary, but also be courteous. Learn how to set limits when needed. Remember that part of your task is structuring the interview to gain important information about the patient's health. A brief summary may help you change the subject yet validate any concerns. "Let me make sure that I understand. You have described many concerns. In particular, I heard about two different kinds of pain, one on your left side that goes into your groin and is fairly new, and one in your upper abdomen after you eat that you have had for months. Let's focus just on the side pain first. Can you tell me what it feels like?"

Finally, do not show impatience. If time runs out, explain the need for a second meeting. Setting a time limit for the next appointment may be helpful. "I know we have much more to talk about. We will continue after lunch. We will have a full hour then."

The Crying Patient

Crying signals strong emotions, ranging from sadness to anger or frustration. If the patient is on the verge of tears, pausing, gentle probing, or responding with empathy gives the patient permission to cry. Usually crying is therapeutic, as is your quiet acceptance of the patient's distress or pain. Offer a tissue and wait for the patient to recover. Make a supportive remark like, "I am glad you were able to express your feelings." Most patients will soon compose themselves and resume the story. Aside from acute grief or loss, it is unusual for crying to escalate and become uncontrollable.

Crying makes many people uncomfortable. If this is true for you, you need to learn how to accept displays of emotion so that as a nurse you can support patients at these significant times.

The Angry or Disruptive Patient

Many patients have reasons to be angry; they may be ill, they may have suffered a loss, they may lack their accustomed control over their own lives, and they may feel powerless in the health care system (Platt & Gordon, 2004). They may direct this anger toward the nurse. It is possible that this hostility is justified—were you late for the appointment, inconsiderate, insensitive, or angry yourself? If so, acknowledge that fact and try to make amends. More often, however, patients displace their anger onto the nurse as a reflection of their frustration or pain.

Accept angry feelings from patients. Allow them to express such emotions without getting angry in return. Avoid joining such patients in their hostility toward another provider or the agency, even when privately you may feel sympathetic. You can validate their feelings without agreeing with their reasons: "I understand that you felt frustrated by the long wait and answering the same questions over and over. Our complex health care system can seem unsupportive when you are not feeling well." After the patient has calmed down, help find steps that will avert such situations in the future. Rational solutions to emotional problems are not always possible, however, and people need time to express and work through their angry feelings.

Some angry patients become overtly disruptive. Few people can disturb the clinic, nursing unit, or emergency department more quickly than patients who are angry, belligerent, or out of control. Before approaching such patients, alert the security staff—as a nurse, maintaining a safe environment is one of your responsibilities. Stay calm, appear accepting, and avoid being confrontational in return. Keep your posture relaxed and nonthreatening and your hands loosely open. At first, do not try to make disruptive patients lower their voices or stop if they are haranguing you or the staff. Listen carefully. Try to understand what they are saying. Once you have established rapport, gently suggest moving to a different location that is more private and will cause less disruption.

The Dying Patient

Nurses care for dying patients of all ages in many settings, including hospitals, nursing homes, hospices, and patient homes. Interviewing and caring for the dying patient can be challenging for all nurses and must be addressed, especially with the student or new nurse. Many students avoid talking about death because of their own discomfort or anxiety. It is important to work through your feelings. Courses, books, and discussion groups on the care of the dying patient help novices understand their feelings as well as the needs of the patient. Basic communication concepts related to the dying patient and appropriate for beginning students are presented below to begin learning.

Dying patients rarely want to talk about their illnesses at every encounter, nor do they wish to confide in everyone they meet. Give them opportunities to talk, and listen, but if they choose to stay at a social level, respect their preference. Remember that illness—even a terminal one—is only a part of the total person. A smile, a touch, an inquiry about a family member, a comment on the day's events, or even some gentle humor affirms and sustains the unique individual for whom you are caring. Communicating effectively means getting to know the whole patient; that is part of the helping process. Frequent symptom assessment is also important to ensure the appropriate comfort measures are carried out in a timely fashion.

Dying patients experience many feelings that can range from denial, anger, sorrow, depression, to regret. Be sensitive to the patient's feelings about dying; watch for cues that the patient is open to talking about them. Make openings for the patient to ask questions: "I wonder if you have any concerns about your illness, your treatment, and what it will be like when you go home?" "What is important for you to do before you die?" "What is important for you to achieve before you die?" Explore these concerns and provide the information the patient requests. Setting up a meeting with the physician, therapist, palliative care or hospice team members, and any spiritual leaders will help everyone understand the patient's issues and develop a cohesive plan of care. Avoid false reassurance. Accepting the patient's feelings, answering questions truthfully, and being present during difficult times will reassure the patient (Gawande, 2014).

Understanding the patient's wishes about treatment at the end of life is an important nursing responsibility. Patients and family members report improved quality of life, decreased hospital visits, and lower medical costs (Ludwick et al., 2018). Failing to establish communication about end-of-life decisions is viewed as a flaw in nursing care. Patients at admission to the hospital, skilled nursing facilities, or nursing homes are usually asked whether they have advance directives or a durable power of attorney for health care. Review the patient's medical record to see if this information has been collected. If there is no record of the patient's wishes, the condition of the patient often determines what needs to be discussed. For hospitalized patients who are acutely ill, discussions about what the patient wants to have done in the event of cardiac or respiratory arrest should be initiated with the patient and/or family. Often this is led by the attending physician, but the nurse may need to begin the process with the health care team as well as helping the patient or family understand what each option means.

A do-not-resuscitate (DNR) order is a medical order written by a doctor with the patient's consent. It instructs health care providers to not perform cardiopulmonary resuscitation (CPR) if a patient's breathing stops or if the patient's heart stops beating. An advance directive is a document by which a person makes provisions for health care decisions in the event that in the future, the person becomes unable to make those decisions. These may include the use of CPR, ventilators, dialysis, artificial feeding and/or hydration, and antibiotics. A durable power of attorney for health care is a legal document that designates an agent or proxy to make health care decisions if the patient is no longer able to make them.

Concept Mastery Alert

Durable Power of Attorney for Health Care and Advance Directives

Durable power of attorney for health care and advance directives can be easily confused. Someone who has durable power of attorney for health care is able to act as a proxy to make health care decisions when a patient is unable to do so. An advance directive is a document that outlines the patient's health care wishes if the patient is unable to do so.

Asking about advance directives, a durable power of attorney for health care, or DNR status is difficult when you have no previous relationship with the patient or lack knowledge of the patient's values and life experience. Because the media often gives patients an unrealistic view of the effectiveness of CPR, ask, "What do you know about cardiopulmonary resuscitation?" If the patient is not familiar with CPR, work with the physician to educate the patient and family about the likely success of CPR and its side effects (e.g., fractured ribs). Assure the patient that relieving pain and taking care of other spiritual and physical needs will be a priority.

Hospice care begins when treatment for a disease is stopped, and it is clear the patient is not going to survive the illness. Hospice nurses help the patient and family make end-of-life decisions, complete tasks, and provide pain relief and nursing care. Patients with a terminal disease who only have months to live may benefit from the continuity of care that hospice services provide. Many patients and families are unaware of these services. Investigate hospice services in your area so you can explain how hospice can help your patient.

The LGBTQIA Patient

Sexual orientation and gender identity are important to consider when communicating with patients. When interviewing a patient who identifies as part of the lesbian, gay, bisexual, transgender, queer/questioning, intersex, and asexual (LGBTQIA) community, do not assume their gender identity by the way they look, dress, or act. Ask the patient what name they prefer to use, and verify whether it is the same as the name in the patient medical record. Ask the patient what pronouns they prefer used; these may include "she," "he," "they," "zie," and "hir." Do not assume the patient's partner is a "wife," "husband," "boyfriend," etc., until you clarify the relationship and the partner's preferred pronouns (Thomson & Katz-Wise, 2020). If pertinent to the reason for seeking care, ask the transgender patient whether they have had surgery or are taking hormone treatments.

LGBTQIA

L – Lesbian
G – Gay
B – Bisexual
T – Transgender
Q – Queer/questioning
I – Intersex
A – Asexual

The terminology continues to evolve but the constant is to use the terms your patient prefers and be respectful in your interactions.

If the patient seems uncomfortable and unwilling to share personal information, try to make the environment more welcoming. Emphasize that high-quality care will be given to all patients, regardless of race, gender, sexuality, or religion. Be empathetic and open-minded during the interview. You might say, "Out of respect for my patient's right to self-identify, I ask all patients what gender pronoun they'd prefer I'd use for them. What pronoun would you like me to use for you? How do you identify your gender? In order to help assess your health risks relating to your reason for being here, can you tell me your history with hormone use or gender-affirming surgery?" (GLMA, 2020; Kersey-Matusiak, 2019; Keuroghlian et al., 2017).

The Interview across a Language Barrier

Many people in the United States do not speak English as their primary language, and the command of English for many more is less than fluent. Of people in the United States, 22% speak a language other than English at home (United States Census Bureau, 2020). Of foreign-born U.S. residents, 85% speak a language at home other than English (Gambino et al., 2014). This group of people are less likely to have access to regular primary or preventive care and more likely to report problems with care or even experience medical errors. Learning to work with qualified interpreters is both cost-effective and important for optimal care (Clarke et al., 2019; Hadziabdic et al., 2009).

The U.S. Department of Health and Human Services Office of Minority Health sponsors the "Think Cultural Health" website to provide a guide to providing effective communication and language assistance services to advance health equity for patients who are members of minority groups at every point of contact in the health care system. This site offers many resources for nurses and is available at https://hclsig.thinkculturalhealth.hhs.gov/.

If your patient speaks a different language, make every effort to find a professional medical interpreter. A few broken words and gestures are no substitutes for the full story. There is a difference between an interpreter and a translator. An *interpreter* is a specialist in converting oral information from one language to another, while a *translator* specializes in converting written information from one language to another. The ideal interpreter is a neutral person who is familiar with both languages and cultures. Recruiting family members or friends to serve as interpreters can be hazardous; confidentiality and cultural norms may be violated, meanings may be distorted, and transmitted information may be incomplete. Untrained interpreters may try to speed up the interview by telescoping lengthy replies into a few words, losing much of what may be significant detail (Mikkelson, 2019).

Before beginning the patient interview, meet with the medical interpreter, establish rapport, and review the topics and goals for each section of the history. Explain that you need the interpreter to translate everything, not to condense or summarize. After going over your plans, arrange the room so that you have easy eye contact and nonverbal communication with the patient. The patient should be the focus of the interview. The interpreter's positioning can be influenced by whether the interpretation is signed or spoken, the patient's cultural boundaries, the reason for the interview, and the physical configuration of the room. Often, interpreters position themselves slightly behind the patient to maximize the transparency of the interpreted session (The National Council on Interpreting in Health Care, 2003). Let the patient know that everything said will be interpreted throughout the session. *Make your questions clear, short, and simple.* Speak directly to the patient, asking questions like, "How long have you been sick?" rather than "How long has the patient been sick?" Respect cultural beliefs that the patient expresses. The interpreter may be able to serve as a cultural broker and help explain any pertinent cultural beliefs of the patient or the family. Thank both the patient and interpreter at the end of the interview (Keuroghlian et al., 2017).

When available, bilingual written questionnaires are invaluable, especially for the review of systems. First, however, be sure that patients can read in their language; otherwise, ask for help from the interpreter. In some clinical settings, there are speakerphone translators; use them if there are no better options.

The Patient with Low Literacy

Before giving written instructions, assess the patient's ability to read. Literacy levels are highly variable, and marginal reading skills are more prevalent than commonly believed. Explore the many reasons people do not read; they may include language barriers, learning disorders, poor vision, or lack of education. Some patients feel uncomfortable about disclosing their reading deficits. Asking about educational level may be helpful, but practical approaches are more fruitful. Ask, "How comfortable are you with filling out medical forms?" or ask the patient to read whatever instructions you have written. Another rapid screen is to hand the patient a written text upside down—most patients who read will turn the page around immediately. Lack of reading skill may explain why the patient has not taken medications as prescribed or adhered to recommended treatments. Respond sensitively, and do not confuse the degree of literacy with level of intelligence (Welch, 2014).

The Patient with Impaired Hearing

Communicating with a person who has hearing loss can present many of the same challenges as communicating with patients who speak different languages. The deaf community is a distinct cultural group with its own language. It is important to find out the patient's preferred method of communicating. Patients may use American Sign Language, a unique language with its own syntax, various other combinations of signs, and speech. Ask when the hearing loss occurred relative to the patient's development of speech and what schools the patient attended. These questions help determine whether the patient identifies with the deaf culture or the hearing culture. If the patient prefers sign language, find an interpreter and use the principles identified in the section on "The Interview across the Language Barrier" (Fig. 3-7). Written questionnaires are also useful. Time-consuming handwritten questions and answers may be the only solution at times, though literacy skills may also be an issue.

Hearing deficits vary. If the patient has a hearing aid, make sure the patient is using it and it is working. For patients with unilateral hearing loss, sit

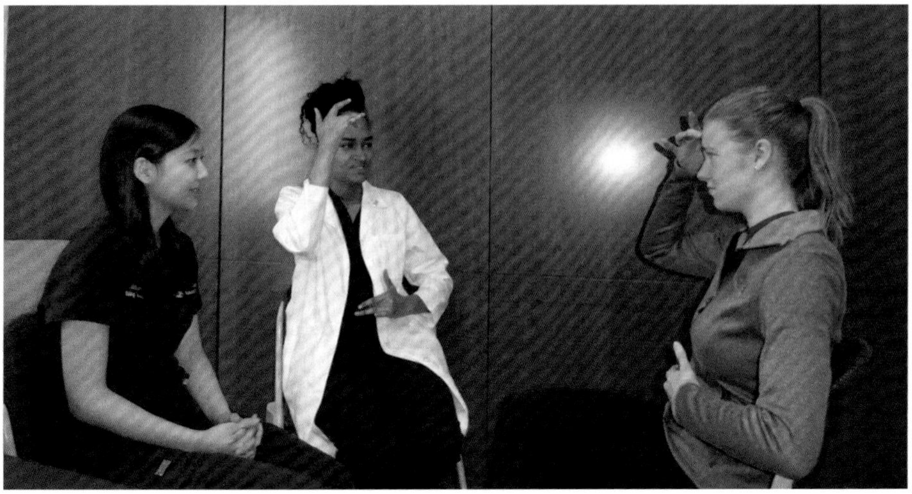

FIGURE 3-7 Patients with impaired hearing may use American Sign Language, a unique language with its own syntax, various other combinations of signs, and speech.

on the hearing side. A person who is *hard of hearing* may not be aware of the problem, a situation you will have to tactfully address. Eliminate background noise such as television or hallway conversation. For patients who have partial hearing or can read lips, face them directly in good light. Patients should wear glasses or contact lenses as needed to better see visual cues that help them understand you.

Begin by getting your patient's attention. Speak clearly at a normal volume and rate, but drop your voice to a lower pitch. Use facial expressions and gestures. Avoid letting your voice trail off at the ends of sentences, covering your mouth or looking down at papers while speaking. Even the best lip readers comprehend only a percentage of what is said, so having patients repeat information back is important. If the patient asks you to repeat a question, rephrase it instead of repeating it since different words may be more easily understood. At the end of the interview, provide printed instructions for the patient to take home (American Speech-Language-Hearing Association [ASHA], 2020; Funk et al., 2018).

The Patient with Impaired Vision

When meeting a patient who is blind or has low vision, introduce yourself in your normal voice tone, and explain who you are and why you are there. If the room is unfamiliar, orient the patient to the surroundings and report if anyone else is present. If you leave the room and return, announce yourself again. If the patient has a guide dog, ask permission to greet the animal. Direct questions and comments to the patient and not to a third party. Walk over to the side of the bed or chair and continue the conversation with the patient, staying in one place while obtaining the patient history. It may be helpful to adjust the light. Encourage visually impaired patients to wear glasses or contact lenses whenever possible. Use more verbal explanations because postures and gestures are unseen. Read aloud what you write or enter in the medical record. Ask the patient what format is best for handouts or take-home materials (e.g., recorded, Braille, large print [18-point type], via e-mail). Say "goodbye" before leaving the room so the patient is not left talking to an empty room or figuring out what happens next.

The Patient with Cognitive Disabilities

Patients with moderate cognitive disabilities can usually give adequate histories. If you suspect a disability, however, pay special attention to the patient's school record and ability to function independently. How far has the patient gone in school? If they did not finish, why? What kind of courses have they taken? How did they do? Has any testing been done? Are they living alone? Do they need assistance with activities such as transportation or shopping? The sexual history is equally important and often overlooked. Find out if the patient is sexually active and provide information about pregnancy or sexually transmitted infections as needed.

If you are unsure about the patient's level of disability, shift to the mental status examination and assess simple calculations, vocabulary, memory, and abstract thinking.

See Chapter 19, "Mental Status and Mental Health Assessment."

For patients with severe cognitive disabilities, you may have to turn to the family or caregivers for the history. Identify the person who accompanies the patient, but always show interest in the patient first. Establish rapport, make eye contact if culturally appropriate, and engage in simple conversation. Ask if the patient uses alternative or augmentative communication (AAC) (ASHA, 2020; Hemsley et al., 2012). Avoid "talking down" or condescending behavior. The patient, family members, caregivers, or friends will notice and appreciate your respect.

CLINICAL TIP

Augmentative and alternative communication (AAC) includes all forms of communication (other than oral speech), such as facial expressions or gestures, use of symbols or pictures, or writing. People with severe speech or language problems may use special augmentative aids, such as picture and symbol communication boards or electronic devices.

The Patient with Personal Problems

Patients may ask you for advice about personal problems that fall outside the range of your clinical expertise. Should the patient quit a stressful job, for example, or move out of state? Instead of responding, ask what alternatives the patient has considered, related pros and cons, and available support systems and resources. Letting the patient talk through the problems is more therapeutic than giving your own opinions.

Sexuality in the Nurse–Patient Relationship

Nurses occasionally find themselves physically attracted to their patients. Similarly, patients may make sexual overtures or exhibit flirtatious behavior toward nurses. The emotional and physical intimacy of the nurse–patient relationship may lend itself to these sexual feelings.

If you become aware of such feelings in yourself, accept them as a normal human response, and bring them to a conscious level to keep them from affecting your professional behavior. Denial can increase the risk of responding inappropriately. *Any* sexual contact or romantic relationship with patients is *unethical* and *illegal*; keep your relationship with the patient professional, and seek help if you need it (American Nurses Association, 2020).

Sometimes, nurses meet patients who act in seductive manners or make sexual advances. It is tempting to ignore this behavior, hoping it will go away. It is your responsibility to ensure that your demeanor with the patient remains professional at all times. Calmly but firmly make it clear that your relationship is professional, not personal. If unwelcome overtures continue, leave the room and find a chaperone before continuing the interview.

ETHICS OF INTERVIEWING

A chapter on interviewing would not be complete without mention of the ethics related to patient information. The potential power of the nurse–patient communication calls for guidance beyond one's innate sense of morality (American Nurses Association, 2020). Ethics are a set of principles crafted through reflection and discussion to define what is right and wrong. Medical ethics guide professional behavior. The principle of **confidentiality** is of paramount importance in the nurse–patient relationship. The nurse is obligated to protect patient information. Simply deleting the patient's name from a story may not be adequate protection. For example, a student may tell a friend a baby was born today with club feet at ABC hospital. If only one baby was born on this day at ABC hospital, the baby can be identified.

Information may only be shared with appropriate health care team members. At the start of the interview, the patient should be told with whom the information will be shared. Do not agree to a patient's request not to reveal a piece of information with anyone before you know what the information is. Should such a request be made, tell the patient that if the information revealed is harmful to the patient or another person, then you are obligated to share it with appropriate authorities. It is also inappropriate for you to review the charts of patients for whom you are not caring. Confidentiality is a key quality that fosters the nurse–patient relationship and facilitates quality health care.

Bibliography

CITATIONS

American Nurses Association. (2020). *Nursing code of ethics.* Nursebooks.org. Retrieved April 27, 2020, from https://www.nursingworld.org/coe-view-only

American Speech-Language-Hearing Association (ASHA). (2020). *Augmentative and alternative communication (AAC).* Retrieved May 21, 2020, from http://www.asha.org/public/speech/disorders/AAC/

Antai-Otong, D. (2007). *Nurse-client communication: A life span approach.* Jones and Bartlett.

Bershad, D. (2019). Motivational interviewing: A communication best practice. *American Nurse Today, 14*(9), 96–98.

Carr, D. D. (2017). Motivational interviewing supports patient-centered-care and communication. *J of NY State Nurses Association, 45*(1), 39–43.

Cerrato, P. (2013). *Do your EHR manners turn patients off? medscape business of medicine.* Retrieved April 10, 2020, from http://www.medscape.com/viewarticle/809237

Clarke, S. K., Jaffe, J., & Mutch, R. (2019). Overcoming communication barriers in refugee health care. *Pediatric Clinics North America, 66*(3), 669–686.

Drobny, S. D. (2017). Making patients partners in real-time electronic charting. *American Journal of Nursing, 117*(4), 11.

Funk, A., Garcia, C., & Mullen, T. (2018). Understanding the hospital experience of older adults with hearing impairment. *American Journal of Nursing, 118*(6), 28–34.

Gambino, C. P., Acosta, Y. D., & Grieco, E. M. (2014). *English-speaking ability of the foreign = born population in the United States: 2012. U.S. Census Bureau.* Retrieved April 18, 2020, from https://www2.census.gov/library/publications/2014/acs/acs-26.pdf

Gawande, A. (2014). *Being mortal: medicine and what matters in the end.* Metropolitan Books/Henry Holt & Co.

GLMA. (2020). *Cultural competence webinar series: Gay and quality healthcare for lesbian, gay, bisexual & transgender people: A four-part webinar series. Part 2: Creating a welcoming and safe environment for LGBT people and families.* Retrieved April 24, 2020, from http://www.glma.org/index.cfm?fuseaction=page.viewPage&pageID=1031&nodeID=1

Hadziabdic, E., Heikkilä, K., Albin, B., & Hjelm, K. (2009). Migrants'perceptions of using interpreters in health care. *International Nursing Review, 56*(4), 461–468.

Hastings, C. (1989). The lived experiences of the illness: making contact with the patient. In: P. Benne & J. Wrubel (Eds.). *The primacy of caring: stress and coping in health and illness.* Addison-Wesley.

Health Information Privacy – HIPPA for Professionals. (2020). *U.S. Department of Health and Human Services.* Retrieved April 27, 2020, from https://www.hhs.gov/hipaa/for-professionals/index.html

Hemsley, B., Balandin, S., & Worrall, L. (2012). Nursing the patient with complex communication needs: time as a barrier and a facilitator to successful communication in hospital. *Journal of Advanced Nursing, 68*(1), 116–126.

Kersey-Matusiak, G. (2019). *Delivering culturally competent nursing care: working with diverse and vulnerable populations* (2nd ed.). Springer Publishing Co.

Keuroghlian, A. S., Ard, K. L., & Makadon, H. J. (2017). Advancing health equity for lesbian, gay, bisexual and transgender (LGBT) people through sexual health education and LGBT-affirming health care environments. *Sexual Health, 4*(1), 119–122.

Kleinman, A., Eisenberg, L., & Good, B. (1978). Culture, illness, and care: clinical lessons from anthropological and cross-cultural research. *Annals of Internal Medicine, 88*(2), 251–258.

Lein, C., & Wills, C. E. (2007). Using patient-centered interviewing skills to manage complex patient encounters in primary care. *Journal of the American Academy of Nurse Practitioners, 19*(5), 215–220.

Ludwick, R., Baughman, K. R., Jarjoura, D., & Kropp, D. J. (2018). Advance Care Planning: An exploration of the beliefs, self-efficacy, education and practices of RNs and LPNs. *American Journal of Nursing, 118*(12), 26–32.

Mikkelson, H. (2019). *The art of working with interpreters: A manual for healthcare professionals.* Retrieved April 28, 2020, from https://acebo.myshopify.com/pages/the-art-of-working-with-interpreters-a-manual-for-health-care-professionals

Platt, F. W., & Gordon, G. H. (2004). *Field guide to the difficult patient interview.* Wolters Kluwer.

Riley, J. B. (2020). *Communication in nursing* (9th ed.). Mosby Elsevier.

Sheldon, L. K., & Foust, J. (2014). *Communication for nurses: Talking with patients* (3rd ed.). Jones and Bartlett.

Stokowski, L. (2013). *Electronic nursing documentation: Charting new territory. Medscape nurses.* Retrieved April 10, 2020, from http://www.medscape.com/viewarticle/810573_1

The National Council on Interpreting in Health Care. (2003). *Guide to interpreter positioning in health care settings.* Retrieved April 26, 2020, from http://www.ncihc.org/assets/documents/workingpapers/NCIHC%20Working%20Paper%20-%20Guide%20to%20Interpreter%20Positioning%20in%20Health%20Care%20Settings.pdf

Thomson, K., & Katz-Wise, S. (2020). *Gender identity & pronoun use: A guide for pediatric health care professionals, 2017. Boston Children's Hospital.* Retrieved April 24, 2020, from https://notes.childrenshospital.org/clinicians-guide-gender-identity-pronoun-use/

United States Census Bureau. (2020). *American fact finder. Language spoken at home 2017.* Retrieved April 18, 2020, from https://data.census.gov/cedsci/all?q=Language%20Spoken%20at%20Home&hidePreview=false&t=Language%20Spoken%20at%20Home&tid=ACSST1Y2018.S1601

Welch, J. (2014). Building a foundation for brief motivational interviewing: communication to promote health literacy and behavior change. *Journal of the American Academy of Nurse Practitioners, 45*(12), 566–572.

ADDITIONAL REFERENCES

Carlson, C., Howe, T., Pedersen, C., & Yoder, L. H. (2020). Caring for visually impaired patients in the hospital: A multidisciplinary quality improvement project. *American Journal of Nursing, 120*(5), 48–55.

Ferguson, L. F., Ward, H., Card, S., Sheppard, S., & McMurtry, J. (2013). Putting the "patient" back into patient-centered care: An education perspective. *Nurse Education in Practice, 13*(4), 283–287.

National Center for Education Statistics. U.S. Dept. of Education. (2020). Adult Literacy in the United States. Retrieved May 21, 2020, from https://nces.ed.gov/datapoints/2019179.asp

Noordman, J., van der Weijden, T., & van Dulmen, S. (2014). Effects of video-feedback on the communication, clinical competence and motivational interviewing skills of practice nurses: a pre-test posttest control group study. *Journal of Advanced Nursing*, *70*(10), 2272–2283.

Noyes, R., & Clancy, J. (2016). The Dying Role: Its Relevance to Improved Patient Care. *Psychiatry*, *79*(1), 199–205.

O'Hagan, S., Manias, E., Elder, C., Pill, J., Woodward-Kron, R., McNamara, T., Webb, G., & McColl, G. (2014). What counts as effective communication in nursing? Evidence from nurse educators' and clinicians' feedback on nurse interactions with simulated patients. *Journal of Advanced Nursing*, *70*(6), 1344–1355.

Refugee Health Technical Assistance Center. (2020). Best Practices for Communicating Through an Interpreter. Retrieved May 21, 2020, from https://refugeehealthta.org/access-to-care/language-access/best-practices-communicating-through-an-interpreter/

Wittenberg-Lyles, E., Goldsmith, J., & Ragan, S. I. (2010). The COMFORT Initiative: Palliative nursing and the centrality of communication. *Journal of Hospice Palliative Nursing*, *12*(5), 282–292.

4 THE HEALTH HISTORY

KEY TERMS

comprehensive health assessment	focused or problem-oriented assessment	follow-up history
emergency history		health history
		source of history

Learning Objectives

The student will:

1. Explain the four types of histories and when each is used.
2. Describe and obtain the components of a comprehensive health history.
3. Adapt the history keeping sensitive topics in mind.

This chapter explains how to obtain a patient health history. All history information is considered subjective data. Consider the **health history** a chance for the patient to tell their "story" (Fig. 4-1).

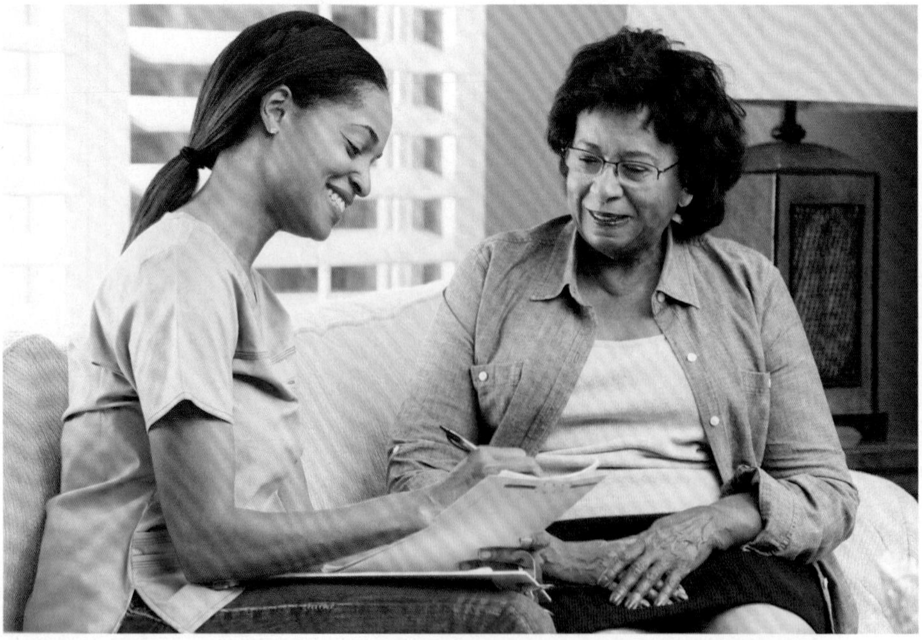

FIGURE 4-1 The health history is a chance for the patient to tell their "story" in their words.

TYPES OF PATIENT HEALTH HISTORIES

How much history to gather varies based on the purpose of the patient encounter. The admission of a new patient to a clinic, hospital, long-term care facility, or visiting nurse agency usually requires a **comprehensive health assessment**. This history provides the nurse with a full picture of the patient's health status, as well as health promotion and risk reduction needs. The comprehensive history includes the patient's current health problems, past history, family history, a review of body systems, and health patterns. It provides a basis for assessing patient concerns, health status, risk factors, and health promotion.

A **focused or problem-oriented assessment** is appropriate in many situations, especially when the patient is known to the nurse or health care facility. For example, this may be useful for a patient hospitalized for surgery who develops shortness of breath postoperatively or a college student visiting the university health services for a sore throat. Here the nurse focuses on gathering information mostly on the patient's current problem. The patient's symptoms, age, and this history will determine the extent of the physical examination needed; it is likely smaller in scope than a comprehensive health assessment (Table 4-1).

TABLE 4-1 The Health History: Comprehensive or Focused?

Comprehensive Assessment	Focused Assessment
• Is appropriate for new patients in all settings • Provides fundamental and personalized knowledge about the patient • Strengthens the nurse–patient relationship • Provides baselines for future assessments • Creates a platform for health promotion through education and counseling	• Is appropriate for established patients, especially during routine or urgent care visits • Addresses focused concerns or symptoms • Assesses symptoms restricted to a specific body system

A **follow-up history** is a form of a focused assessment (Fig. 4-2). The patient is returning to have a problem evaluated after treatment, or a second-shift nurse may be following up on a problem identified by a nurse on an earlier shift. Here the nurse gathers data to evaluate whether the treatment plan was successful.

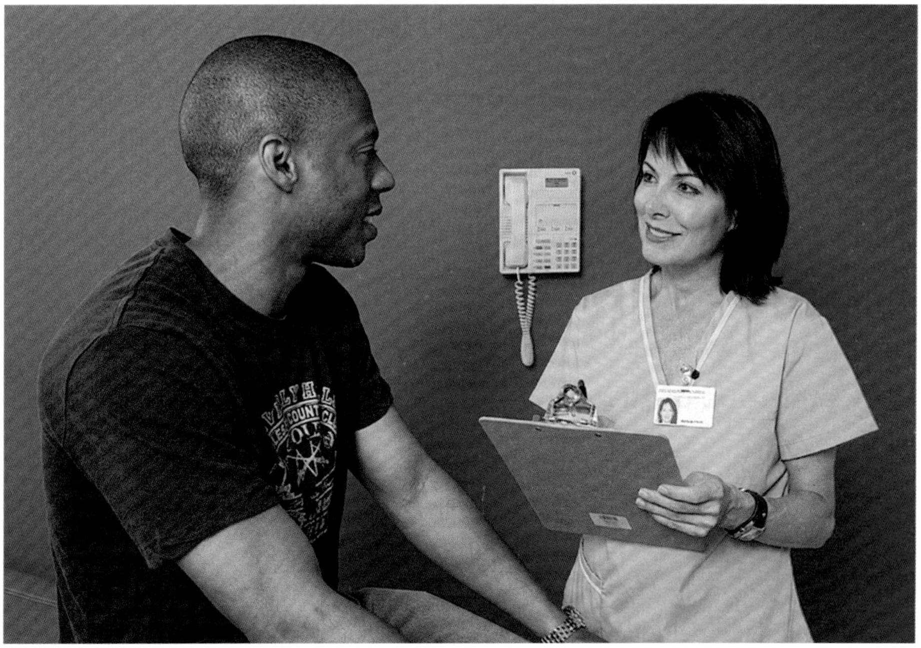

FIGURE 4-2 Obtaining a follow-up history.

A medical emergency generates a fourth type of data collection, the **emergency history**. The data collection is focused on the patient's emergent problem with a systematic prioritization of need based on the patient's presentation. Rapid assessment is performed in life-threatening situations, for example, assessment of circulation, airway, and breathing (CAB) when cardiac arrest is suspected.

Mastery of all the components of the comprehensive history provides proficiency and the ability to select the elements most pertinent to the patient encounter.

THE COMPREHENSIVE ADULT HEALTH HISTORY

Overview

The seven components of the *comprehensive adult health history* are:

See Chapter 23, "Assessing Children: Infancy through Adolescence" for *comprehensive pediatric health histories.*

- Identifying data and source of the history
- Chief complaint(s)
- History of present illness (HPI)
- Past history
- Family history
- Review of systems
- Health patterns

As described in Chapter 3, "Interviewing and Communication," the health history may not spring forth in this order. The interview is more fluid. Follow the *patient's* cues to elicit the patient's narrative of illness, provide empathy, and strengthen rapport. For the documentation, transform the patient's language and story into the seven components of the history familiar to all members of the health care team. This restructuring can organize clinical reasoning and provide a template for identification of patient problems.

Review the features of the components of the adult health history described in Table 4-2, then study the more detailed explanations that follow.

Initial Information

Date and Time of History

The date is always important. Be sure to document the time the history was obtained.

Identifying Data

Identifying data include age, gender, birth date, marital or relationship status, occupation, and any other biographic data appropriate to the agency.

TABLE 4-2 Overview: Components of the Adult Health History

Identifying data	• *Identifying data*—includes age, date of birth, gender, occupation, marital or relationship status, education level, primary language spoken and read • *Source of the history*—usually the patient, but can be a family member or friend, letter of referral, or the medical record • If appropriate, establish *source of referral*, because a written report may be needed
Reliability	This may vary according to the patient's memory, trust, and mood. Note whether the patient or other source appears reliable when giving the history. If judged unreliable, provide reason why.
Chief complaint(s)	The one or more symptoms or concerns causing the patient to seek care
History of present illness	• Elaborates on the *chief complaint*; describes how each symptom developed • Includes patient's thoughts and feelings about the illness • Pulls in relevant portions of the *review of systems* called "pertinent positives and negatives" (see section "Pertinent Positives and/or Negatives") • May include *medications, allergies,* and habits of *smoking* and *alcohol,* which are frequently pertinent to the present illness
Past history	• Lists childhood illnesses • Lists adult illnesses with dates for at least three categories: medical, surgical, and psychiatric • Includes health maintenance practices such as immunizations, screening tests, lifestyle issues, and home safety • Includes risk factors
Family history	• Outlines or diagrams age and health or age and cause of death of siblings, parents, grandparents, and children • Documents presence or absence of specific illnesses in family (e.g., hypertension, coronary artery disease)
Review of systems	Documents presence or absence of common symptoms related to each major body system
Health patterns	Documents personal/social history

Knowledge of the patient's education level and primary language will help the nurse assess the patient's health literacy level. The **source of history** can be the patient (primary source) or a family member, friend, health care provider, or the medical record (secondary sources). Designating the source helps the nurse and reader assess the type of information provided and possible biases.

CLINICAL TIP

Health literacy is the degree to which individuals have the capacity to obtain, process, and understand basic health information and services needed to make appropriate health decisions (National Network of Libraries of Medicine, 2020). If a formal assessment would be beneficial, there are tools that may be used to assess an individual's health literacy available from the Agency for Healthcare Research and Quality (Health Literacy Measurement Tools [Revised], 2020).

Reliability

Document the reliability of the person providing the information. For example, "The patient is vague when describing symptoms, and details are confusing" or "The patient appears reliable." This judgment reflects the quality of the information provided by the patient and is usually made at the end of the interview.

Chief Complaint(s)

Make every attempt to quote the patient's own words. For example, "My stomach hurts and I feel awful." Sometimes patients have no specific complaints. Report their goals instead. For example, "I have come for my regular check-up" or "I've been admitted for a thorough evaluation of my heart." In the hospital setting, the chief complaint may be the same as the admitting diagnosis, but do not assume this is always true. The patient may have other concerns or problems.

History of Present Illness

The history of present illness section is a complete, clear, and chronologic account of the problems prompting the patient to seek care. The narrative should include the onset of the problem, the setting in which it developed, its manifestations, and any treatments (Box 4-1). The HPI should reveal the patient's responses to the symptoms and the effect the illness has had on daily living.

BOX 4-1 KEY ELEMENTS OF THE HISTORY OF PRESENT ILLNESS

- Seven attributes of each principal symptom
- Self-treatment for the symptom by the patient or family
- Past occurrences of the symptom(s)
- Pertinent positives and/or negatives from the review of systems
- Risk factors or other pertinent information related to the symptom

Seven Attributes of a Symptom

Remember the mnemonic "OLD CART" from Chapter 2 that may help the novice history taker gather all the symptom attributes:

1. *O*nset. When did (does) it start? Setting in which it occurs, including environmental factors, personal activities, emotional reactions, or other circumstances that may contribute to the illness.
2. *L*ocation. Where is it? Does it radiate?
3. *D*uration. How long does it last?
4. *C*haracteristic symptoms. What is it like? How severe is it? (For pain, ask a rating on a scale of 1 to 10.)
5. *A*ssociated manifestations. Have you noticed anything else that accompanies it?

6. *R*elieving/exacerbating factors. Is there anything that makes it better or worse?
7. *T*reatment. What have you done to treat this? Was it effective?

See Chapter 2, "Critical Thinking and Clinical Judgment in Health Assessment" for a more complete list of questions for each attribute.

Self-Treatment

Be sure to ask what over-the-counter (OTC), prescribed medication, or other treatments (e.g., ice packs or alternative therapies) the patient has tried to alleviate symptoms. If the patient has already tried the typical first course of treatment and it has failed, the provider will need to consider either more advanced treatment or an alternative diagnosis. For example, if the patient complains of heartburn that was unrelieved by an antacid, the problem may be cardiac in origin rather than gastrointestinal.

Past Occurrences of the Symptom

The patient may have had the same or similar problems in the past. Inquire about this and ask what treatment(s) were previously used and the results.

Pertinent Positives and/or Negatives

Pertinent positives and/or negatives from the review of systems related to the chief complaint should be sought (e.g., a history of asthma in a patient with difficulty breathing). These data may help differentiate diagnoses and individualize nursing interventions.

Risk Factors or Other Pertinent Information

Risk factors or other pertinent information related to the symptom is frequently relevant, such as risk factors for coronary artery disease in a patient with chest pain or current medications that may have side effects similar to the complaint.

Past History

The five key elements of the *past history* are listed in Box 4-2.

BOX 4-2 KEY ELEMENTS OF THE PAST HISTORY

- Allergies
- Medications
- Childhood illnesses
- Adult illnesses
- Health maintenance

Allergies

Allergies to medications, foods, insects, and/or environmental factors, such as pollens should be noted. Be sure to record the specific reaction to each allergen, for example, rash, nausea, anaphylaxis, and others.

Medications

Medications, including name, dose and route, and frequency of use, are included. Also list home remedies, nonprescription OTC drugs, vitamins, mineral or herbal supplements, oral contraceptives, and medicines borrowed from family members or friends. If the patient is unsure, ask them to bring in all medications to see exactly what is taken. Medication reconciliation is important in preventing prescribing errors (e.g., prescribing the same drug under two different names, detecting drug interactions or drug/herbal interactions, recognizing changes in clinical signs or symptoms related to drug therapy). Medication reconciliation is usually done upon admission to the hospital or other medical facility.

Concept Mastery Alert

Allergic Responses and Adverse Effects

When obtaining information from the patient about medications, it is extremely important to ask about and document all adverse effects and all allergic responses to medications that the patient reports. An adverse effect is not the same as an allergic reaction. A patient who has experienced an adverse effect may still receive the medication if the need for the medication is greater than the risk of the adverse effect. In most cases, if a patient experiences an allergic reaction to a medication, this prevents the patient from ever receiving the medication again.

Childhood Illnesses

Childhood illnesses, such as measles, rubella, mumps, whooping cough, chickenpox, rheumatic fever, scarlet fever, and polio, are included in the past history section. Also included are any chronic childhood illnesses, such as asthma.

Adult Illnesses

Adult illnesses should be included in each of the following areas:

- *Medical:* Chronic or genetic illnesses such as diabetes, hypertension, hepatitis, asthma, cancer, sickle cell disease or HIV; should include dates and reasons for hospitalizations
- *Surgical:* Dates, reasons for surgery, and types of operations or treatments
- *Accidents:* Type, dates, treatment, and residual disability of major accidents
- *Psychiatric:* Illness and time frame, hospitalizations, and treatments

Health Maintenance

The *health maintenance* section includes several factors:

- *Immunizations:* Ask whether the patient has received vaccines for tetanus, pertussis, diphtheria, polio, measles, mumps, rubella, influenza, COVID-19, varicella (chickenpox) or herpes zoster (shingles), hepatitis A and B, *Haemophilus influenzae* type b (Hib), human papillomavirus (HPV), meningitis, and pneumonia. Include the dates of original and booster immunizations. The Centers for Disease Control and Prevention updates vaccine recommendations yearly for different age groups. To obtain the most current recommendations, go to http://www.cdc.gov/vaccines/schedules/index.html.
- *Screening tests:* These may include tuberculin tests, cholesterol tests, stool for occult blood, Pap smears, and mammograms. Include the results and

the dates the tests were performed. Alternatively, screening tests may be asked about during and documented in the review of systems.

- *Safety measures:* Nurses should ask about the use of seat belts in cars, smoke/carbon monoxide detectors, sports helmets or padding, and so forth.

- *Risk factors:*

Tobacco:	Do you use or have you ever used tobacco? Do you smoke or chew tobacco? Do you use electronic cigarettes (vape)? At what age did you start? How many packs per day (ppd) do you smoke? How many ppd in the past? How many times a day do you smoke or vape?
Environmental hazards:	Are you exposed to any hazards in your home or work environment?
Substance use:	Do you use or have you ever used marijuana, cocaine, heroin, amphetamines, methylphenidate (Ritalin) or other recreational drugs? Do you drink high-energy (high-caffeine) drinks? What kind and how much?
Alcohol:	How much alcohol do you drink per sitting and per week?

CLINICAL TIP

For patients over 50 years of age, ask if they have had the shingles vaccine. If they say yes, ask whether they had the Shingrix or Zostavax vaccine. The Shingrix vaccine is preferred and recommended by the CDC for adults 50 years and older. The Zostavax vaccine can be given to adults 60 years and older if they are allergic to Shingrix.

Alcohol and Drugs

Many nurses hesitate to ask patients about use of alcohol and drugs, whether prescribed or illegal. Misuse of alcohol or drugs often directly contributes to symptoms and the need for care and treatment. In 2018, an estimated 53.2 million Americans aged 12 or older were current illicit drug users. This estimate represents 19.4% of the population aged 12 or older (Substance Abuse and Mental Health Services Administration [SAMHSA)], 2018). Recreational drugs include marijuana/hashish, cocaine (including crack), heroin, hallucinogens, inhalants, and methamphetamine. Patients may also misuse prescription stimulants, tranquilizers, sedatives, and/or pain relievers.

In 2018, 24.5% or 67.1 million people aged 12 or older reported binge alcohol drinking in the past 30 days. Heavy drinking was reported by 16.6 million people aged 12 or older. Among young adults aged 18 to 25, the rate of binge drinking was 34.9% or about 11.9 million young adults, and the rate of heavy drinking was 9.0% or 3.1 million young adults (SAMHSA, 2018).

Despite the high prevalence of substance use disorders, they remain underdiagnosed. Because of the high incidence, nurses should routinely ask about current and past use of alcohol or drugs, patterns of use, and family history (Boucek et al., 2019; Cheal et al., 2014; Monico et al., 2019). Adolescents and older adults should also be assessed for drug or alcohol misuse.

Alcohol

Questions about alcohol and other drugs follow naturally after questions about cigarettes. "What do you like to drink?" or "Tell me about your use of alcohol" are good opening questions that avoid the easy yes-or-no response. Remember to assess what the patient considers alcohol; some patients do not use this term for wine or beer. Two additional questions—"Have you ever had a drinking problem?" and "When was your last drink?"—along with a drink within 24 hours are suspicious for problem drinking. To detect problem drinking, use a well-validated short screening tool that does not take much time. The Alcohol Use Disorders Identification Test-Concise (AUDIT-C) is a brief reliable test to identify individuals with alcohol use disorders or dependence (Fig. 4-3) (Frank et al., 2008; Salisbury-Afshar & Fleming, 2019; U.S. Preventive Services Task Force, 2018a).

AUDIT-C

Please circle the answer that is correct for you.

1. How often do you have a drink containing alcohol?					**SCORE**
Never (0)	Monthly or less (1)	Two to four times a month (2)	Two to three times per week (3)	Four or more times a week (4)	______
2. How many drinks containing alcohol do you have on a typical day when you are drinking?					
1 or 2 (0)	3 or 4 (1)	5 or 6 (2)	7 to 9 (3)	10 or more (4)	______
3. How often do you have six or more drinks on one occasion?					
Never (0)	Less than Monthly (1)	Monthly (2)	Two to three times per week (3)	Four or more times a week (4)	______
TOTAL SCORE Add the number for each question to get your total score.					______

The AUDIT-C is scored on a scale of 0 to 12 (scores of 0 reflect no alcohol use). In men, a score of 4 or more is considered positive; in women, a score of 3 or more is considered positive. Generally, the higher the AUDIT-C score, the more likely it is that the patient's drinking is affecting their health and safety.

FIGURE 4-3 The AUDIT-C. (AUDIT-C was developed by the U.S. Department of Veterans Affairs. It is an adaptation of the AUDIT tool developed by WHO. Babor, T. F., Higgins-Biddle, J. C., Saunders, J. B., & Monteiro, M. G. (2001). *Audit: The alcohol use disorders identification test* (2nd ed.) © World Health Organization 2001. https://www.who.int/publications-detail/audit-the-alcohol-use-disorders-identification-test-guidelines-for-use-in-primary-health-care)

Illicit Drugs

As with alcohol, questions about drugs should be more focused in order to get answers that distinguish use from misuse. A good opening question is, "Have you ever used any drugs other than those required for medical reasons?" From there, either ask specifically about patterns of use (last use, how often, substances used, amount) or inquire about modes of consumption.

Useful questions may include "Have you ever injected a drug?" and "Have you ever smoked or inhaled a drug?" "Have you ever taken a pill for non-medical reasons?" As choices of drugs of abuse change, it is important to stay up to date about the most current hazards and risks from overdose.

Once you identify substance abuse, continue further with questions like, "Are you always able to control your use of drugs?" "Have you had any bad reactions? What happened?" "Any drug-related accidents, injuries, or arrests? Job or family problems?" and "Have you ever tried to quit? Tell me about it."

Family History

The family history is an important part of the patient history. An accurate family history can identify diseases that the patient is at increased risk of developing. Early and routine screening as well as education on diet and lifestyle changes can be incorporated into the patient's plan of care. Patients should also be encouraged to keep their own record of diseases and causes of death in the family. Family history tools, both electronic and printed, are available to assist the patient with this (Fig. 4-4).

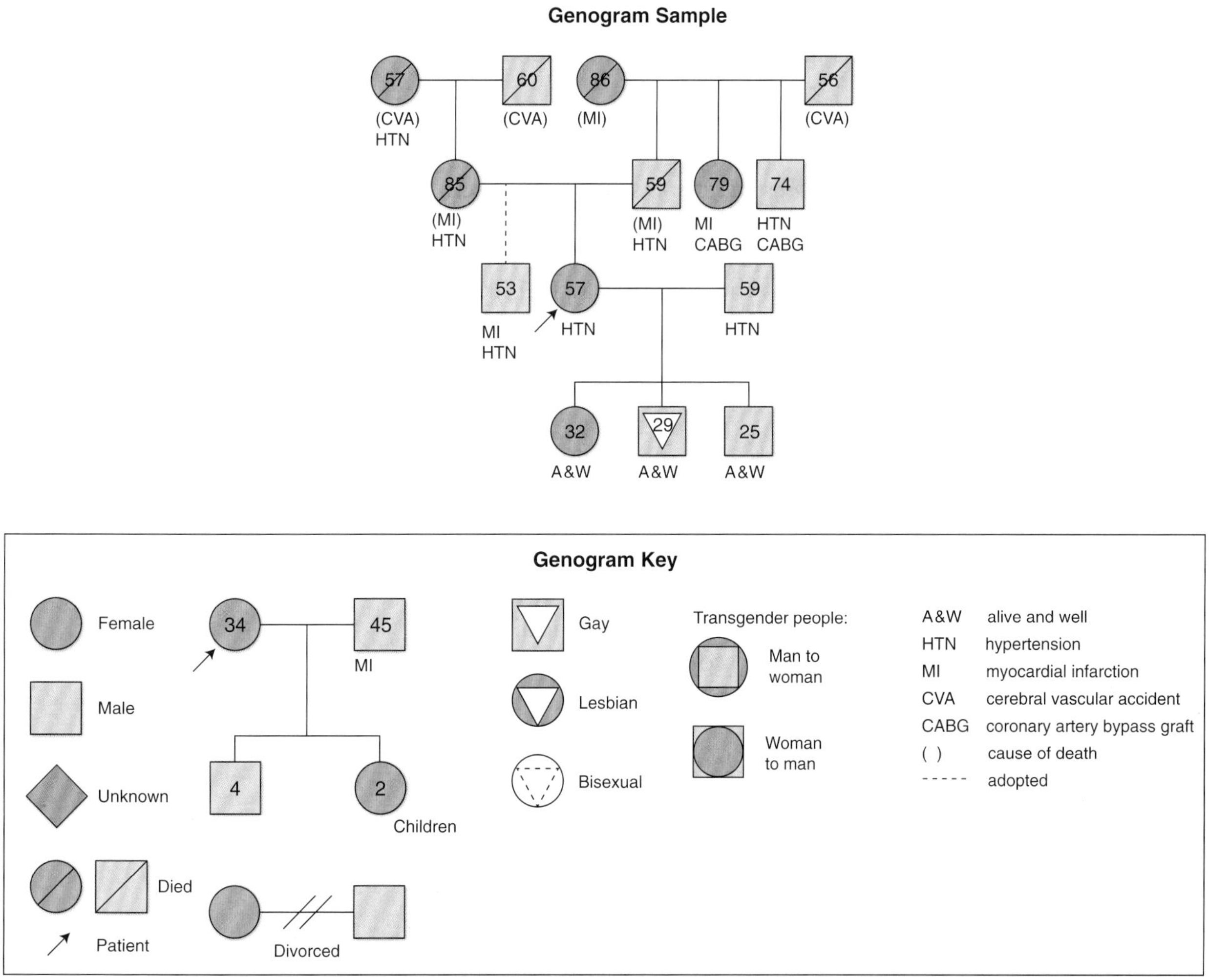

FIGURE 4-4 A genogram is a diagram of the family history.

CLINICAL TIP

Family history tools available on the web include the U.S. Surgeon General's My Family Health Portrait (https://phgkb.cdc.gov/FHH/html/index.html) and the Utah Health Family Tree (http://www.health.utah.gov/genomics/familyhistory/toolkit.html).

Under family history, the nurse records the age and health or age and cause of death of each immediate relative, including parents, grandparents, siblings, children, and grandchildren. *In addition, each of the following conditions should be reviewed with the patient to determine whether they are present or absent in the family:* hypertension, coronary artery disease, elevated cholesterol levels, stroke, diabetes, thyroid or renal disease, arthritis, tuberculosis, asthma or lung disease, headache, seizure disorder, mental illness, suicide, substance abuse, cancer and the site, genetic diseases and allergies, as well as symptoms reported by the patient. Be sure to ask if there are any other diseases not mentioned. The family history may be documented in written or electronic format per agency protocol. A genogram is a diagram of the family history. It provides a visual record that allows the provider to quickly identify disease patterns within the family. Using a genogram while taking notes during the history is a quick, accurate way to remember the information provided by the patient. See Figure 4-4 for an example.

Review of Systems

Understanding and using questions in the *review of systems* section are often challenging for beginning students. Think about asking a series of questions going from "head to toe." It is helpful to prepare the patient for the questions to come by saying, "The next part of the history may feel like a hundred questions, but it is important and needs to be thorough." Most review of systems questions pertain to *symptoms,* but on occasion, some nurses also include questions about diseases like pneumonia or tuberculosis.

Start with a fairly general question as you address each of the different systems. This focuses the patient's attention and allows you to shift to more specific questions about systems that may be of concern. Examples of starting questions are "How are your ears and hearing?" "How about your lungs and breathing?" "Any trouble with your heart?" "How is your digestion?" and "How about your bowels?" Note that the need for additional questions will vary depending on the patient's age, complaints, and general state of health and your clinical judgment.

The review of systems questions may uncover problems that the patient has overlooked, particularly in areas unrelated to the *present illness.* Significant health events, such as a major prior illness or a parent's death, require full exploration. Remember that *major health events should be recorded under the present illness or past history sections in your documentation.* Keep your technique flexible. Interviewing the patient yields various findings that you organize into formal written format only after the interview and examination are completed.

Listed next is a standard series of review of systems questions. As you gain experience, the yes-or-no questions placed at the end of the interview will take no more than several minutes. Remember to pause after each symptom to give the patient time to respond. Do not use medical terms with the patient; for example, say "blurred vision" instead of "diplopia."

- General: Usual weight, recent weight change, any clothes that fit more tightly or loosely than before; weakness, fatigue, or fever
- Skin: Rashes, lumps, sores, itching, dryness, changes in color; changes in hair or nails; changes in size or color of moles
- Head, eyes, ears, nose, throat (HEENT):
    - *Head:* Headache, head injury, dizziness, lightheadedness
    - *Eyes:* Vision, glasses or contact lenses, last examination, pain, redness, excessive tearing, double or blurred vision, spots, specks, flashing lights, glaucoma, cataracts
    - *Ears:* Hearing, tinnitus, vertigo, earaches, infection, discharge; if hearing is decreased, use or nonuse of hearing aids
    - *Nose and sinuses:* Frequent colds; nasal stuffiness, discharge, or itching; hay fever; nosebleeds; sinus trouble
    - *Throat (or mouth and pharynx):* Condition of teeth and gums; bleeding gums; dentures if any and how they fit; last dental examination; sore tongue; dry mouth; frequent sore throats; hoarseness
- Neck: Swollen glands; goiter; lumps, pain, or stiffness in the neck
- Breasts: Lumps, pain, or discomfort; nipple discharge; self-examination practices; last examination by a health care provider; last mammogram
- Respiratory: Cough; sputum (color, quantity); hemoptysis, dyspnea, wheezing, pleurisy, tuberculosis (TB) testing; may include asthma, bronchitis, emphysema, pneumonia, COVID-19, and TB
- Cardiovascular: Heart trouble, high blood pressure, rheumatic fever, heart murmurs; chest pain or discomfort; palpitations, dyspnea, orthopnea, paroxysmal nocturnal dyspnea, edema; results of past electrocardiograms or other cardiovascular tests
- Gastrointestinal:
    - Trouble swallowing, heartburn, appetite, nausea
    - Bowel movements, stool color and size, change in bowel habits, pain with defecation, rectal bleeding, black or tarry stools, hemorrhoids, constipation, diarrhea

  - Abdominal pain, food intolerance, excessive belching, or passing of gas
  - Jaundice, liver, or gallbladder trouble; hepatitis; last colonoscopy

- Peripheral vascular: Muscle pain with walking (intermittent claudication); leg cramps; varicose veins; past clots in the veins; swelling in calves, legs, or feet; color change in fingertips or toes during cold weather; swelling with redness or tenderness

- Urinary: Frequency of urination, polyuria, nocturia, urgency, burning or pain during urination, hematuria, urinary infections, kidney or flank pain, kidney stones, ureteral colic, suprapubic pain, incontinence; in males, reduced caliber or force of the urinary stream, hesitancy, dribbling

- Reproductive:
  - *Male:*
    - Hernias, discharge from or sores on the penis, testicular pain or masses, scrotal pain or swelling, history of sexually transmitted infections (STIs) and their treatments
    - Sexual habits, sexual preference, gender identity; sexual interest, function, satisfaction, birth control methods, condom use, and problems; concerns about HIV infection; HPV infection, vaccine; history of sexual abuse
  - *Female:*
    - Age at menarche; regularity, frequency, and duration of periods; amount of bleeding; bleeding between periods or after intercourse; date of last menstrual period; dysmenorrhea
    - Age at menopause, menopausal symptoms, postmenopausal bleeding
    - Vaginal discharge, itching, sores, lumps, STIs, and treatments
    - Number of pregnancies, number and type of deliveries, number of abortions (spontaneous and induced), complications of pregnancy, birth control methods
    - Sexual habits, sexual preference, gender identity; sexual interest, function, satisfaction, and any problems, including dyspareunia; concerns about HIV infection; HPV infection, vaccine; history of sexual abuse
    - If the patient was born before 1971, exposure to diethylstilbestrol (DES) from maternal use during pregnancy

CLINICAL TIP
Maternal DES use during pregnancy is linked to vaginal and cervical carcinoma.

- Musculoskeletal: Muscle or joint pain, stiffness, arthritis, gout, backache; if present, location of affected joints or muscles, any swelling, redness, pain, tenderness, stiffness, weakness, or limitation of motion or activity; timing of symptoms (e.g., morning or evening), duration, and any history of trauma; neck or low back pain; joint pain with systemic features such as fever, chills, rash, anorexia, weight loss, or weakness
- Psychiatric: Nervousness; tension; mood, including depression, anxiety, posttraumatic stress disorder, memory change, suicide attempts
- Neurologic: Headache, dizziness, vertigo; fainting, blackouts, seizures, weakness, paralysis, numbness or loss of sensation, tingling or "pins and needles" feeling; tremors or other involuntary movements; changes in mood, attention, or speech; changes in orientation, memory, insight, or judgment
- Hematologic: Anemia, easy bruising or bleeding, past transfusions, transfusion reactions
- Endocrine: Thyroid issues, heat or cold intolerance, excessive sweating, excessive thirst or hunger, polyuria, change in glove or shoe size

Health Patterns

The *health patterns* section provides a guide for gathering personal/social history from the patient and daily living routines that may influence health and illness (Table 4-3).

TABLE 4-3 Health Patterns

Health Pattern	Sample Questions
Self-perception, self-concept:	
Describes self-concept and perceptions of self (e.g., body image, feeling state, self-esteem, personal identity, and social identity)	How would a friend describe you? How do you feel about your ability to handle ___? If you could change anything about yourself, what would you change?
Value-belief:	
Describes patterns of values, beliefs (including spiritual), or goals that guide choices or decisions	What is your source of strength and hope? Is religion or a higher power significant to you? Describe how.

(continued)

TABLE 4-3 **Health Patterns** *(Continued)*

Health Pattern	Sample Questions
Activity-exercise:	
Describes pattern of exercise, activity, leisure, and recreation	Describe your exercise routine or activities. Describe your leisure and recreation activities. Have you experienced any change in your activities due to your illness?
Sleep-rest:	
Describes patterns of sleep, rest, and relaxation	At what time do you usually retire and awaken? Do you feel rested?
Nutrition:	
Describes pattern of food and fluid consumption	Describe a typical day's diet. Are you on any special diet?
Role-relationship:	
Describes pattern of role interactions and relationships. Includes roles, family functioning and problems, and work and neighborhood environment	Who lives with you? Describe the relationships you have with your family and friends. Who provides support for you? Describe your job. What is your neighborhood like? Do you feel safe?
Coping-stress-tolerance:	
Describes general coping pattern and its effectiveness in terms of stress tolerance	What are the current stressors in your life? What do you do to reduce stress?

SENSITIVE TOPICS THAT CALL FOR SPECIFIC APPROACHES

Nurses talk with patients about many subjects that are emotionally charged. Even seasoned clinicians are affected by societal taboos enveloping certain subjects: abuse of alcohol or drugs, sexual practices, death and dying, financial concerns, racial and ethnic bias, family interactions, domestic violence, psychiatric illnesses, physical deformities, bowel function, and others. Many of these topics trigger strong personal responses related to familial, cultural, and societal value systems. Mental illness, drug use during pregnancy, and sexual practices are examples of issues that may evoke biases that can affect the patient interview. This section explores challenges to the nurse in several of these sensitive areas.

Box 4-3 outlines several basic principles that can help guide your response to sensitive topics. Look into strategies for becoming more comfortable

BOX 4-3 GUIDELINES FOR BROACHING SENSITIVE TOPICS

- *The single most important rule is to be nonjudgmental.* The nurse's role is to learn about the patient and help the patient achieve better health. Disapproval of behaviors or elements in the health history will only interfere with this goal.
- *Explain why you need to know certain information.* This makes patients less apprehensive. For example, say to patients, "Because sexual practices put people at risk for certain diseases, I ask all of my patients the following questions."
- Find opening questions for sensitive topics and learn the specific kinds of information needed for your assessments.
- Finally, consciously acknowledge whatever discomfort you are feeling. Denying your discomfort may lead you to avoid the topic altogether.

with sensitive areas. Examples include reading about these topics in nursing, medical, and lay literature; talking to selected colleagues and teachers openly about your concerns; taking courses that help you explore your own feelings and reactions; and ultimately, reflecting on your own life experience. Take advantage of all these resources. Whenever possible, listen to experienced nurses, and then practice similar discussions with your own patients (Fig. 4-5).

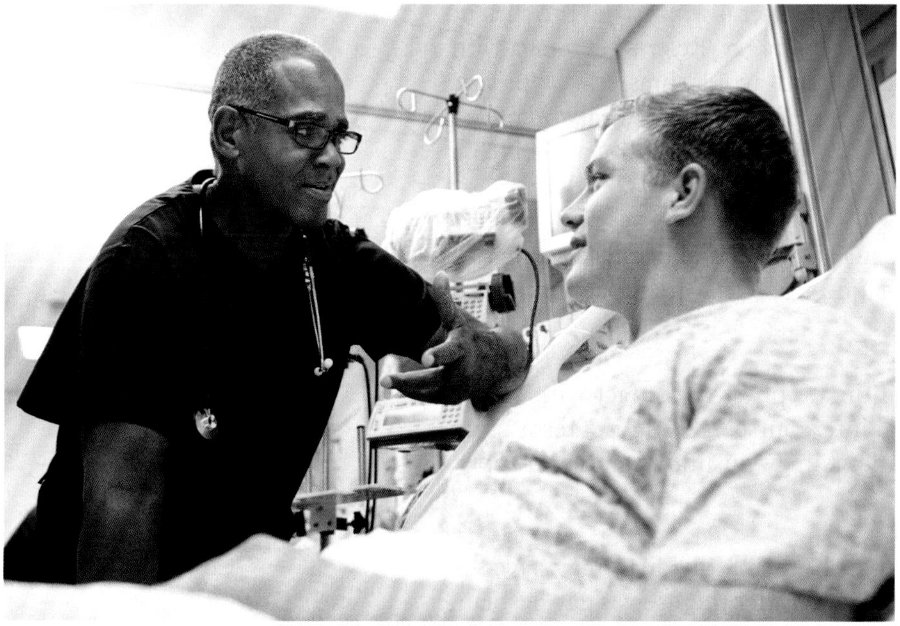

FIGURE 4-5 The nurse talks with the patient about various topics.

The Sexual History

Many patients have questions or concerns about sexuality that they would discuss more freely if asked directly about sexual health. Asking questions about sexual behavior can be lifesaving. Sexual behaviors determine risks for pregnancy and STIs; good interviewing helps prevent or reduce these risks. Sexual practices may be directly related to the patient's symptoms and integral to both diagnosis and treatment. Acceptance of all patients is important. LGBTQIA individuals face health disparities linked to societal stigma, discrimination, and denial of their civil and human rights (HealthyPeople.gov, 2020). Additionally, sexual dysfunction may result from use of medication or from misinformation that, if recognized, can be readily addressed.

You can introduce questions about sexual behavior at multiple points in an interview. If the chief complaint involves genitourinary symptoms, include questions about sexual health as part of "expanding and clarifying" the patient's story. You can ask these questions as part of the review of systems. You can bring them into discussions about health maintenance along with diet, exercise, and screening tests, or as part of lifestyle issues or important relationships covered in the personal and social history section. Do not forget this area of inquiry just because the patient is elderly or has a disability, a chronic illness, a same-sex partner, or no partner.

An orienting sentence or two is often helpful: "To assess your risk for various diseases, I need to ask you some questions about your sexual health and practices" or "I routinely ask all patients about their sexual functioning." For more specific complaints you might state, "To figure out why you have this discharge and what we should do about it, I need to ask some questions about your sexual activity." Try to be matter-of-fact in your style; the patient will be likely to follow your lead. *Use specific language.* Refer to genitalia with explicit words such as "penis" or "vagina" and avoid phrases like "private parts." Choose words that the patient understands or explain what you mean, for example, "By intercourse, I mean when a man inserts his penis into a woman's vagina."

See specific questions in Chapter 21, "Reproductive Systems."

In general, ask about both specific sexual behaviors and satisfaction with sexual function. Here are examples of questions that help patients reveal their concerns:

- "When was the last time you had intimate physical contact with someone? Did that contact include sexual intercourse?" Using the term "sexually active" can be ambiguous. Patients may misunderstand and reply, "No, I just lie there."
- "Do you have sex with men, women, or both?" Individuals may have sex with persons of the same gender yet not consider themselves gay, lesbian, or bisexual. Some gay and lesbian patients have had sex with the opposite gender. Your questions should always be about the behaviors.
- "How many sexual partners have you had in the last 6 months? In the last 5 years? In your lifetime?" Again, these questions give the patient an easy opportunity to acknowledge multiple partners. Ask also about routine use of condoms. "Do you use condoms? How often?"
- It is important to ask all patients, "Do you have any concerns about sexually transmitted infections (STIs), HIV infection, or AIDS?" even if no explicit risk factors are evident.

- "Do you have someone you can talk with about your sexual behaviors/encounters? If you experience a sexual encounter that is forced, violent, or otherwise unpleasant, do you know to whom you can turn?"

Note that these questions make no assumptions about marital status, sexual preference, or attitudes toward pregnancy or contraception. Listen to each of the patient's responses, and ask additional questions as indicated. To elicit information about sexual behaviors, you will need to ask more specific and focused questions than in other parts of the interview.

The Mental Health History

Cultural constructs of mental and physical illness vary widely, causing marked differences in acceptance and attitudes. Think how easy it is for patients to talk about diabetes and taking insulin compared with discussing schizophrenia and using psychotropic medications. Ask open-ended questions initially. "Have you ever had any problem with emotional or mental illnesses?" Then move to more specific questions such as "Have you ever visited a counselor or psychotherapist?" "Have you ever been prescribed medication for emotional issues?" "Have you or has anyone in your family ever been hospitalized for an emotional or mental health concerns?"

For patients with depression or cognitive disorders such as schizophrenia, a careful history of the illness is in order. Depression is common worldwide but still remains underdiagnosed and undertreated, therefore routine screening is recommended. Be sensitive to reports of mood changes or symptoms such as fatigue, unusual tearfulness, appetite or weight changes, insomnia, and vague somatic complaints. Two opening screening questions are: "Over the past 2 weeks, have you felt down, depressed, or hopeless?" and "Over the past 2 weeks, have you felt little interest or pleasure in doing things?" (Lakkis & Mahmassani, 2015). If the patient seems depressed, also ask about thoughts of suicide: "Have you ever thought about hurting yourself or ending your life?" As with chest pain, you must evaluate severity—like angina, depression is potentially lethal.

For further approaches, see Chapter 19, "Mental Status and Mental Health Assessment."

Many patients with schizophrenia or other psychotic disorders can function in the community and tell you about their diagnoses, symptoms, hospitalizations, and current medications. You should investigate their symptoms and assess any effects on mood or daily activities.

Family Violence

Violence is a serious public health problem. Because of the high prevalence of physical, sexual, and emotional abuse, many authorities recommend the routine screening of all female patients for domestic violence (Nelson et al., 2012). However, men can also be victims of violence. Other patients at increased risk are children and the elderly (U.S. Preventive

Services Task Force, 2018b; Centers for Disease Control and Prevention [CDC], 2020). As with other sensitive topics, start this part of the interview with general "normalizing" questions: "Because abuse is common in many people's lives, I ask about it routinely." "Are there times in your relationships that you feel unsafe or afraid?" "Some people tell me that someone at home is hurting them in some way. Is this true for you?" "Within the last year, have you been hit, kicked, punched, or otherwise hurt by someone you know? If so, by whom?" As with other segments of the history, use a pattern that goes from general to specific and less difficult to more difficult.

Physical abuse—often not mentioned by either victim or perpetrator—should be considered in the following situations:

- If injuries are unexplained, seem inconsistent with the patient's story, are concealed by the patient, or cause embarrassment
- If the patient has delayed getting treatment for trauma
- If there is a past history of repeated injuries or "accidents"
- If the patient or person close to the patient has a history of alcohol or drug abuse
- If the partner tries to dominate the interview, will not leave the room, or seems unusually anxious or solicitous

When abuse is suspected, it is important to spend part of the encounter alone with the patient. Use the transition to the physical examination as a reason to ask the other person to leave the room. If the patient is also resistant, do not force the situation, potentially placing the victim in jeopardy. Be attuned to diagnoses that have a higher association with abuse, such as pregnancy.

Child abuse is unfortunately also common. Asking parents about their approaches to discipline is a routine part of well-child care. You can also ask parents how they cope with a baby who will not stop crying or a child who misbehaves: "Most parents get upset when their baby cries (or their child has misbehaved). How do you feel when your baby cries?" "What do you do when your baby won't stop crying?" "Do you have any fears that you might hurt your child?" Find out how other caregivers or companions handle these situations as well.

DOCUMENTING THE HEALTH HISTORY

Today, documentation of the patient's health history is frequently computerized. The record must be accurate and thorough, no matter the type of documentation system used. A sample written documentation of the history can be seen in Chapter 2, "Critical Thinking and Clinical Judgment in Health Assessment."

BIBLIOGRAPHY

CITATIONS

Boucek, L., Kane, I., Lindsay, D. L., Hagle, H., Salvio, K., & Mitchell, A. M. (2019). Screening, brief intervention, and referral to treatment (SBIRT) education of residential care nursing staff: Impact on staff and residents. *Geriatric Nursing*, *40*(6), 553–557.

Centers for Disease Control and Prevention (CDC). (2020). *Violence prevention.* Retrieved June 5, 2020, from http://www.cdc.gov/violenceprevention/index.html

Cheal, N. E., McKnigh-Eily, L., & Weber, M. K. (2014). Alcohol screening and brief intervention: a clinical solution to a vital public health issue. *American Nurse Today*, *9*(9), 34–35.

Frank, D., DeBenedetti, A. F., Volk, R. J., Williams, E. C., Kivlahan, D. R., & Bradley, K. A. (2008). Effectiveness of the AUDIT-C as a screening test for alcohol misuse in three race/ethnic groups. *Journal of General Internal Medicine*, *23*(6), 781–787.

Health Literacy Measurement Tools (Revised). (2020). *Agency for Healthcare Research and Quality.* Retrieved May 4, 2020, from https://www.ahrq.gov/health-literacy/quality-resources/tools/literacy/index.html

Healthy People.gov. (2020). *Lesbian, gay, bisexual, and transgender health.* Retrieved June 4, 2020, from https://www.healthypeople.gov/2020/topics-objectives/topic/lesbian-gay-bisexual-and-transgender-health

Lakkis, N. A., & Mahmassani, D. M. (2015). Screening instruments for depression in primary care: a concise review for clinicians. *Postgraduate Medicine*, *127*(1), 99–106.

Monico, L. B., Mitchell, S. G., Dusek, K., Gryczynski, J., Schwartz, R. P., Oros, M., Hosler, C., O'Grady, K. E., & Brown, B. S. (2019). A comparison of screening practices for adolescents in primary care: After implementation of screening, brief intervention, and referral to treatment. *Journal of Adolescent Health*, *65*(1), 46–50.

National Network of Libraries of Medicine. (2020). *Health literacy definition.* Retrieved May 4, 2020, from https://nnlm.gov/initiatives/topics/health-literacy

Nelson, H. D., Bougatsos, C., & Blazina, I. (2012). Screening women for intimate partner violence: a systematic review to update the U.S. Preventive Services Task Force recommendation. *Annals of Internal Medicine*, *156*(11), 796–808, W-279, W-280, W-281, W-282.

Salisbury-Afshar, E., & Fleming, M. (2019). Identification of and treatment for unhealthy alcohol use in primary care settings. *American Family Physician*, *99*(12), 733–734.

Substance Abuse and Mental Health Services Administration (SAMHSA). (2019). *Key Substance Use and Mental Health Indicators in the United States, 2018.* National Survey on Drug Use and Health: Summary of National Findings, HHS Publication No. PEP19-5068.

U.S. Preventive Services Task Force. (2018a). Screening for Intimate Partner Violence, Elder Abuse, and Abuse of Vulnerable Adults US Preventive Services Task Force Final Recommendation Statement. *JAMA: The Journal of the American Medical Association*, *320*(16), 1678–1687.

U.S. Preventive Services Task Force. (2018b). Screening and Behavioral Counseling Interventions to Reduce Unhealthy Alcohol Use in Adolescents and Adults: Recommendation Statement. *JAMA: The Journal of the American Medical Association*, *320*(18), 1899–1909.

ADDITIONAL REFERENCES

Health Promotion and Counseling

Centers for Disease Control and Prevention. *Vaccines and immunizations.* Retrieved May 4, 2020, from http://www.cdc.gov/vaccines/

Knox, J., Hasin, D. S., Larson, F. R. R., & Kranzler, H. R. (2019). Prevention, screening, and treatment for heavy drinking and alcohol use disorder. *The Lancet Psychiatry*, *6*(12), 1054–1067.

National Guideline Clearinghouse. *Agency for Healthcare Research and Quality (AHRQ).* Retrieved May 4, 2020, from http://www.ahrq.gov/clinic/

National Institution on Alcohol Abuse and Alcoholism. *Alcohol Screening and Brief Intervention for Youth: A Practitioner's Guide.* Retrieved May 4, 2020, from https://www.niaaa.nih.gov/publications/clinical-guides-and-manuals/alcohol-screening-and-brief-intervention-youth/resources

National Institution on Alcohol Abuse and Alcoholism. *Alcohol Use Disorders Identification Test (AUDIT).* Retrieved May 4, 2020, from https://pubs.niaaa.nih.gov/publications/audit.htm

Substance Abuse and Mental Health Services Administration (SAMHSA). (2018). Retrieved May 4, 2020, from https://www.samhsa.gov/

5 CULTURAL AND SPIRITUAL ASSESSMENT

KEY TERMS

biases	culture	race
cultural competence	culture-bound syndromes	religion
cultural humility	ethnicity	spirituality
		values

Learning Objectives

The student will:

1. Explain why culture is important in the health assessment process.
2. Define cultural competence and cultural humility.
3. Demonstrate behaviors that show sensitivity to a patient's culture during the assessment process.
4. Explain the difference between spirituality and religion.
5. Explain why the patient's spiritual needs should be assessed.
6. Use a spiritual assessment tool to assess a patient's spiritual needs.

CULTURE AND SPIRITUALITY

Patients do not live in isolation; they are part of families, communities, ethnic groups, religious groups, and cultures. To accurately assess patients' health needs, the nurse must assess patients within the contexts of the patients' backgrounds. Global migration has greatly increased the challenges of providing health care to patients with varying health care beliefs, practices, and needs different from those of the health care provider (Kersey-Matusiak, 2019). Culture and ethnicity contribute to interpersonal communication styles as well as health beliefs, values, and practices. Culture shapes not only patients' beliefs but also nurses' (Fig. 5-1). Spirituality is the aspect of humanity that refers to the way individuals seek and express meaning and purpose and the way they experience their connectedness to the moment,

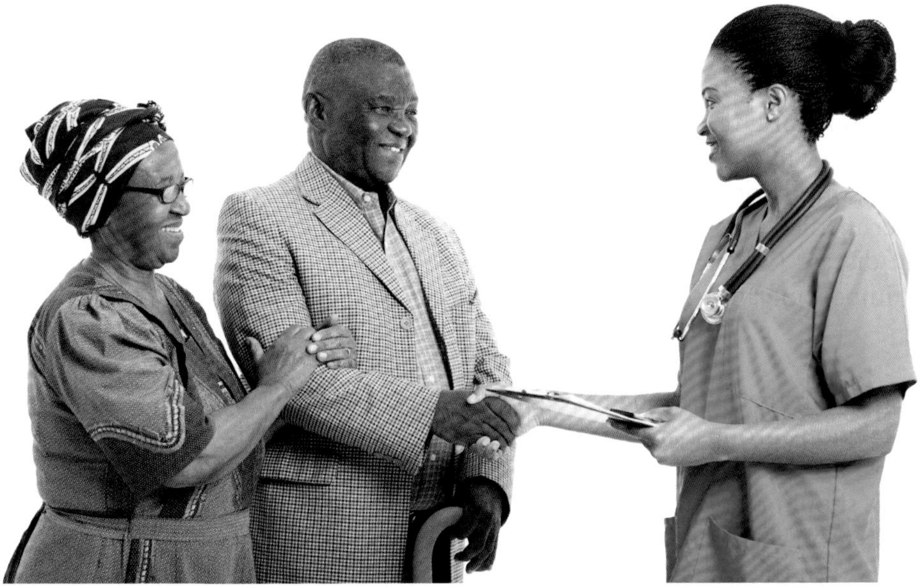

FIGURE 5-1 Nurses work with many patients of cultures different from their own.

the self, others, nature, and the significant or sacred (Pulchaski et al., 2009). This chapter will discuss the importance of culture and spirituality in relation to health assessment.

CULTURAL ASSESSMENT

Cultural assessment is part of the foundation for every patient's plan of care. It provides valuable data for setting mutual goals, planning care, intervening, and evaluating the care (Andrews et al., 2019). Cultural assessment is a systematic, comprehensive examination of individuals, families, groups, and communities regarding their health-related cultural beliefs, values, and practices.

There are many definitions of culture. Purnell (2013) defines culture as "the totality of socially transmitted behavioral patterns, arts, beliefs, values, customs, lifeways, and all other products of human work and thought characteristic of a population of people that guide their worldview and decision making." In other words, **culture** is the system of shared ideas, rules, and meanings that influences how we view the world, experience it emotionally, and behave in relation to other people. It can be viewed as the "lens" through which we perceive and make sense of the world we inhabit. The meaning of culture is broader than that of the term **ethnicity**. An ethnic group is composed of "individuals who self-identify membership with or belong to a group with shared values, ancestry, and experiences" (Leininger & McFarland, 2002; McFarland & Wehbe-Alamah, 2019). **Race**, on the other hand, is a socially constructed concept of dividing people into populations or groups on the basis of various sets of physical characteristics, usually based on genetic ancestry. Most biologists and anthropologists today do not recognize race as a biologically valid classification, in part because there is more genetic variation within groups than between them. However, research in genetics, genomics, and epigenetics has expanded dramatically and has had a profound influence on the health of people around the world. Humans are more alike than different genetically—only 0.1% of human DNA varies from another person—but these genetic variations explain why susceptibility to common diseases differs among individuals and populations. It also provides the knowledge needed to safely administer medications and counsel patients regarding the preventions and risk of disease (Giger, 2017). Knowledge of a patient's genetic background is important and should be identified during the history.

Culture is not limited to ethnic or minority groups; everyone has a culture. For example, LGBTQIA individuals, religious groups, and teenagers may identify with the culture of these groups. Likewise, deaf individuals recognize a connection to this culture. Nurses should recognize and be sensitive to the cultural needs of all patients (Kersey-Matusiak, 2019; Wichinski, 2015). Culture can be further defined as the thoughts, communications, actions, customs, beliefs, values and institutions of racial, ethnic, religious or social groups. Culture defines how health care information is received; how rights and protections are exercised; what is considered to be a health problem; how symptoms and concerns about the problem are expressed; who should provide treatment for the problem; and what type of treatment should be given. The U.S. Department of Health and Human Services has developed the Healthy People 2030 goals that will continue the Healthy People 2020 goals of improving overall health of Americans and reducing health disparities among ethnic or cultural groups in the United States (Healthy People, 2020). In order to accomplish this, the Office of Minority Health (OMH) created the *National Standards for Culturally and Linguistically Appropriate Services (CLAS) in Health and Health Care* (Box 5-1). The principal standard is "Provide effective, equitable, understandable, and respectful quality care and services that are responsive to diverse cultural health beliefs and practices, preferred languages, health literacy, and other communication needs" (U.S. Department of Health and Human Services, 2009).

LGBTQIA stands for lesbian, gay, bisexual, transgender, queer/questioning, intersex, and asexual.

Nursing has long recognized and practiced holistic care of the patient, and attention to culture is a part of caring for the whole patient. The nurse communicates with and cares for people of many different cultures. One does not have to be well versed in every culture to provide culturally appropriate care, but one must be open and sensitive to other cultures. Ellis Fletcher created the concept of *cultural sensibility*, "a deliberative proactive behavior by health care providers who examine cultural situations through thoughtful reasoning, responsiveness, and discreet [attentive, considerate, and observant] interactions" (Fletcher, 2015). One first identifies one's own biases, prejudices, and stereotypes about different cultures, races, or ethnicity. The nurse then uses reflective thinking to analyze interactions and events in order to develop cultural awareness.

The term **cultural competence** recognizes the need for a set of skills necessary to care for people of different cultures. However, cultural competence

BOX 5-1 THE NATIONAL STANDARDS FOR CULTURALLY AND LINGUISTICALLY APPROPRIATE SERVICES IN HEALTH AND HEALTH CARE

Principal Standard

1. Provide effective, equitable, understandable, and respectful quality care and services that are responsive to diverse cultural health beliefs and practices, preferred languages, health literacy, and other communication needs.

Governance, Leadership, and Workforce

2. Advance and sustain organizational governance and leadership that promotes CLAS and health equity through policy, practices, and allocated resources.
3. Recruit, promote, and support a culturally and linguistically diverse governance, leadership, and workforce that are responsive to the population in the service area.
4. Educate and train governance, leadership, and workforce in culturally and linguistically appropriate policies and practices on an ongoing basis.

Communication and Language Assistance

5. Offer language assistance to individuals who have limited English proficiency and/or other communication needs, at no cost to them, to facilitate timely access to all health care and services.
6. Inform all individuals of the availability of language assistance services clearly and in their preferred language, verbally and in writing.
7. Ensure the competence of individuals providing language assistance, recognizing that the use of untrained individuals and/or minors as interpreters should be avoided.
8. Provide easy-to-understand print and multimedia materials and signage in the languages commonly used by the populations in the service area.

Engagement, Continuous Improvement, and Accountability

9. Establish culturally and linguistically appropriate goals, policies, and management accountability, and infuse them throughout the organizations' planning and operations.
10. Conduct ongoing assessments of the organization's CLAS-related activities and integrate CLAS-related measures into assessment measurement and continuous quality improvement activities.
11. Collect and maintain accurate and reliable demographic data to monitor and evaluate the impact of CLAS on health equity and outcomes and to inform service delivery.
12. Conduct regular assessments of community health assets and needs and use the results to plan and implement services that respond to the cultural and linguistic diversity of populations in the service area.
13. Partner with the community to design, implement and evaluate policies, practices, and services to ensure cultural and linguistic appropriateness.
14. Create conflict- and grievance-resolution processes that are culturally and linguistically appropriate to identify, prevent, and resolve conflicts or complaints.
15. Communicate the organization's progress in implementing and sustaining CLAS to all stakeholders, constituents, and the general public.

U.S. Department of Health and Human Services, Office of Minority Health. Think Cultural Health. https://thinkculturalhealth.hhs.gov/clas/standards

must not be reduced to knowledge of a static set of traits and beliefs for particular ethnic groups that is applied to every member of the group. In reality, there are subgroups and variations within all cultural groups. For example, there are many subcultures among Hispanic and Asian people. In addition, culture is ever-changing and always being revised as group members interact with each other and the world around them.

Campinha-Bacote (2010) developed a model of cultural competence that defines culture as a process, not a state. Nurses see themselves *becoming* culturally competent, not *being* culturally competent. Campinha-Bacote sees "cultural desire" as the motivation the nurse needs to "want to" and not "need to" become culturally aware, culturally knowledgeable, and culturally skillful and to seek cultural encounters. One becomes culturally competent by "genuinely seeking cultural encounters, obtaining cultural knowledge, conducting culturally sensitive assessments, and being humble to the process of cultural awareness" (Campinha-Bacote, 2010).

Tervalon and Murray-Garcia (1998) developed the concept of cultural humility when caring for patients from culturally diverse backgrounds. **Cultural humility** is defined as a "process that requires humility as individuals continually engage in self-reflection and self-critique as lifelong learners and reflective practitioners" (Tervalon & Murray-Garcia, 1998). It is a process that includes "examining cultural beliefs and cultural systems of both patients and nurses to locate the points of cultural dissonance or synergy that contribute to patients' health outcomes" (Foronda, 2020; Tervalon & Murray-Garcia, 1998). It calls for health providers to reduce the power imbalance that exists in caregiver–patient relationships and maintain mutually respectful and dynamic partnerships with patients.

Yancu and Farmer (2017) note that the concept of cultural competence implies a product, while cultural humility is a process. They believe the two concepts complement each other and using both will improve care of diverse cultural populations. Campinha-Bacote proposes a new term, "competemility" (a combination of *compete*nce and hu*mility*), to emphasize the synergistic relationship of cultural competence and cultural humility (Fitzgerald & Campinha-Bacote, 2019).

It is clear there is overlap among theorists, but *self-reflection* is a common denominator. Begin your self-reflection by answering the following questions:

1. Am I aware of my biases? Prejudices? Stereotypes?
2. Am I comfortable interacting with people from different cultures?
3. Do I seek out experiences with other cultures?
4. Do I seek out opportunities to learn about other cultures?
5. Do I respect the beliefs of individuals from other cultures?
6. Do I know how to access language interpreter services for patients?

Bias: A preference or an inclination, especially one that inhibits impartial judgment, for example, the attitudes or feelings that we attach to perceived differences in other cultures

Prejudice: A disapproving or negative attitude that is not rooted in fact or accurate information

Stereotype: A uniform image of one group that is believed by another group; a fixed, overgeneralized belief about a particular group or class of people

Now read the following case studies, and observe how cultural differences and unconscious bias can unwittingly lead to poor communication and disrupt the quality and outcomes of patient care.

CASE STUDY

Scenario 1

A 28-year-old man from Ghana who recently moved to the United States complained to a friend about U.S. medical care. He had gone to the clinic because of fever and fatigue. He described being weighed, having his temperature taken, and having a cloth wrapped tightly—to the point of pain—around his arm. The nurse, a 36-year-old woman from Washington, D.C., had asked the patient many questions, examined him, and asked to take blood, which the patient had refused. The patient's final comment was, "and she didn't even give me chloroquine!" This had been his primary reason for seeking care. The patient was expecting few questions, no examination, and treatment for malaria, which is what fever usually indicates in his former community.

In this example, cross-cultural miscommunication is understandable and thus less threatening to explore. Consider the next case study, as this occurs in many clinical interactions in which unconscious bias leads to miscommunication.

CASE STUDY

Scenario 2

A 16-year-old high school student came to the local youth health center because of painful menstrual cramps that were interfering with concentrating at school. She was dressed in a tight top and short skirt and had multiple facial piercings. The health care provider asked the following questions: "Are you passing all of your classes? What kind of job do you want after high school? What kind of birth control do you want?" The patient felt pressured into accepting birth control pills from a prescribing provider, even though she had clearly told the nurse she had never had intercourse and planned to wait to become sexually active until after she got married. She was an honor student planning to go to college, but the nurse did not ask about these goals. The chief complaint of cramps was dismissed as minor, when the provider said, "Oh you can just take some ibuprofen. Cramps usually get better as you get older." The patient does not want to take the birth control pills that were prescribed, nor does she want to seek health care soon again. She experienced the encounter as an aggressive interrogation and therefore did not trust the health care provider. In addition, the nurse's questions made assumptions about the patient's life and did not show respect for her health concerns. Even though the provider pursued some important psychosocial domains, the patient received ineffective health care because of conflicting cultural values and nurse bias.

In both of these cases, the failure stems from mistaken assumptions or biases. In the first case, the nurse did not consider the patient's belief about his symptoms and expectations for care. In the second case, the nurse allowed stereotypes to dictate the agenda instead of listening to the patient and respecting her as an individual, without digging deeper, potentially missing an underlying pathology that could explain the patient's menstrual cramps. Each of us has our own cultural background and biases. These do not simply fade away as we become nurses. We must continually learn about different cultures and how to therapeutically interact with each person as a respected individual with a wide array of cultural influences.

Avoid letting personal impressions about cultural groups turn into stereotyping rather than understanding. For example, you may hear that Hispanic patients are more dramatic when they express pain or that Asian patients are stoic. Recognize these are stereotypes. Evaluate each patient with pain as an individual, being aware of your reaction to the patient's communication style. Work on becoming aware of your own values and biases, developing communication skills that transcend cultural differences, and building therapeutic partnerships based on respect for each patient's life experience. This framework, described in the next section, will allow you to approach each patient as a unique individual.

THE THREE DIMENSIONS OF CULTURAL HUMILITY

The three dimensions of cultural humility include:

- *Self-awareness:* Learn about your own biases—we all have them.
- *Respectful communication:* Work to eliminate assumptions about what is "normal." Learn directly from your patients; they are the experts on their own cultures, needs, and illnesses.
- *Collaborative partnerships:* Build your patient relationships on respect and mutually acceptable plans.

Self-Awareness

Start by exploring your own cultural identity:

1. How do you describe yourself in terms of ethnicity, class, region or country of origin, religion, and political affiliation? Don't forget the characteristics that could be areas of change for an individual such as life roles, sexual orientation, gender, or physical ability.
2. With what aspects of your family of origin do you identify, and how are you different from your family of origin?
3. How do these identities influence your beliefs and behaviors?

A more challenging task is to bring our own values and biases to a conscious level. **Values** are the standards we use to measure our own and others' beliefs and behaviors. **Biases** are the attitudes or feelings that we attach to perceived differences. Being attuned to difference is normal; in fact, in

> *Concept Mastery Alert*
>
> **Self-Examination**
>
> Before beginning a cultural assessment of a patient, the nurse must conduct a self-examination to determine any personal biases and prejudices that may exist unintentionally. This self-examination allows the nurse to become fully aware of possible unacknowledged feelings and beliefs. This is an important first step. Once this is accomplished, the nurse can gain knowledge and an awareness of the culture's health practices.

the distant past, reacting to differences may have preserved life. Instinctively knowing members of one's own group is a survival skill that we may have outgrown as a society but that is still actively, if unconsciously, at work.

Feeling guilty about our biases makes it hard to recognize and acknowledge them. Start with less threatening constructs, like the way an individual relates to time, a culturally determined phenomenon. Are you always on time—a positive value in the Western culture? Or do you tend to run a little late? How do you feel about people whose habits are opposite to yours? Next time you attend a meeting or class, notice who is early, on time, or late. Is it predictable? Think about the role of physical appearance. Do you consider yourself thin, midsize, or heavy? How do you feel about your weight? What does prevailing U.S. culture teach us to value in physique? How do you feel about people who have different weights?

Respectful Communication

Given the complexity of global society, no one can possibly know the health beliefs and practices of every culture and subculture. Let your patients be the experts on their own unique cultural perspectives. Even if patients have trouble describing their values or beliefs, they can often respond to specific questions. Find out about the patient's cultural background. Review the section "Explore the Patient's Perspective" in Chapter 3, "Interviewing and Communication" for questions to use. Maintain an open, respectful, and inquiring attitude. "What did you hope to get from this visit?" If you have established rapport and trust, patients will be willing to teach you. Be aware of questions that contain assumptions. And always be ready to acknowledge your areas of ignorance or bias. "I don't know a lot about Ghana. What would have happened at a clinic there if you had these concerns?" Or with the second patient scenario, and with much more difficulty, it would be appropriate to say, "I mistakenly made assumptions about you that are not right. I apologize. Would you be willing to tell me more about yourself and your future goals?"

The RESPECT Model can provide a guide for effective cross-cultural communication (Fig. 5-2).

Learning about specific cultures, especially those living in your geographic area, is valuable because it helps you provide culturally appropriate nursing care to patients from other cultures. A complete review of cultural health beliefs and practices is beyond the scope of this text. You must search out resources to expand your knowledge, and this should be a lifelong learning subject. College courses, books, and conferences on culture are helpful resources. Go to movies filmed in different countries to better understand the perspective of different cultures. Learn about the health concerns of different ethnic groups. Investigate the barriers to health care in your community. Most importantly, be open to learning from each patient. Do not assume that your impressions about a given cultural group apply to the individual before you.

The RESPECT Model

What is most important in considering the effectiveness of your cross-cultural communication, whether it is verbal, nonverbal, or written, is that you remain open and maintain a sense of respect for your patients. The RESPECT Model can help you remain effective and patient-centered in all of your communication with patients.

Rapport
- Connect on a social level.
- See the patient's point of view.
- Consciously suspend judgment.
  Recognize and avoid making assumptions.

Empathy
- Remember the patient has come to you for help.
- Seek out and understand the patient's rationale for their behaviors and illness.
- Verbally acknowledge and legitimize the patient's feelings.

Support
- Ask about and understand the barriers to care and compliance.
- Help the patient overcome barriers.
- Involve family members if appropriate.
- Reassure the patient you are and will be available to help.

Partnership
- Be flexible.
- Negotiate roles when necessary.
- Stress that you are working together to address health problems.

Explanations
- Check often for understanding.
- Use verbal clarification techniques.

Cultural competence
- Respect the patient's cultural beliefs.
- Understand that the patient's views of you may be defined by ethnic and cultural stereotypes.
- Be aware of your own cultural biases and preconceptions.
- Know your limitations in addressing health issues across cultures.
- Understand your personal style and recognize when it may not be working with a given patient.

Trust
- Recognize that self-disclosure may be difficult for some patients.
- Consciously work to establish trust.

Guide to Providing Effective Communication and Language Assistance Services
www.ThinkCulturalHealth.hhs.gov

OMH U.S. Department of Health and Human Services Office of Minority Health

THINK CULTURAL HEALTH

FIGURE 5-2 The RESPECT Model. (Reprinted from the Office of Minority Health, 2020; adapted with permission from Mutha, S., Allen, C., & Welch, M. (2002). *Toward culturally competent care: A toolbox for teaching communications strategies*. Center for Health Professions, University of California, San Francisco.)

CLINICAL TIP

Consider various barriers to health care to your patient and their family, for example, costs of appointments/medicines, lack of health insurance, distance between home and clinic/hospital, lack of a car, poor English skills, and lack of understanding of Western medical care.

Under the Department of Health and Human Services, the OMH sponsors *Culturally Competent Nursing Care: A Cornerstone of Caring,* an engaging e-learning program designed to help you build knowledge and skills related to cultural and linguistic competency. Find it at https://ccnm.thinkculturalhealth.hhs.gov/. The National Center for Cultural Competence at Georgetown University also provides multiple resources and tools available at: http://nccc.georgetown.edu/.

Collaborative Partnerships

Through continual work on self-awareness and seeing through the "lens" of others, the nurse lays the foundation for the collaborative relationship that best supports the patient's health. Communication based on trust, respect, and the nurse's willingness to reexamine assumptions allows patients to be more open to expressing views that diverge from the dominant culture. They may have strong feelings such as anger or shame. As the nurse, you must be willing to listen to and validate these feelings, and not let your own feelings of discomfort or time pressure prevent you from exploring painful areas. You must be willing to reexamine your beliefs about what is the "right approach" to clinical care in any given situation. Make every effort to be flexible and creative as you develop shared plans that reflect the patients' knowledge about their best interests congruent with their beliefs and effective clinical care.

Transcultural Perspectives on the Health History

Culture impacts history taking in multiple ways. Knowledge of the cultural or ethnic groups in your practice region will help you better understand and interpret the patient's needs. Knowledge of categories of dissonance will help the novice recognize potential problems. Time in social conversation, use of silence, distance between the interviewer and client, eye contact, modesty, use of touch, and gestures vary by culture. A patient's nonverbal communication may confuse a novice nurse when it is different from the nurse's communication style. It can be disconcerting working with a person whose culture reverses nodding the head for "yes" and shaking the head for "no," as is the case in Bulgaria. Experiencing discomfort or frustration during the history may be a clue that there is cultural dissonance. It is best to stop and clarify the situation with the patient.

Cultural and ethnic variations (Box 5-2) may be evident during the physical examination, and some of these will be noted in the text during the system examinations.

BOX 5-2 CULTURAL VARIATIONS IN COMMUNICATION

- Time spent in social conversation before discussing the purpose of the visit
- Amount of time the patient and nurse are comfortable with silence or "no one talking"
- Distance between the interviewer and client; comfort with interpersonal space
- Eye contact—varies from none to continuous; avoidance of eye contact is considered a sign of respect in some cultures
- Comfort with being touched: For example, shaking hands when greeting a new patient is not done in some cultures, and touch between different sexes is not permissible
- Gestures while talking—some cultures "talk with their hands" while others are still
- Modesty, especially during examination

THE HEALTH ASSESSMENT

Aspects of culture relevant to health assessment include (Kersey-Matusiak, 2019; McFarland & Wehbe-Alamah, 2019):

1. Communication and language
2. Family structure
3. Family roles and organization
4. Social networks
5. Educational background and learning style
6. Nutrition
7. Childbearing and child-rearing practices
8. High-risk behaviors
9. Health care beliefs and practices
10. Health care practitioners
11. Spirituality and religion

A full cultural assessment can be quite lengthy and take more time than the nurse has on admission. The questions in Box 5-3 will provide the nurse with basic essential information.

BOX 5-3 CULTURAL ASSESSMENT

Culture and Language

How would you like to be addressed?
Do you consider yourself a part of any cultural group(s)?
Where were you born? Where have you lived since then and when (during what years)?
What language do you speak at home? What other languages do you speak? What language do you prefer for communicating with health care providers?
How well do you understand, speak, and read English?

Spirituality

Do you practice a particular religion?
What prayers, rituals, and/or diet would you like to continue in the hospital?
Would you like a spiritual leader to be notified that you are here?

Nutrition

What foods do you prefer? When and where do you eat meals?
Do you prefer any special foods during illness or certain religious seasons (e.g., Lent or Ramadan)?
Are there any foods prohibited by your cultural or religion that you would like us to know?

Reason for Hospitalization

What do you think caused your illness?
What do you call this illness?

Family

Who belongs to your family?
Who is the decision maker on health issues in your family?

Nursing Care

What interventions would be used for this illness in your culture?
How do you feel about health care providers of a different sex or culture?

BOX 5-4 TRANSCULTURAL PERSPECTIVES FOR THE HEALTH HISTORY

Introduction

It is generally better to begin the interview using formal titles. Ask the patient how they would like to be addressed. Inquire what language the patient speaks if it is not English.

Source

Note whether an interpreter was used for the history and indicate their relationship to the patient and a contact phone number. See Chapter 3, "Interviewing and Communication," for more information on working with an interpreter.

Reason for Seeking Care

Patients may interpret their symptoms per their cultural view, as did the man from Ghana in the case study. There are also culture-bound syndromes, which are illnesses defined by a particular culture but that have no corresponding illness in Western medicine. Use a question at the end of the interview, such as, "What did you hope to get from this visit?" to identify potential disconnects between patient and nurse or additional concerns the patient may have.

Self-Treatment

Be sure to ask what treatment the patient has used already and whether it helped. Traditional or alternative medicine remedies should be clarified.

Medications

When asking about medications, include herbal remedies and medicines from alternative health care providers. For example, Ayurvedic medicine is a system of traditional medicine native to India and practiced in other parts of the world as a form of alternative medicine.

Family and Social History

Family is important in all cultures, but definitions of family and who is included in the family may vary among cultures. In the history, note the family structure and who the decision makers are for the family, especially for health care issues.

Review of Systems

Ask about health promotion activities for each system as these may vary. One may also ask about symptoms of diseases commonly seen in the patient's ethnic or genetic background.

Data from Andrews, M. A., Boyle, J. S., & Collins, J. (2019). *Transcultural concepts in nursing care* (8th ed). Lippincott Williams & Wilkins.

Be aware that some languages have different versions; for example, Chinese may be Mandarin, Cantonese, or another dialect.

An example of a culture-bound syndrome is "mal ojo" or "evil eye" in Spanish. Mal ojo occurs when someone is the recipient of someone else's ill wishes. Symptoms may include fever, malaise, anorexia, vomiting and irritability. To the patient or parent of a child, these are real events and must be taken seriously. Referral to a healer of the patient's culture may be the best option.

Transcultural perspectives for the health history are presented in Box 5-4. Biocultural variations in the physical examination will be noted in the body systems chapters of this textbook.

SPIRITUAL ASSESSMENT

Many definitions of spirituality have been proposed. The difficulty in defining spirituality may lie in the lack of conceptual clarity of the term (Kersey-Matusiak, 2019; Sessanna et al., 2007). Spirituality is a dimension of culture, and it is culture-specific in how it is viewed. Nurses and researchers of Western culture have tried to separate spirituality from religion, but this may do a disservice to non-Western cultures, in which spirituality rises from religious beliefs or exposure to a religious culture. An estimated 84%

of the world is religious, and for these people, religion is the basis of spirituality (Sherwood, 2018). Spirituality is a vital human experience shared by all humans; atheists and nonpractitioners may still have spiritual dimensions as well. Purnell (2013) broadly defines **spirituality** as "all behaviors that give meaning to life and provide strength to the individual." Buck (2006) defines spirituality as "that most human of experiences that seeks to transcend self and find meaning and purpose through connection with others, nature and/or a Supreme Being, which may or may not involve religious structures or traditions." **Religion** may be described as a system of beliefs or a practice of worship.

When an individual's sense of purpose or meaning of life is threatened for example a cancer diagnosis, spiritual distress may result (Nolan et al., 2020). It may also be a response to illness or the loss of a relative or friend. Refer to the Table 5-1 to review examples of possible losses a person may experience. Nursing care includes assessment of the patient's spiritual needs and implementation of care related to these needs. Analyses in a nurse's case plan may include psychosocial/spiritual needs. In addition, The Joint Commission on Accreditation of Healthcare Organizations (JCAHO) requires the administration of a spiritual assessment as part of its accreditation standards. JCAHO mandates spiritual assessments in hospitals, home care organizations, long-term care facilities, and certain behavioral health care organizations (Hessel, 2009; Hodge, 2006; JACHO, 2019).

Spiritual distress results when the patient experiences a disruption in the life principle that pervades a person's being and integrates and transcends one's biologic and psychological nature. Listen to the patient's concerns. Encourage the patient to talk about what fears, concerns, or losses they are experiencing. Ask the patient what has helped them cope with such issues in the past. Provide resources available for the patient to use, for example, supportive care resources, a spiritual leader, or cognitive behavioral therapy (Nolan et al., 2020).

The generalist nurse is not prepared to provide intense spiritual counseling, just as they do not provide intense nutrition counseling or physical therapy. However, the nurse may provide spiritual care by supporting the patient's practice of spirituality such as prayer or meditation; being present during unpleasant experiences; listening to the patient share fears, thoughts, or distress; providing opportunities for the patient to practice religious rituals; or referring the patient to a religious leader of the patient's choice.

The nurse approaches spiritual assessment in two tiers. Patients will not discuss deep concerns until a trusting relationship has been built with the nurse. During the first meeting, the nurse obtains a brief assessment of general information, such as the patient's religion and whether the patient would like a religious leader to be informed of the hospitalization. Does the patient have any rituals or prayers to be continued in the hospital? Nursing care schedules can be arranged to allow time for prayer during the day. Explaining to the patient that research has shown a connection between physical health and spiritual comfort will help the patient understand why questions about spirituality are being asked. The patient's diagnosis may cause fears or concerns. The nurse can ask, "Do you have any concerns or fears because of your diagnosis?" The patient may not be ready to discuss the feelings aroused by the illness. By providing an opening for discussion, the nurse communicates willingness to listen when the patient wishes to discuss spiritual concerns.

Concept Mastery Alert

Discussing Religion and Spirituality

While the admission assessment includes asking about religious affiliation, it is best if the nurse waits until a trusting relationship has been established to ask about deeper questions regarding religion and spirituality. Patients are not likely to discuss deep concerns until the nurse has earned the patient's trust.

TABLE 5-1 Loss History

Losses of Other People—through Death	Loss of Other People—through:
• Parent(s) • Spouse/partner • Sibling • Child • Grandchild • Grandparent(s) • Friend • Relative	• Separation • Divorce • Geographic move • Job loss • Retirement • Miscarriage • Drug abuse
Loss of Self	**Personal Attributes—Developmental Losses**
• Physical illness • Divorce • Spouse's/partner's death • Job loss • Retirement • Substance abuse • Mental illness • Abortion • Surgery • Physical/emotional abuse • Sexual abuse	• Loss of fertility • Loss of mobility • Loss of vision • Loss of hearing • Loss of natural hair color • Loss of hair • Loss of skin tone
Social Role	**Abstract Losses**
• Loss of job • Loss of partner and social contacts • Loss of status in society	• Hopes • Dreams • Faith • Childhood • Humor • Femininity/virility • Identity
Concrete Losses	**Aspects to Consider**
• Personal possessions • Money • Pet • Job • Stocks, bonds • Residence	• Immediate reaction to the loss • Feelings at the time of loss • The client's age at the time of loss • What did the client remember most about the experience? • Coping mechanisms • Support systems • To what did the client find most difficult to adjust?

Adapted from Ginette, G. Ferszt, PhD, RN, PMHCNS-BC, FAAN Professor, College of Nursing, University of Rhode Island. Personal Communication.

Listening is an important part of being *present* with a patient. Nursing *presence* "is a holistic and reciprocal exchange between the nurse and patient that involves a sincere connection and sharing of human experience through active listening, attentiveness, intimacy and therapeutic touch, spiritual exploration, empathy, caring and compassion, and recognition of the patient's psychological, psychosocial, and physiologic needs" (Hessel, 2009). Nursing presence is often what patients value most from the nurse.

Observe the patient's nonverbal cues that may indicate the patient is distressed, such as little or no affect, pitch of voice, posture, facial expression, crying, or inappropriate anger. Sitting with the patient and reflecting back to the patient what the nurse sees may encourage the patient to express concerns. "I noticed that after the doctor discussed your diagnosis you have been very quiet and appear sad. Do you have any concerns?" The key nursing action here is to *listen,* not talk. Rather, allow the patient to talk. Use the techniques discussed in Chapter 3 to encourage the patient to express feelings and concerns. The patient may make statements that reflect spiritual distress such as "Why did I get cancer?" "I'm a burden to my family," and "I just don't know what to do." These statements should be addressed. Again, let the patient do the talking. The nurse should not offer solutions; rather, the nurse should use the interviewing techniques to help the patient identify the problem and resources used in the past to cope with problems: "What helps you cope?" "What are your sources of strength and hope?" "Who are your support persons?" If more help is needed, the nurse can refer the patient to a specialist.

Stoll's (1979) guidelines for spiritual assessment (Box 5-5) provide an outline for the novice to begin assessing a patient's spiritual needs.

BOX 5-5 STOLL'S GUIDELINES FOR SPIRITUAL ASSESSMENT

Concept of God or Deity

1. Is religion or God significant to you? If yes, can you describe how?
2. Is prayer helpful to you? What happens when you pray?
3. Does a God or deity function in your personal life? If yes, can you describe how?
4. How would you describe your God or what you worship?

Sources of Hope and Strength

1. Who is the most important person to you?
2. To whom do you turn when you need help? Are they available?
3. In what ways do they help?
4. What are your sources of strength and hope?
5. What helps the most when you are afraid or need special help?

Religious Practices

1. Do you feel your faith (or religion) is helpful to you? If yes, would you tell me how?
2. Are there any religious practices that are important to you?
3. Has being sick (or what has happened to you) made any difference in your practice of praying or religious practices?
4. What religious books or symbols are helpful to you?

Relation between Spiritual Beliefs and Health

1. What has bothered you most about being sick (or what is happening to you)?
2. What do you think is going to happen to you?
3. Has being sick (or what has happened to you) made any difference in your feelings about God or the practice of your faith?
4. Is there anything that is especially frightening or meaningful to you now?

With permission from Stoll, R. I. (1979). *Guidelines for spiritual assessment. American Journal of Nursing, 79*(9), 1574–1577.

Incorporating cultural and spiritual assessment into one's nursing practice may seem awkward at first. Like other nursing skills, this becomes easier with practice and experience. Practice the assessments with your classmates or friends and relatives, where you may feel more comfortable. Knowledge of the patient's cultural and spiritual needs can make the difference between successful and poor health care. You can build patient and family trust and understanding of health care in the United States; this will help ensure patients follow directions and continue to seek medical care in the future.

Bibliography

CITATIONS

Andrews, M. A., Boyle, J. S., & Collins, J. W. (2019). *Transcultural concepts in nursing care* (8th ed.). Lippincott Williams & Wilkins.

Buck, H. G. (2006). Spirituality: concept analysis and model development. *Holistic Nursing Practice, 20*(6), 288–292.

Campinha-Bacote, J. (2010). The process of cultural competence in the delivery of healthcare services. Retrieved May 8, 2020, from http://transculturalcare.net/the-process-of-cultural-competence-in-the-delivery-of-healthcare-services/

Fitzgerald, E., & Campinha-Bacote, J. (2019). Cultural competemility: a paradigm shift in the cultural competence versus cultural humility debate—Part 1. *Online Journal of Issues in Nursing, 24*(1).

Fletcher, S. N. E. (2015). *Cultural sensibility in health care.* Sigma Theta Tau International.

Foronda, C. (2020). A theory of cultural humility. *Journal of Transcultural Nursing, 31*(1), 7–12.

Giger, J. N. (2017). *Transcultural nursing: Assessment & intervention* (7th ed.). Elsevier.

Healthy People. (2020). Office of disease prevention and health promotion. Retrieved February 20, 2020, from http://www.healthypeople.gov/2020/about/foundation-health-measures/Disparities

Hessel, J. A. (2009). Presence in nursing practice: a concept analysis. *Holistic Nursing Practice, 23*(5), 276–281.

Hodge, D. (2006). A template for spiritual assessment: a review of the JACHO requirements and guidelines for implementation. *Social Work, 51*(4), 317–326.

JACHO. (2019). Medical record spiritual assessment. Retrieved May 8, 2020, from https://www.jointcommission.org/standards/standard-faqs/critical-access-hospital/provision-of-care-treatment-and-services-pc/000001669/

Kersey-Matusiak, G. (2019). *Delivering culturally competent nursing care: Working with diverse and vulnerable populations* (2nd ed.). Springer Publishing.

Leininger, M. M., & McFarland, M. R. (2002). *Transcultural nursing: Concept theories, research and practice* (3rd ed.). McGraw-Hill.

McFarland, M. R., & Wehbe-Alamah, H. B. (2019). Leininger's theory of culture care diversity and universality: an overview with a historical retrospective and a view toward the future. *Journal of Transcultural Nursing, 30*(6), 540–557.

Mutha, S., Allen, C., & Welch, M. (2002). *Toward culturally competent care: A toolbox for teaching communication strategies.* Center for Health Professions, University of California.

Nolan, T. S., Browning, K., Vo, J. B., Meadows, R. J., & Paxton, R. J. (2020). Assessing and managing spiritual distress in cancer survivorship. *American Journal of Nursing, 120*(1), 40–47.

Pulchaski, C., Ferrell, B., Virani, R., Otis-Green, S., Baird, P., Bull, J., Chochinov, H., Handzo, G., Nelson-Becker, H., Prince-Paul, M., Pugliese, K., & Sulmasy, D. (2009). Improving the quality of spiritual care as a dimension of palliative care: the report of the consensus conference. *Journal of Palliative Medicine, 12*(10), 885–904.

Purnell, L. D. (2013). *Transcultural health care: a culturally competent approach* (4th ed.). Davis FA.

Sessanna, L., Finnell, D., & Jezewski, M. A. (2007). Spirituality in nursing and health related literature: a concept analysis. *Journal of Holistic Nursing, 25*(4), 252–262.

Sherwood, H. (2018). Religion: why faith is becoming more and more popular. The Guardian. Retrieved May 8, 2020, from https://www.theguardian.com/news/2018/aug/27/religion-why-is-faith-growing-and-what-happens-next

Tervalon, M., & Murray-Garcia, J. (1998). Cultural humility versus cultural competence: a critical distinction in defining physician training outcomes in multicultural education. *Journal of Health Care for the Poor and Underserved, 9*(2), 117–125.

U.S. Department of Health and Human Services. (2009). Office of Minority Health. Think Cultural Health. Retrieved September 1, 2020, from https://thinkculturalhealth.hhs.gov/clas/standards

Wichinski, K. A. (2015). Providing culturally proficient care for transgender. *Nursing, 45*(2), 58–73.

Yancu, C. N., & Farmer, D. F. (2017). Product or process: Cultural competence or cultural humility? *Palliative Medicine and Hospice Care Open Journal, 3*(1), e1–e4.

ADDITIONAL REFERENCES

Spiritual Care

Biro, A. L. (2012). Creating conditions for good nursing by attending to the spiritual. *Journal of Nursing Management, 20*(8), 1002–1011.

Caldeira, S., & Timmins, F. (2015). Editorial: Time as presence and opportunity: the key to spiritual care in contemporary nursing practice. *Journal of Clinical Nursing, 24*(17–18), 2355–2356.

Hansbrough, W. B., & Georges, J. M. (2019). Validation of the presence of nursing scale using data triangulation. *Nursing Research, 68*(6), 439–444.

Hodge, D. (2015). Administering a two-stage spiritual assessment in healthcare settings: a necessary component of ethical and effective care. *Journal of Nursing Management, 23*(1), 27–38.

Narayan, M. C. (2010). Culture's effects on pain assessment and management. *American Journal of Nursing, 110*(4), 38–47.

Nelson, R. (2016). Spirituality: Part of nursing practice, but too often neglected. *American Journal of Nursing, 116*(9), 19–20.

Reinert, K. G., Campbell, J. C., Bandeen-Roche, K., Sharps, P., & Lee, J. (2015). Gender and race variation in the intersection of religious involvement, early trauma, and adult health. *Journal of Nursing Scholarship, 47*(4), 318–327.

Tanyi, R. A. (2006). Spirituality and family nursing: spiritual assessment and interventions for families. *Journal of Advanced Nursing, 53*(3), 287–294.

Culture

Beard, K. V., Gwanmesia, E., & Miranda-Diaz, G. (2015). Culturally competent care: using the ESFT model in nursing. *American Journal of Nursing, 115*(6), 58–62.

McEvoy, M. (2003). Culture and spirituality as an integrated concept in pediatric care. *MCN: The American Journal of Maternal Child Nursing, 25*(1), 39–43.

McFarland, M. R., & Wehbe-Alamah, H. B. (2015). *Leininger's culture care diversity and universality* (3rd ed.). Jones and Bartlett.

Miller, S. (2009). Cultural humility is the first step to becoming global care providers. *Journal of Obstetric, Gynecologic, & Neonatal Nursing, 38*(1), 92–93.

Myers, V. A. (2013). *What if I say the wrong thing?* ABA Publishing.

National Center for Cultural Competence. Georgetown University. Self Assessments. Retrieved March 3, 2021, from https://nccc.georgetown.edu/assessments/

Shen, Z. (2015). Cultural competence models and cultural competence assessment instruments in nursing: a literature review. *Journal of Transcultural Nursing, 26*(3), 308–321.

6 PHYSICAL EXAMINATION: GETTING STARTED

KEY TERMS

physical examination | standard precautions | tangential lighting

Learning Objectives

The student will:

1. Describe how to individualize the physical examination approach based on the patient's overall needs and the environment.
2. Select an environment that enhances the accuracy of the physical examination.
3. Discuss the environmental features necessary to ensure patient safety and comfort during a physical examination.
4. Describe and use the equipment for performing a physical examination.
5. Identify safety precautions when conducting the physical examination.

Indicate the correct order of and how to use the four cardinal techniques.

Once you understand the patient's concerns and have elicited a careful history, the physical examination can then be performed. When learning about physical assessment, students often want to proceed directly to the examination; however, the collection of subjective information during history taking assists the focus of the examination accordingly (Fig. 6-1). At first, you may feel unsure of your skills and how the patient will relate to you. With practice, your skills in physical examination will grow, and you will gain confidence. Through study and repetition, the examination will soon flow more smoothly, and the attention will shift from technique and how to handle instruments to what you hear, see, and feel. Touching the patient's body will seem more natural, and you will learn ways to minimize the patient's discomfort. Before long, you will gain proficiency, and what once took between 1 and 2 hours will take considerably less time. You will continually hone these important relational and clinical skills throughout your practice.

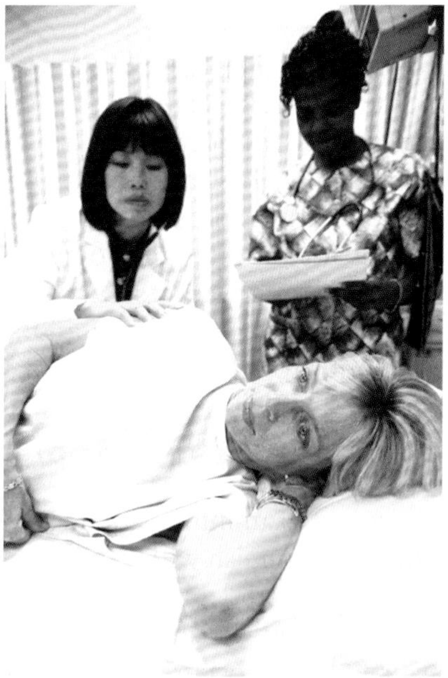

FIGURE 6-1 A thorough health history helps guide the nurse's physical examination.

The **physical examination** is a process to obtain objective data from the patient. The subjective data in the health history is obtained prior to the examination and will assist the nurse with navigating a complex examination. Each body system connects to another. A finding in one system may not be an isolated finding. For example, the patient who presents with a chief complaint of blurred vision may be having vision changes because of age, an injury, a retina or macular affliction, or changes due to hyperglycemia (Fig. 6-2). The purpose of the physical examination is to determine changes in a patient's health status and plan how to respond to a problem as well as promote healthy lifestyles and well-being. A decision to perform a comprehensive or a focused assessment is described in Chapter 4, "The Health History," and is made on an individual basis.

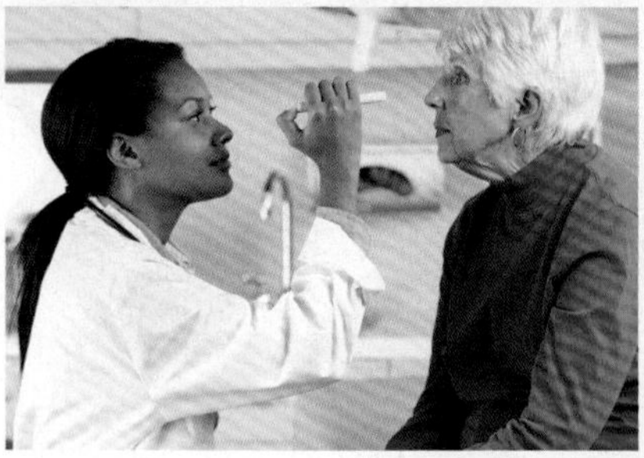

FIGURE 6-2 A chief complaint of blurred vision can indicate many different changes.

THE COMPREHENSIVE ADULT PHYSICAL EXAMINATION

Beginning the Examination: Setting the Stage

As new practitioners, the impetus is to dive in and begin the physical examination. However, as in anything worthwhile, preparation is paramount (Box 6-1).

BOX 6-1 PREPARING FOR THE PHYSICAL EXAMINATION

- Reflect on your approach to the patient.
- Adjust the lighting and the environment.
- Check that the equipment is available and in working order.
- Make the patient comfortable.
- Choose the sequence of examination.

Before beginning the physical examination, think through your approach to the individual patient, professional demeanor, and how to make the patient feel comfortable and relaxed. Review the measures that promote the patient's physical comfort and safety, making any necessary adjustments in the lighting and surrounding environment. Refer to specific accommodations for various age groups found in Chapter 23, "Assessing Children: Infancy through Adolescence," and Chapter 24, "Assessing Older Adults." Remember to gather the equipment and review the patient chart, if available, prior to entering the room.

Reflecting on Your Approach to the Patient

When first examining patients, feelings of insecurity are inevitable, but these will soon diminish with experience. As you enter the room, identify yourself as a nursing student. Appear calm and organized, even when you may feel inexperienced. It is common to forget part of the examination, especially at first. If that occurs, simply examine that area out of sequence. It is not unusual to go back to the patient and ask to check one or two items that might have been overlooked or may need additional attention.

Beginners will need to spend more time than experienced nurses on select portions of the examination, such as the fundoscopic examination or cardiac auscultation. To avoid alarming the patient, warn the patient ahead of time by saying, for example, "I would like to spend extra time listening to your heart and the heart sounds, but this doesn't mean I hear anything wrong." Many patients view the physical examination with some anxiety. They feel vulnerable, physically exposed, apprehensive about possible pain, and uneasy about what the nurse may find. At the same time, they appreciate your concern about their health and respond to your attention. With these considerations in mind, the skillful nurse is thorough without wasting time, systematic but flexible, and gentle yet not afraid to cause discomfort should it be required. The skillful nurse examines each region of the body and at the same time is aware of the whole patient, notes any wince or worried glance, and shares information that calms, explains, and reassures.

As a beginner, *avoid interpreting your findings.* You are not the patient's primary health care provider, and your inferences may be premature or incorrect. As you grow in experience and responsibility, sharing findings will become more appropriate. If the patient has specific concerns, discuss them with your faculty. At times, you may discover abnormalities such as an ominous mass or a deep ulceration. Always avoid showing distaste, alarm, or other negative reactions. Keeping your verbal and nonverbal communication in check is paramount. If you find anything that is unusual or disturbing, always talk with your clinical instructor.

Adjusting the Lighting and the Environment

Nurses practice in a variety of settings, and flexibility and creativity are warranted to ensure adequate lighting and an environment conducive for physical examination and patient care (Fig. 6-3). Several environmental factors

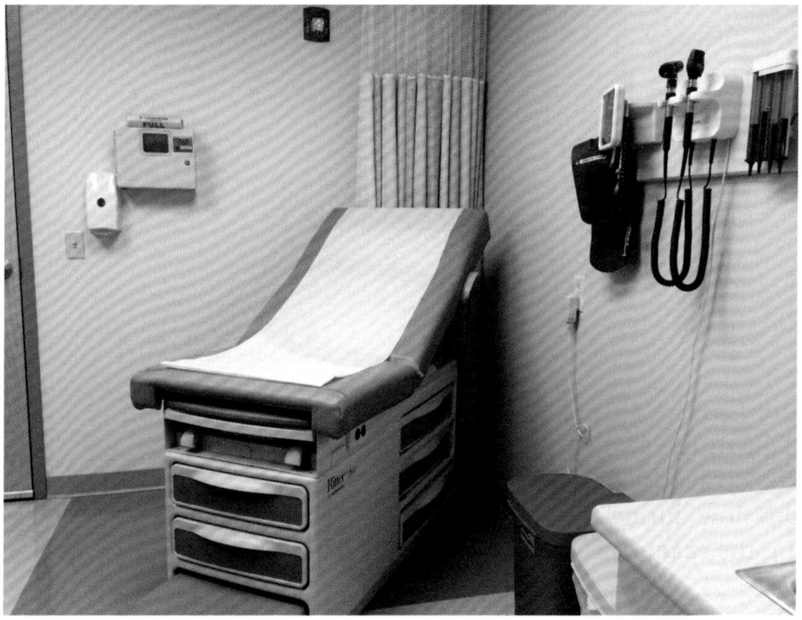

FIGURE 6-3 A clean, well-lit examination room ready for a new patient.

affect the caliber of each examination. For best results, it is important to "set the stage" so that both you and the patient are comfortable. Awkward positioning for either of you impairs detection of physical findings. Take the time to adjust the bed to a convenient height, and ask the patient to move toward you or turn over or shift position whenever this makes examining selected areas of the body more visible and accessible. Be sure to lower the bed when you are finished.

Good lighting and a quiet environment make a difference in what you see and hear but may be hard to arrange. Do the best you can. If a television interferes with auscultating heart sounds, politely ask the patient to lower the volume and remember to thank the patient as you leave.

Tangential lighting (Fig. 6-4A) is optimal for inspecting structures such as the jugular venous pulse, the thyroid gland, and the apical impulse of the heart. It casts light across body surfaces that shows contours, elevations, and depressions, whether moving or stationary, into sharper relief. When light is perpendicular to the surface or diffuse (Fig. 6-4B), shadows are reduced and subtle undulations across the surface are lost. Experiment with focused, tangential lighting across the tendons on the back of your hand; try to see the pulsations of the radial artery at your wrist.

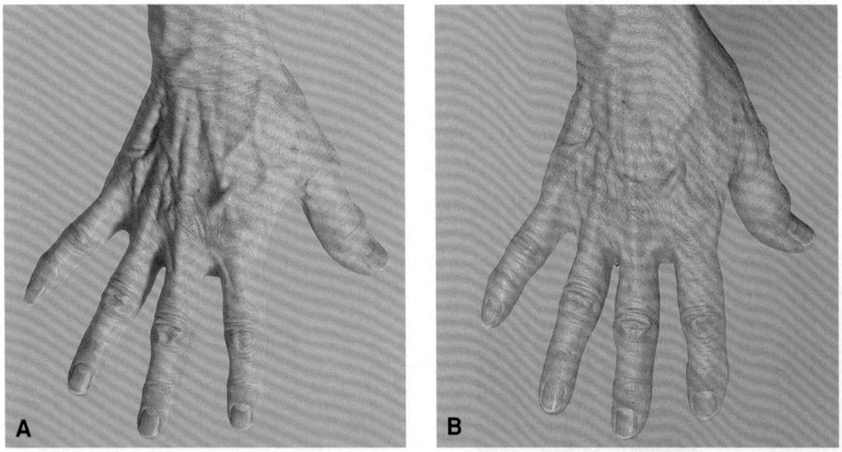

FIGURE 6-4 Tangential lighting (**A**) is useful for seeing variations in body surfaces while perpendicular lighting (**B**) reduces shadows.

Checking Your Equipment

Prior to the start of the physical examination, collect all necessary equipment and supplies and ensure all are in working order (Box 6-2). For example, check the batteries in the penlight and otoscope or ophthalmoscope to confirm they turn on. This ensures a smooth flow during the examination and avoids having to leave the patient during the examination to search for equipment.

BOX 6-2 LIST OF EQUIPMENT FOR PHYSICAL EXAMINATION

- Hand sanitizer
- Examination gloves
- Alcohol wipes

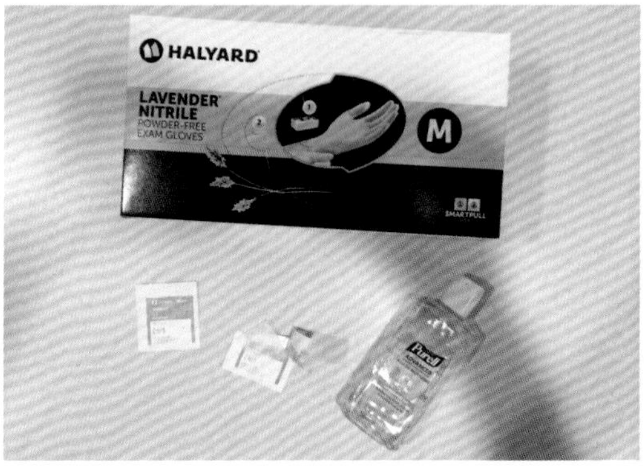

- Paper and pen, or computer
- Draw sheet or drape
- Stadiometer
- Scale
- Examination light/gooseneck lamp
- Thermometer
- Watch with a second hand
- Sphygmomanometer
- Stethoscope
- Pulse oximeter
- Doppler
- Ophthalmoscope
- Otoscope/speculums
- Nasal speculum
- Scents for testing sense of smell (e.g., mint, coffee, or alcohol swab if other scents are not available)
- Snellen chart or visual acuity card to test distant vision
- Near vision card

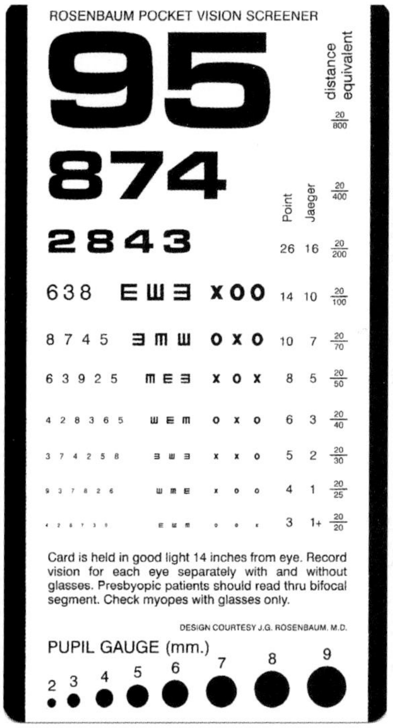

(continued)

BOX 6-2 LIST OF EQUIPMENT FOR PHYSICAL EXAMINATION (*Continued*)

- Opaque card
- Penlight
- Tongue depressors
- 2 × 2 gauze pads
- Cup of water
- Ruler and flexible tape measure, preferably marked in centimeters

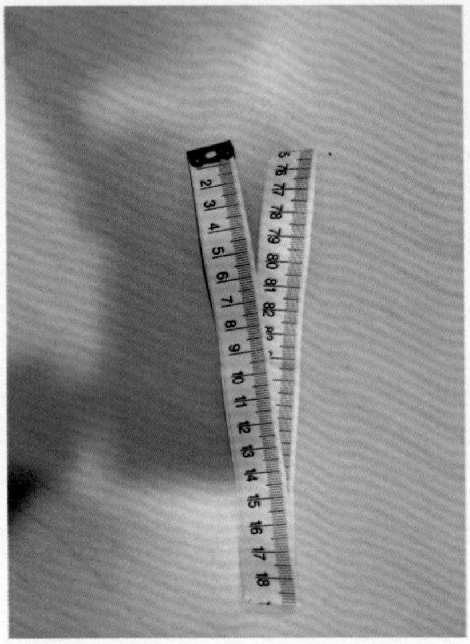

- Goniometer
- Scoliometer
- Reflex hammer
- Tuning forks, 128 and 512 Hz
- Q-tips, paper clips, or other disposable objects for testing sense of touch
- Cotton
- Mini-mental status examination tool

Pictures and basic details about specific equipment are provided in Box 6-3 with additional information in the corresponding systems chapters on how the equipment will facilitate your examination of the patient. Specific equipment is necessary for each component of the physical examination.

Familiarity of each piece of equipment is necessary for specific techniques and will be explained in more detail in corresponding chapters.

Observing Standard and Universal Precautions

Prior to beginning the physical examination and working with patients, study the Centers for Disease Control and Prevention (CDC) guidelines to protect patients and examiners from the spread of infectious disease. These precautions can be found at the CDC website. Advisories for standard and methicillin-resistant *Staphylococcus aureus* (MRSA) precautions and for universal precautions are briefly summarized here (CDC, 2018, 2019a, 2019b, 2020a, 2020b; Broussard, 2021).

BOX 6-3 **EXPLANATION OF EQUIPMENT AND INSTRUMENTS FOR THE PHYSICAL EXAMINATION**

- Stadiometer: Measures height and must be installed at the correct height and mounted to the wall to achieve accurate measurements
- Scale: Measures weight and needs to be calibrated per institutional policy
- Ophthalmoscope: Visualizes the interior of the eye, especially the retina

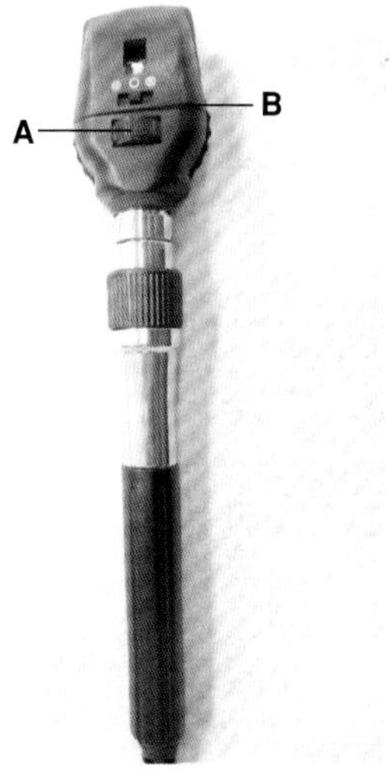

This side of the ophthalmoscope faces the patient. **A.** Indicates the wheel used to change the size and color of the light emitted from this side. **B.** Indicates the wheel used to change the diopter focus.

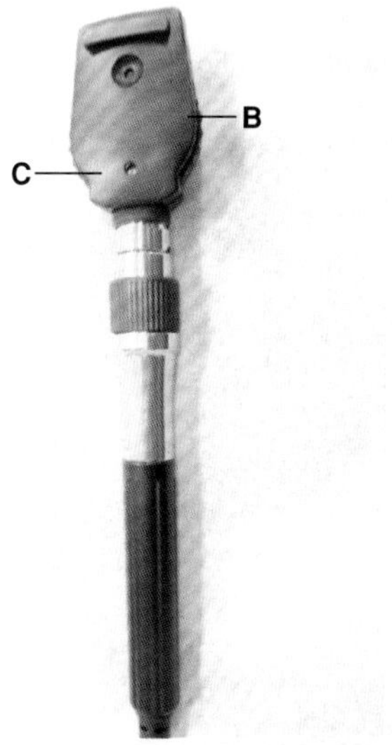

This side of the ophthalmoscope faces the nurse; the top ridge of the scope rests against the nurse's eyebrow. **B.** Indicates the wheel that changes the diopter focus. **C.** Shows the indicator of diopters.

- Otoscope: Visualizes the ear canal and eardrum
- Speculum: Cone-shaped attachment that attaches to the otoscope to examine the ear

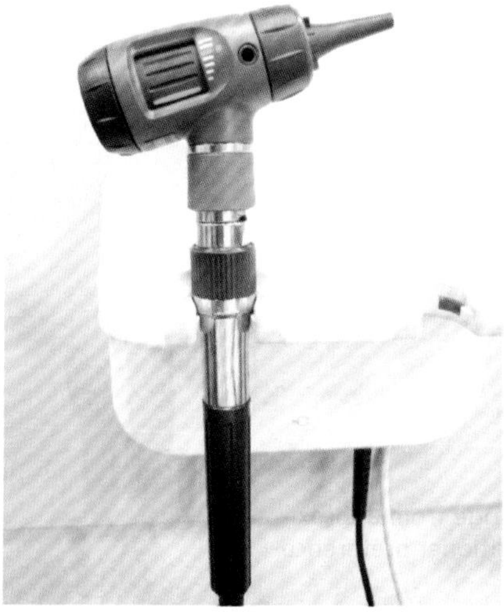

(*continued*)

BOX 6-3 EXPLANATION OF EQUIPMENT AND INSTRUMENTS FOR THE PHYSICAL EXAMINATION (*Continued*)

- Nasal speculum: Opens the nasal passage to visualize inside the nose
- Snellen chart or visual acuity card: Tests distant vision
- Near vision card: Tests near vision
- Opaque card: Covers the eye not being examined
- Penlight: Provides additional light for viewing various areas of the body and checking the eyes
- Tongue depressors: Used for mouth examination
- 2 × 2 gauze pads: Used during tongue examination
- Examination light/gooseneck lamp: Provides additional lighting

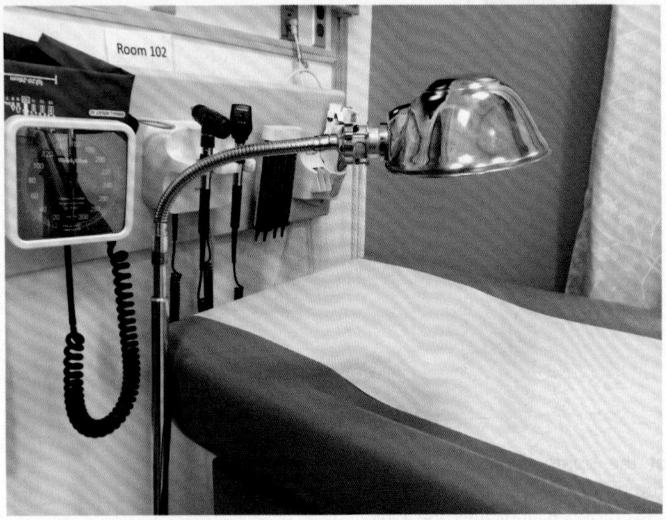

- Thermometer: Measures temperature

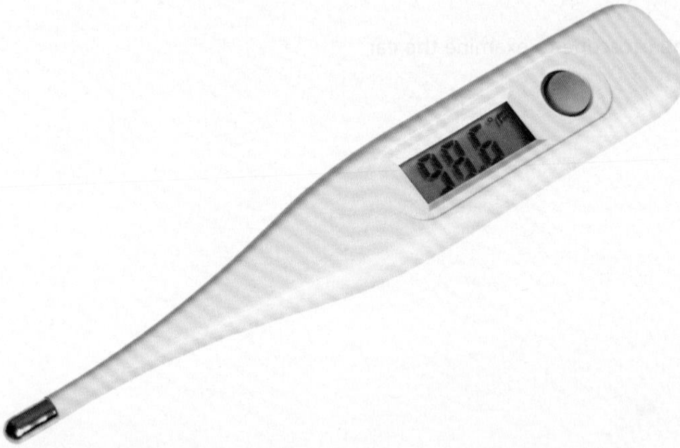

- Watch with a second hand: Calculates respiration and pulse rates
- Sphygmomanometer: Measures blood pressure
- Stethoscope with the following characteristics:
  - Stethoscopes range in length from 22 to 31 in. The tubing can range from approximately 17 to 22 in in length and should be chosen based on practitioner preference and comfort.

BOX 6-3 **EXPLANATION OF EQUIPMENT AND INSTRUMENTS FOR THE PHYSICAL EXAMINATION (*Continued*)**

- Ear tips should fit snugly and painlessly. To get this fit, choose ear tips of the proper size, align the earpieces with the angle of the ear canals, and adjust the spring of the connecting metal band to a comfortable tightness.

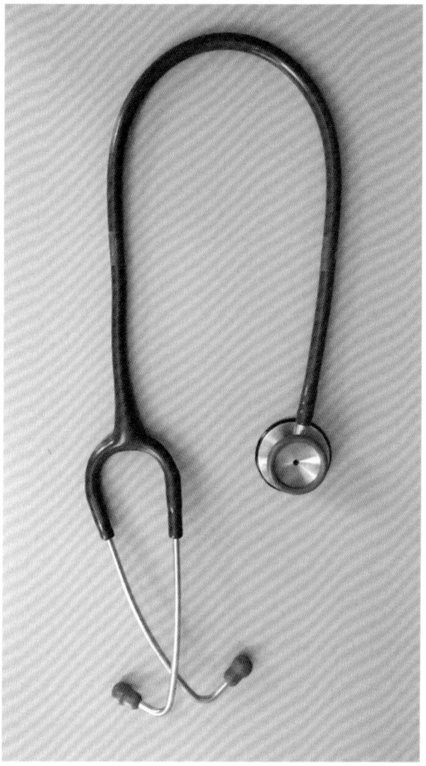

- A bell and a diaphragm: The disk at the end of the stethoscope is the bell and diaphragm.
  The bell (A) is the smaller, cupped side of the stethoscope, and transmits lower-pitched sounds. The diaphragm (B) is the larger, flatter side of the stethoscope, and this transmits higher-pitched sounds. By rotating the disk at the end of the stethoscope, you can change from the bell to the diaphragm as needed. By tapping lightly on the disk, you can determine which side is open for sound transmission. If you own a stethoscope that has the bell and diaphragm on the same side, then you will press firmly to use the diaphragm and barely press at all to use the bell.

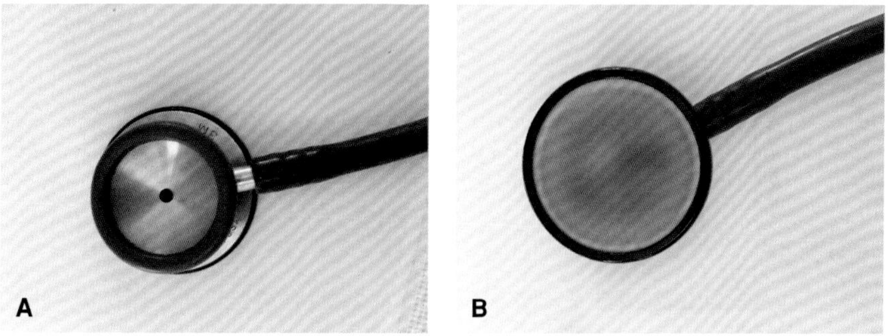

(continued)

BOX 6-3 **EXPLANATION OF EQUIPMENT AND INSTRUMENTS FOR THE PHYSICAL EXAMINATION (*Continued*)**

- Pulse oximeter: Measures oxygen saturation
- Doppler: Detects blood flow and pulses
- Reflex hammer: Tests strength of a reflex

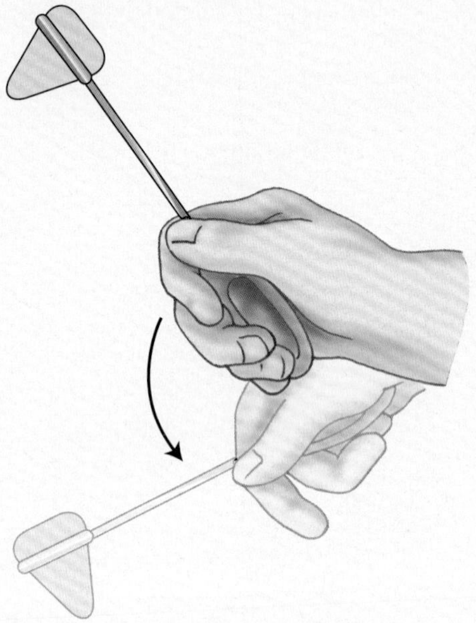

- Tuning forks: Two-pronged with tines that form a U-shape; tests vibration (128 Hz) and sound (512 Hz). The frequency is found on the front of the tuning fork.

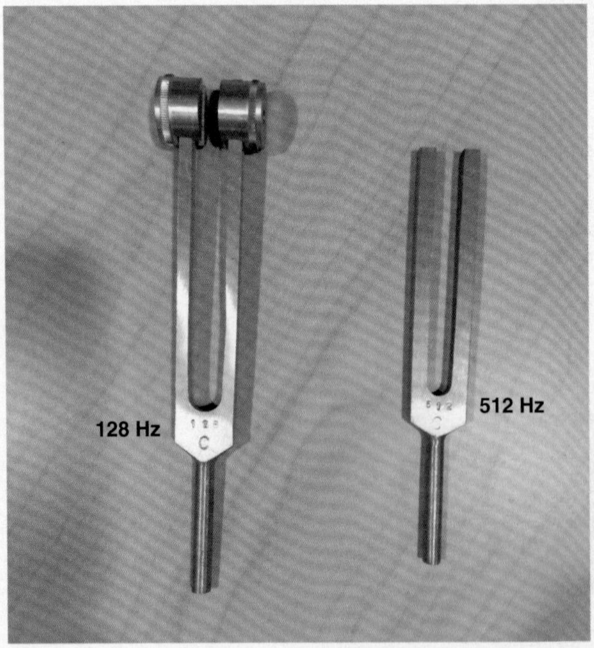

BOX 6-3 EXPLANATION OF EQUIPMENT AND INSTRUMENTS FOR THE PHYSICAL EXAMINATION (*Continued*)

- Q-tips, paper clips, or other disposable objects: Tests ability to discriminate touch sensation
- Cotton: Tests the sense of light touch
- Q-tip or broken tongue blade: Tests the sense of sharp touch

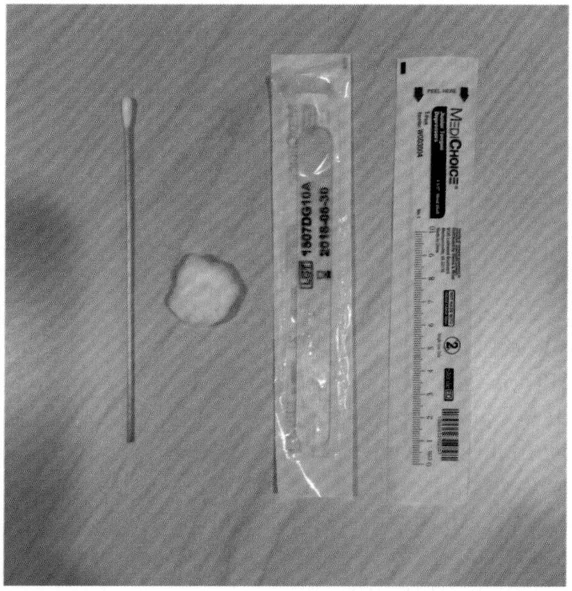

- Substances with distinct odors (e.g., vanilla and coffee): Test for sensory perception of smell and taste
- Two test tubes (optional): Test temperature sensation

Standard precautions are based on the principle that all blood, body fluids, secretions, excretions (except sweat), nonintact skin, and mucous membranes may contain transmissible infectious agents. These practices apply to all patients in any setting. They include hand hygiene; use of personal protective equipment (gloves, gowns, and mouth, nose, and eye protection); safe injection practices; safe handling of contaminated equipment or surfaces; respiratory hygiene and cough etiquette; patient isolation criteria; and precautions relating to equipment, toys, solid surfaces, and laundry handling. Because hand hygiene practices have been shown to reduce the transmission of norovirus, *Cryptosporidium,* and *Clostridioides difficile* (CDC, 2018, 2019a, 2019b, 2020a, 2020b), the CDC hygiene recommendations are summarized in Box 6-4. White coats and stethoscopes also harbor bacteria and should be cleaned frequently. Stethoscopes should be cleaned before and after use with every patient (Bearman et al., 2014; Batista et al., 2019).

Concept Mastery Alert

Gloves and the Chain of Infection

Gloves, which are used during patient care for numerous reasons, are essential in preventing a nurse's hands from becoming a vehicle for the transmission of organisms from one patient to another. The nurse puts on gloves to care for a patient, then removes the gloves, discarding them appropriately and performing hand hygiene. These actions disrupt the chain of infection. Gloves do not limit a nurse's exposure to body fluids and secretions. Rather, they prevent it.

Universal precautions are a set of guidelines designed to prevent parenteral, mucous membrane, and noncontact exposures of health care workers to blood-borne pathogens, including human immunodeficiency virus (HIV) and hepatitis B virus (HBV). Immunization with the hepatitis B

BOX 6-4 THE CENTERS FOR DISEASE CONTROL AND PREVENTION KEY RECOMMENDATIONS FOR HAND HYGIENE

1. Key situations in which hand hygiene should be performed include:
   a. Before touching a patient, even if gloves will be worn
   b. Before exiting the patient's care area after touching the patient or the patient's immediate environment
   c. After contact with blood, body fluids or excretions, or wound dressings
   d. Prior to performing an aseptic task (e.g., placing an intravenous line, preparing an injection)
   e. If hands will be moving from a contaminated body site to a clean body site during patient care
   f. After glove removal
2. Use soap and water when hands are visibly soiled (e.g., blood, body fluids) or after caring for patients with known or suspected infectious diarrhea (e.g., *Clostridium difficile,* norovirus). Otherwise, the preferred method of hand decontamination is with an alcohol-based hand rub (CDC, 2020b; Food and Drug Administration, 2018; Batista et al., 2019).

vaccine for health care workers with exposure to blood is an important adjunct to universal precautions. The following fluids are considered potentially infectious: all blood and other body fluids containing visible blood, semen, and vaginal secretions; and cerebrospinal, synovial, pleural, peritoneal, pericardial, and amniotic fluids. Protective barriers include gloves, gowns, aprons, masks, and protective eyewear. All health care workers should follow the precautions for safe injections and prevention of injury from needle sticks, scalpels, and other sharp instruments and devices. Report to your health service immediately if such injury occurs (CDC, 2018, 2019a, 2020b).

Making the Patient Comfortable

Patient Privacy and Comfort

Access to the patient's body is a unique and time-honored privilege in the role of the nurse. Showing sensitivity for privacy and patient modesty must be ingrained in your professional behavior to convey respect for the patient's vulnerability. Close nearby doors, draw the curtains in the hospital or examining room, and wash your hands thoroughly before the examination begins.

During the examination, be aware of the patient's feelings and any discomfort. Respond to the patient's facial expressions and ask, "Are you OK?" or "Is this painful?" to elicit unexpressed worries or sources of pain. Adjusting the angle of the bed or examining table, rearranging the pillows, or adding blankets for warmth demonstrates that you are attentive to the patient's well-being.

Draping the Patient

You will acquire the art of *draping the patient* (Box 6-5) with the gown or draw sheet as you learn each segment of the examination in the chapters ahead.

BOX 6-5 TIPS FOR DRAPING THE PATIENT

- *Your goal is to visualize one area of the body at a time.* This preserves the patient's modesty and helps you focus on the area being examined.
- With the patient sitting, auscultate the lungs with the gown untied in back.
- For the breast examination, uncover the right breast and keep the left chest draped. Redrape the right chest, then uncover the left chest and proceed to examine the left breast and heart.
- For the abdominal examination, only the abdomen should be exposed. Adjust the gown to cover the chest and place the sheet or drape at the inguinal area.
- To help the patient prepare for potentially awkward segments, briefly describe the plan before starting, for example, "Now I am going to move your gown so I can check the pulse in your groin area."

Courteous Clear Instructions

Make sure the instructions to the patient at each step in the examination are courteous and clear. For example, "I would like to examine your abdomen now, so please lie down." Let the patient know if you anticipate they may experience discomfort.

Keeping the Patient Informed

As you proceed with the examination, talk with the patient to see if they want to know about your findings. Is the patient curious about the lung findings or your method for assessing the liver or spleen? Tell the patient the results of the vital signs and use this as a teaching moment.

When you have completed the examination, tell the patient your general impressions and what to expect next. For hospitalized patients, make sure the patient is comfortable and safe, and rearrange the immediate environment to the patient's satisfaction. To promote safety and prevent falls, be sure to lower the bed, place the side table and personal items within reach, and raise the bed rails. As you leave, clean your equipment, dispose of any waste materials, and wash your hands.

THE CARDINAL TECHNIQUES OF EXAMINATION

Before you begin the examination, study the four cardinal techniques of examination. Plan your sequence and scope of examination and how you will position the patient.

The physical examination relies on four classic techniques: inspection, palpation, percussion, and auscultation (Table 6-1). You will learn in later chapters about additional maneuvers that are important in amplifying physical diagnosis, such as having the patient lean forward to better detect the murmur of aortic regurgitation or balloting the patella to check for joint effusion.

These four techniques—inspection, palpation, percussion, and auscultation—will *always* be used in this order in all systems with the exception of the abdomen. During the abdominal examination, the sequence will be inspection, auscultation, percussion, and palpation. Auscultation follows inspection so as not to increase bowel motility with palpation.

Concept Mastery Alert

Palpation versus Percussion

Both palpation and percussion can require the nurse to use their hands. Palpation includes tactile pressure from the palmar fingers or finger pads to assess areas of skin elevation, depression, warmth, or tenderness; lymph nodes; pulses; and contours and sizes of organs and masses. Percussion involves tapping body parts to produce sound waves that enable the examiner to assess the density of underlying structures.

TABLE 6-1 Cardinal Techniques of Examination

Technique	Description	Demonstration
Inspection	Close observation of the details of the patient's appearance, behavior, and movement such as facial expression; mood; body build and conditioning; skin conditions such as petechiae or ecchymoses; eye movements; pharyngeal color; symmetry of thorax; height of jugular venous pulsations; abdominal contour; lower extremity edema; gait	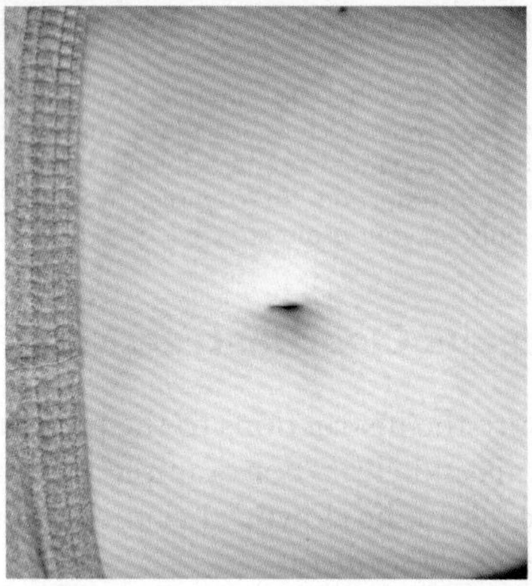
Palpation	Tactile pressure from the palmar fingers or finger pads to assess areas of skin elevation, depression, warmth, or tenderness; lymph nodes; pulses; contours and sizes of organs and masses; crepitus in the joints The metacarpal/phalangeal joint or ulnar surface of the hand is used to detect vibration.	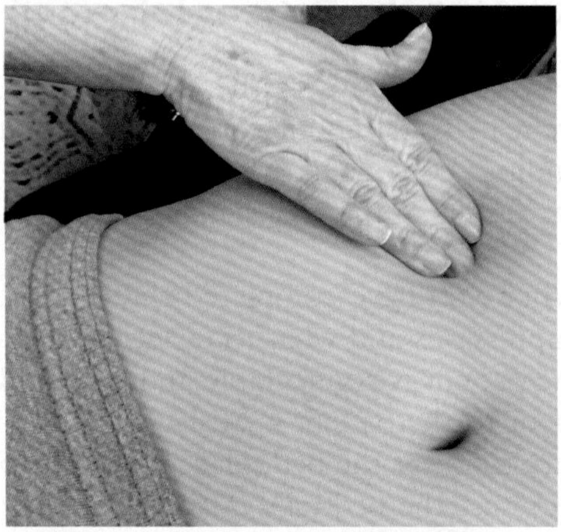
Percussion	Use of the striking or *plexor finger*, usually the third, to deliver a rapid tap or blow against the distal *pleximeter finger*, usually the distal third finger of the left hand laid against the surface of the chest or abdomen, to evoke a sound wave such as resonance or dullness from the underlying tissue or organs, including size and density This sound wave also generates a tactile vibration against the pleximeter finger.	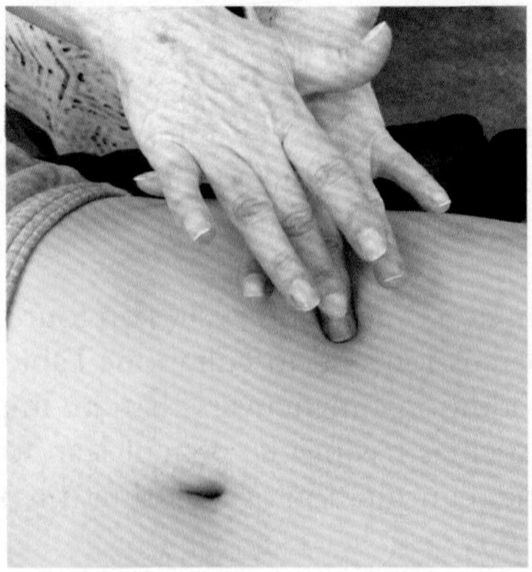

Technique	Description	Demonstration
Auscultation	Use of the diaphragm and bell of the stethoscope to detect the characteristics of heart, lung, and bowel sounds, including location, timing, duration, pitch, and intensity For the heart, this involves sounds from closure of the four valves, extra sounds from blood flow into the atria and ventricles, and murmurs. Auscultation also permits detection of bruits or turbulence over arterial vessels.	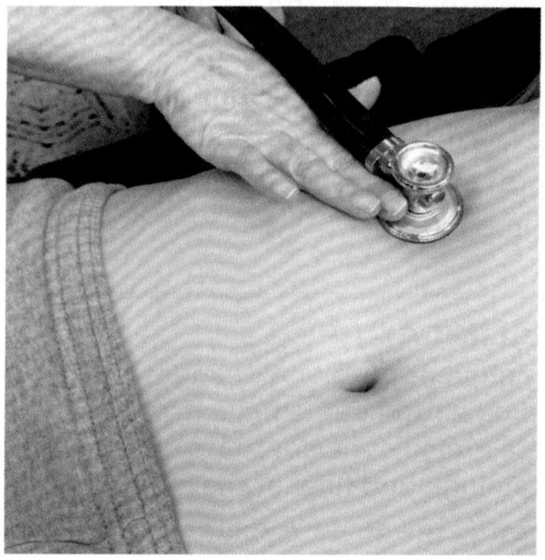

SEQUENCE OF EXAMINATION

The key to a thorough and accurate physical examination is developing a systematic sequence of examination. Organize your comprehensive or focused examination around four general goals:

- Maximizing the patient's comfort
- Maintaining patient safety
- Avoiding unnecessary changes in position
- Enhancing clinical accuracy and efficiency

Patients can be nervous during physical examinations related to the examination itself or to the possible findings. As a new practitioner, you may also feel nervous. With practice, you will become more self-assured. Initially, practice in the lab with friends posing as simulated patients. This repetition will enhance your skills, and this confidence will also help allay patient anxiety. Additionally, maintain a person's privacy by pulling the curtain, draping the person to decrease exposure and to prevent chilling. Watch the patient's nonverbal communication for indications of pain or uneasiness. Answer questions and talk with the patient, indicating what you plan to do and your findings.

Patient safety is paramount. This may take multiple forms, from the initial washing of hands to moving on and off the examination table using fall prevention techniques or remembering to clean equipment, especially your stethoscope's bell and diaphragm with an alcohol swab, before and after each use (CDC, 2020a, 2020b; Food and Drug Administration, 2018; Sahiledengle, 2019).

In general, move from "head to toe." Avoid examining the patient's feet, for example, before checking the face or mouth. You will quickly see that some segments of the examination are best assessed when the patient is sitting, such as examination of the head and neck and the thorax and lungs, while others are best obtained with the patient supine, such as the abdominal examination. You want to optimize the time with your patient in one position and avoid unnecessary changes in position, which may be difficult for some patients.

CLINICAL TIP

Frequent positional changes in a patient with shortness of breath may alter breathing patterns, or a patient with joint pain may experience increased pain. Both of these examples demonstrate the importance of limiting unnecessary changes and maintaining good flow of the physical examination.

Examining the patient from the patient's *right side* and moving to the opposite side or foot of the bed or examining table only as necessary is recommended in physical examination. This is the standard position for the physical examination and has several advantages compared with the left side: estimates of jugular venous pressure are more reliable, the palpating hand rests more comfortably on the apical impulse, the right kidney is more frequently palpable than the left, and examining tables are frequently positioned to accommodate a right-side approach (Fig. 6-5).

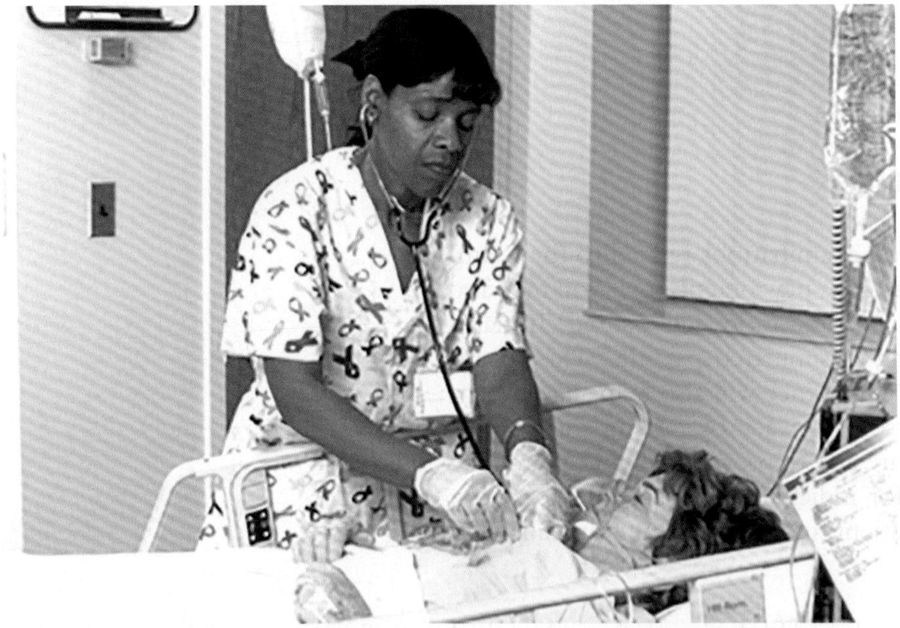

FIGURE 6-5 Much of the examination occurs on the patient's right side as this facilitates a number of physiologic advantages. (Reprinted with permission from Clin-Sims, Wolters Kluwer.)

Left-handed students are encouraged to adopt right-sided positioning, even though at first it may seem awkward. It may still be easier to use the left hand for percussing or for holding instruments such as the otoscope or reflex hammer.

As you study the body systems in the upcoming chapters and review the techniques associated with each examination, you will begin to understand the components of the physical examination. Once you have learned how to examine each body system, you will methodically formulate the composition and flow of the head-to-toe physical examination. Chapter 22, "Putting the Physical Examination All Together," has a detailed list of how to incorporate the systems with limited position changes while maintaining continuity of the examination. The culmination of the course is the ability to incorporate the skills learned and perform a head-to-toe physical examination, keeping in mind patient safety and comfort and thoroughness of the examination. At first, you may need notes to remind you what to look for, but over time, this sequence will become habit.

Bibliography

CITATIONS

Batista, I. R., Prates, A. C. L., Santos, B. S., Araújo, J. C. C., Bonfim, Y. C. O., Pimenta Rodrigues, M. V., Morceli, G., Polettini, J., Cavalleri, A. C., Winkelstroter, L. K., & Pereira, V. C. (2019). Determination of antimicrobial susceptibility and biofilm production in Staphylococcus aureus isolated from white coats of health university students. *Annals of Clinical Microbiology and Antimicrobials*, *18*(1), 37. https://doi.org/10.1186/s12941-019-0337-6

Bearman, G., Bryant, K., Leekha, S., Mayer, J., Munoz-Price, L. S., Murthy, R., Palmore, T., Rupp, M. E., & White, J. (2014). Healthcare personnel attire in non-operating-room settings. *Infection Control and Hospital Epidemiology*, *35*(2), 107–121.

Broussard, I. M., & Kahwaji, C. I. (2021). Universal precautions. [Updated 2020 Dec 20]. In: StatPearls [Internet]. Treasure Island (FL): StatPearls Publishing. https://www.ncbi.nlm.nih.gov/books/NBK470223/

Centers for Disease Control and Prevention. (2018). Core infection prevention and control practices for safe healthcare delivery in all settings—Recommendations of the HICPAC. Retrieved May 22, 2020, from https://www.cdc.gov/hicpac/recommendations/core-practices.html

Centers for Disease Control and Prevention. (2019a). Hand hygiene in healthcare settings. Retrieved May 22, 2020, from http://www.cdc.gov/handhygiene/

Centers for Disease Control and Prevention. (2019b). Information about MRSA for healthcare and patients. Retrieved May 22, 2020, from http://www.cdc.gov/mrsa/healthcare/patient/

Centers for Disease Control and Prevention. (2020a). Hand hygiene recommendations: Guidance for healthcare providers about hand hygiene and COVID-19. Retrieved May 22, 2020, from https://www.cdc.gov/coronavirus/2019-ncov/hcp/hand-hygiene.html

Centers for Disease Control and Prevention. (2020b). Handwashing: Clean hands save lives. Retrieved May 22, 2020, from https://www.cdc.gov/handwashing/index.html

Food and Drug Administration. (2018). Safety and effectiveness for health care antiseptics: Topical antimicrobial drug products for over-the-counter human use. Retrieved May 22, 2020, from https://www.federalregister.gov/documents/2017/12/20/2017-27317/safety-and-effectiveness-of-health-care-antiseptics-topical-antimicrobial-drug-products-for

Sahiledengle, B. (2019). Stethoscope disinfection is rarely done in Ethiopia: What are the associated factors? *PloS One*, *14*(6), e0208365. https://doi.org/10.1371/journal.pone.0208365

ADDITIONAL READINGS

Blenkharn, J. I. (2020). Rigid infection prevention and control rules and religious discrimination: An uncomfortable juxtaposition? *Journal of Infection Prevention*, *21*(1), 35–39. https://doi.org/10.1177/1757177419884690

Craft, J., Hudson, P., Plenderleith, M., Wirihana, L., & Gordon, C. (2013). Commencing nursing students' perceptions and anxiety of bioscience. *Nurse Education Today*, *33*(11), 1399–1405. https://doi.org/10.1016/j.nedt.2012.10.020

Davies, R. H., & Rees, B. (2010). In praise of the physical examination. Include "eyeballing" the patient. *BMJ (Clinical Research Ed.)*, *340*, c291.

De Lott, L. B., Panarelli, J. F., Samimi, D., Petrilli, C., Snyder, A., Kuhn, L., Saint, S., Chopra, V., & Whipple, K. M. (2019). Patient preferences for physician attire in ophthalmology practices. *Journal of Academic Ophthalmology*, *11*(1), e36–e42. https://doi.org/10.1055/s-0039-1688913

Douglas, C., Windsor, C., & Lewis, P. (2015). Too much knowledge for a nurse? Use of physical assessment by final-semester nursing students. *Nursing & Health Sciences*, *17*(4), 492–499. https://doi.org/10.1111/nhs.12223

Flinkman, M., Leino-Kilpi, H., Numminen, O., Jeon, Y., Kuokkanen, L., & Meretoja, R. (2017). Nurse competence scale: A systematic and psychometric review. *Journal of Advanced Nursing*, *73*(5), 1035–1050. https://doi.org/10.1111/jan.13183

Haun, N., Hooper-Lane, C., & Safdar, N. (2016). Healthcare personnel attire and devices as fomites: A systematic review. *Infection Control and Hospital Epidemiology*, *37*(11), 1367–1373. https://doi.org/10.1017/ice.2016.192

Herrle, S., Corbett, E., Fagan, M., Moore, C. G., & Elnicki, D. M. (2011). Bayes' theorem and physical examination: Probability assessment and diagnostic decision-making. *Academic Medicine*, *86*(5), 618–627.

Jayarajah, U., Athapathu, A. S., Jayawardane, B., Prasanth, S., & Seneviratne, S. N. (2019). Hygiene practices during clinical training: Knowledge, attitudes and practice among a cohort of South Asian Medical students. *BMC Medical Education [Electronic Resource]*, *19*(1), 157. https://doi.org/10.1186/s12909-019-1582-2.

Kampf, G., Todt, D., Pfaender, S., & Steinmann, E. (2020). Persistence of coronaviruses on inanimate surfaces and their inactivation with biocidal agents. *The Journal of Hospital Infection*, *104*(3), 246–251. https://doi.org/10.1016/j.jhin.2020.01.022

Kohtz, C., Brown, S. C., Williams, R., & O'Connor, P. A. (2017). Physical assessment techniques in nursing education: A replicated study. *Journal of Nursing Education*, *56*(5), 287–291. https://doi.org/10.3928/01484834-20170421-06

Kratzel, A., Todt, D., V'kovski, P., Steiner, S., Gultrom, M., Thao, T. T. N., Ebert, N., Holwerda, M., Steinmann, J., Niemeyer, D., Dijkman, R., Kampf, G., Drosten, C., Steinmann, E., Thiel, V., & Pfaender, S. (2020). Inactivation of severe acute respiratory syndrome coronavirus 2 by WHO-recommended hand rub formulations and alcohols. *Emerging Infectious Diseases*, *26*(7), 1592–1595. https://doi.org/10.3201/eid2607.200915external icon

Murdoch, N. L., Bottorff, J. L., & McCullough, D. (2014). Simulation education approaches to enhance collaborative healthcare: A best practices review. *International Journal of Nursing Education Scholarship*, *10*:/j/ijnes.2013.10.issue-1/ijnes-2013-0027/ijnes-2013-0027.xml. https://doi.org/10.1515/ijnes-2013-0027

Murdoch, N. L., Epp, S., & Vinek, J. J. (2017). Teaching and learning activities to educate nursing students for interprofessional collaboration: A scoping review. *Interprof Care*, *31*(6), 744–753. https://doi.org/10.1080/13561820.2017.1356807

Noon, A. (2014). The cognitive processes underpinning clinical decision in triage assessment: a theoretical conundrum? *International Emergency Nursing*, *22*(1), 40–46.

Numminen, O., Leino-Kilpi, H., Isoaho, H., & Meretoja, R. (2016). Newly graduated nurses' occupational commitment and its associations with professional competence and work-related factors. *Journal of Clinical Nursing*, *25*(1–2), 117–126. https://doi.org/10.1111/jocn.13005

Numminen, O., Meretoja, R., Ihoaho, H., & Leino-Kilpi, H. (2013). Professional competence of practicing nurses. *Journal of Clinical Nursing*, *22*(10), 1411–1423.

Padilha, M. J., Machado, P. P., Ribeiro, A., Ramos, J., & Costa, P. (2019). Clinical virtual simulation in nursing education: randomized controlled trial. *Journal of Medical Internet Research [Electronic Resource]*, *21*(3), 1–9. https://doi.org/10.2196/11529

Unsworth, J., Tucker, G., & Hindmarsh, Y. (2015). Man versus machine: the importance of manual blood pressure measurement skills amongst registered nurses. *Journal of Hospital Administration*, *4*(6), 61–67.

Vergehese, A., & Horwitz, R. I. (2009). In praise of the physical examination. *Bmj (Clinical Research Ed.)*, *339*, b5448.

Vikke, H. S., & Giebner, M. (2016). POSAiDA: presence of Staphylococcus aureus/MRSA and Enterococcus/VRE in Danish ambulances. A cross-sectional study. *BMC Research Notes*, *9*, 194. https://doi.org/10.1186/s13104-016-1982-x

Yamauchi, T. (2001). Correlation between work experiences and physical assessment in Japan. *Nursing & Health Sciences*, *3*(4), 213–224. https://doi.org/10.1046/j.1442-2018.2001.00091.x

Zambas Shelaine, I., Smythe Elizabeth, A., & Jane, K. M. (2016). The consequences of using advanced physical assessment skills in medical and surgical nursing: A hermeneutic pragmatic study. *International Journal of Qualitative Studies on Health and Well-being*, *11*(1), 32090. https://doi.org/10.3402/qhw.v11.32090

7 GENERAL SURVEY INCLUDING VITAL SIGNS AND PAIN

KEY TERMS

auscultatory gap	hypertension	pain
diastole	Korotkoff sounds	systole
general survey	orthostatic hypotension	vital signs

Learning Objectives

The student will:

1. Identify the components of the general survey.
2. Identify appropriate subjective questions based on initial observations.
3. Demonstrate how to measure blood pressure, pulse, respiration, and temperature.
4. Discuss variations in vital signs and the possible causes.
5. Perform and document a pain assessment using information from the health history and the physical examination.
6. Describe the different types of pain.
7. Discuss health promotion related to vital sign assessment and knowledge of baseline parameters.

The "General Survey" section provides an overview of the nurse's initial patient assessment prior to exploring each system in detail. The objective observation of the patient begins with the first moments of the encounter and continues throughout the history and physical examination. The nonverbal cues collected during the **general survey** enable the nurse to select appropriate subjective questions for the individual patient to garner more information. Many factors are assessed, such as the patient's general appearance, apparent state of health, demeanor, facial expression or affect, grooming, posture, and gait (Fig. 7-1). Height and weight would also be assessed with the general survey and will be covered in detail in Chapter 8, "Nutrition and Hydration."

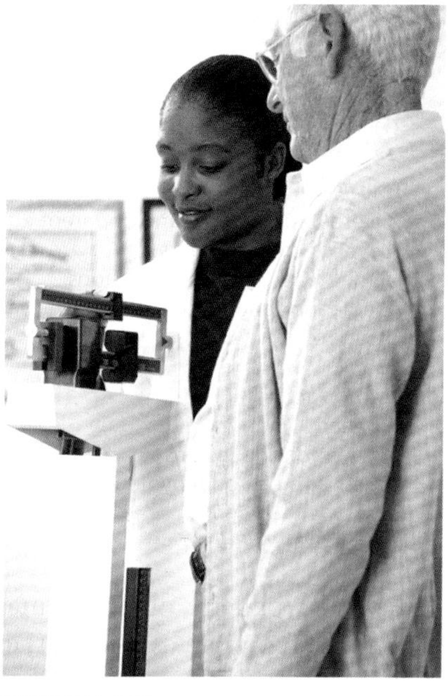

FIGURE 7-1 The nurse assesses many aspects during the general survey.

As the assessment skills of the nurse become more attuned to individual patients, the distinguishing features of each patient are depicted so well in documentation that a colleague could almost envision the person.

Many factors contribute to the patient's makeup, such as age, genetic composition, childhood illnesses, culture, and gender identity and expression. In addition, social determinants of health (SDOHs), that is, where people work, live, play, and learn are multifactorial (Centers for Disease Control and Prevention [CDC], 2020b). Areas with poor SDOHs often have low socioeconomic status, insufficient housing, and unsafe neighborhoods (Hahn et al., 2018). These limitations adversely affect health because, for example, individuals may be unable to exercise outside due to safety issues or they have little access to stores or pharmacies with necessary food and other resources. These conditions need to be addressed to improve quality of life and health. Recall that the patient's socioeconomic status may affect many of the characteristics you assess, including blood pressure, posture, mood and alertness, facial coloration, dentition, condition of the tongue and gingiva, color of the nail beds, muscle bulk, and more.

Recapture the observations you have been making since the first moments of your interaction with a patient and refine them throughout your assessment (Box 7-1). Does the patient hear you when greeted in the waiting room or examination room? Do they rise with ease? Walk easily or stiffly? If hospitalized when you first meet, what is the patient doing—sitting up and enjoying television? Lying in bed? What occupies the bedside table? Is it a magazine? An uneaten meal? A stack of "get well" cards? A Bible or a Koran? An emesis basin? Nothing at all? Each of these observations may raise one or more tentative hypotheses about the patient to consider during future assessments.

BOX 7-1 GENERAL SURVEY—INITIAL OBSERVATIONS

Physical Appearance and Apparent State of Health and Mood

- Overall appearance and apparent age
- Level of consciousness
- Facial features and expressions
- Demeanor and affect
- Posture
- Gait
- Motor activity
- Speech
- Skin color and lesions
- Dress and personal hygiene

The **vital signs** are objective measurements and are completed as part of the initial step in an assessment, especially in emergent situations. The vital signs include blood pressure, heart rate, respiratory rate, and temperature.

A keen understanding of the anatomy and physiology associated with each vital sign, how the values can be affected, and how to interpret the findings is important for each nurse. This will assist in figuring out the urgency of the situation and in comparing the parameters from baseline. The vital signs are also indicators of health outcomes, hospital readmissions, and use of resources (Sapra et al., 2020).

GENERAL SURVEY

Apparent State of Health

Try to make a general judgment based on observations throughout the encounter. Support it with the significant details. Does the patient look their age? Appear ill? Unhappy? Fatigued?

Level of Consciousness

Is the patient awake, alert, and responsive to you and others in the environment? If not, promptly assess the level of consciousness. Orientation can be checked by asking about person, place, time, and situation (see Chapter 19, "Mental Status and Mental Health Assessment").

Facial Expression

Observe the patient's facial expression at rest, during conversation, during the physical examination, and when interacting with others. Watch closely for eye contact. Is it natural? Sustained and unblinking? Quickly averted? Absent?

Are the movements of the face symmetric? Is there *ptosis*? An uneven smile?

Check the patient for the stare of hyperthyroidism; the immobile face of Parkinson disease; or the flat or sad effect of depression. Decreased eye contact may be cultural, or it may suggest anxiety, fear, or sadness. Asymmetry of the face could indicate a stroke, palsy, or injury to the cranial nerve.

Posture, Gait, Motor Activity, and Speech

What is the patient's preferred posture? Assess the patient before calling their name in the waiting room. How is the patient sitting? Does the position or nonverbal communication change when you are in the room with the patient?

CLINICAL TIP
Patients often prefer sitting upright when they have left-sided heart failure and leaning forward with arms propped up when they have chronic obstructive pulmonary disease (COPD).

Is the patient restless or quiet? How often does the patient change positions? How fast or slow are their movements?

Anxious patients appear agitated and restless. Patients in pain often avoid movement.

Is there any apparent involuntary motor activity? Are some body parts immobile? Which ones?

Look for tremors, other involuntary movements, or paralysis. See Chapter 20, "The Nervous System," Table 20-11, "Tremors and Involuntary Movements."

Does the patient walk smoothly with comfort, self-confidence, and balance, or is there a limp or discomfort, fear of falling, loss of balance, or any indication of a movement disorder? Does the patient use an assistive device like a cane, walker, or brace to ambulate?

See Chapter 20, "The Nervous System," Table 20-4, "Abnormalities of Gait and Posture." An impaired gait increases the risk of falls.

Is the patient's speech articulate? Garbled? Rapid or slow?

Fatigue is a nonspecific symptom with many causes. It refers to a sense of weariness or loss of energy that patients may describe in various ways: "I don't feel like getting up in the morning," "I don't have any energy," "I just feel blah," "I'm all done in," "I can hardly get through the day," "By the time I get to the office, I feel as if I've done a day's work." Because fatigue is a normal response to hard work, sustained stress, or grief, try to elicit the life circumstances in which it occurs. Fatigue unrelated to such situations requires further investigation.

Use open-ended questions to explore the attributes of the patient's fatigue and encourage the patient to fully describe what they are experiencing. Important clues about etiology often emerge from a good psychosocial history, exploration of sleep patterns, and a thorough review of systems.

Fatigue is a common symptom of depression and anxiety states, but it may also indicate infections (e.g., hepatitis, mononucleosis, tuberculosis); endocrine disorders (e.g., hypothyroidism, adrenal insufficiency, diabetes mellitus); heart failure; chronic disease of the lungs, kidneys, or liver; electrolyte imbalance; moderate to severe anemia; postural orthostatic tachycardia syndrome (POTS); malignancies; nutritional deficits; and medication side effects.

Weakness is different from fatigue. It denotes a demonstrable loss of muscle power and will be discussed later with other neurologic symptoms (see Chapter 20, "The Nervous System").

Weakness, especially if localized in a neuroanatomic pattern, suggests possible neuropathy or myopathy.

Odors of the Body and Breath

Odors can be important diagnostic clues, such as the fruity odor of diabetes or the scent of alcohol. (For the scent of alcohol, the AUDIT-C questions in Chapter 4, "The Health History," will help you determine possible misuse.)

Breath odors may indicate alcohol, acetone (diabetes), pulmonary infections, uremia, or liver failure.

Never assume that alcohol on a patient's breath explains changes in mental status or neurologic findings.

These changes may have serious but treatable causes such as hypoglycemia, subdural hematoma, or postictal state.

Skin Color and Obvious Lesions

Inspect for any changes in skin color, scars, plaques, or nevi (see Chapter 9, "The Integumentary System").

Pallor, cyanosis, jaundice, rashes, bruises, or any changes should be assessed in greater detail.

Dress, Grooming, and Personal Hygiene

How is the patient dressed? Is the clothing appropriate for the temperature and weather? Is it clean, properly buttoned, and zipped? Are there rips or excessive stains on the clothing? Does it fit? How is the condition of the clothing? How does it compare with clothing worn by people of comparable age and social group? The patient's clothing may provide information about the patient's social or cultural background.

Excess clothing may reflect the cold intolerance of hypothyroidism; hide a skin rash or scars from self-mutilation or needle marks; mask anorexia; or signal personal lifestyle preferences.

Has the patient added additional holes on the belt to enlarge it? To make it smaller?

Altering a belt may indicate weight gain or weight loss.

Take note of the patient's shoes. Are there holes or cut-outs? Is the patient wearing slippers? Are the laces tied?

CLINICAL TIP
Holes in shoes or slippers may indicate gout, bunions, or other painful foot conditions. Shoes that are worn out can contribute to foot and back pain, calluses, falls, and infection. Untied laces or slippers may suggest edema.

Is the patient wearing any unusual jewelry? Do they have any body piercing? Tattoos? When and where were they obtained?

CLINICAL TIP
Copper bracelets may suggest joint pain. Piercings or tattoos may appear on any part of the body.

Note the patient's hair, fingernails, and use of makeup. They may be clues to the patient's personality, culture, self-regard, or lifestyle.

CLINICAL TIP
Overgrown hair or lack of nail hygiene may suggest the length of a possible illness or change in circumstances. Bitten fingernails may reflect stress. Yellowing of the index and middle finger may indicate a smoking habit.

Do personal hygiene and grooming seem appropriate to the patient's age, lifestyle, occupation, culture, and socioeconomic group? These are norms that vary widely.

Neglected appearance may imply depression or dementia but should only be compared with the patient's norm, not with the nurse's expectation.

Signs of Distress

- Cardiac or respiratory distress: Is the patient clutching the chest? Do you see pallor, diaphoresis, labored breathing, wheezing, coughing, shortness of breath, or the patient sitting in a tripod position?
- Pain: Do you see grimacing, crying, or diaphoresis? Is the patient holding, favoring, or protecting a body part or area of the body?
- Anxiety or depression: Do you see anxious facial expressions; fidgety movements; cold, moist palms; inexpressive or flat affect; poor eye contact; or psychomotor slowing? See Chapter 19, "Mental Status and Mental Health Assessment."

THE VITAL SIGNS

Vital signs are an integral part of the assessment. These include the blood pressure, heart rate, respiratory rate, and temperature. These important measurements may be completed at the start of the physical examination. If any vital sign is not within the normal parameters, then rechecking during the cardiovascular or respiratory system examinations is prudent.

During the assessment, check the blood pressure and pulse. To check the pulse, the heart rate can be assessed by counting the radial pulse with your fingers, or the apical pulse with your stethoscope at the cardiac apex. Keep contact with the patient as if still checking the pulse, and then count the respiratory rate without alerting the patient, as breathing patterns may unconsciously change if the patient knows breaths are being counted. The temperature may be taken at various anatomic sites; the ideal site depends on the individual patient and the equipment available. Further details on techniques for ensuring accuracy of the vital signs are provided later in the chapter. It is important to know the normal parameters for vital signs and to be aware of the patient's baseline vitals to quickly decipher during your assessment if changes are significant.

See Chapter 14, "The Cardiovascular System," Table 14-5, "Variations and Abnormalities of the Apical Impulse," and Chapter 13, "The Respiratory System," Table 13-5, "Abnormalities in Rate and Rhythm of Breathing."

Blood Pressure

Monitoring Blood Pressure

More than 100 million Americans, or nearly half of all adults in the United States, have elevated blood pressure (CDC, 2020a). Close to half a million deaths are connected to high blood pressure as the primary or contributing cause, which translates into almost 1,300 deaths per day (CDC, 2020a). **Hypertension** varies among different demographic groups, but those with unfavorable SDOHs experience disproportionately high rates, expected to continue to rise in the upcoming years (American Heart Association, 2020). Detection and management are integral to patient care. High blood pressure varies by sex and race, however uncontrolled blood pressure disproportionately correlates with SDOHs, and the statistics are predicted to climb in upcoming years (American Heart Association, 2020). More men (47%) than women (43%) have high blood pressure. Of non-Hispanic Black adults, 54% have hypertension compared to 46% of non-Hispanic White adults, 39% of non-Hispanic Asian adults, and 36% of Hispanic adults (American Heart Association, 2020).

The American Heart Association has outlined seven goals for improving heart health, and healthy blood pressure is an important part of that. The goals include maintaining blood pressure; keeping blood sugar levels low; maintaining cholesterol levels in healthy ranges; participating in regular exercise; avoiding excess weight; eating a healthy diet; and quitting or never smoking (Muntner et al., 2019).

Screening at office visits or health fairs often detects elevated blood pressure. Follow-up and confirmation of an elevated reading has moved into the home environment. Studies have shown that home and ambulatory blood pressure monitoring confirms more cardiovascular disease and end-organ damage than do office measurements (see Chapter 14, "The Cardiovascular System") (Hahn et al., 2018).

Attention to accuracy of both the equipment and the technique and detail in the reading of blood pressure is crucial. Errors in blood pressure measurement can increase the risk of unnecessary treatment or misdiagnosis (Pappaccogli et al., 2019). Blood pressure devices may be aneroid, hybrid, or electronic, and there are international protocols for evaluating their accuracy.

CLINICAL TIP

Self-monitoring of blood pressure by well-instructed patients using approved devices improves blood pressure control, especially when it is done two times daily on the upper arm with automatic readouts (Myers et al., 2018; Reboussin et al., 2018).

Choice of Blood Pressure Cuff (Sphygmomanometer)

Take the time to choose a cuff of appropriate size for your patient's arm (Fig. 7-2). Follow the guidelines in Table 7-1, and advise your patients about how to choose the best cuff for home use and the need to have it recalibrated routinely. Educate patients on the best options, and make them aware that although the wrist and finger monitors are popular, they are less accurate. Patients at home need to be able to demonstrate correct technique to insure accurate readings.

The width of the inflatable bladder of the cuff should be about 40% of the upper arm circumference. The length of the inflatable bladder should be about 80% of upper arm circumference (almost long enough to circle the arm).

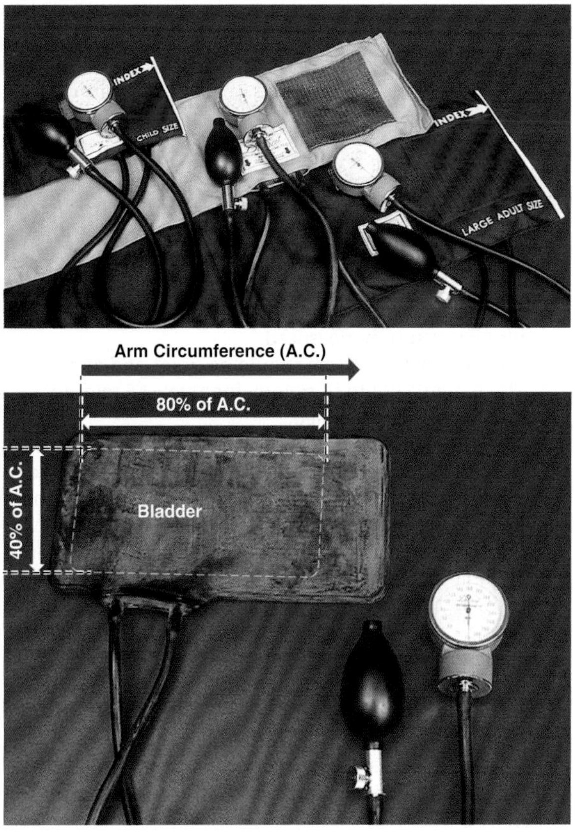

FIGURE 7-2 Different blood pressure cuff sizes.

TABLE 7-1 Selecting the Correct Size Blood Pressure Cuff for Adults

Usual Cuff Size	Arm Circumference (cm)
Small adult	22–26
Adult	27–34
Large adult	35–44
Adult thigh	45–52

Source: Saugel, B., Dueck, R., & Wagner, J. Y. (2014). Measurement of blood pressure. *Best Practice & Research. Clinical Anaesthesiology*, *28*(4), 309–322. https://doi.org/10.1016/j.bpa.2014.08.001

CLINICAL TIP
If the cuff is too *small* (narrow), the blood pressure will read *high.* If the cuff is too *large* (wide), the blood pressure will read *low* on a small arm and *high* on a large arm (Wohlfahrt et al., 2020).

Technique for Measuring Blood Pressure

Before assessing the blood pressure, take several steps to make sure your measurement will be accurate (Box 7-2). Proper technique is important and reduces the inherent variability arising from the patient or examiner, the equipment, and the procedure itself (Vischer & Burkard, 2017).

BOX 7-2 STEPS TO ENSURE ACCURATE BLOOD PRESSURE MEASUREMENT

- The patient should avoid smoking, exercise, or caffeine for 30 minutes before the blood pressure is measured.
- The examination room should be quiet and at a comfortable temperature.
- The patient should sit quietly for at least 5 minutes in a chair with both feet flat on the floor and legs uncrossed.
- The arm selected should be accessible and without clothing, fistulas for dialysis, scars near the brachial artery that was accessed for a deep vein intravenous line, or lymphedema from axillary node dissection or radiation therapy.
- Palpate the brachial artery to confirm that it has a viable pulse.
- Position the arm so that the brachial artery at the antecubital crease is *at heart level*—roughly level with the fourth interspace at its junction with the sternum.
- If the patient is seated, rest the arm on a table a little above the patient's waist.

CLINICAL TIP
If the brachial artery is *below* heart level, the blood pressure will be higher. If the brachial artery is *higher,* the blood pressure will be lower (Kallioinen et al., 2017).

Measuring Blood Pressure

Blood pressure is the measurement of the pressure on the walls of the blood vessels. **Systole** is the pressure in the arteries when the left ventricle contracts, and **diastole** is the pressure in the arteries when the heart muscle rests and refills with blood.

A. Position the cuff and the arm.

- The arm is exposed (without clothing) and positioned at heart level.
- The feet are uncrossed and if the patient is sitting, the feet are placed on the floor.
- Select the correct size blood pressure cuff.
- Center the fully deflated cuff bladder over the brachial artery.
- The lower border of the cuff should be about 2.5 cm above the antecubital crease.
- Secure the cuff snugly and evenly.

CLINICAL TIP
A loose cuff or a bladder that balloons outside the cuff leads to falsely high readings.

B. Estimate the systolic pressure and add 30 mm Hg.

- To determine how high to raise the cuff pressure, first estimate the systolic pressure by palpation.
- As you feel the brachial artery with the fingers of one hand, inflate the cuff until the brachial pulse disappears, and then inflate another 20 to 30 mm Hg more.
- Deflate the cuff (the manometer should fall 2 to 3 mm Hg/sec), and note when the palpable pulse reappears. This is the estimated systolic blood pressure.
- Deflate the cuff promptly and completely and wait 15 to 30 seconds.

C. Position the stethoscope over the brachial artery.

- Clean the portion of your stethoscope that will be in contact with the patient with an alcohol wipe.

- Place the diaphragm (or bell) of the stethoscope lightly over the brachial artery, taking care to make an air seal with its full rim (Liu et al., 2016).

- Pump up the cuff and add 30 mm Hg to the palpated pulse found on the previous step. Use of this sum as the target for subsequent inflations prevents discomfort from unnecessarily high cuff pressures. It also avoids the occasional error caused by an **auscultatory gap**—a silent interval that may be present between the systolic and the diastolic pressures (Fig. 7-3).

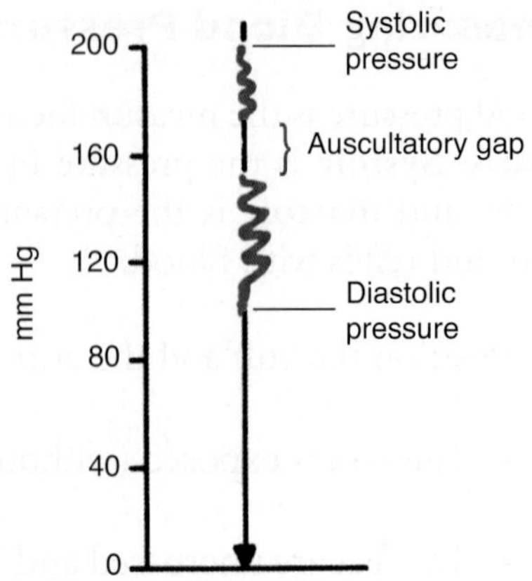

FIGURE 7-3 The auscultatory gap occurs between the systolic and diastolic pressures.

CLINICAL TIP

An unrecognized auscultatory gap may lead to serious underestimation of systolic pressure (150 instead of 200 in Fig. 7-3) or overestimation of diastolic pressure. If you find an auscultatory gap, record your findings completely (e.g., 200/98 with an auscultatory gap from 170 to 150). An auscultatory gap is associated with arterial stiffness and atherosclerotic disease (Pan et al., 2017).

- **Korotkoff sounds** are heard when the blood pressure cuff changes the sounds of the blood flowing through the artery. The sounds can be heard using either the bell or the diaphragm. Both sides of the stethoscope have similar results, and each is reliable (Kohlman-Trigoboff, 2015). The practitioner may choose a bell or diaphragm as long as they can hear the sounds clearly.

- Do not allow the stethoscope to touch the cuff or clothing (Fig. 7-4).

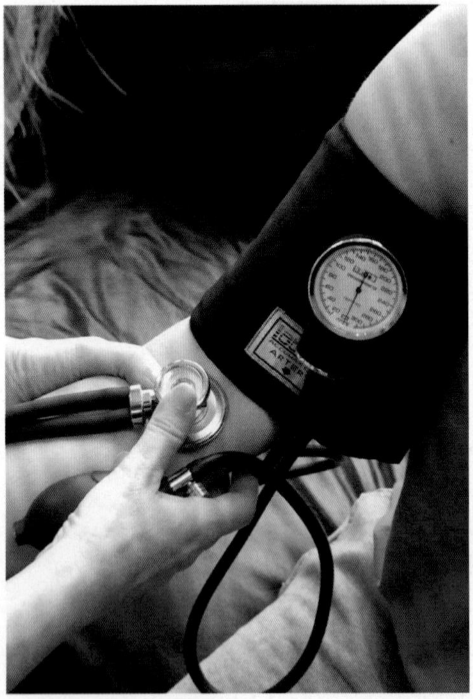

FIGURE 7-4 Allowing the stethoscope to touch the cuff or clothing can skew findings.

D. Identify the systolic blood pressure.

- Deflate the cuff slowly at a rate of about 2 mm Hg/sec.
- Note the level at which you hear the sounds of at least two consecutive beats. The first sound is the *systolic* pressure (Fig. 7-5).

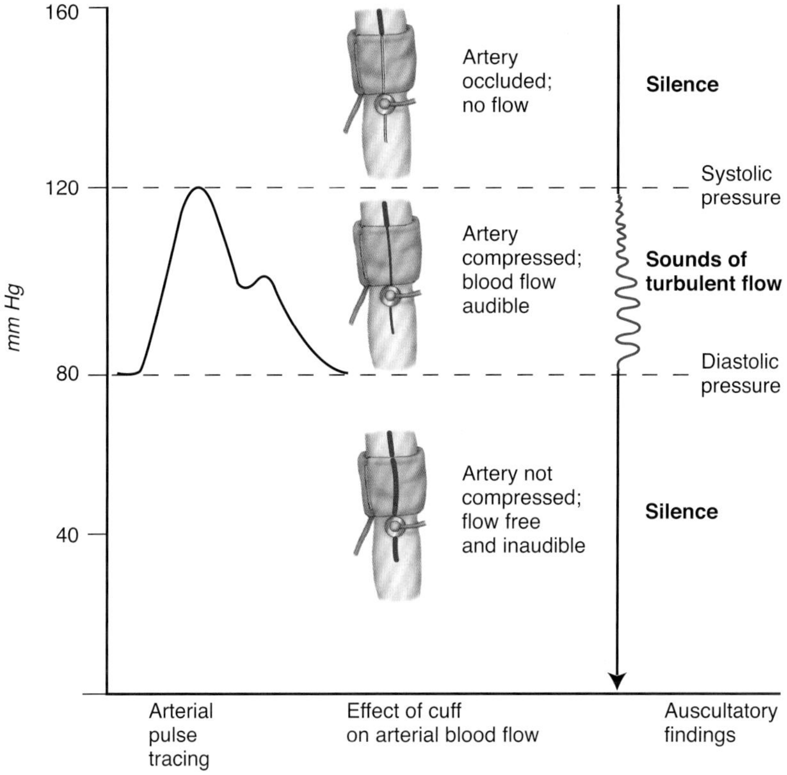

FIGURE 7-5 The first two consecutive heart sounds indicate the systolic pressure.

E. Identify the diastolic blood pressure.

- Listen for the last sound.
- To confirm the disappearance point, listen as the pressure falls another 10 to 20 mm Hg.
- Then deflate the cuff rapidly to zero.
- The disappearance point, which is usually only a few mm Hg below the muffling point, provides the best estimate of true *diastolic* pressure.

In some people, the muffling point and the disappearance point are further apart. Occasionally, as in aortic regurgitation, the sounds never disappear. If the difference is 10 mm Hg or greater, record both figures (e.g., 154/80/68).

F. Average two or more readings.

- Read both the systolic and the diastolic levels to the nearest 2 mm Hg (Wohlfahrt et al., 2020).
- Wait at least 2 minutes and repeat.
- Average your readings.
- If the first two readings differ by more than 6 mm Hg, take additional readings.

By making the sounds less audible, venous congestion may produce artificially low systolic and high diastolic pressures.

CLINICAL TIP
Make sure the numbers face you directly. Avoid slow or repetitive inflations of the cuff, because the resulting venous congestion can cause false readings.

G. Measure blood pressure in both arms at least once. Normally, there may be a difference in pressure of 4 mm Hg and sometimes up to 10 mm Hg. Subsequent readings should be made on the arm with the higher pressure.

Pressure difference of more than 10 mm Hg occurs in subclavian steal syndrome, aortic dissection, and supravalvular aortic stenosis and should be investigated.

Blood pressure cuff selection is important. Attention to cuff size is crucial to alleviate incorrect readings which can result in inaccurate treatment. If the correct cuff is not available, one should be ordered to accommodate the patient's size. Inconsistencies can result in falsely high or falsely low readings (Table 7-2).

TABLE 7-2 Errors that Result in False Readings

Falsely High Readings	Falsely Low Readings
Cuff or bladder too small (short or narrow)	Cuff or bladder too large (wide)
Cuff too loose or uneven	Pressing stethoscope too tightly against pulse
Arm below heart level	Arm above heart level
Arm not supported	Repeating assessments too quickly
Inflating or deflating cuff too slowly (high diastolic)	Inaccurate level of inflation
Deflating too quickly (low systolic and high diastolic)	

Classifications of Blood Pressure

High Blood Pressure

The American College of Cardiology and the American Heart Association provide guidelines for the management of hypertension. Current classifications of hypertension include both stage 1 and stage 2 (Table 7-3) (Whelton et al., 2018). Note that either the systolic or diastolic component may be high.

TABLE 7-3 Classification of Normal and Abnormal Blood Pressure

Category	Systolic (mm Hg)		Diastolic (mm Hg)
Normal	<120	and	<80
Elevated	120–129	and	<80
Hypertension			
Stage 1	130–139	or	80–89
Stage 2	≥140	or	≥90

Blood pressure should be documented as normal, elevated, or stage 1 or stage 2 hypertension. The mean of two or more properly measured, seated blood pressure readings taken during two or more office visits is recommended for diagnosis of hypertension (Pappaccogli et al., 2019; Saugel et al., 2014). Blood pressure measurement should be verified in the contralateral arm (Yano et al., 2015).

CLINICAL TIP
Assessment of hypertension also includes its effects on target "end organs"—the eyes, heart, brain, and kidneys. Look for hypertensive retinopathy, left ventricular hypertrophy, and neurologic deficits suggesting stroke. Renal assessment requires urinalysis and blood tests of renal function.

When the systolic and diastolic levels fall in different categories, use the higher category. For example, 170/84 mm Hg indicates stage 2 hypertension, and 126/86 mm Hg indicates stage 1 hypertension. In *isolated systolic hypertension*, systolic blood pressure is 130 mm Hg or greater, and diastolic blood pressure is less than 80 mm Hg.

Treatment of isolated systolic hypertension in patients 60 years of age or older reduces mortality and complications from cardiovascular disease (Jordan et al., 2020).

Low Blood Pressure

Interpret relatively low levels of blood pressure in light of past readings and the patient's present clinical state.

CLINICAL TIP
A pressure of 106/70 mm Hg would usually be considered normal but could also indicate significant hypotension if past pressures have been high.

If indicated, assess *orthostatic hypotension*, common in older adults. Measure blood pressure and heart rate in two positions—*supine* after the patient is resting from 3 to 10 minutes, then within 3 minutes once the patient *stands up*. Normally, as the patient rises from the horizontal to the standing position, systolic pressure drops slightly or remains unchanged while diastolic pressure rises slightly. **Orthostatic hypotension** is a drop in systolic blood pressure of at least 20 mm Hg or in diastolic blood pressure of at least 10 mm Hg within 3 minutes of standing (Metzler et al., 2013; Spångfors et al., 2019).

See Chapter 24, "Assessing Older Adults."

CLINICAL TIP
Causes of orthostatic hypotension include medications, moderate or severe blood loss, prolonged bed rest, and diseases of the autonomic nervous system.

Special Circumstances

Weak or Inaudible Korotkoff Sounds

Consider technical problems, such as erroneous placement of the stethoscope, failure to make full skin contact with the bell, or diaphragm and venous engorgement of the patient's arm from repeated inflations of the cuff. Also consider the possibility of shock or vascular disease.

When you cannot hear any Korotkoff sounds, you may be able to estimate the systolic pressure by palpation. Alternative methods such as Doppler techniques or direct arterial pressure tracings may be necessary.

To intensify Korotkoff sounds, one of the following methods may be helpful:

- Raise the patient's arm before and while you inflate the cuff. Then lower the arm and determine the blood pressure.
- Inflate the cuff. Ask the patient to make a fist several times, and then determine the blood pressure.

Arrhythmias

Irregular rhythms produce variations in pressure and therefore unreliable measurements. Ignore the effects of an occasional premature contraction (Bunkenborg et al., 2016). With frequent premature contractions or atrial fibrillation, determine the average of several observations and note the measurements are approximate. Ambulatory monitoring for 2 to 24 hours is recommended (Geerse et al., 2019).

CLINICAL TIP
Detection of an irregular rhythm suggests *atrial fibrillation.* For all irregular patterns, obtain an electrocardiogram (ECG) to identify the type of rhythm (Montrivade et al., 2020).

White Coat Hypertension

"White coat hypertension" describes hypertension in people whose blood pressure measurements are higher in the physician's office than at home or in more relaxed settings. This phenomenon occurs in 10% to 25% of patients, especially women and anxious individuals, and may last for several visits. Try to relax the patient or use remote telehealth to remeasure the blood pressure later in the encounter. Home monitoring has been used effectively to diagnose white coat hypertension and prevent inappropriate treatment.

Home or ambulatory hypertension, unlike white coat or isolated office hypertension, signals increased risk of cardiovascular disease (Lambe et al., 2017; O'Brien & Marshall, 2015; Roerecke et al., 2019)

The Obese or Very Thin Patient

For the *obese arm,* use a cuff that is 15 cm in width. If this cuff is too short despite a large circumference, use a thigh cuff or a longer cuff. If the arm circumference is greater than 50 cm and not amenable to use of a thigh cuff, wrap an appropriately sized cuff around the forearm, hold the forearm at heart level, and feel for the radial pulse (Lambe et al., 2017). Other options include using a Doppler probe at the radial artery or an oscillometric device. For the *very thin arm,* consider using a pediatric cuff.

CLINICAL TIP
Using a small cuff overestimates systolic blood pressure in obese patients (Pan et al., 2017).

The Hypertensive Patient with Systolic Blood Pressure Higher in the Arms than the Legs

Coarctation of the aorta in children or adults generally presents with systolic hypertension, greater in the arms than the legs. Assess blood pressure in the legs and "femoral delay" at least once in every hypertensive patient.

Compare blood pressures in the arms and legs. Compare the volume and timing of the radial and femoral pulses. Normally, volume is equal and the pulses occur simultaneously.

Coarctation of the aorta is a narrowing of the thoracic aorta, usually distal to the left subclavian artery. Compare blood pressures in the arms and legs. In healthy patients, the systolic blood pressure should be 5 to 10 mm higher in the lower extremities than in the arms. Coarctation of the aorta and occlusive aortic disease are distinguished by hypertension in the upper extremities and low blood pressure in the legs and by diminished or delayed femoral pulses (Lin et al., 2018).

Heart Rate and Rhythm

Examine the arterial pulses, the heart rate and rhythm, and the amplitude and contour of the pulse wave.

Heart Rate

The radial pulse is commonly used to assess the heart rate. With the pads of your index and middle fingers, compress the radial artery until a maximal pulsation is detected (Fig. 7-6). If the rhythm is regular and the rate seems normal, count the rate for 30 seconds and multiply by 2. If the rate is unusually fast or slow, however, count it for 60 seconds. The normal range is 60 to 100 beats per minute (Aladin et al., 2014).

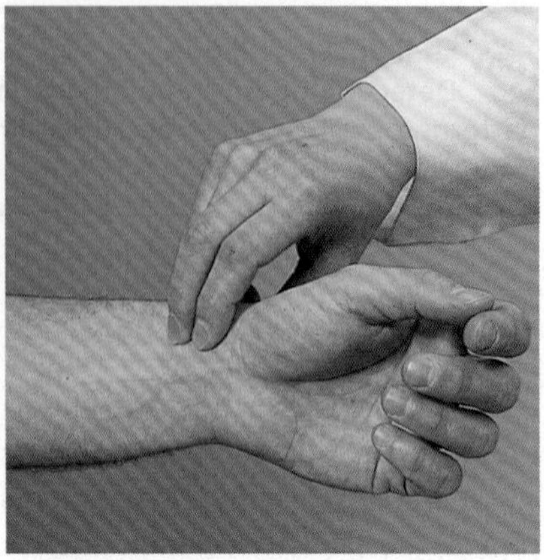

FIGURE 7-6 Pulse can be measured by palpating the radial artery with the index and middle fingers.

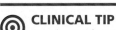

CLINICAL TIP
An elevated resting heart rate is associated with increased risk of cardiovascular disease and mortality (Johansson, 2019).

Rhythm

Begin by palpating the radial pulse. If there are any irregularities, assess the rhythm at the cardiac apex by listening with your stethoscope. Premature beats of low amplitude may not be transmitted to the peripheral pulses and the heart rate can be seriously underestimated. Is the rhythm regular or irregular? If irregular, try to identify a pattern: (1) Do early beats appear in a basically regular rhythm? (2) Does the irregularity vary consistently with respiration? (3) Is the rhythm totally irregular?

See Chapter 14, "The Cardiovascular System," Table 14-1, "Selected Heart Rates and Rhythms."

See Chapter 15, "The Peripheral Vascular System and Lymphatic System," Table 15-5, "Abnormalities of Arterial Pulse and Pressure Waves."

If the radial pulse is irregular or the patient's condition calls for a more precise pulse rate, then an apical pulse should be assessed for 1 minute. The examiner places the stethoscope at the apex (fifth intercostal space at the midclavicular line) and auscultates the S_1 and S_2, noting the rate and rhythm. An ECG should be checked to determine the rhythm.

Concept Mastery Alert

Irregular Distal Pulse

Novice nurses may assume that when a distal pulse is irregular, they should check the radial pulse on the patient's other wrist. However, the preferred follow-up is to assess an apical pulse for 1 minute. The examiner places the stethoscope at the apex (fifth intercostal space at the midclavicular line) and auscultates the S_1 and S_2, noting rate and rhythm. An ECG should be checked to determine the rhythm.

Respiratory Rate and Rhythm

Observe the *rate, rhythm, depth,* and *effort of breathing*. Count the number of respirations (one respiration includes an inspiration and an expiration) in 1 minute either by visual inspection or by subtly listening over the patient's trachea with your stethoscope during your examination of the head and neck or chest. Normally, adults take 12 to 20 breaths per minute in a quiet, regular pattern. An occasional sigh is normal. Check to see if expiration is prolonged.

See Chapter 13, "The Respiratory System," Table 13-5, "Abnormalities in Rate and Rhythm of Breathing."

CLINICAL TIP
Prolonged expiration is common in COPD.

Temperature

Body temperature varies and is affected both externally and internally. Everyday clinical practice relies on noninvasive routes such as the oral, tympanic membrane, rectal, axillary, temporal artery measurements as well as no-touch thermometers. These devices use electronic and/or infrared technology (Cardona-Morrell et al., 2016).

Oral Temperature

Oral temperature is the method used the most as it is both easy and reliable. The average oral temperature, usually quoted at 37°C (98.6°F), fluctuates considerably. In the early morning hours, it may fall as low as 36.6°C (97.7°F), and in the late afternoon or evening, it may rise as high as 37.5°C (99.5°F) (Exergen Manual, 2020).

To take an oral temperature, place the disposable cover over the probe and insert the thermometer under the tongue into the posterior sublingual pocket (Fig. 7-7). Ask the patient to close both lips, and then watch closely for the digital readout. An accurate temperature recording usually takes about 10 seconds. Note that hot or cold liquids and even smoking can alter the temperature reading. In these situations, it is best to delay measuring the temperature for 10 to 15 minutes. Due to breakage and/or mercury exposure, glass thermometers are largely being replaced by electronic thermometers; however, mercury glass thermometers may still be used in homes. These thermometers take approximately 3 minutes to register.

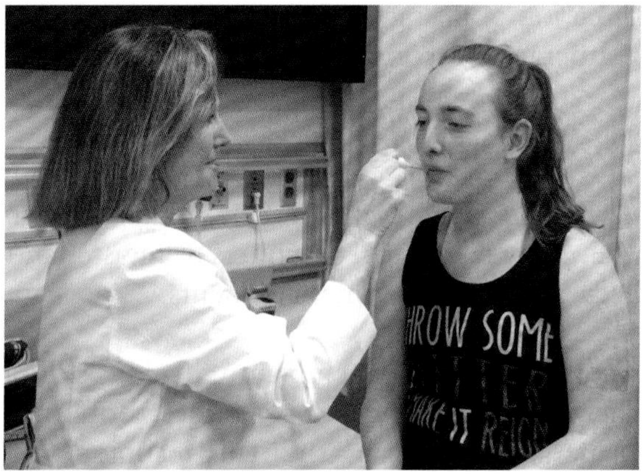

FIGURE 7-7 Oral temperature is measured with the thermometer under the tongue.

Taking oral temperatures is not recommended when patients are unconscious, restless, or unable to close their mouths. Temperature readings may be inaccurate, and thermometers may be broken by unexpected movements of the patient's jaws. The other options available should be chosen based on individual situations and availability.

CLINICAL TIP

Rapid respiratory rates tend to increase the discrepancy between oral and rectal temperatures. In these situations, rectal, tympanic, temporal, or axilla temperatures are more reliable.

Tympanic Membrane Temperature

Tympanic membrane temperature is also commonly used, though it can be more variable than oral or rectal temperatures. Studies vary in methodology but suggest that in adults, *oral and temporal artery temperatures* correlate more closely with the pulmonary artery temperature, about 0.5°C lower (O'Brien & Marshall, 2015; Roerecke et al., 2019). Alternatively, the tympanic membrane shares the same blood supply as the hypothalamus, where temperature regulation occurs in the brain. Accurate temperature readings

Concept Mastery Alert

Tympanic Membrane Temperature

The tympanic membrane temperature is the most reliable core body temperature measurement that can be done without invasive monitoring devices. The tympanic membrane is supplied by a tributary of the internal carotid artery that supplies the hypothalamus, the body's thermoregulatory center, or the area where temperature regulation occurs in the brain.

require access to the tympanic membrane. This is an increasingly common practice and is quick, safe, and reliable if performed properly. Make sure the external auditory canal is free of cerumen, which lowers temperature readings. Place the cover on and position the probe in the canal so that the infrared beam is aimed at the tympanic membrane. Wait 2 to 3 seconds until the digital temperature reading appears.

Rectal Temperature

Rectal temperature is the most inconvenient method, but it measures the temperature internally and is therefore the most accurate.

To measure temperature this way, select a rectal thermometer probe (usually red). Place the disposable cover over the probe and lubricate it. Ask the patient to lie on one side with the hip flexed, and insert the thermometer about 3 to 4 cm (1.5 in) through the anus and into the rectum, in a direction pointing to the umbilicus. Wait about 10 seconds for the digital temperature recording to appear.

Axillary Temperature

Axillary temperatures are *lower* than oral temperatures by approximately 1°F. They take 5 to 10 minutes to register and are generally considered less accurate than other measurements.

To take an axillary temperature, place a probe cover over the electronic thermometer probe and place the thermometer in the middle of the axilla while adducting the arm. This technique is convenient and can be used with unconscious patients. It is not recommended for patients with rapid temperature changes as it lags behind rapid core changes.

Temporal Artery Temperature

A temporal artery thermometer measures the blood flow through the superficial temporal artery, which branches off the external carotid artery and lies within a millimeter of the skin surface of the forehead and behind the earlobes. Place the probe against the center of the forehead and depress the infrared scanning button. Continue holding the button and slowly slide the probe midline across the forehead to the hairline (not down the side of the face). Move the probe from the forehead and touch behind the earlobe. Release the button, and the temperature will be visible on the display (Levy et al., 2018).

No-Touch Thermometers

Newer no-touch thermometers increased in popularity with the COVID-19 pandemic. The non-contact infrared thermometers (NCITs) decrease the risk of contamination and spreading disease. They are easy and quick to use. Correct technique is important to accurately assess temperature. The person cannot move as the thermometer is aimed perpendicular to the forehead. Sunlight, certain face wipes, and cosmetics can impede temperatures as can lack of clear visibility of the forehead due to head coverings or hair.

Fever, Chills, and Night Sweats

Fever or *pyrexia* refers to an abnormal elevation in body temperature (see Table 7-4 for normal temperature ranges).

Hyperpyrexia refers to extreme elevation in temperature, above 41.1°C (106°F).

TABLE 7-4 Temperature Routes and Normal Ranges

	0–2 Years (°F)	3–10 Years (°F)	11–65 Years (°F)	65 Years and Older (°F)
Oral	n/a	95.9–99.5	97.6–99.6	96.4–98.5
Tympanic Membrane	97.5–100.4	97.0–100.0	96.6–99.7	96.4–99.5
Rectal	97.9–100.4	97.9–100.4	98.6–100.6	97.1–99.2
Axillary	94.5–99.1	96.6–98.0	95.3–98.4	96.0–97.4
Temporal and No-Touch	97.9–100.7	97.9–100.3	97.9–100.1	97.9–100.1
Core	97.5–100.0	97.5–100.0	98.2–100.2	96.8–98.8

Ask about fever if patients have an acute or chronic illness. Find out whether the patient has used a thermometer to measure the temperature. Bear in mind that errors in technique can lead to unreliable information. Has the patient felt feverish or unusually hot, noted excessive sweating, or felt chilly and cold? Try to distinguish between subjective *chilliness* and a *shaking chill* with shivering throughout the body and chattering of teeth.

CLINICAL TIP
Recurrent shaking chills suggest more extreme swings in temperature and systemic *bacteremia.*

Feeling cold, goosebumps, and shivering accompany a rising temperature, while feeling hot and sweating accompany a falling temperature. Normally, the body temperature rises during the day and falls during the night. When fever exaggerates this swing, *night sweats* may occur. Malaise, headache, and pain in the muscles and joints often accompany fever.

Feelings of heat and sweating also accompany menopause. Night sweats may also occur with tuberculosis and malignancy.

Fever has many causes. Focus your questions on the timing of the illness and its associated symptoms. Become familiar with patterns of infectious diseases that may affect your patient. Inquire about travel, contact with sick people, or other unusual exposures. Be sure to inquire about medications because they may cause fever. In contrast, recent ingestion of aspirin, acetaminophen, corticosteroids, and nonsteroidal antiinflammatory drugs (NSAIDs) may mask fever and affect the temperature recorded at the time of the physical examination.

CLINICAL TIP
Causes of fever include infection; trauma, such as surgery or crush injuries; malignancy; blood disorders, such as acute hemolytic anemia; drug reactions; and immune disorders, such as collagen vascular disease.

Hypothermia

Hypothermia refers to an abnormally low temperature below 35°C (95°F) rectally. The chief cause of hypothermia is exposure to cold. Other predisposing causes include reduced movement as in paralysis, interference with vasoconstriction as from sepsis or excess alcohol intake, starvation, hypothyroidism, or hypoglycemia. Elderly people are especially susceptible to hypothermia and also less likely to develop fever.

ACUTE AND CHRONIC PAIN

Pain is a subjective finding and requires frequent assessment. At one point, pain had been labeled the "fifth vital sign," but the opioid crisis resulted in this concept falling out of favor (Institute of Medicine, 2011). Pain assessment is commonly missed, and when pain is noted, it is often not effectively managed. Pain is a frequent motivator for people to seek health care. Each year, approximately 100 million Americans report persistent, chronic pain, which is often underassessed and undertreated (Gordon, 2015). A comprehensive approach to guide physical examination and management should be adopted in practice, as pain is a leading cause of disability and contributes significantly to health care costs.

Referred pain and visceral pain are discussed in further detail in Chapter 16, "The Gastrointestinal and Renal Systems."

Assessing Acute and Chronic Pain

Pain is subjective; only the patient can describe what is occurring, and it can be both sensory and emotional. It is unpleasant and may or may not be associated with tissue damage. Pain is both complex and multifactorial. It involves sensory, emotional, and cognitive processing, but it can lack a specific physical etiology (Gordon, 2015).

Acute pain is usually associated with a physical cause and is triggered in the nervous system to alert the body to injury, disease, or inflammation. Acute pain arises quickly, can be severe, and is short-lived. This temporary, normal protective feature aids in preventing additional injury and resolves after treatment and healing takes place (Dahlhamer et al., 2018).

Chronic pain has different characteristics: it is not associated with cancer or other medical conditions that persist for more than 3 to 6 months; it lasts more than 1 month beyond the course of an acute illness or injury; and/or it recurs at intervals of months or years (Holleran, 2020; Peters et al., 2017;

Chronic pain may be a spectrum disorder related to mental health and somatic conditions. See Chapter 19, "Mental Status and Mental Health Assessment."

Walk & Poliak-Tunis, 2016). More than 40% of patients with chronic pain report that their pain is poorly controlled (National Institutes of Health, 2020). Pain affects more Americans than do cancer, heart disease, and diabetes combined (Gordon, 2015). In other words, chronic or persistent pain is ongoing, and it can affect every aspect of life.

Adopt a multidisciplinary measurement-based approach to assessing the patient's pain, carefully listening to the patient's description of the many features of pain and contributing factors. Pain is subjective, and only the patient can really tell you how severe it is. Use one of the multiple accepted screening tools available (Dehghani et al., 2014).

Onset

When did the pain begin? How? Does it occur at a specific time of day?

Location

Ask the patient to point to the pain, because lay terms may not be specific enough to localize the site of origin. Also ask about any radiation of the pain.

Duration

Is it constant? Does it come and go? Is it acute? Chronic? Persistent? Or is it breakthrough pain?

Characteristic Symptoms

Assessing the severity of the pain is especially important. Patient reporting is the underlying component of most pain assessments, of which there are many tools. Use a consistent method to determine severity, based on your practice site guidelines. The tool must be valid, reliable and sensitive for the first and subsequent interactions (Boitor et al., 2016). When using your current tool, ensure it is suitable for the individual patient especially if they have a sensory or cognitive deficit (Allred & Healy, 2020), are unable to express pain due to cultural practice or beliefs, or if they find it difficult to follow the tool due to educational level, language barrier, or other communication difference (Givler et al., 2020).

Samples of scales used in practice to assess pain severity include:

- *Visual analog scale (VAS):* A 110-mm long vertical or horizontal line; explain to the patient that each line stands for a degree of pain starting at one end on the left or on top with no pain and ending with severe pain on the far right or bottom. Ask the patient to point to the level of pain on the scale (McCaffery & Pasero, 1999).
- *Numeric rating scale (NRS):* Using a scale with 0 being no pain and 10 being the worst pain imaginable, a person notes their pain on the point scale (Wong & Baker, 1988).

- *Verbal pain rating scale:* Using verbalization on a scale to describe pain may include words like "no pain," "mild," "moderate," "severe," and "worst pain imaginable."

- *Combinations of pain scales include:* the Wong-Baker Faces Pain Scale (http://wongbakerfaces.org) used for children as well as patients with language barriers or cognitive impairment (Pain Assessment Screening Tool & Outcomes Registry [PASTOR], 2020) and the Defense & Veterans Pain Rating Scale (DVPRS) tool (Fig. 7-8), which is part of a larger chronic pain assessment called the PASTOR (Melzack, 2005). Each of these tools has a face for a person who is happy and does not have any pain, correlating with a 0 and progressing up the pain scale to a 10, which is unimaginable pain that hurts badly. Ask the patient to choose the face that correlates best to the pain (Melzack, 2005).

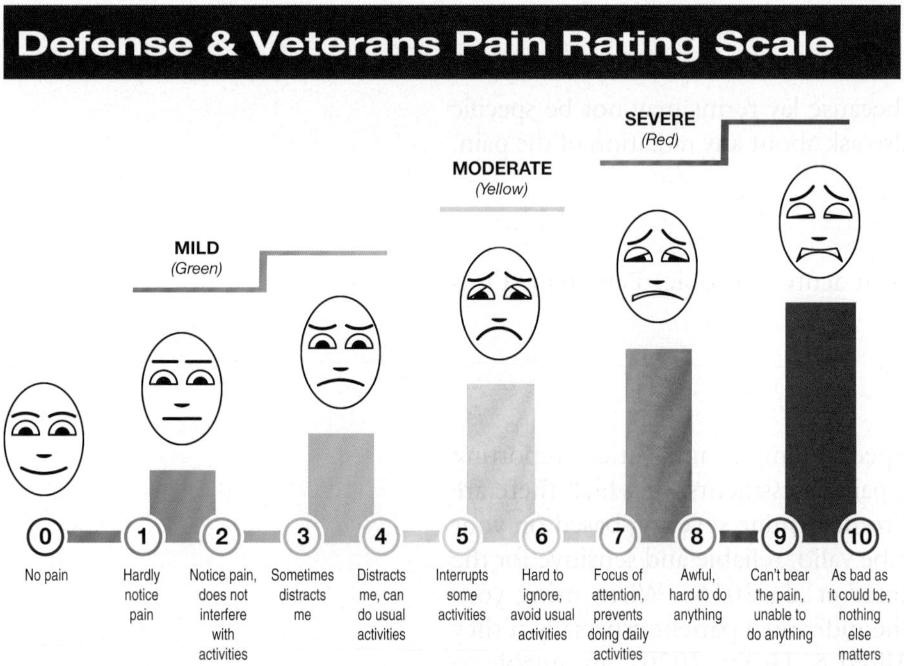

FIGURE 7-8 The DVPRS tool is an example of a combination pain scale. (Reprinted from Defense & Veterans Center for Integrative Pain Management; http://www.dvcipm.org.)

Multidimensional tools like the Brief Pain Inventory and the McGill Pain Questionnaire are also available; these take longer to administer but address the effects of pain on the patient's activity level (Nuckols et al., 2014).

Also ask the patient the following questions:

- Describe the pain. Is it sharp? Dull? Burning?

- Does it follow a particular pattern?

- Is it related to an injury or a particular movement? Stressful event?

Associated Manifestations

Does anything occur when you experience the pain? Nausea? Vomiting? Headaches? Burning? Itching?

Relieving Factors

What makes the pain better? Worse?

See Chapter 3, "Interviewing and Communication."

Treatments

Be sure to ask about any treatments that the patient has tried, including medications, physical therapy, and alternative medicines and if these were prescribed for them or if they are taking somebody else's prescription. A comprehensive medication history helps identify drugs that interact with analgesics and/or reduce their efficacy. It may also help identify misuse of drugs, including opioids (Dowell et al., 2016; Tsao et al., 2012).

Identify any comorbid conditions such as arthritis, diabetes, HIV/AIDS, substance abuse, sickle cell disease, or psychiatric disorders. These can have significant effects on the patient's experience of pain (Vergeld & Utesch, 2020).

Chronic pain is the leading cause of disability and impaired performance at work. Inquire about the effects of pain on the patient's daily activities, mood, sleep, work, and sexual activity.

Health Disparities

Be aware of the well-documented health disparities in pain treatment and delivery of care, which range from lower use of analgesics in emergency rooms for Black and Hispanic patients to disparities in the use of analgesics for cancer, postoperative, and low-back pain (Bateman & Carvalho, 2019). Studies show that clinician stereotypes, language barriers, and unconscious clinician biases in decision making all contribute to these disparities (Mainka et al., 2015). Critique your own communication style, be aware of nonverbal cues, seek information and best practice standards, and improve your techniques of patient education and empowerment as first steps in ensuring uniform and effective pain management.

See the Institute of Medicine report, *Relieving Pain in America: A Blueprint for Transforming Prevention, Care, Education, and Research* (Gordon, 2015).

CLINICAL TIP

Nonverbal cues may include wincing, sweating, protectiveness of painful area, facial grimacing, clutching a side rail, or unusual posture favoring one limb or body area.

Types of Pain

Be familiar with advances in the scientific understanding of pain processes. Review the summary of types of pain in Box 7-3 to aid in your understanding of caring for patients in pain.

BOX 7-3 TYPES OF PAIN

Nociceptive or somatic pain	Pain related to tissue damage is termed *nociceptive* or *somatic.* Nociceptive pain can be either acute and remitting or chronic and persistent. This form of pain is mediated by the afferent A-delta and C-fibers of the sensory system that respond to noxious stimuli and is modulated by both neurotransmitters and psychological processes. Modulating neurotransmitters include endorphins, histamines, acetylcholine, and monoamines like serotonin, norepinephrine, and dopamine. These afferent nociceptors can be sensitized by inflammatory mediators (Zhang & Bao, 2006).
Neuropathic pain	Pain resulting from direct injury to the peripheral or central nervous system is termed *neuropathic.* Over time, neuropathic pain may become independent of the inciting injury, become burning, lancinating, or shock-like in quality, persisting beyond healing from the initial injury. Mechanisms postulated to evoke neuropathic pain include central nervous system brain or spinal cord injury from stroke or trauma; peripheral nervous system disorders causing entrapment or pressure on spinal nerves, plexuses, or peripheral nerves; and referred pain syndromes with increased or prolonged pain responses to inciting stimuli. These triggers appear to induce changes in pain signal processing through "neuronal plasticity," leading to pain that persists beyond healing from the initial injury (Sullivan et al., 2016).
Psychogenic and idiopathic pain	*Psychogenic pain* relates to the many factors that influence the patient's report of pain; these can include psychiatric conditions like anxiety or depression, personality and coping style, cultural norms, and social support systems. *Idiopathic pain* is pain without an identifiable etiology.

Pain Management

Management of pain is complex and can be challenging. Treatment of pain requires sophisticated knowledge of nonopioid, opioid, and adjuvant analgesics and modalities of behavioral and physical therapy, which are beyond the scope of this book. More recently, health care providers have become more attentive to the care and management of patients who experience chronic pain. Nurses may be reluctant to administer narcotics because of fear of inducing addiction. Use of validated screening tools for opioid use disorder assessment in patients with pain and an awareness of one's own perspective and biases in regard to pain control are important (O'Brien & Dodd, 2020; Wald & Garber, 2018).

When evaluating the efficacy of treatment, focus on the four As to monitor patient outcomes:

- Analgesia
- Activities of daily living
- Adverse effects
- Aberrant drug-related behaviors

RECORDING YOUR FINDINGS

The documentation of the physical examination begins with a general description of the patient's appearance based on the general survey. As a novice practitioner, you may initially use sentences to describe your findings. As you progress in your practice, you will use the boxes provided in the electronic health record in conjunction with phrases in the comment boxes. The style in the case study contains phrases appropriate for most write-ups.

Choose vivid and graphic adjectives, as if you are painting a picture in words. Avoid clichés such as "well developed" or "well nourished" or "in no acute distress," because these are nondescript and could apply to any patient. You want to convey the special features of the individual patient.

Record the vital signs taken at the time of the examination. They are preferable to those taken earlier in the day by other providers.

CASE STUDY

Recording the Physical Examination—The General Survey and Vital Signs

"Mrs. Mary Scott, a 36-year-old woman, well groomed, fit, and cheerful. Height 5′6″, weight 140 lb, T 37.5°C oral, P 72 and regular, R 16 even, BP 120/80 R arm sitting, 118/76 L arm sitting."

or

"Mr. Edward Jones, an 82-year-old man who looks pale and chronically ill. He is alert and maintaining eye contact but unable to speak more than two or three words at a time due to shortness of breath. He has intercostal muscle retraction when breathing and sits upright in bed. He is thin, with diffuse muscle wasting. Height 6′0″, weight 157 lb, T 101.2°F tympanic, P 108 and irregular, R 32 shallow/labored, BP 160/95 R arm sitting."

Suggests exacerbation of COPD.

HEALTH PROMOTION AND COUNSELING

Blood Pressure

Monitoring a patient's blood pressure at home may be necessary, and it is important for the nurse to verify that it is correctly done. If a manual blood pressure is measured, it is important to assess the environment for noise levels to ensure the reading is taken in a quiet room. Check to ensure the correct cuff size is available and the person is able to apply the cuff or has a caregiver who is able to correctly place the cuff. Generating a list of approved electronic instruments or sphygmomanometers for home testing is helpful, and those covered by insurance should be included. Home sphygmomanometers should be checked periodically for accuracy by simultaneously taking and comparing the readings with an office or clinic sphygmomanometer (Picone et al., 2020).

Everyone should be aware of their baseline vital signs. Notifying a health care provider of deviations is important, especially for patients who are monitoring blood pressure for a specific reason. Documentation of vital signs along with associated symptoms that occur at that time, for example, shortness of breath while walking up a flight of stairs, can be recorded in a journal or tracked using a smart phone.

Pulse

A patient taking certain cardiac medications will need to take their own pulse rate prior to taking the medication and be aware of potential side effects. They need to know at what parameters to hold the medication and when to call the health care provider. Also, patients should take a pulse rate prior to and after exercise to determine the reaction to exercise.

Teach patients how to check *one* carotid pulse by lightly placing two to three fingers on the site and counting for 1 minute. Recording the rate, rhythm, and depth is important after the assessment.

Respirations

Explain to the person assessing the respirations at home that this includes a full inspiration and a full expiration for a full minute, which is measured with a watch with a second hand. Recording the rate, rhythm, and depth is important after the assessment.

Temperature

Educate patients or their caregivers on how to correctly take a temperature, the normal ranges, and when to notify a health care provider. Review the various routes and instruments necessary and have them demonstrate the skill.

Patients should be aware of the risk factors for heatstroke, such as excessive exercise in hot, humid weather conditions; poor ventilation on hot days; decreased fluid intake; and sudden exposure to hot climates. Patients also need to be aware of the risk factors for hypothermia when there is prolonged exposure to cold temperatures. Thermometers generally used to measure fevers will not register temperatures as low as hypothermia (core 95°F [35°C]).

Bibliography

CITATIONS

Aladin, A. I., Whelton, S. P., Al-Mallah, M. H., Blaha, M. J., Keteyian, S. J., Juraschek, S. P., Rubin, J., Brawner, C. A., & Michos, E. D. (2014). Relation of resting heart rate to risk for all-cause mortality by gender after considering exercise capacity (the Henry Ford exercise testing project). *American Journal of Cardiology, 114*(11), 1701–1706. https://doi.org/10.1016/j.amjcard.2014.08.042

Allred, K., & Healy, P. (2020). R7 perceptions of behavioral pain assessment tools and pain outcomes in non-verbal patients: A pilot survey. *Pain Management Nursing, 21*(2), 220. https://doi.org/10.1016/j.pmn.2020.02.061

American Heart Association. (2020). My Life Check | Life's Simple 7. Retrieved June 10, 2020, from https://www.heart.org/en/healthy-living/healthy-lifestyle/my-life-check–lifes-simple-7

Bateman, B. T., & Carvalho, B. (2019). Addressing racial and ethnic disparities in pain management in the midst of the opioid crisis. *Obstetrics and Gynecology, 134*(6), 1144–1146. https://doi.org/10.1097/AOG.0000000000003590

Boitor, M., Fiola, J. L., & Gélinas, C. (2016). Validation of the critical-care pain observation tool and vital signs in relation to the sensory and affective components of pain during mediastinal tube removal in postoperative cardiac surgery intensive care unit adults. *Journal of Cardiovascular Nursing, 31*(5), 425–432. https://doi.org/10.1097/JCN.0000000000000250

Bunkenborg, G., Poulsen, I., Samuelson, K., Ladelund, S., & Åkeson, J. (2016). Mandatory early warning scoring–implementation evaluated with a mixed-methods approach. *Applied Nursing Research, 29*, 168–176. https://doi.org/10.1016/j.apnr.2015.06.012

Cardona-Morrell, M., Prgomet, M., Turner, R. M., Nicholson, M., & Hillman, K. (2016). Effectiveness of continuous or intermittent vital signs monitoring in preventing adverse events on general wards: a systematic review and meta-analysis. *International Journal of Clinical Practice, 70*(10), 806–824. https://doi.org/10.1111/ijcp.12846

Centers for Disease Control and Prevention (CDC). (2020a). Facts about hypertension. Retrieved June 10, 2020, from https://www.cdc.gov/bloodpressure/facts.htm.

Centers for Disease Control and Prevention (CDC). (2020b). Social determinants of health. Retrieved June 8, 2020, from https://www.cdc.gov/socialdeterminants/index.htm

Dahlhamer, J., Lucas, J., Zelaya, C., Nahin, R., Mackey, S., DeBar, L., Kerns, R., Von Korff, M., Porter, L., & Helmick, C. (2018). Prevalence of chronic pain and high-impact chronic pain among adults—United States, 2016. *Morbidity and Mortality Weekly Report, 67*(36), 1001–1006. https://doi.org/10.15585/mmwr.mm6736a2

Dehghani, H., Tavangar, H., & Ghandehari, A. (2014). Validity and reliability of behavioral pain scale in patients with low level of consciousness due to head trauma hospitalized in intensive care unit. *Archives of Trauma Research, 3*(1), e18608. https://doi.org/10.5812/atr.18608

Dowell, D., Haegerich, T. M., & Chou, R. (2016). CDC Guideline for Prescribing Opioids for Chronic Pain–United States, 2016. *JAMA, 315*(15), 1624–1645. https://doi.org/10.1001/jama.2016.1464

Geerse, C., van Slobbe, C., van Triet, E., & Simonse, L. (2019). Design of a care pathway for preventive blood pressure monitoring: Qualitative study. *JMIR Cardio, 3*(1), e13048. https://doi.org/10.2196/13048

Givler, A., Bhatt, H., & Maani-Fogelman, P. A. (2020). The importance of cultural competence in pain and palliative care. [Updated 2020 June 1]. In: *StatPearls [Internet]*. StatPearls Publishing. https://www.ncbi.nlm.nih.gov/books/NBK493154/

Gordon, D. B. (2015). Acute pain assessment tools: Let us move beyond simple pain ratings. *Current Opinion Anaesthesiology, 28*(5), 565–569. https://doi.org/10.1097/ACO.0000000000000225

Hahn, R., Truman, B., & Williams, D. (2018). Civil rights as determinants of public health and racial and ethnic health equity: Health care, education, employment, and housing in the United States. *Population Health, 4*, 17–24. https://doi.org/10.1016/j.ssmph.2017.10.006

Holleran, R. (2020). 3D Managing Chronic Pain the ED. *Pain Management Nursing, 21*(2), 211. https://doi.org/ 10.1016/j.pmn.2020.02.025

Institute of Medicine. (2011). Committee on Advancing Pain Research, Care, and Education. Relieving Pain in America: A Blueprint for Transforming Prevention, Care, Education, and Research. National Academies Press.

Johansson, A. (2019). Core temperature-The intraoperative difference between esophageal versus nasopharyngeal temperatures and the impact of prewarming, age, and weight. *Aana Journal, 87*(1), 6.

Jordan, J., Ricci, F., Hoffmann, F., Hamrefors, V., & Fedorowski, A. (2020). Orthostatic hypertension: Critical appraisal of an overlooked condition. *Hypertension, 75*(5), 1151–1158. https://doi.org/10.1161/HYPERTENSIONAHA.120.14340

Kallioinen, N., Hill, A., Horswill, M. S., Ward, H. E., & Watson, M. O. (2017). Sources of inaccuracy in the measurement of adult patients' resting blood pressure in clinical settings: a systematic review. *Journal of Hypertension, 35*(3), 421–441. https://doi.org/10.1097/HJH.0000000000001197

Kohlman-Trigoboff, D. (2015). The missing vital sign: The significance of bilateral arm blood pressures. *Journal of Vascular Nursing, 33*(3), 127–130. https://doi.org/10.1016/j.jvn.2015.06.003

Lambe, K., Currey, J., & Considine, J. (2017). Emergency nurses' decisions regarding frequency and nature of vital sign assessment. *Journal of Clinical Nursing, 26*(13–14), 1949–1959. https://doi.org/10.1111/jocn.13597

Levy, N., Sturgess, J., & Mills, P. (2018). "Pain as the fifth vital sign" and dependence on the "numerical pain scale" is being abandoned in the US: Why? *British Journal of Anaesthesia, 120*(3), 435–438. https://doi.org/10.1016/j.bja.2017.11.098

Lin, T. T., Wang, C. L., Liao, M. T., & Lai, C. L. (2018). Agreement between automated and human measurements of heart rate in patients with atrial fibrillation. *Journal of Cardiovascular Nursing, 33*(5), 492–499. https://doi.org/10.1097/JCN.0000000000000486

Liu, C., Griffiths, C., Murray, A., & Zheng, D. (2016). Comparison of stethoscope bell and diaphragm, and of stethoscope tube length, for clinical blood pressure measurement. *Blood Pressure Monitoring, 21*(3), 178–183. https://doi.org/10.1097/MBP.0000000000000175

Mainka, T., Maier, C., & Enax-Krumova, E. K. (2015). Neuropathic pain assessment: update on laboratory diagnostic tools. *Current Opinion Anaesthesiology, 28*(5), 537–545. https://doi.org/10.1097/ACO.0000000000000223

McCaffery, M., & Pasero, C. (1999). *Pain: Clinical Manual.* Mosby; 16.

Melzack, R. (2005). The McGill pain questionnaire: from description to measurement. *Anesthesiology, 103*(1), 199–202. https://doi.org/10.1097/00000542-200507000-00028

Metzler, M., Duerr, S., Granata, R., Krismer, F., Robertson, D., & Wenning, G. K. (2013). Neurogenic orthostatic hypotension: pathophysiology, evaluation, and management. *Journal of Neurology, 260*(9), 2212–2219. https://doi.org/10.1007/s00415-012-6736-7

Montrivade, S., Chattranukulchai, P., Siwamogsatham, S., Vorasettakarnkij, Y., Naeowong, W., Boonchayaanant, P., Sakulsupsiri, A., Ariyachaipanich, A., Lertsuwunseri, V., Rungpradubvong, V., Satitthummanid, S., Puwanant, S., Prechawat, S., Srimahachota, S., Chaipromprasit, J., Buddhari, W., Boonyaratavej, S., Sitthisook, S., Buranakitjaroen, P., … Sangwatanaroj, S. (2020). Hypertension subtypes among Thai hypertensives: An analysis of Telehealth-assisted instrument in home blood pressure monitoring Nationwide Pilot Project. *International Journal of Hypertension, 2020*, 3261408. https://doi.org/10.1155/2020/3261408

Muntner, P., Shimbo, D., Carey, R. M., Charleston, J. B., Gaillard, T., Misra, S., Myers, M. G., Ogedegbe, G., Schwartz, J. E., Townsend, R. R., Urbina, E. M., Viera, A. J., White, W. B., & Wright, J. T., Jr. (2019). Measurement of blood pressure in humans: A scientific statement from the American Heart Association. *Hypertension, 73*(5), e35–e66. https://doi.org/10.1161/HYP.0000000000000087

Myers, M. G., Asmar, R., & Staessen, J. A. (2018). Office blood pressure measurement in the 21st century. *Journal of Clinical Hypertension (Greenwich, Conn.), 20*(7), 1104–1107. https://doi.org/10.1111/jch.13276

National Institutes of Health. Pain Management. (2020). Research Portfolio Online Reporting Tools (RePORT). Retrieved March 13, 2021, from https://report.nih.gov/

Nuckols, T. K., Anderson, L., Popescu, I., Diamant, A. L., Doyle, B., Capua, P. Di., & Chou, R. (2014). Opioid prescribing: a systematic review and critical appraisal of guidelines for chronic pain. *Annals of Internal Medicine, 160*(1), 38–47. https://doi.org/10.7326/0003-4819-160-1-201401070-00732

O'Brien, M., & Dodd, P. (2020). 1E Improving the image of pain care through advanced nursing practice. *Pain Management Nursing, 21*(2), 210. https://doi.org/10.1016/j.pmn.2020.02.017

O'Brien, P., & Marshall, A. C. (2015). Coarctation of the aorta. *Circulation, 131*(9), e363–e365. https://doi.org/10.1161/CIRCULATIONAHA.114.008821

Pain Assessment Screening Tool and Outcomes Registry (PASTOR). (2020). Defense & veterans center for integrative pain management. Retrieved June 12, 2020, from http://www.dvcipm.org/clinical-resources/pain-assessment-screening-tool-and-outcomes-registry-pastor

Pan, F., He, P., Liu, C., Li, T., Murray, A., & Zheng, D. (2017). Variation of the Korotkoff stethoscope sounds during blood pressure measurement: analysis using a convolutional neural network. *IEEE J Biomed Health Inform, 21*(6), 1593–1598. https://doi.org/10.1109/JBHI.2017.2703115

Pappaccogli, M., Di Monaco, S., Perlo, E., Burrello, J., D'Ascenzo, F., Veglio, F., Monticone, S., & Rabbia, F. (2019). Comparison of automated office blood pressure with office and out-off-office measurement techniques. *Hypertension, 73*(2), 481–490. https://doi.org/10.1161/HYPERTENSIONAHA.118.12079

Peters, M. L., Smeets, E., Feijge, M., van Breukelen, G., Andersson, G., Buhrman, M., & Linton, S. J. (2017). Happy despite pain: A Randomized controlled trial of an 8-week internet-delivered positive psychology intervention for enhancing well-being in patients with chronic pain. *Clinical Journal of Pain, 33*(11), 962–975. https://doi.org/10.1097/AJP.0000000000000494

Picone, D. S., Deshpande, R. A., Schultz, M. G., Fonseca, R., Campbell, N. R., Delles, C., Hecht Olsen, M., Schutte, A. E., Stergiou, G., Padwal, R., Zhang, X., & Sharman, J. E. (2020). Nonvalidated home blood pressure devices dominate the online marketplace in Australia. *Hypertension, 75*(6), 1593–1599. https://doi.org/10.1161/HYPERTENSIONAHA.120.14719

Reboussin, D. M., Allen, N. B., Griswold, M. E., Guallar, E., Hong, Y., Lackland, D. T., MillerIII, E. R., Polonsky, T., Thompson-Paul, A. M., & Vupputuri, S. (2018). 2017 ACC/AHA/AAPA/ABC/ACPM/AGS/ APhA/ASH/ASPC/NMA/PCNA Guideline for the Prevention, Detection, Evaluation, and Management of High Blood Pressure in Adults American College of Cardiology Foundation and American Heart Association, Inc. Retrieved June 10, 2020, from https://healthmetrics.heart.org/wp-content/uploads/2017/11/2017-Guideline-for-the-Prevention-Detection-Evaluation-and-Management-of-High-Blood-Pressure-in-Adults-Slide-Set.pdf

Roerecke, M., Kaczorowski, J., & Myers, M. G. (2019). Comparing automated office blood pressure readings with other methods of blood pressure measurement for identifying patients with possible hypertension: A systematic review and meta-analysis. *JAMA Internal Medicine, 179*(3), 351–362. https://doi.org/10.1001/jamainternmed.2018.6551

Sapra, A., Malik, A., & Bhandari, P. (2020). Vital sign assessment. In: *StatPearls*. StatPearls Publishing.

Saugel, B., Dueck, R., & Wagner, J. Y. (2014). Measurement of blood pressure. *Best Practice & Research. Clinical Anaesthesiology, 28*(4), 309–322. https://doi.org/10.1016/j.bpa.2014.08.001

Spångfors, M., Bunkenborg, G., Molt, M., & Samuelson, K. (2019). The National Early Warning Score predicts mortality in hospital ward patients with deviating vital signs: A retrospective medical record review study. *Journal of Clinical Nursing, 28*(7–8), 1216–1222. https://doi.org/10.1111/jocn.14728

Sullivan, D., Lyons, M., Montgomery, R., & Quinlan-Colwell, A. (2016). Exploring opioid-sparing multimodal analgesia options in trauma: A Nursing perspective. *Journal of Trauma Nursing*, *23*(6), 361–375. https://doi.org/10.1097/JTN.0000000000000250

Temporal artery thermometer: exergen instructions for use. (2020). Exergen manual. Retrieved June 11, 2020, from www.exergen.com/medical/PDFs/tat2000cmanual.pdf.

Tsao, J. C., Plankey, M. W., & Young, M. A. (2012). Pain, psychological symptoms and prescription drug misuse in HIV: A literature review. *Journal of Pain Management*, *5*(2), 111–118.

Vergeld, V., & Utesch, T. (2020). Pain-related self-efficacy among people with back pain: A systematic review of assessment tools. *Clinical Journal of Pain*, *36*(6), 480–494. https://doi.org/10.1097/AJP.0000000000000818

Vischer, A. S., & Burkard, T. (2017). Principles of blood pressure measurement—Current techniques, office vs ambulatory blood pressure measurement. *Advances in Experimental Medicine and Biology*, *956*, 85–96. https://doi.org/10.1007/5584_2016_49

Wald, A., & Garber, C. E. (2018). A review of current literature on vital sign assessment of physical activity in primary care. *Journal of Nursing Scholarship*, *50*(1), 65–73. https://doi.org/10.1111/jnu.12351

Walk, D., & Poliak-Tunis, M. (2016). Chronic pain management: An overview of taxonomy, conditions commonly encountered, and assessment. *Medical Clinics of North America*, *100*(1), 1–16. https://doi.org/10.1016/j.mcna.2015.09.005

Whelton, P. K., Carey, R. M., Aronow, W. S., Charleston, J. B., Gaillard, T., Misra, S., Myers, M. G., Ogedegbe, G., Schwartz, J. E., Townsend, R. R., Urbina, E. M., Viera, A. J., White, W. B., & Wright, J. T., Jr. (2018). 2017 ACC/AHA/AAPA/ABC/ACPM/AGS/APhA/ASH/ASPC/NMA/PCNA Guideline for the Prevention, Detection, Evaluation, and Management of High Blood Pressure in Adults: A Report of the American College of Cardiology/American Heart Association Task Force on Clinical Practice Guidelines. *Journal of the American College of Cardiology*, *71*(19), e127–e248. https://doi.org/10.1016/j.jacc.2017.11.006

Wohlfahrt, P., Cífková, R., Kraj oviechová, A., Šulc, P., Bruthans, J., Linhart, A., Filipovský, J., Mayer, O., & Widimský, J., Jr. (2020). Comparison of three office blood pressure measurement techniques and their effect on hypertension prevalence in the general population. *Journal of Hypertension*, *38*(4), 656–662. https://doi.org/10.1097/HJH.0000000000002322

Wong, D. L., & Baker, C. M. (1988). Pain in children: comparison of assessment scales. *Pediatric Nursing*, *14*(1), 9–17.

Yano, Y., Stamler, J., Garside, D. B., Daviglus, M. L., Franklin, S. S., Carnethon, M. R., Liu, K., Greenland, P., & Lloyd-Jones, D. M. (2015). Isolated systolic hypertension in young and middle-aged adults and 31-year risk for cardiovascular mortality: the Chicago Heart Association Detection Project in Industry study. *Journal of the American College of Cardiology*, *65*(4), 327–335. https://doi.org/10.1016/j.jacc.2014.10.060

Zhang, X., & Bao, L. (2006). The development and modulation of nociceptive circuitry. *Current Opinion in Neurobiology*, *16*(4), 460–466. https://doi.org/10.1016/j.conb.2006.06.002

8 NUTRITION AND HYDRATION

KEY TERMS

body mass index (BMI) nutritional status stadiometers

Learning Objectives

The student will:

1. Assess the nutritional status of an individual through a nutrition history and physical examination.
2. Identify individuals at risk for malnutrition or overnutrition.
3. Differentiate between normal and abnormal nutrition assessment findings.
4. Identify individuals with dehydration or overhydration.
5. Provide nutrition and exercise counseling to maintain or improve patients' health.

Nutritional status is a key element of overall health. Good nutrition is important for every body system. Poor nutrition may be a problem in itself (e.g., lack of vitamin D can cause rickets), or it may exacerbate an underlying disease, such as diabetes or cardiovascular disease. Low protein reserves will impede healing (e.g., from surgery). Poor nutrition in children may delay growth and contribute to cognitive issues in school. Problems with nutrition may be the result of many factors.

Weight gain occurs when caloric intake exceeds caloric expenditure over time and typically appears as increased body fat. Hypothyroidism may cause weight gain by reducing body metabolism. Weight gain may also reflect abnormal accumulation of body fluids. When the retention of fluid is mild, the fluid may not be visible, but several pounds of fluid may indicate edema.

Weight loss is an important symptom with many causes. Mechanisms include decreased intake of food for such reasons as anorexia (lack or loss of appetite for food), dysphagia (difficulty or discomfort in swallowing), vomiting, diarrhea, inability to absorb nutrients from the gastrointestinal tract, increased metabolic needs, allergies to foods, problems with chewing, dislike of foods, and/or peer pressure. Poor food choices, inability to cook or poor cooking habits, lack of access to food stores, or lack of financial resources may also cause nutrition problems. The nurse sorts through the data the patient provides to identify underlying issues and creates a plan of care. If the nurse finds the patient needs more testing or intense counseling, the patient should be referred to a nurse practitioner, physician, or registered dietician. Table 8-1 outlines the eating disorders anorexia nervosa, bulimia nervosa, and binge eating disorder.

Causes of weight loss include gastrointestinal diseases; endocrine disorders (diabetes mellitus, hyperthyroidism, adrenal insufficiency); chronic infections; malignancy; chronic cardiac, pulmonary, or renal failure; depression; and anorexia nervosa (see Table 8-1).

TABLE 8-1 Clinical Features of Eating Disorders

It is difficult to determine the specific number of people who experience eating disorders since many people do not seek treatment. These severe disturbances are often difficult to detect, especially in teens wearing baggy clothes or in individuals who binge and then induce vomiting or evacuation. Current research suggests that a genetic–environmental interaction may contribute to the development of eating disorders. It is important to be familiar with the three principal eating disorders—anorexia nervosa, bulimia nervosa, and binge eating disorder. These conditions are characterized by distorted perceptions of body image and weight. Early detection is important, because prognosis improves when treatment occurs in the early stages of these disorders.

Anorexia Nervosa	Bulimia Nervosa	Binge Eating Disorder

• Restricted calories with significantly low BMI
• Terror of gaining weight, viewing self as fat even when emaciated
• Frequently starving but in denial; lacking insight
• Often brought in by family members
• Initial symptoms may be failure to make expected weight gains in childhood or adolescence, amenorrhea in women, loss of libido or potency in men.
• Additional features supporting diagnosis: self-induced vomiting or purging, excessive exercise, and use of appetite suppressants and/or diuretics
• Comorbidities include: major depressive disorder, bipolar disorder, anxiety disorders, and substance abuse disorders
• Biologic or medical complications:
  • *Skin:* hair loss, Russell sign, lanugo, yellowing
  • *Endocrine:* amenorrhea, hypercortisolemia, hypoglycemia, osteoporosis, euthyroid hypothyroxinemia
• *Cardiovascular disorders:* bradycardia, tachycardia, hypotension, arrhythmias, cardiomyopathy, electrocardiogram changes
• *Fluid/electrolyte:* dehydration, hypokalemia, hypochloremia, acidosis/alkalosis, hypomagnesia, increased blood urea nitrogen
	• Repeated binge eating followed by the use of inappropriate compensatory behavior to prevent weight gain, including self-induced vomiting; misuse of laxatives, diuretics, or other medications; fasting; and/or excessive exercise
	• Level of severity is based on the number of inappropriate compensatory behaviors
	• Often occurs with normal weight
	• Overeating at least once a week during a 3-mo period; large amounts of food consumed in short period (approximately 2 h)
	• Preoccupation with eating; craving and compulsion to eat; lack of control over eating; alternating with periods of starvation
	• Dread of fatness but may be obese
	• Comorbidities include major depressive disorder, bipolar disorder, and substance abuse disorders
	• Triggers for binging may include stress, poor self-image, and restricted dieting.
	• Biologic complications:
	  • *Skin:* hair loss, Russell sign
	  • *Endocrine:* None reported
	  • *Cardiovascular disorders:* hypotension, tachycardia, arrhythmias, electrocardiogram changes, cardiomyopathy
	  • *Fluid/electrolyte:* dehydration, hypokalemia, hypochloremia, acidosis/alkalosis
		• Binge eating disorder is the most common eating disorder.
		• Repeated binge eating episodes during which a person feels a loss of control and marked distress over his or her eating
		• Unlike bulimia nervosa, binge eating episodes are not followed by purging, excessive exercise, or fasting.
		• Usually overweight or obese
		• Eating unusually large amounts of food in a specific amount of time, such as a 2-h period
		• Eating even when full or not hungry
		• Eating quickly during binge episodes
		• Eating until uncomfortably full
		• Eating alone or in secret to avoid embarrassment
		• Feeling distressed, ashamed, or guilty about eating patterns
		• Frequently dieting, possibly without weight loss
		• Gastrointestinal complications:
		  • Constipation
		  • Stomach cramps
		  • Acid reflux
		  • Stomach rupture

(continued)

TABLE 8-1 Clinical Features of Eating Disorders (*Continued*)

Anorexia Nervosa	Bulimia Nervosa	Binge Eating Disorder
• *Musculoskeletal:* muscle wasting, osteoporosis, osteopenia, fracture risk • *Gastrointestinal:* constipation, diarrhea, esophageal rupture, dental enamel erosion, gastric dilation or rupture, esophageal rupture • *Other:* Weakness, cachexia	• *Musculoskeletal:* osteopenia • *Gastrointestinal:* acid reflux disorder, pancreatitis, parotid gland swelling, erosion of dental enamel, sensitive teeth with increased decay, inflamed sore throat, intestinal distress from laxative abuse • *Other:* weakness, fatigue	

Sources: NIH & National Institute of Mental Health. Eating disorders. Retrieved July 10, 2020, from https://www.nimh.nih.gov/health/topics/eating-disorders/index.shtml; National Eating Disorder Association. Binge eating disorder. Retrieved July 10, 2020, from https://www.nationaleatingdisorders.org/learn/by-eating-disorder/bed; NIH & Medline Plus. Eating disorders. Retrieved July 10, 2020, from https://medlineplus.gov/eatingdisorders.html#cat_79; Psychiatric Association. (2013). *DSM-5: Diagnostic and statistical manual of mental disorders* (5th ed.). American Psychiatric Association; Halter, M. J. (2018). *Varcarolis' foundations of psychiatric-mental health nursing* (8th ed.). Elsevier.

Severe vitamin or mineral deficiencies or lack of protein, carbohydrates, or fats will produce characteristic signs and symptoms. However, it is preferred to recognize the potential deficiency in the patient's diet before signs and symptoms occur. For example, when a patient reports lactose intolerance, the nurse should assess the diet for adequate intake of calcium and vitamin D through nonmilk foods and supplements before signs of rickets develop.

CLINICAL TIP

Weight loss with relatively high food intake suggests *diabetes mellitus, hyperthyroidism,* or *malabsorption.* Also consider binge eating (bulimia) with clandestine vomiting.

Nutritional status is assessed at most nurse–patient encounters. A general screening assessment is done during a complete health assessment. If the patient's chief complaint involves nutrition or if the general screening finds unusual results, an in-depth nutrition assessment should be done. Patients admitted to long-term care facilities and patients with problems that require good nutrition to heal, such as pressure injuries, should be thoroughly assessed. The U.S. Department of Agriculture's (USDA) *ChooseMyPlate* website (www.choosemyplate.gov) is a tool to help individuals analyze their diets and set goals for healthier diets. The nurse can use the site with a patient to demonstrate how to perform a diet analysis and track individual progress. The website includes nutrition tips, nutrition information for various populations, print materials, interactive tools, and links to other nutrient and physical activity information.

Poverty, old age, social isolation, physical disability, emotional or mental impairment, lack of teeth, ill-fitting dentures, alcoholism, and drug abuse increase the likelihood of malnutrition.

For tools for assessing the older adult, see Figures 8-1 and 8-2 and the Mini Nutritional Assessment (MNA) in Chapter 24, "Assessing Older Adults."

Figures 8-1 and 8-2 show two screening tools to identify individuals at risk for nutritional deficits.

Nutrition Screening Checklist		
I have an illness or condition that made me change the kind and/or amount of food I eat.	Yes (2 pts)	________
I eat fewer than two meals per day.	Yes (3 pts)	________
I eat few fruits or vegetables, or milk products.	Yes (2 pts)	________
I have three or more drinks of beer, liquor, or wine almost every day.	Yes (2 pts)	________
I have tooth or mouth problems that make it hard for me to eat.	Yes (2 pts)	________
I don't always have enough money to buy the food I need.	Yes (4 pts)	________
I eat alone most of the time.	Yes (1 pt)	________
I take three or more different prescribed or over-the-counter drugs each day.	Yes (1 pt)	________
Without wanting to, I have lost or gained 10 lb in the last 6 months.	Yes (2 pts)	________
I am not always physically able to shop, cook, and/or feed myself.	Yes (2 pts)	________
	TOTAL	________
Instructions. Check "yes" for each condition that applies, then total the nutritional score. For total scores of 3-5 points (moderate risk) or 6 points or more (high risk), further evaluation is needed (especially for older adults).		

FIGURE 8-1 The American Academy of Family Physicians nutrition screening checklist. (Adapted from Nutrition Screening—American Academy of Family Physicians. Bagley B. (1998). Nutrition and health. *American Academy of Family Physicians*, *57*(5), 933–934. Retrieved June 30, 2020, from http://www.aafp.org/afp/980301ap/edits.html)

Dietary Intake Screening		
	Portions Consumed by Patient	**Recommended per day**
Vegetables		2 ½ c
Fruits		2 c
Grains, cereals, bread group		6 oz
Dairy group		3 c-eq
Meat/meat substitute group (protein foods)		5 ½ oz
Sugars, fats, snack foods		—
Soft drinks		—
Alcoholic beverages		Men ≤ 2 Women ≤ 1
Instructions. Ask the patient for a 24-hour dietary recall (or a 2-day dietary intake) before completing the form.		

FIGURE 8-2 A dietary intake screening tool. (Adapted from 2020–2025 Dietary Guidelines for Americans. https://www.dietaryguidelines.gov/resources/2020-2025-dietary-guidelines-online-materials)

Hydration status is critical to every patient's health. Underhydration or overhydration may accompany disease, medical treatment, and environmental conditions. The patient can die or suffer serious complications if alterations in hydration are not recognized immediately. It is the nurse who most closely monitors the patient's hydration status. Conditions that contribute to dehydration include exposure to excessive heat, exercise in heat, decreased mobility, inability to drink (e.g., a patient who is comatose), medications such as diuretics, vomiting and/or diarrhea, burn injuries, and hemorrhage. Conditions that contribute to overhydration include heart failure, kidney failure, liver disease, increased sodium intake, and excess intravenous fluid.

Signs and symptoms of hydration and nutrition problems are reflected in multiple body systems, including the integumentary, respiratory, cardiovascular, peripheral vascular, gastrointestinal, and musculoskeletal systems. As you read the body system chapters, note the signs and symptoms of nutrition or hydration deficits or excess. For summaries of the signs and symptoms of nutrition and hydration disorders, see the section "Evaluating Nutritional Disorders" and Box 8-1, "Assessment of Dehydration and Overhydration."

BOX 8-1 ASSESSMENT OF DEHYDRATION AND OVERHYDRATION

Dehydration: Deficient Fluid Volume

- Symptoms
  - Thirst
  - Diaphoresis
  - Vomiting/diarrhea
- Signs
  - Short-term weight loss
  - Dry mucous membranes/eyes
  - Sunken eyes
  - Decreased skin turgor
  - Fever
  - Decreased blood pressure and pulse pressure
  - Increased pulse rate and decreased pulse amplitude
  - Decreased urine output and increased specific gravity
  - Decrease in venous filling
  - Alteration in mental status
  - Weakness
- Contributing factors
  - Exposure to excessive heat
  - Exercise in heat
  - Decreased mobility
  - Inability to drink
  - Older age
  - Medications—diuretics
  - Burns
  - Hemorrhage
  - Vomiting/diarrhea
  - Fever

Overhydration: Excess Fluid Volume

- Signs
  - Short-term weight gain
  - Edema
  - Increased blood pressure
  - Decreased or bounding pulse
  - Jugular vein distention
  - S_3 heart sound
  - Fine crackles in lungs
  - Dyspnea
  - Alteration in mental status
  - Urine output and urine-specific gravity may be decreased or increased depending on diagnosis
- Contributing factors
  - Heart failure
  - Kidney failure
  - Liver disease
  - Increased sodium intake
  - Intravenous fluid overload

EVALUATING NUTRITIONAL DISORDERS

Table 8-2 can help you interpret your nutritional assessment findings. Each body system is listed with signs and symptoms of nutritional concerns and the implications for each.

TABLE 8-2 Nutritional Concerns by Body System

Body System or Region	Sign or Symptom	Implications
General	Weakness and fatigue	Anemia or electrolyte imbalance
	Weight loss	Decreased calorie intake, increased calorie use, or inadequate nutrient intake or absorption
Skin, hair, and nails	Dry, flaky skin	Vitamin A, vitamin B complex, or linoleic acid deficiency
	Dry skin with poor turgor	Dehydration
	Rough, scaly skin with bumps	Vitamin A deficiency
	Petechiae or ecchymoses	Vitamin C or K deficiency
	Sore that will not heal	Protein, vitamin C, or zinc deficiency
	Thinning, dry hair	Protein deficiency
	Spoon-shaped, brittle, or ridged nails	Iron deficiency
Eyes	Night blindness; corneal swelling, softening, or dryness; Bitot spots (gray triangular patches on the conjunctiva)	Vitamin A deficiency
	Red conjunctiva	Riboflavin deficiency
Throat and mouth	Cracks at the corner of the mouth	Riboflavin or niacin deficiency
	Magenta tongue	Riboflavin deficiency
	Beefy, red tongue	Vitamin B_{12} deficiency
	Soft, spongy, bleeding gums	Vitamin C and K deficiencies
	Swollen neck (goiter)	Iodine deficiency
Cardiovascular	Edema	Protein deficiency
	Tachycardia, hypotension	Fluid volume deficit
Gastrointestinal	Ascites (accumulation of fluid in the peritoneal cavity)	Protein deficiency
Musculoskeletal	Bone pain and bow leg	Vitamin D or calcium deficiency
	Muscle wasting	Protein, carbohydrate, and fat deficiency
Neurologic	Altered mental status	Dehydration and thiamine or vitamin B_{12} deficiency
	Paresthesia (sensation of numbness, prickling, or tingling)	Vitamin B_{12}, pyridoxine, or thiamine deficiency

THE HEALTH HISTORY

In the general assessment, the nurse assesses nutrition during the "review of systems" (ROS) and "health patterns" section. Under the ROS, the patient is asked about weight changes, fatigue, allergies, and problems in the gastrointestinal system, which may signal nutrition problems. Under health patterns, the patient's nutrition and exercise patterns are discussed. These may also help the nurse identify a patient problem with nutrition (see Chapter 4, "The Health History").

Common or Concerning Symptoms

Symptoms that may immediately elicit concerns about nutritional status include:

- Changes in weight, usually unintended
- Anorexia
- Changes in the senses of taste or smell
- Difficulty chewing or swallowing

Changes in Weight

Changes in weight result from changes in body tissues or changes in body fluid.

CLINICAL TIP
Rapid changes in weight over only a few days suggest an increase or decrease in body fluids, not tissues.

Begin with broad open-ended questions, such as, "Tell me about your weight gain (loss)." Use the "OLD CART" mnemonic to ask follow-up questions.

- *Onset:* When did you notice the change in your weight? When do you think it began?
- *Location:* Is the weight gain (or loss) distributed over your whole body or in a particular area?

CLINICAL TIP
Weight gain or swelling in the lower legs may indicate water retention due to cardiac or peripheral vascular disease, not a nutrition problem.

- *Duration:* Has the gain (or loss) been consistent? In spurts? Have you alternated between gaining and losing weight?

- *Characteristic symptoms:* How much weight have you gained (or lost)? How does your weight compare to a year (or 6 months) ago? Have you experienced increased hunger (or anorexia) during this time? Do you have difficulty chewing? Has your sense of smell changed? Taste?

- *Associated manifestations:* Do you tire easily? Do you often feel cold? Is your skin drier than usual? Are your ankles swollen? Have you noticed a change in the fit of your clothes? Have you changed your diet during this time? Have you changed your exercise routines or patterns of living? Who cooks for you? Who shops for you? Have you noticed any change in your teeth? Dentures?

- *Relieving factors:* Has anything helped you lose (or gain) weight?

- *Treatment:* Have you tried any diets or supplements to lose (or gain) weight?

Follow up on other symptoms in a similar fashion.

Be sure to ask the patient about food allergies or intolerances, such as lactose intolerance. Ask about chronic illnesses in the patient and family, as these may be related to the possible nutritional problems.

If an in-depth nutrition assessment is needed, a nutrition history form is helpful. Questions for one such form are outlined in Table 8-3.

TABLE 8-3 Nutrition History

Assessment Area	Sample Questions
Food pattern	How many meals and snacks do you eat a day?
	Which is the biggest meal?
	How many meals do you eat outside the home? Where are they eaten?
	Are you on any special diet or fad diet?
	Do you use food supplements, for example, protein shakes? If yes, which ones?
	Have you ever eaten a large amount of food in a short time or felt you could not control what or how much you are eating?
Personal food preferences	Are there any foods you particularly like or dislike?
	Are there any foods you feel are harmful or beneficial?
	Do you have any cultural or religious requirements or preferences?

(*continued*)

The patient who consumes large quantities of food in a short time or cannot control how much food they eat may have binge eating disorder (NIH & National Institute of Diabetes and Kidney Disorders, 2016, December).

TABLE 8-3 Nutrition History (*Continued*)

Assessment Area	Sample Questions
Food preparation	Who does the cooking? How are the foods prepared? What type of oil do you use for frying (saturated or unsaturated)? What spices or condiments do you commonly use?
Finances	Do you have enough money for food? Would you eat any differently if more money was available for food? Do you use any supplementary financial program?
Accessibility	Who does the shopping? When? Where? How close is your preferred grocery store? Do you have transportation to the store?
Patient health	Do you have any trouble with chewing or digesting food? How often do you have a bowel movement? Do you take any nutritional supplements or vitamins? What type? How much? Do you have any food allergies or food intolerances? What medications do you take? In what dose? How often? Do you drink alcohol? What type? How much? Per day? Per week? Do you smoke? How many packs per day? Please rate your stress level on a scale of 1 to 10 (1 being low stress and 10 being extremely stressed). Does the stress affect your appetite? Have you ever been tested for anemia or had your cholesterol level tested? What were the results? Are you happy with your health? Do you have an eating disorder? Heart disease? Osteoporosis? Diabetes? Obesity? Gastrointestinal disorder?
Exercise pattern	Describe your exercise on a typical day (or week).
Body image	Are you satisfied with your weight? What would you change about your body if you could?
Family health	Is there any heart disease, osteoporosis, diabetes, obesity, or gastrointestinal disorders in the family?
Family dietary patterns	Does anyone in the family eat a special diet? Does your family eat meals together? How often? Is mealtime a social time?

In addition to the nutrition history, the nurse should collect a sample food intake record. The nurse can ask the patient for a 24-hour recall of food and beverage intake. This is efficient if the patient can accurately remember the types and quantities of what they consumed. If time allows, the patient can be given a sheet to record a 2-day diet intake or a weekly diary. The nurse can help the patient analyze the record at a later appointment. If the patient is hospitalized or in a long-term care facility, the nurse can use the patient intake record.

PHYSICAL EXAMINATION

Signs of poor nutrition may occur in any body system. Usually by the time a sign appears the condition is fairly severe. See Table 8-2, "Nutritional Concerns by Body System."

The nurse looks for signs of nutritional problems and hydration problems during the general head-to-toe physical examination. For example, assessment of the skin for nutritional deficits begins with the general survey and continues as one moves through the examination from head to toe. When a full patient examination is not necessary, the nurse can systematically look for signs of nutrition or hydration problems.

General Survey

Begin the physical examination with the patient's *height and weight* and vital signs. Note the patient's *body frame.* Is it small, medium, or large? The patient's **body mass index (BMI)** can be calculated from the height and weight. See the section, "Calculating the BMI."

The proportion of weight to height can indicate whether the patient is overweight or underweight. Note that individuals with large muscle mass may have a falsely high BMI. This must be taken into account before assuming the patient is obese or overweight.

Height Measurement

To measure the patient's height:

1. Have the patient remove their shoes and hat.

Also have patient undo hair styles or remove hair pieces or ornaments that add any height, if possible.

2. Use a **stadiometer** attached to the wall.
3. The patient should stand facing away from the wall with a straight back and the heels, hips, shoulders, and occiput aligned (Fig. 8-3).

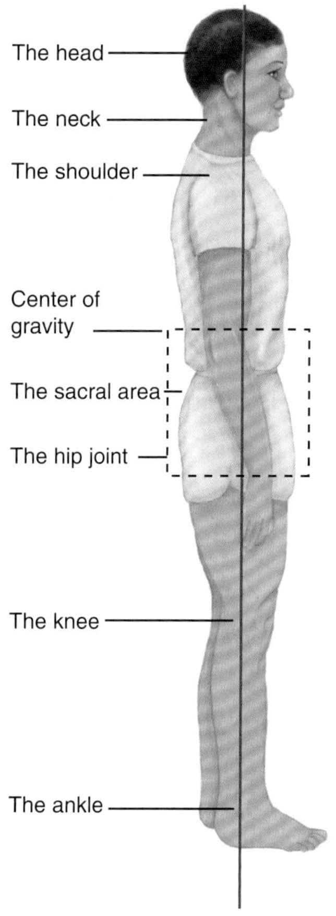

FIGURE 8-3 Ensuring proper alignment results in the most accurate height measurement.

4. The patient's head, back, buttocks, and heels should be against the wall.
5. Record the patient's height.
6. All children younger than 2 years should have their body length measured supine on a length measuring board. Height, using stadiometers, can only be used after age 2 and for individuals 3 years and older, provided they are able to stand. See Chapter 23, "Assessing Children: Infancy through Adolescence."

Weight Measurement

The balance beam scale or a standing electronic scale may be used in health care settings for patients who can stand up (Fig. 8-4). There are digital chair and bed scales for infants and patients unable to stand on a scale. Read the instructions for such scales.

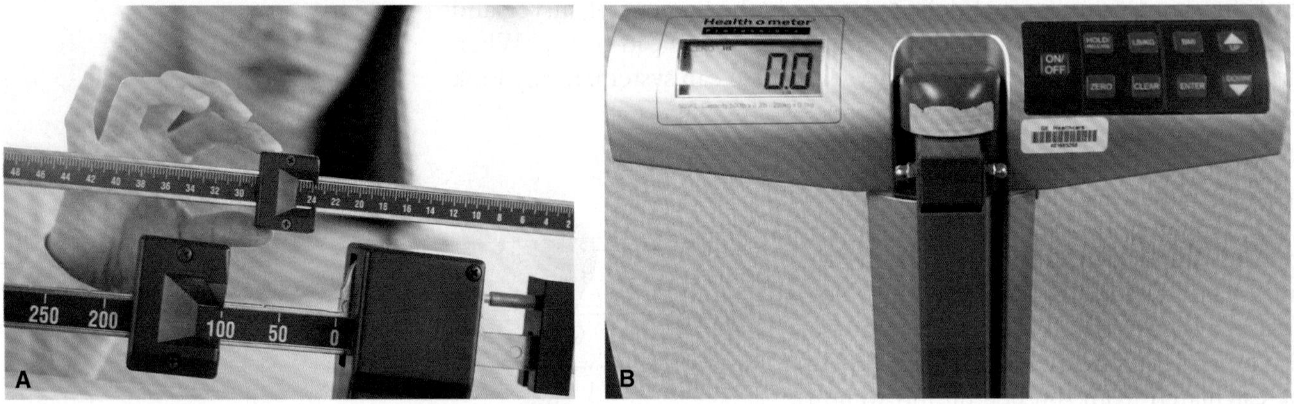

FIGURE 8-4 **A.** A balance beam scale. (tmcphotos/Shutterstock) **B.** A standing electronic scale.

Weight can vary during the day. If serial weights are needed, the patient should be weighed at the same time in the morning on the same scale and in the same clothing. In the hospital, this is often the hospital gown.

For the balance beam scale:

1. First zero the balance beam.
   a. Be sure the movable weights are at zero.
   b. If necessary, move the counter weights until the pointer is balanced in the middle at zero.
2. Have the patient remove shoes and outer clothing for a one-time weight.
3. The patient should step on the scale facing the balance beam.
4. Slide the large weight forward first. When the pointer is overbalanced downward, slide the large weight back to the previous notch.
5. Slide the small weight forward until the beam is balanced.
6. Read and document weight.

Individuals who have problems concerning weight, such as an eating disorder, may prefer to face away from the measurement beam.

Skin, Hair, and Nails

Thoroughly inspect the skin for dryness, flaking, cracking, or sores that will not heal. Assess skin color and turgor. See Chapter 9, "The Integumentary System." Inspect the hair for texture, thinning, and loss of color. Check the nails for shape and brittleness.

See Table 8-2, "Nutritional Concerns by Body System."

CLINICAL TIP
A pale color in fair-skinned patients or pale palms and mucous membranes in dark-skinned patients may indicate anemia. Turgor recoil greater than 3 seconds may indicate dehydration. Vitamin deficiencies may cause changes in skin, hair, and nails.

Head, Ears, Eyes, Nose, and Throat (HEENT)

Inspect the face for dark circles under the eyes.

CLINICAL TIP
Allergies may cause circles.

Inspect the mucous membranes for dryness, color, and intactness. Note cracking at the corners of the mouth, bleeding gums, and changes in tongue color. Look for an enlarged thyroid gland.

CLINICAL TIP
Dry membranes and sunken eyes indicate dehydration. Pale membranes may indicate anemia. Bleeding gums, cracking, and color changes may indicate vitamin deficiencies. An enlarged thyroid may indicate lack of iodine or thyroid malfunction.

Respiratory

Assess lung sounds for adventitious sounds. Fine crackles may indicate fluid overload in cardiac failure or pulmonary edema.

Cardiovascular and Peripheral Vascular

Measure blood pressure and pulse rate and amplitude. Assess peripheral vein filling. Tachycardia, a weak pulse and decreased blood pressure can indicate dehydration, while an increased jugular venous distention and increased blood pressure may mean overhydration. Flat veins with hands or feet dependent may indicate dehydration; full veins when hands and feet are elevated may indicate overhydration.

Inspect arms and legs for edema, petechiae, and ecchymoses. Petechiae and ecchymoses may be due to a lack of vitamin C or K. Edema may be secondary to a protein deficiency, fluid retention in cardiac failure, or venous stasis in peripheral vascular disease.

Petechiae are minute hemorrhagic spots in the skin, which do not blanch with pressure. They are a sign of blood leaking from capillaries under the skin. Ecchymoses are flat, blue or purple patches measuring 1 cm or more in diameter; they are caused by blood leaking into the skin.

Gastrointestinal

Observe for distention and ascites. Abdominal distention and ascites may be due to protein deficiency liver disease and low albumin.

Ascites is the accumulation of fluid in the peritoneal cavity, causing abdominal swelling.

Measure waist circumference. Place the tape measure over bare skin just above the hip bones (Fig. 8-5). Have the patient take a breath and measure the waist after exhalation.

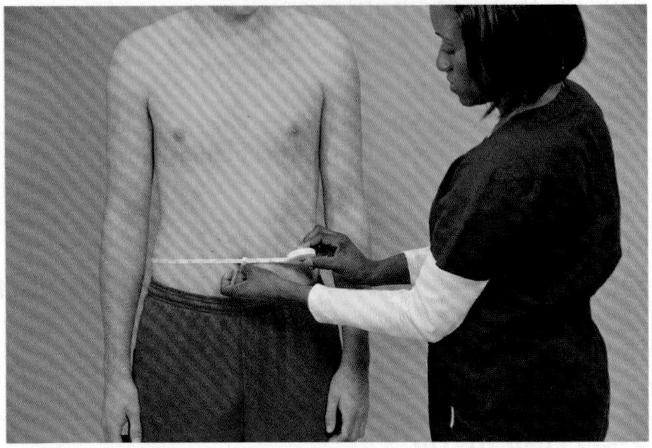

FIGURE 8-5 Measuring waist circumference.

CLINICAL TIP
The waist circumference indicates central body fat. Waist circumference greater than 40 in in men and greater than 35 in in women is related to an increased risk for cardiovascular disease and type 2 diabetes (NHLBL, 2013; NIDDKD, 2016).

Musculoskeletal

Note muscle wasting or flaccidity (loss of muscle tone), bone pain, and bowing of tibia. Measure arm circumference. Muscle wasting and flaccidity may be secondary to protein deficiency. Lack of vitamin D can cause bone pain and bowing of the legs.

Neurologic

Note changes in mental status, irritability, inability to concentrate, or paresthesias. Dehydration and lack of vitamins may cause these symptoms.

Paresthesia is a skin sensation that is described as tingling, tickling, pricking, burning, or numbing.

Calculating the BMI

Use the patient's measurements of height and weight to calculate the BMI. Body fat consists primarily of adipose in the form of triglycerides and is stored in subcutaneous, interabdominal, and intramuscular fat deposits that are difficult to measure directly. The BMI incorporates estimated but more accurate measures of body fat than weight alone. Note that BMI criteria for overweight and obesity are not rigid points but rather guidelines for estimating increasing risks to patient health and well-being from both excess and low weights. For older adults, there is a disproportionate risk for undernutrition.

CLINICAL TIP
More direct and accurate measures of body fat are obtained by measuring skinfold thickness, bioelectrical impedance, underwater weighing, and dual energy x-ray absorptiometry (DEXA). However, these methods require specific equipment and training. The BMI is moderately correlated with these methods. When patients require a more precise fat measurement than what the BMI indicates, they should be referred to a specialist for more accurate measurement.

The *waist-hip* ratio is also another indirect indicator of obesity. One divides the waist circumference by the hip circumference to obtain the ratio. Low risk for women is a ratio of 0.80 or lower and for men 0.95 or lower.

The correlation between BMI and body fat is fairly strong, but even if two people have the same BMI, their level of body fat may differ. At the same BMI,

- women tend to have more body fat than men.
- Black people have less body fat than White people.
- Asian people have more body fat than White people.
- older people, on average, tend to have more body fat than younger adults.
- athletes have less body fat than non-athletes (CDC, 2020a).

BMI standards are derived from two surveys: the National Health Examination Survey, consisting of three survey cycles between 1960 and 1970, and the National Health and Nutrition Examination Survey, conducted over three cycles between the 1970s and the 1990s.

There are several ways to obtain the BMI, as shown in Table 8-4. Choose the method most suited to your practice. The NIH and the NHLBI

TABLE 8-4 Calculating Body Mass Index

BMI Calculation Setup

1. Use the BMI table below.
   a. Find the patient's height in inches in the first column.
   b. Move across the height row to the column with the patient's weight in pounds.
   c. Follow the weight column up to the BMI number.
2. Use the "BMI calculator" from NIH at https://www.nhlbi.nih.gov/health/educational/lose_wt/BMI/bmicalc.htm.
3. Calculate the BMI using one of the following formulas:

Unit of Measure	Method of Calculation
Weight in *pounds*, height in *inches*	$\text{BMI} = \frac{\text{Weight (Pound)}}{\text{Height}^2\ (\text{Inches}^2)} \times 703$ Example: Weight = 150 lb, Height = 5 ft 5 in (65 in) Calculation: [150 ÷ (1.65)^2 × 703 = 24.96]
Weight in *kilograms*, height in *meters*	$\text{BMI} = \frac{\text{Weight (Kilogram)}}{\text{Height}^2\ (\text{Meters}^2)}$ Example: Weight = 68 kg, Height = 165 cm (1.65 m) Calculation: 68 ÷ (1.65)^2 = 24.98

(continued)

TABLE 8-4 Calculating Body Mass Index (*Continued*)

Body Mass Index Table

	Normal							Overweight							Obese						
BMI	19	20	21	22	23	24	25	26	27	28	29	30	31	32	33	34	35	36	37	38	39
Height (inches)	Body Weight (pounds)																				
58	91	96	100	105	110	115	119	124	129	134	138	143	148	153	158	162	167	172	177	181	186
59	94	99	104	109	114	119	124	128	133	138	143	148	153	158	163	168	173	178	183	188	193
60	97	102	107	112	118	123	128	133	138	143	148	153	158	163	168	174	179	184	189	194	199
61	100	106	111	116	122	127	132	137	143	148	153	158	164	169	174	180	185	190	195	201	206
62	104	109	115	120	126	131	136	142	147	153	158	164	169	175	180	186	191	196	202	207	213
63	107	113	118	124	130	135	141	146	152	158	163	169	175	180	186	191	197	203	208	214	220
64	110	116	122	128	134	140	145	151	157	163	169	174	180	186	192	197	204	209	215	221	227
65	114	120	126	132	138	144	150	156	162	168	174	180	186	192	198	204	210	216	222	228	234
66	118	124	130	136	142	148	155	161	167	173	179	186	192	198	204	210	216	223	229	235	241
67	121	127	134	140	146	153	159	166	172	178	185	191	198	204	211	217	223	230	236	242	249
68	125	131	138	144	151	158	164	171	177	184	190	197	203	210	216	223	230	236	243	249	256
69	128	135	142	149	155	162	169	176	182	189	196	203	209	216	223	230	236	243	250	257	263
70	132	139	146	153	160	167	174	181	188	195	202	209	216	222	229	236	243	250	257	264	271
71	136	143	150	157	165	172	179	186	193	200	208	215	222	229	236	243	250	257	265	272	279
72	140	147	154	162	169	177	184	191	199	206	213	221	228	235	242	250	258	265	272	279	287
73	144	151	159	166	174	182	189	197	204	212	219	227	235	242	250	257	265	272	280	288	295
74	148	155	163	171	179	186	194	202	210	218	225	233	241	249	256	264	272	280	287	295	303
75	152	160	168	176	184	192	200	208	216	224	232	240	248	256	264	272	279	287	295	303	311
76	156	164	172	180	189	197	205	213	221	230	238	246	254	263	271	279	287	295	304	312	320

Conversion formulas: 2.2 lb = 1 kg; 1.0 in = 2.54 cm; 100 cm = 1 m.

Source: CDC. (2020, September 17). Healthy weight, nutrition, and physical activity. About adult BMI. http://www.cdc.gov/healthyweight/assessing/bmi/adult_bmi/#Interpreted; Reprinted from National Institutes of Health and National Heart, Lung, and Blood Institute: Clinical Guidelines on the Identification, Evaluation and Treatment of Overweight and Obesity in Adults: The Evidence Report. June 1998. Retrieved June 12, 2020, from http://www.nhlbi.nih.gov/health/educational/lose_wt/BMI/bmi_tbl.htm. *For BMI greater than 35 go to Body Mass Index Table 2 at: https://www.nhlbi.nih.gov/health/educational/lose_wt/BMI/bmi_tbl2.htm

caution that people who are very muscular, for example body builders, may have a high BMI but still be healthy (NHLBI, 2013). Likewise, the BMI for people with low muscle mass and reduced nutrition may appear to have a "healthy" BMI, though it is not healthy for them.

If the BMI is 35 or higher, measure the patient's *waist circumference.* With the patient standing, measure the waist just above the hip bones. The patient may have excess body fat if the waist measures:

- 35 in or more for women
- 40 in or more for men

HEALTH PROMOTION AND COUNSELING

Important Topics for Health Promotion and Counseling

Important health promotion topics related to nutritional status include:

- Optimal weight, nutrition, and diet
- Exercise
- Hydration

Optimal Weight, Nutrition, and Diet

Fewer than half of U.S. adults maintain a healthy weight, with a BMI between 18.5 and 24.9. Obesity has increased in every segment of the U.S. population, regardless of age, gender, ethnicity, or socioeconomic status (National Heart, Lung and Blood Institute, 2013). Review the statistics about the rising prevalence of obesity nationally and worldwide in Box 8-2. Table 8-5 outlines the implications of obesity.

BOX 8-2 OBESITY AT A GLANCE

- According to the National Center for Health Statistics, 73.6% of adults ages 20 or older are overweight or obese (Fryar et al., 2021a).
- In younger populations, 35.4% of children ages 2–19 years were overweight or obese (Fryar et al., 2021b).
- The prevalence of being overweight or obese varies by ethnic and socioeconomic groups (CDC, 2019).
- Overweight and obesity increase risk of heart disease, numerous types of cancers, type 2 diabetes, stroke, arthritis, sleep apnea, infertility, and depression.
- More than 80% of people with type 2 diabetes (CDC, 2020c) and 20% of people with hypertension or elevated cholesterol are overweight or obese.
- Obesity is increasing worldwide: Although being poor in the world's poorest countries is associated with underweight and malnutrition, being poor in a middle-income country adopting a Western lifestyle is associated with increased risk of obesity (Ng et al., 2014).

TABLE 8-5 Obesity-Related Risk Factors and Diseases

Cardiovascular
- Hypertension
- Congestive heart failure
- Cor pulmonale
- Varicose veins
- Pulmonary embolism
- Coronary artery disease

Endocrine
- Metabolic syndrome
- Type 2 diabetes
- Dyslipidemia
- Polycystic ovary syndrome/androgenicity
- Amenorrhea/infertility/menstrual disorders

Gastrointestinal
- Gastroesophageal reflux disease (GERD)
- Nonalcoholic fatty liver disease (NAFLD)
- Cholelithiasis
- Hernias
- Cancer: colon, pancreas, esophagus, liver

Genitourinary
- Urinary stress incontinence
- Obesity-related glomerulopathy
- Hypogonadism (male)
- Cancer: breast, cervical, ovarian, uterine pregnancy complications
- Nephrolithiasis, chronic renal disease

Integumentary
- Striae distensae (stretch marks)
- Status pigmentation of legs
- Lymphedema
- Cellulitis
- Intertrigo, carbuncles
- Acanthosis nigricans/skin tags

Musculoskeletal
- Hyperuricemia and gout
- Immobility
- Osteoarthritis (knees, hips)
- Low back pain

Neurologic
- Stroke
- Idiopathic intracranial hypertension
- Meralgia paresthetica

Psychological
- Depression/low self-esteem
- Body image disturbance
- Social stigmatization

Respiratory
- Dyspnea
- Obstructive sleep apnea
- Hypoventilation syndrome
- Hypoventilation syndrome/pickwickian syndrome
- Pulmonary embolism
- Asthma

Sources: NHLBI. (n.d.). Overweight and obesity. Signs, symptoms and complications. https://www.nhlbi.nih.gov/health-topics/overweight-and-obesity; CDC. (2020, September 17). The health effects of overweight and obesity. https://www.cdc.gov/healthyweight/effects/index.html; Norris, T. L. (2019). *Porth's pathophysiology: Concepts of altered health status* (10th ed.). Wolters Kluwer.

To promote optimal patient weight and nutrition, adopt the four-step approach outlined in Box 8-3. Even reducing weight by 5% to 10% can improve blood pressure, lipid levels, and glucose tolerance, reducing the risk of diabetes or hypertension.

BOX 8-3 FOUR STEPS TO PROMOTE OPTIMAL WEIGHT AND NUTRITION

- Measure BMI and waist circumference; identify risk of overweight and obesity.
- Assess dietary intake.
- Assess the patient's motivation to change.
- Provide counseling about nutrition and exercise.

Take advantage of the resources available for patient assessment and counseling summarized in the following sections. Review the role of weight in the growing prevalence of *metabolic syndrome,* discussed further in Chapter 14, "The Cardiovascular System."

Step 1: Measure the BMI and Assess Risk Factors

Classify the BMI according to the national guidelines in Table 8-6. If the BMI is *higher than 25,* assess the patient for *additional risk factors* for heart disease and other obesity-related diseases: hypertension, high low-density lipoprotein (LDL) cholesterol, low high-density lipoprotein (HDL) cholesterol, high triglycerides, high blood glucose, family history of premature heart disease, physical inactivity, and smoking. Patients with a BMI over 25 and two or more risk factors should pursue weight loss, especially if the waist circumference is high.

TABLE 8-6 Classification of Overweight and Obesity by BMI

	Obesity Class	BMI (kg/m²)
Underweight		<18.5
Normal		18.5–24.9
Overweight		25.0–29.9
Obesity	I	30.0–34.9
	II	35.0–39.9
Extreme obesity	III	≥40

Source: CDC. (2020, March 3). Defining adult overweight and obesity. https://www.cdc.gov/obesity/adult/defining.htm

CLINICAL TIP

Adults with a BMI greater than 25, men with waist circumferences greater than 40 in, and women with waist circumferences greater than 35 in are at increased risk for heart disease and obesity-related diseases. Measuring the waist-to-hip ratio (waist circumference divided by hip circumference) may be a better risk predictor for individuals older than 75 years. Ratios greater than 0.95 in men and greater than 0.80 in women are considered elevated.

Step 2: Assess Dietary Intake

Obtain a nutrition history and a diet intake record. Analyze the patient's intake record. The USDA's *ChooseMyPlate* is an excellent resource to help you analyze the patient's intake record and can be easily accessed online (Fig. 8-6).

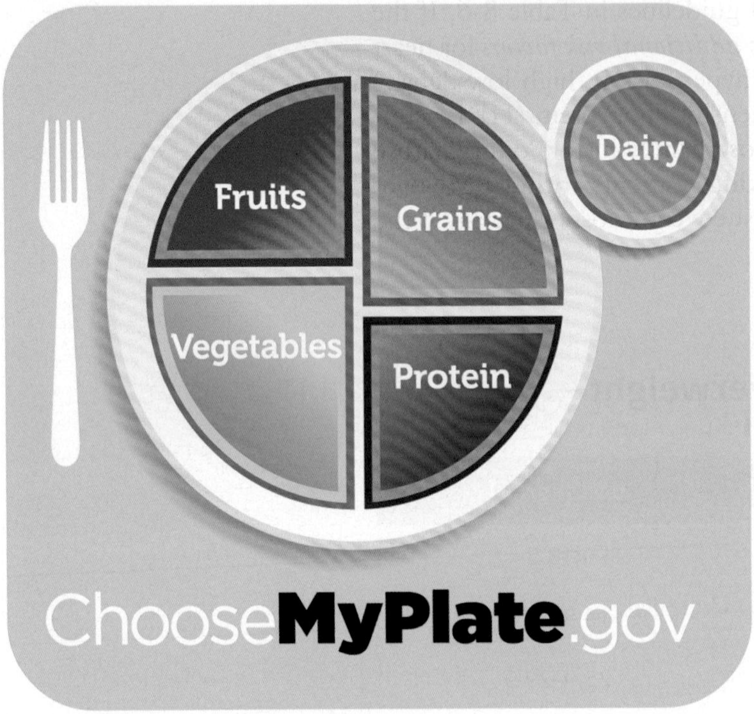

FIGURE 8-6 The USDA's ChooseMyPlate can help health care providers and patients evaluate dietary intake.

Step 3: Assess the Patient's Motivation to Change

Assess the patient's readiness to make the lifestyle changes that promote weight loss. Prochaska's model of change helps the nurse tailor interventions to the patient's stage of readiness (Table 8-7).

Step 4: Provide Counseling about Nutrition and Exercise

Advising patients about diet and weight loss is important, especially in light of the many often contradictory dieting options in the popular press. The following four resources provide excellent guidelines for counseling patients:

- U.S. Department of Health and Human Services and U.S. Department of Agriculture. Dietary Guidelines for Americans 2020–2025. https://www.dietaryguidelines.gov
- USDA ChooseMyPlate. What is MyPlate. https://www/myplate.gov/eat-healthy/what-is-myplate

TABLE 8-7 Obesity: Stages of Change Model and Assessing Readiness

Stage	Characteristic	Patient Verbal Cue	Appropriate Intervention(s)	Sample Dialogue
Precontemplation	Unaware of problem, no interest in change	"I'm not really interested in weight loss. It's not a problem."	Provide information about health risks and benefits of weight loss.	"Would you like to read some information about the health aspects of obesity?"
Contemplation	Aware of problem, beginning to think of changing	"I know I need to lose weight, but with all that's going on in my life right now, I'm not sure I can."	Help resolve ambivalence, and discuss barriers.	"Let's look at the benefits of weight loss, as well as what you may need to change."
Preparation	Realizes benefits of making changes and thinking about how to change	"I have to lose weight, and I'm planning to do that."	Teach behavior modification; provide education	"Let's take a closer look at how you can reduce some of the calories you eat and how to increase your activity during the day."
Action	Actively taking steps toward change	"I'm doing my best. This is harder than I thought."	Provide support and guidance with a focus on the long term.	"It's terrific that you're working so hard. What problems have you had so far? How have you solved them?"
Maintenance	Initial treatment goals reached	"I've learned a lot through this process."	Relapse control	"What situations continue to tempt you to overeat? What can be helpful for the next time you face such a situation?"

Sources: American Medical Association. Roadmaps for Clinical Practice—Case Studies in Disease Prevention and Health Promotion—Assessment and Management of Adult Obesity: A Primer for Physicians. Communication and Counseling Strategies. Booklet 8. Chicago, November 2003; Adapted from Prochaska, J. O., & DiClemente, C. C. (1986). Toward a comprehensive model of change. In W. R. Miller (Ed.). *Treating addictive behaviors* (pp. 3–27). Plenum.

- NHLBI Publications and Resources. Aim for a Healthy Weight: Keep an Eye on Portion Size (Z Card). https://www.nhlbi.nih.gov/health-topics/all-publications-and-resources/aim-healthy-weight-keep-eye-portion-size-z-card
- Iowa Department of Public Health. (2007). The secret to serving size is in your hand. https://idph.iowa.gov/Portals/1/Files/WIC/svg_size_engligh.pdf

Diet recommendations hinge on assessment of the patient's motivation and readiness to lose weight and individual risk factors. The CDC (2020b) recommends the following general guidelines:

- A 10% weight reduction over 6 months, or a decrease of 500 to 1,000 kcal/day, for overweight and obese adults.
- A weight loss goal of 1/2 to 1 lb per week because more rapid weight loss does not lead to better results at 1 year (CDC, 2020a).

These guidelines recommend low-calorie diets of 1,200 to 1,500 kcal per day for women and 1,500 to 1,700 kcal per day for men. Interventions that combine nutrition education, diet, and exercise with behavioral therapy are most likely to succeed. The USDA's *Dietary Guidelines for Americans* cite evidence supporting the role of moderate physical activity in weight loss and weight loss maintenance programs. Moderate physical activity enhances and may assist with maintenance of weight; it increases cardiorespiratory fitness; and it may decrease abdominal fat (U.S. Department of Health and Human Services & U.S. Department of Agriculture, 2020).

If the BMI falls *below 18.5*, be concerned about eating disorders or other medical conditions. These conditions are summarized in Table 8-1.

Once you have assessed food intake, nutritional status, and motivation to adopt healthy eating behaviors or lose weight, give patients the recommendations for healthy eating patterns from the *Dietary Guidelines for Americans 2020–2025*, as summarized in Box 8-4.

Concept Mastery Alert

Anorexia Nervosa and Bulimia Nervosa

When completing a nutritional history, the nurse needs to be alert for findings that may suggest anorexia nervosa. Patients with anorexia nervosa are preoccupied with controlling their environments so that they limit the number of calories ingested and perform exercise to lose even those limited calories. They have a low BMI and other physical symptoms related to starvation. This is in contrast to patients with bulimia nervosa, who may be of normal weight or even overweight and are preoccupied with eating, often engaging in binge eating followed by purging.

BOX 8-4 RECOMMENDATIONS FOR HEALTHY EATING PATTERNS

- Consume a variety of foods within and among the basic food groups while staying within calorie requirements
- A healthy diet includes:
  - A variety of vegetables from all subgroups—dark green, red, and orange; legumes (beans and peas); starchy vegetables; and any other vegetables
  - Fruits, especially whole fruits
  - Grains, at least half of which are whole grains
  - Fat-free or low-fat dairy, including milk, yogurt, cheese, and/or fortified soy beverages
  - A variety of protein foods, including seafood, lean meats and poultry, eggs, legumes (beans and peas), and nuts, seeds, and soy products
  - Oils, monosaturated or unsaturated
  - Limit saturated fats and trans fats as well as added sugars.
  - Limit sodium to 2,300 mg per day for children 14 years and older.
  - Use spices or herbs, such as dill, chili powder, paprika, or cumin, and lemon or lime juice to add flavor without adding salt.
- If you drink alcoholic beverages, do so in moderation: one drink per day for women and two drinks per day for men.
- Maintain moderate physical activity for at least 30 minutes each day, for example, walking 3 to 4 mph.

Source: U.S. Department of Agriculture and U.S. Department of Health and Human Services. (2020, December). *Dietary Guidelines for Americans, 2020–2025* (9th ed.). https://www.dietaryguidelines.gov/

Assess adolescent females and women of childbearing age for adequate intake of iron and folic acid. Assist adults older than 50 years to identify foods rich in vitamin B_{12} and calcium. Advise older adults and those with dark skin or low exposure to sunlight to increase intake of vitamin D. Table 8-8 outlines common sources of key nutrients.

TABLE 8-8 **Nutrition Counseling: Sources of Nutrients**

Nutrient	Food Source
Calcium	Dairy foods such as yogurt, milk, and natural cheeses
	Breakfast cereal, fruit juice with calcium supplements
	Dark green, leafy vegetables such as collards, turnip, and mustard greens; kale; bok choy
	Sardines
Iron	Clams, mussels, oysters, sardines, anchovies
	Lean meat, dark turkey meat
	Iron-fortified cereals
	Spinach, peas, lentils, turnip greens, artichokes
	Enriched and whole-grain bread
	Dried prunes and raisins
Folate	Cooked dried beans and peas
	Oranges, orange juice
	Dark green, leafy vegetables; spinach, mustard greens
	Liver
	Black-eyed peas, lentils, okra, chickpeas, peanuts
	Folate-fortified cereals
Vitamin D	Vitamin D–fortified milk, orange juice, and cereals
	Cod liver oil, swordfish, salmon, herring, mackerel, tuna, trout
	Egg yolk
	Mushrooms

Sources: Adapted from U.S. Department of Agriculture and U.S. Department of Health and Human Services. (2020, December). *Dietary Guidelines for Americans, 2020–2025* (9th ed.). https://www.dietaryguidelines.gov/; Choose MyPlate.gov. Retrieved July 2, 2020, from http://www.choosemyplate.gov/index.htm; Dietary Supplements, National Institutes of Health. *Dietary supplement fact sheets: Calcium; vitamin D*. Retrieved March 20, 2021 from http://ods.od.nih.gov/factsheets/list-all/

Blood Pressure and Diet

Evidence shows that regular and frequent exercise, decreased sodium intake, increased potassium intake, and maintenance of a healthy weight reduce the risk for developing hypertension and help lower blood pressure in adults who are already hypertensive. Explain to patients that most dietary sodium comes from salt (sodium chloride). The recommended daily allowance (RDA) of sodium is less than 2,300 mg, approximately

1 tsp per day. However, individuals with hypertension, diabetes, or chronic kidney disease; those who are 51 or older; and/or those of African American heritage should consume no more than 1,500 mg sodium per day (American Heart Association, 2020; Cogswell et al., 2016; Fulgoni et al., 2014). Patients need to read food labels closely, especially the nutrition facts panels. Low-sodium foods are those with sodium listed at less than 5% of the RDA of 2,300 or less. For nutritional interventions to reduce the risk for cardiac disease, refer to Chapter 14, "The Cardiovascular System." Table 8-9 identifies foods to increase and decrease in the patient's diet.

TABLE 8-9 Patients with Hypertension: Recommended Changes in Diet

Dietary Change	Food Source
Increase foods high in potassium	Baked white or sweet potatoes, cooked greens such as spinach
	Bananas, plantains, many dried fruits, orange juice
Decrease foods high in sodium	Canned foods (soups, tuna fish)
	Pretzels, potato chips, pickles, olives
	Many processed foods (frozen dinners, ketchup, mustard)
	Batter-fried foods
	Table salt, including for cooking

Source: Adapted from U.S. Department of Agriculture and U.S. Department of Health and Human Services. (2020, December). *Dietary Guidelines for Americans, 2020–2025* (9th ed.). https://www.dietaryguidelines.gov/

Exercise

Fitness is a key component of both weight control and weight loss. Adults should do at least 2 hours and 30 minutes each week of aerobic physical activity at a moderate level or 1 hour and 15 minutes each week of aerobic physical activity at a vigorous level. An example of a moderate-intensity activity is walking briskly, 3 mph or faster (Hew-Butler et al., 2015). However, research has shown that if a middle-aged or older woman with a normal BMI wants to maintain her weight over an extended period, she must engage in the equivalent of 60 minutes per day of physical activity at a moderate intensity (Shanks, 2010). Patients can increase exercise by such simple measures as parking farther away from their places of work or using stairs instead of elevators. A safe goal for weight loss is 1/2 to 2 lb per week. Box 8-5 lists more examples of moderate and vigorous activities.

BOX 8-5 MODERATE AND VIGOROUS EXERCISE

A 154-lb man (5 ft, 10 in) will use up approximately the number of calories listed doing each activity below. *Those who weigh more will use more calories, and those who weigh less will use fewer.* The calorie values listed include both calories used by the activity and calories used for normal body functioning.

Activities	**Approximate Calories Used by a 154-lb Man**	
Moderate Physical Activities	**In 1 hour**	**In 30 minutes**
Hiking	370	185
Light gardening/yard work	330	165
Dancing	330	165
Golf (walking and carrying clubs)	330	165
Bicycling (<10 mph)	290	145
Walking (3 1/2 mph)	280	140
Weight training (general light workout)	220	110
Stretching	180	90
Vigorous Physical Activities	**In 1 hour**	**In 30 minutes**
Running/jogging (5 mph)	590	295
Bicycling (more than 10 mph)	590	295
Swimming (slow freestyle laps)	510	255
Aerobics	480	240
Walking (4 1/2 mph)	460	230
Heavy yard work (chopping wood)	440	220
Weight lifting (vigorous effort)	440	220
Basketball (vigorous)	440	220

Source: CDC. (2020, October 28). Healthy weight, nutrition and physical activity. How many calories are used in typical activities? https://www.cdc.gov/healthyweight/physical–activity/index.html

Hydration

According to the *Report of the Dietary Guidelines Advisory Committee on the Dietary Guidelines for Americans*, "In order to prevent dehydration, water must be consumed daily (CDC, 2021). Healthy individuals who have routine access to fluids and who are not exposed to heat stress consume adequate water to meet their needs." Purposeful drinking may be warranted for individuals who are exposed to heat stress or who perform sustained vigorous physical activity in hot temperatures. Current guidelines recommend athletes use their thirst as a guide to regulate their intake of fluids, because purposeful over-drinking of water or low-sodium sports drinks can lead to hyponatremia (CDC, 2021).

The older adult is at increased risk of morbidity and mortality from dehydration. In view of the ongoing obesity epidemic, individuals are encouraged to drink water and other fluids with few or no calories. The complexity of the human fluid regulatory mechanisms and interindividual differences are the primary reasons why a consensus on a daily water requirement has not been reached. It is believed that the combination of thirst and usual drinking behaviors, especially the consumption of fluids with meals, is sufficient to maintain normal hydration (Armstrong & Johnson, 2018; CDC, 2021).

Individuals with limited ability to obtain fluids for themselves, such as persons with disabilities, older adults in nursing homes, or persons confined to a bed, are at increased risk for dehydration. These patients' hydration status should be assessed at least daily and appropriate fluids provided.

BIBLIOGRAPHY

American Heart Association. (2020). How much sodium should I eat per day? Retrieved July 2, 2020, from https://www.heart.org/en/healthy-living/healthy-eating/eat-smart/sodium/how-much-sodium-should-i-eat-per-day

Armstrong, L. E., & Johnson, E. C. (2018). Water intake, water balance, and the elusive daily water requirement. *Nutrients, 10*(12), 1928.

CDC. (2019). Overweight and obesity. Data and statistics. https://www.cdc.gov/obesity/data/index.html

CDC. (2020a). Healthy weight. How good is BMI as an indicator of body fatness? https://www.cdc.gov/healthyweight/assessing/bmi/adult_bmi/index.html

CDC. (2020b). Healthy weight. Losing weight: What is a healthy weight loss? https://www.cdc.gov/healthyweight/losing_weight/index.html

CDC. (2020c). National Diabetes Statistics Report 2020. https://www.cdc.gov/diabetes/pdfs/data/statistics/national-diabetes-statistics-report.pdf

CDC. (2021). Water and nutrition. https://cdc.gov/healthywater/drinking/nutrition/index.html

Cogswell, M. E., Mugavero, K., Bowman, B. A., & Frieden, T. R. (2016). Dietary sodium and cardiovascular disease risk—Measurement matters. *New England Journal of Medicine, 375*(6), 580–586.

Fryar, C. D., Carroll, M. D., & Afful, J. (2021a, January 29). Prevalence of overweight, obesity, and severe obesity among adults aged 20 and over: United States, 1960–1962 through 2017–2018. *NCHS Health E-Stats.* https://www.cdc.gov/nchs/data/hestat/obesity-adult-17-18/obesity-adult.htm

Fryar, C. D., Carroll, M. D., & Afful, J. (2021b, January 29). Prevalence of Overweight, Obesity, and Severe Obesity Among Children and Adolescents Aged 2–19 Years: United States, 1963–1965 through 2017–2018. https://www.cdc.gov/nchs/data/hestat/obesity-child-17-18/obesity-child.htm

Fulgoni, V. L. 3rd, Agarwal, S., Spence, L., & Samuel, P. (2014). Sodium intake in US ethnic subgroups and potential impact of a new sodium reduction technology: NHANES dietary modeling. *Nutrition Journal, 13*(1), 120. https://doi.org/10.1186/1475-2891-13-120

Hew-Butler, T., Rosner, M. H., Fowkes-Godek, S., Dugas, J. P., Hoffman, M. D., Lewis, D. P., Maughan, R. J., Miller, K. C., Montain, S. J., Rehrer, N. J., Roberts, W. O., Rogers, I. R. A., Siegel, J., Stuempfle, K. J., Winger, J. M., & Verbalis, J. G. (2015). Statement of the Third International Exercise-associated Hyponatremia Consensus Development Conference Carlsbad, California, 2015. *Clinical Journal of Sport Medicine, 25*, 303–320.

National Heart Lung, and Blood Institute. (2013, November). Managing overweight and obesity in adults: Systematic evidence review from the obesity expert panel: the evidence report. https://www.nhlbi.nih.gov/health-topics/managing-overweight-obesity-in-adults

National Heart, Lung and Blood Institute. (2013, February 13). Calculate body mass index. http://www.nhlbi.nih.gov/health/educational/wecan/healthy-weight-basics/body-mass-index.htm

National Institute of Diabetes and Digestive and Kidney Diseases. (2016, December). Risk factors for type 2 diabetes. https://www.niddk.nih.gov/health-information/diabetes/overview/risk-factors-type-2-diabetes

National Institute of Diabetes and Digestive and Kidney Disorders. (2016, June). Binge eating disorder. https://www.niddk.nih.gov/health-information/weight-management/binge-eating-disorder/definition-facts

Ng, M., Fleming, T., Robinson, M., Thomson, B., Graetz, N., Margono, C., Mullany, E. C., Biryukov, S., Abbafati, C., Abera, S. F., Abraham, J. P., Abu-Rmeileh, N. M. E., Achoki, T., AlBuhairan, F. S., Alemu, Z. A., Alfonso, R., Ali, M. K., Ali, R., Guzman, N. A., … Gakidou, E. (2014). Global, regional, and national prevalence of overweight and obesity in children and adults during 1980–2013: a systematic analysis for the Global Burden of Disease Study 2013. *Lancet, 384*(9945), 766–781.

Shanks, L. J. (2010, March 23). 60 minutes of exercise per day needed for middle-aged women to maintain weight. *Harvard Gazette: Health & Medicine.* https://news.harvard.edu/gazette/story/2010/03/60-minutes-of-exercise-per-day-needed-for-middle-aged-women-to-maintain-weight/

U.S. Department of Agriculture and U.S. Department of Health and Human Services. (2020, December). *Dietary Guidelines for Americans, 2020–2025* (9th ed.). https://www.dietaryguidelines.gov/

ADDITIONAL REFERENCES

Budd, G. M., & Peterson, J. A. (2014). The obesity epidemic, Part 1: Understanding the origins. *American Journal of Nursing, 114*(12), 40–45.

Budd, G. M., & Peterson, J. A. (2015). The obesity epidemic, Part 2: Nursing assessment and intervention. *American Journal of Nursing, 115*(1), 38–46.

UNIT 2

Body Systems

9 THE INTEGUMENTARY SYSTEM

KEY TERMS

acral	integumentary system	pressure injury
adipose tissue	jaundice	sebaceous glands
dermis	lesion	subcutaneous tissue
edema	nonpitting edema	sweat glands
epidermis	pitting edema	turgor

Learning Objectives

The student will:

1. Explain the functions of the integumentary system.
2. Identify the structures of the skin, nails, and hair.
3. Obtain history of the integumentary system.
4. Describe the equipment necessary to perform an integumentary examination.
5. Appropriately prepare and position the patient for the integumentary examination.
6. Correctly perform an integumentary examination.
7. Accurately describe primary, secondary, and vascular lesions.
8. Identify risk factors for pressure injuries.
9. Correctly perform an assessment for pressure injury risk using the Braden scale.
10. Discuss risk reduction and health promotion strategies to prevent skin cancer.
11. Identify risk factors for skin cancer.

Intact and functioning skin is essential for the life and health of the patient. The skin is the largest and heaviest organ of the body, accounting for approximately 16% of body weight and covering an area of roughly 1.2 to 2.3 m^2.

Nursing assessment of the **integumentary system** is frequently superficial, unless the patient has a significant problem, such as third-degree burns. A thorough integumentary assessment requires time; turning heavy, unconscious, or uncooperative patients in order to perform the assessment may be difficult during a busy shift. For the nurse, assessment of the skin is much more than discovering skin lesions or diseases. Examination of the skin can reveal signs of systemic diseases, medication side effects, dehydration, overhydration, or physical abuse; allow early identification of potentially cancerous lesions and risk factors for pressure injury formation; and identify the need for hygiene and health promotion education.

ANATOMY AND PHYSIOLOGY

The skin keeps the body in homeostasis despite daily assaults from the environment. The skin:

1. *provides a barrier* protecting the body from:
   a. injury secondary to mechanical, chemical, thermal, and ultraviolet (UV) light sources.
   b. penetration by microorganisms.
   c. loss of water and electrolytes, thereby preventing dehydration.
2. *regulates body temperature* by allowing heat dissipation through sweat glands and heat storage through subcutaneous insulation.
3. *synthesizes vitamin D* from cholesterol by the action of UV light.
4. *allows sensory perception* via end sensory organs for touch, pain, temperature, and pressure.
5. *provides nonverbal communication,* such as posture, facial movements, or vasomotor responses such as blushing.
6. *provides identity* through skin color and facial features.
7. *allows wound repair* through cell replacement of surface injuries.
8. *allows excretion of metabolic wastes,* such as electrolytes, minerals, sugar, or uric acid.

Hair, nails, and sebaceous and sweat glands are considered appendages of the skin. The skin and its appendages undergo many changes during aging. See Chapter 24, "Assessing Older Adults," to review normal and abnormal changes of the skin with aging.

Skin

The skin contains three layers: the epidermis, the dermis, and the subcutaneous tissues (Fig. 9-1).

The most superficial layer, the **epidermis,** is thin, devoid of blood vessels, and divided into two layers: an outer, horny layer of dead keratinized cells and an inner, cellular layer where both melanin and keratin are formed. Migration from the inner layer to the top layer takes approximately 1 month.

The epidermis depends on the underlying **dermis** for its nutrition. The dermis is well supplied with blood. It contains connective tissue, sebaceous glands, sweat glands, and hair follicles. It merges below with **subcutaneous,** or **adipose tissue,** also known as fat.

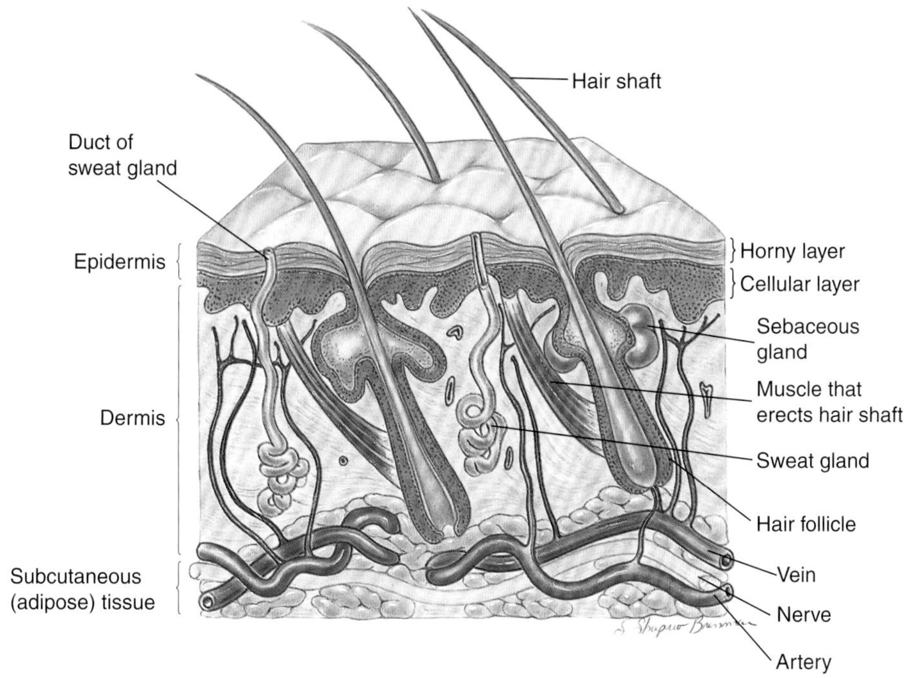

FIGURE 9-1 Structures of the skin.

The color of healthy skin depends primarily on four pigments: melanin, carotene, oxyhemoglobin, and deoxyhemoglobin. The amount of *melanin,* the brownish pigment of the skin, is genetically determined and is increased by exposure to sunlight. *Carotene* is a golden yellow pigment that exists in subcutaneous fat and in heavily keratinized areas such as the palms and soles.

Another yellow color in the skin may be jaundice due to deposition of bilirubin in the skin. Liver disease, biliary duct obstruction, or increased destruction of red blood cells increases serum bilirubin, which is then deposited in the skin. Jaundice is easiest to observe in the sclera, nails, palms, and soles. See Chapter 16, "The Gastrointestinal and Renal Systems," for further discussion of jaundice.

Hemoglobin, which circulates in the red cells and carries most of the oxygen of the blood, exists in two forms. *Oxyhemoglobin,* a bright red pigment, predominates in the arteries and capillaries. An increase in blood flow through the arteries to the capillaries causes a reddening of the skin (e.g., with blushing), while the reverse usually produces pallor. The skin of light-colored people is normally redder on the palms, soles, face, neck, and upper chest.

As blood passes through the capillary bed, oxyhemoglobin loses its oxygen to the tissues and changes to *deoxyhemoglobin*—a darker and somewhat bluer pigment. An increased concentration of deoxyhemoglobin in cutaneous blood vessels gives the skin a bluish cast known as *cyanosis.*

There are two types of cyanosis. If the oxygen level in the arterial blood is low, cyanosis is *central* and indicates decreased oxygenation in the patient. If the oxygen level is normal, cyanosis is *peripheral.* Peripheral cyanosis occurs when cutaneous blood flow decreases and slows, and tissues extract more oxygen than usual from the blood. Peripheral cyanosis may be a response to anxiety or a cold environment.

Skin color is also affected by the scattering of light reflected back through the cloudy superficial layers of the skin or vessel walls. This scattering makes the color look more blue and less red. The bluish color of a subcutaneous vein results from this effect; it appears much bluer than the venous blood obtained on venipuncture.

Hair

Adults have two types of hair: *vellus hair,* which is short, fine, inconspicuous, and relatively unpigmented; and *terminal hair,* which is coarser, thicker, more conspicuous, and usually pigmented. Scalp hair and eyebrows are examples of terminal hair.

Nails

Nails protect the distal ends of the fingers and toes (Fig. 9-2). The firm, rectangular, and usually curving *nail plate* gets its pink color from the vascular *nail bed* to which the plate is firmly attached. Note the white moon, or *lunula,* and the white free edge of the nail plate. Roughly one fourth of the nail plate (the *nail root*) is covered by the proximal nail fold. The *cuticle* extends from the fold and functioning as a seal, protects the space between the fold and the plate from external moisture. *Lateral nail folds* cover the sides of the nail plate. Note that the angle between the proximal nail fold and nail plate is normally less than 180 degrees.

Fingernails grow approximately 0.1 mm daily; toenails grow more slowly.

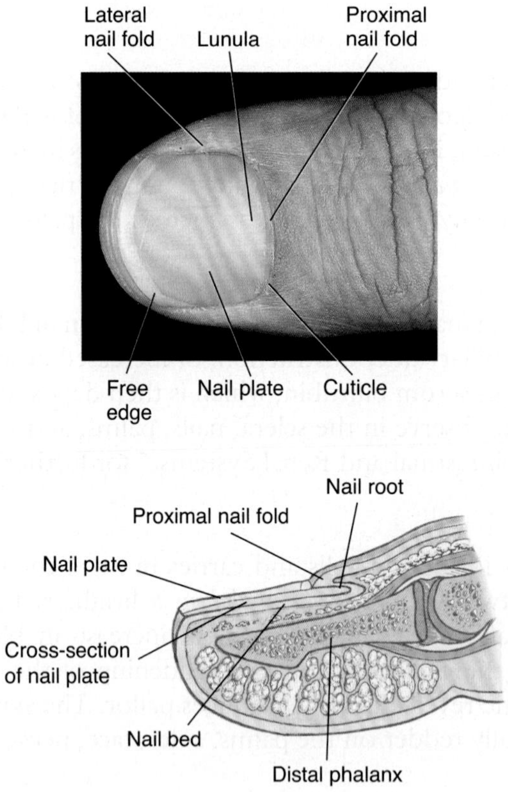

FIGURE 9-2 Structures of the nail.

Sebaceous Glands and Sweat Glands

Sebaceous glands produce *sebum,* a fatty substance secreted onto the skin surface through the hair follicles. These glands are present on all skin surfaces except the palms and soles. The sebum lubricates hair and skin and reduces water loss through the skin.

Sweat glands are of two types: eccrine and apocrine. The *eccrine glands* are widely distributed, open directly onto the skin surface, and by their sweat production, help control body temperature. In contrast, the *apocrine glands* are found chiefly in the axillary and genital regions, usually open into hair follicles, and are stimulated by emotional stress. Bacterial decomposition of apocrine sweat is responsible for adult body odor.

THE HEALTH HISTORY

The purpose of the integumentary history is to identify and of the following:

- Diseases of the skin
- Systemic diseases that have skin manifestations (Table 9-1)
- Physical abuse
- Risk for pressure injuries
- Risk for skin cancer
- Need for health promotion education regarding the skin

Common or concerning symptoms identified in an integumentary system history are listed in Box 9-1.

The patient with an integumentary issue will frequently state the problem when asked the purpose of the visit. The nurse can use the "OLD CART" mnemonic to ask follow-up questions in order to obtain a full description of the condition. For example, if the patient reports a rash, ask:

- *Onset:* When did it start?
  Have you started any new medications or changed existing medications?
  Have you been out of the country recently?
  Have you ever had similar symptoms in the past?
- *Location:* Where is it located?
  Has it changed size or spread to another part of your body?
- *Duration:* How long have you had the rash?
  Does it come and go?
- *Characteristic symptoms:* Describe your rash.
  What did it first look like?
  Has it changed?

Many contagious diseases present with skin rashes, for example, rubeola, rubella, and varicella.

TABLE 9-1 Diseases and Related Integumentary Changes

Addison disease	Hyperpigmentation of skin and mucous membranes
Chronic renal disease	Pallor, xerosis, pruritus, hyperpigmentation, uremic frost, metastatic calcification in the skin, calciphylaxis, "half and half" nails, hemodialysis-related skin disease
Cushing disease	Striae, skin atrophy, purpura, ecchymoses, telangiectasias, acne, moon facies, buffalo hump, hypertrichosis
Diabetes	Diabetic dermopathy, acanthosis nigricans, neuropathic ulcers, peripheral vascular disease
Disseminated intravascular coagulation	Skin necrosis, petechiae, ecchymoses, hemorrhagic bullae, purpura fulminans
Dyslipidemias	Xanthomas (tendon, eruptive, and tuberous), xanthelasma (may occur in healthy people)
Hypothyroidism	Dry, rough, and pale skin; coarse and brittle hair; myxedema; alopecia (lateral third of the eyebrows to diffuse); skin cool to touch; thin and brittle nails
Hyperthyroidism	Warm, moist, soft, and velvety skin; thin and fine hair; alopecia; vitiligo; pretibial myxedema (in Graves disease); hyperpigmentation (local or generalized)
Kawasaki disease	Mucosal erythema (lips, tongue, and pharynx), strawberry tongue, cherry red lips, polymorphous rash (primarily on trunk), erythema of palms and soles with later desquamation of fingertips
Liver disease	Jaundice, spider angiomas, and other telangiectasias, palmar erythema, Terry nails, pruritus, purpura, caput medusae
Meningococcemia	Pink macules and papules, petechiae, hemorrhagic petechiae, hemorrhagic bullae, purpura fulminans
Peripheral vascular disease	Dry, scaly, shiny atrophic skin; dystrophic, brittle toenails; cool skin; hairless shins; ulcers; pallor; cyanosis; gangrene
Pregnancy (not a disease; physiologic changes)	Melasma, increased pigmentation of areolae, linea nigra, palmar erythema, varicose veins, striae, spider angiomas, hirsutism, pyogenic granuloma
Systemic lupus erythematosus	Photosensitivity, malar (butterfly) rash, discoid rash, alopecia, vasculitis, oral ulcers, Raynaud phenomenon
Thrombocytopenic purpura	Petechiae, ecchymoses
Viral Exanthems	
Coxsackie A (hand, foot, and mouth)	Oral ulcers; macules, papules, and vesicles on hands, feet, and buttocks
Erythema infectiosum (fifth disease)	Erythema of cheeks ("slapped cheeks") followed by erythematous, pruritic, reticulated (net-like) rash that starts on trunk and proximal extremities (rash worsens with sun, fever, and temperature changes)
Roseola infantum (HHV-6)	Erythematous, maculopapular, discrete rash (often fever present) that begins on head and spreads to involve trunk and extremities, petechiae on soft palate
Rubella (German measles)	Erythematous, maculopapular, discrete rash (often fever present) that begins on head and spreads to involve trunk and extremities, petechiae on soft palate
Rubeola (measles)	Erythematous, maculopapular rash that begins on head and spreads to involve trunk and extremities (lesions become confluent on face and trunk, but are discrete on extremities), Koplik spots on buccal mucosa
Varicella (chickenpox)	Generalized, pruritic, vesicular (vesicles on an erythematous base, "dew drop on a rose petal") rash begins on trunk and spreads peripherally, lesions appear in crops and are in different stages of healing
Herpes zoster (shingles)	Pruritic, vesicular rash (vesicles on an erythematous base) in a dermatomal distribution

Source: Hall, J. C., & Hall, B. J. (2017). *Sauer's manual of skin diseases* (11th ed.). Lippincott Williams & Wilkins.

BOX 9-1	COMMON OR CONCERNING SYMPTOMS
Rash	Lesions
Nonhealing lesions	Bruising (ecchymosis)
Moles	Hair loss
Growths	Nail changes

- *Associated manifestations:* Does it itch?
  Is there any discharge?
- *Relieving/exacerbating factors:* Have you used or done anything that seems to make it better?
  Does anything make it worse?
- *Treatment:* Have you put anything on it to treat it?

If the patient does not offer a specific complaint, be sure to ask about each of the symptoms listed in Box 9-1. Start with broad open-ended questions:

"Have you noticed any changes in your skin? Your hair? Your nails?"
"Have you had any rashes? Sores? Lumps? Itching?"

Even subtle changes in moles or skin lesions may indicate cancerous changes and need follow-up. Ask, "Do you have any moles you are concerned about or that you have noticed any change at all? Any new moles?" If the patient reports such moles, ask how they have changed and pursue any personal or family history of melanoma or skin cancer.

Past History

Questions regarding the patient's history may include:

- Do you have any skin diseases such as melanoma, eczema, or psoriasis?
- Do you have diabetes or peripheral vascular disease?
- Do you have any allergies or food sensitivities?
- Have you ever had a severe sunburn? How many second-degree sunburns have you experienced?
- Have you ever been on corticosteroid medications for more than 2 weeks?
- What prescribed or over-the-counter medications do you take?
- What immunizations have you had?

Family History

Questions to ask regarding the patient's history may include:

- Do any family members have the same or similar symptoms?
- Has anyone in your family had melanoma, eczema, or psoriasis or skin biopsies?
- Does anyone in your family have allergies?

Lifestyle and Personal Habits

Questions to ask regarding the patient's lifestyle and personal habits may include:

- Describe your bathing and shampooing routines. Have you changed product brands recently?
- Do you wear false nails, wigs, hair extensions, and/or false eyelashes?
- Do you go to a nail salon or gym?
- How much sun exposure do you receive daily?
- How often do you use sunscreen? What sun protective factor (SPF) value of sunscreen do you use?
- Do you perform skin self-examinations? How often?
- Are you exposed to any chemicals or radiation at home or work?
- What are your hobbies?
- Describe a typical day's diet.

PHYSICAL EXAMINATION

Equipment needed for a physical examination of the integumentary system includes:

- Good lighting
- Ruler or measuring tape
- Magnifying glass
- Gloves

The examination of the skin, hair, and nails begins with the general survey and continues throughout the physical examination. Make sure the patient wears a gown that allows close inspection of all anterior and posterior skin surfaces. A sheet can be used to maintain privacy and cover the parts of the body not being examined. Wash your hands, and explain the examination to the patient.

CLINICAL TIP
Patients at risk for skin cancer may not request a skin examination, so the general physical examination is an important opportunity to look for melanomas and other skin cancers, especially in hard-to-see areas such as the back and posterior legs.

Inspect the entire skin surface in good light, preferably natural light or artificial light that resembles it. Correlate your findings with observations of the mucous membranes, especially when assessing skin color, because diseases may appear in both areas. Techniques for examining these membranes are described in Chapter 11, "The Eyes," and Chapter 12, "Ears, Nose, Mouth, and Throat."

Artificial light often distorts colors and masks jaundice.

Skin

Inspect and palpate the skin, noting the characteristics in the following sections.

Color

Skin color will vary according to genetic background and may have fair, olive, tan, brown, or golden hues. Color change may be general, affecting all the skin or localized, confined to an area, for example, the right forearm (Table 9-2). Patients may notice a change in their skin color before the nurse does. Ask patients if they have noted any changes to their skin color? Follow up with "OLD CART" if the patient responds affirmatively.

Look for increased pigmentation, loss of pigmentation, or redness of the skin. Is it generalized or local? If local, indicate its location.

Assess for cyanosis or pallor. Look for the red color of oxyhemoglobin versus the pallor in its absence. These are best observed where the horny layer of the epidermis is thinnest and causes the least scatter—the fingernails, the lips, and the mucous membranes, particularly those of the mouth and the palpebral conjunctiva. In dark-skinned people, inspecting the palms and soles may also be useful.

CLINICAL TIP
Pallor results from decreased redness in *anemia* and decreased blood flow, as occurs in fainting or arterial insufficiency.

Causes of *central cyanosis* include advanced lung disease, congenital heart disease, and hemoglobinopathies. Genetic disorders involving hemoglobin include sickle cell disease and thalassemia.

TABLE 9-2 Skin Color Changes

General Changes

Cyanosis

Cyanosis is the somewhat bluish color that is visible in these toenails and toes. Compare this color with the normally pink fingernails and fingers of the same patient. Impaired venous return in the leg caused this example of peripheral cyanosis. Cyanosis, especially when slight, may be hard to distinguish from normal skin color.

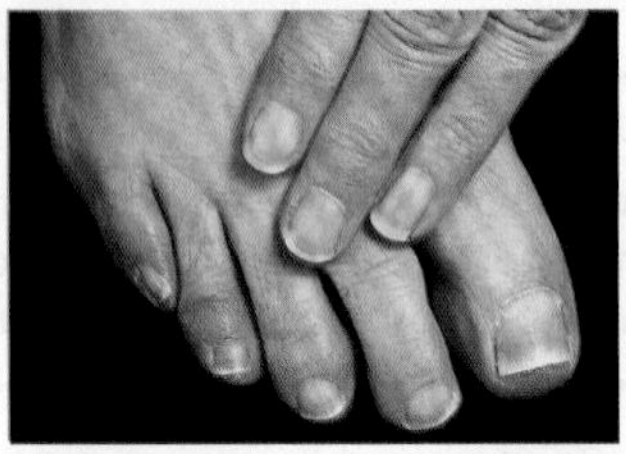

Erythema

The red hue caused by increased blood flow results in the "slapped cheeks" of *erythema infectiosum* (also called "fifth disease").

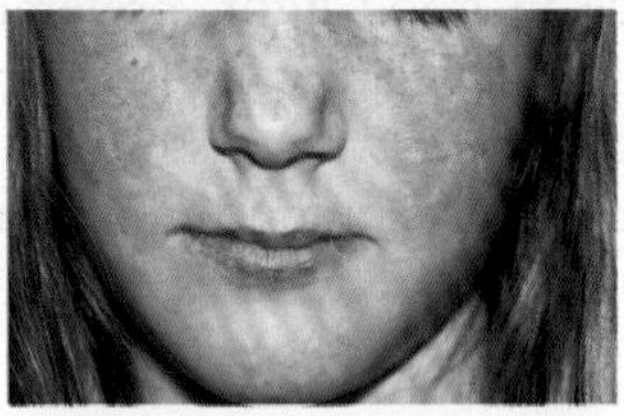

Carotenemia

The yellowish palm of carotenemia is compared with a normally pink palm, sometimes a subtle finding. Unlike jaundice, carotenemia does not affect the sclera, which remains white. The cause is a diet high in carrots and other yellow vegetables or fruits. Carotenemia is not harmful but indicates the need for assessing dietary intake.

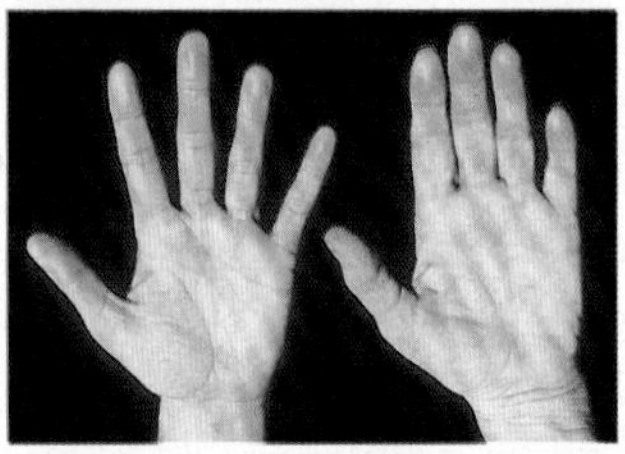

Jaundice

Jaundice makes the skin diffusely yellow. Contrast this patient's skin color with the examiner's hand. Jaundice is seen most easily and reliably in the sclera, as shown here. It may also be visible in mucous membranes. Causes include *liver disease* and *hemolysis of red blood cells.*

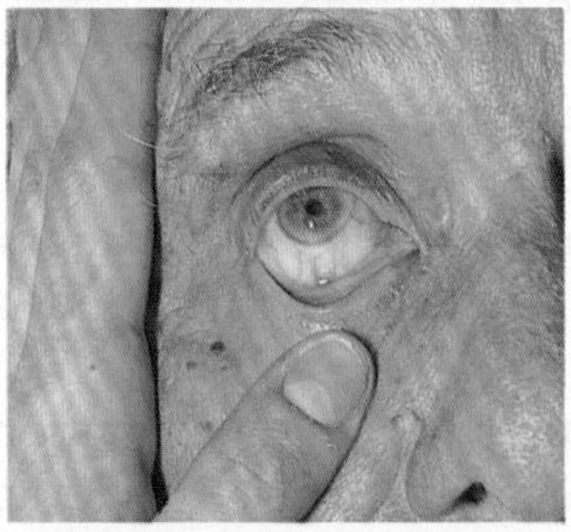

Local Changes

Café-Au-Lait Spot

A café-au-lait spot is slightly but uniformly pigmented macule or patch with a somewhat irregular border, usually 0.5–1.5 cm in diameter and benign. Six or more such spots, each with a diameter greater than 1.5 cm, however, suggest neurofibromatosis. (The small, darker macules are unrelated.)

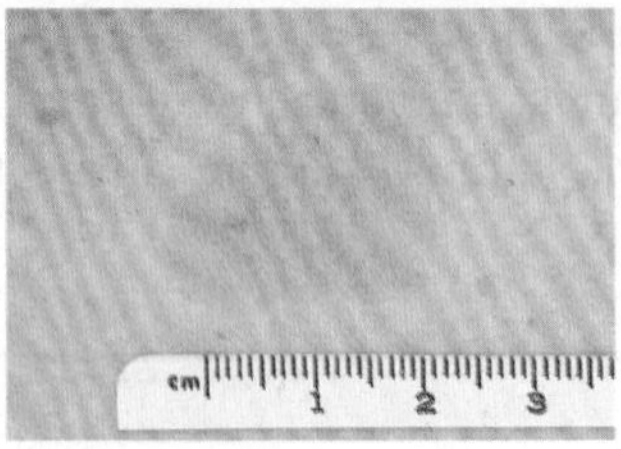

Vitiligo

In vitiligo, depigmented macules appear on the face, hands, feet, extensor surfaces, and other regions and may coalesce into extensive areas that lack melanin. The brown pigment is normal skin color; the pale areas are vitiligo. The condition may be hereditary. These changes may be distressing to the patient.

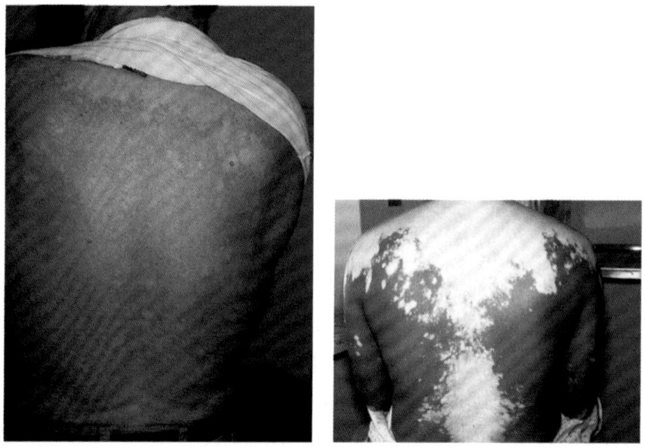

Tinea Versicolor

This is a common superficial fungal infection of the skin, causing hypopigmented, slightly scaly macules on the trunk, neck, and upper arms (short-sleeved shirt distribution). They are easier to see in darker skin and in some people; they are more obvious after tanning. In lighter skin, macules may look reddish or tan instead of pale.

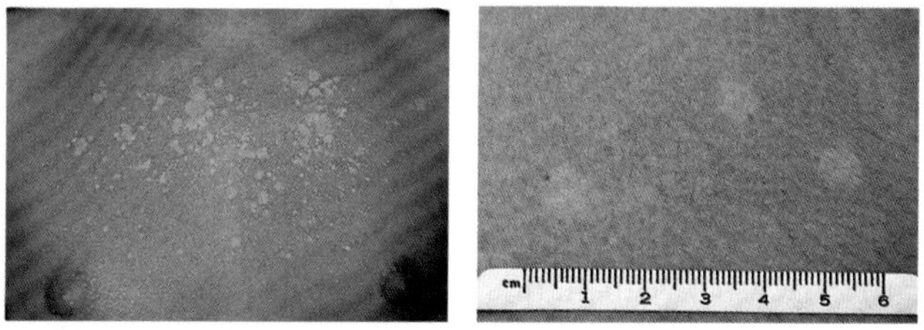

Acanthosis Nigricans

This is a skin condition characterized by areas of dark, velvety discoloration in body folds and creases. The affected skin can become thickened. Acanthosis nigricans is most often seen in the armpits, groin, and neck. It is frequently associated with obesity and diabetes.

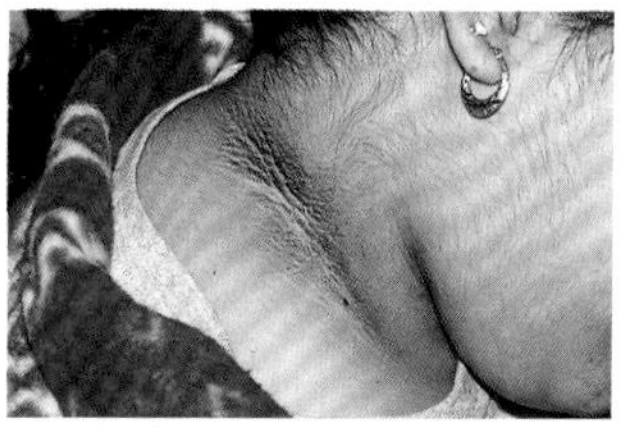

Sources of photos: *Tinea Versicolor*—Ostler, H. B., Mailbach, H. I., & Hoke, A. W. (2004). *Diseases of the eye and skin: A color atlas*. Lippincott Williams & Wilkins; *Vitiligo, Erythema*—Goodheart, H. P. (2003). *Goodheart's photoguide of common skin disorders: Diagnosis and management* (2nd ed.). Lippincott Williams & Wilkins.

Central cyanosis is best identified in the lips, oral mucosa, and tongue. The lips, however, may turn blue in the cold, and melanin in the lips may simulate cyanosis in darker-skinned people.

Cyanosis of the nails, hands, and feet may be central or peripheral in origin. Anxiety or a cold examining room may cause peripheral cyanosis.

CLINICAL TIP

Cyanosis in *congestive heart failure* is usually peripheral, reflecting decreased blood flow, but in *pulmonary edema,* it may also be central. *Venous obstruction* may cause peripheral cyanosis.

Look for the yellow color of **jaundice** in the sclera. Do not confuse a normal scleral yellow pigmentation in dark-skinned individuals with jaundice. Rather, observe the hard palate with a bright light for jaundice. Jaundice may also appear in the palpebral conjunctiva, lips, undersurface of the tongue, tympanic membrane, and skin. Pressing the skin over a bony prominence and observing the color when your finger is removed will accentuate the yellow hue.

CLINICAL TIP
Jaundice suggests liver disease or excessive hemolysis of red blood cells.

For the yellow color that accompanies high levels of carotene, look at the palms, soles, and face.

Moisture

Note excessive dryness, sweating, and oiliness. Skin should be dry to touch without flaking or cracking. Perspiration may appear on the face, hands, axillae, or skin folds in response to a warm environment; increased metabolic activity, such as fever or exercise; and anxiety or pain. Excessive dryness, often accompanied by flaking, or excessive sweating (diaphoresis) may indicate a problem. Carefully inspect skin folds where moisture may cause skin breakdown.

Dryness may indicate hypothyroidism. Oiliness is associated with acne. Dry skin with parched cracked lips, dry mucous membranes, and lack of tears indicate dehydration.

Temperature

Use the backs of your hands to make this assessment (Fig. 9-3). In addition to identifying generalized warmth or coolness of the skin, note the temperature of any areas with increased pigmentation or erythema.

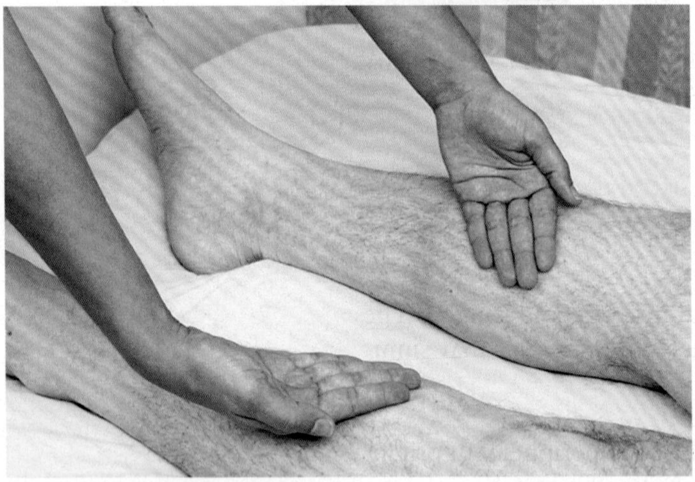

FIGURE 9-3 Use the dorsum (back) of your hand to assess skin temperature.

CLINICAL TIP
Generalized warmth may indicate *fever* and/or *hyperthyroidism while* coolness can indicate *hypothyroidism.* Local warmth may indicate inflammation or cellulitis.

Texture

Note the roughness or smoothness of the skin. Normal skin feels smooth and firm with an even surface.

Roughness may be a finding with *hypothyroidism;* a velvety texture can indicate *hyperthyroidism.*

Mobility and Turgor

Lift a fold of skin below the clavicle, the forearm, or on the abdomen and note the ease with which it lifts up (*mobility*) and the speed with which it returns into place (**turgor**). Normally the skin promptly returns into place.

Do not test turgor on the dorsal surface of the hand in the older adult; this will result in a false-positive finding due to loss of subcutaneous tissue. Decreased mobility is a finding with edema and *scleroderma, while* decreased turgor can indicate dehydration.

Edema

The presence of excess fluid in the interstitial spaces is **edema.** It may be localized due to an injury or may be the result of a systemic problem (e.g., heart failure). Systemic edema most often occurs in the dependent portions of the body, the feet, legs, and sacral area. The skin appears puffy and feels tight. Mobility is decreased and cyanosis or jaundice in the skin is obscured.

Edema may be pitting or nonpitting. In **pitting edema** the interstitial water is mobile and can be translocated with the pressure exerted by a finger (Fig. 9-4). A "pit" or depression is left for 5 to 30 seconds. The degree of pitting is measured on a 1 to 4 scale (Table 9-3).

See Chapter 15, "The Peripheral Vascular System and Lymphatic System," for a further discussion of edema.

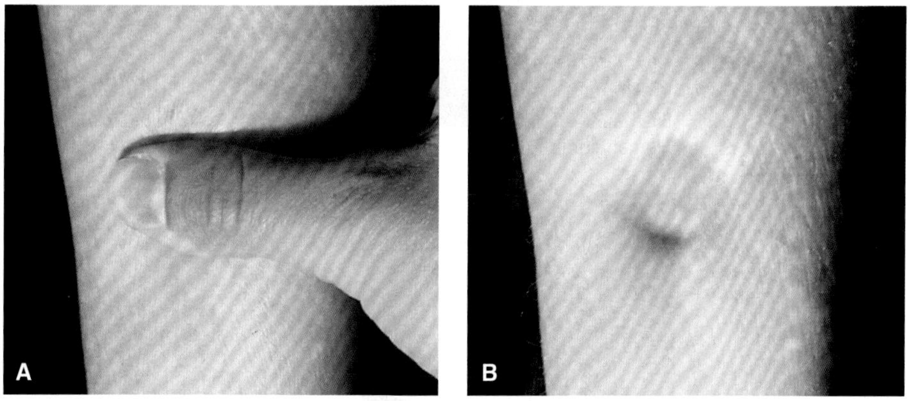

FIGURE 9-4 **A.** The nurse can translocate fluid in the edema by exerting pressure with a finger. **B.** The resultant "pitting" demonstrates the interstitial fluid has moved away from the pressure. (Reprinted with permission from Strayer, D. S., Saffitz, J. E., & Rubin, E. (2020). *Rubin's pathology: Mechanisms of human disease* (8th ed.). Wolters Kluwer.)

TABLE 9-3 Pitting Edema Scale

Scale	Depression (mm)	Duration of Rebound
1+	2	Immediately
2+	4	Fewer than 15 sec
3+	6	Up to 30 sec
4+	8	More than 30 sec

Nonpitting edema reflects a condition in which serum proteins have accumulated in the interstitial space with the water and coagulated. This is frequently seen with local infection or trauma and is called *brawny edema*.

Lesions

Inspect the skin for lesions. A **lesion** is a circumscribed pathologic alteration of the skin. Lesions may be classified as primary (*initial lesions;* Table 9-4), secondary (*lesions that arise from primary lesions;* Table 9-5), and vascular lesions (Table 9-6). Document the following characteristics of any lesion(s).

TABLE 9-4 Primary Skin Lesions

Flat Lesions (Nonpalpable Lesions with Local Changes in Skin Color)

Macule—Less than 1.0 cm

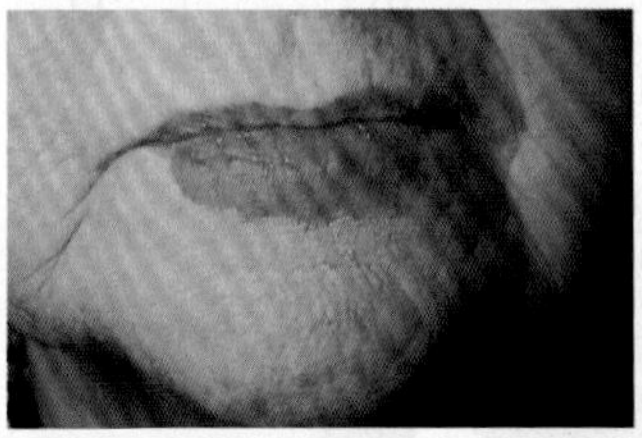
Hemangioma.

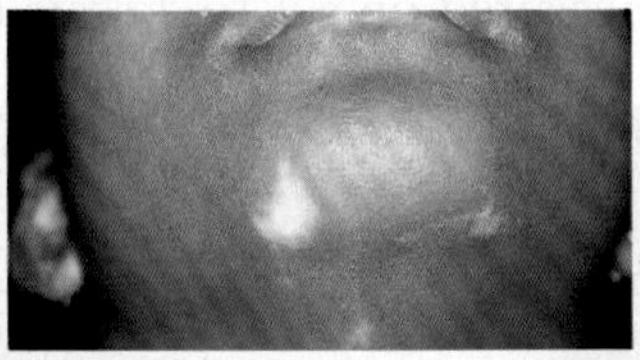
Vitiligo.

Patch—1.0 cm or larger

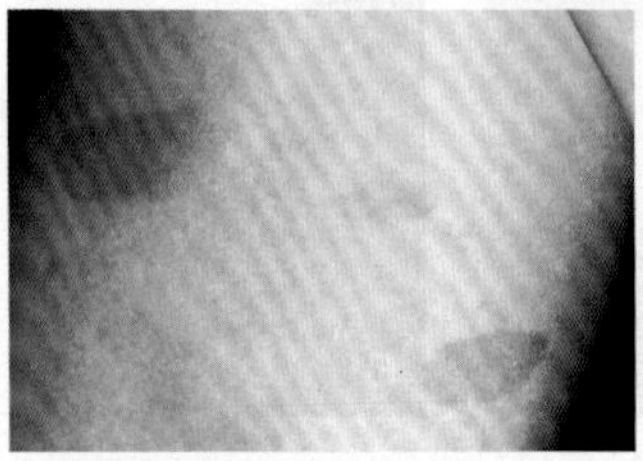
Café-au-lait spot.

Palpable Elevated Lesions and Solid Masses

Plaque—Elevated superficial lesion 1.0 cm or larger, often formed by coalescence of papules

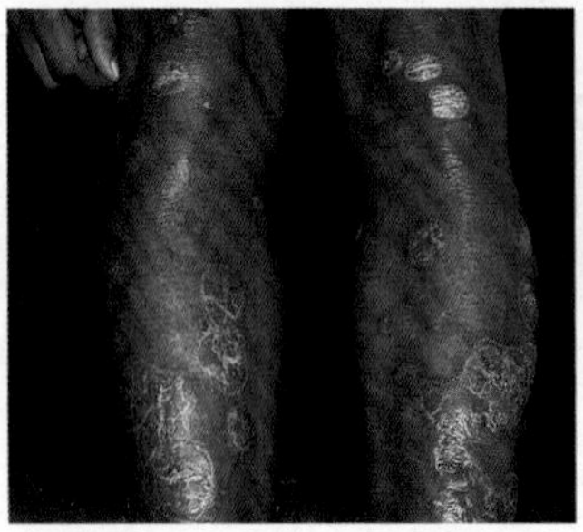
Psoriasis.

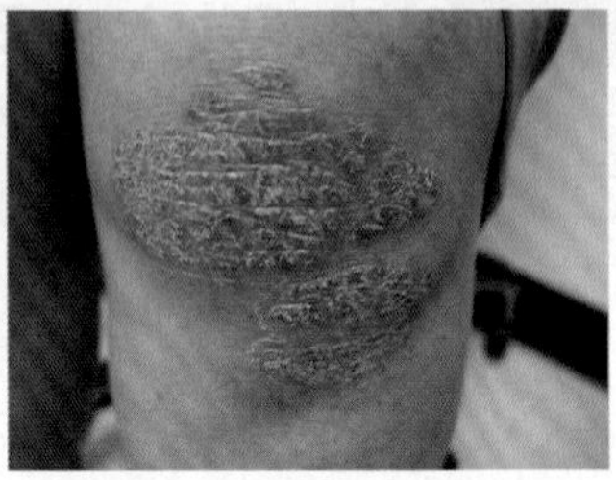
Psoriasis.

Palpable Elevated Lesions and Solid Masses (*continued*)

Papule—Less than 1.0 cm

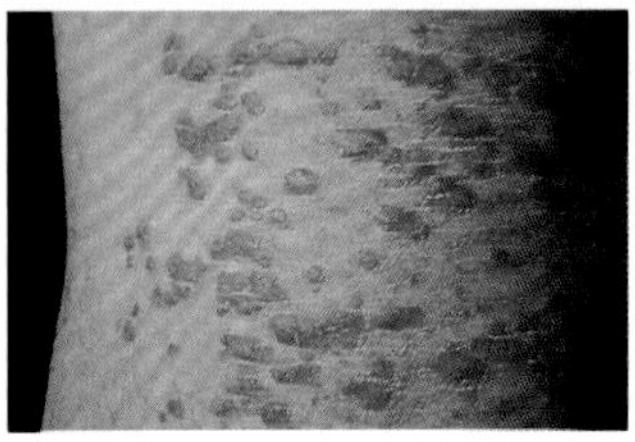

Psoriasis.

Nodule—Marble-like lesion larger than 0.5 cm, often deeper and firmer than a papule

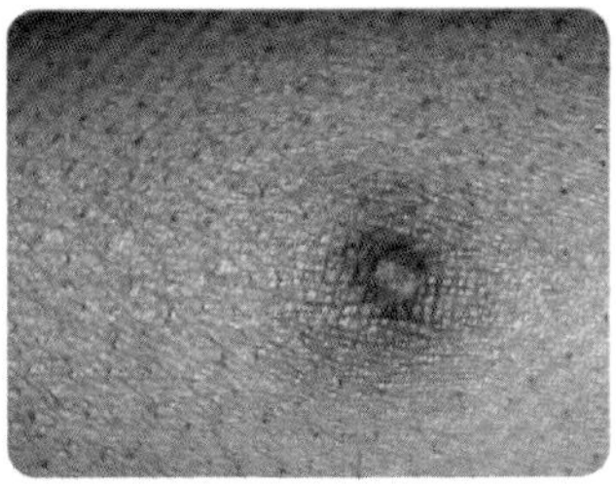

Dermatofibroma.

Cyst—Nodule filled with expressible material, either liquid or semisolid

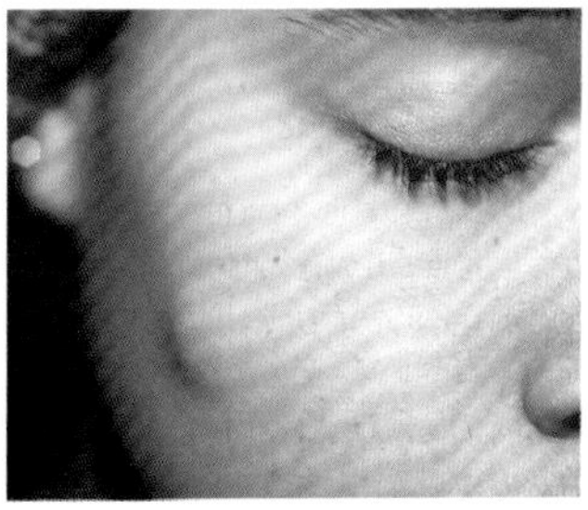

Epidermal inclusion cyst.

Wheal—A somewhat irregular, often reddish or deeper brown on patients with dark complexions, superficial area of localized skin edema

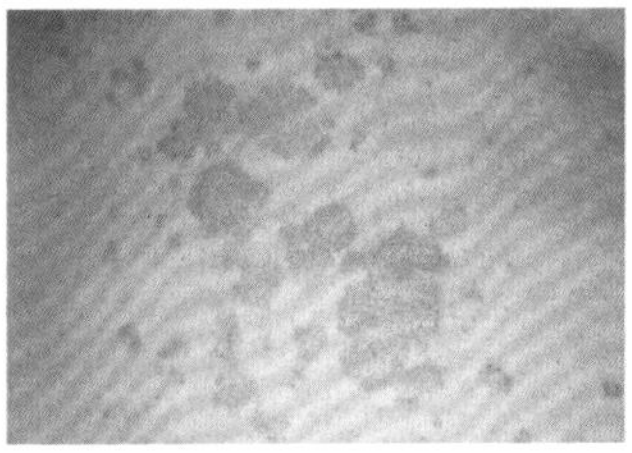

Urticaria.

Palpable Elevated Fluid-Filled, Round or Oval Lesions (Blisters)

Vesicle—Less than 1.0 cm; filled with serous fluid

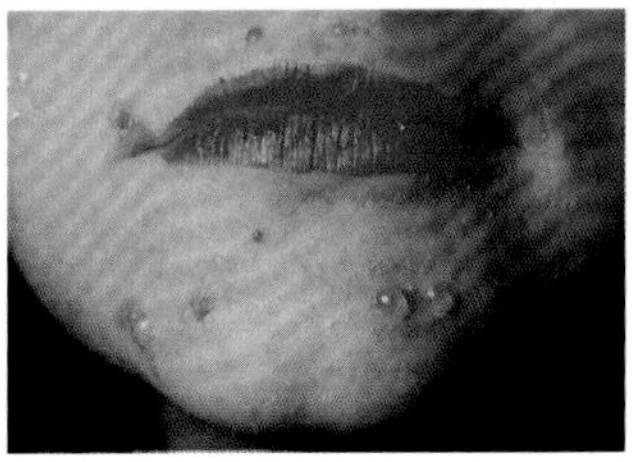

Herpes simplex.

(continued)

TABLE 9-4 Primary Skin Lesions (*Continued*)

Palpable Elevated Fluid-Filled, Round or Oval Lesions (Blisters) (*continued*)

Bulla—1.0 cm or larger; filled with serous fluid

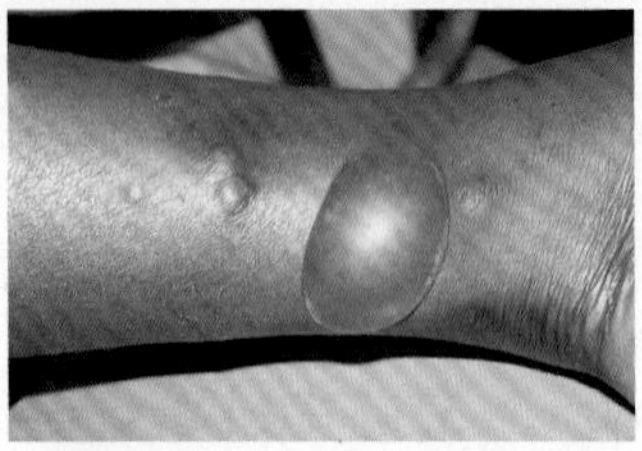

Insect bite.

Pustule—Filled with pus

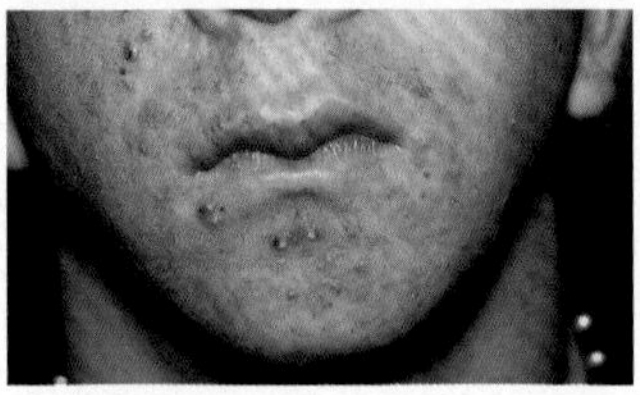

Acne.

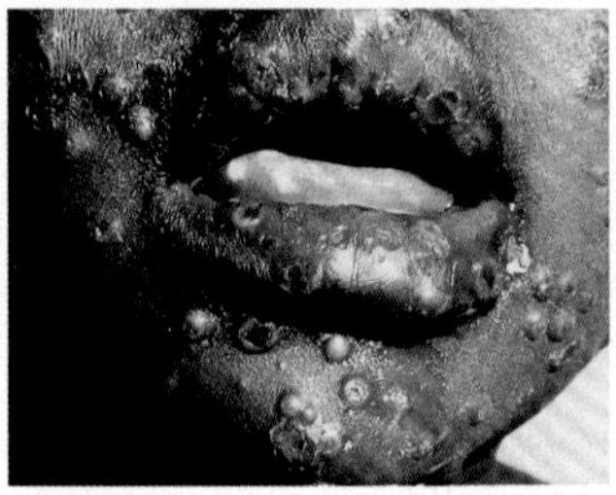

Smallpox.

Burrow—A minute, slightly raised tunnel in the epidermis, commonly found on the finger webs and on the sides of the fingers. It looks like a short (5–15 mm), linear or curved gray line and may end in a tiny vesicle. Skin lesions include small papules, pustules, lichenified areas, and excoriations. With a magnifying lens, look for the *burrow* of the mite that causes scabies.

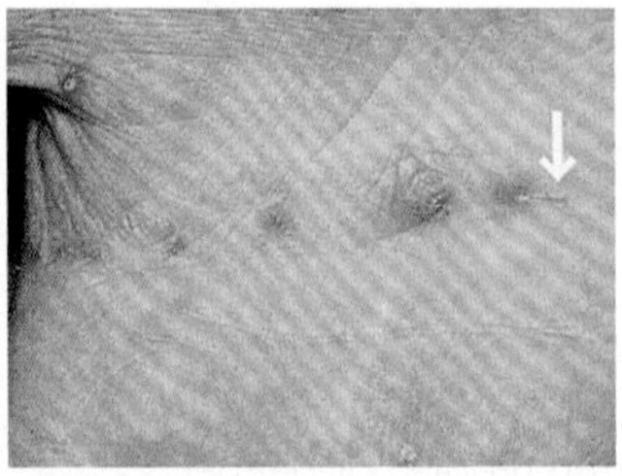

Scabies.

Sources of photos: *Hemangioma, Café-au-Lait Spot, Psoriasis* [bottom], *Herpes Simplex*— Lugo-Somolinos, A., McKinley-Grant, L., Goldsmith, L., Papier, A., & Adigun, C. (2011). *VisualDx: Essential dermatology in pigmented skin*. Wolters Kluwer; *Psoriasis [right]*—Image provided by Stedman's; *Dermatofibroma*—Reprinted with permission from Lugo-Somolinos, A., McKinley-Grant, L., Goldsmith, L., Papier, A., & Adigun, C. (2011). *VisualDx: Essential dermatology in pigmented skin*. Wolters Kluwer; *Smallpox*—Ostler, H. B., Mailbach, H. I., & Hoke, A. W. (2004). *Diseases of the eye and skin: A color atlas*. Lippincott Williams & Wilkins; *Vitiligo, Epidermal Inclusion Cyst, Urticaria, Insect Bite, Acne, Scabies*—Goodheart, H. P. (2003). *Goodheart's photoguide of common skin disorders: Diagnosis and management* (2nd ed.). Lippincott Williams & Wilkins.

TABLE 9-5 Secondary Skin Lesions

Scales—Flakes of dead exfoliated epidermis; color may be white, gray, or silvery. Texture may be fine or thick

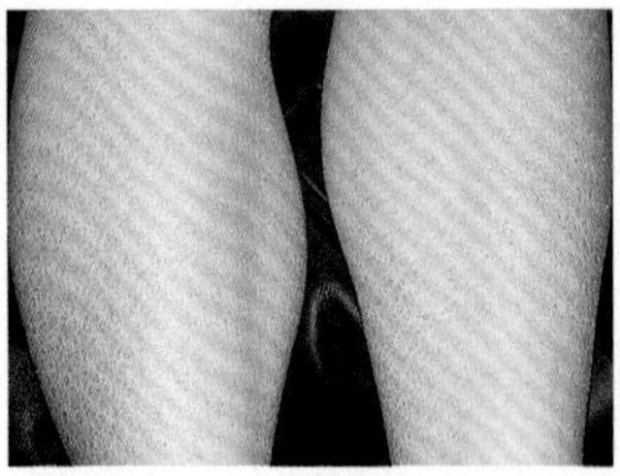

Ichthyosis vulgaris.

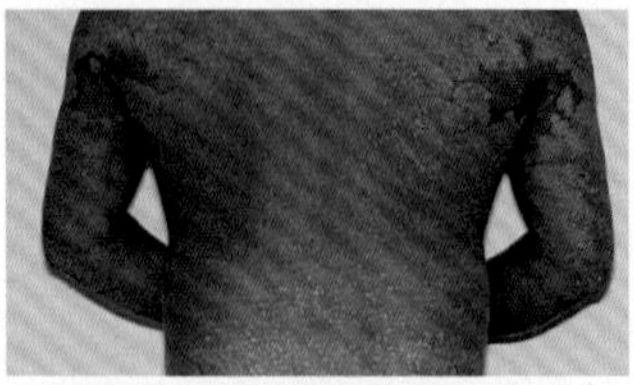

Dry skin.

Crust—The dried residue of skin exudates such as serum, pus, or blood; can be red-brown, orange, or yellow

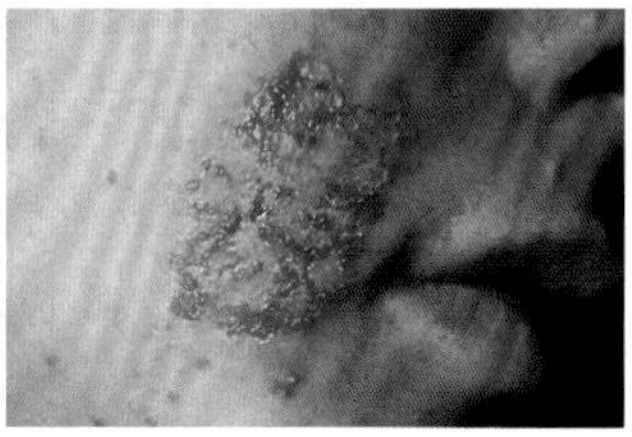

Impetigo.

Lichenification—Visible and palpable thickening of the epidermis and roughening of the skin with increased visibility of the normal skin furrows (often from chronic rubbing)

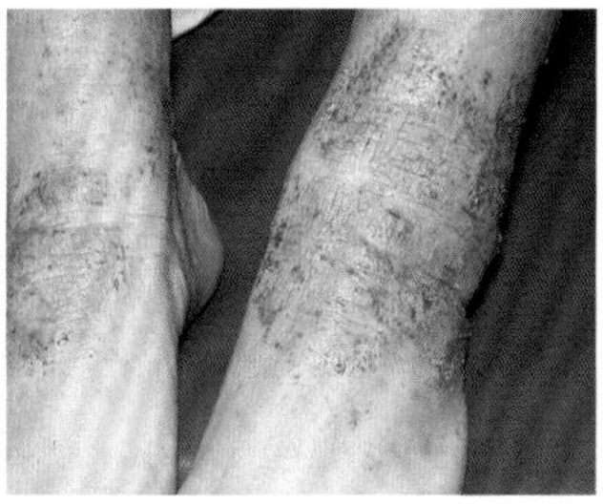

Neurodermatitis.

Scars—Flat connective tissue left after an injury or disease heals; can be red or purple initially; older scars can fade to silver or white

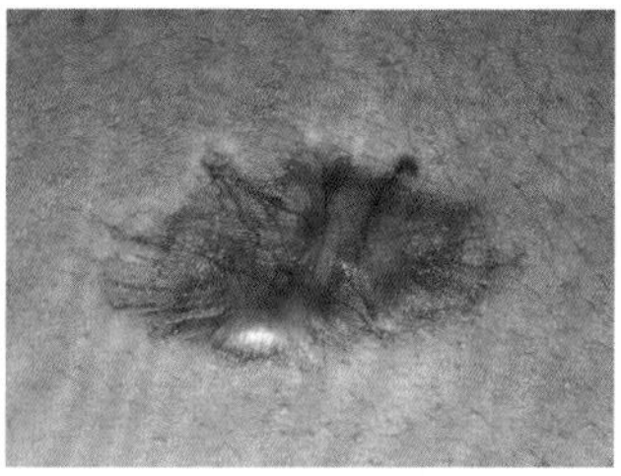

Hypertrophic scar from steroid injections.

Keloid—Hypertrophic scarring that extends beyond the borders of the initiating injury

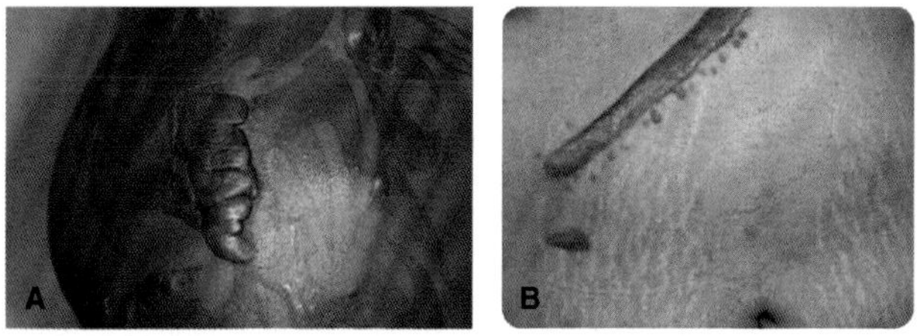

A. Keloid Secondary to Tattoos. **B.** Keloid on the Abdomen.

Erosion—Nonscarring wearing away of the superficial epidermis; surface is moist but does not bleed

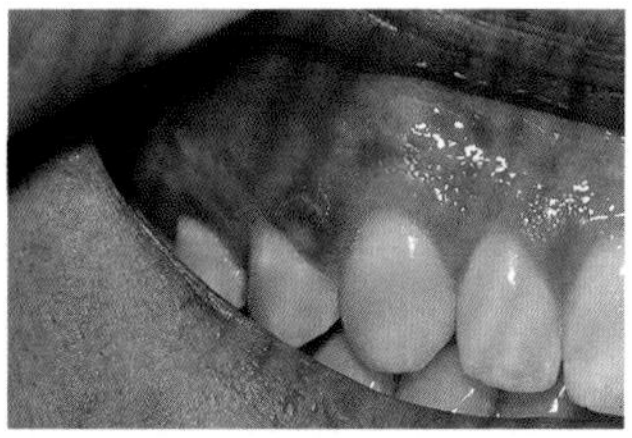

Aphthous stomatitis, moist area after the rupture of a vesicle, as in chickenpox.

(*continued*)

TABLE 9-5 Secondary Skin Lesions (*Continued*)

Excoriation—Linear or punctate erosions caused by scratching	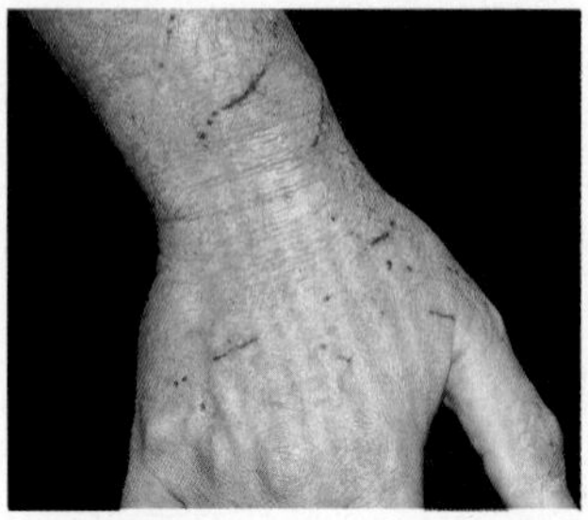 Cat scratches.
Fissure—A linear crack in the skin, often resulting from excessive dryness	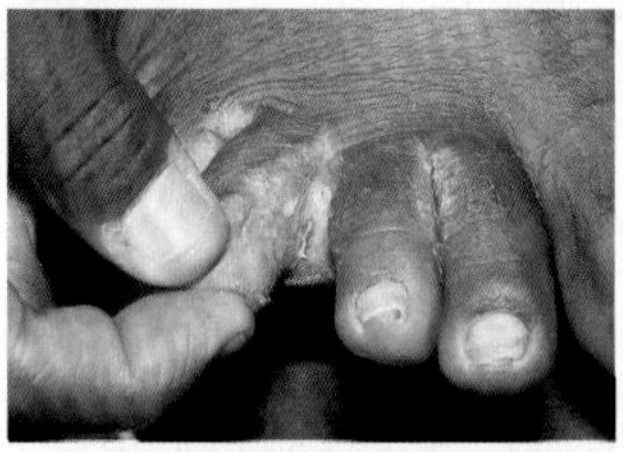 Athlete's foot.
Ulcer—A deeper loss of epidermis and dermis; may bleed and scar	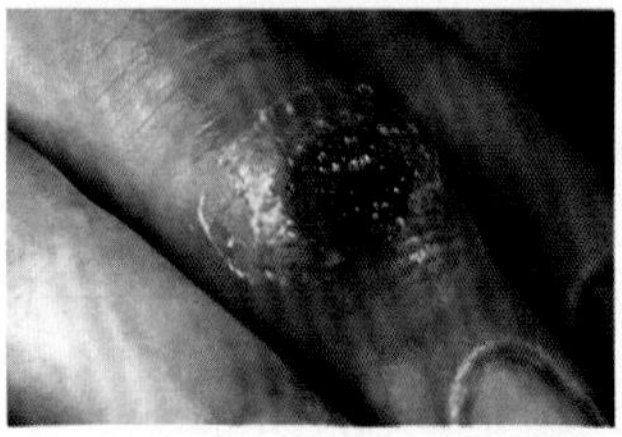 Stasis ulcer of venous insufficiency, syphilitic chancre.

Sources of photos: *Erosion, Excoriation, Fissure*—Goodheart, H. P. (2003). *Goodheart's photoguide of common skin disorders: Diagnosis and management* (2nd ed.). Lippincott Williams & Wilkins; *Ichthyosis, Dry Skin, Hypertrophic Scar*—Goodheart, H. P. (2003). *Goodheart's photoguide of common skin disorders: Diagnosis and management* (2nd ed.). Lippincott Williams & Wilkins; *Impetigo*—Hall, J. C. (2006). *Sauer's manual of skin diseases* (9th ed.). Lippincott Williams & Wilkins; *Keloid Secondary to Tattoos*—Hall, J. C., & Hall, B. J. (2017). *Sauer's manual of skin diseases* (11th ed.). Wolters Kluwer; *Keloid on the Abdomen*—Lugo-Somolinos, A., McKinley-Grant, L., Goldsmith, L., Papier, A., & Adigun, C. (2011). *Visual Dx: Essential dermatology in pigmented skin*. Wolters Kluwer; *Lichenification*—Goodheart, H. P. (2003). *Goodheart's photoguide of common skin disorders* (2th ed.). Lippincott Williams & Wilkins; *Ulcer*—Centers for Disease Control and Prevention.

TABLE 9-6 Vascular and Purpuric Lesions of the Skin

	Vascular Lesions		
	Spider Angioma[a]	**Spider Vein**[a]	**Cherry Angioma**
Example	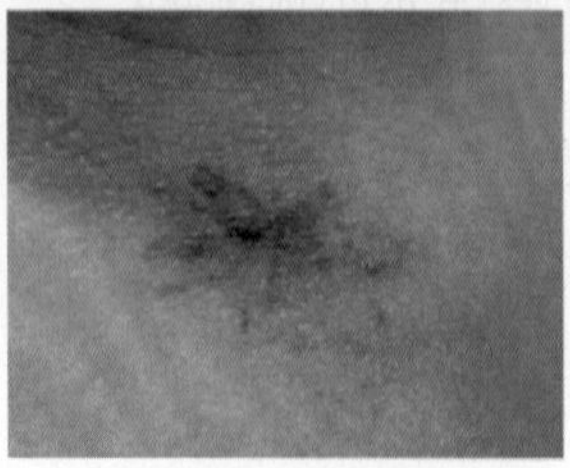	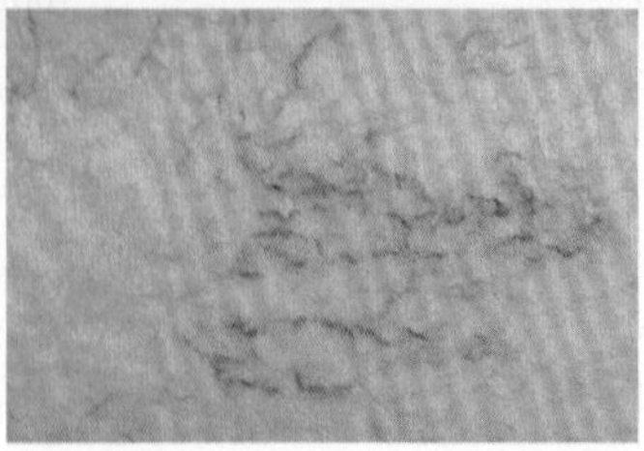	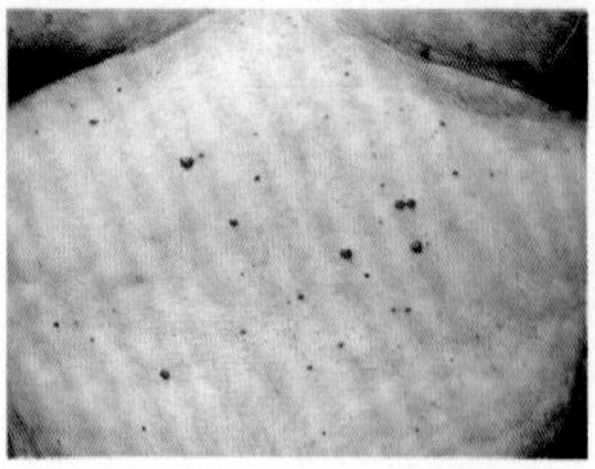

Color and Size	Fiery red; from very small to 2 cm	Bluish; size variable from very small to several inches	Bright or ruby red; may become brownish with age; 1–3 mm
Shape	Central body, sometimes raised, surrounded by erythema and radiating legs	Variable; may resemble a spider or be linear, irregular, cascading	Round, flat or sometimes raised, may be surrounded by a pale halo
Pulsatility and Effect of Pressure	Often seen in center of the spider when pressure with a glass slide is applied; pressure on the body causes blanching of the spider	Absent; pressure over the center does not cause blanching, but diffuse pressure blanches the veins	Absent; may show partial blanching, especially if pressure applied with edge of a pinpoint
Distribution	Face, neck, arms, and upper trunk; almost never below the waist	Most often on the legs, near veins; also on the anterior chest	Trunk; also extremities
Significance	Usually normal; solitary or few. If numerous in telangiectatic mats, may indicate liver disease. Also seen in pregnancy, vitamin B deficiency.	Often accompanies increased pressure in the superficial veins, as in varicose veins	None; increases in size and numbers with aging

Purpuric Lesions

	Petechia / Purpura	Ecchymosis
Example	Petechia 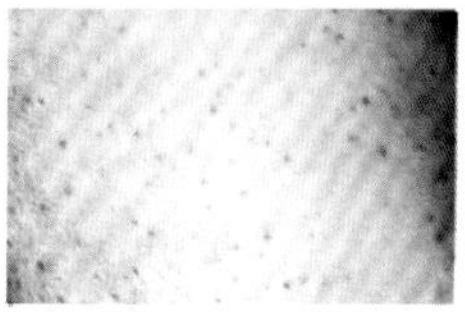 Purpura 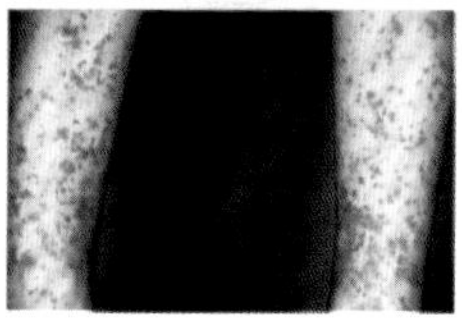	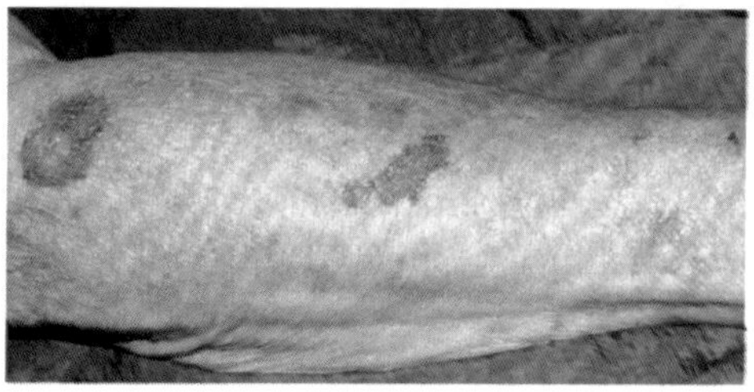
Color and Size	Deep red or reddish purple; petechia, 1–3 mm; purpura, larger	Purple or purplish blue fading to green, yellow, and brown with time. Variable size, larger than petechiae, >3 mm
Shape	Rounded, sometimes irregular; flat	Rounded, oval, or irregular; may have a central subcutaneous flat nodule (a hematoma)
Pulsatility and Effect of Pressure	Absent; no effect from pressure	Absent; no effect from pressure
Distribution	Variable	Variable
Significance	Blood outside the vessels; if on dorsal forearms, usually *actinic purpura* from chronic sun exposure; may indicate a bleeding disorder or if petechiae, emboli to skin; palpable purpura in *vasculitis*	Blood outside the vessels; often secondary to bruising or trauma; also seen in bleeding disorders

[a]These are telangiectasias, or dilated small vessels that look red or bluish.
Sources of photos: *Petechia*—CDC; *Purpura*—CDC/Mr. Gust; *Spider Angioma*—Barankin Collection, Wolters Kluwer, 2005.

Color

Is the color uniform or variegated? Use "skin-colored" to describe a lesion that is the same shade as the patient's skin. For red lesions or rashes, blanch the lesion by pressing it firmly with your finger or a glass slide to see if the redness temporarily blanches then refills.

Blanching lesions are *erythematous* and suggest inflammation.

Size

Use a ruler to measure each lesion in millimeters or centimeters. For oval lesions, measure the short axis.

Elevation

Flat means you *cannot palpate the lesion with eyes closed.* Raised, or pedunculated (attached to a stalk, e.g., a skin tag) lesions could be felt with the eyes closed.

Number

Lesions can be solitary or multiple. If there are multiple lesions, how many? Also consider estimating the total number of each type of lesion you are describing.

Texture

Palpate the lesion to see if it is smooth, fleshy, *verrucous* (wart-like), or *keratotic* (scaling).

Scaling can be greasy, like *seborrheic dermatitis* or *seborrheic keratoses,* dry and fine like *tinea pedis,* or hard and keratotic like *actinic keratoses* or *squamous cell carcinoma.*

Types of Skin Lesions

Types of skin lesions include:

- *Macule:* Flat, colored spot on the skin (e.g., freckle)
- *Papule:* Small bump or pimple
- *Vesicle:* Small blister containing serous fluid
- *Nevus:* Mole or birthmark

Shape and Pattern

Are the lesions round, oval, linear, clustered, *annular* (in a ring), *arciform* (in an arc), bull's eye, geographic, or *serpiginous* (serpent- or worm-like) (Table 9-7)? Are they dermatomal, covering a skin band that corresponds to a sensory nerve root (*dermatome*)? See Chapter 20, "The Nervous System."

TABLE 9-7 Skin Lesions—Patterns and Shapes

Linear lesions appear as a straight line.

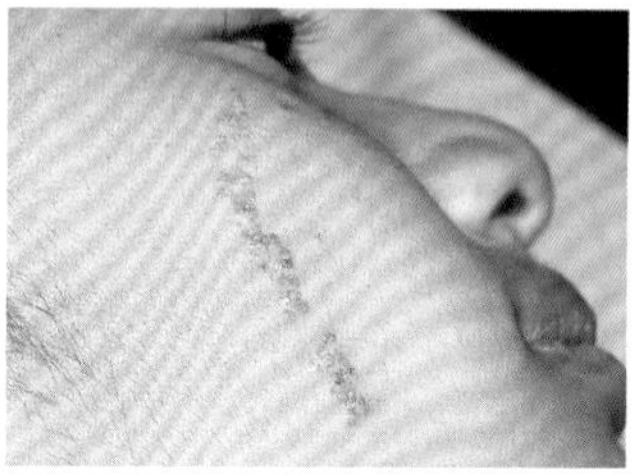

Linear epidermal nevus.

Geographic areas of one color with variably scalloped borders interface with another color.

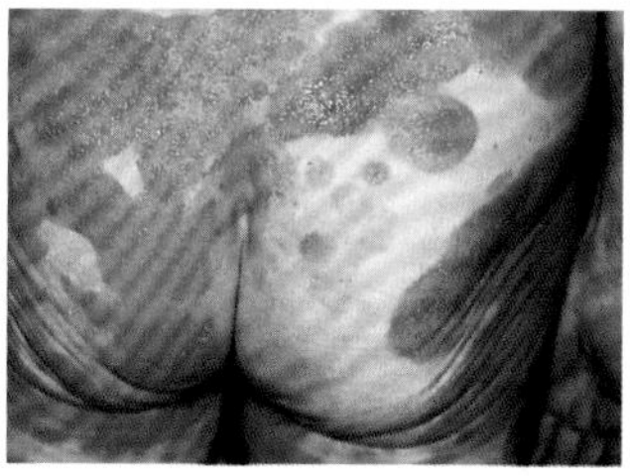

Mycosis fungoides.

Clustered lesions are grouped.

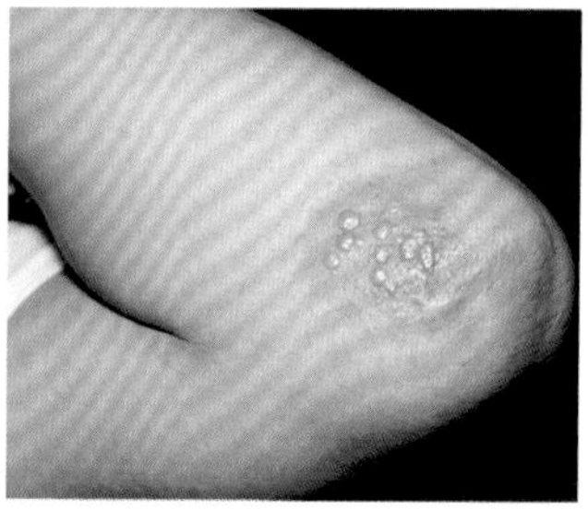

Herpes simplex.

Serpiginous lesions appear to creep from one part to another. The margin has a wavy or serpentine border.

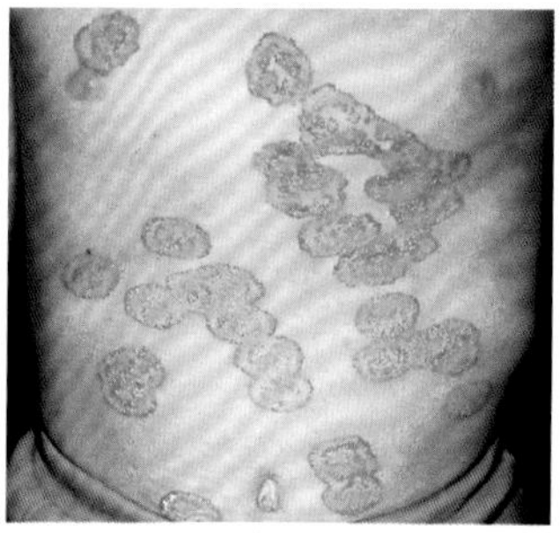

Tinea corporis.

Annular and *arciform* lesions have a circular shape.

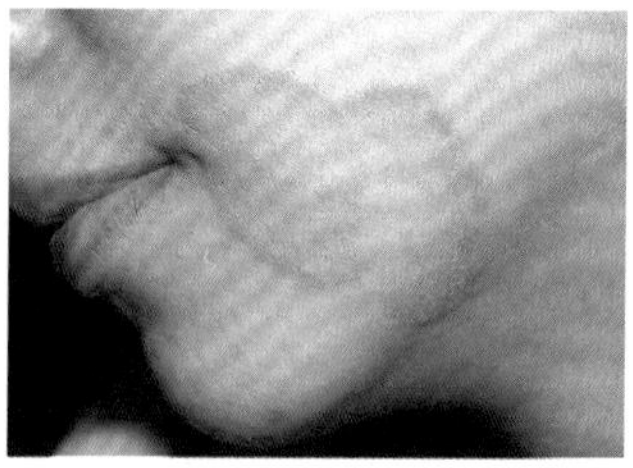

Annular lesion of tinea faciei (ringworm).

(*continued*)

TABLE 9-7 Skin Lesions—Patterns and Shapes (*Continued*)

Confluent lesions are lesions that run together.

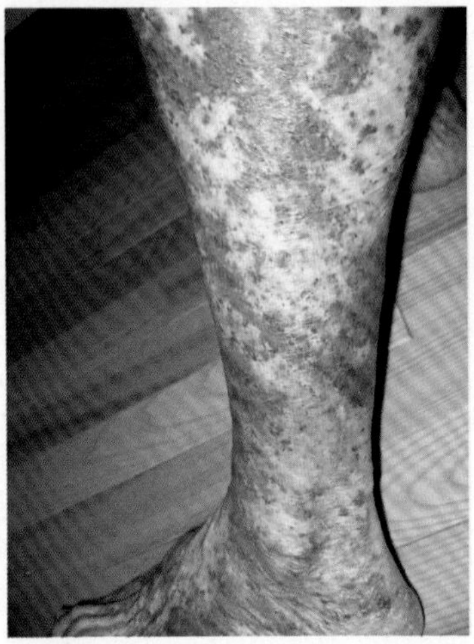

Small-vessel vasculitis.

Target lesions have a bull's eye appearance.

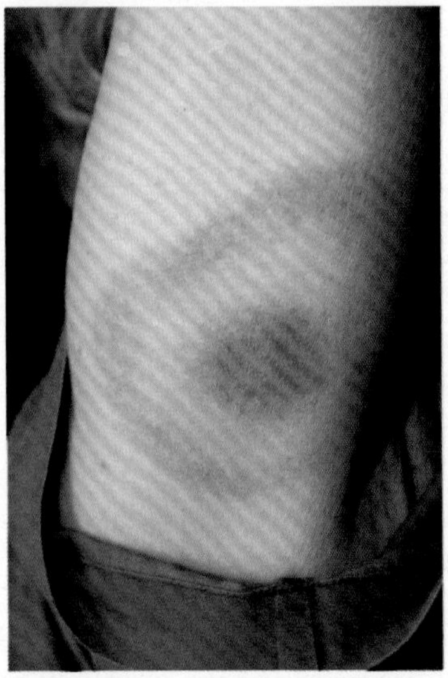

Lyme disease.

Zosteriform lesions follow a nerve dermatome. See dermatome maps in Chapter 20, "The Nervous System."

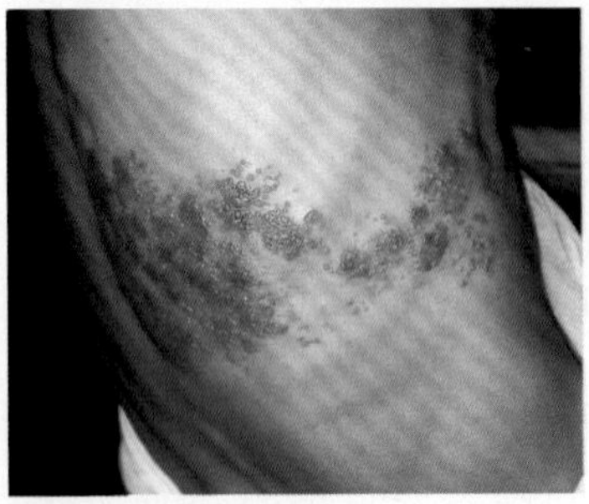

Herpes zoster (shingles).

Sources of photos: *Herpes Zoster*—Reprinted with permission from Goodheart, H. P. (2003). *Goodheart's photoguide of common skin disorders* (2nd ed.). Lippincott Williams & Wilkins; *Linear Epidermal Nevus, Herpes Simplex, Tinea Faciale*—Goodheart, H. P. (2003). *Goodheart's photoguide of common skin disorders: Diagnosis and management* (2nd ed.). Lippincott Williams & Wilkins; *Lyme disease*—Engleberg, N. C., Dermody, T., & DiRita, V. (2012). *Schaechter's mechanisms of microbial disease* (5th ed.). Wolters Kluwer | Lippincott Williams & Wilkins; *Mycosis Fungoides, Tinea Corporis*—Hall, J. C., & Hall, B. J. (2017). *Sauer's manual of skin diseases* (11th ed.). Wolters Kluwer; *Small-Vessel Vasculitis*—Marder, V. J., Aird, W. C., Bennett, J. S., Schulman, S., & White, G. C., II. (2012). *Hemostasis and thrombosis* (6th ed.). Wolters Kluwer | Lippincott Williams & Wilkins.

CLINICAL TIP
Vesicles in a unilateral dermatomal pattern are typical of herpes zoster.

Anatomic Location and Distribution

The nurse should note the anatomic location and distribution over the body (Table 9-8). Are the lesions generalized or localized? Do they, for example, involve the exposed surfaces, the *intertriginous* or skin-fold areas, extensor or flexor areas, or **acral** (peripheral) areas? Do they involve areas exposed to specific allergens or irritants, such as wrist bands, rings, or industrial chemicals?

Many skin diseases have typical distributions. *Acne* typically affects the face, upper chest, and back (Table 9-9); *psoriasis typically affects* the knees and elbows (among other areas); and *Candida* infections typically affect the intertriginous areas.

Evaluating the Patient with Decreased Mobility

People with decreased mobility or who are hospitalized, especially when they are emaciated, elderly, or neurologically impaired, are particularly susceptible to skin damage and ulceration. **Pressure injuries** result when sustained compression obliterates arteriolar and capillary blood flow to the skin (Table 9-10). Injuries may also result from the *shearing forces* created by bodily movements. When a person slides down in bed from a partially sitting position or is dragged rather than lifted up from a supine position, for example, the movements may distort the soft tissues of the buttocks and close off the arteries and arterioles. Friction and moisture further increase the risk.

Assess every patient by carefully inspecting the skin that overlies the sacrum, buttocks, greater trochanters, knees, and heels. Roll the patient onto one side to see the sacrum and buttocks. Inspect the skin folds where moisture promotes maceration and skin breakdown.

Concept Mastery Alert

Evaluating Pressure Injury Care

Improved patient outcomes related to pressure injuries is crucial. If a patient develops a pressure injury but it does not show signs of healing, the nurse must first evaluate the patient's current outcomes and the current measures being used to determine which are effective and which are ineffective. Then the nurse needs to revise the patient's plan of care, modifying or adjusting the ineffective measures to meet the patient's needs and thus improve the patient's outcome.

CLINICAL TIP
Local redness of the skin warns of impending necrosis, although some deep pressure injuries develop without antecedent redness.

It is easier to prevent pressure injuries than to heal them. Every patient with decreased mobility and all hospitalized patients should be assessed for the risk factors that lead to pressure injuries. The risk factors may then be mitigated to prevent pressure injuries. The Braden Scale is a simple effective tool that evaluates levels of risk for injury development in the patient (Fig. 9-5). With its high reliability, predictive validity, and ease of use, the Braden Scale can be used to assess patients as often as every shift if needed (Bergstrom & Braden, 2002). Six factors are rated using a matrix scoring system: sensory

TABLE 9-8 Skin Lesions—Anatomic Location and Distribution

Document the anatomic location of lesions and their distribution, for example, "discrete round red macule on dorsum of foot," or "scattered brown papules across upper posterior chest."

Documentation	Location and Distribution	Example
Red, oval papules across anterior and posterior torso	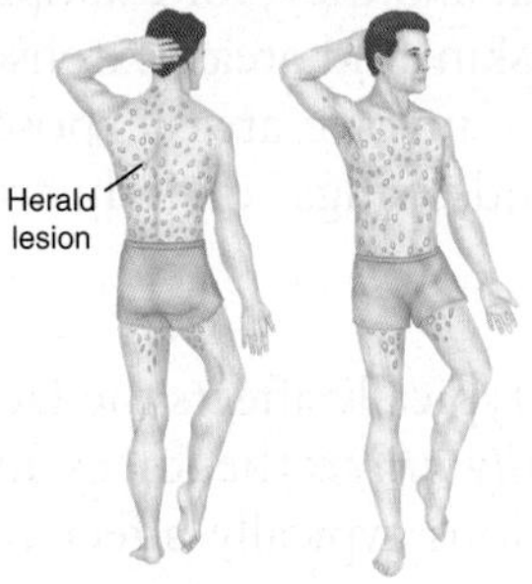	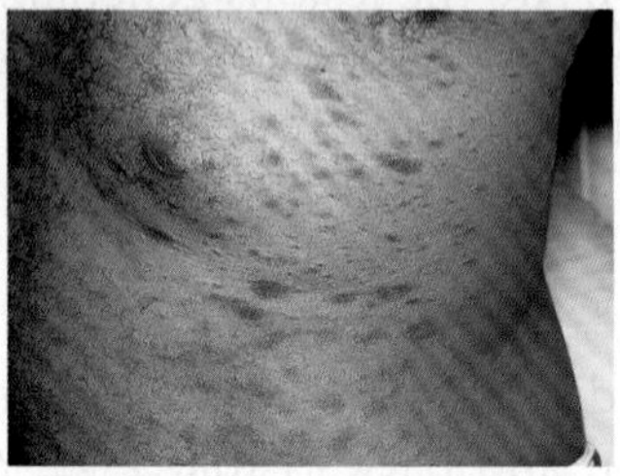 Pityriasis rosea.
Silvery scaly patches on the extensor surfaces (see *arrows*)	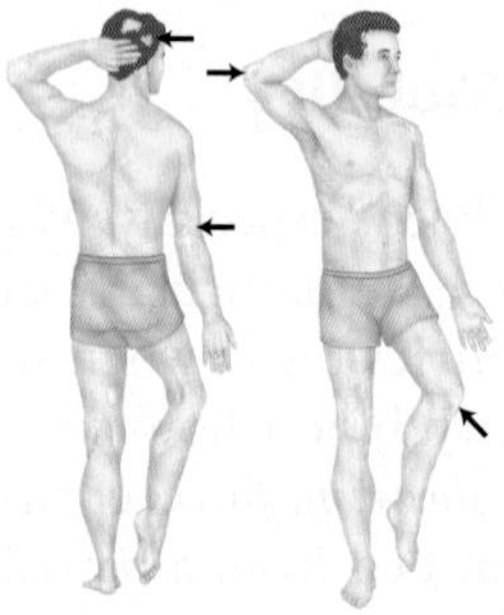	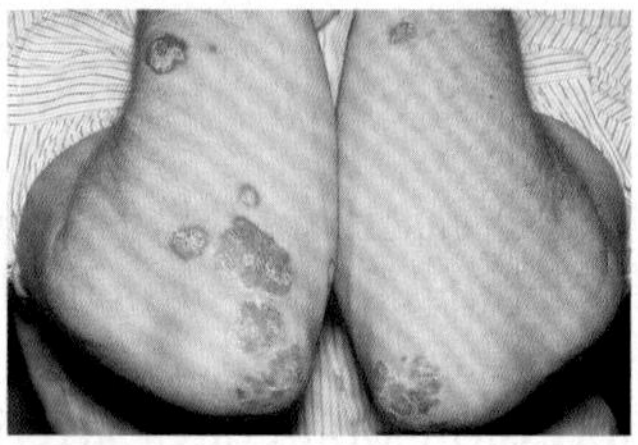 Psoriasis.
Tan, flat, scaly lesions across upper anterior and posterior torso	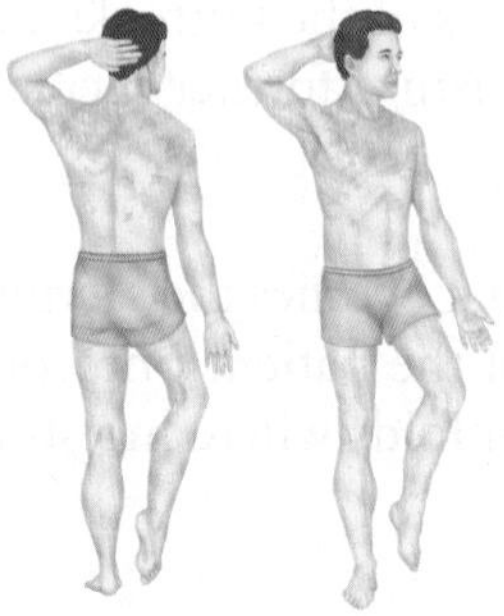	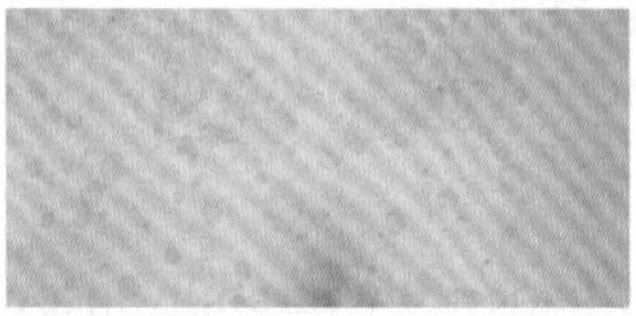 Tinea versicolor.
Silvery, scaly patches mainly on flexor surfaces (see *arrows*)	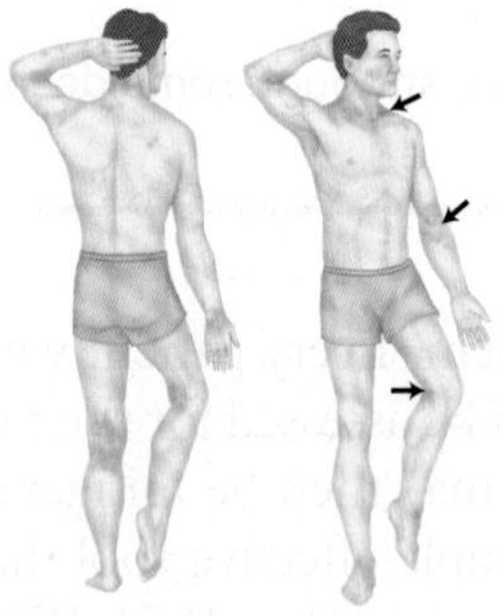	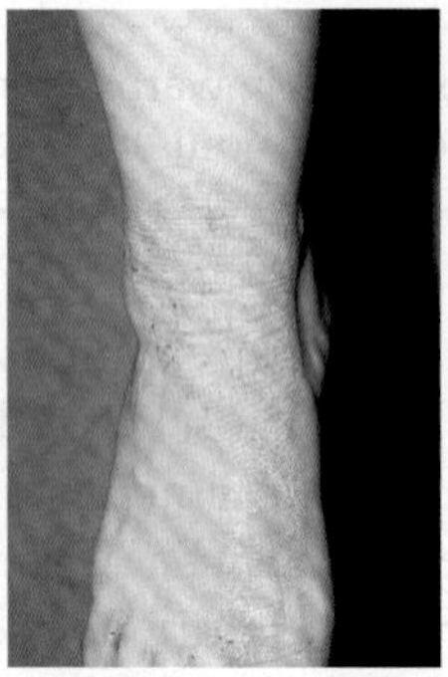 Atopic eczema.

Drawings adapted from Hall, J. C., & Hall, B. J. (2017). *Sauer's manual of skin diseases* (11th ed.). Wolters Kluwer.

TABLE 9-9 Acne Vulgaris—Primary and Secondary Lesions

Acne vulgaris is the most common cutaneous disorder in the United States, affecting more than 85% of adolescents (American Academy of Dermatology Association, 2020a).

Acne is a disorder of the pilosebaceous follicle that involves proliferation of the keratinocytes at the opening of the follicle; increased production of sebum, stimulated by androgens, which combines with keratinocytes to plug the follicular opening; growth of *Propionibacterium acnes,* an anaerobic diphtheroid normally found on the skin; and inflammation from bacterial activity and release of free fatty acids and enzymes from activated neutrophils (American Academy of Dermatology Association, 2020a). Cosmetics, humidity, heavy sweating, and stress are contributing factors.

Lesions appear in areas with the greatest number of sebaceous glands, namely, the face, neck, chest, upper back, and upper arms. They may be primary, secondary, or mixed.

Primary Lesions

Mild acne—Open and closed comedones, occasional papules

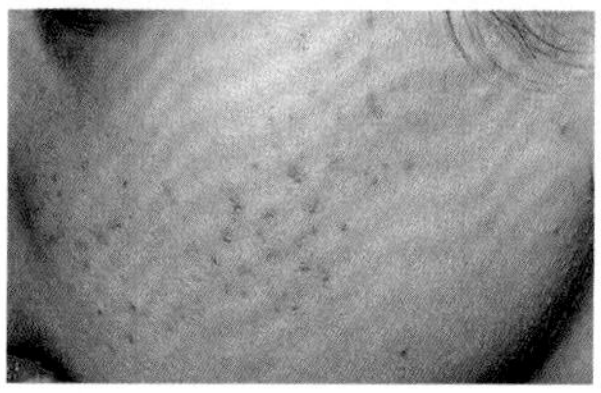

Moderate acne—Comedones, papules, pustules

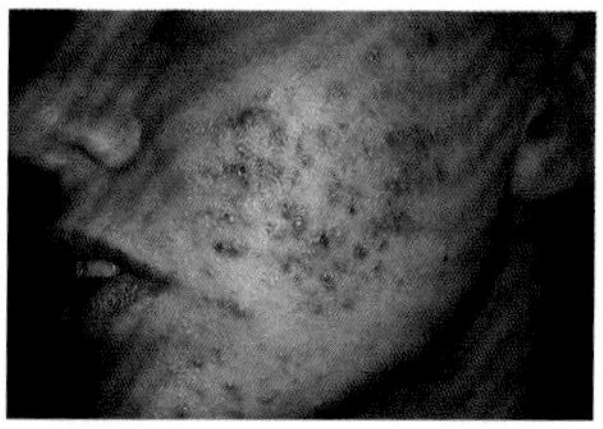

Severe cystic acne

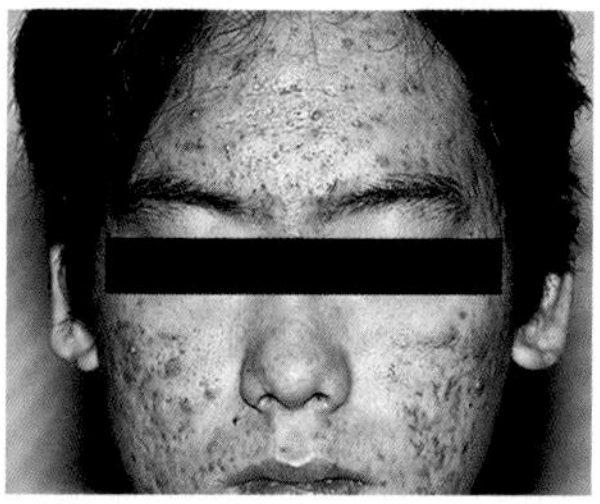

Secondary Lesions

Acne with pitting and scars

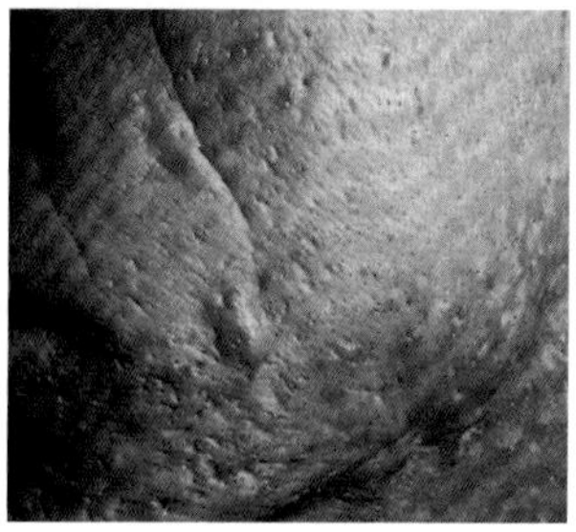

Sources of photos: *Mild acne, Severe cystic acne*—Goodheart, H. P. (2003). *Goodheart's photoguide of common skin disorders: Diagnosis and management* (2nd ed.). Lippincott Williams & Wilkins; *Moderate Acne, Acne With Pitting and Scars*—Hall, J. C., & Hall, B. J. (2017). *Sauer's manual of skin diseases* (11th ed.). Wolters Kluwer.

TABLE 9-10 Pressure Injuries

Pressure (decubitus) injuries usually develop over bony prominences subject to unrelieved pressure, resulting in ischemic damage to underlying tissue. Prevention is important: inspect the skin thoroughly for early warning signs of erythema that blanches with pressure, especially in patients with risk factors.

Pressure injuries form most commonly over the sacrum, ischial tuberosities, greater trochanters, and heels. A commonly applied staging system, based on depth of destroyed tissue, is illustrated below. Note that necrosis or eschar must be débrided before injuries can be staged. Injuries with bases covered with eschar or sloughing tissue are "unstageable." Additionally, injuries may not progress sequentially through the six stages (Edsberg et al., 2016; National Pressure Ulcer Advisory Panel, 2020).

Inspect injuries for signs of infection (drainage, odor, cellulitis, or necrosis). Fever, chills, and pain suggest underlying osteomyelitis. Address the patient's overall health, including comorbid conditions such as vascular disease, diabetes, immune deficiencies, collagen vascular disease, malignancy, psychosis, or depression; nutritional status; pain and level of analgesia; risk for recurrence; psychosocial factors such as learning ability, social supports, and lifestyle; and evidence of polypharmacy, overmedication, or abuse of alcohol, tobacco, or illicit drugs (Patton, 2005).

Risk Factors for Pressure Injuries

- Decreased mobility, especially if accompanied by increased pressure or movement causing friction or shear stress
- Decreased sensation, from brain or spinal cord lesions or peripheral nerve disease
- Decreased blood flow from hypotension or microvascular disease such as diabetes or atherosclerosis
- Fecal or urinary incontinence
- Presence of fracture
- Poor nutritional status or low albumin

Stage 1 Pressure Injury: Nonblanchable Erythema of Intact Skin

Intact skin with a localized area of nonblanchable erythema, which may appear differently in darkly pigmented skin. Presence of blanchable erythema or changes in sensation, temperature, or firmness may precede visual changes. Color changes do not include purple or maroon discoloration; these may indicate deep tissue pressure injury.

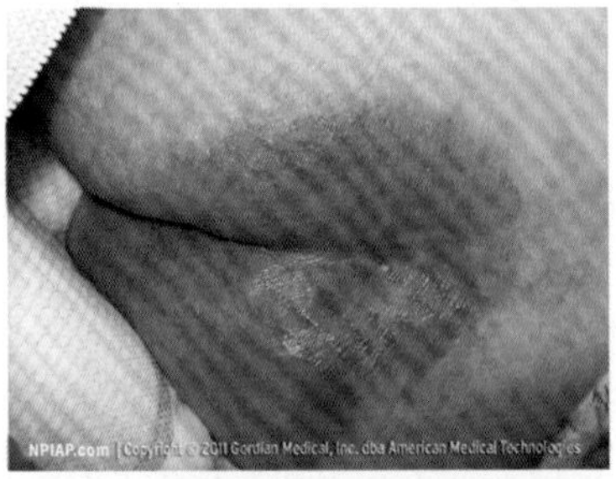

Stage 2 Pressure Injury: Partial-Thickness Skin Loss with Exposed Dermis

Partial-thickness loss of skin with exposed dermis. The wound bed is viable, pink or red, moist, and may also present as an intact or ruptured serum-filled blister. Adipose (fat) is not visible and deeper tissues are not visible. Granulation tissue, slough, and eschar are not present. These injuries commonly result from adverse microclimate and shear in the skin over the pelvis and shear in the heel. This stage should not be used to describe moisture-associated skin damage (MASD) including incontinence-associated dermatitis (IAD), intertriginous dermatitis (ITD), medical adhesive–related skin injury (MARSI), or traumatic wounds (skin tears, burns, abrasions).

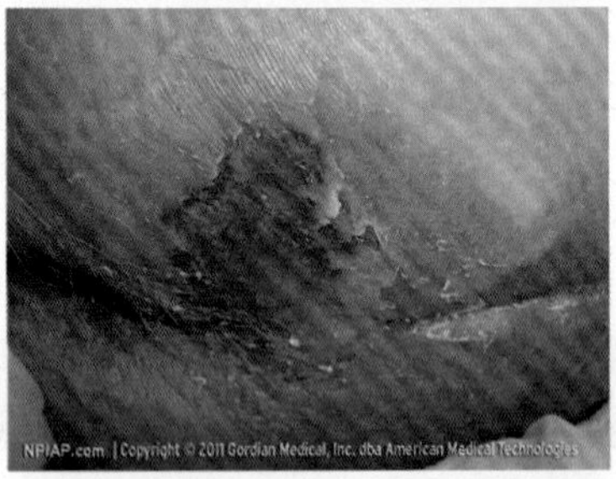

Stage 3 Pressure Injury: Full-Thickness Skin Loss

Full-thickness loss of skin, in which adipose (fat) is visible in the ulcer and granulation tissue and epibole (rolled wound edges) are often present. Slough and/or eschar may be visible. The depth of tissue damage varies by anatomical location; areas of significant adiposity can develop deep wounds. Undermining and tunneling may occur. Fascia, muscle, tendon, ligament, cartilage, and/or bone are not exposed. If slough or eschar obscures the extent of tissue loss this is an unstageable pressure injury.

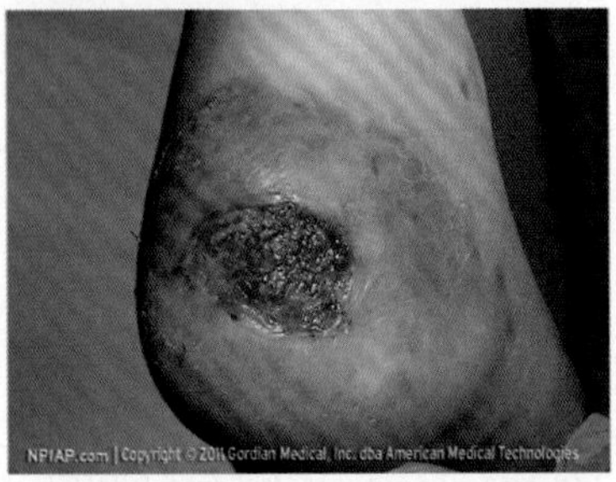

Stage 4 Pressure Injury: Full-Thickness Skin and Tissue Loss

Full-thickness skin and tissue loss with exposed or directly palpable fascia, muscle, tendon, ligament, cartilage, or bone in the ulcer. Slough and/or eschar may be visible. Epibole (rolled edges), undermining and/or tunneling, often occur. Depth varies by anatomical location. If slough or eschar obscures the extent of tissue loss this is an unstageable pressure injury.

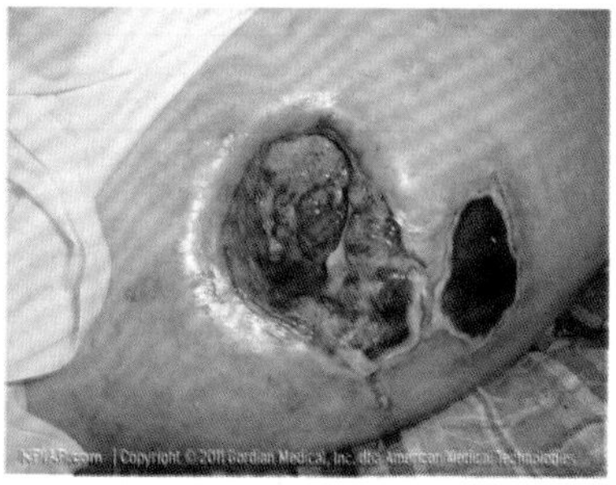

Unstageable Pressure Injury: Obscured Full-Thickness Skin and Tissue Loss

Full-thickness skin and tissue loss in which the extent of tissue damage within the ulcer cannot be confirmed because it is obscured by slough or eschar. If slough or eschar is removed, a stage 3 or stage 4 pressure injury will be revealed. Stable eschar (i.e., dry, adherent, intact without erythema or fluctuance) on the heel or ischemic limb should not be softened or removed.

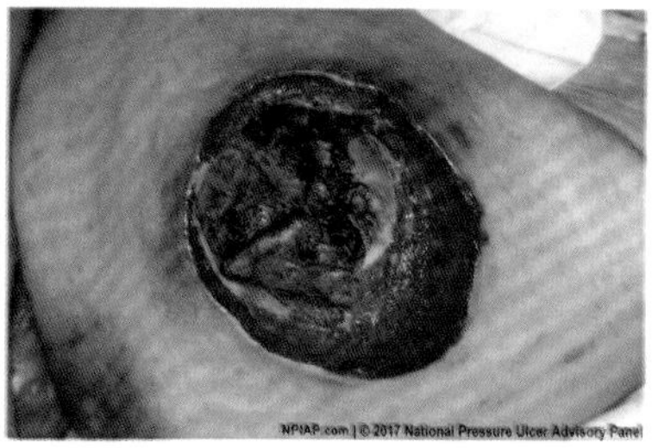

Deep Tissue Pressure Injury: Persistent Nonblanchable Deep Red, Maroon, or Purple Discoloration

Intact or nonintact skin with localized area of persistent nonblanchable deep red, maroon, purple discoloration or epidermal separation revealing a dark wound bed or blood-filled blister. Pain and temperature change often precede skin color changes. Discoloration may appear differently in darkly pigmented skin. This injury results from intense and/or prolonged pressure and shear forces at the bone–muscle interface. The wound may evolve rapidly to reveal the actual extent of tissue injury, or may resolve without tissue loss. If necrotic tissue, subcutaneous tissue, granulation tissue, fascia, muscle, or other underlying structures are visible, this indicates a full-thickness pressure injury (unstageable, stage 3 or stage 4). Do not use DTPI to describe vascular, traumatic, neuropathic, or dermatologic conditions.

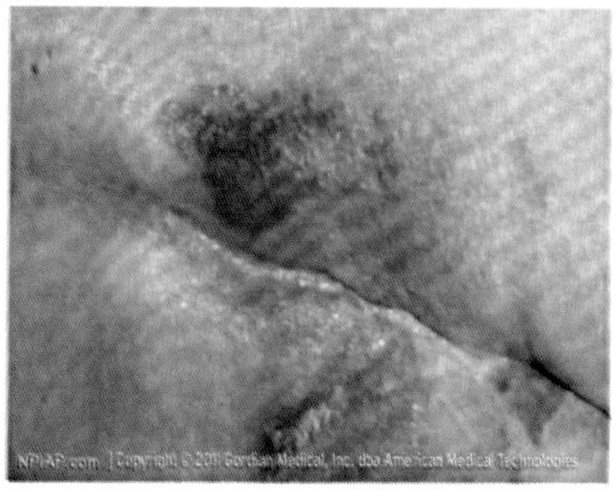

Medical Device–Related Pressure Injury: This Describes an Etiology

Medical device–related pressure injuries result from the use of devices designed and applied for diagnostic or therapeutic purposes. The resultant pressure injury generally conforms to the pattern or shape of the device. The injury should be staged using the staging system.

Mucosal Membrane Pressure Injury

Mucosal membrane pressure injury is found on mucous membranes with a history of a medical device in use at the location of the injury. Due to the anatomy of the tissue, these ulcers cannot be staged.

Source: Used with permission from the National Pressure Injury Advisory Panel (NPIAP). Copyright 2021 NPIAP.

The Braden Scale for Predicting Pressure Sore Risk©								
Patient's Name ____________________		Evaluator's Name ____________________		Date of Assessment				
SENSORY PERCEPTION Ability to respond meaningfully to pressure-related discomfort	**1. Completely Limited** Unresponsive (does not moan, flinch, or grasp) to painful stimuli due to diminished level of consciousness or sedation OR Limited ability to feel pain over most of body	**2. Very Limited** Responds only to painful stimuli Cannot communicate discomfort except by moaning or restlessness OR Has a sensory impairment which limits the ability to feel pain or discomfort over half of body	**3. Slightly Limited** Responds to verbal commands but cannot always communicate discomfort or the need to be turned OR Has some sensory impairment which limits ability to feel pain or discomfort in one or two extremities	**4. No Impairment** Responds to verbal commands Has no sensory deficit that would limit the ability to feel or voice pain or discomfort				
MOISTURE Degree to which skin is exposed to moisture	**1. Constantly Moist** Skin is kept moist almost constantly by perspiration, urine, etc. Dampness is detected every time patient is moved or turned	**2. Very Moist** Skin is often, but not always moist. Linen must be changed at least once a shift	**3. Occasionally Moist:** Skin is occasionally moist, requiring an extra linen change approximately once a day	**4. Rarely Moist** Skin is usually dry, linen only requires changing at routine intervals				
ACTIVITY Degree of physical activity	**1. Bedfast** Confined to bed	**2. Chairfast** Ability to walk severely limited or nonexistent Cannot bear own weight and/or must be assisted into chair or wheelchair	**3. Walks Occasionally** Walks occasionally during day but for very short distances with or without assistance Spends majority of each shift in bed or chair	**4. Walks Frequently** Walks outside room at least twice a day and inside room at least once every 2 hours during waking hours				
MOBILITY Ability to change and control body position	**1. Completely Immobile** Does not make even slight changes in body or extremity position without assistance	**2. Very Limited** Makes occasional slight changes in body or extremity position but unable to make frequent or significant changes independently	**3. Slightly Limited** Makes frequent though slight changes in body or extremity position independently	**4. No Limitation** Makes major and frequent changes in position without assistance				
NUTRITION Usual food intake pattern	**1. Very Poor** Never eats a complete meal Rarely eats more than half of any food offered Eats two servings or less of protein (meat or dairy products) per day Takes fluids poorly Does not take a liquid dietary supplement OR Is NPO and/or maintained on clear liquids or intravenous fluids for more than 5 days	**2. Probably Inadequate** Rarely eats a complete meal and generally eats only about half of any food offered Protein intake includes only three servings of meat or dairy products per day Occasionally will take a dietary supplement OR Receives less than optimum amount of liquid diet or tube feeding	**3. Adequate** Eats over half of most meals Eats a total of four servings of protein (meat, dairy products) per day Occasionally will refuse a meal but will usually take a supplement when offered OR Is on a tube feeding or TPN regimen which probably meets most nutritional needs	**4. Excellent** Eats most of every meal; never refuses a meal Usually eats a total of our or more servings of meat and dairy products Occasionally eats between meals Does not require supplementation				
FRICTION AND SHEAR	**1. Problem** Requires moderate to maximum assistance in moving Complete lifting without sliding against sheets is impossible. Frequently slides down in bed or chair, requiring frequent repositioning with maximum assistance Spasticity, contractures, or agitation leads to almost constant friction	**2. Potential Problem** Moves feebly or requires minimum assistance During a move, skin probably slides to some extent against sheets, chair, restraints, or other devices. Maintains relatively good position in a chair or bed most of the time but occasionally slides down	**3. No Apparent Problem** Moves in bed and in chair independently and has sufficient muscle strength to lift up completely during move Maintains good position in bed or chair					

NPO, nothing by mouth; TPN, total parenteral nutrition

FIGURE 9-5 The Braden Scale. The Braden Scale was developed prior to "pressure injury" becoming the preferred terminology. () 2021 Health Sense Ai. All rights reserved. All copyrights and trademarks are the property of Health Sense Ai or their respective owners or assigns.)

perception, moisture, activity, mobility, nutrition, and friction and shear. A lower score indicates that the patient has a lower functional level and is at higher risk for injury formation. Levels of risk for developing pressure injuries are rated according to the following scores:

- 19 to 23: Not at risk
- 15 to 18: Mild risk
- 13 to 14: Moderate risk
- 10 to 12: High risk
- 9 or lower: Very high risk

Hair

Inspect and palpate the hair. Note its quantity, distribution, and texture.

Alopecia refers to hair loss—diffuse, patchy, or total. Sparse hair may occur with *hypothyroidism while* fine, silky hair may occur with *hyperthyroidism.*

The color of the hair depends on the amount of melanin present and varies from pale blond to black. Graying occurs with aging and may begin in the 20s. Texture varies from silky fine to coarse and thick, straight to varying degrees of curly. As people age, hair tends to feel coarser and drier. However, if such changes occur over a few weeks or months, it may indicate a systemic disease or poor nutrition.

The amount of hair tends to decrease with aging in both men and women. Male pattern baldness is considered a normal change. Table 9-11 illustrates different types of hair loss.

Inspect the scalp for lesions, flaking, and parasites by separating the hair at 1-in to 2-in intervals with your fingers or a swab.

Inspect the body, axillae, and pubic hair for amount and distribution as well as parasites. Loss of hair on the legs may indicate peripheral artery disease, while changes in pubic or axilla hair may indicate hormonal problems.

Nails

Inspect and palpate the fingernails and toenails. Note their color and shape and any lesions. Nails should be pink with white lunulae; smooth and firm in texture; rounded in shape with a 160-degree angle between the nail base and skin (Fig. 9-6); and firmly attached to the nail bed. Longitudinal bands of pigment may

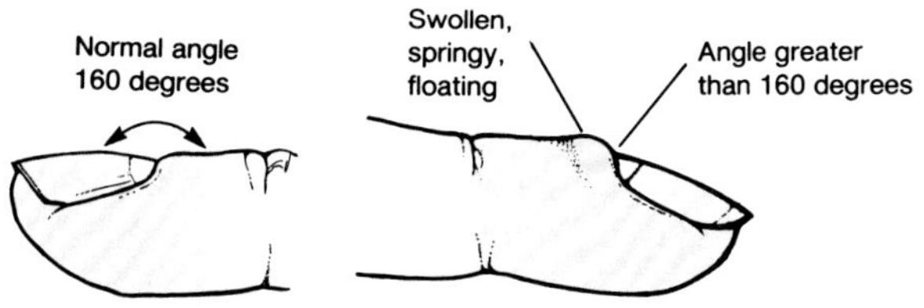

FIGURE 9-6 There should be a 160-degree angle between the nail base and the skin.

be seen in the nails of people who have darker skin (Fig. 9-7). Examples of findings in or near the nails are illustrated in Table 9-12.

Inspect the nail for abnormalities. Note the nail angle.

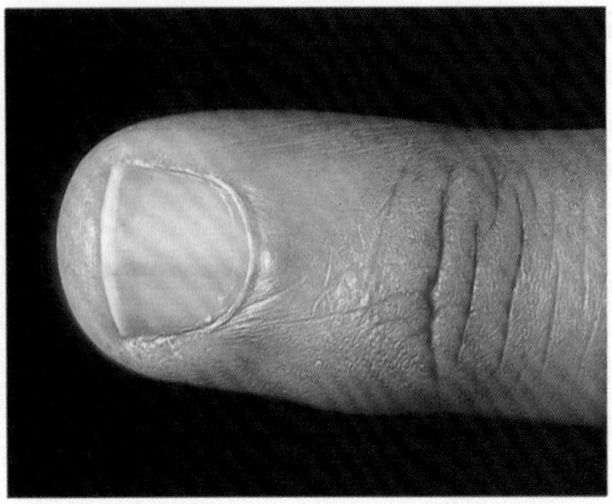

FIGURE 9-7 Longitudinal bands of pigment apparent in the nail of a darker-skinned person.

TABLE 9-11 Hair Loss

Alopecia Areata

Clearly demarcated round or oval patches of hair loss, usually affecting young adults and children. There is no visible scaling or inflammation.

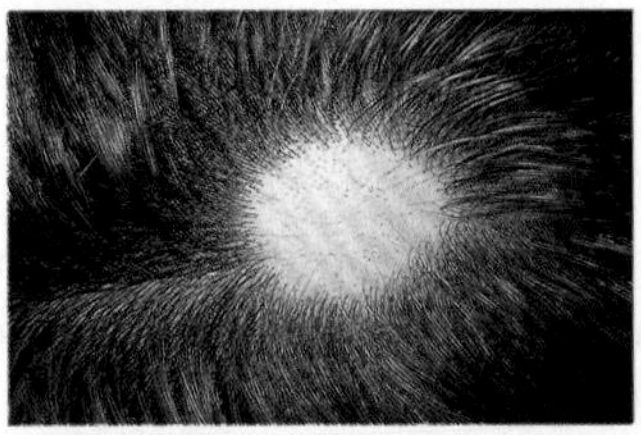

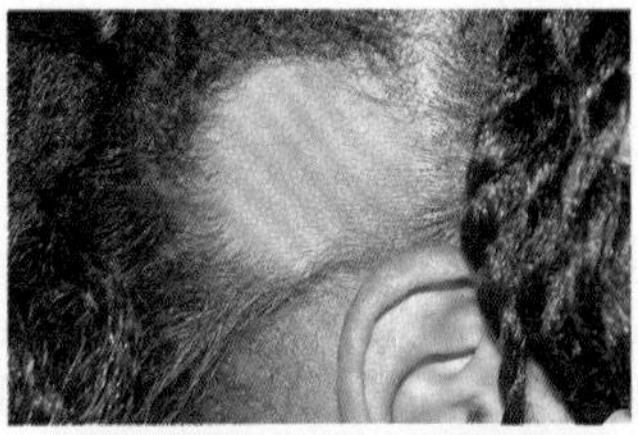

Trichotillomania

Hair loss from pulling, plucking, or twisting hair. Hair shafts are broken and of varying lengths. More common in children, often in settings of family or psychosocial stress.

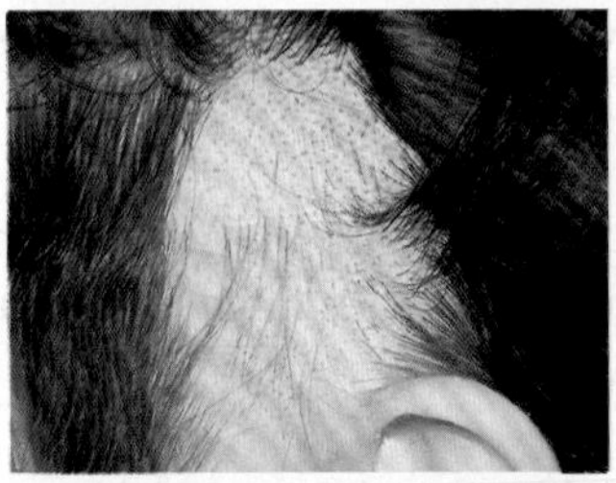

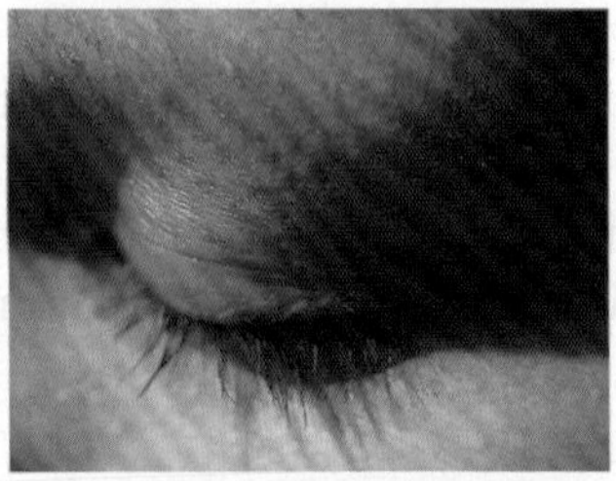

Tinea Capitis ("Ringworm")

Round scaling patches of alopecia. Hairs are broken off close to the surface of the scalp. Usually caused by fungal infection from *tinea tonsurans*. Mimics seborrheic dermatitis.

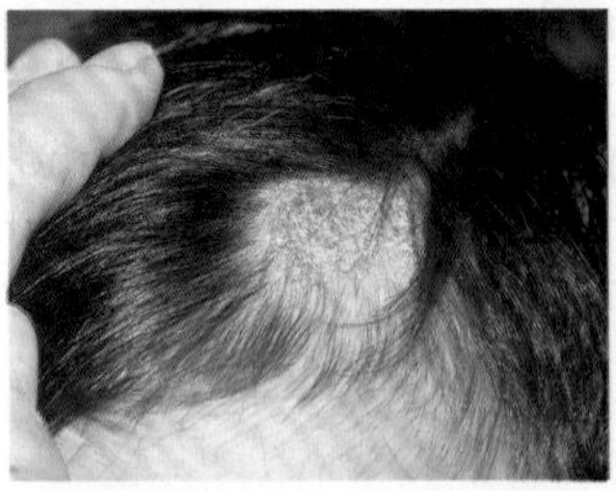

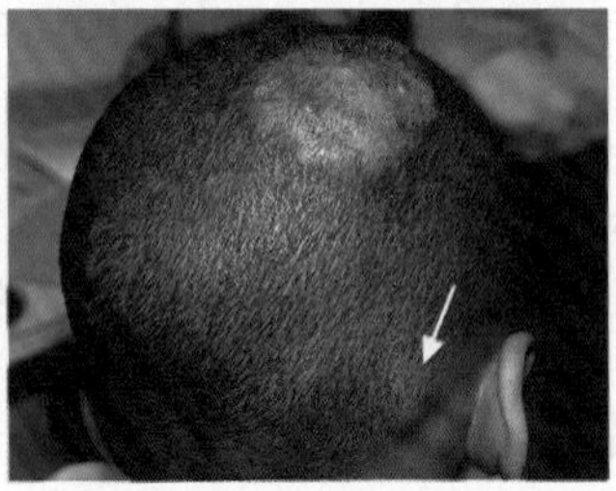

Sources of photos: *Alopecia Areata* [right], *Tinea Capitis*—Goodheart, H. P. (2003). *Goodheart's photoguide of common skin disorders: Diagnosis and management* (2nd ed.). Lippincott Williams & Wilkins; *Alopecia Areata [left]*—Rosdahl, C. B., & Kowalski, M. T. (2011). *Textbook of basic nursing* (10th ed.). Wolters Kluwer; *Trichotillomania [left]*—Hall, J. C. & & Hall, B. J. (2017). *Sauer's manual of skin diseases* (11th ed.). Wolters Kluwer; *Trichotillomania* [right]—Ostler, H. B., Mailbach, H. I., & Hoke, A. W. (2004). *Diseases of the eye and skin: A color atlas*. Lippincott Williams & Wilkins.

TABLE 9-12 Findings in or Near the Nails

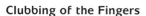

Paronychia

A superficial infection of the proximal and lateral nail folds adjacent to the nail plate. The nail folds are often red, swollen, and tender. Represents the most common infection of the hand, usually from *Staphylococcus aureus* or *Streptococcus* species, and may spread until it completely surrounds the nail plate. Creates a felon if it extends into the pulp space of the finger. Arises from local trauma due to nail biting, manicuring, or frequent hand immersion in water.

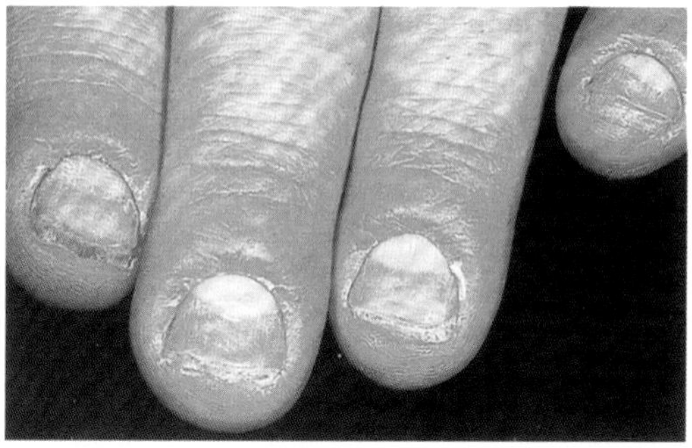

Clubbing of the Fingers

Clinically a bulbous swelling of the soft tissue at the nail base, with loss of the normal angle between the nail and the proximal nail fold. The angle increases to 180 degrees or more, and the nail bed feels spongy or floating. The mechanism is still unknown but involves vasodilatation with increased blood flow to the distal portion of the digits and changes in connective tissue, possibly from hypoxia, changes in innervation, genetics, or a platelet-derived growth factor from fragments of platelet clumps. Seen in congenital heart disease, interstitial lung disease and lung cancer, inflammatory bowel diseases, and malignancies (Spicknall et al., 2005).

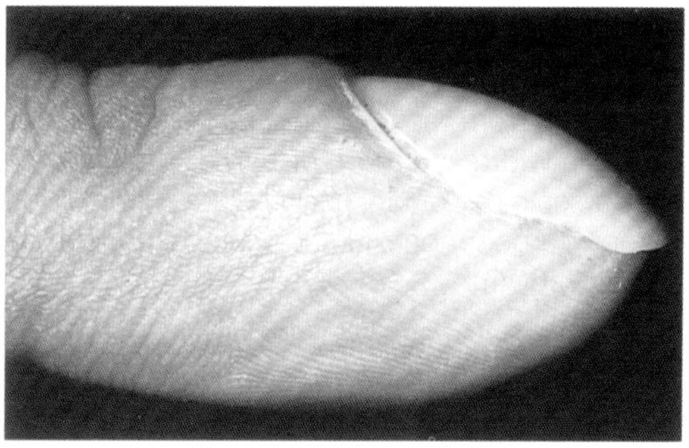

Onycholysis

A painless separation of the whitened opaque nail plate from the pinker translucent nail bed. Starts distally and progresses proximally, enlarging the free edge of the nail. Local causes include trauma from excess manicuring, psoriasis, fungal infection, and allergic reactions to nail cosmetics. Systemic causes include diabetes, anemia, photosensitive drug reactions, hyperthyroidism, peripheral ischemia, bronchiectasis, and syphilis.

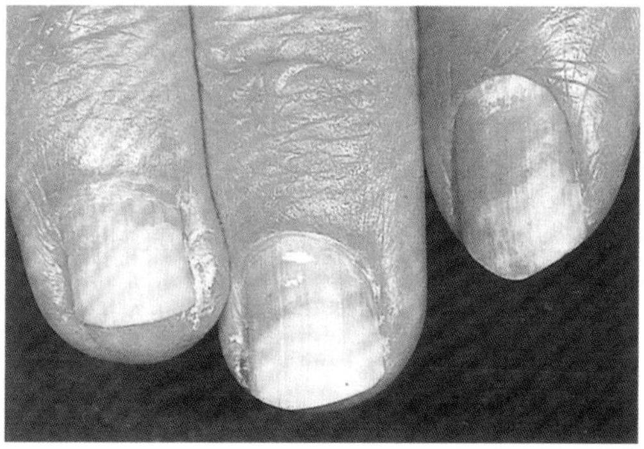

Terry Nails

Nail plate turns white with a ground-glass appearance, a distal band of reddish brown, and obliteration of the lunula. Commonly affects all fingers, though may appear in only one finger. Seen in liver disease, usually cirrhosis, congestive heart failure, and diabetes. May arise from decreased vascularity and increased connective tissue in nail bed.

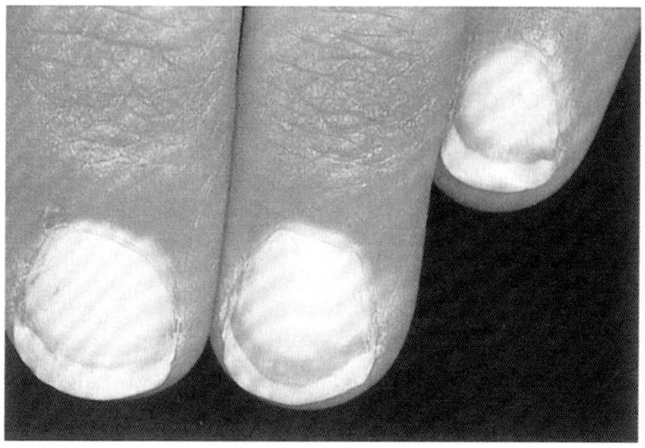

(continued)

TABLE 9-12 Findings in or Near the Nails *(Continued)*

White Spots (Leukonychia)

Trauma to the nails is commonly followed by nonuniform white spots that grow slowly out with the nail. Spots in the pattern illustrated are typical of overly vigorous and repeated manicuring. The curves in this example resemble the curve of the cuticle and proximal nail fold.

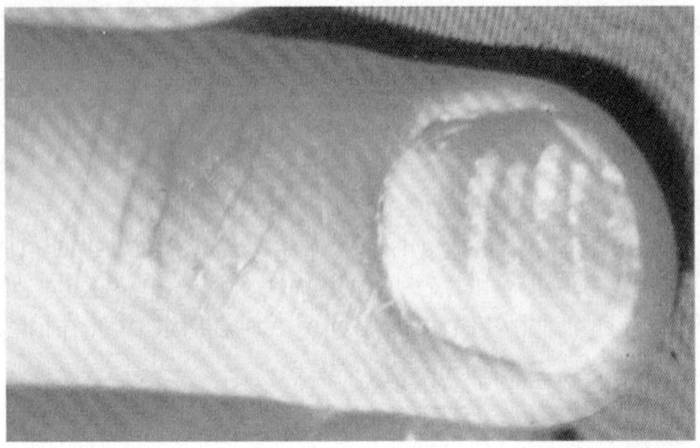

Transverse White Bands (Mees Lines)

Curving transverse white bands that cross the nail parallel to the lunula. Arising from the disrupted matrix of the proximal nail, they vary in width and move distally as the nail grows out. Seen in arsenic poisoning, heart failure, Hodgkin disease, chemotherapy, carbon monoxide poisoning, and leprosy (Fawcett et al., 2004).

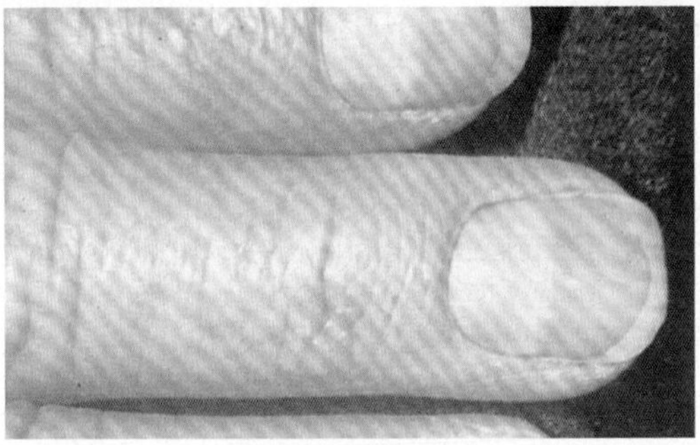

Transverse Linear Depressions (Beau Lines)

Transverse depressions of the nail plates, usually bilateral, resulting from temporary disruption of proximal nail growth from systemic illness. As with Mees lines, timing of the illness may be estimated by measuring the distance from the line to the nail bed (nails grow approximately 1 mm every 6–10 days). Seen in severe illness, trauma, and cold exposure if Raynaud disease is present (Bergstrom & Braden, 2020; Fawcett et al., 2004; Hanford et al., 1995).

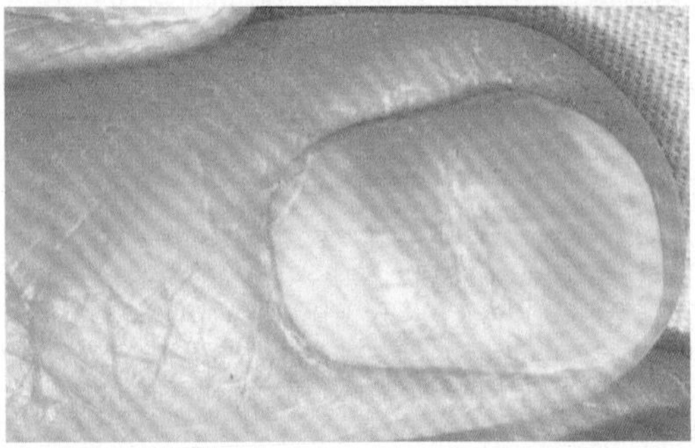

Pitting

Punctate depressions of the nail plate caused by defective layering of the superficial nail plate by the proximal nail matrix. Usually associated with psoriasis but also seen in Reiter syndrome, sarcoidosis, alopecia areata, and localized atopic or chemical dermatitis (Fawcett et al., 2004).

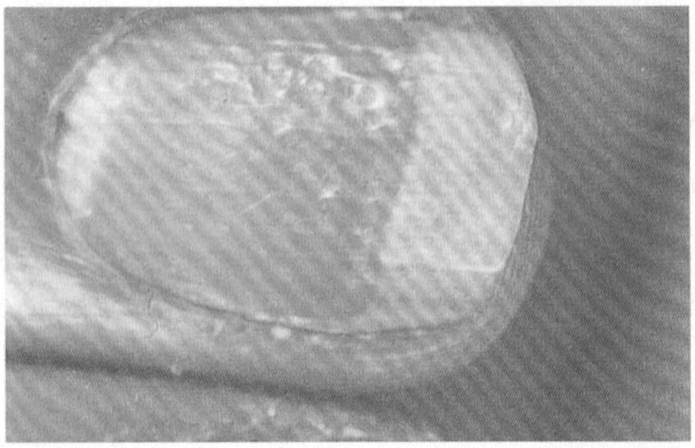

Sources of photos: *Clubbing of the Fingers, Paronychia, Onycholysis, Terry Nails*—Habif, T. P. (1990). *Clinical dermatology: A color guide to diagnosis and therapy* (2nd ed.). CV Mosby; *White Spots, Transverse White Lines, Beau Lines*—Sams, W. M., Jr, & Lynch, P. J. (1990). *Principles and practice of dermatology*. Churchill Livingstone.

RECORDING YOUR FINDINGS

Note that initially you may use sentences to describe your findings; later you will use phrases. Box 9-2 contains phrases appropriate for most write-ups.

BOX 9-2 RECORDING THE PHYSICAL EXAMINATION OF THE SKIN—EXAMPLES

Color pink. Skin warm and moist. Nails without clubbing or cyanosis. No suspicious nevi. No rash, petechiae, or ecchymoses.

OR

Marked facial pallor with circumoral cyanosis. Palms cold and moist. Cyanosis in nail beds of fingers and toes. One raised blue-black nevus, 1 × 2 cm, with irregular border on right forearm. No rash.

Suggests central cyanosis or possible melanoma

OR

Facial ruddiness. Skin icteric. Three spider angiomas over anterior torso. Palmar erythema. Single pearly papule with depressed center and telangiectasias, 1 × 1 cm, on posterior neck above collar line. No suspicious nevi. Nails with clubbing but no cyanosis.

Suggests possible liver disease or basal cell carcinoma

HEALTH PROMOTION AND COUNSELING

Important topics for health promotion and counseling regarding the integumentary system include:

- Skin cancer prevention
- Risk factors for skin cancers
- Avoidance of excessive sun exposure and artificial tanning lamps
- Use of sunscreen

Nurses play an important role in educating patients about early detection of suspicious moles, protective measures for skin care, and the hazards of excessive sun exposure. Skin cancers are the most common cancers in the United States (American Academy of Dermatology Association, 2020). They are caused by a combination of genetic predisposition and UV radiation exposure. Fair-skinned individuals are at the highest risk.

Almost all skin cancers are one of three types:

- *Basal cell carcinomas,* arising in the lowest, or basal, level of the epidermis, account for most of skin cancers. These cancers arise in sun-exposed areas, usually on the head and neck. They are pearly white and translucent, tend to grow slowly, and rarely metastasize.
- *Squamous cell carcinomas,* arise in the upper layer of the epidermis. These cancers are often crusted and scaly with a red, inflamed, or ulcerated appearance; they can metastasize (American Cancer Society, 2020c).

- *Melanomas,* arising from the pigment-producing melanocytes in the epidermis that give the skin its color, is the most lethal type due to its high rate of metastasis and high rate of mortality at advanced stages; the vast majority of skin cancer deaths are from melanoma (American Cancer Society, 2020b). Melanoma is now the fifth most frequently diagnosed cancer in men and the seventh most frequently diagnosed in women. In the United States in 2019, the estimated lifetime risk for melanoma was one in 38 for White Americans, one in 167 for Hispanic Americans, and one in 1,000 for African Americans (American Cancer Society, 2020b).

A fourth type of skin cancer is *Merkel cell carcinoma (MCC),* a rare type that unfortunately looks harmless. It usually starts on areas of skin exposed to the sun, especially the face, neck, arms, and legs, but it can occur anywhere on the body. It can be mistaken for an insect bite, sore, cyst, stye, or pimple. Look for lesions that **grow quickly** (within in a few weeks or months); are **pink, red, or purple; feel painless;** and usually develop on the head or neck. The majority of people who develop MCC are over 50 years of age and have light-color skin (American Academy of Dermatology Association, 2020c; American Cancer Society, 2020a).

Types of skin tumors are described and illustrated in Table 9-13.

Risk Factors for Melanoma

Educate patients about *risk factors for melanoma* (Box 9-3). Early detection of melanoma, when 3 mm or less, significantly improves prognosis.

BOX 9-3 RISK FACTORS FOR MELANOMA

- Personal or family history of previous melanoma
- Atypical or dysplastic moles (moles that change in size or color)
- Male gender
- 50 or more common moles
- Red or light hair
- Light eye or skin color, especially skin that freckles or burns easily
- *Actinic keratosis* (horny overgrowth of the skin) and/or *solar lentigines* (acquired brown macules on sun-exposed areas)
- Ultraviolet radiation from heavy sun exposure, sun lamps, or tanning booths
- Severe blistering sunburns, especially in childhood
- *Congenital melanocytic nevi* (moles present at birth, especially large moles)
- Immunosuppression, for example, from HIV or chemotherapy

American Academy of Dermatology Association. (n.d.). *Skin Cancer: Risk Factors.* https://www.aad.org/media/stats-skin-cancer; Centers for Disease Control & Prevention [CDC], 2020; National Institutes of Health [NIH], National Cancer Institute, 2020.

CLINICAL TIP

The *Melanoma Risk Assessment Tool* developed by the National Cancer Institute, available at http://www.cancer.gov/melanomarisktool can be used to help patients self-assess their risk for melanoma. It assesses an individual's 5-year risk of developing melanoma based on geographic location, gender, race, age, history of blistering sunburns, complexion, number and size of moles, freckling, and sun damage (NIH, National Cancer Institute, 2020).

TABLE 9-13 Skin Tumors

Actinic Keratosis

Superficial, flattened papules covered by a dry scale. Often multiple; can be round or irregular; pink, tan, or grayish. Appear on sun-exposed skin of older, fair-skinned people. Though benign, one of every 1,000 per year develops into squamous cell carcinoma (suggested by rapid growth, induration, redness at the base, and ulceration). Keratoses on face and hand, typical locations, are shown.

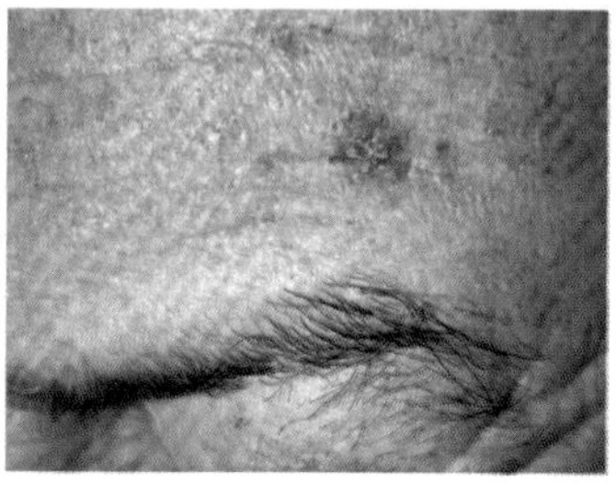

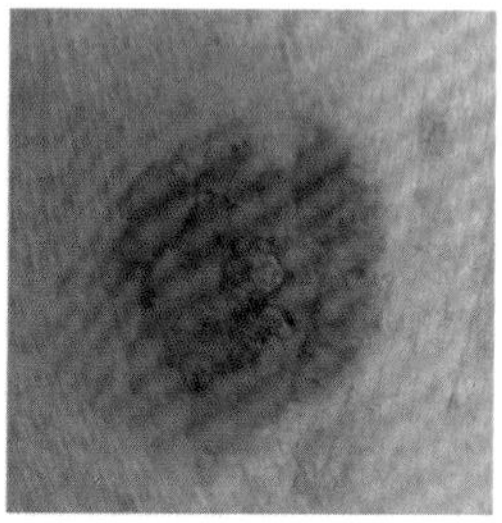

Seborrheic Keratosis

Common, benign, yellowish to brown raised lesions that feel slightly greasy and velvety or warty and have a "stuck on" appearance. Typically multiple and symmetrically distributed on the trunk of older people, but may also appear on the face and elsewhere. In Black people, often younger women, may appear as small, deeply pigmented papules on the cheeks and temples (dermatosis papulosa nigra).

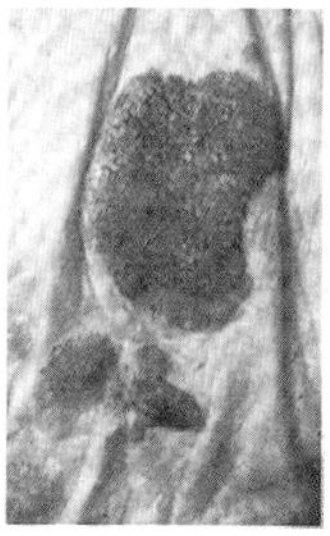

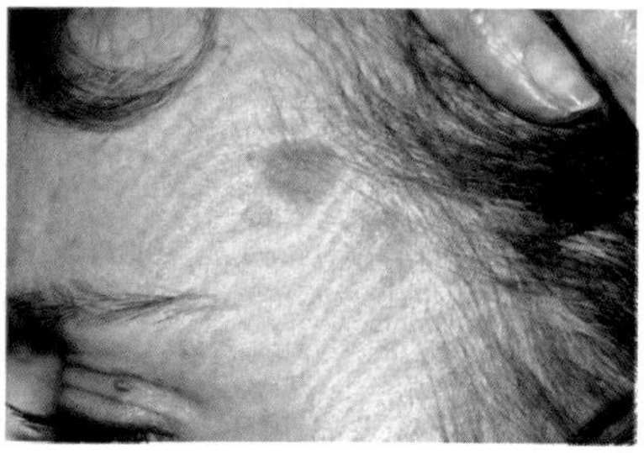

Basal Cell Carcinoma

A basal cell carcinoma, though malignant, grows slowly and seldom metastasizes. It is most common in fair-skinned adults 40 y or older, and usually appears on the face. An initial translucent nodule spreads, leaving a depressed center and a firm, elevated border. Telangiectatic vessels are often visible.

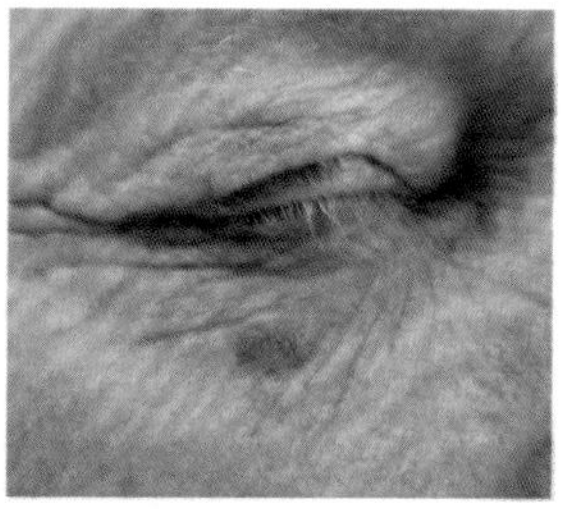

Squamous Cell Carcinoma

Usually appears on sun-exposed skin of fair-skinned adults older than 60 y. May develop in an actinic keratosis. Usually grows more quickly than a basal cell carcinoma, is firmer, and looks redder. The face and the back of the hand are often affected, as shown here.

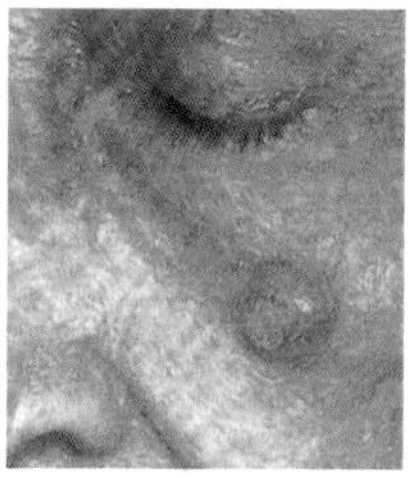

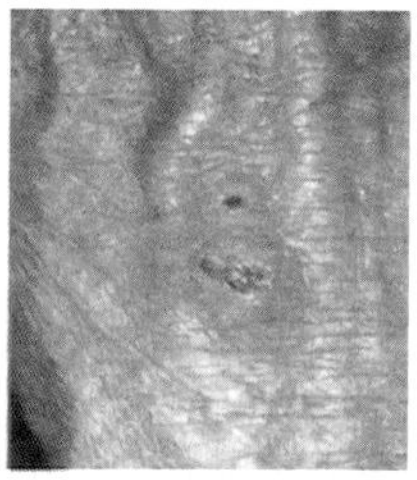

Merkel Cell Carcinoma

Usually appears on sun-exposed skin of fair-skinned older adults, especially the face, neck, arms, and legs. It can be mistaken for an insect bite, sore, cyst, stye, or pimple. Look for lesions that grow quickly (within a few weeks or months), are pink, red, or purple, feel painless.

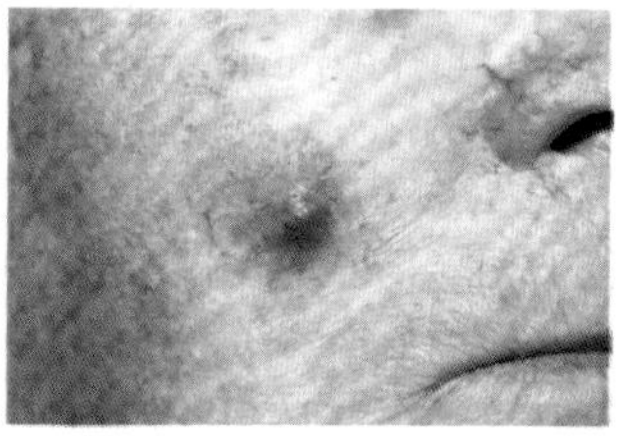

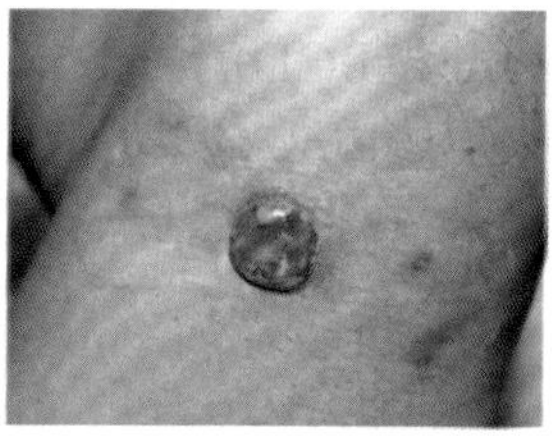

Sources of photos: *Actinic Keratosis [left]*—Edward, S., & Yung, A. (2011). *Essential dermatopathology*. Lippincott Williams & Wilkins; *Actinic Keratosis [right]—Stedman's medical dictionary for the health professions and nursing* (7th ed.). Wolters Kluwer, 2011; *Seborrheic Keratosis [right]*—Goodheart, H. P. (2003). *Goodheart's photoguide of common skin disorders* (2nd ed). Lippincott Williams & Wilkins; *Basal Cell Carcinoma*—Bickley, L. S., Szilagyi, P. G., Hoffman, R. M., & Soriano, R. P. (2020). *Bates' guide to physical examination and history taking* (13th ed.). Wolters Kluwer; *Squamous Cell Carcinoma [left]*—Weber, J., & Kelley, J. (2003). *Health assessment in nursing* (2nd ed.). Lippincott Williams & Wilkins; *Squamous Cell Carcinoma [right]*—CDC/Bob Craig; *Seborrheic Keratosis [left]*—Goodheart, H. P. (2003). *Goodheart's photoguide of common skin disorders* (2nd ed). Lippincott Williams & Wilkins; *Merkel Cell Carcinoma [left]*—Elder, D. E., Elenitsas, R., Rubin, A. I., Ioffreda, M., Miller, J., Miller, III, O. F., & Yun, S. K. (2021). *Atlas of dermatopathology: Synopsis and Atlas of Lever's histopathology of the skin* (4th ed.). Wolters Kluwer; *Merkel Cell Carcinoma [right]*—Craft, N., Fox, L. P., Goldsmith, L. A., Papier, A., Birnbaum, R., & Mercurio, M. G. (2010). *VisualDx: Essential adult dermatology*. Lippincott Williams & Wilkins.

Preventing Skin Cancer

Avoiding Ultraviolet Radiation and Tanning Beds

Increasing lifetime sun exposure correlates directly with increasing risk of skin cancer. In the case of melanoma, it seems that intermittent acute sun exposure leading to sunburn results in a higher risk than does cumulative sun exposure (CDC, 2020). The best defense against skin cancers is to avoid UV radiation exposure by limiting time in the sun, avoiding the mid-day sun, using sunscreen, and wearing sun-protective clothing with long sleeves and hats with wide brims.

Advise patients to avoid indoor tanning, especially children, teens, and young adults. Use of indoor tanning beds, especially before age 35, increases risk of melanoma by as much as 75%.

In 2009, the International Agency for Research on Cancer classified UV-emitting tanning devices as "carcinogenic to humans" (El Ghissassi et al., 2009; WHO, 2020). Better options for tanning include self-tanning products or sprays in conjunction with sunscreen.

Regular Use of Sunscreen to Prevent Skin Cancer

There are many myths about sunscreen. A landmark study in 2011 demonstrated that the regular use of sunscreen decreases the incidence of melanoma (Green et al., 2011). Advise patients to use at least an SPF of 30 with broad-spectrum protection. Everyone should reapply every 2 hours and after swimming or sweating. For water exposure, patients should use water-resistant sunscreens.

Free information about protection and proper use of sunscreen are available from the American Academy of Dermatology and the Skin Cancer Foundation (CDC, 2020; Skin Cancer Foundation, 2015).

Skin Cancer Screening

Clinician Screening

Although the U.S. Preventive Services Task Force found insufficient evidence (grade I) to recommend routine skin cancer screening by health care providers, it does advise clinicians to "remain alert for skin lesions with malignant features" during routine physical examinations and references the ABCDE criteria (Box 9-4) (American Academy of Dermatology Association, 2020; American Cancer Society, 2010; NIH, National Cancer Institute, 2020; U.S. Preventive Services Task Force, 2016; Wolff et al., 2009). The American Cancer Society and the American Academy of Dermatology recommend *full-body examinations* for patients over age 50 or at high risk, since melanoma can appear in any location (American Academy of Dermatology Association, 2015). High-risk patients are those with a personal or family history of multiple or dysplastic nevi or previous melanoma. Both new and changing nevi should be closely examined, since at least half of melanomas newly arise from isolated melanocytes rather than preexisting nevi. Also take advantage of "opportunistic screening" when assessing other body systems, such as the respiratory system, or when bathing a patient.

BOX 9-4 ABCDEs FOR EARLY RECOGNITION OF POSSIBLE MELANOMA

- A for *a*symmetry of one side of mole compared to the other
- B for irregular *b*orders, especially ragged, notched, scalloped, or blurred
- C for *c*olor, especially varying colors from one area to the next, such as shades of tan, brown, or black, or areas of white, red, or blue
- D for *d*iameter ≥6 mm or different from others, especially if changing, itching, or bleeding
- E for *e*volving or changing rapidly in size, shape, or color (The most sensitive criterion, this history may prompt biopsy of a benign-appearing lesion.)

Adding "EFG" will help detect aggressive nodular melanomas because they are often:

- E for *e*levated
- F for *f*irm to palpation
- G for *g*rowing progressively over several weeks

Patient Screening

The American Academy of Dermatology recommends regular self-examination of the skin using the techniques outlined in Box 9-5. Instruct patients with risk factors for skin cancer and melanoma, especially those with a history of high sun exposure, prior or family history of melanoma, 50 or more moles, and/or more than five to 10 atypical moles, to perform regular self-skin examinations. The patient will need a full-length mirror, a handheld mirror, and a well-lit room that provides privacy. Teach the patient the ABCDE-EFG method (Box 9-4) for assessing moles, and show the patient photos of benign and malignant nevi such as those in Table 9-14.

Approximately half of melanomas are initially detected by patients or their partners.

BOX 9-5 PATIENT INSTRUCTIONS FOR THE SKIN SELF-EXAMINATION

Examine your body front and back in the mirror, then the right and left sides with arms raised.

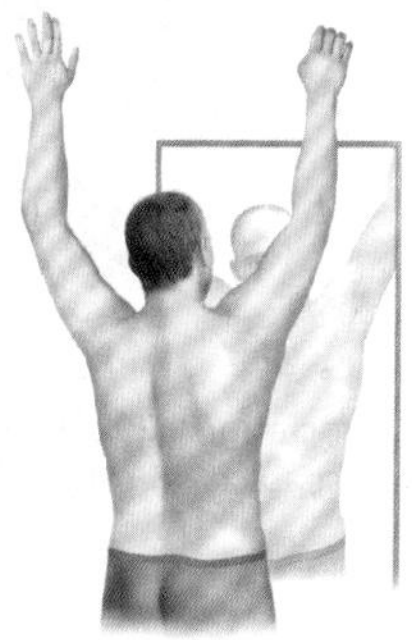

Bend elbows and look carefully at the forearms, upper underarms, and palms.

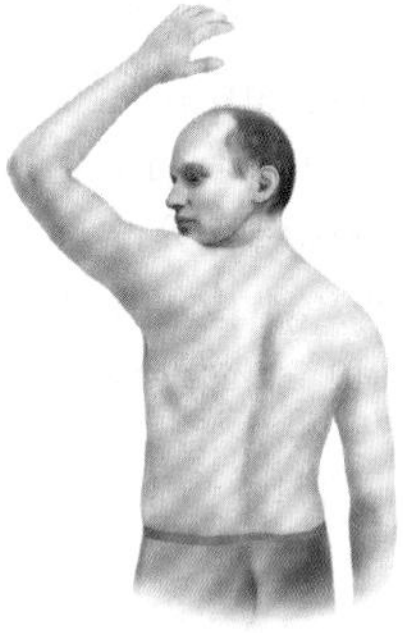

(continued)

BOX 9-5 PATIENT INSTRUCTIONS FOR THE SKIN SELF-EXAMINATION (*Continued*)

Look at the backs of your legs and feet, the spaces between your toes, and the soles.

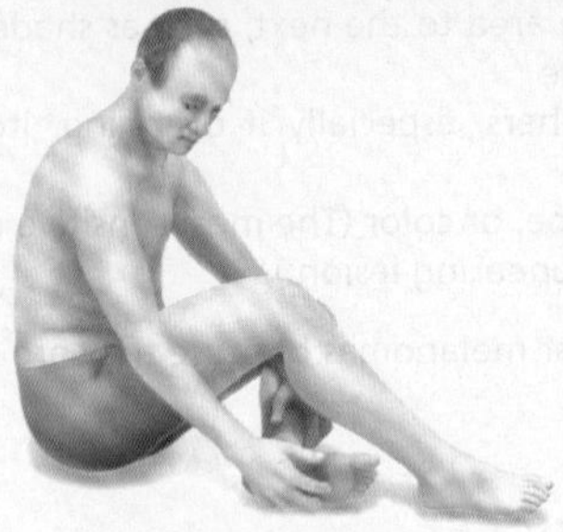

Examine the back of your neck and scalp with a hand mirror. Part your hair for a closer look.

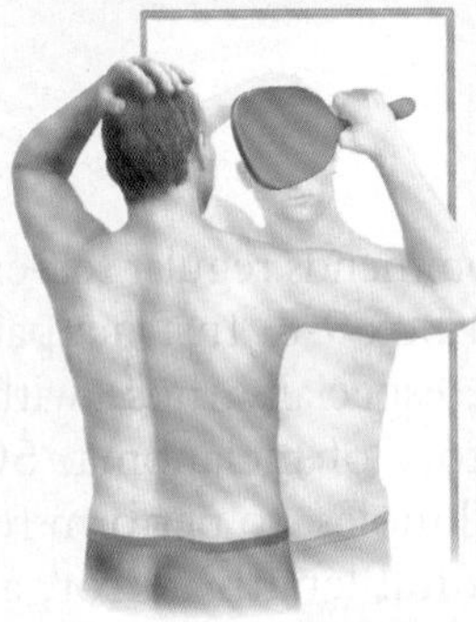

Finally, check your back and buttocks with a hand mirror.

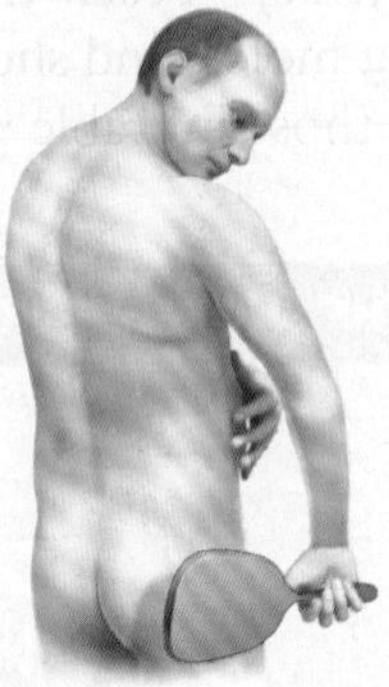

Source: Adapted from American Academy of Dermatology Association. (2021). *Detect skin cancer: How to perform a self skin exam*. https://www.aad.org/public/diseases/skin-cancer/find/check-skin

Inspecting Moles

Patients and clinicians who find moles should apply the *ABCDE-EFG method* to screen for melanoma. Sensitivity ranges from 43% to 97% and specificity from 36% to 100% (Abbasi et al., 2004). Any suspicious mole or skin lesion should be referred to a dermatologist for follow-up. Patients who examine their skin regularly are more likely to have less invasive melanomas if detected. See Table 9-14.

TABLE 9-14 Benign and Malignant Nevi

Benign Nevus

The *benign nevus,* or common mole, usually appears in the first few decades. Several nevi may arise at the same time, but their appearances usually remain unchanged. Note the following typical features and contrast them with those of atypical nevi and melanoma:

- Round or oval shape
- Sharply defined borders
- Uniform color, especially tan or brown
- Diameter <6 mm
- Flat or raised surface

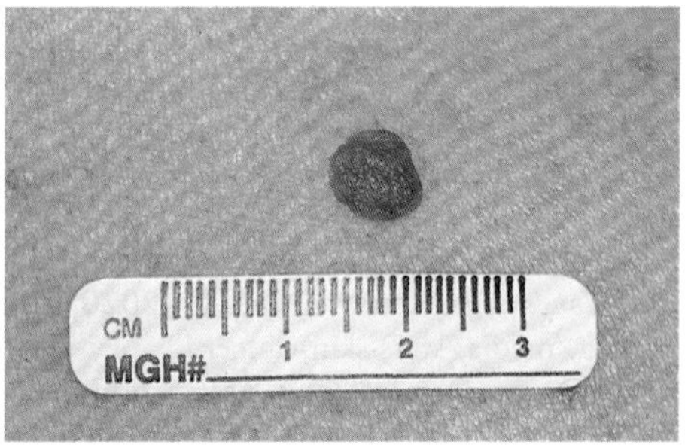

Changes in these features raise the specter of *atypical (dysplastic) nevi,* or melanoma. Atypical nevi are varied in color but often dark and larger than 6 mm, with irregular borders that fade into the surrounding skin. Look for atypical nevi primarily on the trunk. They may number more than 50–100.

Malignant Melanoma

Learn the ABCDE-EFG of melanoma from these reference standard photographs from the American Cancer Society:

- *Asymmetry* (Fig. A)
- Irregular *borders,* especially notching (Fig. B)
- Variation in *color,* especially mixtures of black, blue, and red (Figs. B,C)
- *Diameter* >6 mm (Fig. C)
- *Evolving*, a mole changing in size, shape, or color.
- E for elevated
- F for firm to palpation
- G for growing progressively over several weeks

Review *melanoma risk factors* such as intense year-round sun exposure, blistering sunburns in childhood, fair skin that freckles or burns easily (especially if blond or red hair), family history of melanoma, and nevi that are changing or atypical, especially if the patient is older than 50 y. Changing nevi may have new swelling or redness beyond the border, scaling, oozing, or bleeding, or sensations such as itching, burning, or pain. On darker skin, look for melanomas under the nails, on the hands, or on the soles of the feet.

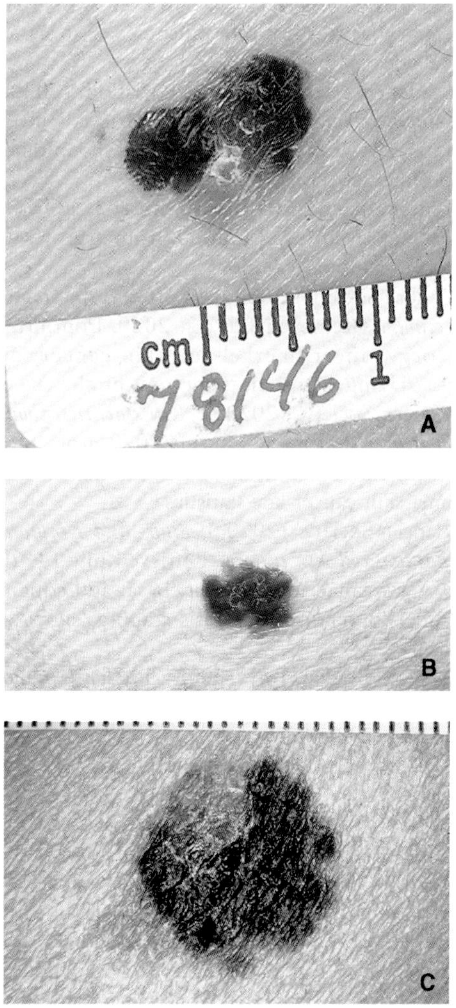

Source: Courtesy of American Cancer Society; American Academy of Dermatology Association.

Bibliography

CITATIONS

Abbasi, N. R., Shaw, H. M., Rigel, D. S., Friedman, R. J., McCarthy, W. H., Osman, I., Kopf, A. W., & Polsky, D. (2004). Early diagnosis of cutaneous melanoma: Revisiting the ABCD criteria. *JAMA: The Journal of the American Medical Association, 292*(22), 2771–2776.

American Academy of Dermatology Association. (2020). *Skin cancer: Incidence rates.* Retrieved July 11, 2020, from https://www.aad.org/media/stats-skin-cancer

American Academy of Dermatology Association. (2021). *Skin cancer: Risk factors.* https://www.aad.org/media/stats-skin-cancer

American Academy of Dermatology Association. (2015). *Skin cancer.* Retrieved October 19, 2015, from https://www.aad.org/media-resources/stats-and-facts/conditions/skin-cancer

American Academy of Dermatology Association. (2020a). *Acne clinical guideline.* Retrieved July 14, 2020, from https://www.aad.org/media/news-releases/acne-guidelines

American Academy of Dermatology Association. (2020b). *What to look for: ABCDEs of melanoma.* Retrieved July 9, 2020, from https://www.aad.org/public/diseases/skin-cancer/find/at-risk/abcdes

American Academy of Dermatology Association. (2020c). *Merkel cell carcinoma: Signs and symptoms.* Retrieved July 12, 2020, from https://www.aad.org/public/diseases/skin-cancer/types/common/merkel-cell/symptoms

American Cancer Society. (2010). *Skin cancer prevention and early detection.* Retrieved July 14, 2020, from http://www.cancer.org/cancer/skincancer/index

American Cancer Society. (2020a). *Signs and symptoms of Merkel cell carcinoma.* Retrieved July 12, 2020, from https://www.cancer.org/cancer/merkel-cell-skin-cancer/detection-diagnosis-staging/signs-and-symptoms.html

American Cancer Society. (2020b). *Key statistics about melanoma skin cancer.* Retrieved July 11, 2020, from http://www.cancer.org/cancer/skincancer-melanoma/detailedguide/melanoma-skin-cancer-key-statistics

American Cancer Society. (2020c). *Signs and symptoms of basal and squamous cell skin cancers.* Retrieved July 14, 2020, from https://www.cancer.org/cancer/basal-and-squamous-cell-skin-cancer/detection-diagnosis-staging/signs-and-symptoms.html

Bergstrom, N., & Braden, B. J. (2002). Predictive validity of the Braden Scale among Black and White subjects. *Nursing Research, 51*(6), 398–403.

Braden, B. J., & Bergstrom, N. (2020). *The Braden Scale for predicting pressure sore risk.* Retrieved July 15, 2020, from http://www.bradenscale.com/products.htm

Centers for Disease Control & Prevention (CDC), Division of Cancer Prevention and Control. (2020). *What are the risk factors for skin cancer?* Retrieved July 11, 2020, from http://www.cdc.gov/cancer/skin/basic_info/risk_factors.htm

Edsberg, L. E., Black, J. M., Goldberg, M., McNichol, L., Moore, L., & Sieggreen, M. (2016). Revised national pressure ulcer advisory panel pressure injury staging system: Revised pressure injury staging system. *Journal of Wound, Ostomy, and Continence Nursing, 43*(6), 585–597.

El Ghissassi, F., Baan, R., Straif, K., Grosse, Y., Secretan, B., Bouvard, V., Benbrahim-Tallaa, L., Guha, N., Freeman, C., Galichet, L., & Cogliano, V.; WHO International Agency for Research on Cancer Monograph Working Group. (2009). A review of human carcinogens—part D: Radiation. *The Lancet Oncology, 10*(8), 751–752.

Fawcett, R. S., Lindford, S., & Stulberg, D. L. (2004). Nail abnormalities: Clues to systemic disease. *American Academy of Family Physicians, 69*(6), 1418–1425.

Green, A. C., Williams, G. M., Logan, V., & Strutton, G. M. (2011). Reduced melanoma after regular sunscreen use: Randomized trial follow-up. *Journal of Clinical Oncology, 29*(3), 257–263.

Hall, J. C., & Hall, B. J. (2017). *Sauer's manual of skin diseases* (11th ed.). Lippincott Williams & Wilkins.

Hanford, R. R., Cobb, M. W., & Banner, N. T. (1995). Unilateral Beau's lines associated with a fractured and immobilized wrist. *Cutis; Cutaneous Medicine for the Practitioner, 56*(5), 263–264.

National Institutes of Health (NIH), National Cancer Institute. (2020). *Skin cancer prevention (PDQ®)—Health professional version.* https://www.cancer.gov/types/skin/hp/skin-prevention-pdq.

National Institutes of Health (NIH), National Cancer Institute. (2020a). *Skin cancer screening—health professional version.* https://www.cancer.gov/types/skin/hp/skin-screening-pdq#_9_toc.

National Institutes of Health (NIH), National Cancer Institute. (2020b). *Melanoma risk assessment tool.* Retrieved July 9, 2020, from http://www.cancer.gov/melanomarisktool

National Pressure Ulcer Advisory Panel. (2020). *Pressure injury stages.* Retrieved July 15, 2020, from https://npiap.com/page/PressureInjuryStages

Patton, R. M. (2005). Is diagnosis of pressure ulcers within an RN's scope of practice? *American Nurse Today, 5*(1), 20.

Skin Cancer Foundation. (2015). *Sun protection.* Retrieved October 19, 2015, from http://www.skincancer.org/prevention/sun-protection

Spicknall, K. E., Zirwas, M. J., & English, J. C., 3rd. (2005). Clubbing: An update on diagnosis, differential diagnosis, pathophysiology, and clinical relevance. *Journal of the American Academy of Dermatology, 52*(6), 1020–1028.

U.S. Preventive Services Task Force. (2016). Screening for skin cancer. Recommendation statement. *JAMA: The Journal of the American Medical Association, 316*(4), 429–435.

WHO. (2020). *Artificial tanning devices: Public health interventions to manage sunbeds.* Retrieved July 16, 2020, from https://www.who.int/publications/i/item/artificial-tanning-devices

Wolff, T., Tai, E., & Miller, T. (2009). Screening for skin cancer: An update of the evidence for the U.S. Preventive Services Task Force. *Annals of Internal Medicine, 150*(3), 194–198. Retrieved July 14, 2020, from http://www.ncbi.nlm.nih.gov/books/NBK34051

ADDITIONAL READINGS

American Cancer Society. *Be safe in the sun*. (2020). Retrieved July 12, 2020, from https://www.cancer.org/healthy/be-safe-in-sun.html

Davis, J. L. (2018). Stamp out skin tears: Skin tear assessment, management, and prevention. *American Nurse Today, 13*(6), 37–40.

Habif, T. P. (2016). *Clinical dermatology: A color guide to diagnosis and therapy* (6th ed.). Mosby.

Palese, A., Zammattio, E., Zuttion, R., Ferrario, B., Ponta, S., Gonella, S., & Comoretto, R. (2020). Avoidable and unavoidable pressure injuries among residents living in nursing homes: A retrospective study. *Journal of Wound, Ostomy, and Continence Nursing, 47*(3), 230–235.

Pressure injuries…Prevention across the acute-care continuum. *American Nurse Today*. May 2018 Supplement.

Spader, C. (2018). Preventing pressure injuries in medical-surgical patients. *American Nurse Today, 13*(6), 41–42.

U.S. Preventive Services Task Force. (2018). Final Recommendation Statement: Skin Cancer Prevention: Behavioral Counseling. https://www.uspreventiveservicestaskforce.org/uspstf/recommendation/skin-cancer-counseling. *JAMA: The Journal of the American Medical Association, 319*(11), 1134–1142.

10 THE HEAD AND NECK

KEY TERMS

adenopathy	lymphadenopathy	traumatic brain injury
concussions	headaches	facies
euphoria	prodrome	

Learning Objectives

The student will:

1. Identify the basic structures and functions of the head and neck.
2. Collect an accurate health history of the head and neck.
3. State questions used during the assessment of a patient with a headache.
4. Perform the physical examination techniques to evaluate the head and neck.
5. Document the physical examination results.
6. Identify the measures for prevention of traumatic brain injury.

The head and neck contain the cranium, face, sensory organs, neck, thyroid gland, and lymph nodes. This chapter is an overview of the head, also known as the cranium. Each of these sequential areas will be addressed with additional anatomic detail followed by the assessment, including an example of subjective health history questions and objective physical examination techniques.

ANATOMY AND PHYSIOLOGY OF THE HEAD

The head portion of the body consists of the skull and face. Regions of the head take their names from the underlying bones of the skull: the frontal, parietal, temporal, and occipital areas. Knowing this anatomy helps locate and describe physical findings (Fig. 10-1). The face is the anterior portion of the head and encompasses the sensory organs, which are the focus of Chapter 11, "The Eyes," and Chapter 12, "Ears, Nose, Mouth, and Throat." Additional systems coincide with the head and neck and are addressed in future chapters, including cranial nerves in Chapter 20, "The

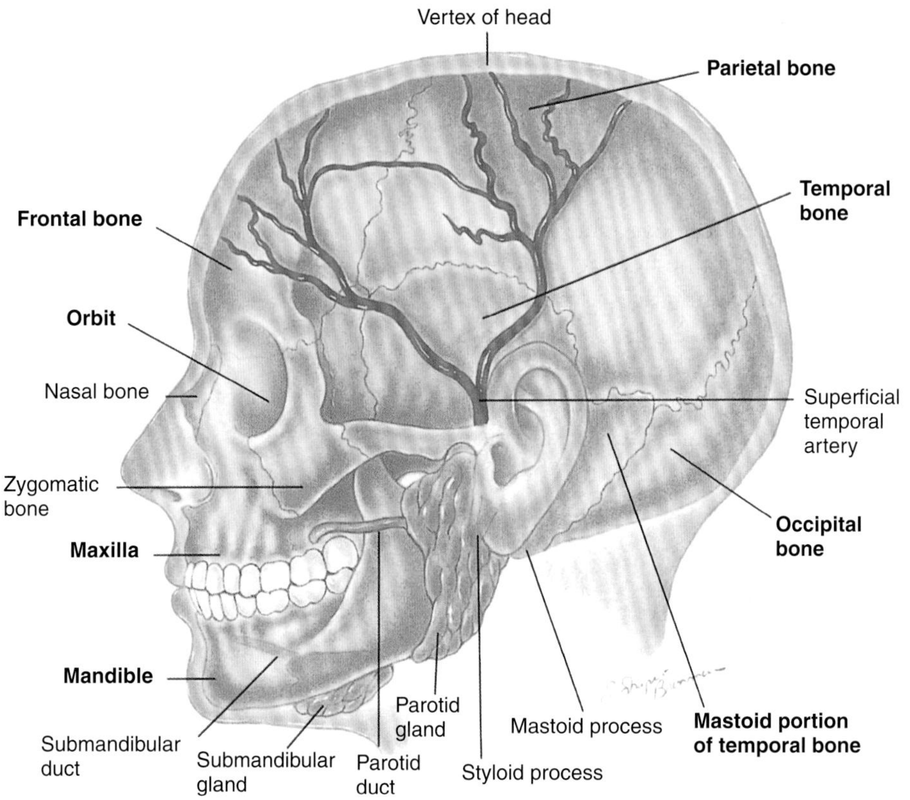

FIGURE 10-1 Structures of the skull.

Nervous System," cervical vertebrae in Chapter 18, "The Musculoskeletal System," and the blood supply to the head and neck in Chapter 15, "The Peripheral Vascular System and Lymphatic System."

HEALTH HISTORY OF THE HEAD

Common or concerning symptoms identified during the health history of the head are listed in Box 10-1.

BOX 10-1 COMMON OR CONCERNING SYMPTOMS OF THE HEAD

Headache
Head injury
Head or neck surgery
Traumatic brain injury

Headache

Headaches are one of the most common complaints in clinical practice, with close to 50% of the adult population experiencing symptoms in the previous year (World Health Organization, 2011, 2016). Multiple factors can contribute to headaches including medical (e.g., migraines, hypertension, medication side effects), emotional (e.g., stress, anxiety), physical (e.g., injury) or environmental (e.g., the weather) (World Health Organization, 2016). Although there are varying types, degrees, and causes, headaches are a global issue that knows no boundaries and impacts people of all ages, races, socioeconomic statuses, and locations (World Health Organization, 2011, 2016).

Tension headaches are one of the most common types of headaches, though many individuals self-treat this type of headache. Migraine headaches are by far the most frequent cause of headaches seen in office practice, as migraines are often the most debilitating, lasting anywhere from 4 hours up to 3 days (Buse et al., 2019; Collaborators GBDH, 2018). Every headache warrants careful evaluation for life-threatening causes such as meningitis, subdural or intracranial hemorrhage, or tumor. It is important to elicit a full description of the headache and all attributes of the patient's pain. Is the headache one-sided or bilateral? Severe with sudden onset? Steady or throbbing? Continuous or intermittent (comes and goes)?

Primary headaches have no identifiable underlying cause (Table 10-1). *Secondary headaches* arise from other conditions; some of these may endanger the patient's life (Table 10-2) (World Health Organization, 2011).

TABLE 10-1 Primary Headaches

Headaches are classified as *primary,* without underlying pathology, or *secondary,* with a serious underlying cause often warranting urgent attention. Secondary headaches are more likely to occur after age 50 with a sudden severe onset and should be ruled out before making the diagnosis of a primary headache (Khokhar et al., 2017). About 90% of headaches are primary headaches and fall into four categories: tension, migraine, cluster, and chronic daily headache. The features of tension, migraine, and cluster headaches are highlighted below. *Chronic daily headache* is not a diagnosis but rather a category containing preexisting headaches that have been transformed into more pronounced forms of migraines, chronic tension type headaches, and medication overuse headaches, and they last more than 15 days a month for more than 3 months (Kumar et al., 2020). Risk factors include obesity; more than one headache a week; caffeine ingestion; use of headache medications for more than 10 days a month, such as analgesics, ergots, and triptans; and sleep and mood disorders.

	Tension	Migraines	Cluster
Process	Process unclear—possibly heightened central nervous system pain sensitivity Involves pericranial muscle tenderness Etiology also unclear	Neuronal dysfunction, possibly of brainstem origin, involving low serotonin level, spreading cortical depression and trigeminovascular activation Types: with aura, without aura, variants	Process unclear—possibly hypothalamic then trigeminoautonomic activation
Lifetime Prevalence	Most common headache (40%); prevalence about 50%	10% of headaches; prevalence 18% of U.S. adults Affects ~15% of women, 6% of men	<1%, more common in men
Location	Usually bilateral May be generalized or localized to the back of the head and upper neck or to the frontotemporal area	Unilateral in ~70%; bifrontal or global in ~30%	Unilateral, usually behind or around the eye or temple

	Tension	Migraines	Cluster
Quality and Severity	Steady Pressing or tightening Nonthrobbing pain Mild to moderate intensity	Throbbing or aching pain Moderate to severe in intensity Preceded by an aura in up to 30%	Sharp, continuous, intense Severe in intensity
Timing			
Onset	Gradual	Fairly rapid, reaching a peak in 1–2 h	Abrupt; peaks within minutes
Duration	30 min to 7 days	4–72 h	15 min to 3 h
Course	Episodic; may be chronic	Recurrent—usually monthly, but weekly in ~10% Peak incidence early to mid-adolescence	Episodic, clustered in time, with several each day for 4–8 wk and then relief for 6–12 mo
Associated Symptoms	Sometimes photophobia, phonophobia Scalp tenderness Nausea absent	Prodrome: nausea, vomiting, photophobia, phonophobia Aura in 30% Either visual (flickering, zig-zagging lines) or motor (paresthesias of hand, arm, or face, or language dysfunction)	Unilateral autonomic symptoms: lacrimation, rhinorrhea, miosis, ptosis, eyelid edema, conjunctival infection
Triggers/ Factors that Aggravate or Provoke	Sustained muscle tension, as in driving or typing Stress Sleep disturbances	Alcohol, certain foods, or stress may provoke Also menses, high altitude Aggravated by noise and bright light	During attack, sensitivity to alcohol may increase
Factors that Relieve	Possibly massage, relaxation	Quiet, dark room Sleep Sometimes transient relief from pressure on the involved artery	

Sources: Headache Classification Committee of the International Headache Society (IHS). (2013). The International Classification of Headache Disorders, 3rd edition (beta version). *Cephalalgia*, *33*, 629; Lipton, R. B., Bigal, M. E., Steiner, T. J., Silberstein, S. D., & Olesen, J. (2004). Classification of primary headaches. *Neurology*, *63*(3), 427–435; Sun-Edelstein, C., Bigal, M. E., & Rappoport, A. M. (2009). Chronic migraine and medication overuse headache: clarifying the current International Headache Society classification criteria. *Cephalalgia*, *29*, 445; Lipton, R. B., Stewart, W. F., Diamond, S., Diamond, M. L., & Reed, M. (2001). Prevalence and burden of migraine in the United States: Data from the American Migraine Study II. *Headache*, *41*(7), 646–657; Fumal, A., & Schoenen, J. (2008). Tension-type headache: current research and clinical management. *Lancet Neurology*, *7*, 70; Nesbitt, A. D., & Goadsby, P. J. (2012). Cluster headache. *British Medical Journal*, *344*, e2407; Baldwin, G., Breiding, M., & Sleet, D. (2016). Using the public health model to address unintentional injuries and TBI: A perspective from the Centers for Disease Control and Prevention (CDC). *Neurorehabilitation*, *39*(3), 345–349. https://doi.org/10.3233/NRE-161366; Castro, M. R., & Gharib, H. (2005). Controversies in the management of thyroid nodules. *Annals of Internal Medicine*, *142*(11), 926–931; Chu, H. T., Liang, C. S., Lee, J. T., Yeh, T. C., Lee, M. S., Sung, Y. F, & Yang, F. C. (2018). Associations between depression/anxiety and headache frequency in Migraineurs: a cross-sectional study. *Headache*, *58*(3), 407–415. https://doi.org/10.1111/head.13215; Coronado, V. G., Thomas, K. E., Sattin, R. W., Johnson, R. L. (2005). The CDC traumatic brain injury surveillance system: Characteristics of persons aged 65 years and older hospitalized with a TBI. *Journal of Head Trauma Rehabilitation*, *20*(3), 215–228. https://doi.org/10.1097/00001199-200505000-00005; Huh, K. R., Kim, J. Y., Choi, S. H., Yoon, Y. H., Park, S. J., & Lee, E. S. (2020). Comparison of traumatic brain injury patients with brain computed tomography in the emergency department by age group. *Clinical and Experimental Emergency Medicine*, *7*(2), 81–86. https://doi.org/10.15441/ceem.19.076; and International Headache Society. (2018). The international classification of headache disorders. *Cephalalgia*, *38*, 1–211.

TABLE 10-2 Secondary Headaches and Cranial Neuralgias

Type	Process	Location	Quality and Severity
Secondary Headaches			
Analgesic Rebound	Withdrawal of medication	Previous headache pattern	Variable
Headaches from Eye Disorders			
Errors of Refraction (farsightedness and astigmatism, but not nearsightedness)	Probably the sustained contraction of the extraocular muscles and possibly of the frontal, temporal, and occipital muscles	Around and over the eyes; may radiate to the occipital area	Steady, aching, dull
Acute Glaucoma	Sudden increase in intraocular pressure	Pain in and around one eye	Steady, aching, often severe
Headache from Sinusitis	Mucosal inflammation of the paranasal sinuses	Usually frontal sinuses above the eyes or over the maxillary sinus	Aching or throbbing, severity variable; consider possible migraine
Meningitis	Viral or bacterial infection of the meninges surrounding the brain and spinal cord	Generalized	Steady or throbbing, severe
Subarachnoid Hemorrhage—"Thunderclap Headache"	Bleeding from a ruptured cerebral saccular aneurysm; rarely from arteriovenous malformation, mycotic aneurysm	Generalized	Very severe, "the worst of my life"
Brain Tumor	Mass lesion causing displacement of or traction on pain-sensitive arteries and veins or pressure on nerves	Variable, including lobes of brain, cerebellum, brainstem	Aching, steady, dull pain worse on awakening the better after several hours
Giant Cell (Temporal) Arteritis	Transmural lymphocytic vasculitis often involving multinucleated giant cells that disrupts the internal elastic lamina of large-caliber arteries	Localized near the involved artery, most often the temporal artery in those > age 50, women > men (2:1 ratio)	Throbbing, generalized, persistent; often severe

Timing					
Onset	***Duration***	***Course***	**Associated Symptoms**	**Factors that Aggravate or Provoke**	**Factors that Relieve**
Variable	Depends on prior headache pattern	Depends on frequency of "mini-withdrawals"	Depends on prior headache pattern	Fever, carbon monoxide, hypoxia, withdrawal of caffeine, other headache triggers	Depends on cause
Gradual	Variable	Variable	Eye fatigue, "sandy" sensations in eyes, redness of conjunctiva	Prolonged use of the eyes, particularly for close work	Rest of the eyes
Often rapid	Variable, may depend on treatment	Variable, may depend on treatment	Blurred vision, nausea, and vomiting; halos around lights, reddening of eye	Sometimes provoked by mydriatic drops	
Variable	Often daily several hours at a time, persisting until treatment	Often daily in a repetitive pattern	Local tenderness, nasal congestion, discharge, and fever	May be aggravated by coughing, sneezing, or jarring the head	Nasal decongestants, antibiotics
Fairly rapid, usually <24 h; may be sudden onset	Variable, usually days	Viral: usually <1 wk; bacterial: persistent until treatment	Fever, stiff neck, photophobia, change in mental status		Immediate treatment and antibiotics for bacterial meningitis
Sudden onset; can be less than a minute	Variable, usually days	Varies according to presenting severity and level of consciousness; worst if initial coma	Nausea, vomiting, loss of consciousness, neck pain Possible prior neck symptoms from "sentinel leaks"	Rebleeding, ↑ intracranial pressure, cerebral edema	Subspecialty treatments
Variable	Often brief; depends on location and rate of growth	Intermittent but may progress in intensity over a period of days	Seizures, hemiparesis, field cuts, personality changes Also nausea, vomiting, vision change, gait change	May be aggravated by coughing, sneezing, or sudden movements of the head	Subspecialty treatments
Gradual or rapid	Variable	Recurrent or persistent over weeks to months	Tenderness over temporal artery, adjacent scalp; fever (in ~50%), fatigue, weight loss; new headache (~60%), jaw claudication (~50%), visual loss or blindness (~15–20%), polymyalgia rheumatica (~50%)	Movement of neck and shoulders	Often steroids

(continued)

TABLE 10-2 Secondary Headaches and Cranial Neuralgias (*Continued*)

Type	Process	Location	Quality and Severity
Postconcussion Headache	Follows mild acceleration–deceleration traumatic brain injury; may involve axonal, cerebrovascular autoregulatory, neurochemical injury	Often but not always localized to the injured area	Dull, aching, constant; may have features of tension and migraine headaches
Cranial Neuralgias			
Trigeminal Neuralgia (cranial nerve (CN) V)	Vascular compression of CN V, usually near entry to pons leading to focal demyelination, aberrant discharge; 10% with causative intracranial lesion	Cheek, jaws, lips, or gums; trigeminal nerve divisions 2 and 3 > 1	Shock-like, stabbing, burning; severe

Note: Blanks appear in this table when the categories are not applicable or not usually helpful in assessing the problem.

Sources: Headache Classification Committee of the International Headache Society (IHS). (2013). The International Classification of Headache Disorders, 3rd ed. (beta version). *Cephalalgia*, *33*, 629; Schwedt, T. J., Matharu, M. S., & Dodick, D. W. (2006). Thunderclap headache. *Lancet Neurology*, *5*, 621; Van de Beek, D., de Gans, J., Spanjaard, L., Weisfelt, M., Reitsma, J. B., & Vermeulen, M. (2004). Clinical features and prognostic factors in adults with bacterial meningitis. *New England Journal of Medicine*, *351*, 1849; Salvarini, C., Cantini, F., & Hunder, G. G. (2008). Polymyalgia rheumatica and giant cell arteritis. *Lancet*, *372*, 234; Smetana, G. W., & Shmerling, R. H. (2002). Does this patient have temporal arteritis? *JAMA*, *287*, 92; Ropper, A. H., & Gorson, K. C. (2007). Clinical practice. Concussion. *New England Journal of Medicine*, *356*, 166. American College of Physicians. (2012). *Neurology—MKSAP 16*; McCrory, P., Feddermann-Demont, N., Dvořák, J., Cassidy, J. D., McIntosh, A., Vos, P. E., Echemendia, R. J., Meeuwisse, W., & Tarnutzer, A. A. (2017). What is the definition of sports-related concussion: a systematic review. *British Journal of Sports Medicine*, *51*(11), 877–887. https://doi.org/10.1136/bjsports-2016-097393; Taylor, C. A., Bell, J. M., Breiding, M. J., & Xu, L. (2017). Traumatic brain injury-related emergency department visits, hospitalizations, and deaths—United States, 2007 and 2013. *Mmwr Surveillance Summaries*, *66*(9), 1–16. https://doi.org/10.15585/mmwr.ss6609a1; and Winkler, E. A., Yue, J. K., Burke, J. F., Chan, A. K., Dhall, S. S., Berger, M. S., Manley, G. T., & Tarapore, P. E. (2016). Adult sports-related traumatic brain injury in United States trauma centers. *Neurosurgical Focus*, *40*(4), E4. https://doi.org/10.3171/2016.1.FOCUS15613.

Look for "red flags" using the screening mnemonic, "SNOOP," that raises suspicion of worrisome secondary causes:

- *Systemic signs, symptoms, or illness:* "The worst headache of my life;" markedly elevated blood pressure; stiff neck or signs of infection; presence of cancer, HIV, pregnancy, or vomiting
- *Neurologic deficits:* Altered mental status, seizures, or papilledema
- *Onset (new or sudden):* After age 50; acute onset like a "thunderclap"
- *Other associated conditions:* After head trauma; increases with the Valsalva maneuver or position changes; triggered by exercise or awakening from sleep
- *Prior history:* Headaches are different than previous ones in progression, pattern, frequency, and/or severity (Smith, 2018).

The history is critical in determining the focus of the physical examination. Using "OLD CART," ask the patient specifically about symptoms related to the headaches.

Timing					
Onset	*Duration*	*Course*	**Associated Symptoms**	**Factors that Aggravate or Provoke**	**Factors that Relieve**
Within 7 days of the injury up to 3 mo	Weeks to up to a year	Tends to diminish over time	Drowsiness, poor concentration, confusion, memory loss, blurred vision, dizziness, irritability, restlessness, fatigue	Mental and physical exertion, straining, stooping, emotional excitement, alcohol	Rest; medication
Abrupt, paroxysmal	Each jab lasts seconds but recurs at intervals of seconds or minutes	May recur daily for weeks to months then resolve; can be chronic progressive	Exhaustion from recurrent pain	Touching certain areas of the lower face or mouth; chewing, talking, brushing teeth	Medication; neurovascular decompression

Opening questions may include "Have you experienced unusually severe headaches?" or "Have you experienced unusually frequent headaches?"

If the patient noticed unusually severe or frequent headaches, then further assessment with "OLD CART" is helpful.

CLINICAL TIP
The most important attributes are the headaches' severity and chronologic patterns. If a headache is severe and of sudden onset, consider subarachnoid hemorrhage, meningitis, or stroke.

- *Onset:* When did you first notice the headache?

CLINICAL TIP
Migraine and *tension headaches* are episodic and tend to peak over several hours. New and persisting, progressively severe headaches raise concerns of *tumor*, *abscess*, or *mass* (Collaborators GBDH, 2018).

- *Location:* Where do you feel the headache? Can you point to the area(s)?

CLINICAL TIP
Unilateral headache is seen in *migraine and cluster headaches* (Collaborators GBDH, 2018; World Health Organization, 2016). Tension headaches often arise in the temporal areas; cluster headaches may be retroorbital.

- *Duration:* How long has this been going on?
  - Did the headache begin suddenly (in a few minutes or less than an hour) or gradually (over a few hours or days)?
  - Is it temporary or constant?
  - When does the pain begin (morning, evening)? Does it wake you at night?
  - How long do the headaches last?
  - Are they recurring?
  - Is there a pattern?
- *Characteristic symptoms:* Describe what it feels like (throbbing, hammering, squeezing).
- Describe the pain on a scale of 1 to 10 with 1 being minimal pain and 10 being the worst pain you ever felt.
- *Associated manifestations:* Do you notice any other symptoms when this occurs? Blurred vision? Nausea? Vomiting? Dizziness?

CLINICAL TIP
Nausea and vomiting are common with *migraine* but also occur with *brain tumors* and *subarachnoid hemorrhage*.

What happened prior to the headache? Did anything precipitate the pain?

Is there a **prodrome** (an early sign or symptom) of unusual feelings such as **euphoria** (a feeling of elation inappropriate to situation), craving for food, fatigue, or dizziness?

Approximately 60% to 70% of patients with migraine have a prodrome prior to onset; 20% experience an aura, including photophobia, scintillating scotomata (blind spot), or reversible visual and sensory symptoms.

Is there an aura with neurologic symptoms, such as change in vision or numbness or weakness in an arm or leg?

Does anything trigger the headache, like specific foods or drinks, exercise, stress, work, environment, or menstruation?

Is there a history of overuse of analgesics (e.g., ibuprofen), ergotamine, or triptans?

CLINICAL TIP
Consider medication overuse in patients with chronic daily headache taking symptomatic medications more than 2 days a week (D'Amico et al., 2018; World Health Organization, 2016).

Do you have a family or personal history of headaches?

Family history may be positive in patients with migraines.

Did you experience a head injury or brain trauma in the past? When?

- *Relieving factors:* What have you tried to make the headache go away? Have you tried sleep, a dark room, cool compresses, and/or relaxation techniques?
  What has worked the best? What has not worked at all?
  Does anything make it worse?
  How have the headaches affected your daily life and activities?

Ask whether coughing, sneezing, or changing the position of the head has any effect (better, worse, or none) on the headache (Smith, 2018). Such maneuvers may increase pain from a brain tumor or acute sinusitis.

- *Treatment:* Has anyone treated you for headaches in the past, like a physician, nurse practitioner, holistic practitioner, herbalist, acupuncturist, or massage therapist?
  If yes, what type of headache was diagnosed?
  Have you used any medication? If yes, what is the name of the medication, its dosage, and its effect?

Traumatic Brain Injury

Traumatic brain injury (TBI) is a blow to the head or a piercing head injury that interferes with the function of the brain. Not all injuries to the head result in a TBI, and those that do occur span from mild to severe. Mild cases, often known as **concussions**, involve a slight change in mental status or consciousness. Severe cases have extended postinjury changes. The TBI may impact memory, thought processes, movement, personality, vision and/or hearing; it can last from days to years and can in some cases result in death (Centers for Disease Control & Prevention, 2019; Syrenicz et al., 2014).

If the patient has experienced head trauma or brain injury in the past, the nurse should use "OLD CART" to learn more.

- *Onset:* When did this occur? Can you describe what happened?
  Do you remember when you hurt your head?
  Precipitating factors: What happened to cause the TBI? Was there absence of protective equipment or helmet or an environmental cause?
- *Location:* Can you show me where you hurt your head?
- *Duration:* Did you lose consciousness? If yes, for how long?
  Did you fall first or lose consciousness first?
- *Characteristic symptoms:* Did you experience any symptoms prior to the head injury like headache, shortness of breath, chest pain, numbness, or tingling?
  Do you have any medical issues (e.g., cardiac history, diabetes, seizures)?
- *Associated manifestations:* Do you experience vision changes? Nausea or vomiting? Attention span deficits? Dizziness? Confusion? Drainage from the ears, nose, eyes, or mouth? Tremors? Seizures? Gait changes?
- *Relieving factors/strategies:* Discuss prevention of further injury using the information in the "Health Promotion and Counseling" section.
- *Treatment:* Have you done anything to treat the injury?

ANATOMY AND PHYSIOLOGY OF THE NECK

For descriptive purposes, divide each side of the neck into two triangles bounded by the sternocleidomastoid muscle (Fig. 10-2). Visualize the borders of the two triangles as follows:

- The *anterior triangle:* the mandible above, the sternocleidomastoid laterally, and the midline of the neck medially
- The *posterior triangle:* the sternocleidomastoid muscle, the trapezius, and the clavicle; note that a portion of the omohyoid muscle crosses the lower portion of this triangle and can be mistaken for a lymph node or mass.

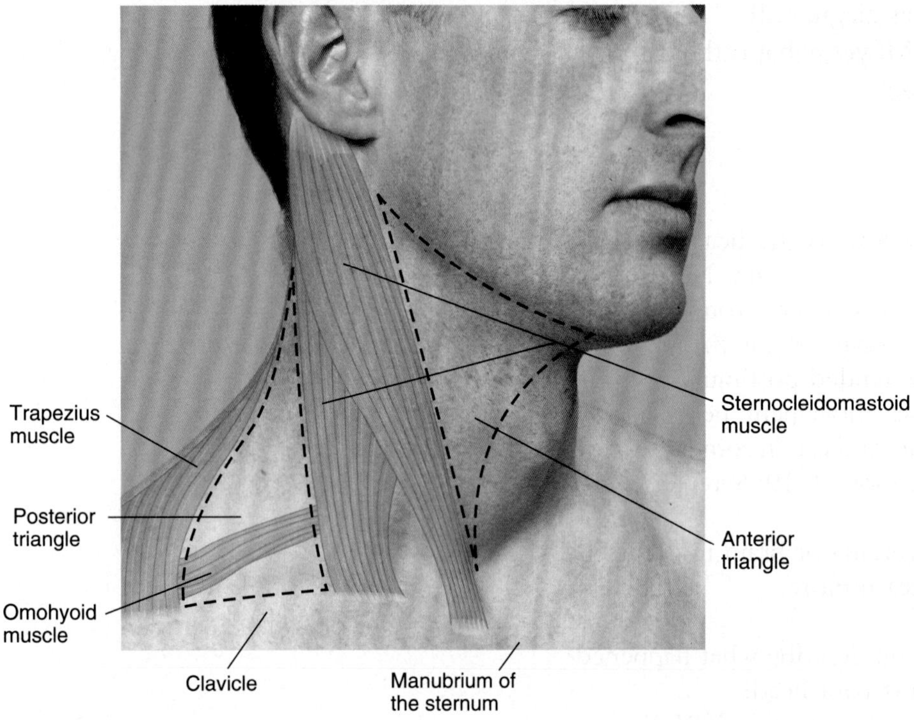

FIGURE 10-2 The neck can be examined by visualizing the anterior and posterior triangles separated by the sternocleidomastoid muscle.

Great Vessels

Under the sternocleidomastoid muscle run the great vessels of the neck (Fig. 10-3): the *carotid artery* and the *internal jugular vein.* The *external jugular vein* passes diagonally over the surface of the sternocleidomastoid and may be helpful when trying to identify jugular venous pressure.

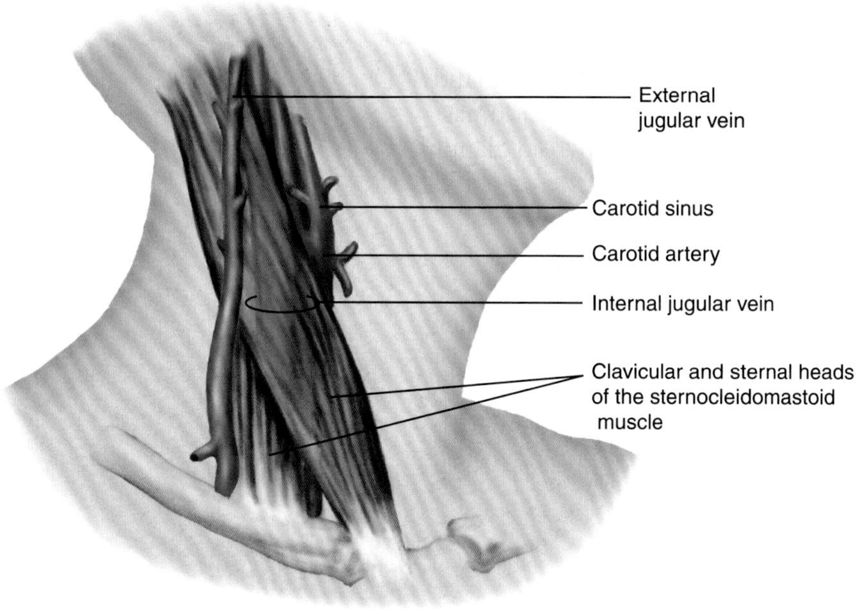

FIGURE 10-3 The great vessels of the neck.

Midline Structures and Thyroid Gland

The midline structures (Fig. 10-4) include: (1) the mobile *hyoid bone* just below the mandible; (2) the *thyroid cartilage* readily identified by the notch on its superior edge; (3) the *cricoid cartilage*; (4) the *tracheal rings*; and (5) the *thyroid gland*.

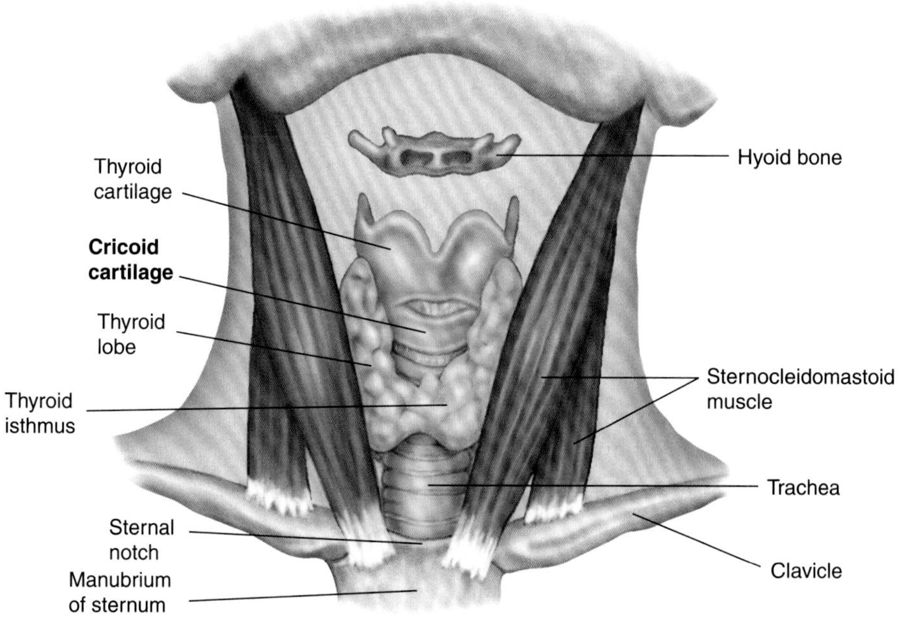

FIGURE 10-4 The midline structures of the neck.

The isthmus of the thyroid gland lies across the trachea below the cricoid cartilage. The lateral lobes of this gland curve posteriorly around the sides of the trachea and the esophagus. Except in the midline, the thyroid gland is covered by thin, strap-like muscles. Of these, only the sternocleidomastoids are visible. Women have larger and more easily palpable thyroid glands than men.

Lymph Nodes

The lymphatic system has many important functions, including maintenance of body fluid levels, absorption of fats from the digestive tract, removal of waste products, and contributions to the immune system. Its function is to detect and eliminate foreign substances. One part of the lymph system is in the head and neck. The nurse needs to be aware of the drainage pattern illustrated in Figure 10-5.

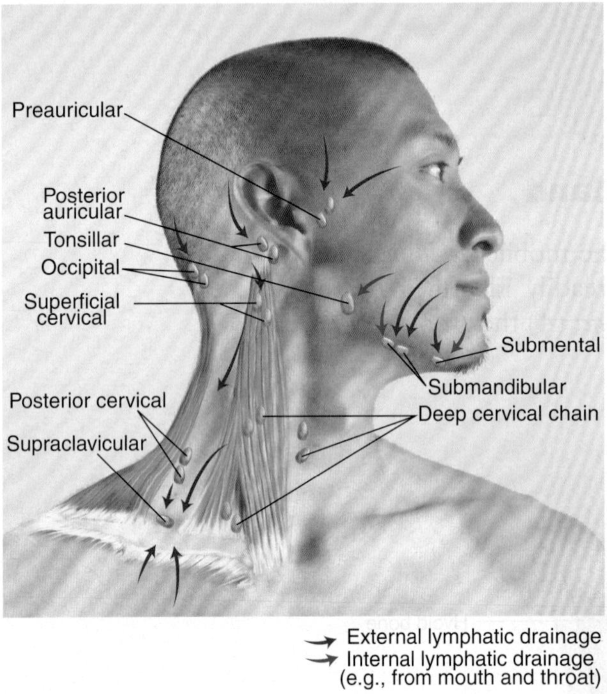

FIGURE 10-5 The lymph nodes and lymphatic drainage pattern of the head and neck.

Knowledge of the lymphatic system is important to a thorough assessment; whenever a malignant or inflammatory lesion is observed, look for involvement of the regional lymph nodes that drain it. Whenever a node is enlarged or tender, look for a source such as infection in the area that it drains.

Ask, "Have you noticed any swollen 'glands' or lumps in your neck?" because patients are more familiar with these lay terms than with "*lymph nodes.*"

Enlarged tender lymph nodes commonly accompany *pharyngitis.*

THE HEALTH HISTORY OF THE NECK

Common or concerning symptoms of the neck are listed in Box 10-2.

BOX 10-2 COMMON OR CONCERNING SYMPTOMS OF THE NECK

Swollen lymph nodes or neck lumps
Enlarged thyroid gland
Hoarseness

If a patient presents with a lump in the neck, explore further using "OLD CART."

- *Onset:* When did you first notice the lump?
- *Location:* Where is the lump?
  Is there more than one lump?
- *Duration:* How long have you had the lump?
- *Characteristic symptoms:* Has the lump changed in size, tenderness, drainage, shape, or consistency?
- *Associated manifestations:* Do you have difficulty swallowing? Have you had any recent infections? Trauma? Radiation? Surgery?
  Do you have a history of smoking? Drinking alcohol? Chewing tobacco?
- *Relieving factors:* Does anything make the lump smaller? Less tender?
  Have you tried compresses at the site?
- *Treatment:* Have you been to a health care provider to address this lump?

Also assess thyroid function, and ask about any evidence of an enlarged thyroid gland or goiter. To evaluate thyroid function, ask about temperature intolerance and sweating. Opening questions include:

With *goiter,* thyroid function may be increased, decreased, or normal.

- Do you prefer hot or cold weather?

CLINICAL TIP
Intolerance to cold, preference for warm clothing and many blankets, and decreased sweating suggest *hypothyroidism*; the opposite symptoms, palpitations, and involuntary weight loss suggest *hyperthyroidism*.

- Do you dress more warmly or less warmly than other people?
- Do you use more or fewer blankets than others at home?
- Do you perspire more or less than others?
- Have you experienced any new palpitations or change in weight?

Note that as people grow older, they sweat less, have less tolerance for cold, and tend to prefer warmer environments.

Hoarseness, which is addressed in Chapter 12, "Ears, Nose, Mouth, and Throat" will frequently arise from the larynx. However, hypothyroidism can cause chronic hoarseness.

PHYSICAL EXAMINATION

Equipment needed for a physical examination of the head and neck include:

- Tangential light
- Cup of water
- Stethoscope

Abnormalities covered by the hair are easily missed, so ask if the patient has noticed anything different or any changes to the scalp or hair. Ask the patient to remove any hair pieces, hair adornments, scarves, or rubber bands. Take into consideration individual cultural practices and personal preferences when examining patients.

The Hair

Note the quantity, distribution, texture, and pattern of loss, if any, of the hair. You may see loose flakes of dandruff. Fine hair accompanies *hyperthyroidism*; coarse hair is found with *hypothyroidism*.

Tiny white ovoid granules that adhere to hairs may be nits (eggs of lice).

The Scalp

Part the hair in several places and look for scaling, lumps, nevi, or other lesions. Redness and scaling may be seen in *seborrheic dermatitis or psoriasis.*

The Skull

Observe the general size and contour of the skull. Note any deformities, depressions, lumps, or tenderness. Learn to recognize the irregularities in a normal skull, such as those near the suture lines between the parietal and occipital bones.

Macrocephaly is an anomaly characterized by a large head in proportion to the body and an underdeveloped brain. The circumference of the head is more than two standard deviations above average for the person's age and sex. *Microcephaly* is an anomaly characterized by a small head in proportion to the body and an underdeveloped brain. The circumference of the head is more than two standard deviations below average for the person's age and sex.

The Face

Note the patient's facial expression and contours. Observe for asymmetry, involuntary movements, edema, and masses. Table 10-3 outlines select **facies** (appearance and expression of the face characteristic of certain conditions).

TABLE 10-3 Selected Facies

Facial Swelling

Cushing Syndrome

The increased adrenal cortisol production of Cushing syndrome produces a round or "moon" face with red cheeks. Excessive hair growth may be present in the mustache and sideburn areas and on the chin.

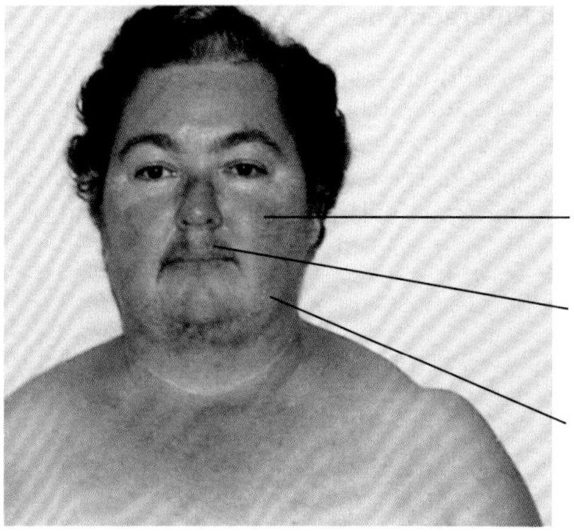

Nephrotic Syndrome

The face is edematous and often pale. Swelling usually appears first around the eyes and in the morning. The eyes may become slitlike when edema is severe.

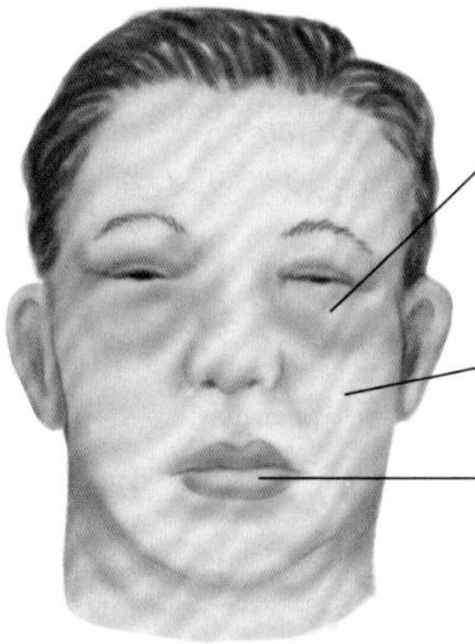

Myxedema

The patient with severe hypothyroidism (*myxedema*) has a dull, puffy facies. The edema, often pronounced around the eyes, does not pit with pressure. The hair and eyebrows are dry, coarse, and thinned. The skin is dry.

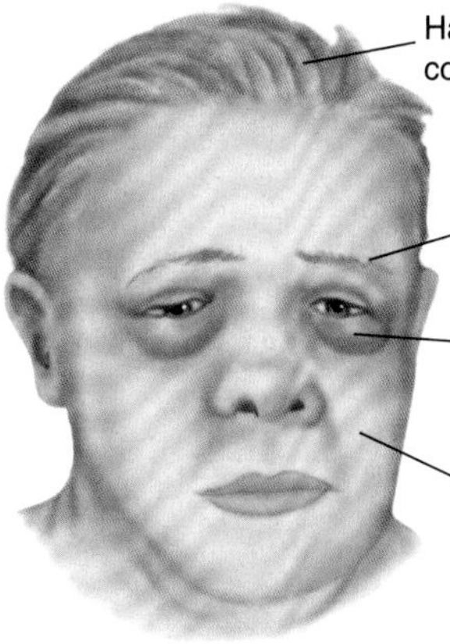

(*continued*)

TABLE 10-3 Selected Facies (*Continued*)

Other Facies

Parotid Gland Enlargement

Chronic bilateral asymptomatic parotid gland enlargement may be associated with obesity, diabetes, cirrhosis, mumps, and other conditions. Note the swellings anterior to the ear lobes and above the angles of the jaw. Gradual unilateral enlargement suggests neoplasm. Acute enlargement is seen in mumps.

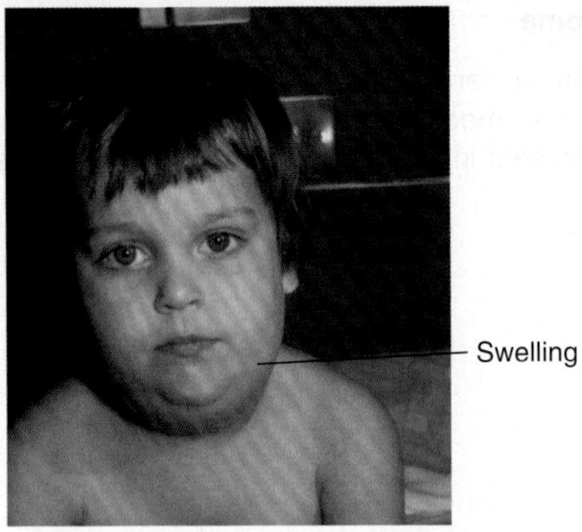

Acromegaly

The increased growth hormone of acromegaly produces enlargement of both bone and soft tissues. The head is elongated, with bony prominence of the forehead, nose, and lower jaw. Soft tissues of the nose, lips, and ears are also enlarged. The facial features appear generally coarsened.

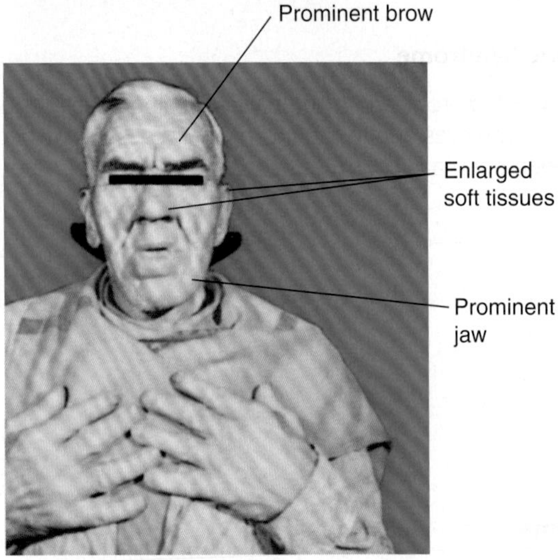

Parkinson Disease

Decreased facial mobility blunts expression. A mask-like face may result, with decreased blinking and a characteristic stare. Since the neck and upper trunk tend to flex forward, the patient seems to peer upward toward the observer. Facial skin becomes oily, and drooling may occur.

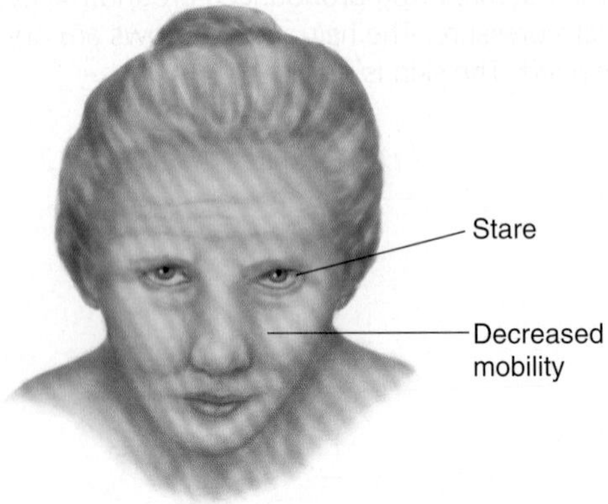

Source: *Cushing Syndrome*—Reprinted with permission from Rubin, R., Strayer, D. S., & Rubin, E. (2012). *Rubin's pathology* (6th ed.). Lippincott Williams & Wilkins.

The Skin

Observe the skin, noting its color, pigmentation, texture, thickness, hair distribution, and any lesions.

CLINICAL TIP
Acne is found in many adolescents. *Hirsutism* (excessive facial hair) occurs in some women with *polycystic ovary syndrome*.

The Neck

Observe the skin of the neck, noting its color, pigmentation, texture, thickness, hair distribution, and any lesions. *Inspect the neck*, noting its symmetry and any masses or scars. Look for enlargement of the parotid or submandibular glands, and note any visible lymph nodes.

A scar of past thyroid surgery is often a clue to under-reported thyroid disease.

The Lymph Nodes

Palpate the lymph nodes. Using the pads of your index and middle fingers, move the skin over the underlying tissues in each area in a circular motion (Fig. 10-6). The patient should be relaxed with the neck flexed slightly forward and if needed, slightly toward the side being examined. You can usually examine both sides at once. For the submental node, however, it is helpful to palpate with one hand in the area behind the mandible.

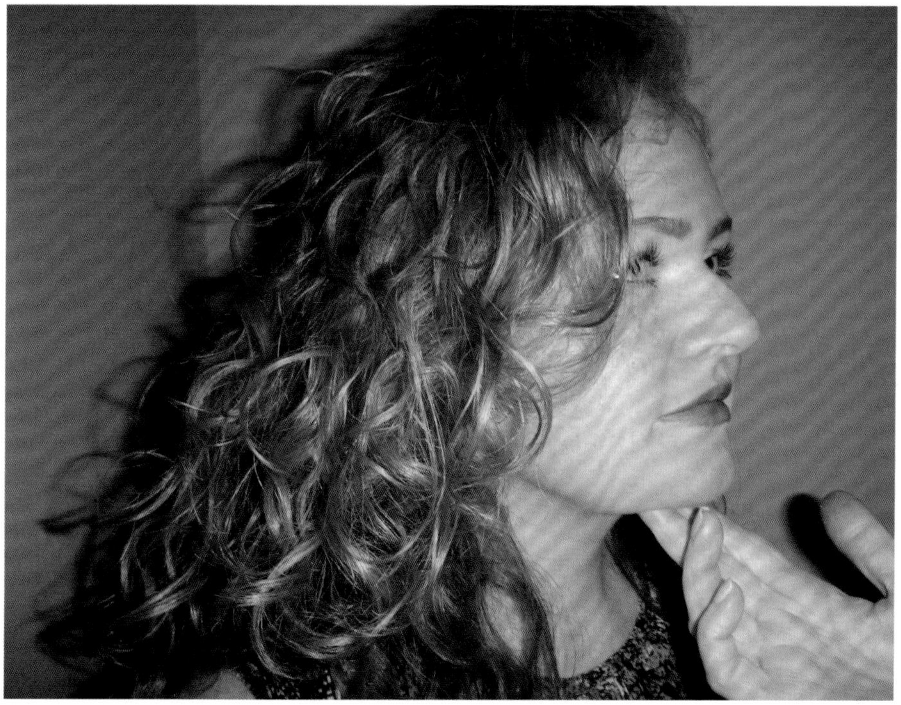

FIGURE 10-6 Palpation of submental node.

Feel in sequence (Fig. 10-7) for the following nodes:

1. *Preauricular*—in front of the ear
2. *Posterior auricular*—superficial to the mastoid process
3. *Occipital*—at the base of the skull posteriorly
4. *Tonsillar*—at the angle of the mandible

A "tonsillar node" that pulsates is really the carotid artery. A small, hard, tender "tonsillar node" high and deep between the mandible and the sternocleidomastoid is probably the styloid process of the temporal bone.

5. *Submandibular*—midway between the angle and the tip of the mandible; these nodes are usually smaller and smoother than the lobulated submandibular gland against which they lie
6. *Submental*—in the midline a few centimeters behind the tip of the mandible
7. *Superficial cervical*—superficial to the sternocleidomastoid
8. *Posterior cervical*—along the anterior edge of the trapezius
9. *Deep cervical chain*—deep to the sternocleidomastoid and often inaccessible to examination; hook your thumb and fingers around either side of the sternocleidomastoid muscle to find them
10. *Supraclavicular*—deep in the angle formed by the clavicle and the sternocleidomastoid

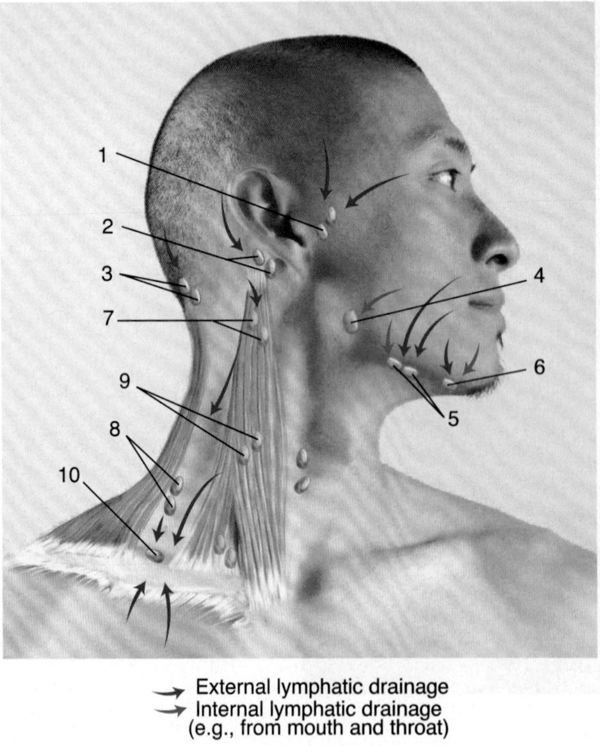

FIGURE 10-7 Sequence for palpating the lymph nodes.

CLINICAL TIP
Enlargement of a supraclavicular node, especially on the left, suggests possible metastasis from a thoracic or an abdominal malignancy.

Begin palpation using the pads of the index and third fingers and palpate the *preauricular nodes* with a gentle rotary motion (Fig. 10-8). Then examine the *posterior auricular* and *occipital* lymph nodes and follow sequentially to *tonsillar*, then *submandibular*. The *submental* is palpated with one hand.

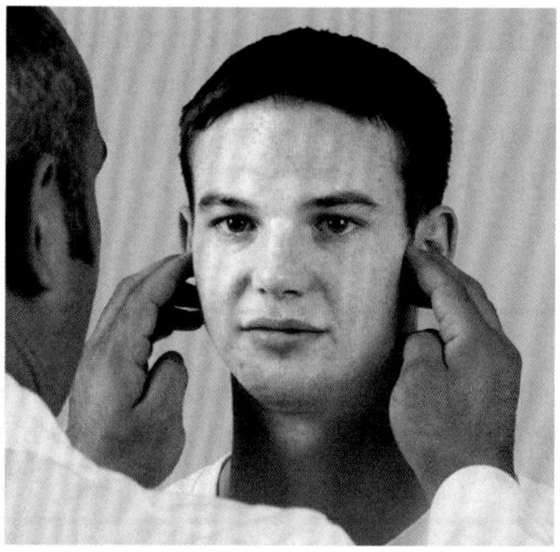
FIGURE 10-8 Use the index and third fingers to palpate the preauricular nodes using a circular motion.

The last lymph nodes in the neck to be palpated are the *superficial cervical* and the *deep cervical chains*, located anterior and superficial to the sternocleidomastoid. Then palpate the *posterior cervical chain* along the trapezius (anterior edge) and along the sternocleidomastoid (posterior edge). Flex the patient's neck slightly forward toward the side being examined. Examine the *supraclavicular* nodes (Fig. 10-9) in the angle between the clavicle and the sternocleidomastoid.

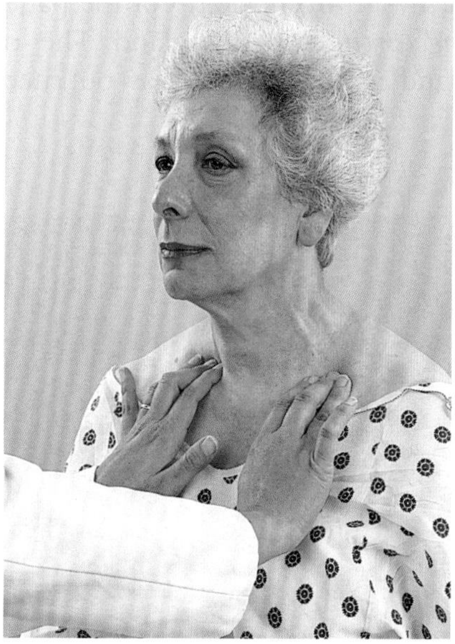
FIGURE 10-9 Palpation of supraclavicular nodes.

Most lymph nodes cannot be palpated. When a node is detected on palpation, note its size, shape, delimitation (discrete or matted together), mobility, consistency, and any tenderness. Small, mobile, discrete, nontender nodes, sometimes termed "shotty," can frequently be found, especially in children.

CLINICAL TIP
Tender nodes suggest inflammation; hard or fixed nodes suggest malignancy.

Enlarged or tender nodes, if unexplained, call for (1) reexamination of the regions they drain and (2) careful assessment of lymph nodes elsewhere so that you can distinguish between regional and generalized **adenopathy/lymphadenopathy** (inflammation or disease of the glands).

Diffuse lymphadenopathy raises suspicion of HIV or AIDS.

Occasionally you may mistake a band of muscle or an artery for a lymph node. You should be able to roll a node in two directions: up and down, and side to side. Neither a muscle nor an artery will pass this test.

The Trachea and the Thyroid Gland

To orient yourself to the neck, identify the thyroid and cricoid cartilages and the trachea below them (Fig. 10-10).

Inspect the trachea for any deviation from its usual midline position. Then *feel for any deviation*. Place your finger along one side of the trachea and note the space between it and the sternocleidomastoid. Compare it with the other side. The spaces should be symmetric.

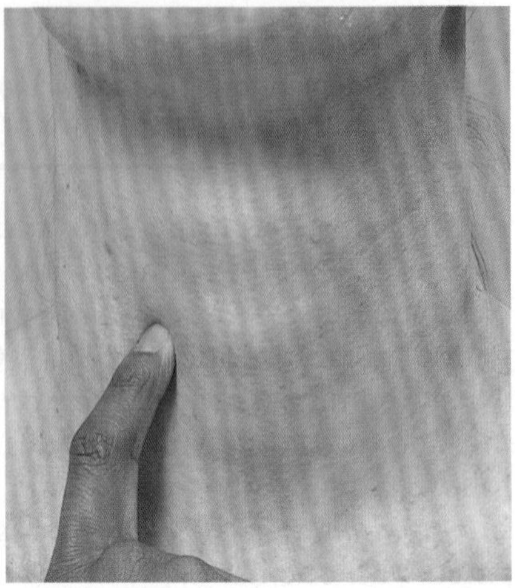

FIGURE 10-10 Identify the thyroid, cricoid cartilages, and the trachea.

CLINICAL TIP
Masses in the neck may push the trachea to one side. Tracheal deviation may also signify important problems in the thorax, such as a mediastinal mass, atelectasis, or a large pneumothorax.

Inspect the neck for the thyroid gland. Tip the patient's head back slightly. Using tangential lighting directed downward from the tip of the patient's chin, *inspect the region below the cricoid cartilage* for the gland. The lower shadowed border of each thyroid gland in Figure 10-11 is outlined by arrows.

Goiter is a general term for an enlarged thyroid gland (Castro & Gharib, 2005; Hegedus, 2004).

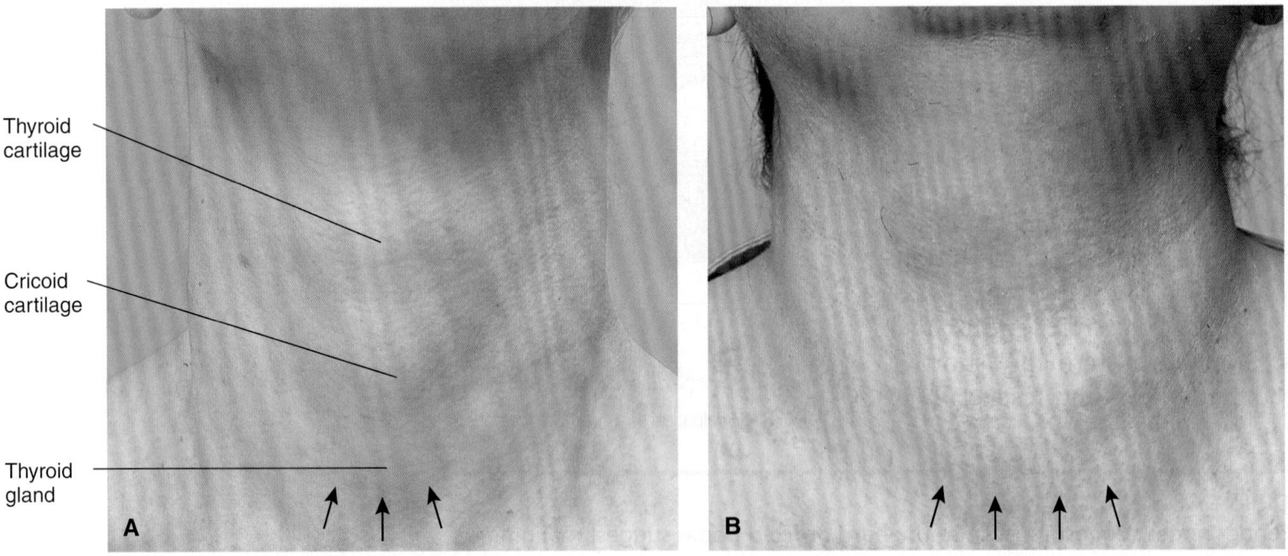

FIGURE 10-11 Use tangential lighting directed downward from the tip of the patient's chin to the lower border of the patient's thyroid. **A.** The normal thyroid at rest. **B.** The enlarged thyroid at rest.

Ask the patient to sip some water and to extend the neck again and swallow. Watch for upward movement of the thyroid gland, noting its contour and symmetry (Fig. 10-12). The thyroid cartilage, the cricoid cartilage,

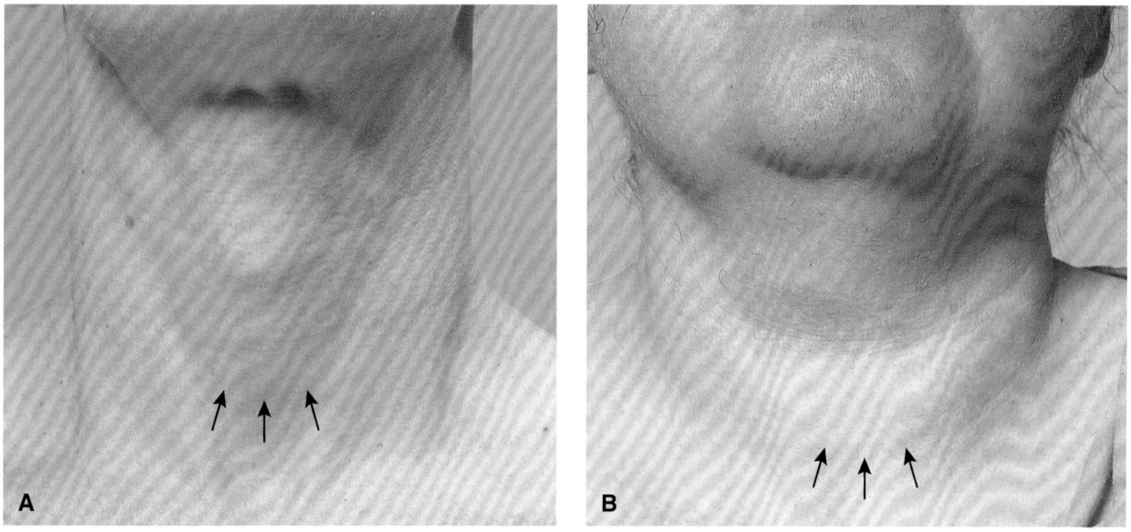

FIGURE 10-12 As the patient swallows, note the contour and symmetry of the thyroid as it moves. Compared to the normal thyroid (**A**), the enlarged thyroid (**B**) looks symmetric upon swallowing.

and the thyroid gland all rise with swallowing and then fall to their resting positions.

Assessment of the thyroid can be done by an anterior or posterior approach (Fig. 10-13). As your skills develop, you will determine which approach is best for you; however, until you become familiar with this examination, check your visual observations with your fingers from in front of the patient and then palpate from the posterior.

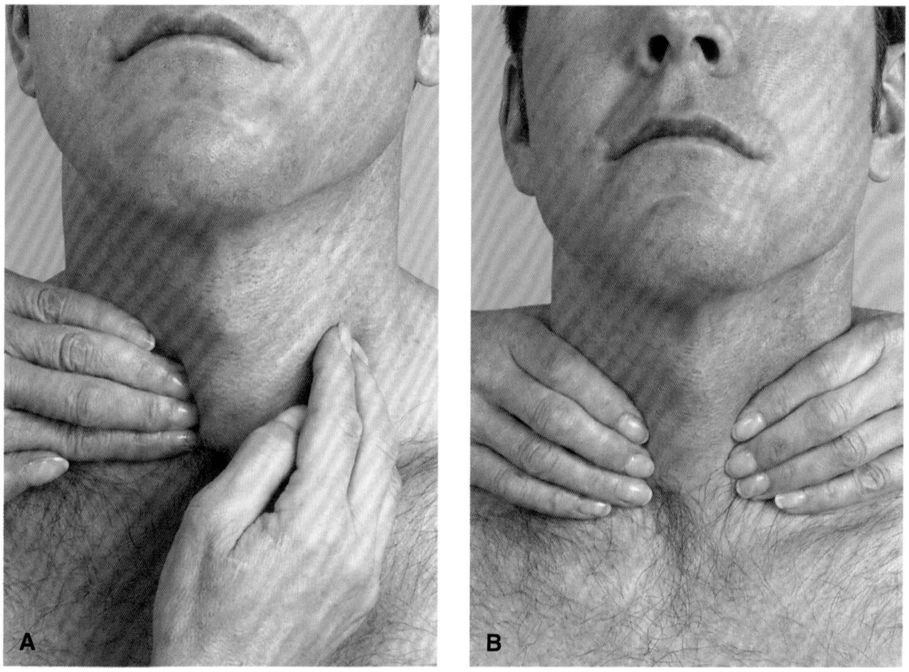

FIGURE 10-13 **A.** Palpating the thyroid with an anterior approach. **B.** Palpating the thyroid with a posterior approach.

Palpating the thyroid gland may seem difficult at first. Use the cues from visual inspection. Find your landmarks—the notched thyroid cartilage and the cricoid cartilage below it. Locate the *thyroid isthmus*, usually overlying the second, third, and fourth tracheal rings.

Adopt good technique, and follow the steps in Box 10-3 for both the anterior and posterior approach. With experience you will become more adept. The thyroid gland is usually easier to feel in a long slender neck than in a short stocky one. In shorter necks, added extension of the neck may help. In some people, however, the thyroid gland is partially or wholly substernal and not amenable to physical examination.

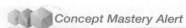

Concept Mastery Alert

Assessing the Thyroid from the Posterior

When assessing the thyroid using the posterior approach, the nurse should ask the patient to flex the neck forward to relax the sternocleidomastoid muscle, making palpation easier. This is the preferred method for both an anterior and posterior assessment of the thyroid.

BOX 10-3 STEPS FOR PALPATING THE THYROID GLAND

- Ask the patient to flex the neck slightly forward to relax the sternocleidomastoid muscles.
- Place the fingers of both hands on the patient's neck so that your index fingers are just below the cricoid cartilage.
- Ask the patient to sip and swallow water as before. Feel for the thyroid isthmus rising up under your finger pads. It is often but not always palpable.
- The lobes are somewhat harder to feel than the isthmus, so practice is needed. The anterior surface of a lateral lobe is approximately the size of the distal phalanx of the thumb and feels somewhat rubbery.
- Note the *size, shape,* and *consistency* of the gland and identify any *nodules* or *tenderness*.
- If the thyroid gland is enlarged, listen over the lateral lobes with a stethoscope to detect a *bruit*, a sound similar to a cardiac murmur but of noncardiac origin.

A localized systolic or continuous bruit may be heard in *hyperthyroidism*.

Although physical characteristics of the thyroid gland, such as size, shape, and consistency, are diagnostically important, assessment of thyroid function depends on symptoms, signs elsewhere in the body, and laboratory tests (Baldwin et al., 2016). Table 10-4 illustrates and outlines thyroid enlargement and function. Table 10-5 outlines symptoms and signs of thyroid dysfunction, and Table 10-6 links different thyroid consistencies with potential causes.

TABLE 10-4 Thyroid Enlargement

Diffuse Enlargement

Includes the isthmus and lateral lobes; there are no discretely palpable nodules. Causes include Graves disease, Hashimoto thyroiditis, and endemic goiter.

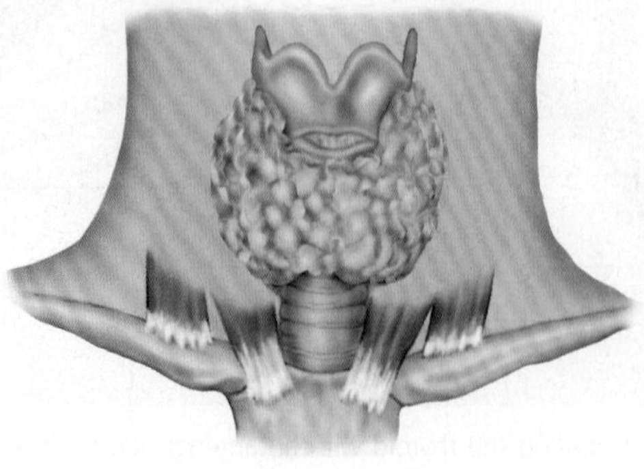

Single Nodule

May be a cyst, a benign tumor, or one nodule within a multinodular gland. It raises the question of malignancy. Risk factors are prior irradiation, hardness, rapid growth, fixation to surrounding tissues, enlarged cervical nodes, and occurrence in males (Syrenicz et al., 2014).

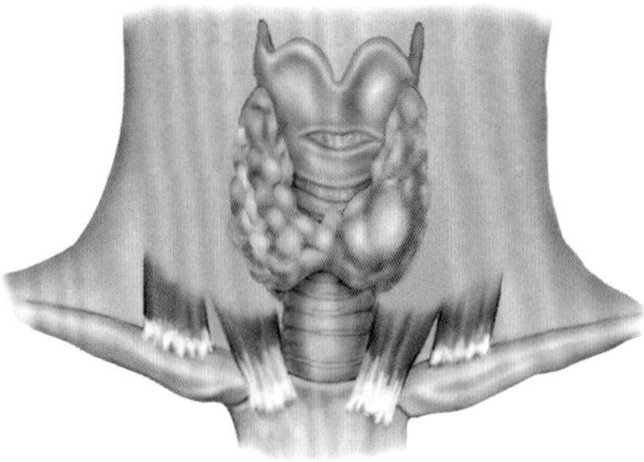

Multinodular Goiter

An enlarged thyroid gland with two or more nodules suggests a metabolic rather than a neoplastic process. Positive family history and continuing nodular enlargement are additional risk factors for malignancy.

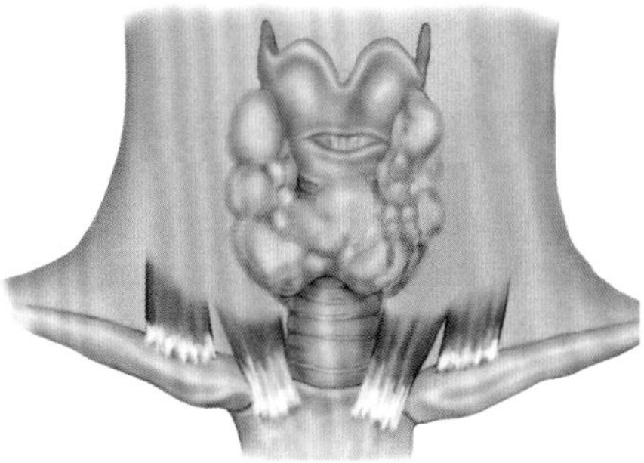

TABLE 10-5 Symptoms and Signs of Thyroid Dysfunction

	Hyperthyroidism	Hypothyroidism
Symptoms	Nervousness	Fatigue, lethargy
	Weight loss despite increased appetite	Modest weight gain with anorexia
	Excessive sweating and heat intolerance	Dry, coarse skin and cold intolerance
	Palpitations	Swelling of face, hands, and legs
	Frequent bowel movements	Constipation
	Muscular weakness of the proximal type and tremor	Weakness, muscle cramps, arthralgias, paresthesias, impaired memory and hearing
Signs	Warm, smooth, moist skin	Dry, coarse, cool skin, sometimes yellowish from carotene, with nonpitting edema and loss of hair
	With Graves disease, eye signs such as stare, lid lag, and exophthalmos	Periorbital puffiness
	Increased systolic and decreased diastolic blood pressures	Decreased systolic and increased diastolic blood pressures
	Tachycardia or atrial fibrillation	Bradycardia and in late stages, hypothermia
	Hyperdynamic cardiac pulsations with an accentuated S_1	Intensity of heart sounds sometimes decreased
	Tremor and proximal muscle weakness	Impaired memory, mixed hearing loss, somnolence, peripheral neuropathy, carpal tunnel syndrome

Source: Syrenicz, A., Koziołek, M., Ciechanowicz, K., Sieradzka, A., Bi czak-Kuleta, A., & Parczewski, M. (2014). New insights into the diagnosis of nodular goiter. *Thyroid Research*, *7*, 6.

TABLE 10-6 Thyroid Consistencies and Associated Conditions

Consistency	Associated Condition
Soft	Graves disease
Firm	Hashimoto thyroiditis Nodules (benign and malignant)
Tender	Thyroiditis

The Carotid Arteries and Jugular Veins

Defer a detailed examination of these vessels until the patient lies down for the cardiovascular examination. Jugular venous distention may be visible in the sitting position, however, and should not be overlooked. You should also be alert to unusually prominent arterial pulsations. See Chapter 14, "The Cardiovascular System" for further discussion.

RECORDING YOUR FINDINGS

Box 10-4 contains examples of documentation of head and neck findings.

BOX 10-4 RECORDING THE PHYSICAL EXAMINATION OF THE HEAD AND NECK—EXAMPLES

Head—The skull is normocephalic/atraumatic (NC/AT). Hair straight, brown, and soft.
Neck—Trachea midline. Neck supple; thyroid isthmus palpable, lobes nonpalpable.
Lymph nodes—No head or neck adenopathy/lymphadenopathy.

OR

Head—The skull is normocephalic/atraumatic. Frontal balding; thin, brown hair.
Neck—Trachea midline. Neck supple; thyroid isthmus midline, lobes palpable but not enlarged.
Lymph nodes—R submandibular and R occipital lymph palpated, 1 × 1 cm, rubbery, nontender, and mobile.

HEALTH PROMOTION AND COUNSELING—PREVENTION OF TRAUMATIC BRAIN INJURY

The Centers for Disease Control and Prevention establishes falls as the leading cause of TBIs in the United States (Centers for Disease Control & Prevention, 2019). TBIs that require hospitalizations vary by age groups; children from birth to 17 years old and adults over the age of 55 incurred TBIs from falls most often while teens and adults between the ages of 15 and 44 were hospitalized more often for TBIs related to motor vehicle accidents (Centers for Disease Control & Prevention, 2019; Syrenicz et al., 2014).

CLINICAL TIP

TBI is a leading cause of death and disability in infants and children. Infants and young children have a malleable, thin skull with sutures that have not fused and a comparatively large head with weak neck muscles, increasing the risk of injury (Centers for Disease Control & Prevention, 2019).

The leading causes of TBI are falls, being hit or struck by an object, and motor vehicle accidents. Teaching patients about prevention of head injuries is paramount.

To decrease the likelihood of falls, suggest the following:

- Install safety features in the home such as grab bars in the bathroom and nonslip mats in the bathtub.
- Avoid the use of throw rugs.
- Remove extension cords from high-traffic areas.
- Use rails on stairs.
- Wear nonslip, well-fitting shoes.
- Install gates on stairs.
- Install window guards.
- Do not use walkers for babies.
- Review medication lists with the health care provider to assess for side effects such as fainting or dizziness, which could lead to falls.

To prevent head injuries in motor vehicle accidents, recommend the following:

- Always use seat belts.
- Ensure children are using car seats or booster seats appropriate for their size and weight.
- Small children should sit in the back seat, especially if the car has a passenger-side airbag.
- Never drive under the influence of alcohol or drugs, including over-the-counter medications that cause drowsiness.
- Use hands-free phones and never text when driving.
- Wear a helmet when riding motorcycles, all-terrain vehicles, motorized scooters, bicycles, horses, or snowmobiles.

CLINICAL TIP
People who experienced a TBI previously are at risk of another and those who do have additional TBIs often take longer to recover from the injury (Chu et al., 2018).

To avoid injuries from being hit by an object, recommend the following:

- Wear helmets when participating in risky activities, such as skiing, snowboarding, skating, batting, and contact sports.
- Place heavy objects on shelves at eye level or lower.
- Avoid dangerous situations or fights.
- Ensure guns and ammunition are locked in separate areas.

Safety and prevention are ongoing, and every possible situation is not addressed here. This is an awareness issue that each individual needs to account for in their own surroundings. Community health nurses can be instrumental with home assessments. They can assist individuals, families, and communities in identifying potential risks and remediations. Box 10-5 lists resources for further TBI prevention teaching.

BOX 10-5 RESOURCES FOR HEADACHE DISORDERS AND PREVENTION OF TRAUMATIC BRAIN INJURIES

Lifting the Burden: The Global Campaign to Reduce the Burden of Headache—who.int/mental_health/neurology/headache/en/

HEADS UP: Education initiative of the CDC to protect children and teens from concussions and other brain injuries—http://www.cdc.gov/headsup/about/index.html

Safe Kids Worldwide: A global organization aimed at keeping kids safe—http://www.safekids.org

Think First: National Injury Prevention Organization—http://www.thinkfirst.org

Brain Injury Association of America—http://www.biausa.org

BIBLIOGRAPHY

CITATIONS

Baldwin, G., Breiding, M., & Sleet, D. (2016). Using the public health model to address unintentional injuries and TBI: A perspective from the Centers for Disease Control and Prevention (CDC). *Neurorehabilitation, 39*(3), 345–349. https://doi.org/10.3233/NRE-161366

Buse, D. C., Greisman, J. D., Baigi, K., & Lipton, R. B. (2019). Migraine progression: a systematic review. *Headache, 59*(3), 306–338. https://doi.org/10.1111/head.13459

Castro, M. R., & Gharib, H. (2005). Controversies in the management of thyroid nodules. *Annals of Internal Medicine, 142*(11), 926–931.

Centers for Disease Control and Prevention. (2019). Surveillance report of traumatic brain Injury-related emergency department visits, hospitalizations, and deaths—United States, 2014. Centers for Disease Control and Prevention, U.S. Department of Health and Human Services.

Chu, H. T., Liang, C. S., Lee, J. T., Yeh, T. C., Lee, M. S., Sung, Y. F, & Yang, F. C. (2018). Associations between depression/anxiety and headache frequency in Migraineurs: a cross-sectional study. *Headache, 58*(3), 407–415. https://doi.org/10.1111/head.13215

Collaborators GBDH. (2018). Global, regional, and national burden of migraine and tension-type headache, 1990–2016: a systematic analysis for the global burden of disease study 2016. *Lancet Neurology*, *17*(11), 954–976. https://doi.org/10.1016/S1474-4422(18)30322-3

Coronado, V. G., Thomas, K. E., Sattin, R. W., Johnson, R. L. (2005). The CDC traumatic brain injury surveillance system: Characteristics of persons aged 65 years and older hospitalized with a TBI. *Journal of Head Trauma Rehabilitation*, *20*(3), 215–228. https://doi.org/10.1097/00001199-200505000-00005

D'Amico, D., Sansone, E., Grazzi, L., Giovannetti, A. M., Leonardi, M., Schiavolin, S., & Raggi, A. (2018). Multimorbidity in patients with chronic migraine and medication overuse headache. *Acta Neurologica Scandinavica*, *138*(6), 515–522. https://doi.org/10.1111/ane.13014

Hegedus, L. (2004). The thyroid nodule. *New England Journal of Medicine*, *351*(17), 1764–1771.

Huh, K. R., Kim, J. Y., Choi, S. H., Yoon, Y. H., Park, S. J., & Lee, E. S. (2020). Comparison of traumatic brain injury patients with brain computed tomography in the emergency department by age group. *Clinical and Experimental Emergency Medicine*, *7*(2), 81–86. https://doi.org/10.15441/ceem.19.076

International Headache Society. (2018). The international classification of headache disorders. *Cephalalgia*, *38*, 1–211.

Khokhar, B., Simoni-Wastila, L., Slejko, J. F., Perfetto, E., Zhan, M., & Smith, G. S. (2017). In-hospital mortality following traumatic brain injury among older medicare beneficiaries, comparing statin users with nonusers. *Journal of Pharmacy Technology*, *33*(6), 225–236. https://doi.org/10.1177/8755122517735656

Kumar, R. G., Ketchum, J. M., Corrigan, J. D., Hammond, F. M., Sevigny, M., & Dams-O'Connor, K. (2020). The longitudinal effects of comorbid health burden on functional outcomes for adults with moderate to severe traumatic brain injury. *Journal of Head Trauma Rehabilitation*, *35*(4), E372–E381. https://doi.org/10.1097/HTR.0000000000000572

McCrory, P., Feddermann-Demont, N., Dvořák, J., Cassidy, J. D., McIntosh, A., Vos, P. E., Echemendia, R. J., Meeuwisse, W., & Tarnutzer, A. A. (2017). What is the definition of sports-related concussion: a systematic review. *British Journal of Sports Medicine*, *51*(11), 877–887. https://doi.org/10.1136/bjsports-2016-097393

Smith, J. H. (2018). Ruling out secondary headache. Practical neurology. A careful history and high degree of suspicion are needed for accurate diagnosis. https://practicalneurology.com/articles/2018-mar-apr/ruling-out-secondary-headache

Syrenicz, A., Koziołek, M., Ciechanowicz, K., Sieradzka, A., Bi czak-Kuleta, A., & Parczewski, M. (2014). New insights into the diagnosis of nodular goiter. *Thyroid Research*, *7*, 6.

Taylor, C. A., Bell, J. M., Breiding, M. J., & Xu, L. (2017). Traumatic brain injury-related emergency department visits, hospitalizations, and deaths—United States, 2007 and 2013. *Mmwr Surveillance Summaries*, *66*(9), 1–16. https://doi.org/10.15585/mmwr.ss6609a1

Winkler, E. A., Yue, J. K., Burke, J. F., Chan, A. K., Dhall, S. S., Berger, M. S., Manley, G. T., & Tarapore, P. E. (2016). Adult sports-related traumatic brain injury in United States trauma centers. *Neurosurgical Focus*, *40*(4), E4. https://doi.org/10.3171/2016.1.FOCUS15613

World Health Organization. (2011). Atlas of headache disorders and resources in the world 2011. Retrieved August 29, 2020, from https://www.who.int/mental_health/management/atlas_headache_disorders/en/

World Health Organization. (2016). Headache disorders. Retrieved March 14, 2021, from https://www.who.int/news-room/fact-sheets/detail/headache-disorders

11 THE EYES

KEY TERMS		
accommodation	convergence	papilledema
amblyopia	direct reaction	photoreceptors
anisocoria	dysconjugate	strabismus
canthus	nystagmus	visual acuity
confrontation	ophthalmoscope	visual field
consensual reaction	palpebral fissure	vitreous humor

Learning Objectives

The student will:

1. Identify the eye's components and their functions.
2. Collect a health history of the eye.
3. Describe the physical examination techniques performed to evaluate the eye and perform a complete eye examination.
4. Demonstrate how to use the ophthalmoscope.
5. Document a complete eye assessment using information from the health history and physical examination.
6. Identify the measures for prevention or early detection of eye disease, infections, or vision loss.

ANATOMY AND PHYSIOLOGY

The eye is the sensory organ of vision and has many critical components, including several cranial nerves. During the assessment, various signs and symptoms signal changes in the eyes. The nurse's role is to detect these changes and work with the health care team to prevent injury or loss of vision.

Eye Structures

The structures of the eye are identified in Figure 11-1. Note that the upper eyelid covers a portion of the iris but does not touch the pupil. The opening

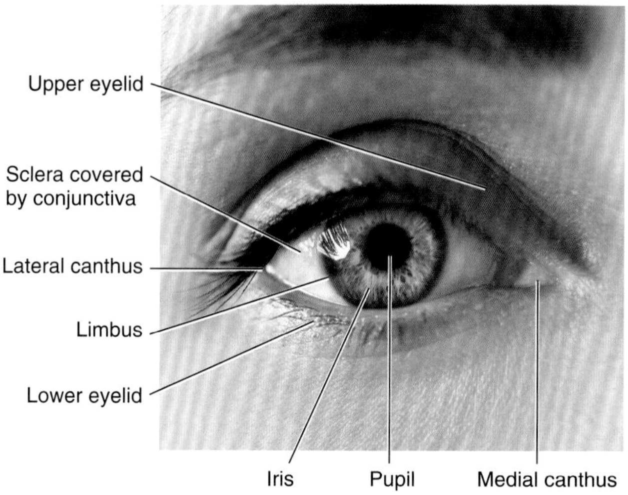

FIGURE 11-1 Structures of the eye (Pixel-Shot/Shutterstock).

between the eyelids is called the **palpebral fissure**. The white sclera may look somewhat darker at its periphery. The *conjunctiva* is a clear mucous membrane with two easily visible components. The *bulbar conjunctiva*, also known as the *sclera*, covers most of the anterior eyeball, adhering loosely to the underlying tissue. The *palpebral conjunctiva* lines the eyelids. The two parts of the conjunctiva merge in a folded recess that permits movement of the eyeball.

"Palpebral" means relating to the eyelids.

Within the eyelids lie firm strips of connective tissue called *tarsal plates.* Each plate contains a parallel row of *meibomian glands*, which open on the lid margin. The *levator palpebrae*, the muscle that raises the upper eyelid, is innervated by the oculomotor nerve, cranial nerve (CN) III. Smooth muscle, innervated by the sympathetic nervous system, also contributes to lid elevation. Figure 11-2 illustrates these structures.

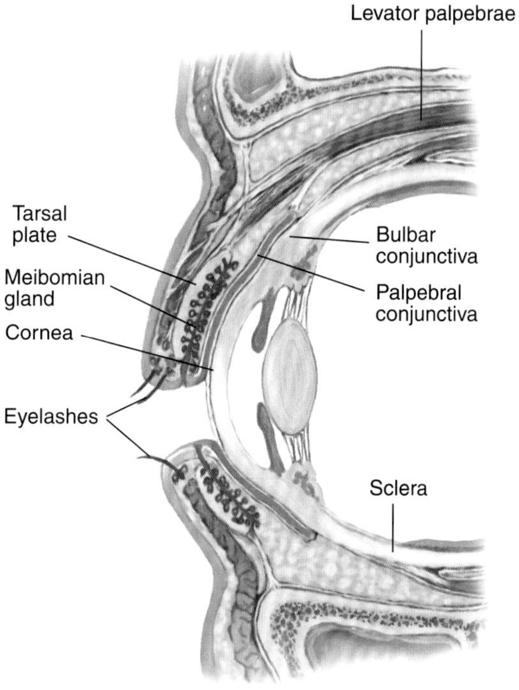

FIGURE 11-2 Sagittal section of the anterior eye with the lids closed.

A film of tear fluid protects the conjunctiva and cornea from drying, inhibits microbial growth, and gives a smooth optical surface to the cornea. This fluid comes from the meibomian glands, conjunctival glands, and lacrimal gland. The *lacrimal gland* lies mostly within the bony orbit, above and lateral to the eyeball (Fig. 11-3).

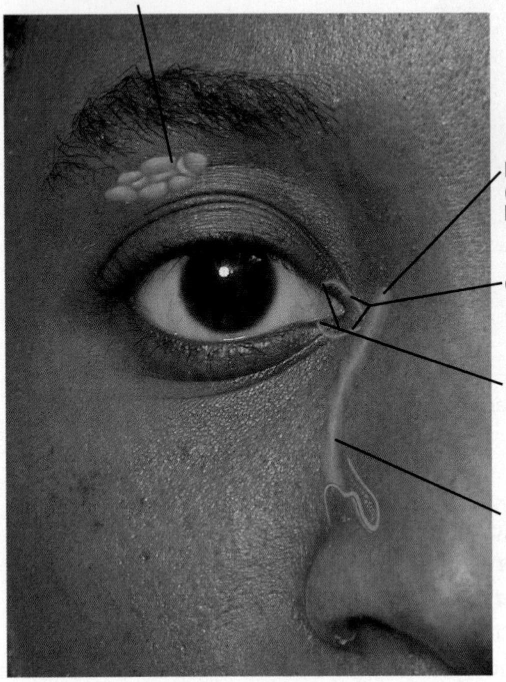

FIGURE 11-3 The lacrimal gland and duct.

The tear fluid spreads across the eye and drains medially through two tiny holes called *lacrimal puncta*. The tears then pass into the *lacrimal sac* and into the nose through the *nasolacrimal duct*. You can easily find a *punctum* atop the small elevation of the lower lid medially. The lacrimal sac rests in a small depression inside the bony orbit and is not visible.

The eyeball is a spherical structure that focuses light on the neurosensory elements within the retina. The muscles of the iris control pupillary size, constricting in bright light and dilating in the dark. Muscles of the *ciliary body* control the thickness of the lens, allowing the eye to focus on near or distant objects.

Vitreous humor is the clear gel that fills the space between the lens and the retina. The aqueous humor is a clear liquid that fills the anterior and posterior chambers of the eye, circulating between the cornea and the lens (Fig. 11-4). Aqueous humor is produced by the *ciliary body*, circulates

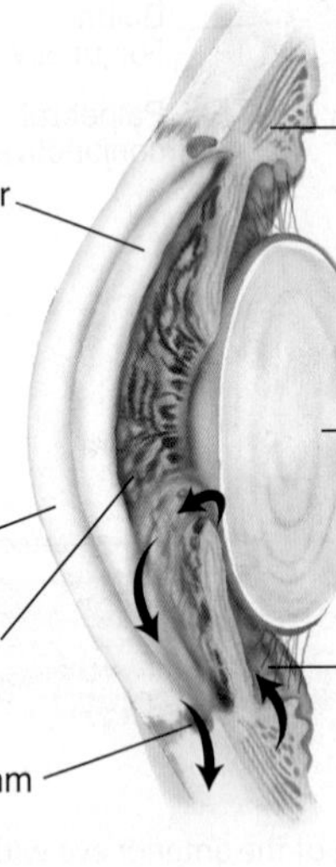

FIGURE 11-4 Circulation of the aqueous humor.

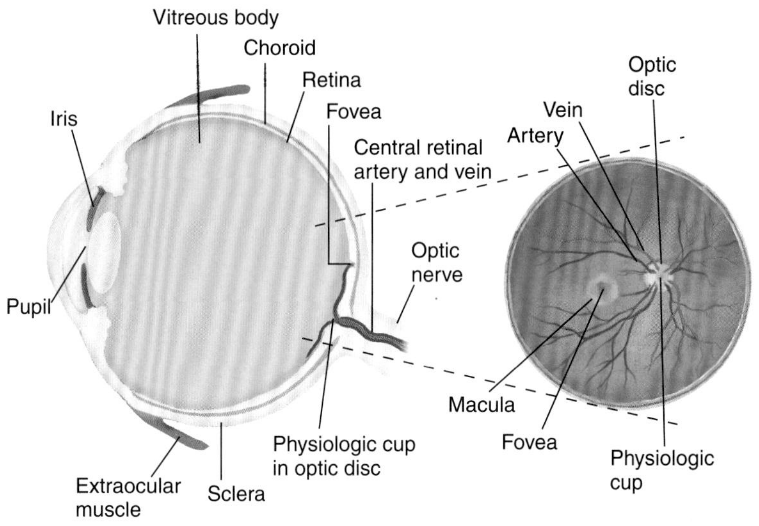

FIGURE 11-5 Cross-section of the right eye showing a portion of the fundus commonly seen with the ophthalmoscope.

from the posterior chamber through the pupil into the anterior chamber, and drains out through the *canal of Schlemm*. This circulatory system helps to control the pressure inside the eye.

The posterior part of the eye seen through an ophthalmoscope is often called the *fundus* of the eye. Structures here include the retina, choroid, fovea, macula, optic disc, and retinal vessels (Fig. 11-5). The entire fundus is not visible at once and as the ophthalmoscope is adjusted, sections of the eye appear. The optic nerve with its retinal vessels enters the eyeball posteriorly. You can find it with an ophthalmoscope at the *optic disc*. When looking into the eye with the ophthalmoscope, it is best to locate the optic disc medially and use this as your landmark. Note the margins of the disc and then locate the arteries and veins. Lateral and slightly inferior to the disc, there is a small depression in the retinal surface that marks the point of central vision. Around it is a darkened circular area called the *fovea*. The roughly circular *macula* (named for a microscopic yellow spot) surrounds the fovea but has no discernible margins. It is unusual to see the normal *vitreous body*, a transparent mass of gelatinous material that fills the eyeball behind the lens. The vitreous body helps maintain the shape of the eye.

Visual Fields

A **visual field** is the entire area seen by an eye when it looks at a central point. Fields are typically diagrammed on circles from the patient's point of view. The center of the circle represents the focus of gaze. The circumference is 90 degrees from the line of the gaze. Each visual field, shown by the white areas in Figure 11-6, is divided into quadrants. Note the fields extend farthest on the temporal sides. Visual fields are normally limited by the brows above, the cheeks below, and the nose medially. A lack of retinal receptors at the optic disc produces an oval blind spot in the normal field of each eye, 15 degrees temporal to the line of gaze.

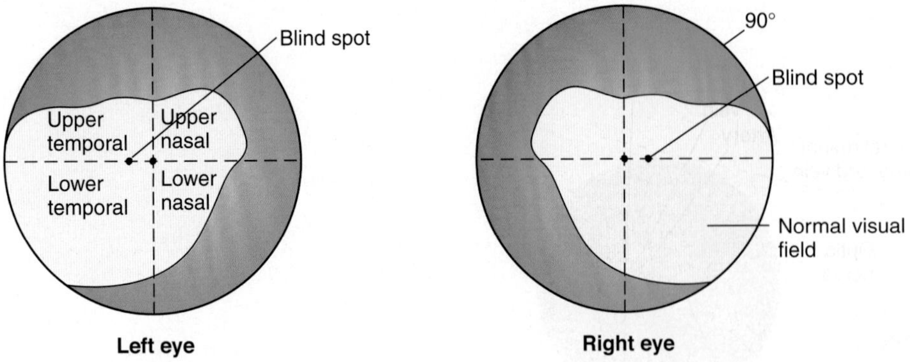

FIGURE 11-6 Visual fields.

When a person is using both eyes, the two visual fields overlap in an area of binocular vision. Laterally, vision is monocular (Fig. 11-7).

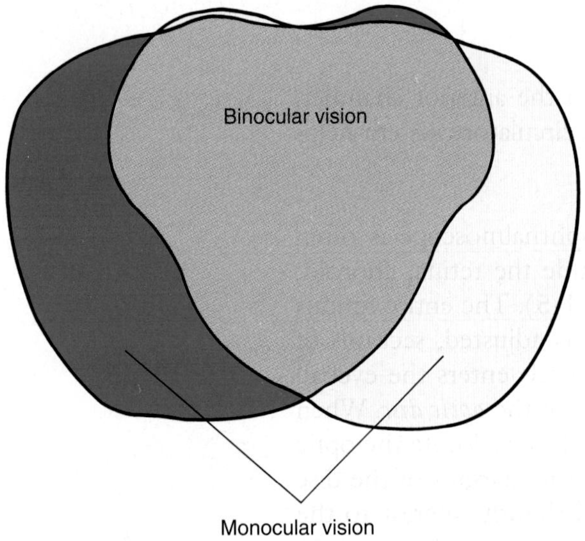

FIGURE 11-7 Monocular and binocular vision.

Visual Pathways

To see an image, light reflected from the image must pass through the pupil and be focused on **photoreceptors** in the retina. The image projected there is upside down and reversed right to left (Fig. 11-8). An image from the upper nasal visual field thus strikes the lower temporal quadrant of the retina.

Nerve impulses, stimulated by light, are conducted through the retina, optic nerve (CN II), and optic tract on each side, then on through a curving tract called the *optic radiation*. This ends in the visual cortex, a part of the occipital lobe.

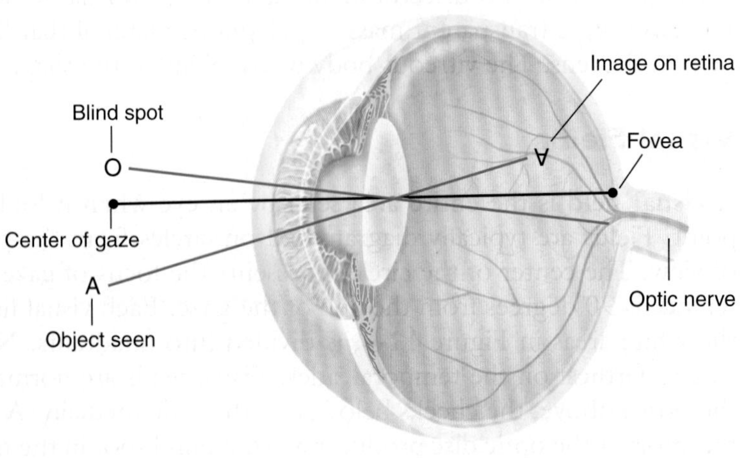

FIGURE 11-8 Visual pathways.

Pupillary Reactions

Pupillary size changes in response to light and to the effort of focusing on a near object.

The Light Reaction

A light beam shining onto one retina causes pupillary constriction both in that eye, termed the *direct reaction* to light, and in the contralateral (opposite) eye, the *consensual reaction* to light (Fig. 11-9). The initial sensory pathways are similar to those described for vision: retina, optic nerve (CN II), and optic tract which diverges in the midbrain. Impulses back to the constrictor muscles are transmitted through the oculomotor nerve, CN III, to the constrictor muscles of the iris of each eye and then transmitted through the oculomotor nerve, CN III.

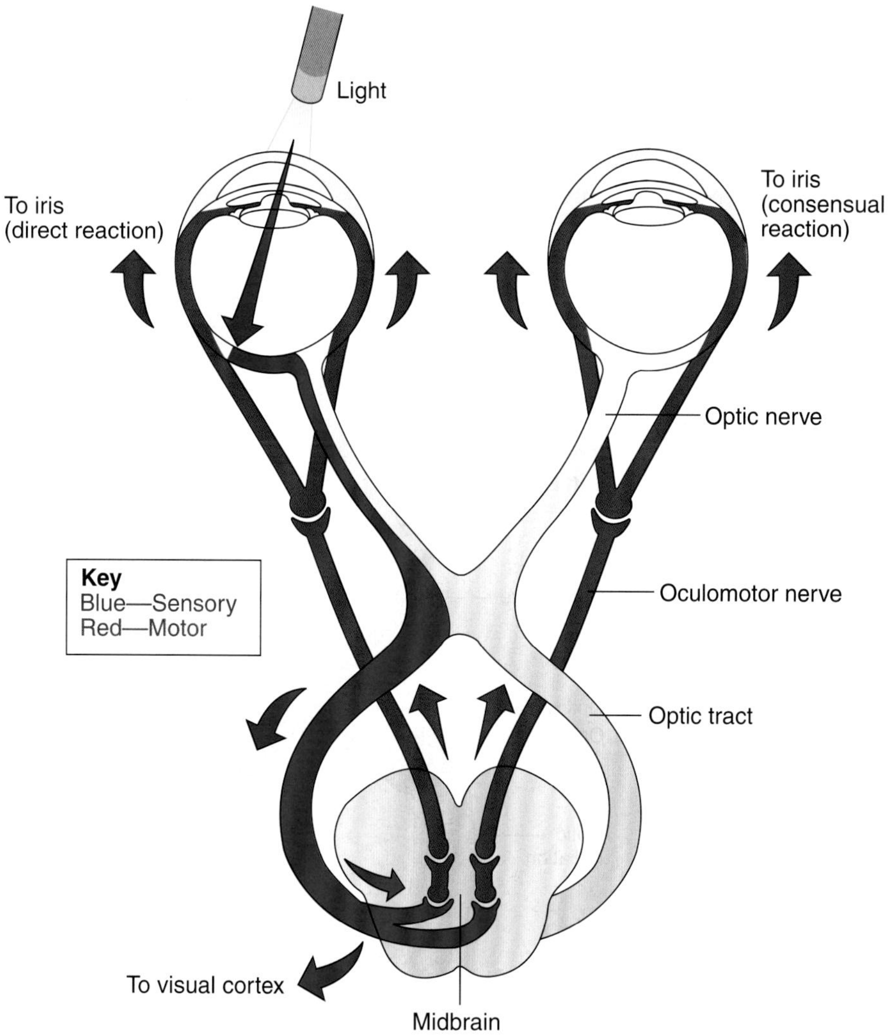

FIGURE 11-9 Pathways of the light reaction.

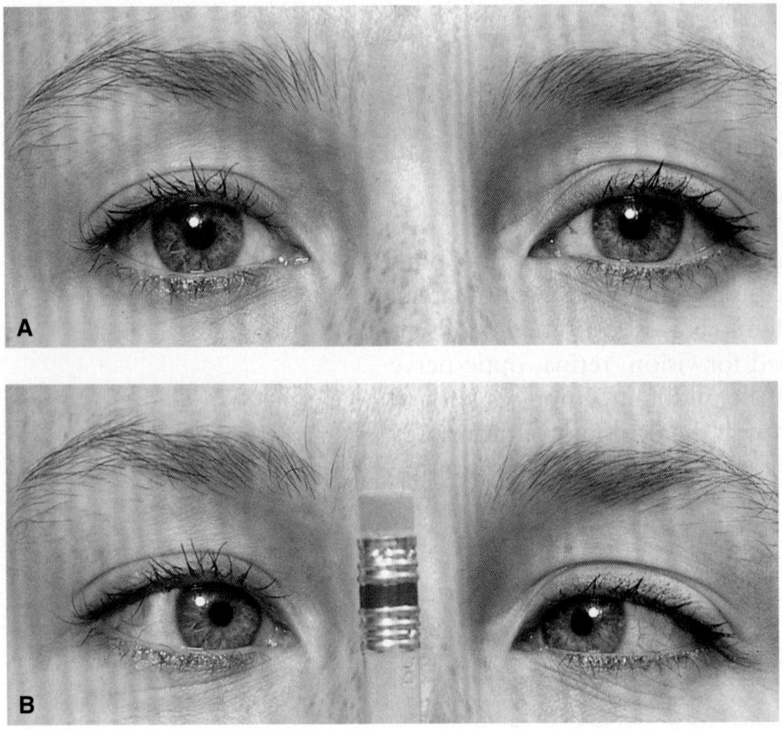

FIGURE 11-10 **A.** Eyes looking straight ahead. **B.** Near reaction with pupil constriction.

The Near Reaction

The near reaction occurs when a person shifts their gaze from a far object to a near one and the pupils constrict (Fig. 11-10). This response, like the light reaction, is mediated by the oculomotor nerve (CN III). At the same time as the *pupillary constriction*, but not a part of it are (1) **convergence** of the eyes, a medial rectus movement; and (2) **accommodation**, an increased convexity of the lenses caused by contraction of the ciliary muscles. In accommodation, the change in shape of the lenses brings near objects into focus, but this is not visible to the examiner.

Autonomic Nerve Supply to the Eyes

Fibers traveling in the oculomotor nerve (CN III) and producing pupillary constriction are part of the parasympathetic nervous system. The iris is also supplied by sympathetic fibers. When these are stimulated, the pupil dilates, and the upper eyelid rises a little, as if from fear. The sympathetic pathway starts in the hypothalamus and passes down through the brainstem and cervical cord into the neck (Fig. 11-11). From there, it follows the carotid artery or its branches into the orbit. A lesion anywhere along this pathway may impair sympathetic effects that dilate the pupil.

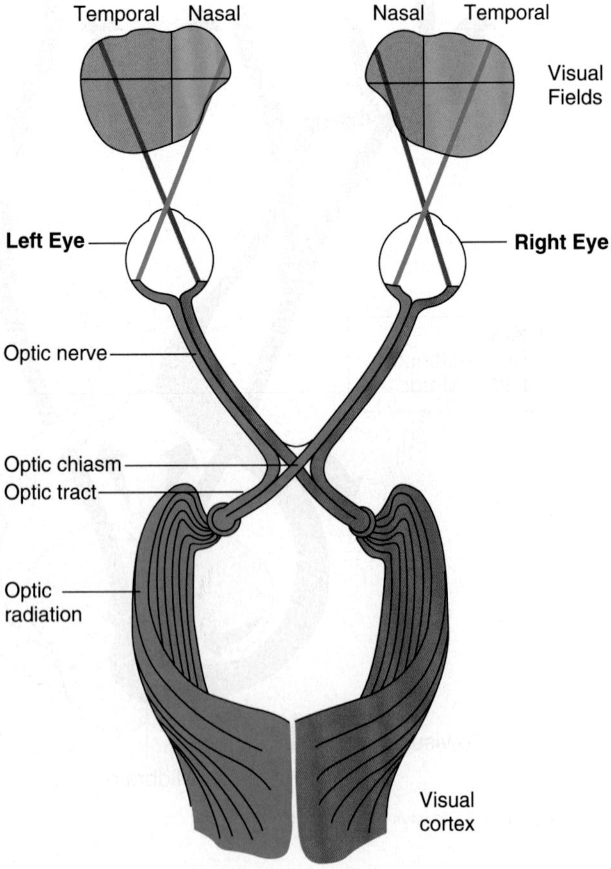

FIGURE 11-11 Visual pathways from the retina to the visual cortex (view from above).

Extraocular Movements

The coordinated action of six muscles, the four rectus (superior, lateral, medial, and inferior) and two oblique (inferior and superior), control the eye. To test the function of each muscle and the nerve that supplies it, ask the patient to move the eye in the direction controlled by that muscle. There are six *cardinal directions*, indicated by the lines in Figure 11-12. When a person looks down and to the right, for example, the right inferior rectus (CN III) is principally responsible for moving the right eye, while the left superior oblique (CN IV) is principally responsible for moving the left. If one of these muscles is paralyzed, the eye will deviate from its normal position in that direction of gaze, and the eyes will no longer appear conjugate, or parallel.

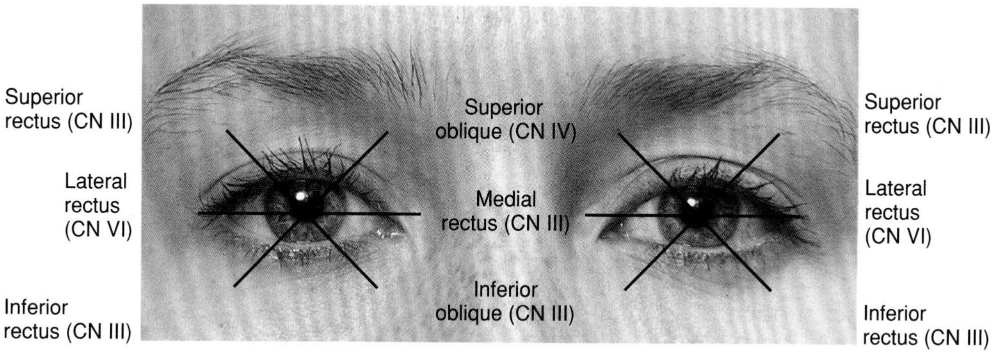

FIGURE 11-12 Six cardinal directions of the gaze.

THE HEALTH HISTORY

Common or concerning symptoms to guide questions while taking a health history of the eyes are listed in Box 11-1.

BOX 11-1 COMMON OR CONCERNING SYMPTOMS

- Changes in vision:
  - Hyperopia
  - Presbyopia
  - Myopia
  - Scotomas
- Double vision or diplopia
- Strabismus
- Blurring
- Redness
- Itching
- Discharge
- Pain
- Tearing
- Edema
- Lesions
- Visual disturbances
- Photophobia
- Use of corrective lenses (i.e., glasses, contact lenses)
- Prosthesis

A scotoma is an area of lost or depressed vision within the visual field and is surrounded by an area of normal vision.

Photophobia or light sensitivity is usually from excess light entering the eye, which may overexcite the photoreceptors in the retina.

The purpose of the health history is to identify changes in the eyes. The nurse should begin the inquiry about the eyes with a broad, open-ended question such as "Have you noticed any changes with your eyes?" The patient may have developed symptoms gradually and learned to live with changes. Older patients may assume vision changes are a part of aging. They may not realize that they could be seeing better and may not answer the questions in the health history relative to the objective assessment revelations. Further investigation is crucial, and more in-depth questioning should be pursued. A more in-depth question might be "Is your vision as good now as previously?"

If changes in vision are revealed, then follow-up with questions:

- Do you experience *difficulty* when looking at something up close or at a distance?

CLINICAL TIP
Difficulty with seeing close objects suggests *hyperopia* (farsightedness) or *presbyopia* (aging vision). Difficulty seeing far objects indicates *myopia* (nearsightedness).

- Is your vision *blurred*? If yes, is the onset sudden or gradual? If sudden and unilateral, is the visual loss painless or painful? Is the entire field of vision blurred or only parts of it?

CLINICAL TIP
If sudden visual loss is *unilateral* and *painless,* consider vitreous hemorrhage from diabetes or trauma, macular degeneration, retinal detachment, retinal vein occlusion, or central retinal artery occlusion.

If vision loss is *painful*, consider causes in the cornea and anterior chamber such as corneal ulcer, uveitis, traumatic hyphema, and acute-angle closure glaucoma (Petsas et al., 2017; Pohl & Tarnutzer, 2018). Optic neuritis from multiple sclerosis may also be painful (Preziosa et al., 2016). Immediate referral may be warranted.

If *bilateral* and *painless*, medications that change refraction such as cholinergics, anticholinergics, and steroids may be contributors. If bilateral and painful, consider chemical or radiation exposures. If the onset of bilateral visual loss is gradual, this usually arises from cataracts or *macular degeneration* (Mandai et al., 2017).

- If the visual field defect is partial, is it central, peripheral, or only on one side?

CLINICAL TIP
Slow central loss may indicate *nuclear cataract* or *macular degeneration* (Mandai et al., 2017). Peripheral loss may indicate advanced *open-angle glaucoma*. One-sided loss may indicate *hemianopsia* or *quadrantic defects.*

- Do lights *flash* across the field of vision?

CLINICAL TIP
Flashing lights with new vitreous floaters suggest detachment of vitreous from the retina. Prompt eye consultation is indicated (Chang, 2017).

- Do *floaters* accompany flashing?
- Does it feel like a curtain is falling?
- Are there *specks* in the vision or areas where you are unable to see scotomas? If so, do they move in the visual field with shifts of your gaze or are they fixed?

Moving specks or strands suggest vitreous floaters; fixed defects suggest lesions in the retina or visual pathways.

- Do you have double vision (*diplopia*)? Are the images side by side (horizontal diplopia) or on top of each other (vertical diplopia)? Does this persist with one eye closed? Which eye is affected?

CLINICAL TIP
One kind of horizontal diplopia is physiologic. Hold one finger upright approximately 6 inches in front of your face, and another finger at arm's length. When you focus on either finger, the image of the other is double. A patient who notices this phenomenon can be reassured. Diplopia in adults may arise from a lesion in the brainstem or cerebellum or from weakness or paralysis of one or more extraocular muscles, as in horizontal diplopia from palsy of cranial nerve (CN) III or VI, or vertical diplopia from palsy of CN III or IV. Diplopia in one eye, with the other closed, suggests a problem in the cornea or lens.

- Do you experience:
  - Excessive tearing?
  - Discharge?
  - Crusting?
  - Redness? (Table 11-1)

CLINICAL TIP
Red, painless eyes are seen with allergies or subconjunctival hemorrhage. A red eye with a gritty sensation is common with viral conjunctivitis. Red, painful eyes are seen with hyphema, episcleritis, acute-angle closure glaucoma, herpes keratitis, presence of a foreign body, fungal keratitis, and sarcoid uveitis (Narayana & McGee, 2015).

- Do you have or have you ever had lesions or growths on your eyelids or eyes?
- Are your eyes painful or uncomfortable when you are in the sun or well-lit places (*photophobia*)?

TABLE 11-1 Red Eyes

	Pattern of Redness	Pain	Vision	Ocular Discharge	Pupil	Cornea	Significance	Illustration
Conjunctivitis	Conjunctival injection: diffuse dilatation of conjunctival vessels with redness that tends to be maximal peripherally	Mild discomfort rather than pain	Not affected except for temporary mild blurring due to discharge	Watery, mucoid, or mucopurulent	Not affected	Clear	Bacterial, viral, and other infections; allergy; irritation	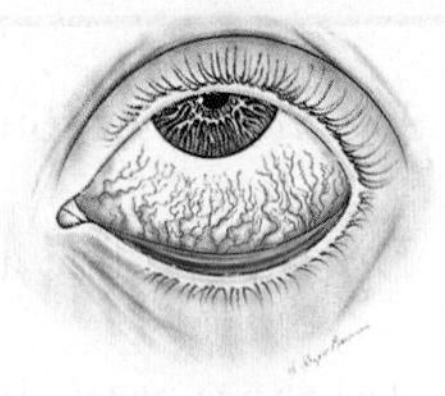
Subconjunctival Hemorrhage	Leakage of blood outside of the vessels, producing a homogeneous, sharply demarcated, red area that fades over days to yellow and then disappears	Absent	Not affected	Absent	Not affected	Clear	Often none; may result from trauma, bleeding disorders, or a sudden increase in venous pressure as from cough	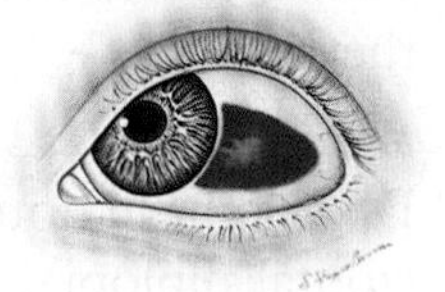
Corneal Injury or Infection	Ciliary injection: dilation of deeper vessels that are visible as radiating vessels or a reddish violet flush around the limbus. Ciliary injection is an important sign of these three conditions but may not be apparent. The eye may be diffusely red instead. Other clues of these more serious disorders are pain, decreased vision, unequal pupils, and a less than perfectly clear cornea.	Moderate to severe, superficial	Usually decreased	Watery or purulent	Not affected unless iritis develops	Changes depending on cause	Abrasions and other injuries; viral and bacterial infections	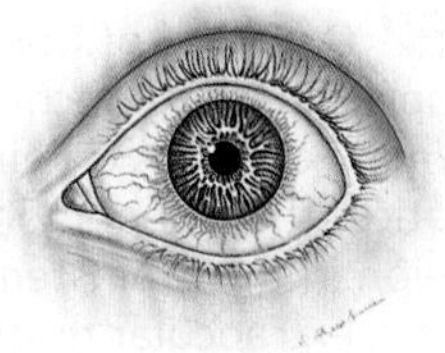
Acute Iritis	Inflammation of the iris	Moderate, aching, deep	Decreased	Absent	May be small and, with time, irregular	Clear or slightly clouded	Associated with many ocular and systemic disorders	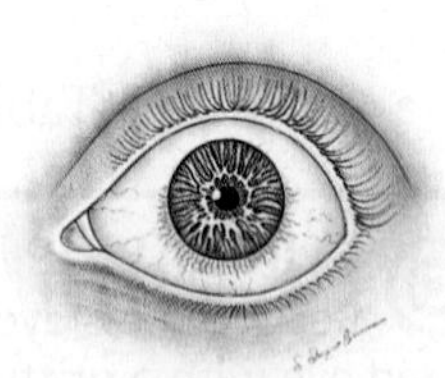
Glaucoma	Dilated vessels especially at the edge of the cornea	Severe, aching, deep	Decreased	Absent	Dilated, fixed	Steamy, cloudy	Acute increase in intraocular pressure—an emergency	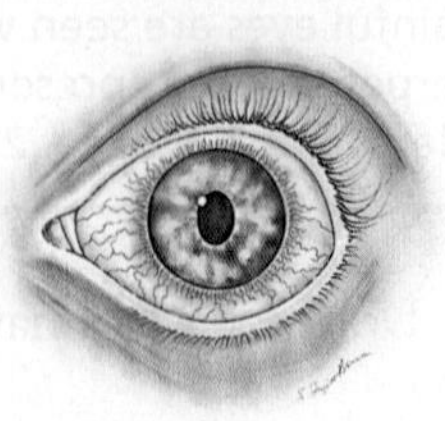

Source: Doshi, R., & Noohani, T. (2020). Subconjunctival hemorrhage. In: *StatPearls*. StatPearls Publishing; Ryder, E. C., & Benson, S. (2020). Conjunctivitis. In: *StatPearls*. StatPearls Publishing.

Eye History

To take a specific history of the eyes, ask:

- Do you have any past history of eye problems or eye disease?
- Do you have a history of:
    - Premature birth?
    - Trauma or injury to the eye?
    - Eye surgery? Was it related to injury, congenital causes, or cosmetic reasons?
    - Eye infections?
    - Strabismus?
    - Amblyopia?
    - Cataracts?
    - Glaucoma?
    - Diabetes?
    - Retinal detachment?
    - Macular degeneration?
    - Blindness?
- When was your last eye examination?
- Have you been tested for color blindness?
- Do you wear glasses or contact lenses?
    - If contact lenses, do you use hard or soft lenses?
    - When did you begin to wear them?
    - Are they corrective or cosmetic?
    - How do you care for your contacts?

- Do you share contacts?
- How long are the contacts in your eye? Day hours? Night hours?

Family History

To obtain relevant family history information, ask if anyone in the family has a history of congenital eye diseases, cataracts, glaucoma, macular degeneration, or diabetes.

Lifestyle Habits

To understand lifestyle habits, ask:

- Do you smoke?
- Do you wear sunglasses?
- Do you use goggles or protective eyewear? When?
- Are you on any medications or drugs that dry out your eyes?

PHYSICAL EXAMINATION

Equipment needed for the physical examination of the eyes includes:

- Eye chart (e.g., Snellen or "E" chart)
- Near vision card (e.g., Rosenbaum or Jaeger)
- Index card or opaque covering
- Penlight
- Ophthalmoscope

Preparation of the Patient

Preparation of the patient and the environment is crucial to obtain correct findings during the eye examination. If the Snellen chart is located outside the examination room, then this portion of the examination should be completed prior to having the patient change into a gown. The area should be well lit and free of distractions. The remainder of the examination will be in a quiet, well-lit room with all necessary equipment in the room.

Components of the eye examination include:

- Vision tests: distal, near, and peripheral
- Inspection of the eyes, eyebrows, lids, conjunctiva, sclera, corneas, lenses, irises, and pupils

- Inspection and palpation of the lacrimal apparatus
- Extraocular movements: assessment of cardinal fields, convergence, corneal light test, cover–uncover test
- Inspection of the fundi, including the optic disc and cup, retina, and retinal vessels

Vision Tests

Visual Acuity Tests

Sight is evaluated using **visual acuity** tests. Various tests are available to use, including the Snellen chart, the "E" chart, and the near vision chart.

Snellen Test

To test the acuity of central vision and the patient's ability to see at a distance, use a well-lit Snellen eye chart (Fig. 11-13). The chart has the largest letters on the top line and the smallest letters on the bottom row. Position the patient 20 feet from the wall chart. Patients who wear glasses or contact lenses other than for reading should wear them for the examination. Ask the patient to cover one eye with an index card (to prevent peeking through the fingers) and to read the smallest line of print possible. Coaxing to attempt the next line may improve performance. A patient who cannot read the largest letter on the top line should be positioned closer to the chart; note the intervening distance. Identify the smallest line of print on which the patient can identify more than half the letters. Record the visual acuity designated at the side of this line and note the number of letters missed. Additionally, note if glasses or contacts were worn. Test each eye separately, and note any misread letters, squinting, or apprehension. During the examination of the second eye, the patient can be asked to read the lines backward or right to left to ensure the letter series is not memorized.

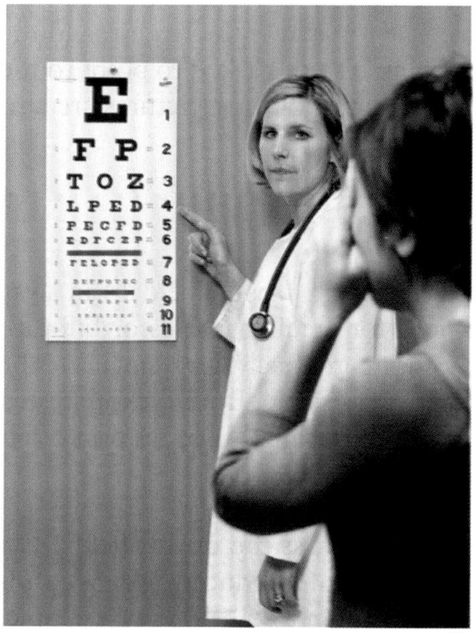

FIGURE 11-13 Assessing visual acuity with a Snellen eye chart.

Visual acuity is expressed as two numbers (e.g., 20/30). The numerator (top number) indicates the distance of the patient from the chart, and this number should always be 20 unless the patient moved closer for testing. The denominator (bottom number) is the distance at which a normal eye can read the line of letters.

An example of documentation might be, "right eye 20/30, left eye 20/30 (–2), with contacts."

Normal vision is 20/20.

Referral to an ophthalmologist should be made if vision is worse than 20/30.

Better-than-normal vision is when the denominator or second number is smaller than the numerator or top number. For example, 20/15 vision is when a person can see from 20 feet (ft) what the normal eye can see from 15 ft.

Legally blind is 20/200. Vision of 20/200 means that at 20 ft, the patient can read print that a person with normal vision could read at 200 ft.

The larger the second number, the worse the vision. "20/40 corrected" means the patient could read the 40 line with glasses (a correction).

The "E" Chart

The "E" chart is used for testing the vision of children or people who are unable to read. It is similar to the Snellen chart in that there are rows with the letter "E" facing different positions. The top row is the largest, and the bottom row is the smallest. The person being tested is asked to point to the direction the "E" is facing. Charts with the letter "C" or pictures are also available for testing.

Myopia (nearsightedness) causes focusing problems for distance vision (Holden et al., 2016).

Near Vision Tests

Test near vision with a special handheld card (e.g., Jaeger) held 14 in away from the eyes. The test identifies the need for reading glasses or bifocals. The card contains paragraphs, and the print gradually gets smaller. The patient is asked to read the smallest paragraph possible. Both eyes are tested at the same time without corrective lenses. Generally, this test is done after the age of 40 as near vision acuity begins to decrease.

When scoring the near test, the numerator is 14, as the card is held 14 in away from the eyes. Normal near vision is 14/14. Reduced near vision is when the denominator, or second number, is larger than 14. For example, 14/20 near vision is when a person has to hold the card at 14 in when others with normal near vision can read it at 20 in.

A Jaegar (J) number is another way for near vision to be rated. The J number delineates the text size read. The J number goes up as the print size goes up. The higher number correlates with decreased near vision:

J1 is the smallest line on the chart = 20/15
J2 = 20/20
J12 = 20/100

Presbyopia (farsightedness) is the impaired near vision found in middle-aged and older people caused by the loss of elasticity of the lens of the eye. Often the patient sees better when the card is farther away.

If there are no charts available, screen visual acuity with any available print (e.g., newspaper) held at 14 inches away from the eyes. If patients cannot read even the largest letters, test their ability to count your upraised fingers and distinguish light (such as your penlight) from the dark.

Peripheral Vision

Visual fields are tested to assess peripheral vision. **Confrontation** is a comparison between the patient and the nurse, provided the nurse has intact peripheral vision, to determine any areas of deficit. The visual fields overlap and should be tested one at a time. The visual field is 180 degrees horizontally and 135 degrees vertically. Screening starts in the temporal fields because most defects involve these areas (Fig. 11-14). Imagine the patient's visual fields projected onto a glass bowl that encircles the front of the patient's head.

Defects in peripheral visual fields may be a sign of normal pressure glaucoma, and the patient should be referred to an ophthalmologist. Patients with normal angle glaucoma have no symptoms until their vision is irreparably damaged.

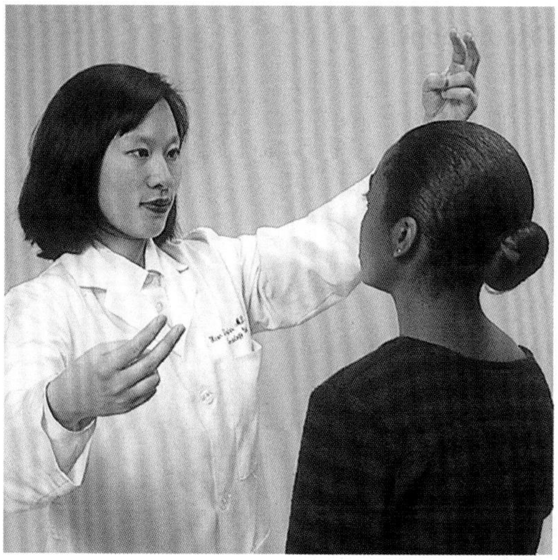

FIGURE 11-14 Assessment of peripheral fields by confrontation.

Field defects that are all or partly temporal are illustrated in Figure 11-15.

To screen for visual field defects by confrontation:

1. Stand or sit directly across from the patient (about 2 ft away).
2. Ask the patient to look with both eyes into your eyes.
3. Spread your arms apart, just behind and lateral to the patient's head.
4. Instruct the patient to point to your wiggling fingers as soon as they are apparent to the patient.
5. Coming from both sides, slowly move the wiggling fingers of both your hands along the imaginary bowl toward the center until the patient points to them.
6. Repeat this pattern in the upper and lower temporal quadrants. Usually, a person sees both sets of fingers at the same time. If so, the fields are usually normal.

Visual field defects are illustrated in Table 11-2.

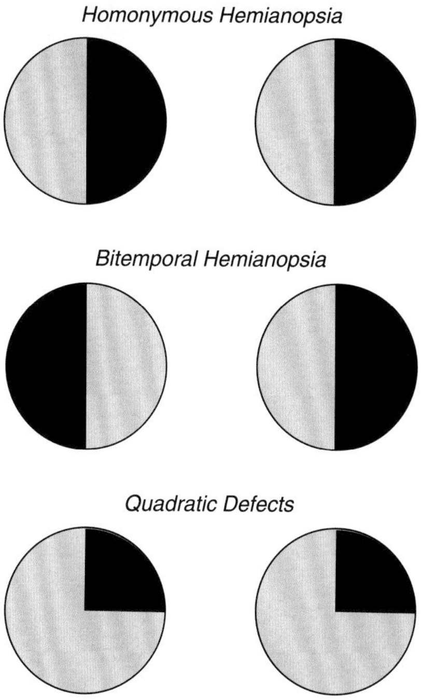

FIGURE 11-15 Temporal field defects.

TABLE 11-2 Visual Field Defects

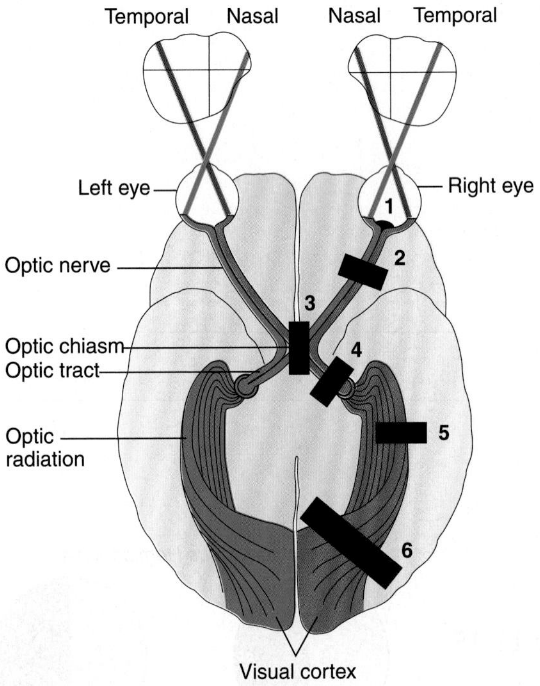

Horizontal Defect

Occlusion of a branch of the central retinal artery may cause a horizontal (altitudinal) defect. Ischemia of the optic nerve also can produce a similar defect.

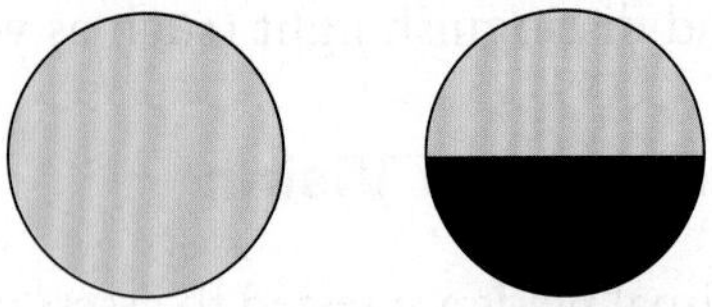

Blind Right Eye (Right Optic Nerve)

A lesion of the optic nerve, and of course of the eye itself, produces unilateral blindness.

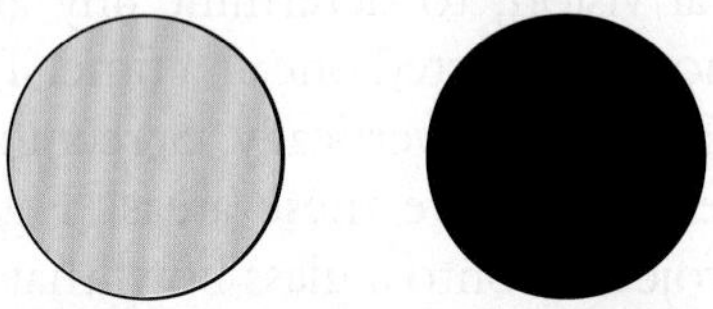

Bitemporal Hemianopsia (Optic Chiasm)

A lesion at the optic chiasm may involve only fibers crossing over to the opposite side. Since these fibers originate in the nasal half of each retina, visual loss involves the temporal half of each field.

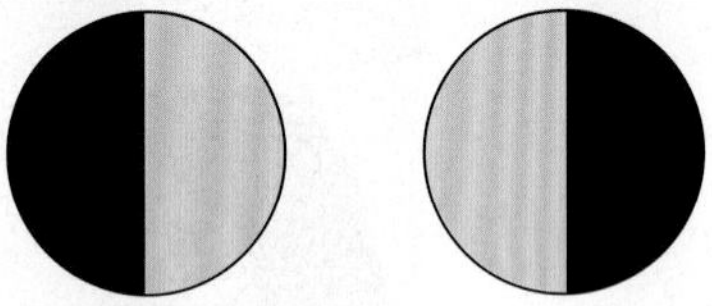

Left Homonymous Hemianopsia (Right Optic Tract)

A lesion of the optic tract interrupts fibers originating on the same side of both eyes. Visual loss in the eyes is therefore similar (homonymous) and involves half of each field (hemianopsia).

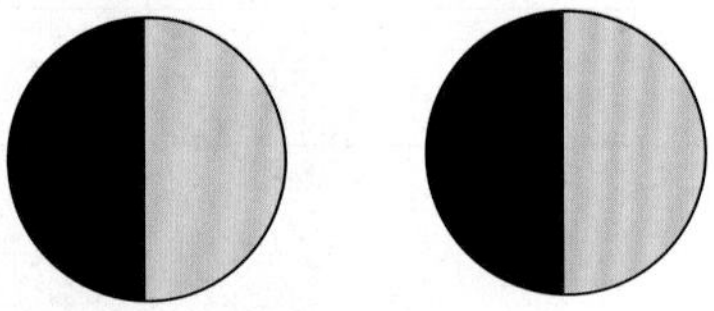

Homonymous Left Superior Quadrantic Defect (Right Optic Radiation, Partial)

A partial lesion of the optic radiation in the temporal lobe may involve only a portion of the nerve fibers, producing a homonymous quadrantic defect.

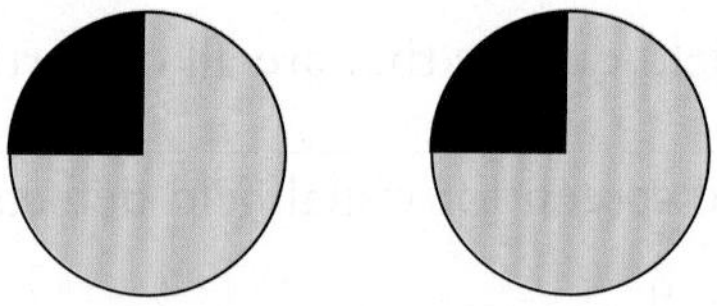

Left Homonymous Hemianopsia (Right Optic Radiation)

A complete interruption of fibers in the optic radiation produces a visual defect similar to that produced by a lesion of the optic tract.

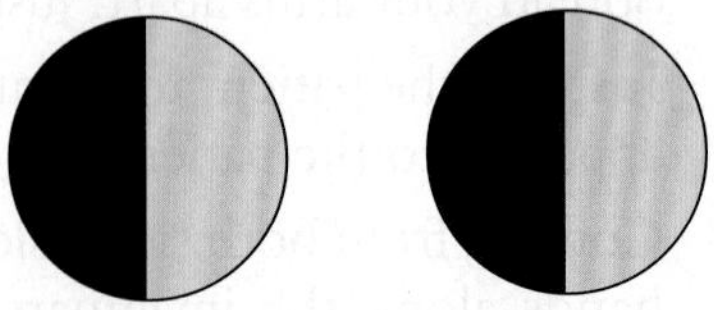

If you find a visual defect, try to establish its boundaries with further testing (Fig. 11-16). Test one eye at a time. Repeat this at several levels to define the border:

1. Stand or sit at eye level approximately 2 ft away from the patient.
2. Testing one eye at a time, ask the patient to cover one eye with a card.
3. With the other eye, the patient looks directly at you.
4. Cover your own eye directly across from the eye the patient has covered.
5. Starting midline above the head, slowly move your wiggling finger from the periphery noting where the patient first responds by saying "now" when they see the finger.
6. Repeat this in several directions or sides and at different levels to define the border. The person should be seeing the wiggling fingers at the same time you do.
7. Repeat the steps with the opposite eye.

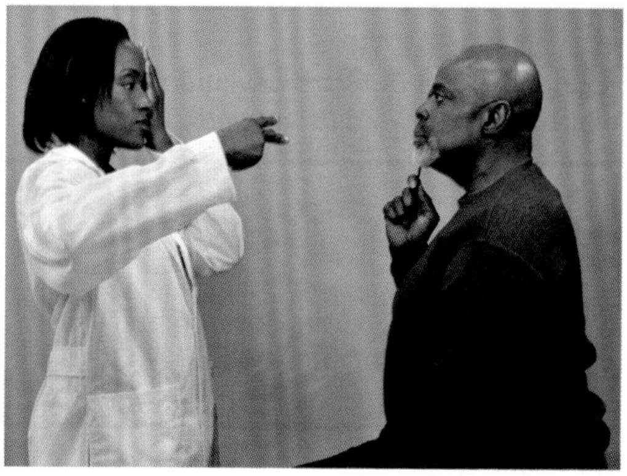

FIGURE 11-16 Additional testing of peripheral fields.

Hemianopsia is when the patient is unable to see in half of the visual field and is generally on one side (Fig. 11-17A). This can occur after a cerebrovascular accident or stroke. The patient is unable to distinguish objects to the side of the visual midline. The loss is contralateral, which is on the opposite side of the brain lesion. A left *homonymous hemianopsia* may thus be established (Fig. 11-17B).

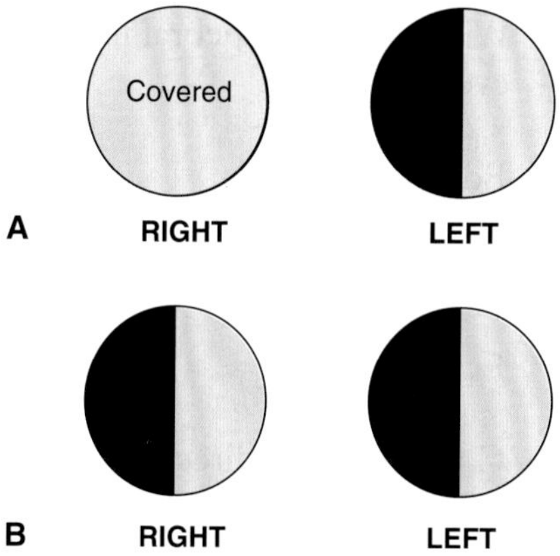

FIGURE 11-17 **A.** One-sided hemianopsia. **B.** Homonymous hemianopsia.

The visual field screening test works with all fields except the temporal field. For this field, start the examination with the wiggling finger behind the patient. In this instance, the examiner will see the finger at all times.

A temporal defect in the visual field of one eye suggests a nasal defect in the other eye. To test this hypothesis, examine the other eye in a similar way, again moving from the anticipated defect toward the better vision.

Small visual field defects and enlarged blind spots require a finer stimulus. Using a small red object such as a red-headed matchstick or the red eraser on a pencil, test one eye at a time. As the patient looks into your eye directly opposite, move the object around in the visual field. The normal blind spot (due to the location of the macula) can be found 15 degrees temporal to the line of gaze—the small red object disappears. Find your own blind spots for practice.

CLINICAL TIP
An enlarged blind spot occurs in conditions affecting the optic nerve such as *glaucoma*, *optic neuritis*, and *papilledema* (Petsas et al., 2017).

The External Eye

Position and Alignment of the Eyes

Stand in front of the patient and survey the eyes for position and alignment. If one or both eyes seem to protrude, assess them from above.

CLINICAL TIP
Inward or outward deviation of the eyes. An abnormal protrusion of the eye, which can be inward or outward, may indicate Graves disease or ocular tumors.

Eyebrows

Inspect the eyebrows, noting their quantity and distribution and any scaliness of the underlying skin.

CLINICAL TIP
Scaliness occurs in seborrheic dermatitis; lateral sparseness occurs in hypothyroidism.

Eyelids

Note the position of the lids in relation to the eyeballs. Inspect for the following:

- Width of the palpebral fissures—open area between the upper and lower eyelids

Upward slanting palpebral fissures are visible in Down syndrome.

- Edema of the lids
- Color of the lids

Red inflamed lid margins occur in *blepharitis,* often with crusting.

- Lesions
- Condition and direction of the eyelashes
- Adequacy with which the eyelids close; look for this especially when the eyes are unusually prominent, when there is facial paralysis, or when the patient is unconscious.

Failure of the eyelids to close exposes the corneas to serious damage.

See Table 11-3 for variations and abnormalities of the eyelids.

Lacrimal Apparatus

Briefly inspect the regions of the lacrimal gland and lacrimal sac for swelling (Table 11-4).

Look for excessive tearing, dryness, or crusting of the eyes. Assessment of dryness may require special testing by an ophthalmologist. To test for nasolacrimal duct obstruction, see the "Special Techniques" section.

CLINICAL TIP
Excessive tearing may be from increased production or impaired drainage of tears. In the first group, causes include conjunctival inflammation and corneal irritation; in the second, causes include ectropion and nasolacrimal duct obstruction.

TABLE 11-3 Variations and Abnormalities of the Eyelids

Ptosis

Ptosis is a drooping of the upper lid. Causes include myasthenia gravis, damage to the oculomotor nerve, and damage to the sympathetic nerve supply (*Horner syndrome*). A weakened muscle, relaxed tissues, and the weight of herniated fat may cause senile ptosis. Ptosis may also be congenital.

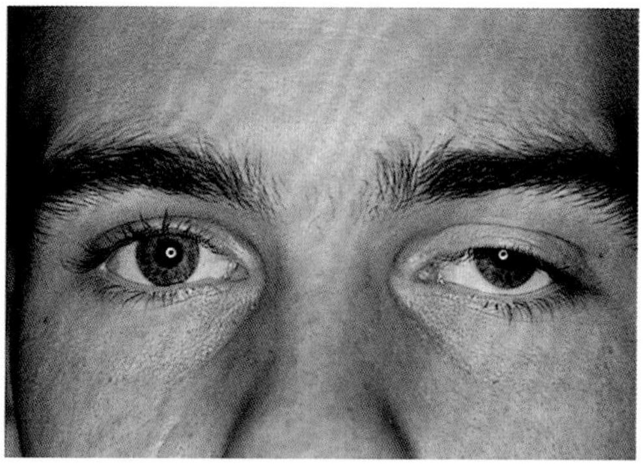

Entropion

Entropion, more common in the elderly, is an inward turning of the lid margin. The lower lashes, which are often invisible when turned inward, irritate the conjunctiva and lower cornea. Asking the patient to squeeze the lids together and then open them may reveal an entropion that is not obvious.

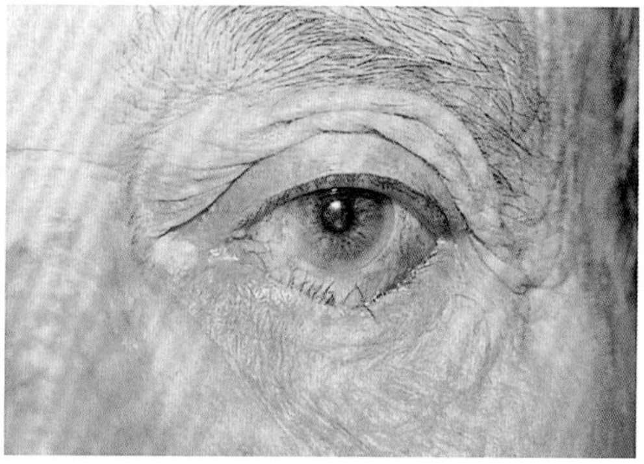

Ectropion

In ectropion, the margin of the lower lid is turned outward, exposing the palpebral conjunctiva. When the punctum of the lower lid turns outward, the eye no longer drains satisfactorily, and tearing occurs. Ectropion is more common in the elderly.

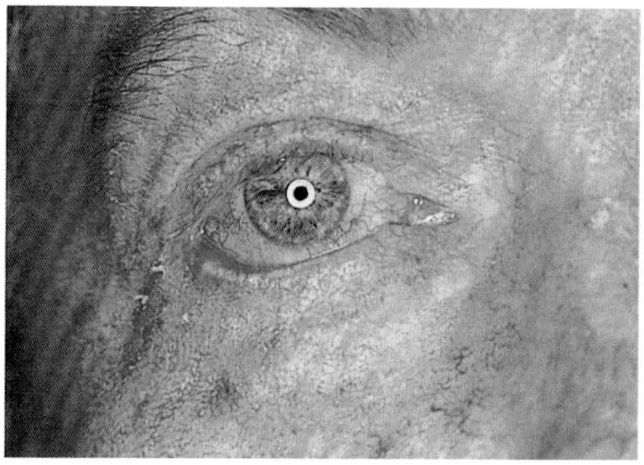

Lid Retraction and Exophthalmos

A wide-eyed stare suggests retracted eyelids. Note the rim of sclera between the upper lid and the iris. Retracted lids and a lid lag are often due to hyperthyroidism.

In exophthalmos, the eyeball protrudes forward. When bilateral, it suggests the infiltrative ophthalmopathy of Graves hyperthyroidism. Edema of the eyelids and conjunctival injection may be associated. Unilateral exophthalmos is seen in Graves disease or a tumor or inflammation in the orbit.

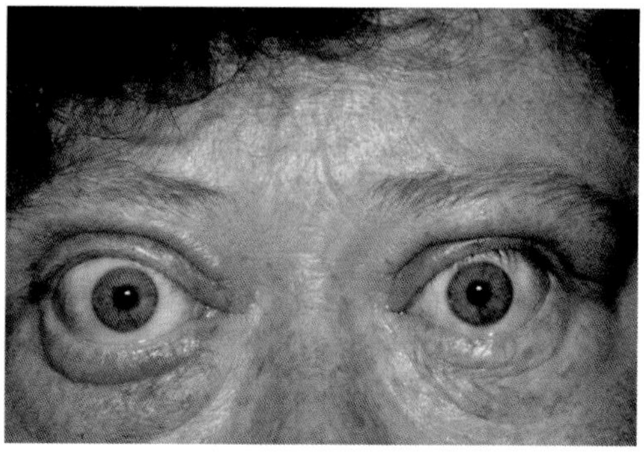

Source of photos: Ptosis, Ectropion, Entropion—Tasman, W., & Jaeger, E., Eds. (2001). *The wills eye hospital atlas of clinical ophthalmology* (2nd ed.). Lippincott Williams & Wilkins.

TABLE 11-4 Lumps and Swellings in and around the Eyes

Pinguecula

A harmless yellowish triangular nodule in the bulbar conjunctiva on either side of the iris. Appears frequently with aging, first on the nasal and then on the temporal side.

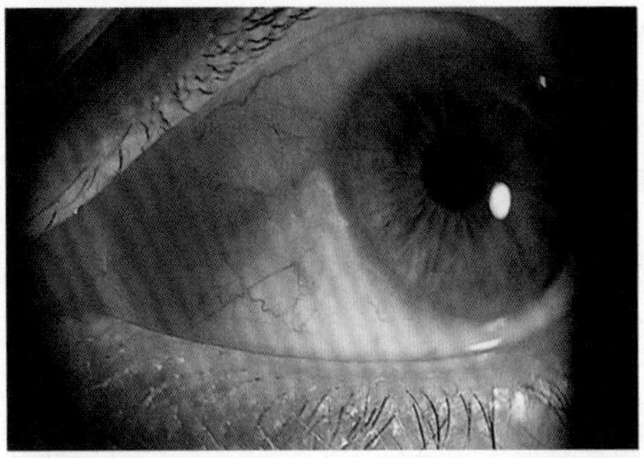

Episcleritis

A localized ocular redness from inflammation of the episcleral vessels. Vessels appear pink and are movable over the scleral surface. May be nodular, as shown, or may show only redness and dilated vessels.

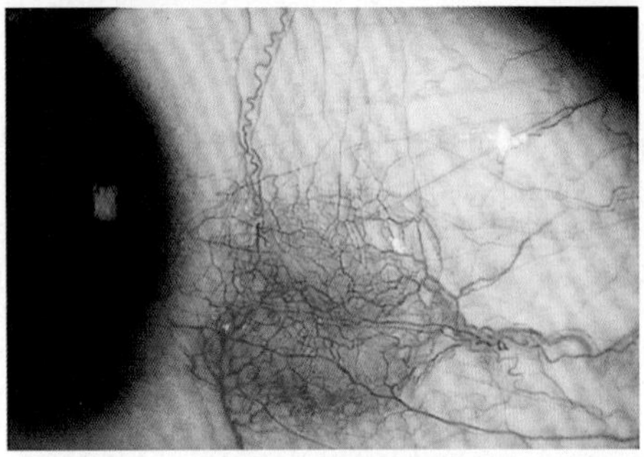

Sty (Hordeolum)

A painful, tender red infection in a gland at the margin of the eyelid

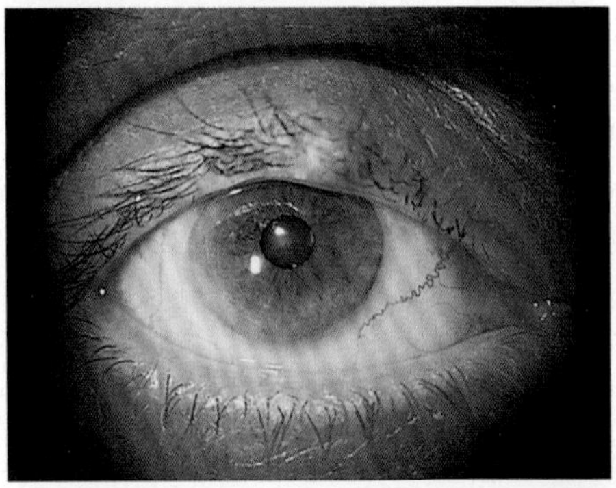

Chalazion

A subacute, nontender, and usually painless nodule involving a meibomian gland. May become acutely inflamed but unlike a sty, usually points inside the lid rather than on the lid margin.

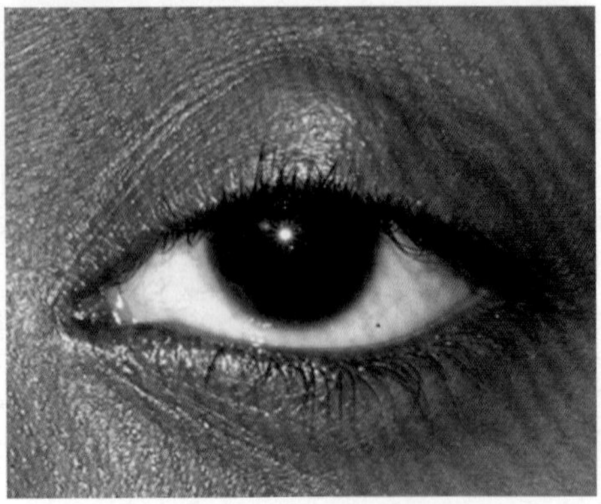

Xanthelasma

Slightly raised, yellowish, well-circumscribed plaques that appear along the nasal portions of one or both eyelids. May accompany lipid disorders.

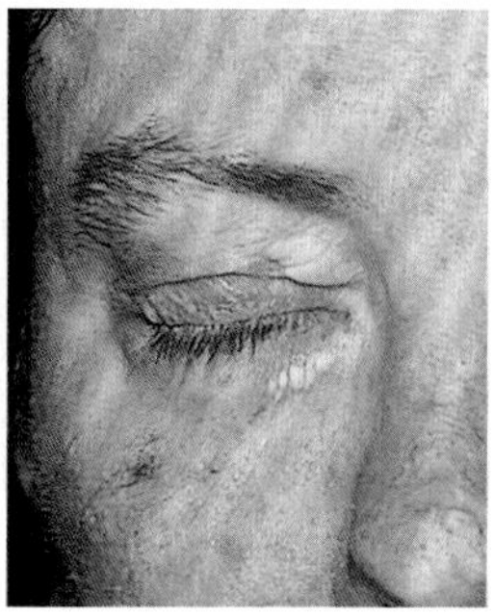

Inflammation of the Lacrimal Sac (Dacryocystitis)

A swelling between the lower eyelid and nose. An *acute* inflammation (illustrated) is painful, red, and tender. *Chronic* inflammation is associated with obstruction of the nasolacrimal duct. Tearing is prominent, and pressure on the sac produces regurgitation of material through the puncta of the eyelids.

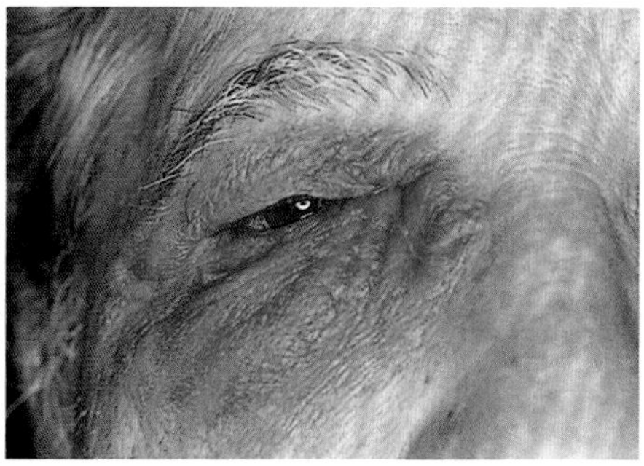

Source of photos: *Pinguecula, Episcleritis, Sty (Hordeolum), Xanthelasma, Inflammation of the Lacrimal Sac (Dacryocystitis)*–Tasman, W., & Jaeger, E., Eds. (2001). *The wills eye hospital atlas of clinical ophthalmology* (2nd ed.). Lippincott Williams & Wilkins; *Chalazion*–Reprinted with permission from Bagheri, N., Wajda, B. N.; Wills Eye Hospital. (2017). *The Wills eye manual: Office and emergency room diagnosis and treatment of eye disease* (7th ed.). Wolters Kluwer.

Conjunctiva and Sclera

Ask the patient to look up as you depress both lower lids with your thumbs, exposing the sclera and conjunctiva (Fig. 11-18). Inspect the sclera and palpebral conjunctiva for color (Fig. 11-19), and note the vascular pattern against the white scleral background. Look for any nodules or swelling.

If you need a fuller view of the eye, rest your thumb and finger on the bones of the cheek and brow, respectively, and spread the lids (Fig. 11-20).

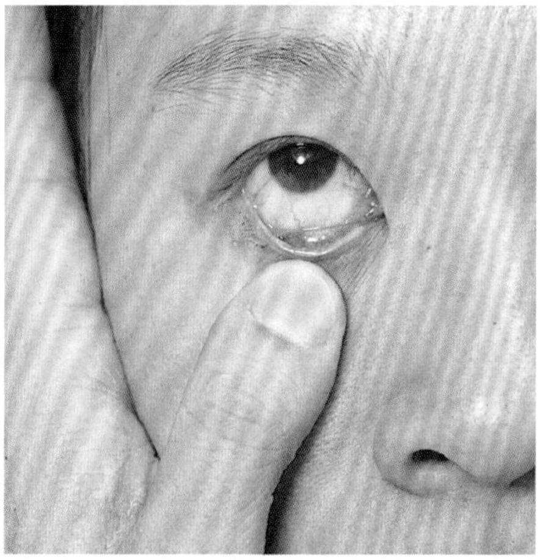

FIGURE 11-18 Assessment of the conjunctiva and sclera.

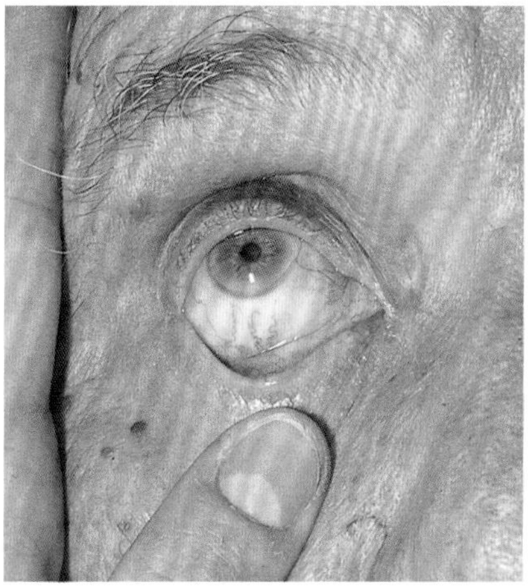

FIGURE 11-19 A yellow sclera indicates jaundice.

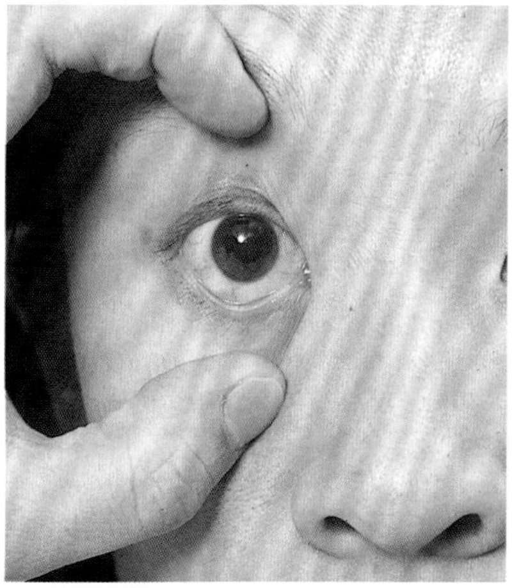

FIGURE 11-20 Full view of the eye.

Ask the patient to look to each side and down. This technique gives you a good view of the sclera and bulbar conjunctiva, but not of the palpebral conjunctiva of the upper lid. For this purpose, you need to evert the lid (see the "Special Techniques" section). Look for any local redness (Fig. 11-21).

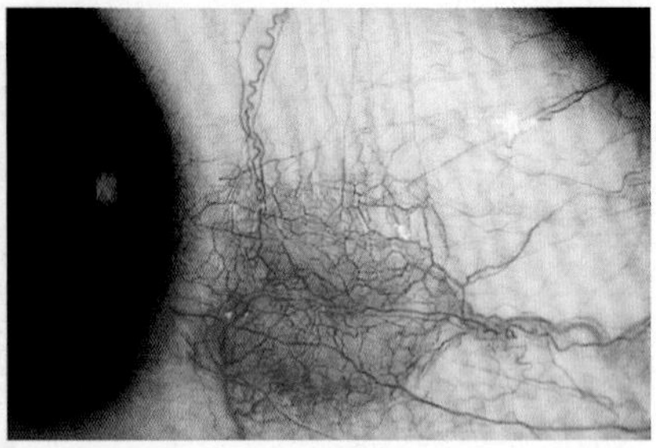

FIGURE 11-21 Local redness from nodular episcleritis. This is often self-limiting in younger adults, and may be seen with rheumatoid arthritis and systemic lupus erythematosus.

For comparisons, see Table 11-1, "Red Eyes."

Cornea and Lens

With oblique lighting, inspect the cornea of each eye for opacities, and note any opacities in the lens that may be visible through the pupil (Table 11-5).

TABLE 11-5 Opacities of the Cornea and Lens

Corneal Arcus

A thin grayish white arc or circle not quite at the edge of the cornea. Accompanies normal aging but also seen in younger people, especially African Americans. In young people, suggests possible hyperlipoproteinemia. Usually benign.

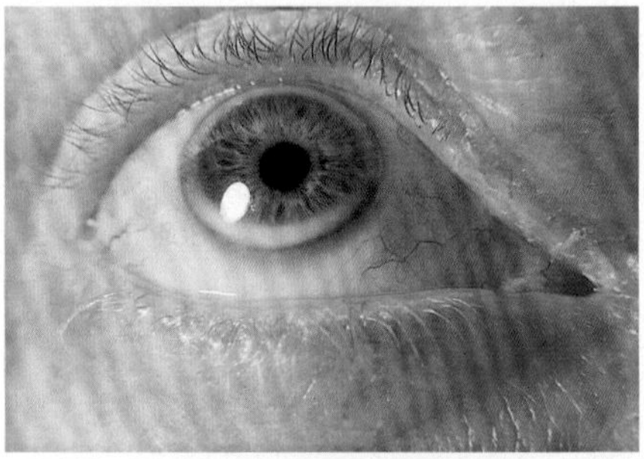

Corneal Scar

A superficial grayish white opacity in the cornea, secondary to an old injury or to inflammation. Size and shape are variable. Do not confuse with the opaque lens of a cataract, visible on a deeper plane and only through the pupil.

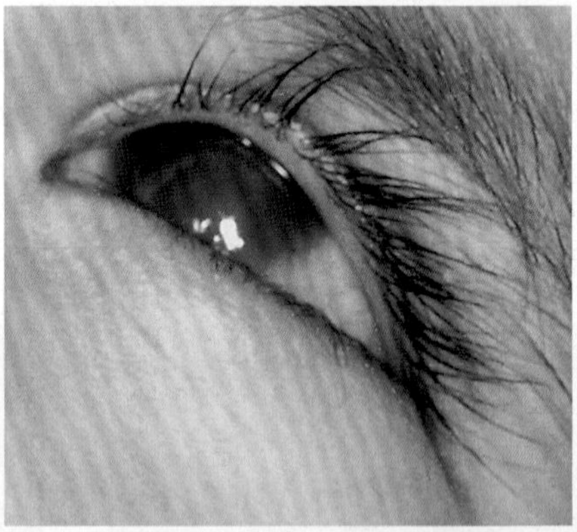

Pterygium

A triangular thickening of the bulbar conjunctiva that grows slowly across the outer surface of the cornea, usually from the nasal side. Reddening may occur. May interfere with vision as it encroaches on the pupil.

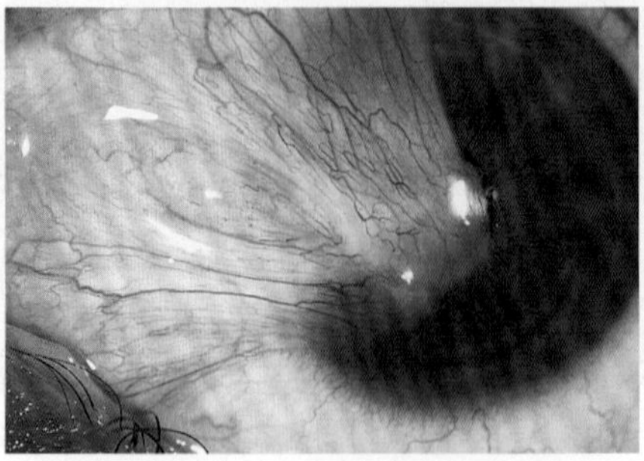

Cataracts

Opacities of the lenses visible through the pupil; most common in old age.

Nuclear Cataract

A nuclear cataract looks gray when seen by a flashlight. If the pupil is widely dilated, the gray opacity is surrounded by a black rim.

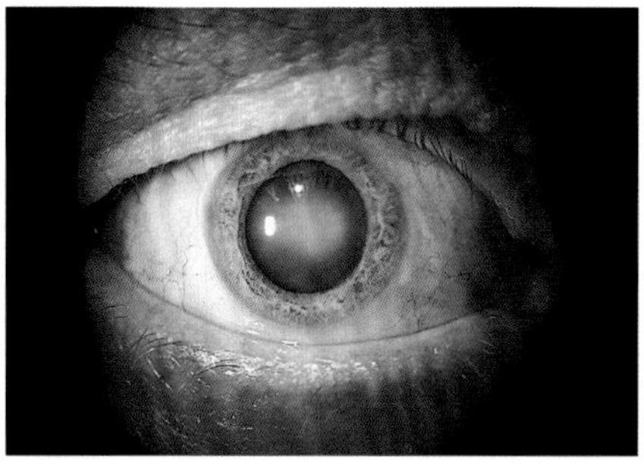

Peripheral Cataract

Produces spoke-like shadows that point inward—gray against black, as seen with a flashlight, or black against red with an ophthalmoscope. A dilated pupil, as shown here, facilitates this observation.

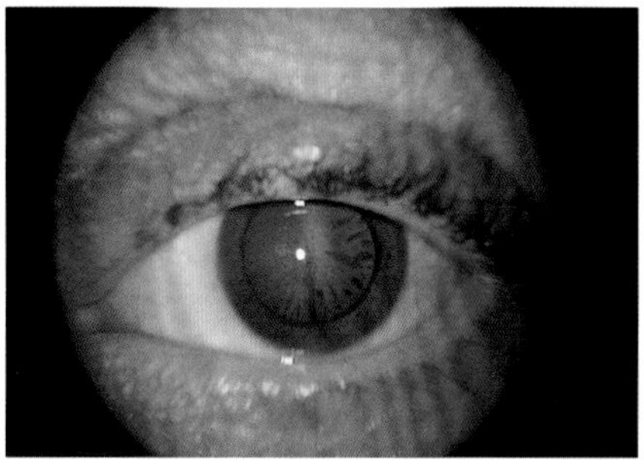

Iris

At the same time, inspect each iris. The markings should be clearly defined. With your light shining directly from the temporal side, look for a crescentic shadow on the medial side of the iris (Fig. 11-22). Because the iris is

Occasionally the iris bows abnormally far forward, forming a narrow angle with the cornea. The light then casts a crescentic shadow.

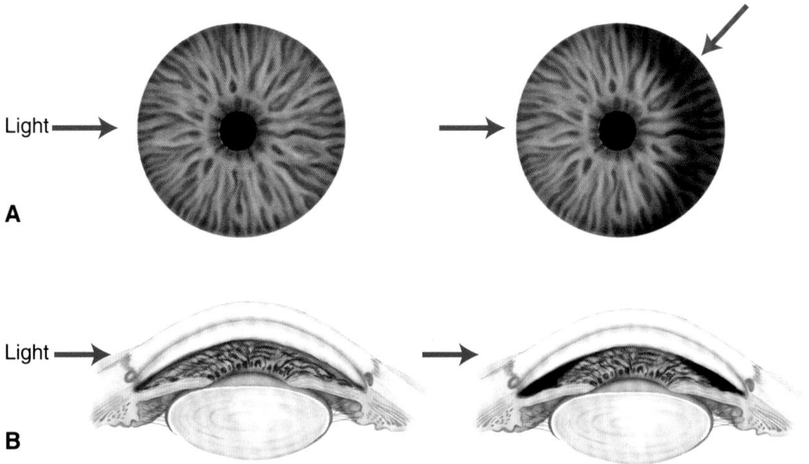

FIGURE 11-22 **A.** The narrow angle increases the risk for acute narrow-angle glaucoma—a sudden increase in intraocular pressure when drainage of the aqueous humor is blocked. **B.** In open-angle glaucoma—the common form of glaucoma—the normal spatial relation between iris and cornea is preserved and the iris is fully lit.

normally fairly flat and forms a relatively open angle with the cornea, this lighting casts no shadow. There are variations in the color of the iris. Many Asian, Hispanic, or Black Americans have brown eyes, and many of European or Scandinavian descent have lighter eye colors.

Pupils

In dim light, inspect the *size*, *shape*, and *symmetry* of each pupil. Measure the pupils with a guide such as a card or a flashlight with black circles of various sizes to facilitate measurement (Fig. 11-23). Document the pupil size and note if the pupils are large (greater than 5 mm), small (less than 3 mm), or unequal.

Miosis refers to constriction of the pupils, *mydriasis* to dilation.

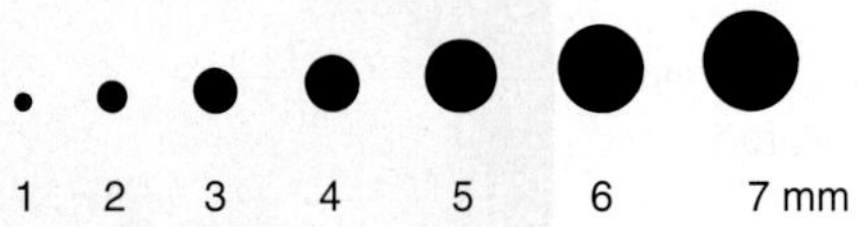

FIGURE 11-23 Pupil size guide.

Anisocoria is a difference in pupil size. This can normally be found in one in five people. Pupillary diameter inequality is generally smaller than 0.5 mm, but it can be up to 1 mm. If pupillary reactions are normal, anisocoria is considered benign. If the change in pupil size is sudden and does not resolve or is in combination with additional symptoms, follow-up with a health care provider is warranted (Table 11-6) (Boyd, 2019).

Compare benign anisocoria with Horner syndrome, oculomotor nerve paralysis, and tonic pupil.

TABLE 11-6 Pupillary Abnormalities

Unequal Pupils *(Anisocoria)*

When anisocoria is greater in bright light than in dim light, the larger pupil cannot constrict properly. Causes include blunt trauma to the eye, open-angle glaucoma, and impaired parasympathetic nerve supply to the iris, as in tonic pupil, oculomotor nerve paralysis, brain injury, or brain tumors. When anisocoria is greater in dim light, the smaller pupil cannot dilate properly, as in Horner syndrome, caused by an interruption of the sympathetic nerve supply. See also Table 20-9, "Pupils in Comatose Patients."

Tonic Pupil *(Adie Pupil)*

Pupil is large, regular, and usually unilateral. Reaction to light is severely reduced and slowed, or even absent. Near reaction, though very slow, is present. Slow accommodation causes blurred vision. Deep tendon reflexes are often decreased.

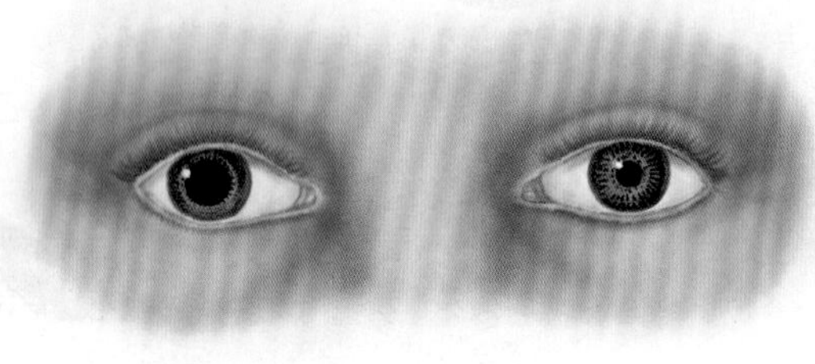

Oculomotor Nerve (CN III) Paralysis

The dilated pupil is fixed to light and near effort. Ptosis of the upper eyelid and lateral deviation of the eye are almost always present.

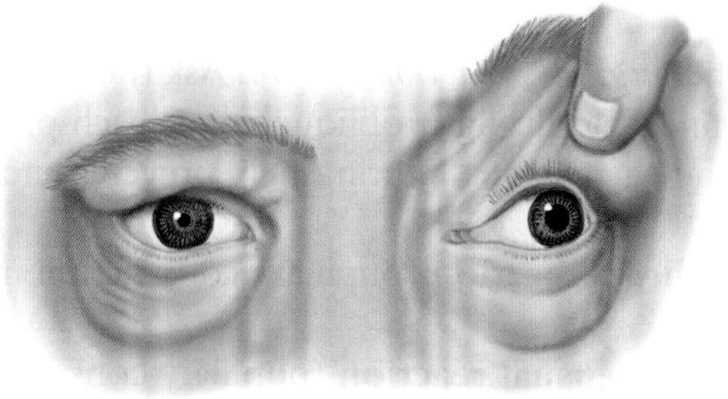

Horner Syndrome

The affected pupil, though small, reacts briskly to light and near effort. Ptosis of the eyelid is present, perhaps with loss of sweating on the forehead. In congenital Horner syndrome, the involved iris is lighter in color than its fellow (*heterochromia*).

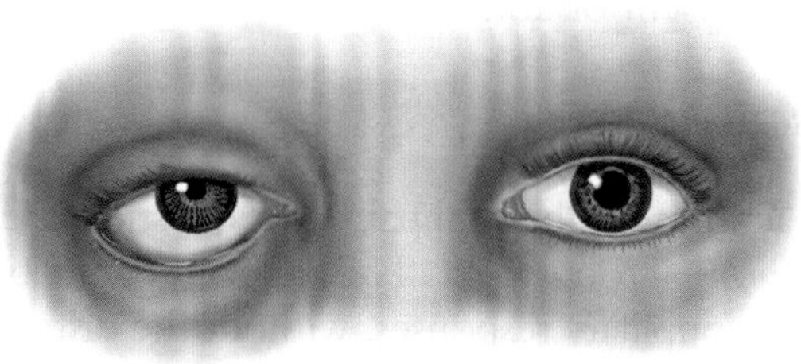

Small, Irregular Pupils

Small, irregular pupils that accommodate but do not react to light indicate *Argyll Robertson pupils* seen in central nervous system syphilis.

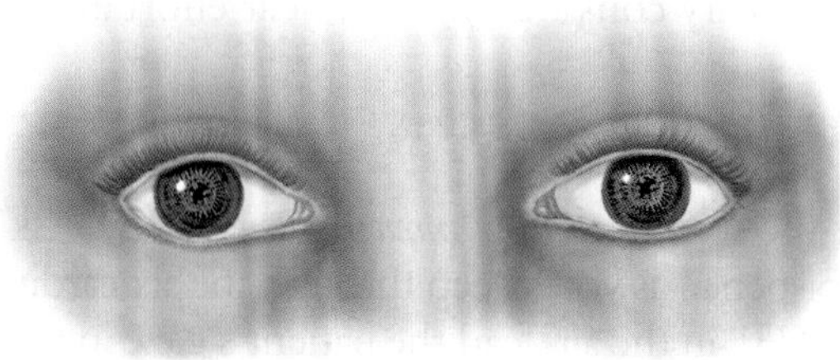

Equal Pupils and One Blind Eye

Unilateral blindness does not cause anisocoria as long as the sympathetic and parasympathetic innervation to both irises is normal. A light directed into the seeing eye produces a direct reaction in that eye and a consensual reaction in the blind eye. A light directed into the blind eye, however, causes no response in either eye.

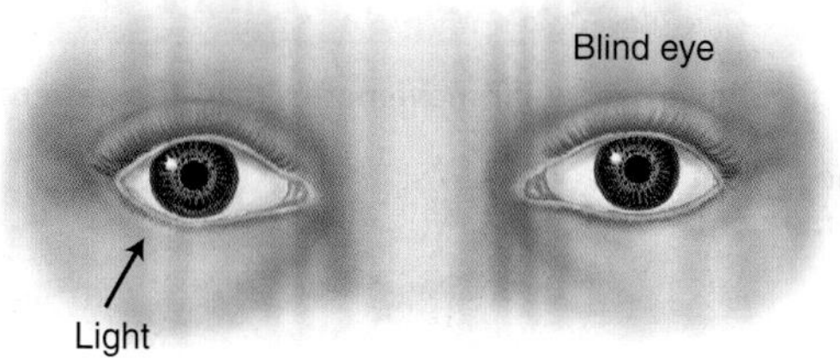

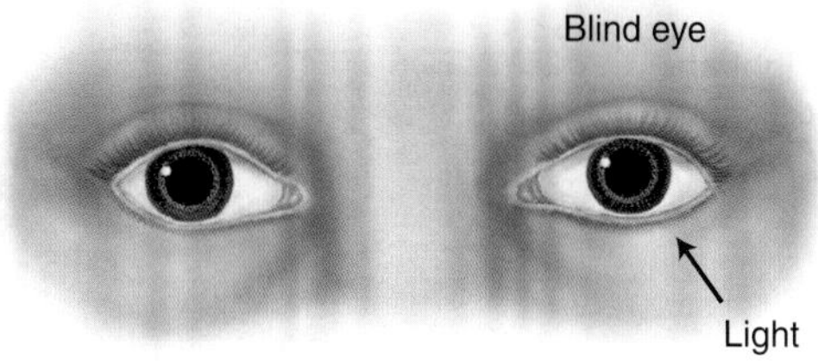

Light Reaction

Test the *pupillary reaction to light.* Ask the patient to look into the distance, and shine a bright light obliquely into each pupil in turn. Both the distant gaze and the oblique lighting help prevent a near reaction. Look for:

- The **direct reaction** (pupillary constriction in the same eye)
- The **consensual reaction** (pupillary constriction in the opposite eye)

Always darken the room and use a bright light before deciding that a light reaction is absent or abnormal.

Near Reaction

If the reaction to light is impaired or questionable, test the *near reaction* in dim and normal room light. Testing one eye at a time makes it easier to concentrate on pupillary responses, without the distraction of extraocular movement. Hold your finger or pencil about 10 cm from the patient's eye. Ask the patient to look alternately at it and into the distance directly behind it. Watch for pupillary constriction with near effort and convergence of the eyes.

Testing the near reaction is helpful in diagnosing Argyll Robertson (p. 275) and tonic (Adie) pupils (p. 274).

Extraocular Muscles

Test the six *extraocular movements (EOMs).* Ask the patient to follow your finger or pencil as you sweep through the six cardinal directions of gaze. Making a wide "H" in the air, lead the patient's gaze in the directions shown in Box 11-2.

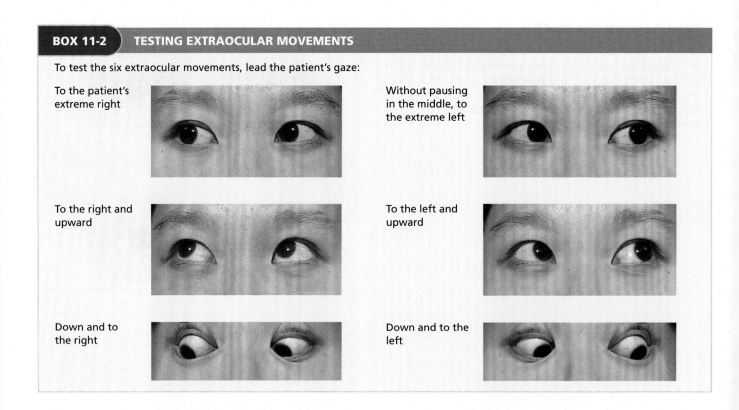

BOX 11-2 TESTING EXTRAOCULAR MOVEMENTS

To test the six extraocular movements, lead the patient's gaze:

To the patient's extreme right

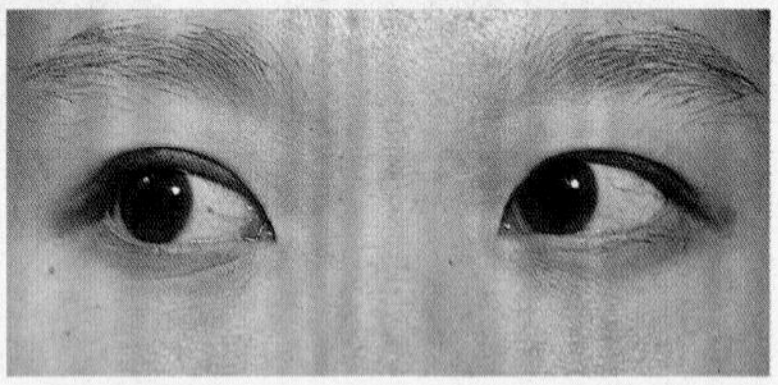

Without pausing in the middle, to the extreme left

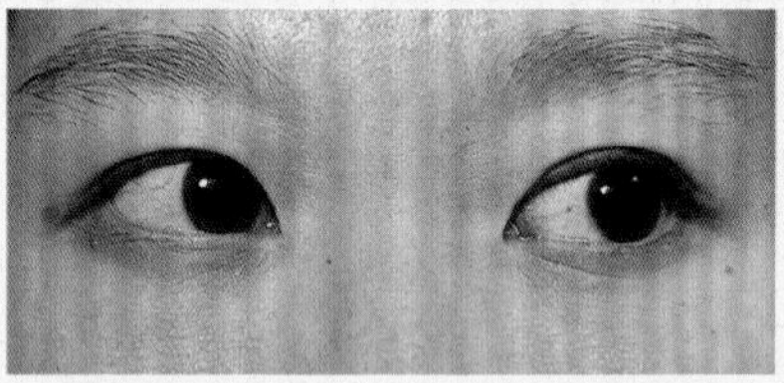

To the right and upward

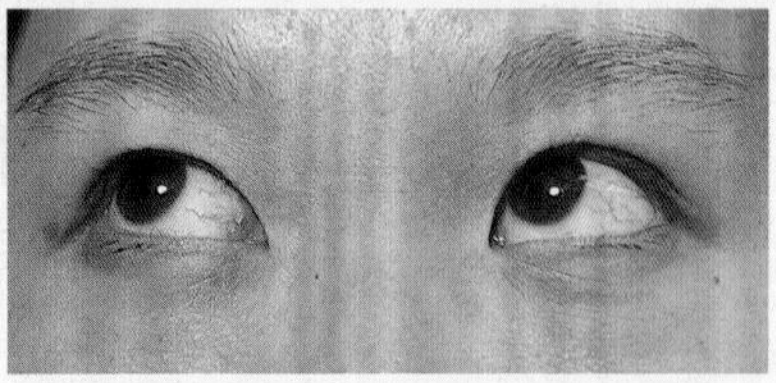

To the left and upward

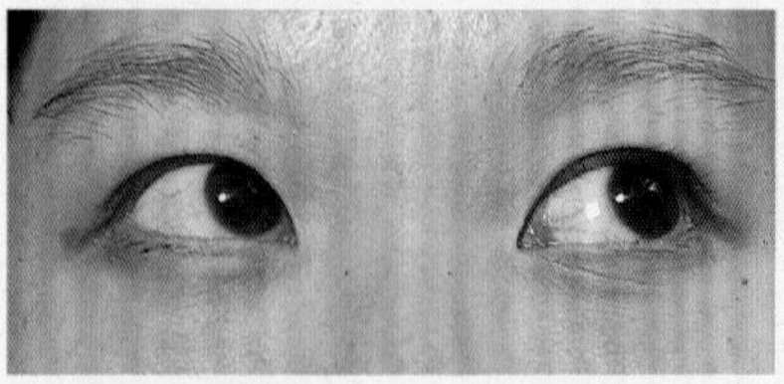

Down and to the right

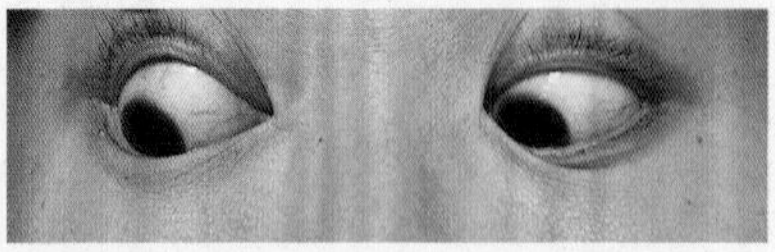

Down and to the left

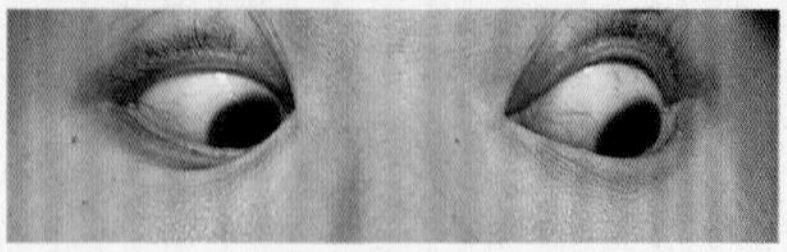

Pause during examination of the upward and lateral gaze to detect *nystagmus*. Move your finger or pencil at approximately 12 to 18 in from the patient. Because middle-aged or older adults may have difficulty focusing on near objects, make this distance greater. Patients should maintain the head midline, but some patients will move their heads to follow your finger. If necessary, hold the head in the proper midline position.

Deviations in movements can signal a brain tumor or injury. The change depends on the location of the lesion or injury. In paralysis of CN VI (Fig. 11-24), the eyes are conjugate in right lateral gaze but not in left lateral gaze.

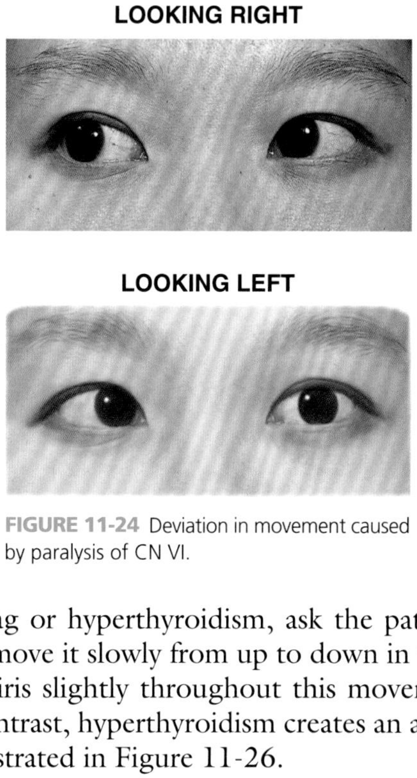

FIGURE 11-24 Deviation in movement caused by paralysis of CN VI.

If you suspect lid lag or hyperthyroidism, ask the patient to follow your finger again as you move it slowly from up to down in the midline. The lid should overlap the iris slightly throughout this movement as depicted in Figure 11-25. In contrast, hyperthyroidism creates an abnormal protrusion of the eyeball as illustrated in Figure 11-26.

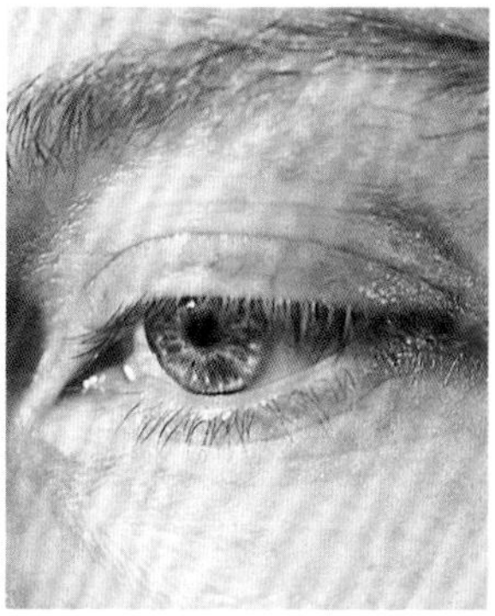

FIGURE 11-25 The lid overlapping the iris.

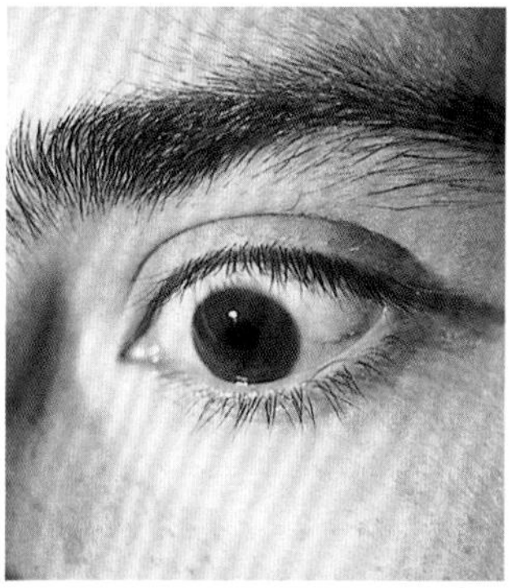

FIGURE 11-26 Note the rim of the sclera from proptosis, an abnormal protrusion of the eyeball in hyperthyroidism, leading to a characteristic "stare" on the frontal gaze.

Assess the extraocular movements, looking for:

- The normal *conjugate movements* of the eyes in each direction. Detect any deviation from normal, or **dysconjugate** gaze (Table 11-7).

TABLE 11-7 Dysconjugate Gaze

There are a variety of gaze abnormality patterns that give nurses clues about developmental disorders and cranial nerve abnormalities.

Developmental Disorders

Developmental dysconjugate gaze is caused by an imbalance in ocular muscle tone. This imbalance has many causes, may be hereditary, and usually appears in early childhood. These gaze deviations are classified according to direction:

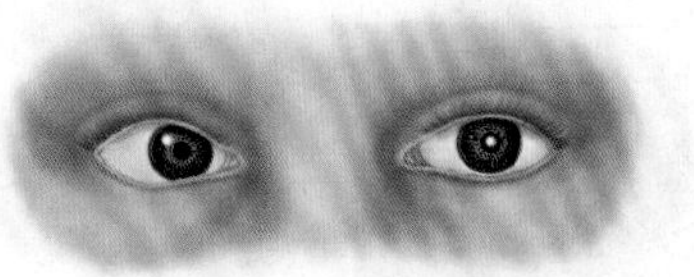

Esotropia (inward deviation).

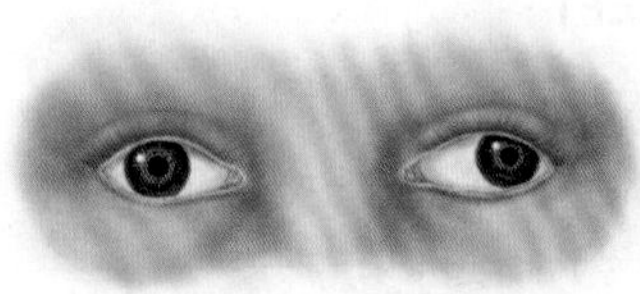

Exotropia (outward deviation).

Cover–Uncover Test

A cover–uncover test may be helpful. Here is what you would see in the right monocular esotropia illustrated above.

Corneal reflections are asymmetric.

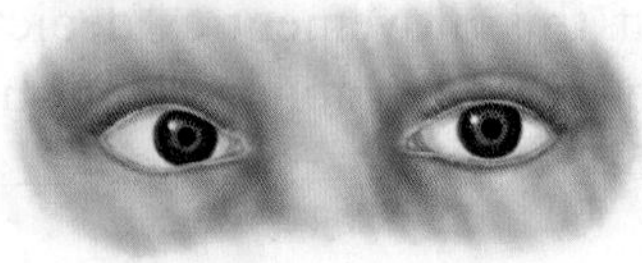

Covered, the right eye moves outward to fix on the light. (The left eye is not seen but moves inward to the same degree.)

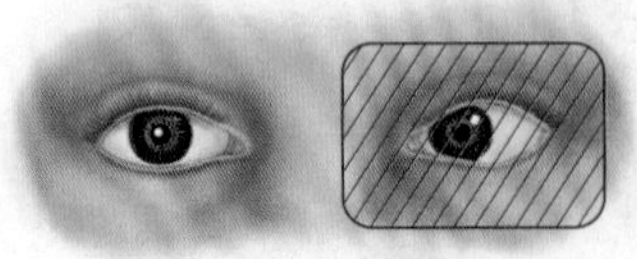

Uncovered, the left eye moves outward to fix on the light. The right eye deviates inward again.

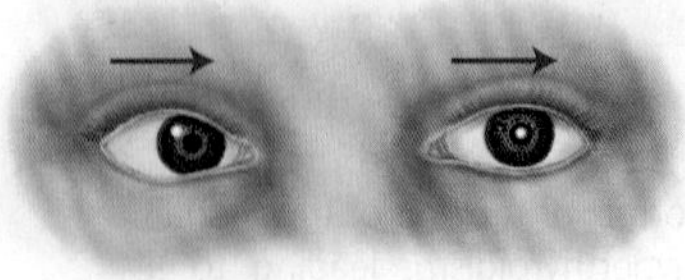

Disorders of Cranial Nerves

New onset of dysconjugate gaze in adult life is usually the result of cranial nerve injuries, lesions, or abnormalities from such causes as trauma, multiple sclerosis, syphilis, and others.

A Left Cranial Nerve VI Paralysis

When looking to the right, eyes are conjugate.

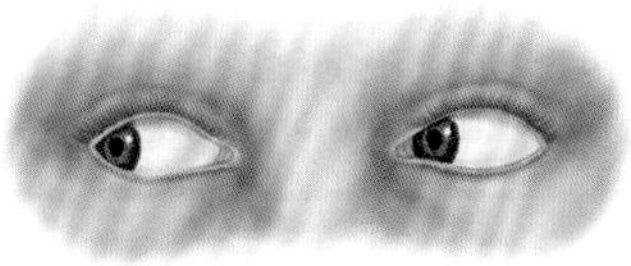

When looking straight ahead, esotropia appears.

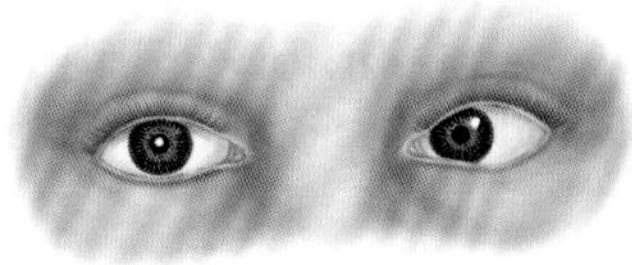

When looking to the left, esotropia is maximum.

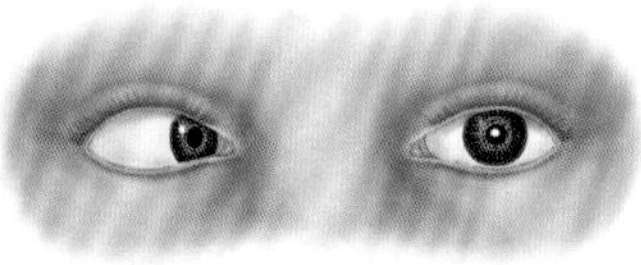

A Left Cranial Nerve IV Paralysis

When looking down and to the right, the left eye cannot look down when turned inward. Deviation is maximum in this direction.

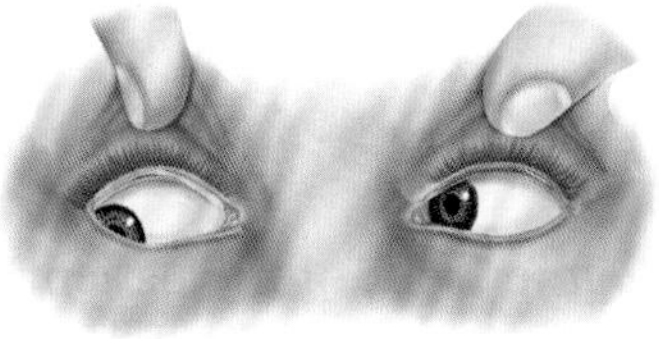

A Left Cranial Nerve III Paralysis

When looking straight ahead, the eye is pulled outward by action of the sixth nerve. Upward, downward, and inward movements are impaired or lost. Ptosis and pupillary dilation may be associated.

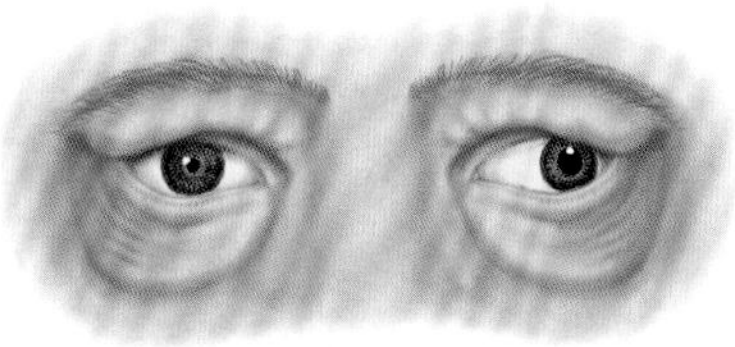

- **Nystagmus**, a fine rhythmic oscillation of the eyes. A few beats of nystagmus on the extreme lateral gaze are normal. If you see it, bring your finger in to within the field of binocular vision and look again. Nystagmus occurs normally when a person watches a rapidly moving object such as a passing train.

CLINICAL TIP
Sustained nystagmus within the binocular field of gaze is seen with various causes, including impairment of vision in early life, disorders of the labyrinth and the cerebellar system, and drug toxicity. See Chapter 20, "The Nervous System."

- *Lid lag* as the eyes move from up to down.

Test for convergence. Ask the patient to follow your index finger or pencil as you move your finger (or a pencil) slowly straight forward to the nose (Fig. 11-27). The converging eyes normally follow the object to within 5 to 8 cm. Test through the entire field.

Poor convergence is common in *hyperthyroidism*.

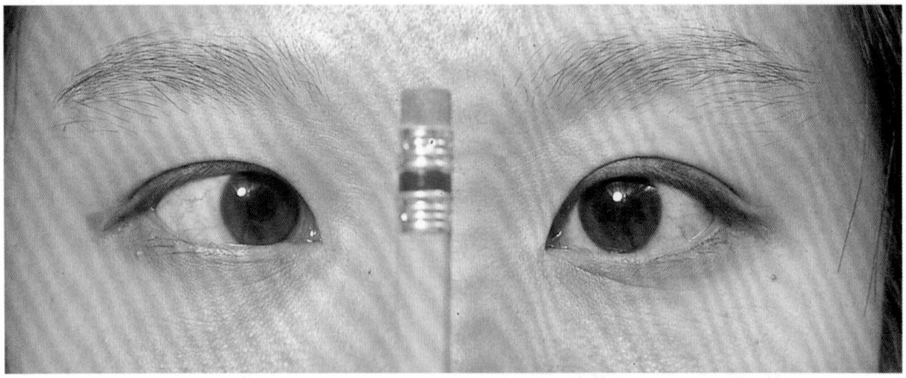

FIGURE 11-27 Convergence.

Examine the *corneal light reflex.* Standing 2 ft in front of the patient, shine a light into the patient's eyes, and ask the patient to look at it. *Inspect the reflections in the corneas.* They should be visible slightly nasal to the center of the pupils (Fig. 11-28).

Asymmetry of the corneal reflections indicates a deviation from normal ocular alignment. A temporal light reflection on one cornea, for example, indicates a nasal deviation of that eye. See Table 11-7, "Dysconjugate Gaze."

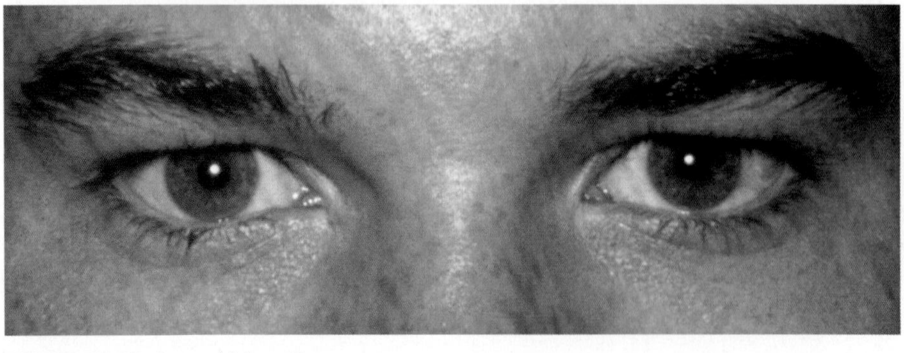

FIGURE 11-28 Corneal light reflex.

A *cover–uncover test* may reveal a slight or latent muscle imbalance not otherwise seen (see Table 11-7 "Dysconjugate Gaze").

Ophthalmoscopic Examination

The nurse would examine the patient's eyes *without dilating the pupils.* The view is therefore limited to the posterior structures of the retina. To see more peripheral structures, to evaluate the macula well, or to investigate unexplained visual loss, ophthalmologists dilate the pupils with mydriatic drops unless this is contraindicated.

Contraindications for mydriatic drops include (1) head injury and coma in which continuing observations of pupillary reactions are essential, and (2) any suspicion of narrow-angle glaucoma.

At first, using the **ophthalmoscope** (Fig. 11-29) may seem awkward, and it may be difficult to visualize the fundus. With patience and practice of proper technique, the fundus will come into view, and the ability to assess important structures such as the optic disc and the retinal vessels becomes easier.

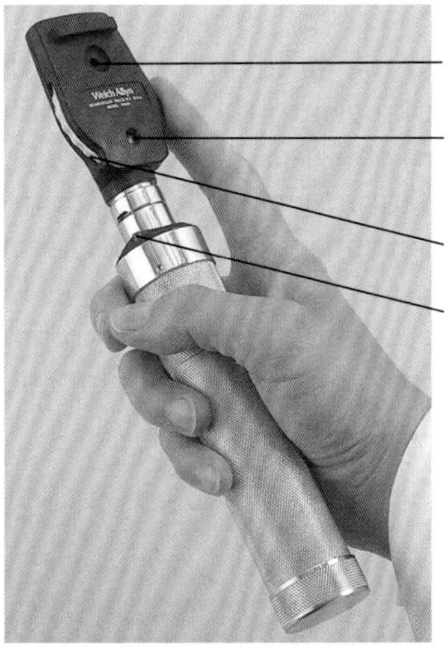

FIGURE 11-29 An ophthalmoscope.

The optic disc's yellowish orange to creamy pink oval or round structure may fill the field of gaze or even exceed it. Of interest, the ophthalmoscope magnifies the normal retina about 15 times and the normal iris about four times. The optic disc actually measures about 1.5 mm. Follow the next steps for this important segment of the physical examination.

Preparing to Examine the Optic Disc

To begin using the ophthalmoscope for assessment, the nurse needs to be aware of how it functions as there are different types. Familiarize yourself with the dials and know how to turn it on. Initially, the scope needs to be set on:

- The brightest light necessary to visualize the retina and blood vessels
- The white light (ignore the other colors)
- The circle (ignore the slits and crosses)
- "0" diopters

If the nurse wears glasses or contact lenses, they can remain on for the examination. If the patient wears glasses they should be removed, though contacts may remain in.

Room lighting should be decreased or turned off without making the room too dark.

Explain to the patient that the ophthalmoscope light will be bright, and it is important focus on a specific point so the eyes do not wander during the examination. Choose a point on the wall over your shoulder that the patient should stare at (you might pick a curtain or determine a spot on the wall behind you). The patient should continue to look in that direction even if you step in the line of view.

Positioning

When looking into the patient's right eye, the nurse holds the scope with the right hand and uses the right eye; when looking into the patient's left eye, the nurse holds the scope with the left hand and uses the left eye. Try to keep your other eye open during the examination. Using the nondominant hand and eye will take practice. It is important to master this, as it decreases the likelihood of the nurse's nose touching the patient's nose. In addition, the hand not holding the scope can brace the thumb and forefinger on the patient's eyebrow to determine the proximity to the patient and to assist with opening the patient's eye if it tends to close.

The Examination

The nurse will shine the light into the patient's eye from 6 in away and at a 15-degree angle and will be able to see the red reflex (Fig. 11-30). Follow this into the eye, resting the ophthalmoscope on your eyebrow and standing about 1.5 to 2 in away from the patient. (It is important to get close to the patient as you will have a wider field of view.) Here, the optic disc, arteries, and veins are visible. If you are unable to visualize the optic disc and vessels, keep your head still and move the diopter dial (which your index finger has been resting on) either way. If the disc becomes clearer, keep turning the dial; if it becomes blurry, then turn the dial in the opposite direction.

Steps for examining the optic disc and the retina are outlined and illustrated in Box 11-3.

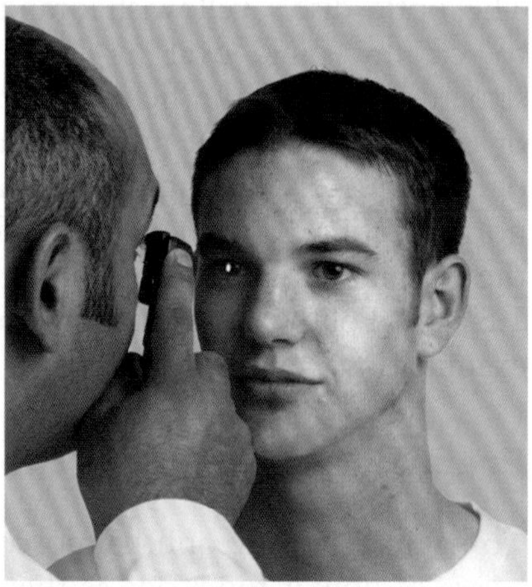

FIGURE 11-30 Examiner at a 15-degree angle from the patient's line of vision, eliciting the red reflex.

BOX 11-3 STEPS FOR EXAMINING THE OPTIC DISC AND THE RETINA

The Optic Disc

- Initially the red reflex comes into view; the nurse needs to be able to look through the red reflex to visualize the arteries and veins.
- Follow the blood vessels as they get wider. Follow the vessels medially toward the nose and look for the round yellowish orange structure described earlier as the optic disc.

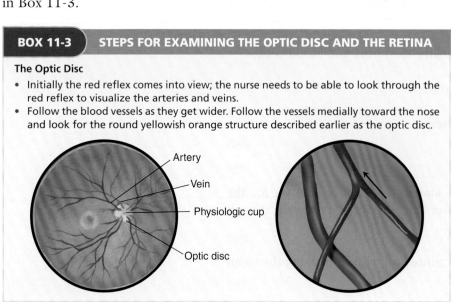

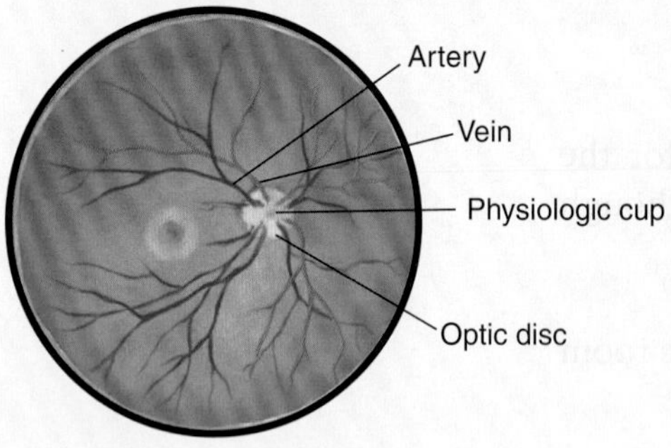

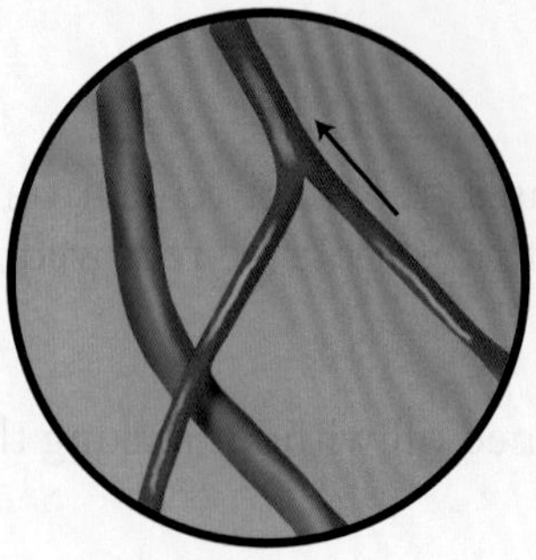

BOX 11-3 STEPS FOR EXAMINING THE OPTIC DISC AND THE RETINA (*Continued*)

- Now, *bring the optic disc into sharp focus* by adjusting the lens of your ophthalmoscope. If both you and the patient have no refractive errors, the retina should be in focus at 0 diopters. If structures are blurred, rotate the lens disc until you find the sharpest focus.

CLINICAL TIP

In a *refractive error*, light rays from a distance do not focus on the retina. In *myopia*, they focus anterior to it and in *hyperopia*, posterior to it. Retinal structures in a myopic eye look larger than normal (Holden et al., 2016).

- For example, if the patient is myopic (nearsighted), rotate the lens disc counterclockwise to the minus diopters (red); in a hyperopic (farsighted) patient, move the disc clockwise to the plus diopters (black). You can correct your own refractive error in the same way.
- *Inspect the optic disc*. Note the following features:
  - *The sharpness or clarity of the disc outline*. The nasal portion of the disc margin may be somewhat blurred, a normal finding.
  - *The color of the disc*, normally yellowish orange to creamy pink. White or pigmented crescents may ring the disc, a normal finding.
  - *The size of the central physiologic cup*, if present. It is usually yellowish white. The horizontal diameter is usually less than half the horizontal diameter of the disc.

CLINICAL TIP

An enlarged cup suggests chronic open-angle glaucoma.

- *The comparative symmetry* of the eyes and findings in the fundi.

Normal variations of the optic disc are outlined in Table 11-8 and abnormalities in Table 11-9.

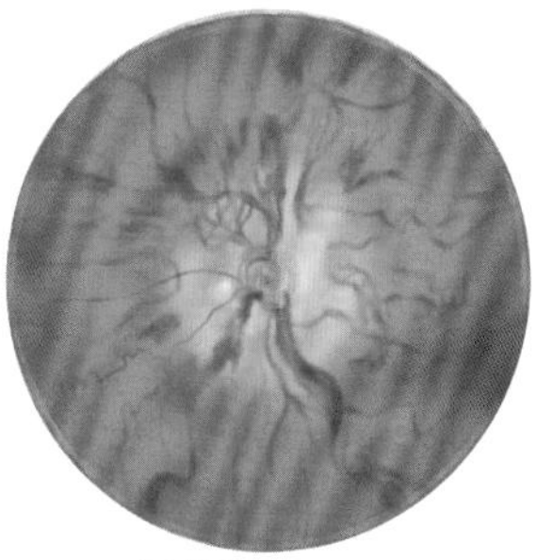

PAPILLEDEMA

Detecting Papilledema

Papilledema describes swelling of the optic disc and anterior bulging of the physiologic cup. Increased intracranial pressure is transmitted to the optic nerve, causing edema of the optic nerve. Papilledema often signals serious disorders of the brain, such as meningitis, subarachnoid hemorrhage, trauma, and mass lesions, so searching for this important disorder is a priority during all your funduscopic examinations.

The Retina—Arteries, Veins, Fovea, and Macula

- *Inspect the retina*, including arteries and veins as they extend to the periphery, arteriovenous crossings, the fovea, and the macula. Distinguish arteries from veins based on the following features. Darker retinas correlate with darker irises. Those with light retinas tend to have better night vision but are more sensitive to bright light (Holmes & Levi, 2018).
- *Follow the vessels peripherally in each of four directions*, noting their relative sizes and the character of the arteriovenous crossings.
- Identify any lesions of the surrounding *retina* and note the size, shape, color, and distribution. As you search the retina, *move your head and instrument as a unit*, using the patient's pupil as an imaginary fulcrum. At first, you may repeatedly lose your view of the retina because your light falls out of the pupil. You will improve with practice.
- Lesions of the retina can be measured in terms of "disc diameters" from the optic disc.

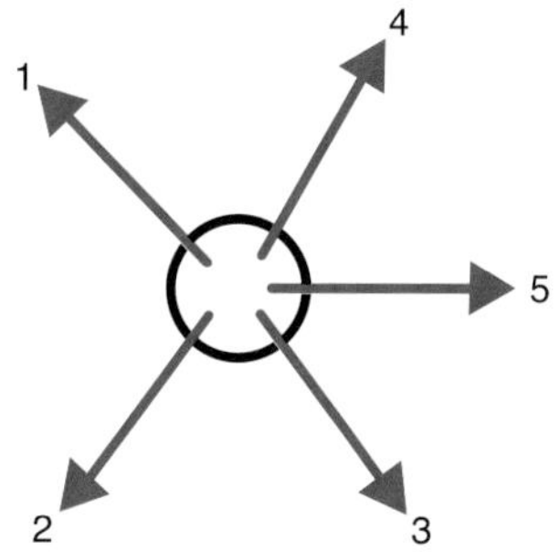

Sequence of inspection from disc to macula in the left eye

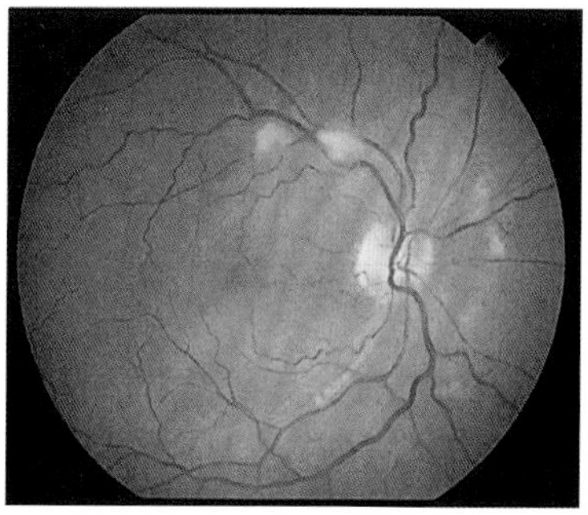

Note the irregular "cotton-wool" patches between 11 and 12 o'clock, 1 to 2 disc diameters from the disc each measures about 1/2 × 1/2 disc diameters.

(*continued*)

BOX 11-3 **STEPS FOR EXAMINING THE OPTIC DISC AND THE RETINA** ***(Continued)***

Tables 11-10, 11-11, and 11-12 outline normal and abnormal fundus and retina findings.

- Inspect the *fovea and surrounding macula.* Direct your light beam laterally or by asking the patient to look directly into the light. Except in older people, the tiny bright reflection at the center of the fovea helps orient you. Shimmering light reflections in the macular area are common in young people.

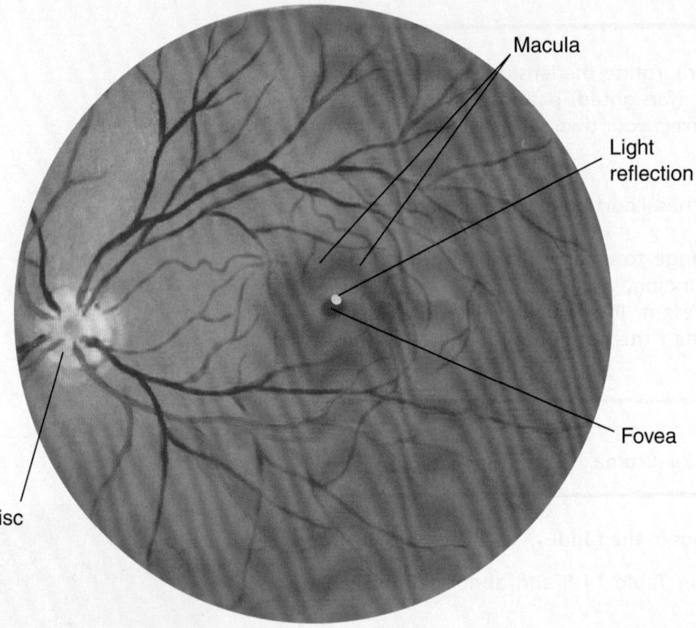

Macular degeneration is an important cause of poor central vision in the elderly. Types include *dry atrophic* (more common but less severe) and *wet exudative,* or neovascular. Undigested cellular debris, called *drusen,* may be hard and sharply defined, as seen below, or soft and confluent with altered pigmentation.

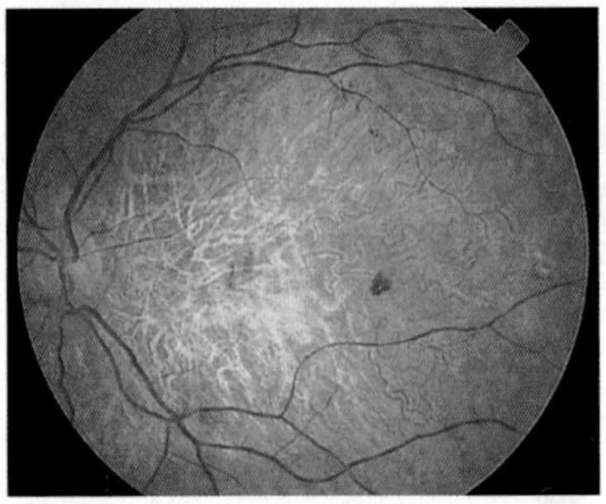

Macular degeneration. Photo from Tasman, W., & Jaeger, E., Eds. (2001). *The Wills Eye hospital atlas of clinical ophthalmology* (2nd ed.). Lippincott Williams & Wilkins.

- *Inspect the anterior structures.* Look for opacities in the *vitreous* or *lens* by rotating the lens disc progressively to diopters of around +10 or +12. This technique allows you to focus on the more anterior structures in the eye. Vitreous floaters may be seen as dark specks or strands between the fundus and the lens. Cataracts are densities in the lens (see Table 11-5).

	Arteries	**Veins**
Color	Light red	Dark red
Size	Smaller (2/3 to 3/4 the diameter of veins)	Larger
Light reflex (*reflection*)	Bright	Inconspicuous or absent

TABLE 11-8 Normal Variations of the Optic Disc

Physiologic Cupping

The physiologic cup is a small whitish depression in the optic disc from which the retinal vessels appear to emerge. Although sometimes absent, the cup is usually visible either centrally or toward the temporal side of the disc. Grayish spots are often seen at its base.

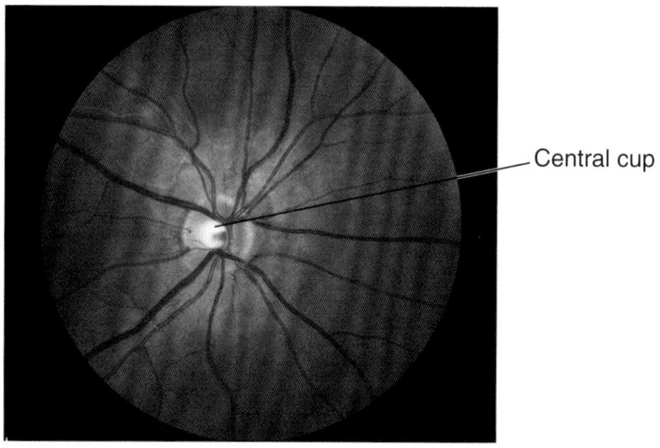

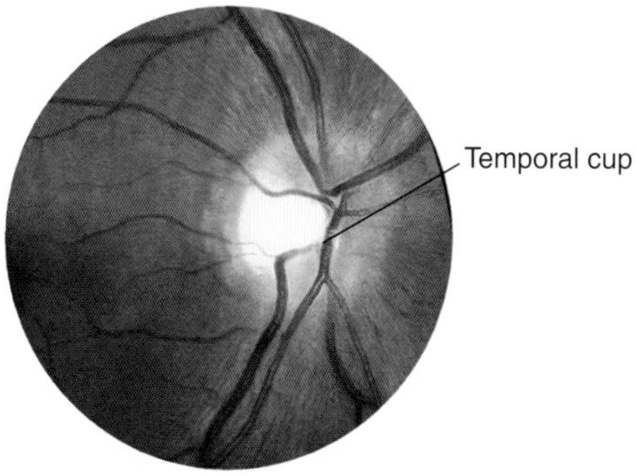

Rings and Crescents

Rings and crescents are often seen around the optic disc. These are developmental variations in which you can glimpse either white sclera, black retinal pigment, or both, especially along the temporal border of the disc. Rings and crescents are not part of the disc itself and should not be included in your estimates of disc diameters.

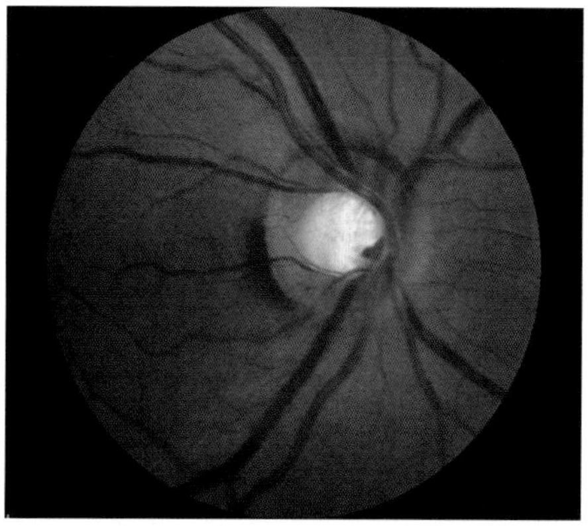

Medullated Nerve Fibers

Medullated nerve fibers are a much less common but dramatic finding. Appearing as irregular white patches with feathered margins, they obscure the disc edge and retinal vessels. They have no pathologic significance.

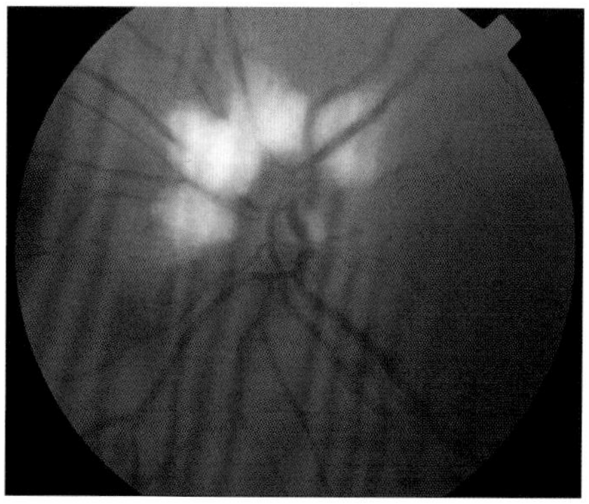

TABLE 11-9 Abnormalities of the Optic Disc

	Process	Appearance	Example
Normal	Tiny disc vessels give normal color to the disc.	Color yellowish orange to creamy pink Disc vessels tiny Disc margins sharp (except perhaps nasally) The physiologic cup is located centrally or somewhat temporally. It may be conspicuous or absent. Its diameter from side to side is usually less than half that of the disc.	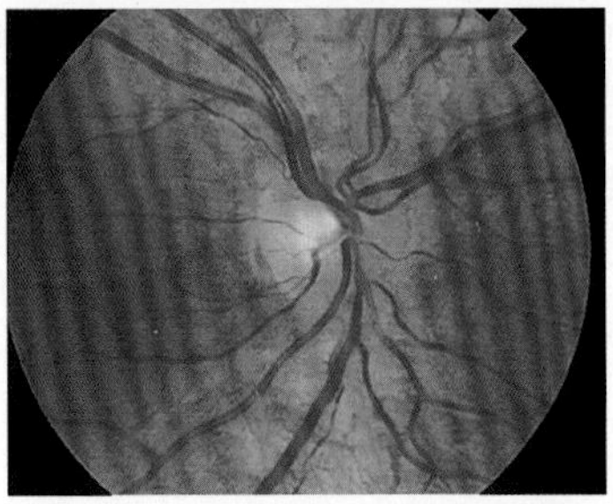
Papilledema	Venous stasis leads to engorgement and swelling.	Color pink, hyperemic Often with loss of venous pulsations Disc vessels more visible, more numerous, curve over the borders of the disc Disc swollen with margins blurred The physiologic cup is not visible.	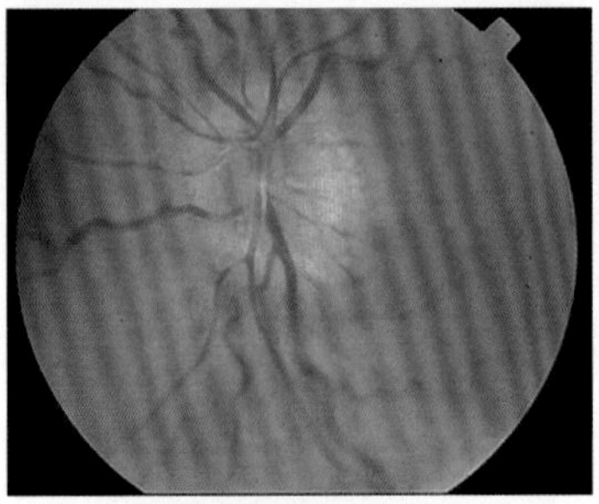
Glaucomatous Cupping	Increased pressure within the eye leads to increased cupping (backward depression of the disc) and atrophy.	The physiologic cup is enlarged, occupying more than half of the disc's diameter, at times extending to the edge of the disc. Retinal vessels sink in and under it, and may be displaced nasally. The base of the enlarged cup is pale.	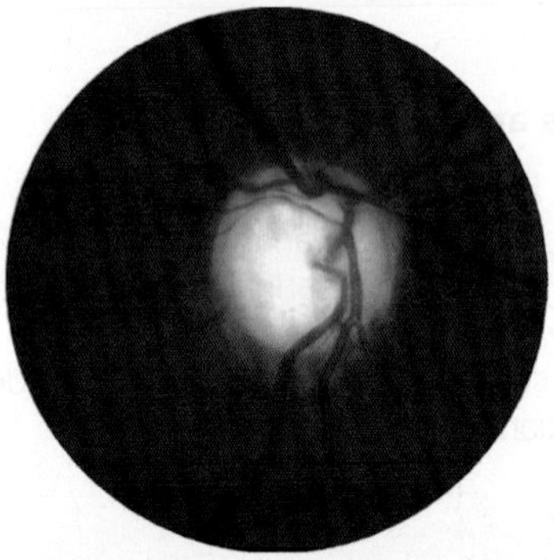
Optic Atrophy	Death of optic nerve fibers leads to loss of the tiny disc vessels.	Color white Tiny disc vessels absent	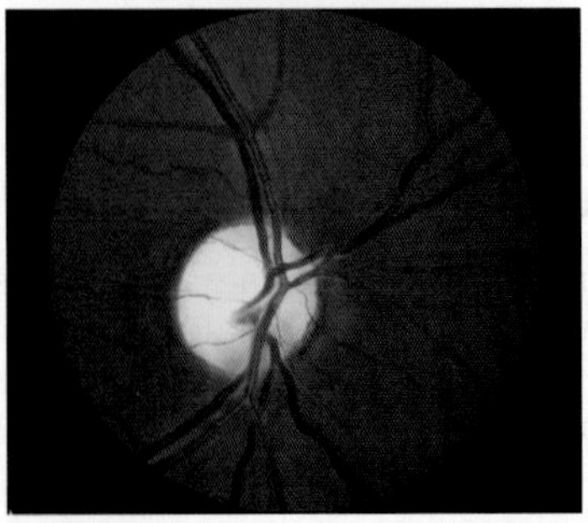

Sources of photos for Normal—Tasman, W., & Jaeger, E., Eds. (2001). *The wills eye hospital atlas of clinical ophthalmology* (2nd ed.). Lippincott Williams & Wilkins; Papilledema, Glaucomatous Cupping, Optic Atrophy—Courtesy of Kenn Freedman, MD.

TABLE 11-10 Ocular Fundi: Normal and Hypertensive Retinopathy

Normal Fundus of a Fair-Skinned Person

Inspect the optic disc. Follow the major vessels in four directions, noting their relative sizes and any arteriovenous crossings, both normal here. Inspect the macular area. The slightly darker fovea is just discernible; no light reflex is visible in this subject. Look for any lesions in the retina. Note the striped, or tessellated, character of the fundus, especially in the lower field, that comes from normal underlying choroidal vessels.

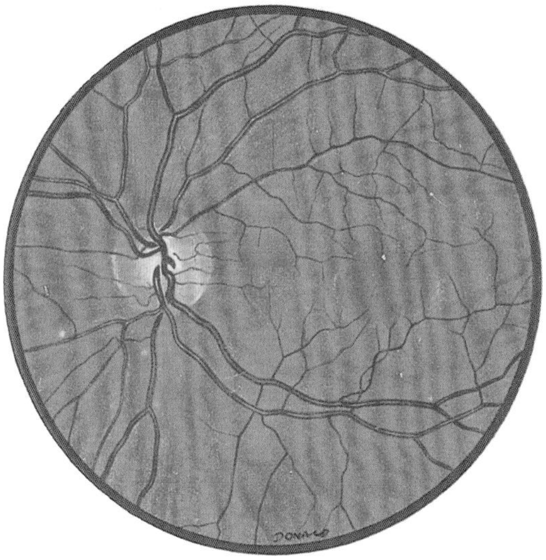

Normal Fundus of a Dark-Skinned Person

Again, inspect the disc, vessels, macula, and retina. The ring around the fovea is a normal light reflection. The color of the fundus has a grayish brown, almost purplish cast, which comes from pigment in the retina and the choroid that characteristically obscures the choroidal vessels; no tessellation is visible. The fundus of a light-skinned person with brunette coloring is redder.

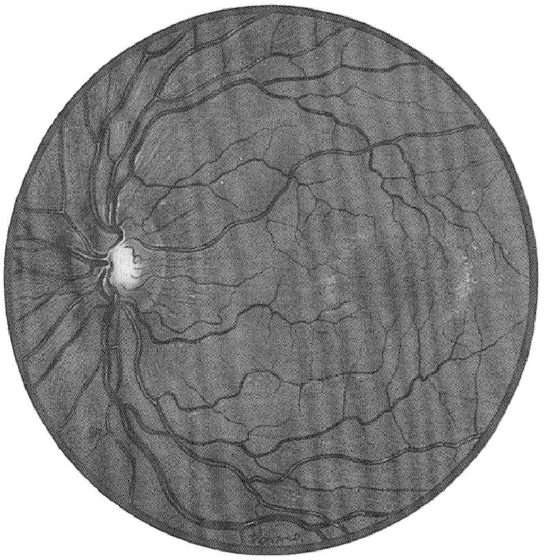

Hypertensive Retinopathy (Modi & Arsiwalla, 2020)

Marked arteriolar–venous crossing changes are seen, especially along the inferior vessels. Copper wiring of the arterioles is present. A cotton-wool spot is seen just superior to the disc. Incidental disc drusen are also present but are unrelated to hypertension.

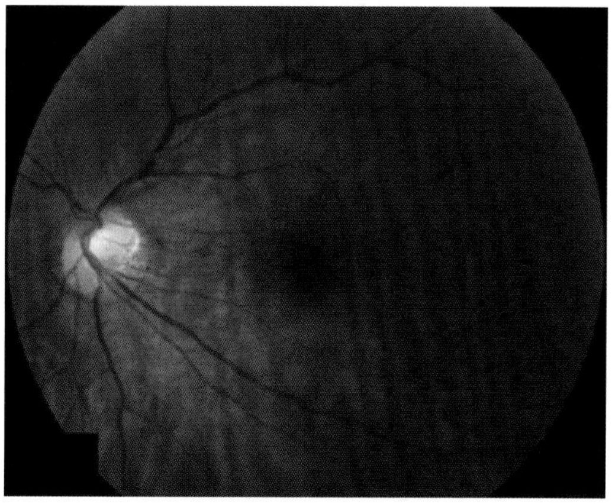

(continued)

TABLE 11-10 Ocular Fundi: Normal and Hypertensive Retinopathy (*Continued*)

Hypertensive Retinopathy with Macular Star

Punctate exudates are readily visible; some are scattered, and others radiate from the fovea to form a macular star. Note the two small, soft exudates about 1 disc diameter from the disc. Find the flame-shaped hemorrhages sweeping toward 7 o'clock and 8 o'clock; a few more may be seen toward 10 o'clock. These fundi show changes typical of accelerated (malignant) hypertension and are often accompanied by a papilledema.

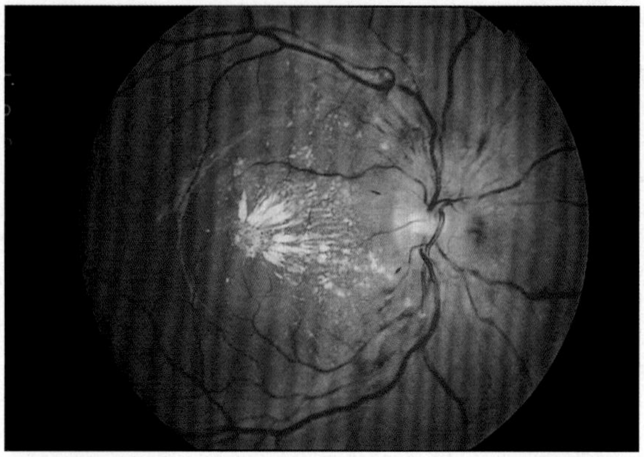

Source of photos: *Hypertensive Retinopathy*—Reprinted with permission from Wu, G. (2010). *Diabetic retinopathy: The essentials*. Wolters Kluwer; *Hypertensive Retinopathy with Macular Star*—Tasman, W., & Jaeger, E., Eds. (2001). *The wills eye hospital atlas of clinical ophthalmology* (2nd ed.). Lippincott Williams & Wilkins; Modi, P., & Arsiwalla, T. (2020). Hypertensive retinopathy. In: *StatPearls*. StatPearls Publishing.

TABLE 11-11 Ocular Fundi: Diabetic Retinopathy

Carefully study the fundi in this series of photographs. They represent a national standard used by ophthalmologists to assess diabetic retinopathy.

Nonproliferative Retinopathy, Moderately Severe

Note tiny red dots or microaneurysms. Note also the ring of hard exudates (white spots) located superotemporally. Retinal thickening or edema in the area of the hard exudates can impair visual acuity if it extends into the center of the macula (detection requires specialized stereoscopic examination).

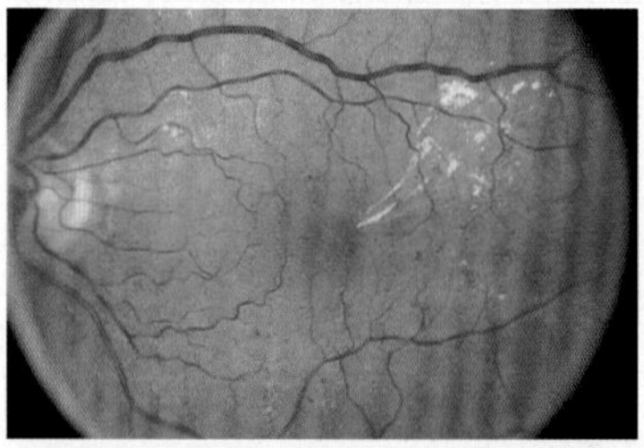

Nonproliferative Retinopathy, Severe

In the superior temporal quadrant, note the large retinal hemorrhage between two cotton-wool patches, beading of the retinal vein just above them, and tiny tortuous retinal vessels above the superior temporal artery.

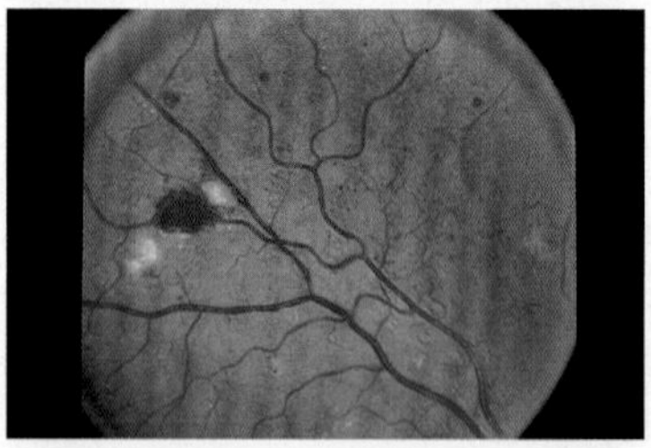

Proliferative Retinopathy with Neovascularization

Note new preretinal vessels arising on the disc and extending across the disc margins. Visual acuity is still normal, but the risk for visual loss is high (photocoagulation reduces this risk by >50%).

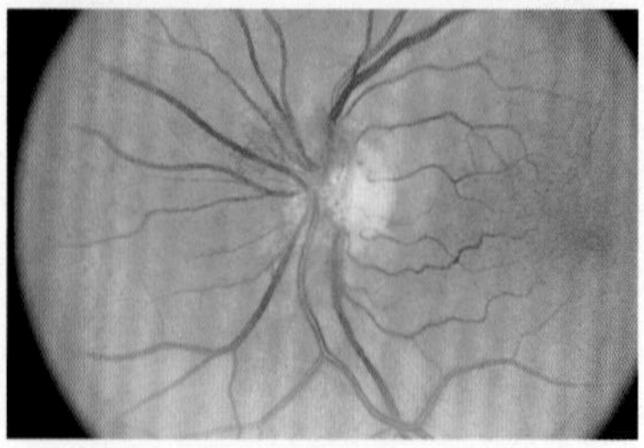

Proliferative Retinopathy, Advanced

This is the same eye, but 2 years later and without treatment. Neovascularization has increased, now with fibrous proliferations, distortion of the macula, and reduced visual acuity.

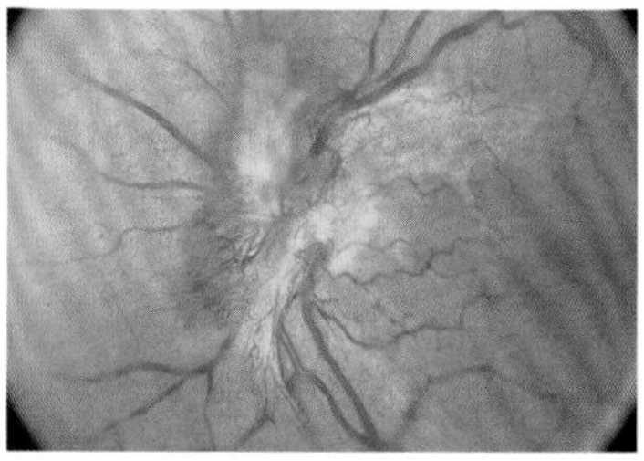

Source of photos: Nonproliferative Retinopathy, Moderately Severe; Proliferative Retinopathy, with Neovascularization; Nonproliferative Retinopathy, Severe; Proliferative Retinopathy, Advanced—Early Treatment Diabetic Retinopathy Study Research Group. Courtesy of MF Davis, MD, University of Wisconsin, Madison; Swain, T., & McGwin, G., Jr. (2020). The Prevalence of eye injury in the United States, estimates from a meta-analysis. *Ophthalmic Epidemiol*, *27*(3), 186–193. https://doi.org/10.1080/09286586.2019.1704794

TABLE 11-12 Retinal Arteries and Arteriovenous Crossings: Normal and Hypertensive

Normal Retinal Artery and Arteriovenous (A-V) Crossing

The normal arterial wall is transparent. Only the column of blood within it can usually be seen. The normal light reflex is *narrow—about one fourth the diameter of the blood column.* Because the arterial wall is transparent, a vein crossing beneath the artery can be seen right up to the column of blood on either side.

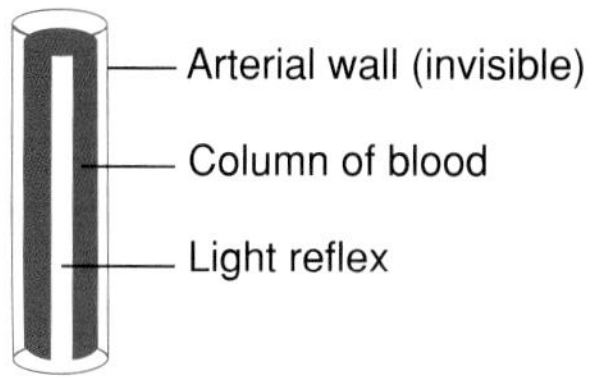

A normal transparent arterial wall.

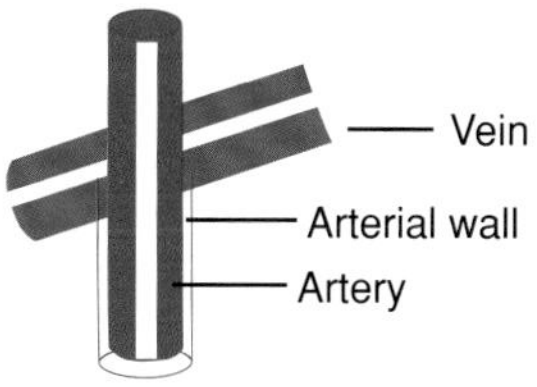

A vein crossing beneath the artery.

Retinal Arteries in Hypertension

In hypertension, the arteries may show areas of focal or generalized narrowing. The light reflex is also narrowed. The arterial wall thickens and becomes less transparent.

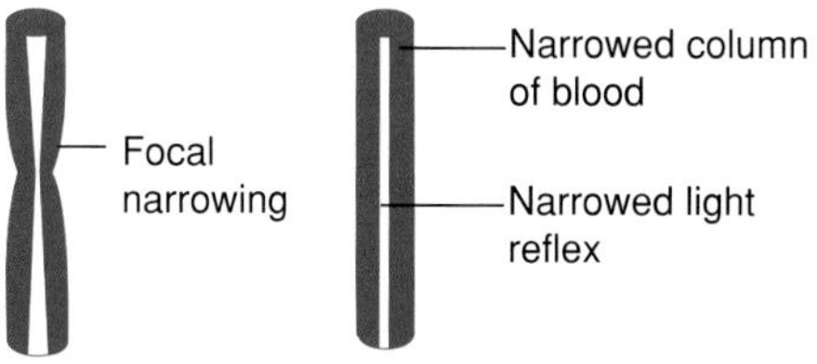

Copper Wiring

Sometimes the arteries, especially those close to the disc, become full and somewhat tortuous and develop an increased light reflex with a bright coppery luster.

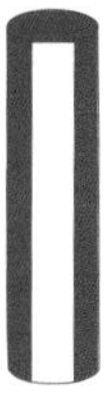

(*continued*)

TABLE 11-12 Retinal Arteries and Arteriovenous Crossings: Normal and Hypertensive (*Continued*)

Silver Wiring

Occasionally a portion of a narrowed artery develops such an opaque wall that no blood is visible within it. It is then called a silver wire artery.

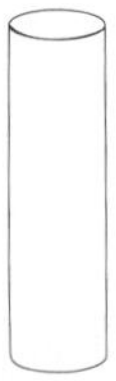

Arteriovenous Crossing

When the arterial walls lose their transparency, changes appear in the arteriovenous crossings. Decreased transparency of the retina probably also contributes to the first two changes shown below.

Concealment or A-V Nicking

The vein appears to stop abruptly on either side of the artery.

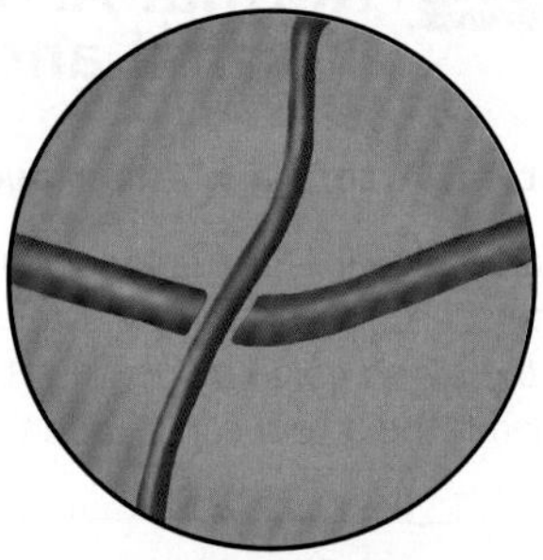

Tapering

The vein appears to taper down on either side of the artery.

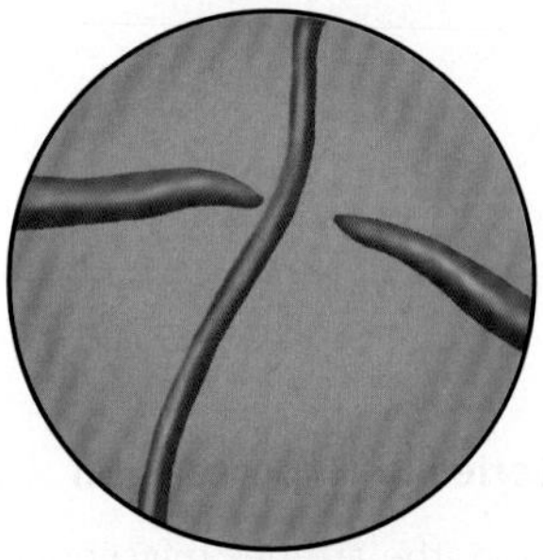

Banking

The vein is twisted on the distal side of the artery and forms a dark, wide knuckle.

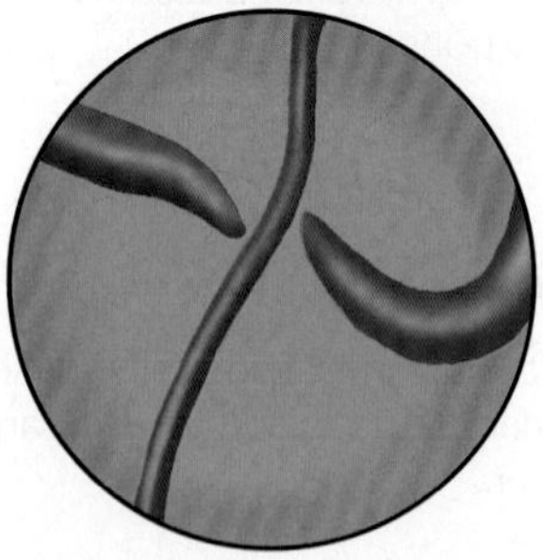

SPECIAL TECHNIQUES

For Nasolacrimal Duct Obstruction

Testing for nasolacrimal duct obstruction helps identify the cause of excessive tearing. Ask the patient to look up. Press on the lower lid close to the medial **canthus**, just inside the rim of the bony orbit—this compresses the lacrimal sac (Fig. 11-31). Look for fluid regurgitated out of the puncta into the eye. Avoid this test if the area is inflamed and tender.

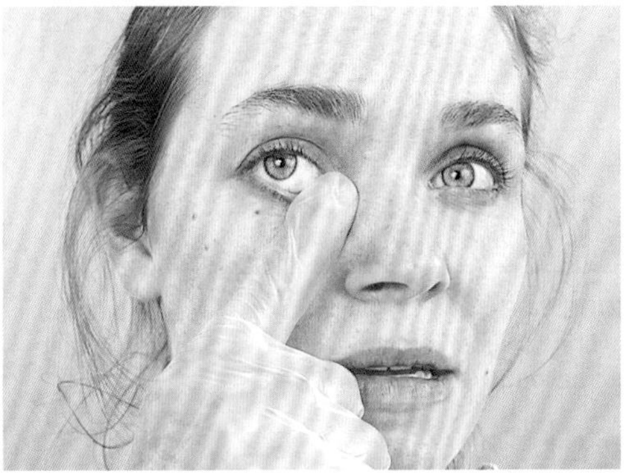

FIGURE 11-31 Assessment of the nasolacrimal duct.

CLINICAL TIP
Discharge of mucopurulent fluid from the puncta suggests an obstructed nasolacrimal duct.

Inspection of the Upper Palpebral Conjunctiva

Adequate examination of the eye in search of a foreign body requires eversion of the upper eyelid. Follow these steps:

- Instruct the patient to look down. Have the patient relax the eyes with reassurance and gentle, assured, and deliberate movements. Raise the upper eyelid slightly so that the eyelashes protrude, and then grasp the upper eyelashes and pull them gently down and forward (Fig. 11-32).

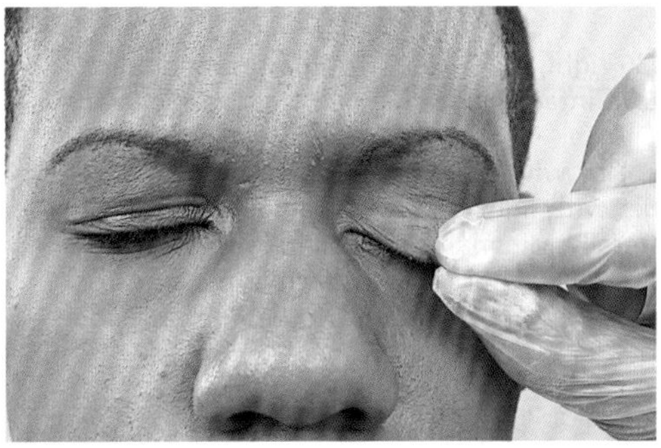

FIGURE 11-32 Grasp the eyelashes, pulling them down and forward.

- Place a small stick such as an applicator or a tongue blade at least 1 cm above the lid margin (and therefore at the upper border of the tarsal plate) (Fig. 11-33). Push down on the stick as you raise the edge of the lid, thus everting the eyelid or turning it “inside out.” Do not press on the eyeball itself.

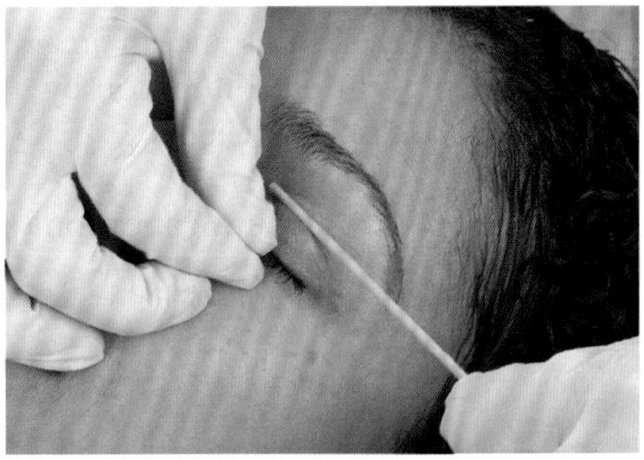

FIGURE 11-33 Place an applicator stick at the upper border of the tarsal plate.

- Secure the upper lashes against the eyebrow and inspect the palpebral conjunctiva (Fig. 11-34). After your inspection, grasp the upper eyelashes and pull them gently forward. Ask the patient to look up. The eyelid will return to its normal position.

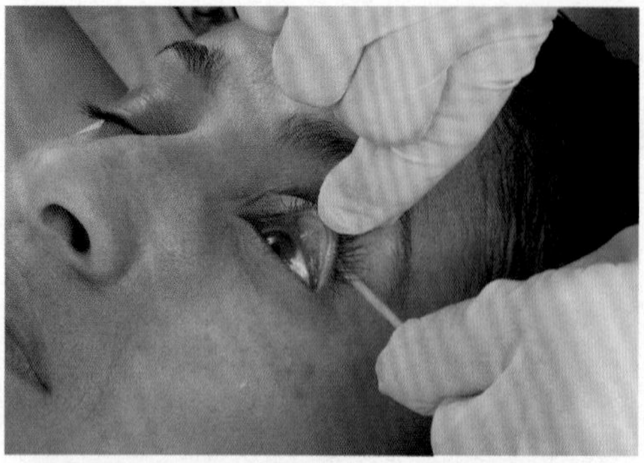

FIGURE 11-34 This view allows you to see the upper palpebral conjunctiva and look for a foreign body that might be lodged there.

RECORDING THE PHYSICAL EXAMINATION OF THE EYE

Box 11-4 includes examples of documentation of eye assessment findings.

BOX 11-4 RECORDING THE EYE EXAM—EXAMPLES

Eyes: near vision—14/14, distal vision—20/20 bilaterally, peripheral vision—visual fields full by confrontation. EOMs intact. No nystagmus. No deviations on cover–uncover test. Convergence to 7 cm.

Thick and equal hair distribution on brows and lids. Lids tan and without lesions. Palpebral fissures equal bilaterally. No edema or ptosis. Lacrimal apparatus nontender, moist without tearing or crusting. Conjunctiva pink and sclera white bilaterally. No opacities in cornea or lens bilaterally. PERRLA. Disc yellowish orange with sharp margins. No hemorrhages or exudates. No arteriolar narrowing.

OR

Eyes: near vision—14/14, distal vision 20/50 right, 20/40 left with glasses, peripheral vision—visual fields full by confrontation. EOMs intact. No nystagmus. No deviations on cover–uncover test. Convergence to 7 cm.

Thin hair distribution on brows and lids. Lids with light greenish, sticky substance matting the lashes. Lacrimal apparatus tender with light greenish drainage bilaterally. Negative lesions. Palpebral fissures equal bilaterally. Minimal edema bilaterally and L ptosis. Conjunctiva reddish and sclera white and cloudy bilaterally. No opacities in cornea or lens bilaterally. PERRLA. Disc yellowish orange with sharp margins. No hemorrhages or exudates. No arteriolar narrowing.

PERRLA: *P*upils *e*qual, *r*ound, and *r*eactive to *l*ight and *a*ccommodation

HEALTH PROMOTION, DISEASE PREVENTION, AND EDUCATION

Vision is a critical sense for experiencing the world around us and an area of importance for health promotion and disease prevention. Education by nurses is vital in maintaining vision and a healthy outlook for clients.

Important topics for health promotion, disease prevention, and education regarding the eye include:

- Vision screening
- Eye protection
- Care of contact lenses

Vision Screening

Changes in vision shift with age. Young children may experience vision changes, and the U.S. Preventive Task Force (USPSTF) recommends vision screening for all children at least once between the ages of 3 and 5 years old to detect amblyopia or its risk factors (Jonas et al., 2017). **Amblyopia**, also known as "lazy eye," affects approximately 3% of preschool children (Holmes & Levi, 2018). This loss of vision is due to an alteration in neural pathways in the developing brain which in turn decreases the visual acuity of the affected eye (Blair et al., 2020). Failure to correct amblyopia during early childhood can result in poor vision for life (Holmes & Levi, 2018).

Strabismus is eye misalignment found most frequently in infants and children up to 5 years old (Gunton et al., 2015). Screening tests for detecting amblyopia and strabismus include simple inspection, the cover–uncover test, corneal light reflex, and visual acuity tests (Blair et al., 2020).

The most common visual change in school-age children, adolescents, and young adults is refractive errors. Most school-age children are screened in school, and young adults present to their health care provider when they have changes in vision or are tested for driving examinations, employment, or physicals. The Snellen vision chart is used for the screening examination.

As aging occurs, cataracts, macular degeneration, and glaucoma become more prevalent (National Academies of Sciences, Engineering, & Medicine; Health, & Medicine Division 2016). These disorders reduce awareness of the social and physical environment and contribute to falls and injuries. To improve detection of visual defects, test visual acuity with a Snellen chart or near vision card. Examine the lens and fundi for clouding of the lens (*cataracts*); mottling of the *macula*; variations in the retinal pigmentation; subretinal hemorrhage or exudate (*macular degeneration*); and change in the size and color of the optic cup or visual field defects (*glaucoma*) (Flint & Tadi, 2020).

Eye Protection

Eye injuries and trauma can occur in the home, during recreational activities, and in a place of employment. Protective eyewear should be used when there is a chance of injury to the eye. Eye injury can result from numerous causes, for example, chemical splashes from cleaning supplies, metal shards or rocks flying when mowing the lawn, sports injuries, body fluids entering the eye, and many more (Swain & McGwin, 2020; Toldi & Thomas, 2020). The activities and environments in which people work and play should be assessed and precautions taken to avoid eye injury and promote healthy habits. Emergency eye care education is important so individuals know how to react when something such as chemicals or a blunt object, enters the eye, or when there is a cut around the eye (Dua et al., 2020; Swain & McGwin, 2020). Additional education includes avoidance of direct sunlight and use of sunglasses to protect the eyes from ultraviolet radiation, and individuals working with chemicals should be taught how to use devices to flush eyes and/or skin if they come into contact with chemicals.

Care of Contact Lenses

Infections can occur and injure the eye if contact lenses are not cared for properly. Patients should remember to wash their hands when inserting or removing lenses, to wear and remove them as prescribed by the health care provider, and to keep them clean and not share them with others. If patients are using solutions, they should discard unused portions at the expiration date. Contact lens wearers may become too familiar with the routine and may need reminders that putting anything into the eye, including contacts, may cause damage if not done correctly. Contact lenses should be inspected by a lens specialist once a year for scratches or damage that can injure the eye.

BIBLIOGRAPHY

CITATIONS

Blair, K., Cibis, G., & Gulani, A. C. (2020). Amblyopia. [Updated 2020 August 10.] In: *StatPearls [Internet]*. StatPearls Publishing. https://www-ncbi-nlm-nih-gov.proxy.library.upenn.edu/books/NBK430890/

Boyd, K. (2019). Visual field testing. American Academy of Ophthalmology. Retrieved September 4, 2020, from https://www.aao.org/eye-health/tips-prevention/visual-field-testing

Chang, S. (2017). Biomedicine: An improved gel for detached retinas. *Nature (London)*, *543*(7645), 319–320.

Doshi, R., & Noohani, T. (2020). Subconjunctival hemorrhage. In: *StatPearls*. StatPearls Publishing.

Dua, H. S., Ting, D. S. J., Al Saadi, A., & Said, D. G. (2020). Chemical eye injury: Pathophysiology, assessment and management. *Eye (Lond)*, *34*(11), 2001–2019. https://doi.org/10.1038/s41433-020-1026-6

Flint, B., & Tadi, P. (2020). Physiology, aging. [Updated 2020 March 21]. In: *StatPearls [Internet]*. StatPearls Publishing. https://www-ncbi-nlm-nih-gov.proxy.library.upenn.edu/books/NBK556106/

Gunton, K. B., Wasserman, B. N., & DeBenedictis, C. (2015). Strabismus. *Primary Care*, *42*(3), 393–407. https://doi.org/10.1016/j.pop.2015.05.006

Holden, B. A., Fricke, T. R., Wilson, D. A., Jong, M., Naidoo, K. S., Sankaridurg, P., Wong, T. Y., Naduvilath, T. J., & Resnikoff, S. (2016). Global prevalence of myopia and high myopia and temporal trends from 2000 through 2050. *Ophthalmology*, *123*(5), 1036–1042. https://doi.org/10.1016/j.ophtha.2016.01.006

Holmes, J. M., & Levi, D. M. (2018). Treatment of amblyopia as a function of age. *Visual Neuroscience*, *35*, E015. https://doi.org/10.1017/S0952523817000220

Jonas, D. E., Amick, H. R., Wallace, I. F., Feltner, C., Schaaf, E. B. V., Brown, C. L., & Baker, C. (2017). Vision Screening in Children Ages 6 Months to 5 Years: A Systematic Review for the U.S. Preventive Services Task Force [Internet]. Agency for Healthcare Research and Quality (US); (Evidence Synthesis, No. 153). https://www.ncbi.nlm.nih.gov/books/NBK487841/

Mandai, M., Watanabe, A., Kurimoto, Y., Hirami, Y., Morinaga, C., Daimon, T., Fujihara, M., Akimaru, H., Sakai, N., Shibata, Y., Terada, M., Nomiya, Y., Tanishima, S., Nakamura, M., Kamao, H., Sugita, S., Onishi, A., Ito, T., Fujita, K., … Takahashi, M. (2017). Autologous induced stem-cell–derived retinal cells for macular degeneration. *The New England Journal of Medicine*, *376*(11), 1038–1046.

Modi, P., & Arsiwalla, T. (2020). Hypertensive retinopathy. In: *StatPearls*. StatPearls Publishing.

Narayana, S., & McGee, S. (2015). Bedside diagnosis of the 'Red Eye': A systematic review. *American Journal of Medicine*, *128*(11), 1220–1224.e1.

National Academies of Sciences, Engineering, and Medicine; Health and Medicine Division. (2016). Board on Population Health and Public Health Practice; Committee on Public Health Approaches to Reduce Vision Impairment and Promote Eye Health; Welp, A., Woodbury, R. B., & McCoy, M. A, et al. (Eds.). *Making Eye Health a Population Health Imperative: Vision for Tomorrow*. National Academies Press (US); Understanding the Epidemiology of Vision Loss and Impairment in the United States. https://www-ncbi-nlm-nih-gov.proxy.library.upenn.edu/books/NBK402366/

Petsas, A., Chapman, G., & Stewart, R. (2017). Acute angle closure glaucoma – A potential blind spot in critical care. *Journal of the Intensive Care Society*, *18*(3), 244–246.

Pohl, H., & Tarnutzer, A. A. (2018). Acute angle-closure glaucoma. *The New England Journal of Medicine*, *378*(10), e14.

Preziosa, P., Comi, G., & Filippi, M. (2016). Optic neuritis in multiple sclerosis: Looking from a patient's. *Neurology*, *87*(3), 338–339.

Ryder, E. C., & Benson, S. (2020). Conjunctivitis. In: *StatPearls*. StatPearls Publishing.

Swain, T., & McGwin, G., Jr. (2020). The Prevalence of eye injury in the United States, estimates from a meta-analysis. *Ophthalmic Epidemiol*, *27*(3), 186–193. https://doi.org/10.1080/09286586.2019.1704794

Toldi, J. P., & Thomas, J. L. (2020). Evaluation and management of sports-related eye injuries. *Current Sports Medicine Reports*, *19*(1), 29–34. https://doi.org/10.1249/JSR.0000000000000677

12 EARS, NOSE, MOUTH, AND THROAT

KEY TERMS

acoustic	hematemesis	tinnitus
aphthous	hemoptysis	turbinate
dysphagia	labyrinth	tympanic
epistaxis	otalgia	vertigo
furuncle	otorrhea	vestibule
helix	presbycusis	

Learning Objectives

The student will:

1. Identify the structures and function of the ear, nose, mouth, and throat.
2. Obtain a health history of the ear, nose, mouth, and throat.
3. Describe the physical examination techniques to evaluate the ear, nose, mouth, and throat.
4. Demonstrate how to use the otoscope.
5. Document a complete ear, nose, mouth, and throat assessment utilizing information from the health history and the physical examination.
6. Identify the measures for prevention or early detection of ear, sinus, and throat infections; hearing loss; and maintenance of oral health.

The ear is the sensory organ of hearing. Critical functions of the ear are hearing and balance. During the assessment there are various signs and symptoms that signal changes in the ears. The nurse's role is to detect changes and work with the health care team to prevent infections, loss of hearing, or loss of balance.

The nose is the sensory organ of smell. The nurse assesses changes in the sense of smell as well as changes in breathing patterns and signs of sinus infections.

The mouth and throat are the first part of the digestive system, and the nurse assesses for changes in taste, eating patterns, and oral hygiene. Voice quality is also assessed. In all components of the system, the nurse assesses the patient for deviations from normal and teaches preventative practices to maintain these sensory organs.

THE EAR

The ear has three compartments: the external ear, the middle ear, and the inner ear.

The External Ear

The *external ear* is composed of the pinna (auricle) and the external ear canal (Fig. 12-1). The pinna consists chiefly of cartilage covered by skin and has a firm elastic consistency. Its prominent curved outer ridge is the **helix**. Parallel and anterior to the helix is another curved prominence, the *antihelix*. Inferiorly is the fleshy projection of the earlobe, or *lobule*. The ear canal opens behind the *tragus*, a triangular nodular area pointing backward over the entrance to the canal.

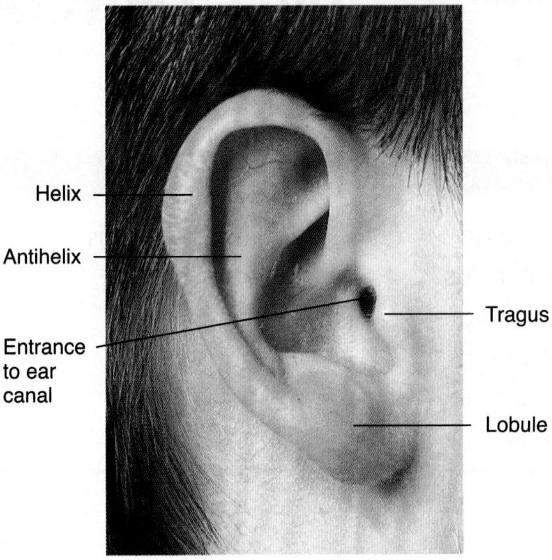

FIGURE 12-1 Landmarks of the external ear.

The function of the pinna is to gather sound waves and funnel them down the ear canal to assist in localization of sound.

The *external ear canal* or the external **acoustic** (sound or hearing) meatus curves inward and is made up of cartilage and bone. Cartilage surrounds the outer two thirds. The skin in this area is hairy and contains glands that produce cerumen (wax). The inner third of the canal is surrounded by bone and lined by thin, hairless skin. Pressure on this latter area causes pain—a point to remember when you examine the ear.

Behind the ear and below the ear canal is the mastoid part of the temporal bone. The lowest portion of this bone, the *mastoid process*, is palpable behind the lobule.

At the end of the ear canal, lies the **tympanic** membrane (TM). The TM is a thin, semitransparent membrane that divides the external and middle ear.

The Middle Ear

The *middle ear* or *tympanic cavity* extends from the TM to the oval window (Fig. 12-2). The middle ear is an air-filled cavity that transmits sound

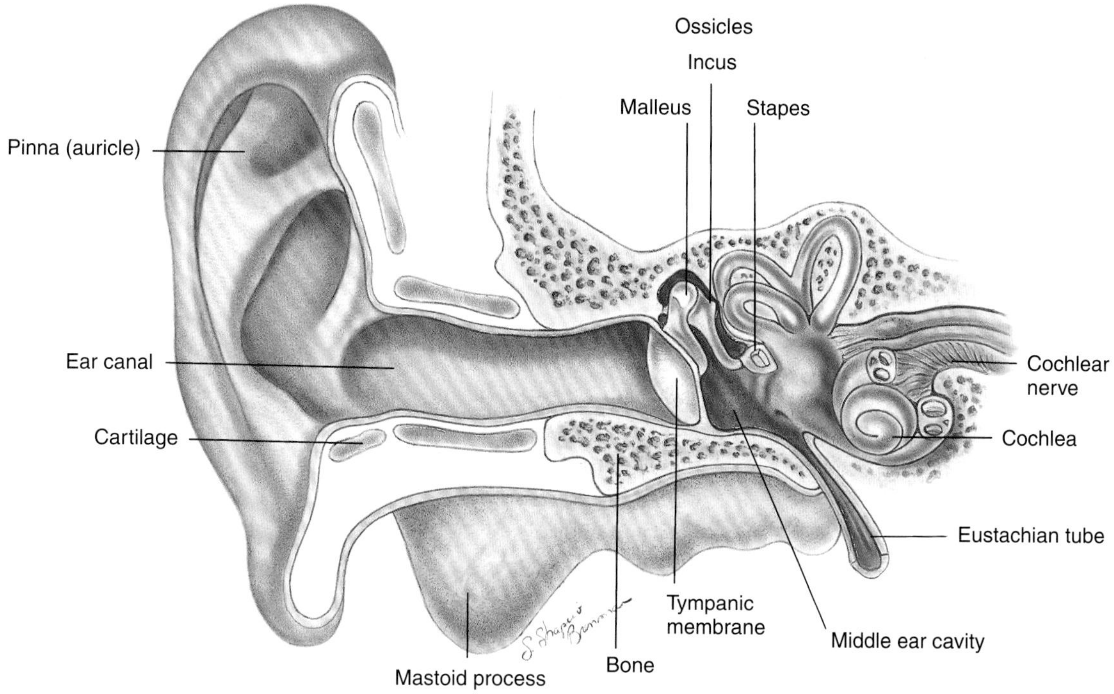

FIGURE 12-2 Landmarks of the middle and inner ear.

by way of three tiny bones, the *ossicles*: the *malleus* (hammer), the *incus* (anvil), and the *stapes* (stirrup). The ossicles transform sound vibrations into mechanical waves for the inner ear. The proximal end of the *Eustachian tube* connects the middle ear to the nasopharynx.

The *malleus* is one of the three ossicles and is attached to the medial TM. The *handle* and the *short process* of the malleus are the two chief landmarks of the TM. From the *umbo*, where the eardrum meets the tip of the malleus, a light reflection called the *cone of light* fans downward and anteriorly. Above the short process lies a small portion of the eardrum called the *pars flaccida*. The remainder of the TM is the *pars tensa*. Anterior and posterior malleolar folds, which extend obliquely upward from the short process, separate the pars flaccida from the pars tensa but are usually invisible unless the eardrum is retracted. A second ossicle, the *incus* can sometimes be seen through the drum and the third ossicle, the *stapes* is not visible.

The Inner Ear

The inner ear includes the *cochlea*, the *semicircular canals*, and the distal end of the *auditory nerve*, which is also known as the *vestibulocochlear nerve*, or acoustic nerve, *cranial nerve (CN) VIII*. Movements of the stapes vibrate the perilymph in the **labyrinth** of the semicircular canals and the hair cells and endolymph in the ducts of the cochlea, producing electrical nerve impulses transmitted by the auditory nerve to the brain. The inner ear functions to conduct sound to the central nervous system and to assist with balance.

Much of the middle ear and all of the inner ear are inaccessible to direct examination. Some inferences concerning their condition can be made, however, by testing auditory function.

Hearing Pathways

The first part of the hearing pathway, from the external ear through the middle ear, is known as the *conductive* phase. The second part of the pathway, involving the cochlea and the cochlear nerve, is called the *sensorineural* phase.

Hearing disorders of the external and middle ear cause *conductive hearing loss.* External ear causes include cerumen impaction, *otitis externa*, trauma, *squamous cell carcinoma*, and benign bony growths such as *exostoses or osteomas.* Middle ear disorders include *otitis media*, congenital conditions, cholesteatomas and otosclerosis, tumors, and perforation of the TM.

Disorders of the inner ear cause *sensorineural hearing loss* from congenital and hereditary conditions, *presbycusis*, viral infections such as *rubella* and *cytomegalovirus*, *Ménière disease*, noise exposure, ototoxic drug exposure, and *acoustic neuroma* (Eggermont, 2017).

Air conduction (Fig. 12-3) describes the normal first phase in the hearing pathway. An alternate pathway, known as *bone conduction*, bypasses the external and middle ear and is used for testing purposes. A vibrating tuning fork, placed on the head, sets the bone of the skull into vibration and stimulates the cochlea directly. In a person with intact hearing, air conduction is more sensitive than bone conduction.

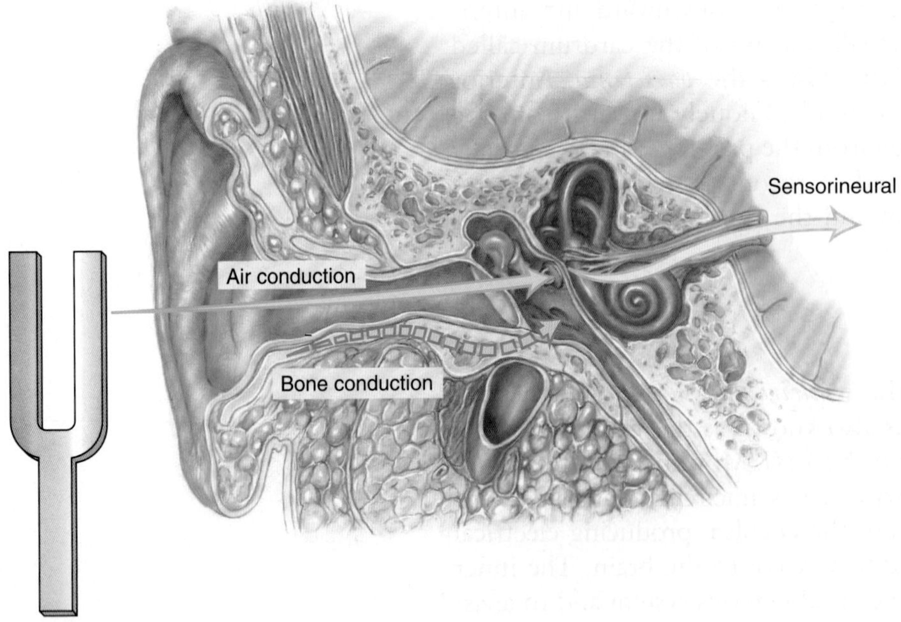

FIGURE 12-3 Air conduction.

Equilibrium

The labyrinth within the inner ear senses the position and movements of the head and helps maintain balance.

THE HEALTH HISTORY OF THE EARS

The purpose of the nursing health history of the ears is to detect changes in the patient's hearing, ears, and balance. The opening questions include "How is your hearing?" and "Have you had any trouble with your ears?"

Common or concerning symptoms related to the ears are listed in Box 12-1.

BOX 12-1 COMMON OR CONCERNING SYMPTOMS OF THE EARS

- Hearing loss
- Earache
- Discharge
- Tinnitus
- Vertigo

If the patient has noticed an ear issue, then further assessment utilizing the mnemonic "OLD CART" is helpful.

Hearing Loss

If the patient reports hearing loss, further explore the issue using "OLD CART."

- *Onset:* When did you first notice the change in your ears and/or hearing?
- *Location:* Does it involve the left ear, right ear, or both ears?
- *Duration:* How long has this been going on?
  - Did it start suddenly or gradually?
  - Is it temporary or constant?
- *Characteristic symptoms:* Do you notice any other symptoms when this occurs?
  - Have you put anything in your ear (e.g., food, dislodged pencil eraser)?
  - Has anything ever crawled or flown into your ear (e.g., bugs)?
  - Do you clean your ears with cotton swabs?
  - Does the inside of your ear ever feel itchy? If so, what do you do when this occurs?
  - Do you scratch the inside of your ear? With what?
- *Associated manifestations:* Does anything else seem to be going on at the same time?
  - Nausea? Dizziness?
  - What happened prior to the hearing loss? Did anything occur before or possibly cause the loss?
- *Relieving factors:* Does anything make it better?
- *Treatment:* Have you seen any other care provider for this?

Also ask about a preexisting history of *hearing loss*.

Hearing loss may also be congenital, from single-gene mutations (Alford & Sutton, 2011).

Try to distinguish *conductive loss*, which results from problems in the external or middle ear, from *sensorineural loss*, which are problems in the inner ear, the cochlear nerve, or its central connections in the brain. People with sensorineural loss have particular trouble understanding speech, often complaining that others mumble; noisy environments make hearing worse. With conductive loss, noisy environments may help. Two questions may be helpful: Does the patient have difficulty understanding others or avoid noisy areas? Does a noisy environment make a difference in the ability of the person to hear?

Symptoms associated with hearing loss, such as earache or vertigo, help when assessing likely causes. In addition, inquire specifically about medications that might affect hearing and ask about sustained exposure to loud noise.

Medications that affect hearing include aminoglycosides, aspirin, nonsteroidal antiinflammatory drugs (NSAIDs), quinine, and furosemide.

Earache

Complaints of an *earache*, or *pain in the ear*, are especially common. Ask about associated fever, sore throat, cough, or concurrent upper respiratory infection (URI). If any of these symptoms occur, there is an increased chance of an ear infection.

Otalgia is also known as ear pain. There are two types of otalgia. Primary otalgia occurs within or around the ear such as *otitis externa*, *otitis media*, *mastoiditis*, *or auricular infections*. Referred otalgia originates in another anatomic structure such as in the mouth, throat, or neck (Harrison & Cronin, 2016; Kim et al., 2015).

If the patient reports earaches, ask:

- *Onset:* When did the last earache occur?
  How often do you have earaches?
- *Location:* Which ear was affected?
- *Duration:* How long did it last?
- *Characteristic symptoms:* Did you have any other symptoms?
- *Associated manifestations:* What additional symptoms were occurring or what might have occurred prior to the earache?
  Did you or anyone around you have a cold, fevers, or chills?
  When was the last time you were swimming? Took a bath? Went in a hot tub? Did you go underwater?
- *Relieving factors:* What relieves the pain?
- *Treatment*: Has this been treated previously or is it being treated now?

Discharge

Ask about *discharge* or **otorrhea** from the ear, especially if it is associated with an earache or trauma.

Cerumen (wax) is normally found in the ear. The earwax tends to be yellowish to dark brown in color and of a sticky consistency. In East Asians or Native North Americans, it is usually drier and whitish to gray in color (Prokop-Prigge et al., 2015). In general, the cerumen falls out of the ear on its own or is removed with washing, but it can build up and block the ear canal. Wax blockage is one of the most common causes of hearing loss.

If the patient reports discharge, ask:

- When did you first notice the discharge?
- In which ear?
- Describe the discharge.
    - Color?
    - Presence of blood?
    - Consistency?
    - Amount?
    - Constant or intermittent drainage?
- Does anything stop the discharge? Has it gotten worse or better?
- Have you noticed any other symptoms?
    - Sore throat?
    - Cough?
    - Respiratory infection?
    - Fever?
    - Dizziness?
    - Headaches?

CLINICAL TIP
Discharge from the ear, if associated with an earache or trauma, is cause for additional assessment. *Acute otitis externa* and *acute or chronic otitis media* with perforation usually present with a yellow-green or purulent discharge. In general, the ear is painful and once a "pop" is felt, drainage occurs and the pain will resolve.

Tinnitus

Tinnitus is a perceived sound that has no external stimulus and is commonly heard as musical ringing or a rushing or roaring noise. It can involve one or both ears. Tinnitus may accompany hearing loss and often remains unexplained, though some causes may include loud noises or a side effect of a medication. Occasionally, popping sounds originate in the temporomandibular joint, or sounds from the neck vessels may be audible.

Tinnitus is a common symptom, increasing in frequency with age. When associated with hearing loss and vertigo, it is suggestive of Ménière disease.

If the patient reports tinnitus, ask:

- When did this begin?
- Is it in the left ear, right ear, or both ears?
- Is it temporary or constant?
- Do you notice any other symptoms when this occurs?

Vertigo

Vertigo refers to the perception that the patient or the environment is rotating or spinning (Table 12-1). These sensations point primarily to a problem in the labyrinths of the inner ear, peripheral lesions of CN VIII, or lesions in its central pathways or nuclei in the brain.

Vertigo is a challenging symptom. Patients differ widely in what they mean by the word "dizzy." "Are there times when you feel dizzy?" is an appropriate first question, but patients often find it difficult to be more specific. Ask "Do you feel unsteady as if you are going to fall or black out?" or "Do you feel the room is spinning or tilting (vertigo)?" Elicit information while clarifying exactly what the patient means. You may need to offer the patient several choices of wording. Ask if the patient feels pulled to the ground or off to one side and if the dizziness is related to a change in body position. Pursue any associated feelings of clamminess or flushing, nausea, or vomiting. Check which medications the patient is taking and if any may be contributing to this feeling.

CLINICAL TIP
Feeling unsteady, lightheaded, or "dizzy in the legs" sometimes suggests a cardiovascular etiology.

A feeling of being pulled suggests true vertigo from an inner ear problem or a central or peripheral lesion of CN VIII.

If the patient reports vertigo or dizziness, ask:

- When did the dizziness begin?
- Is it temporary or constant?
- How long does it last?
- What other symptoms do you experience with it?
- How does it affect your daily life? What activities of daily living are impacted due to the vertigo (e.g., avoiding steps or driving a car)?
- What makes it feel better or go away?
- When was your last ear examination? What were the results? Was any further testing necessary?

Past History

Topics to explore related to the past history of the ears include:

- Congenital hearing loss
- Removal of cerumen
- "Swimmer's ear"

TABLE 12-1 Dizziness and Vertigo

"Dizziness" is a nonspecific term used by patients encompassing several disorders that clinicians must carefully clarify. A detailed history usually identifies the primary etiology. It is important to learn the specific meanings of the following terms or conditions:

- *Vertigo*—a spinning sensation accompanied by nystagmus and ataxia; usually from *peripheral vestibular dysfunction* (~40% of "dizzy" patients) but may be from a *central brainstem lesion* (~10%; causes include atherosclerosis, multiple sclerosis, vertebrobasilar migraine, or transient ischemic attack [TIA])
- *Presyncope*—a near faint from "feeling faint or lightheaded;" causes include orthostatic hypotension, especially from medication, arrhythmias, and vasovagal attacks (~5%)
- *Dysequilibrium*—unsteadiness or imbalance when walking, especially in older patients; causes include fear of walking, visual loss, weakness from musculoskeletal problems, and peripheral neuropathy (up to 15%)
- *Psychiatric*—causes include anxiety, panic disorder, hyperventilation, depression, somatization disorder, and alcohol and substance abuse (~10%)
- *Multifactorial or unknown*—(up to 20%)

	Onset	Duration and Course	Hearing	Tinnitus	Additional Features
Peripheral Vertigo					
Benign Positional Vertigo	Sudden, often when rolling onto the affected side or tilting up the head	Onset a few seconds to <1 min Lasts a few weeks, may recur	Not affected	Absent	Sometimes nausea, vomiting nystagmus
Vestibular Neuronitis (Acute Labyrinthitis)	Sudden	Onset hours to up to 2 wk May recur over 12–18 mo	Not affected	Absent	Nausea, vomiting, nystagmus
Ménière Disease	Sudden	Onset several hours to ≥1 day Recurrent	Sensorineural hearing loss—recurs, eventually progresses	Present, fluctuating	Pressure or fullness in affected ear; nausea, vomiting, nystagmus
Drug Toxicity	Insidious or acute—linked to loop diuretics, aminoglycosides, salicylates, alcohol	May or may not be reversible Partial adaptation occurs	May be impaired	May be present	Nausea, vomiting
Acoustic Neuroma	Insidious from CN VIII compression, vestibular branch	Variable	Impaired, one side	Present	May involve CN V and VII
Central Vertigo	Often sudden (see causes above)	Variable but rarely continuous	Not affected	Absent	Usually with other brainstem deficits—dysarthria, ataxia, crossed motor and sensory deficits

Sources: Chan, Y. (2009). Differential diagnosis of dizziness. *Current Opinion in Otolaryngology & Head and Neck Surgery, 17*, 200; Kroenke, K., Lucas, C. A., Rosengerg, M. L., Scherokman, B., Herbers, J. E. Jr, Wehrle, P. A., & Boggi, J. O. (1992). Causes of persistent dizziness: a prospective study of 100 patients in ambulatory care. *Annals of Internal Medicine, 117*(11), 898–904; Tusa, R. J. (2001). Vertigo. *Neurologic Clinics. 19*, 23–55; Lockwood, A. H., Salvi, R. J., & Burkard, R. F. (2002). Tinnitus. *New England Journal of Medicine, 347*, 904; Babu, S., Schutt, C. A., & Bojrab, D. I. (2019). *Diagnosis and treatment of vestibular disorders*. Springer International Publishing; Carrillo Muñoz, R., Ballve Moreno, J. L., Villar Balboa, I., Rando Matos, Y., Cunillera Puertolas, O., Almeda Ortega, J., Perez, E. R., Curto, X. M., Ripollès, C. R., Farres, N. M., Mendez, A. M., Nova, J. C. G., Santos, M. B., Miñano, J. J. V., Erazo, D. L. P., Sánchez, A. M. H., & Grupo de estudio del vértigo en atención primaria Florida. (2019). Disability perceived by primary care patients with posterior canal benign paroxysmal positional vertigo. *BMC Family Practice*, *20*(1), 156. https://doi.org/10.1186/s12875-019-1035-3; Kovacs, E., Wang, X., & Grill, E. (2019). Economic burden of vertigo: A systematic review. *Health Economics Review*, *9*(1), 37–14. https://doi.org/10.1186/s13561-019-0258-2; and Murray, L. L. A. (2019). Vertigo. *Australasian Journal on Ageing*, *38*(4), 291. https://doi.org/10.1111/ajag.12727

Additional topics to explore related to the past history of the ears include:

- Ear surgery
- Trauma or injury to your ear(s)
- Infection
- Exposure to hazardous noise levels (e.g., work, home, war)
- History of syphilis, rubella, meningitis

Family History

Explore the following issues in the patient's family history:

- Hearing loss
- Allergies
- Smoking or exposure to cigarette smoke

Lifestyle Habits

Relevant lifestyle question to ask include:

- Have you ever been exposed to loud noises?
- What is your occupation? Hobbies (e.g., hunting)?
- Do you attend concerts? Bars? Loud places?
- Do you use headphones or earbuds to listen to music? How often? On what volume level?
- Do you use lawn mower? Power tools? Firearms?
- Do you live near a busy road or train tracks?
- Have you ever used ear plugs or protectors? Do you currently?
- Have you ever used hearing aid(s)? Which ear? Currently? At all times?
- Have you used medications or drugs that interfere with how you hear or cause dizziness? Any medications that cause ototoxicity (e.g., large doses of antibiotics infused rapidly)?

THE NOSE AND PARANASAL SINUSES

The nose has four primary functions:

1. Inspiration and expiration
2. Filtration, warmth, and moisturization of the air exchanged
3. Sensation of smell
4. Resonance of speech

The external anatomy of the nose is illustrated in Figure 12-4.

Approximately the upper third of the nose is supported by bone, the lower two thirds by cartilage. Air enters the nasal cavity through the *anterior naris* on either side, passes into the wider area known as the *vestibule*, and on through the narrow nasal passage to the nasopharynx.

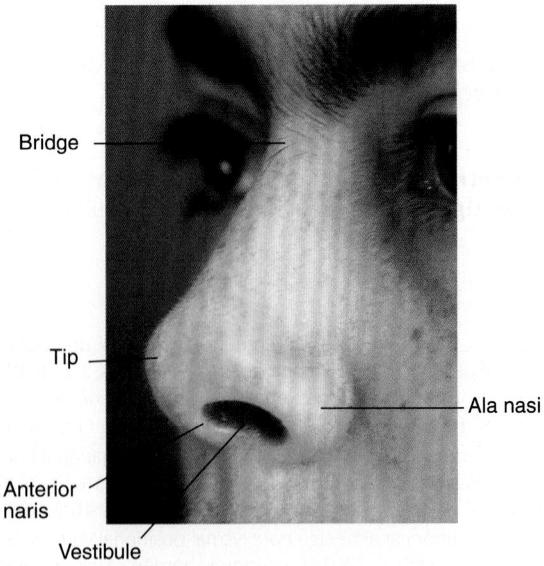

FIGURE 12-4 Landmarks of the external nose.

The medial wall of each nasal cavity is formed by the *nasal septum*, which, like the external nose, is supported by both bone and

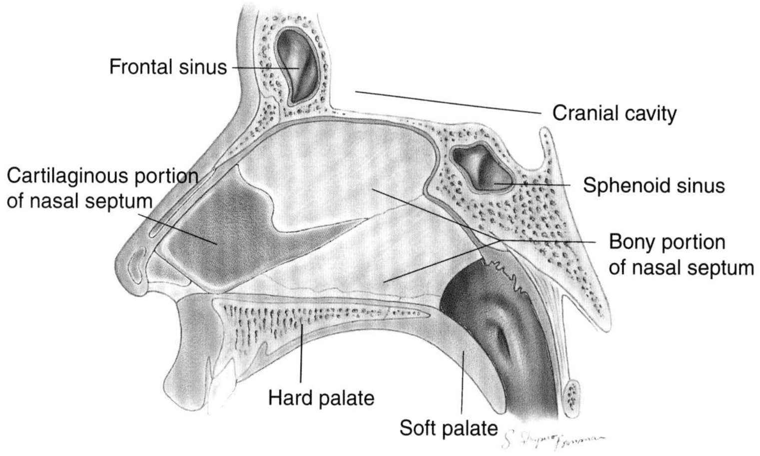

FIGURE 12-5 The medial wall of the left nasal cavity (mucosa not shown).

cartilage (Fig. 12-5). It is covered by a mucous membrane well supplied with blood. The vestibule, unlike the rest of the nasal cavity, is lined with hair-bearing skin, not mucosa.

Laterally, the anatomy is more complex (Fig. 12-6). Curving bony structures, the **turbinates**, covered by a highly vascular mucous membrane protrude into the nasal cavity (Fig. 12-7). Below each turbinate is a groove, or

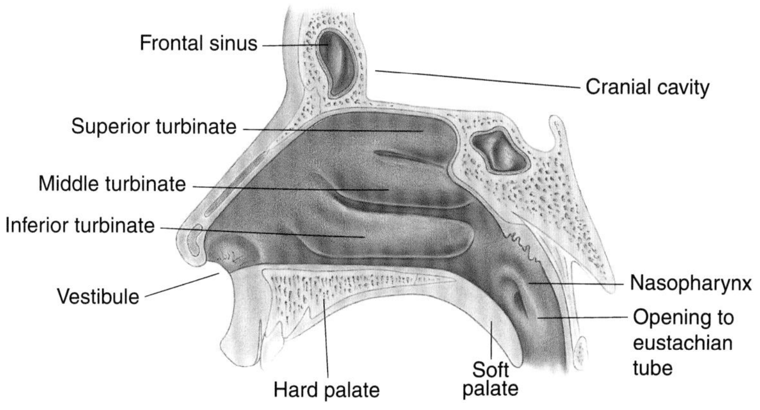

FIGURE 12-6 The lateral wall of the nasal cavity.

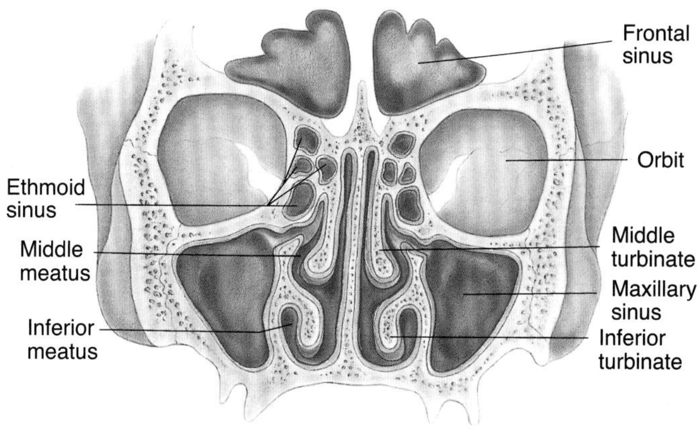

FIGURE 12-7 Anterior cross-section of the nasal cavity.

meatus, each named according to the turbinate above it. The nasolacrimal duct drains into the inferior meatus and most of the paranasal sinus drains into the middle meatus. Their openings are not usually visible.

The additional surface area provided by the turbinates and the overlying mucosa aids the nasal cavities in their principal functions: cleansing, humidification, and temperature control of inspired air.

The *paranasal sinuses* are air-filled cavities within the bones of the skull. Like the nasal cavities into which they drain, they are lined with mucous membranes. The paranasal sinuses are air-filled and make the skull lighter and add to speech resonance. Their locations are illustrated in Figure 12-8. Only the frontal and maxillary sinuses are readily accessible to clinical examination.

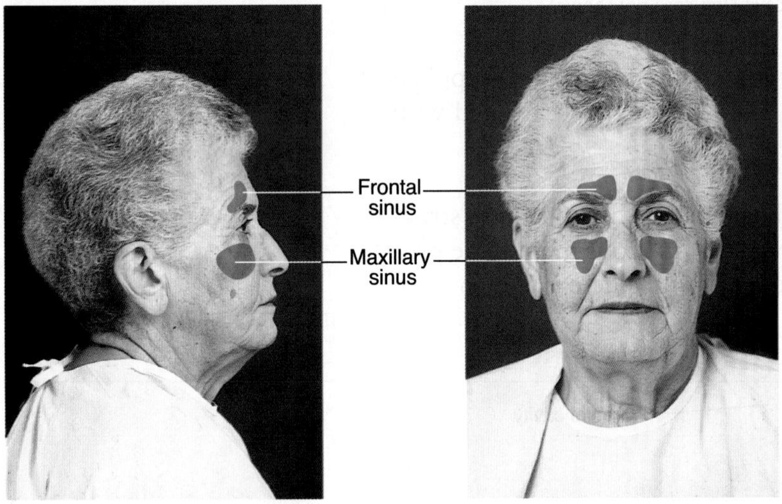

FIGURE 12-8 The paranasal sinuses.

THE HEALTH HISTORY OF THE NOSE AND SINUSES

The purpose of the nursing health history of the nose and sinuses is to detect changes in the patient's breathing, sense of smell, nose, and sinuses. Opening questions include "How is your breathing" and "Have you noticed any changes with your nose or sinuses?"

Common or concerning symptoms identified in a history of the nose and sinuses are listed in Box 12-2.

BOX 12-2 COMMON OR CONCERNING SYMPTOMS OF THE NOSE AND SINUSES

- Rhinorrhea—drainage
- Congestion—difficulty breathing through the nose
- Epistaxis—bleeding
- Change in sense of smell
- Pain

Rhinorrhea refers to drainage from the nose and is often associated with *nasal congestion*, a sense of stuffiness or obstruction. These symptoms are frequently accompanied by sneezing, watery eyes, and throat discomfort as well as by itching in the eyes, nose, and throat (Wheatley & Togias, 2015).

CLINICAL TIP
Causes of rhinorrhea and nasal congestion include *viral infections, allergic rhinitis* ("hay fever"), and *vasomotor rhinitis.* Itching favors an allergic cause.

Assess the chronology of the illness. Do symptoms last for a week or so, especially when common colds and related syndromes are prevalent, or does it occur seasonally when pollens are in the air? Is it associated with specific environmental triggers? What remedies has the patient used? How well do they work? How long were they used?

Environmental triggers or seasonal association suggest *allergic rhinitis.* Excessive use of decongestants can worsen symptoms, causing *rhinitis medicamentosa.*

Rhinorrhea

If the patient reports rhinorrhea, use "OLD CART" to learn more.

- *Onset:* When did you first notice the runny nose?
  Does it occur when pollen is in the air? Or did it occur after you were exposed to others with colds?
  What brings the runny nose on? Are you at a certain place when it occurs? Does it occur at a certain time?
- *Location:* In which side does it occur or is it on both sides?
- *Duration:* How long does it last? A day? A week? A season?
  Does it interfere with sleep? Work? Activities of daily living?
- *Characteristic symptoms:* Describe the runny nose.
  What color is the discharge?
  Consistency?
  Amount?
  Is it constant or does it come and go?
- *Associated manifestations:* Have you noticed any other symptoms?
  Sore throat?
  Cough?
  Cold?
  Fever?
  Headache?
  Tenderness over the sinuses?
- *Relieving factors:* Does anything stop your runny nose? Has it gotten worse or better? Does anything make it better?
- *Treatment:* What remedies have worked? For how long? How well did they work?

Congestion

If the patient reports congestion, ask: Did symptoms appear after an URI? Is there pain upon bending forward? Is there a maxillary toothache? Fever or local headache? Tenderness over the sinuses?

CLINICAL TIP
Together these suggest *acute bacterial sinusitis*. Testing finds at least one bacterial pathogen and often more about 90% of the time (DeMuri et al., 2018; Wald & DeMuri, 2018).

Inquire about drugs that might cause stuffiness. Examples include oral contraceptives, cocaine, and alcohol.

Is the patient's nasal congestion limited to one side? If so, you may be dealing with a different problem that requires careful physical examination. Ask:

Consider a deviated nasal septum, foreign body, or tumor.

- How long have you noticed the congestion on one side?
- Have you injured your nose?
- Do you remember putting anything in your nose?
- Have you had surgery on your nose?
- Do you have a history of polyps? A family history of polyps?

Epistaxis is bleeding from the nose. The blood usually originates from the nose itself but may also come from a paranasal sinus or the nasopharynx. However, in patients who are lying down or have bleeding that originates in posterior structures, blood may pass into the throat instead of out of the nostrils. You must identify the source of the bleeding carefully—is it from the nose, or has it been coughed up or vomited? Assess the site of bleeding, its severity, and associated symptoms. Carefully differentiate epistaxis from **hemoptysis** (coughing up of blood) or **hematemesis** (vomiting of blood), because each has different causes. Is it a recurrent problem? Has there been easy bruising or bleeding elsewhere in the body?

CLINICAL TIP
Local causes of epistaxis include trauma (especially nose picking), inflammation, drying and crusting of the nasal mucosa, tumors, and foreign bodies. Bleeding disorders also may contribute to epistaxis.

If a patient reports epistaxis, ask:

- *Onset:* When did you first notice the bloody nose?
  What caused the bloody nose? Injury? Dry room air? An object?
- *Location:* In which side does it occur or does it occur on both?
- *Duration:* How long does it last? How often do the nosebleeds occur?
- *Characteristic symptoms:* Describe the nosebleeds.
  What color is the blood? Bright red? Black? Dark reddish brown?
  Consistency?
  Amount?
  Constant or intermittent drainage?
- *Associated manifestations:* Have you noticed any other symptoms?
  Injury to the nose?
  Recent surgery—nose or adenoids?
  Inflammation?
  Drying of the mucous membrane?

- *Relieving factors:* What makes the bleeding stop? Is it difficult to stop?
- *Treatment:* Are you taking any nasal steroid medications (e.g., Flonase)?

Assess if the patient is on anticoagulation therapy or aspirin, which interfere with clotting. Nasal sprays, if overused, can contribute to the rebound effect, causing inflammation and congestion.

Change in Sense of Smell

- *Onset:* When did you first notice the change in sense of smell? What triggered this? Was there any illness prior to the change in smell? Injury?
- *Location:* In which side did the change of smell occur? Both?
- *Duration:* Is it constant or intermittent?
- *Characteristic symptoms:* Are there any smells you can detect? Which ones?
- *Associated manifestations:* Have you noticed any other symptoms?
- *Relieving factors:* Does anything relieve this?
- *Treatment:* Have you tried anything to treat this?

Loss of smell and taste has been associated with COVID-19 infection.

Past History

Topics to explore in the patient's past history related to the nose and sinuses include:

- Sinus infections
- URIs
- Allergies
- Trauma or injury
- Nasal or sinus surgery
- Polyps
- Dental history

Family History

Topics to explore in the family history related to the nose and sinuses include:

- Allergies
- Asthma

Lifestyle Habits

Relevant lifestyle topics to explore include:

- Air quality: What is the air quality like at home and at work? How often are air filters changed? How old is your home and work or school site? Do these sites have rugs? How often are they vacuumed or cleaned?
- Pets: What kind of pets do you have? How many? Are they in the house or outside? Do they sleep in bed with you?

- Alcohol: What kind of alcohol do you consume? How much?
- Tobacco use: What kind of tobacco do you use? How often? How many?
- Vape/e-cigarette use: What kind do you use? How often? How long have you used these products?
- Recreational drugs: What kind of drugs do you use? Route? How often?

Snorting cocaine can perforate the nasal mucous membrane. Frequent use can cause chronic rhinitis.

THE MOUTH AND PHARYNX

The *lips* are muscular folds that surround the entrance to the mouth. When opened, the gums (gingiva) and teeth are visible. Note the scalloped shape of the *gingival margins* and the pointed *interdental papillae* (Fig. 12-9).

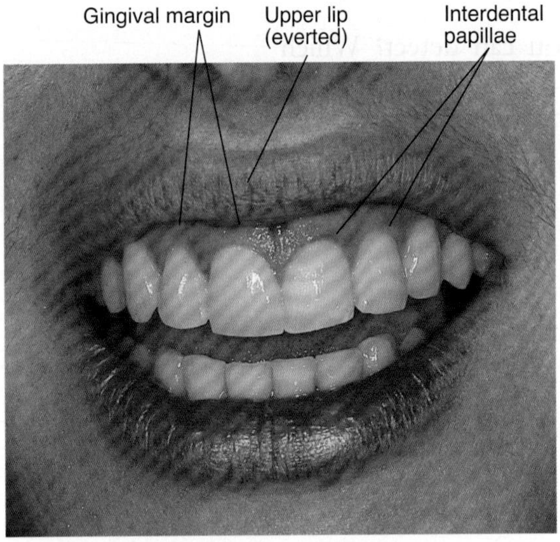

FIGURE 12-9 The lips, gingiva, and teeth.

The *gingiva* is firmly attached to the teeth and to the maxilla and mandible. In lighter-skinned people, the gingiva is pale or coral pink (Fig. 12-10A). In darker-skinned people, it may be diffusely or partly brown, as shown in Figure 12-10B. A midline mucosal fold, called a *labial frenulum*, connects

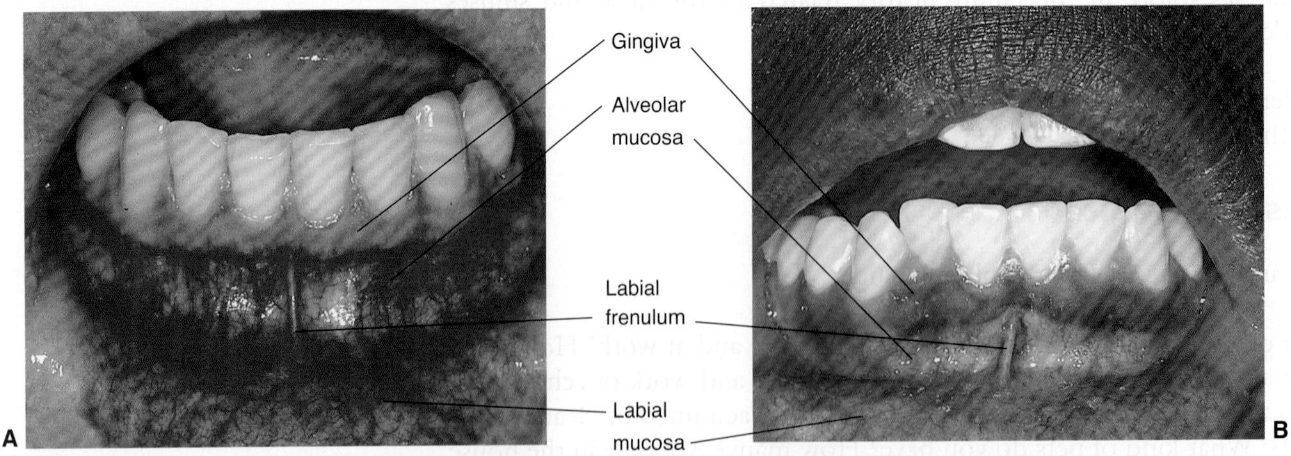

FIGURE 12-10 The gingiva of patient with lighter skin (**A**) and of a patient with darker skin (**B**).

each lip with the gingiva. A shallow *gingival sulcus* between the gum's thin margin and each tooth is not readily visible (but is probed and measured by dentists). Adjacent to the gingiva is the *alveolar mucosa*, which merges with the *labial mucosa* of the lip.

Each tooth, composed chiefly of *dentin*, lies rooted in a bony socket with only its enamel-covered crown exposed (Fig. 12-11). Small blood vessels and nerves enter the tooth through its apex and pass into the pulp canal and pulp chamber.

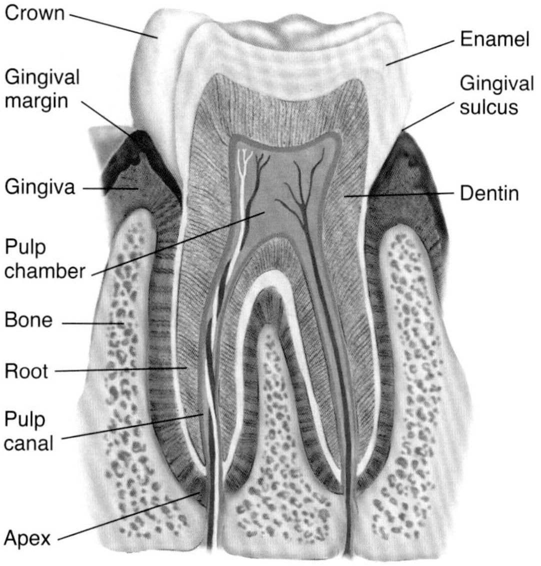

FIGURE 12-11 Structures of the tooth.

Terms designating the 32 adult teeth, 16 in the upper and 16 in the lower jaw, are noted in the labels of Figure 12-12.

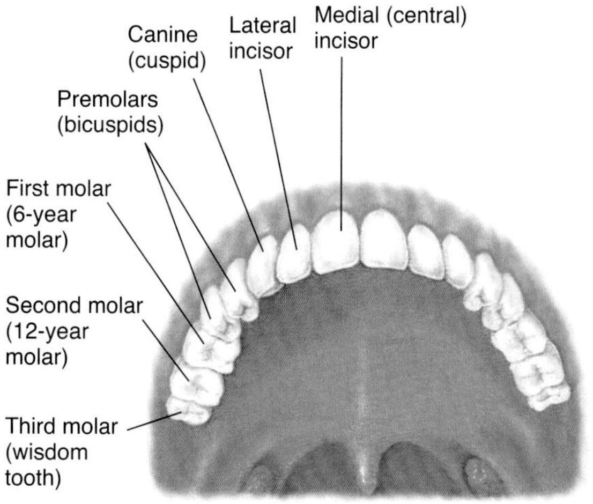

FIGURE 12-12 The types of adult teeth.

The dorsum of the *tongue* is covered with papillae (Fig. 12-13), giving it a rough surface. Some of these papillae look like red dots, which contrast with the thin white coat that often covers the tongue. The undersurface of the tongue has no papillae. Note the midline *lingual frenulum* that connects the tongue to the floor of the mouth and the *ducts of the submandibular gland* (Wharton ducts) that pass forward and medially (Fig. 12-14). They open on papillae that lie on each side of the lingual frenulum. The paired sublingual salivary glands lie just under the floor of the mouth mucosa.

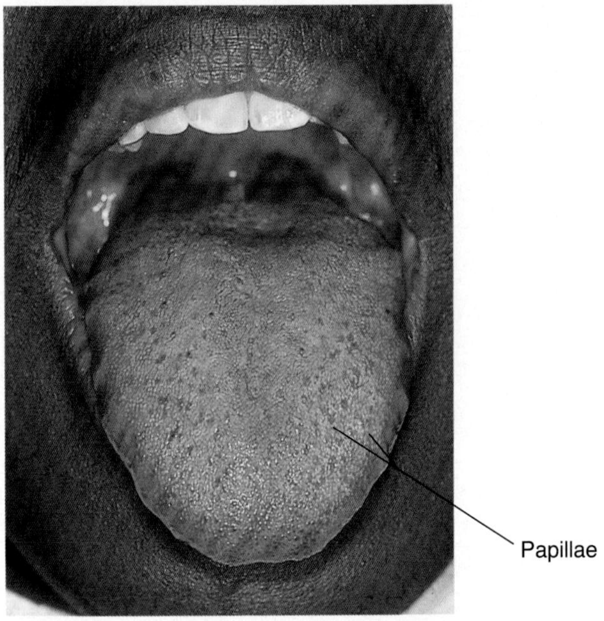

FIGURE 12-13 Papillae visible on the tongue.

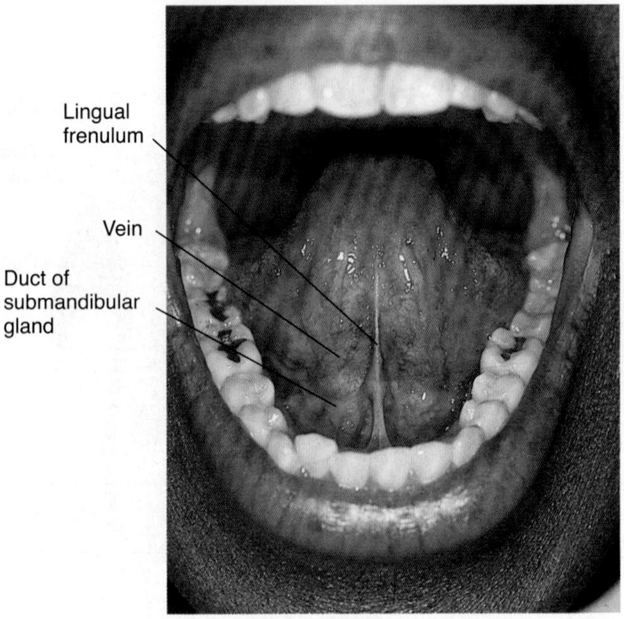

FIGURE 12-14 Structures underneath the tongue.

Above and behind the tongue rises an arch formed by the *anterior* and *posterior pillars*, the *soft palate*, and the *uvula* (Fig. 12-15). A meshwork of small blood vessels may web the soft palate. The *posterior pharynx* is visible in the recess behind the soft palate and tongue.

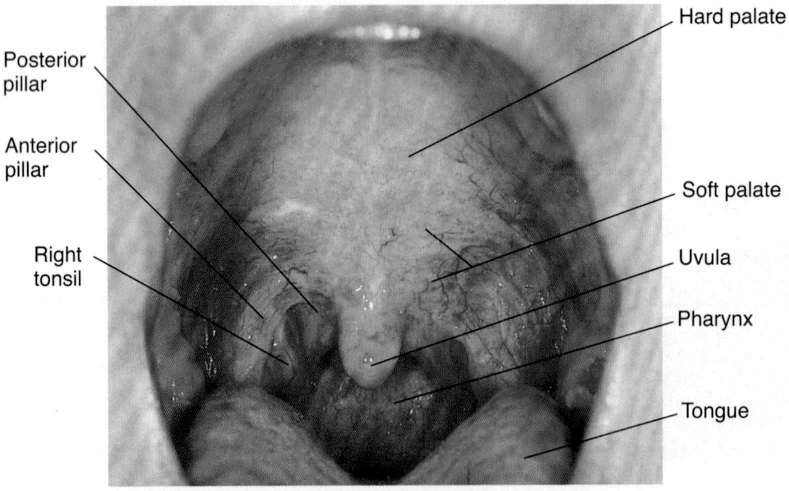

FIGURE 12-15 Structures inside the mouth.

In Figure 12-15, note the right tonsil protruding from the hollowed *tonsillar fossa*, or cavity, between the anterior and posterior pillars. In adults, tonsils are often small or absent, as in the empty left tonsillar fossa here.

The *buccal mucosa* lines the cheeks (Fig. 12-16). Each *parotid duct*, sometimes termed the *Stensen duct*, opens onto the buccal mucosa near the upper second molar. Its location is frequently marked by its own small papilla.

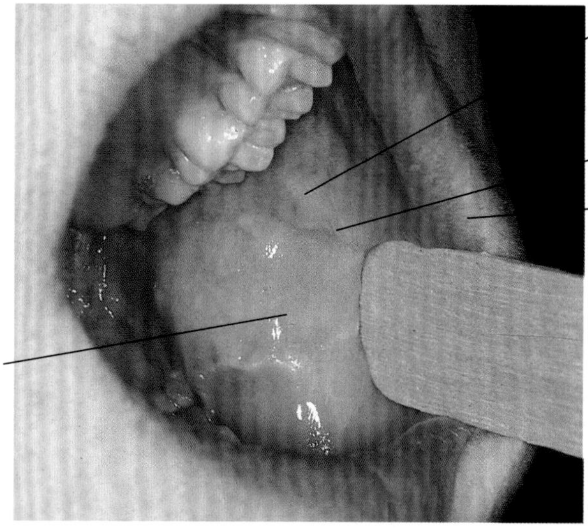

FIGURE 12-16 Examining the buccal mucosa.

THE HEALTH HISTORY OF THE MOUTH AND PHARYNX

The purpose of the nursing health history of the mouth and throat is to detect changes in skin integrity, speech, or swallowing and infection or illness.

Opening questions include "Have you noticed any changes in your mouth or throat?" and "Have you had any difficulty eating or swallowing?"

Common or concerning symptoms identified in a history of the mouth and pharynx are listed in Box 12-3.

BOX 12-3 COMMON OR CONCERNING SYMPTOMS OF THE MOUTH AND THROAT

- Sore throat
- Hoarseness
- Lesions
- Sore tongue
- Bleeding gums
- Toothache
- Dysphagia

Sore throat is a frequent complaint, usually associated with acute upper respiratory symptoms.

CLINICAL TIP
Fever, pharyngeal exudates, and anterior lymphadenopathy, especially in the absence of cough, suggest streptococcal pharyngitis, or strep throat (Centers for Disease Control & Prevention [CDC], 2016; Luo et al., 2019).

Hoarseness refers to an altered quality of the voice, often described as husky, rough, or harsh. The pitch may be lower than before. Hoarseness usually arises from inflammation or infection of the larynx but may also develop as laryngeal lesions which press on the laryngeal nerves (Stachler et al., 2018).

Ask the patient about smoking or inhalation of other irritants, alcohol use, acid reflux, voice use, environmental allergies, and any associated symptoms. Differentiate if the problem is acute or chronic.

Acute hoarseness might be caused by voice overuse or acute viral laryngitis.

Is the problem chronic, lasting more than 2 weeks? Is there prolonged tobacco or alcohol use, cough or hemoptysis, weight loss, or unilateral throat pain?

CLINICAL TIP
If hoarseness lasts over 2 weeks, refer the patient for laryngoscopy and consider causes such as *hypothyroidism*, reflux, vocal cord nodules, head and neck cancers, thyroid masses, and neurologic disorders like *Parkinson disease*, *amyotrophic lateral sclerosis*, and *myasthenia gravis*.

If the patient reports hoarseness, continue the assessment using "OLD CART."

- *Onset:* When did the hoarseness begin? How often do you have hoarseness?
- *Location:* Where in the throat do you feel this?
- *Duration:* How long did it last?
- *Characteristic symptoms:* Did you have any other symptoms?
- *Associated manifestations:* What additional symptoms have occurred or what might have preceded the hoarseness?
  - Did you or anyone around you have a cold? Cough?
  - Did you overuse your voice?
  - Were you in a situation in which you needed to raise your voice or scream (e.g., concert, crowded area, jack hammers)?
  - Do you smoke? Vape? If yes, what do you smoke? How many/much per day and for how long?
  - Are you around others who smoke?
- *Relieving factors:* What relieves the hoarseness?
- *Treatment:* Has this been treated previously? Currently?

A *sore tongue* may result from local lesions as well as systemic illness. If the patient reports a sore tongue, ask for the duration and a description.

Note findings under the tongue, such as aphthous ulcers or atrophic glossitis (see Table 12-8).

Bleeding from the gums is a common symptom of the mouth that may occur, especially when brushing teeth. Ask what type of toothbrush is used. Hard or soft? Ask about local lesions and any tendency to bleed or bruise elsewhere.

Bleeding gums are most often caused by *gingivitis* (inflammation of the gingiva).

Additional questions regarding the mouth and throat include:

- Do you have *bleeding gums*?
  When did this begin?
  Where is the bleeding?
  Was this temporary or is it constant?
  Do you notice any other symptoms when this occurs?
- Do you have a *toothache*?
  When was your last dental examination?
  What were the results?
  Were any further visits necessary?
- Do you have difficulty swallowing (**dysphagia**)?
  When did this begin?
  What brought it on?
  Was it temporary or is it constant?
  What other symptoms do you experience at this time?
  How does it affect your daily life?
  What makes it feel better or go away?
  How has this changed what you eat? How has it changed with whom you eat?
- Do you have a history of lesions in your mouth?
  When did you first notice the lesions?
  Where are the lesions located? Are there any others?
  Describe the lesions. Size? Shape? Color? Discharge? Pain? Relationship to other lesions?
- Have you noticed any other symptoms?
  Itching?
  Cough?
  Cold (respiratory infection)?
  Fever?
  Dizziness?
  Headaches?
  Does anything make these symptoms better?

Past History

Relevant topics for a past history of the mouth and pharynx include:

- Sore throat
- Loss of voice
- Dental, mouth, or throat surgery
- Trauma or injury to teeth, mouth, or throat
- History of infections
- Oral cancer
- Sexually transmitted infection (STI)

Family History

Topics relevant to taking the family history of the mouth and pharynx include:

- Allergies
- Smoking or exposure to smoke
- Stroke
- Tuberculosis

Lifestyle Habits

Lifestyle topics to assess that are relevant to the mouth and pharynx include:

- How many times a day do you brush your teeth?
- Do you floss? How often?
- Do you use tobacco? Cigarettes, e-cigarettes, vapes, cigars, pipes, or chewing tobacco? How many/much do you use per day? When did you start?
- Do you smoke marijuana? Cocaine? Inhale any other product?
- Do you drink alcohol? What kind? How many ounces per day?
- What is your occupation?
- Do you use dental dams during oral sex?

PHYSICAL EXAMINATION OF THE EAR

Equipment needed for a physical examination of the ear includes:

- Tuning fork (512 Hz preferred for hearing assessment)
- Otoscope
- Speculum
- Tongue blade
- Gloves
- Penlight

The Pinna (Auricle)

Inspect the pinna and surrounding tissue for deformities, lumps (Table 12-2), or skin lesions. If ear pain, discharge, or inflammation is present, move the pinna up and down, press the tragus, and press firmly just behind the ear.

CLINICAL TIP
Movement of the pinna and tragus (the "tug test") is painful in acute *otitis externa* (inflammation of the ear canal) but not in *otitis media* (inflammation of the middle ear). Tenderness behind the ear occurs in *otitis media*.

Concept Mastery Alert

Otitis Externa and Otitis Media

Ear pain is a common complaint with otitis externa and otitis media. Although the symptoms of both are similar, there are two significant differences. First, the nurse needs to evaluate pain on movement of the pinna and tragus. A positive finding is closely associated with otitis externa. In addition, the nurse needs to evaluate for a history of exposure to water. Typically, one of the causes of otitis externa is frequent submersion of the ear in water, as would happen with a recent vacation to the beach or swimming.

TABLE 12-2 Lumps on or Near the Ear

Keloid

A firm, nodular, hypertrophic mass of scar tissue extending beyond the area of injury. It may develop in any scarred area but is most common on the shoulders and upper chest. A keloid on a pierced earlobe may have troublesome cosmetic effects. Keloids are more common in darker-skinned people and may recur following treatment.

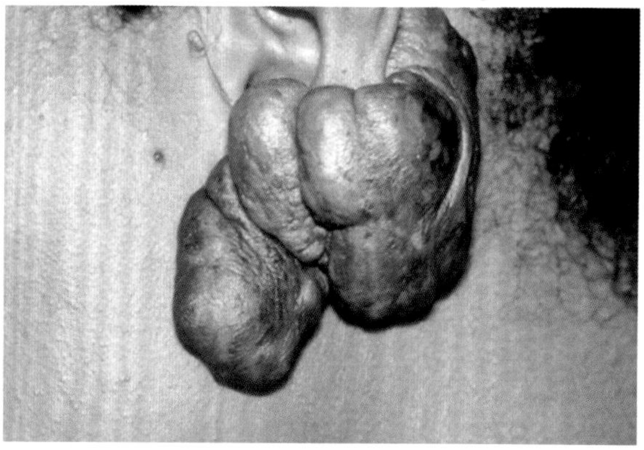

Chondrodermatitis Helicis

This chronic inflammatory lesion starts as a painful, tender papule on the helix or antihelix. Here, the upper lesion is at a later stage of ulceration and crusting. Reddening may occur. Biopsy is needed to rule out carcinoma.

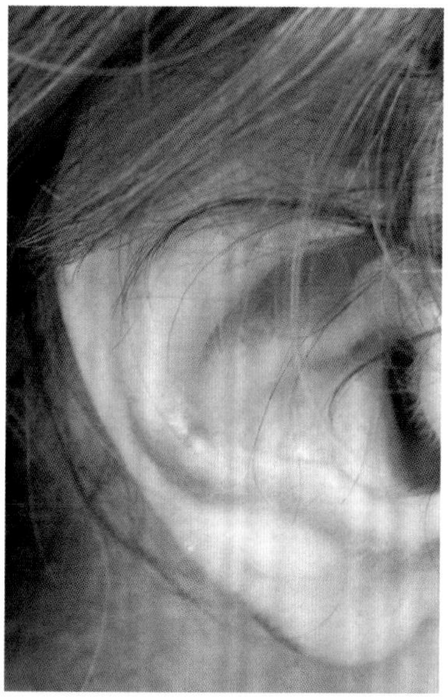

Tophi

A deposit of uric acid crystals characteristic of chronic tophaceous gout. It appears as hard nodules in the helix or antihelix and may discharge chalky white crystals through the skin. It also may appear near the joints, hands, feet, and other areas. It usually develops after chronic sustained high blood levels of uric acid.

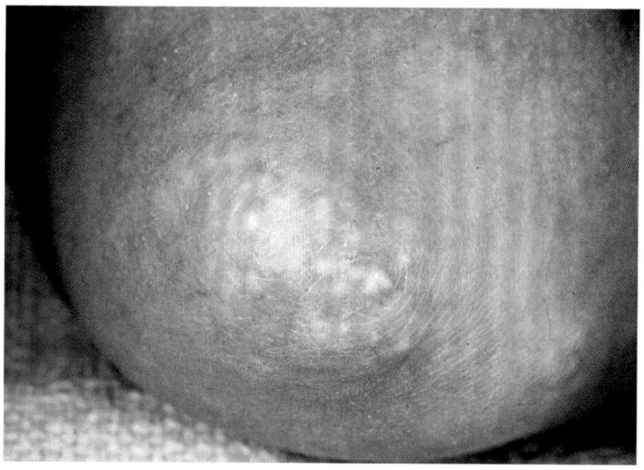

(continued)

TABLE 12-2 Lumps on or Near the Ear (*Continued*)

Basal Cell Carcinoma

Recurrent basal cell carcinoma of the ear.

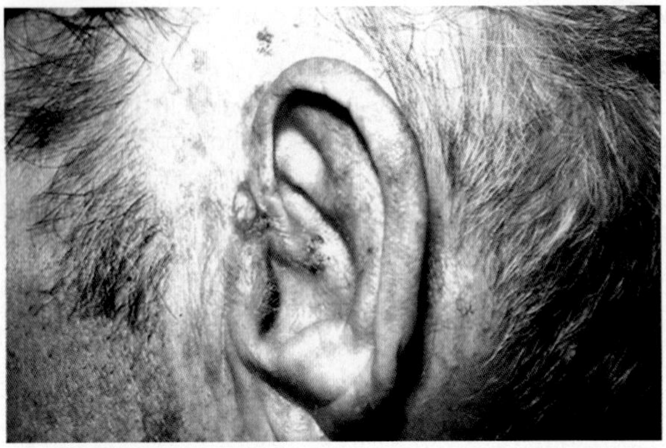

Cutaneous Cyst

Formerly called a *sebaceous cyst*, a dome-shaped lump in the dermis forms a benign closed firm sac attached to the epidermis. A dark dot (blackhead) may be visible on its surface. Histologically, it is usually either (1) an *epidermoid* cyst, common on the face and neck, or (2) a *pilar (trichilemmal)* cyst, common in the scalp. Both may become inflamed.

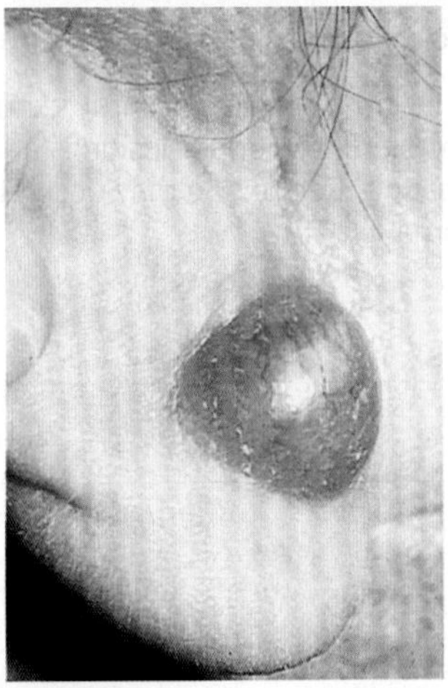

Rheumatoid Nodules

In chronic rheumatoid arthritis, look for small lumps on the helix or antihelix and additional nodules elsewhere on the hands, along the surface of the ulna distal to the elbow, and on the knees and heels. Ulceration may result from repeated injuries. These nodules may antedate the arthritis.

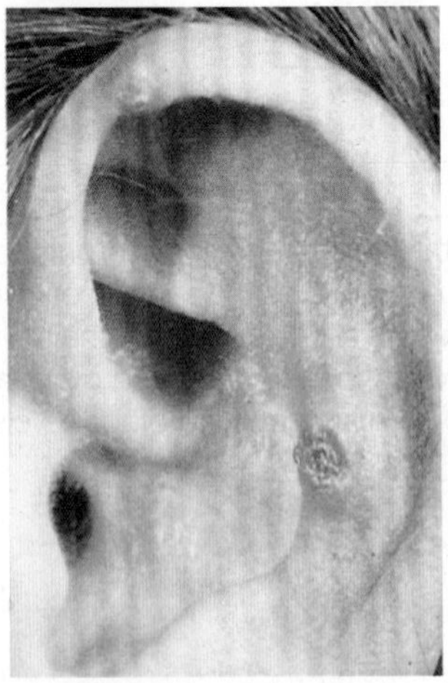

Sources of photos: Keloid—Sams, W. M. Jr, & Lynch, P. J., Eds. (1990). Principles and practice of dermatology. Churchill Livingstone; *Tophi*—Elder, D. E. (2014). *Lever's histopathology of the skin* (11th ed.). Wolters Kluwer; *Cutaneous Cyst*—jaojormami/Shutterstock; *Chondrodermatitis Helicis*—Barankin Collection, Wolters Kluwer, 2005; *Basal Cell Carcinoma*—Hall, J. C., & Hall, B. J. (2017). *Sauer's manual of skin diseases* (11th ed.). Wolters Kluwer; *Rheumatoid Nodules*—Champion, R. H., Burton, J. L., & Ebling, F. J. G., Eds. (1992). *Rook/Wilkinson/Ebling textbook of dermatology* (5th ed.). Blackwell Scientific.

The Ear Canal and Drum

To see the ear canal and drum, use an otoscope with the brightest light and the largest ear speculum that inserts easily into the canal. Position the patient's head so that you can see comfortably through the otoscope. To straighten the ear canal, grasp the pinna firmly but gently and pull it upward, backward, and slightly away from the head (Fig. 12-17).

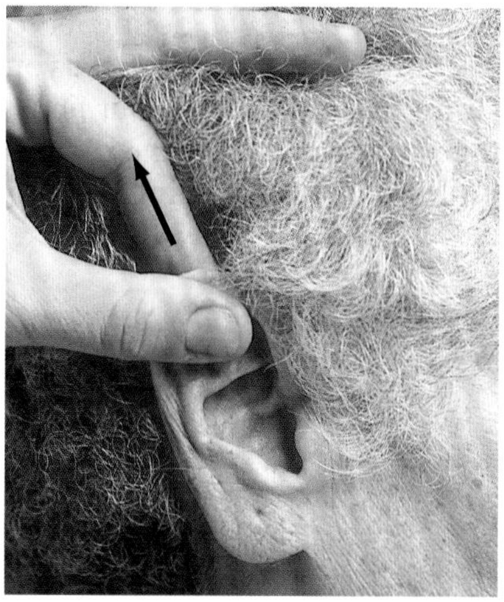

FIGURE 12-17 Straightening the ear canal.

Hold the otoscope handle (Fig. 12-18) in your dominant hand and pull the pinna up and back prior to inserting the otoscope (Fig. 12-19).

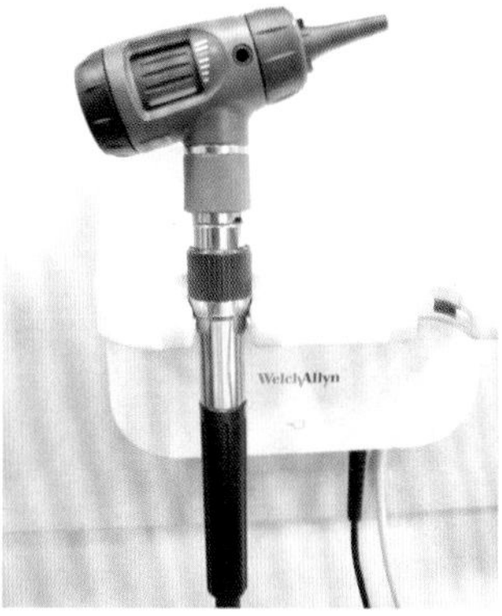

FIGURE 12-18 An otoscope.

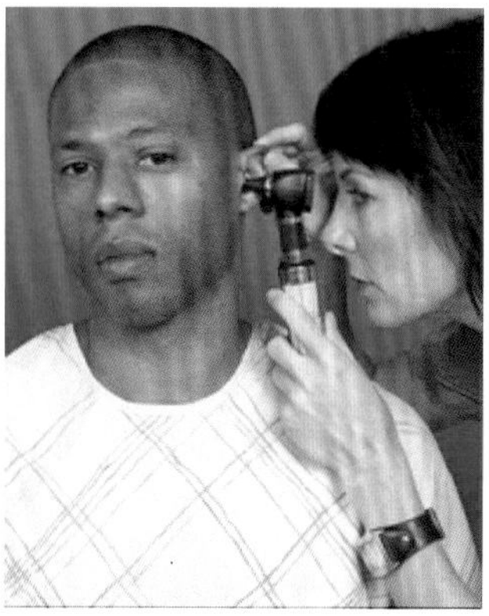

FIGURE 12-19 Using the otoscope. (Reprinted with permission from Timby, B. K., & Smith, N. E. (2017). *Introductory medical-surgical nursing* (12th ed.). Wolters Kluwer.)

Insert the speculum gently into the ear canal, directing it somewhat down and forward and through the hairs, if any, toward the eardrum.

Nontender nodular swellings covered by normal skin deep in the ear canals (Fig. 12-20) suggest *exostoses.* These are nonmalignant overgrowths, which may obscure the drum.

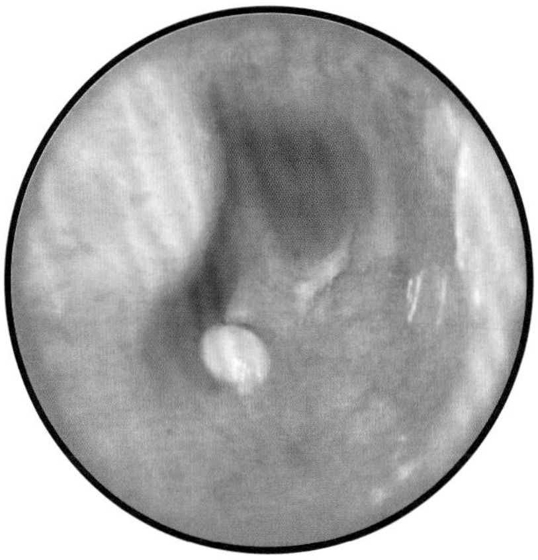

FIGURE 12-20 Exostoses.

Inspect the ear canal, noting any discharge, foreign bodies, redness of the skin (Fig. 12-21), or swelling. Cerumen, which varies in color and consistency from yellow and flaky to brown and sticky or even to dark and hard, may wholly or partly obscure your view.

In acute otitis externa, the canal is often swollen, narrowed, moist, pale, and tender. It may be reddened. In *chronic otitis externa,* the skin of the canal is often thickened, red, and itchy.

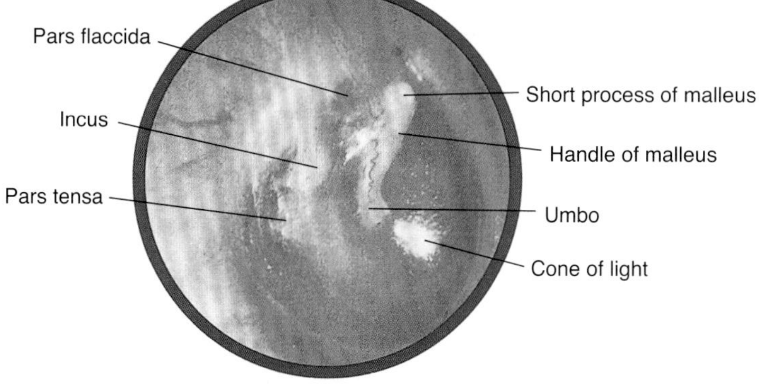

FIGURE 12-21 Acute otitis externa of the right ear canal.

Inspect the eardrum, noting its color and contour. The cone of light—usually easy to see—helps orient you. The examiner is unable to visualize the entire eardrum at once but finds a landmark such as the cone of light and follows upward to see the handle of the malleus. Abnormalities that may be observed in the eardrum are outlined in Table 12-3.

A red bulging drum indicates acute purulent otitis media (Shirai & Preciado, 2019). An amber drum indicates serous effusion.

TABLE 12-3 Abnormalities of the Eardrum

Normal Eardrum (Right)

This normal right eardrum (tympanic membrane) is pinkish gray. Note the malleus lying behind the upper part of the drum. Above the short process lies the *pars flaccida*. The remainder of the drum is the *pars tensa*. From the umbo, the bright cone of light fans anteriorly and downward. Posterior to the malleus, part of the incus is visible behind the drum. The small blood vessels along the handle of the malleus are normal.

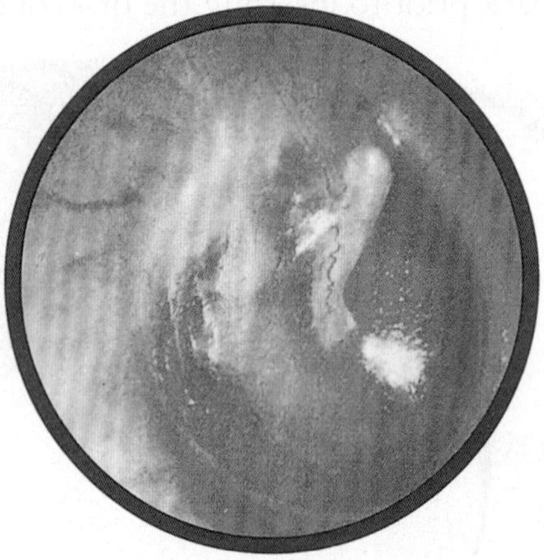

Perforation of the Drum

Perforations are holes in the eardrum that usually result from purulent infections of the middle ear. They may be *central*, if not involving the margin of the drum, or *marginal*, when the margin is involved. The membrane covering the perforation may be notably thin and transparent.

The more common central perforation is illustrated here. A reddened ring of granulation tissue surrounds the perforation, indicating chronic infection. The eardrum itself is scarred, and no landmarks are visible. Discharge from the infected middle ear may drain out through such a perforation. A perforation often closes in the healing process, as in the next photo. There may be associated earache or even hearing loss, especially if the perforations are large.

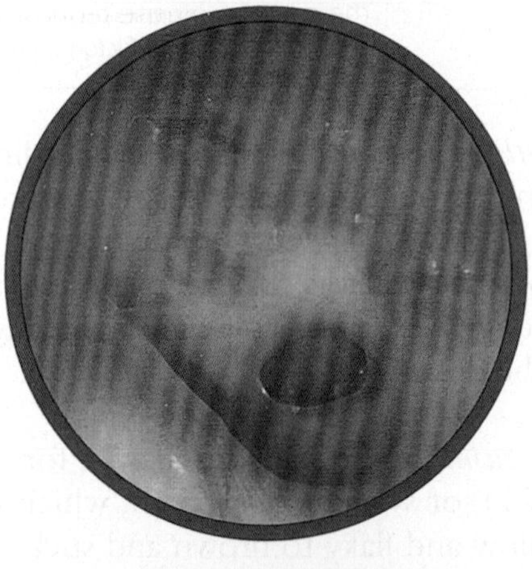

Tympanosclerosis

Tympanosclerosis is a scarring process of the middle ear from otitis media that involves deposition of hyaline and calcium and phosphate crystals in the eardrum and middle ear. When severe, it may entrap the ossicles and cause conductive hearing loss.

In the inferior portion of this left eardrum, note the large, chalky white patch with irregular margins. Other abnormalities in this eardrum include a *healed perforation* (the large oval area in the upper posterior drum) and signs of a *retracted drum*. A retracted drum is pulled medially away from the examiner's eye, and the malleolar folds are tightened into sharp outlines. The short process often protrudes sharply, and the handle of the malleus, pulled inward at the umbo, looks foreshortened and more horizontal.

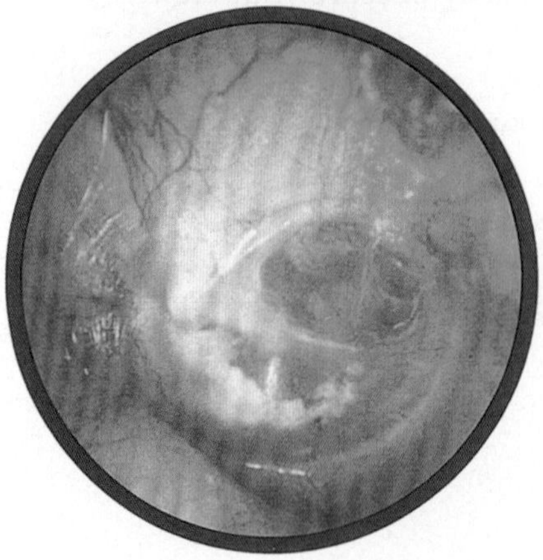

Serous Effusion

Serous effusions are usually caused by viral upper respiratory infections (*otitis media with serous effusion*) or by sudden changes in atmospheric pressure as from flying or diving (*otitic barotrauma*). The eustachian tube cannot equalize the air pressure in the middle ear with that of the outside air. Air is partly or completely absorbed from the middle ear into the bloodstream, and serous fluid accumulates there instead. Symptoms include fullness and popping sensations in the ear, mild conduction hearing loss, and perhaps some pain.

Amber fluid behind the eardrum is characteristic, as in this patient with otic barotrauma. A fluid level, a line between air above and amber fluid below, can be seen on either side of the short process. Air bubbles (not always present) can be seen here within the amber fluid.

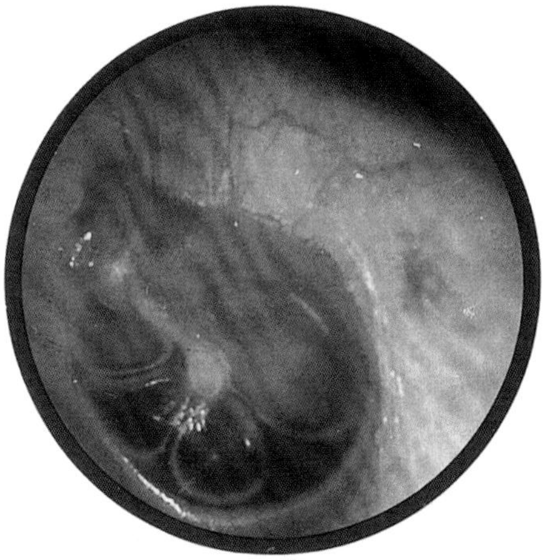

Acute Otitis Media with Purulent Effusion

Acute otitis media with purulent effusion is caused by bacterial infection from *Streptococcus pneumoniae* or *Haemophilus influenzae*. Symptoms include earache, fever, and hearing loss. The eardrum reddens, loses its landmarks, and bulges laterally toward the examiner's eye.

Here the eardrum is bulging, and most landmarks are obscured. Redness is most obvious near the umbo, but dilated vessels can be seen in all segments of the drum. A diffuse redness of the entire drum often develops. Spontaneous rupture (perforation) of the drum may follow with discharge of purulent material into the ear canal.

Hearing loss is of the conductive type. Acute purulent otitis media is much more common in children than in adults.

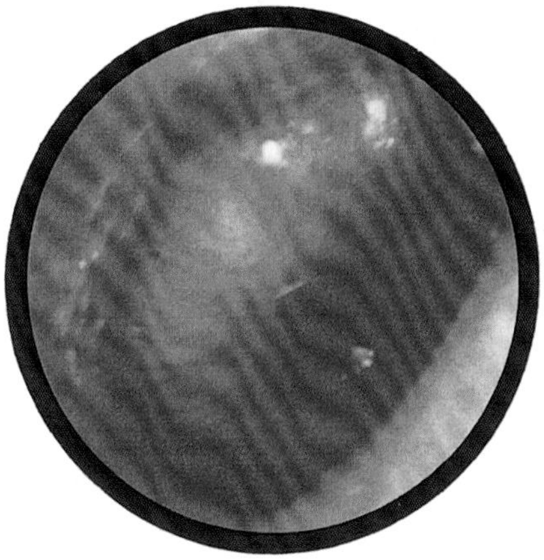

Bullous Myringitis

Bullous myringitis is a viral infection characterized by painful hemorrhagic vesicles that appear on the tympanic membrane, the ear canal, or both. Symptoms include earache, blood-tinged discharge from the ear, and hearing loss of the conductive type.

In this right ear, at least two large vesicles (bullae) are discernible on the drum. The drum is reddened, and its landmarks are obscured.

This condition is caused by mycoplasma, viral, and bacterial otitis media.

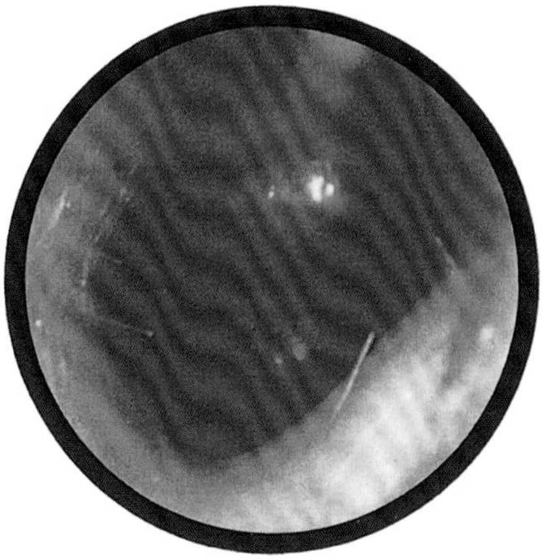

Sources of photos: *Normal Eardrum*—Hawke, M., Keene, M., & Alberti, P. W. (1984). *Clinical otoscopy: A text and colour atlas*. Churchill Livingstone; *Perforation of the Drum, Tympanosclerosis*—Courtesy of Michael Hawke, MD, Toronto, Canada; *Serous Effusion*—Hawke, M., Keene, M., & Alberti, P. W. (1984). *Clinical otoscopy: A text and colour atlas*. Churchill Livingstone; *Acute Otitis Media, Bullous Myringitis*—The Wellcome Trust, National Medical Slide Bank, London, UK and associated copyright holders.

Identify the *handle of the malleus*, noting its position, and inspect the *short process of the malleus.*

An unusually prominent short process and a prominent handle that looks more horizontal suggest a retracted drum.

Gently move the speculum so that you can see as much of the drum as possible, including the *pars flaccida* superiorly and the margins of the *pars tensa*. Look for any perforations. The anterior and inferior margins of the drum may be obscured by the curving wall of the ear canal. An advanced practitioner may evaluate the mobility of the eardrum with a pneumatic otoscope.

A serous effusion, a thickened drum, or purulent otitis media may decrease mobility. Note that with a perforation, there will be no mobility.

Testing Auditory Acuity

A patient who reports difficulty hearing during the subjective questioning is twice as likely to have a hearing deficit; for patients who report normal hearing the likelihood of moderate to severe hearing impairment is only 0.13 (Bagai et al., 2006). In hospitalized patients who have a hearing loss, there is an increased fall rate among those without hearing aids (Tiase et al., 2020).

The *whispered voice test* (Box 12-4) is a reliable screening test for hearing loss if the examiner uses a standard method of testing and exhales before whispering. Sensitivity is 90% to 100% and specificity 70% to 87% (McShefferty et al., 2013). This test detects significant hearing loss of greater than 30 dB. A formal hearing test is still the gold standard (Zhang et al., 2019).

BOX 12-4 WHISPERED VOICE TEST FOR AUDITORY ACUITY

- The patient is sitting, and you stand 2 ft behind so the patient is unable to read your lips.
- Test one ear at a time, starting with the better-hearing ear.
- Using one finger, occlude the non-test ear and slightly rub the tragus in a circular motion preventing sound to transfer to the non-test ear.
- Exhale a full breath before whispering to ensure a quiet voice.
- Whisper a sequence with three numbers/letters, such as "2-K-5." Use a different combination for the other ear.
- Interpretation:
  - *Normal:* Patient repeats initial sequence correctly.
  - *Normal:* Patient responds incorrectly, so test a second time with a different number/letter combination; patient repeats at least three out of the possible six numbers and letters correctly.
  - *Abnormal:* Four of the six possible numbers and letters are incorrect. Conduct further testing by audiometry. (The Weber and Rinne tests are less accurate.) (Zhang et al., 2019)

Testing for Conductive versus Neurosensory Hearing Loss: Tuning Fork Tests

If hearing is diminished and a person has not passed the whisper voice test, try to distinguish between *conductive* and *sensorineural* hearing loss. You need a quiet room and a *512-Hz* tuning fork. These frequencies fall within the range of human speech (500 to 3,000 Hz)—functionally the most important range. Tuning forks with lower pitches may lead to overestimating bone conduction and can also be felt as vibration. Set the fork into light vibration by briskly stroking it between the thumb and index finger or by tapping it on your forearm.

In unilateral *conductive hearing loss*, sound is heard in (lateralized to) the impaired ear. Etiologies include acute otitis media, otosclerosis (abnormal growth of bone in the middle ear), perforation of the eardrum, and obstruction of the ear canal (e.g., cerumen). See Table 12-4, "Patterns of Hearing Loss."

TABLE 12-4 Patterns of Hearing Loss

Conductive Loss

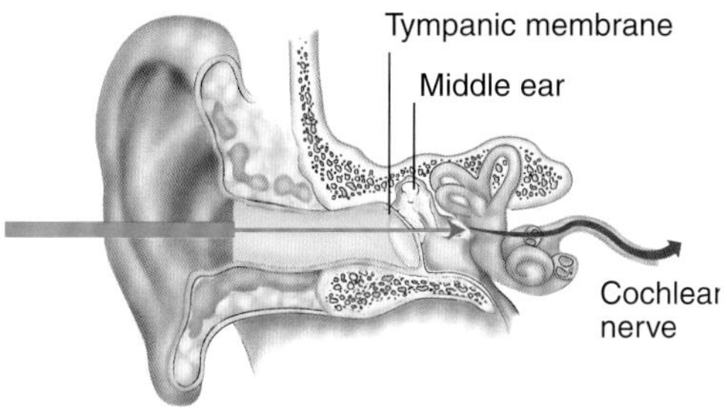

Sensorineural Loss

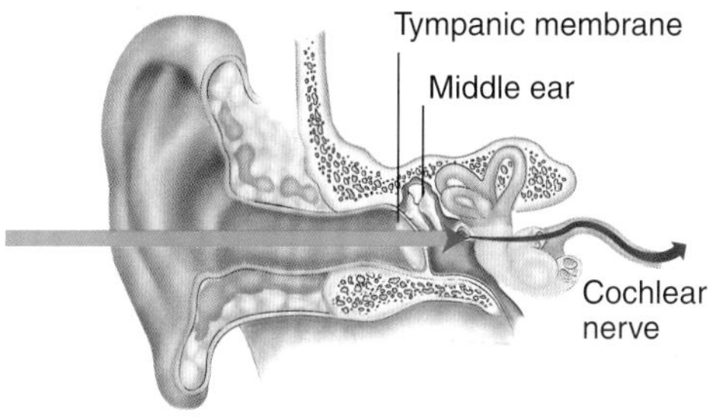

	Conductive Loss	Sensorineural Loss
Pathophysiology	External or middle ear disorder impairs sound conduction to inner ear. Causes include foreign body, *otitis media*, perforated eardrum, and otosclerosis of ossicles.	Inner ear disorder involves cochlear nerve and neuronal impulse transmission to the brain. Causes include loud noise exposure, inner ear infections, trauma, tremors, congenital and familial disorders, and aging.
Usual Age of Onset	Childhood and young adulthood up to age 40	Middle or later years
Ear Canal and Drum Effects	• Abnormality usually visible, except in otosclerosis • Little effect on sound • Hearing seems to improve in noisy environment • Voice becomes soft because inner ear and cochlear nerve are intact	• Problem not visible. • Higher registers are lost, so sound may be distorted. • Hearing worsens in noisy environment. • Voice may be loud because hearing is difficult.
Weber Test *(in unilateral hearing loss)*	• Tuning fork at vertex • Sound lateralizes to *impaired ear*—room noise not well heard, so detection of vibrations *improves*.	• Tuning fork at vertex • Sound lateralizes to *good ear*—inner ear or cochlear nerve damage impairs transmission to affected ear.
Rinne Test	• Tuning fork at external auditory meatus then on mastoid bone • Bone conduction longer than or equal to air conduction ($BC \geq AC$). While air conduction through the external or middle ear is impaired, vibrations through bone bypass the problem to reach the cochlea.	• Tuning fork at external auditory meatus then on mastoid bone • Air conduction longer than bone conduction ($AC > BC$). The inner ear or cochlear nerve is less able to transmit impulses regardless of how the vibrations reach the cochlea. The normal pattern prevails.

Tuning forks are used in the Weber and Rinne tests.

- *Test for lateralization (Weber test).* Place the base of the lightly vibrating tuning fork firmly on top of the patient's head or on the mid-forehead (Fig. 12-22).
  - Ask where the patient hears the sound. Is it on one or both sides? Normally the vibration is heard in the midline or equally in both ears. If nothing is heard, try again, pressing the fork more firmly on the head.
  - Restrict this test to patients with unilateral hearing loss since patients with normal hearing may lateralize (hear sound on one side), and patients with bilateral conductive or sensorineural deficits will not lateralize.

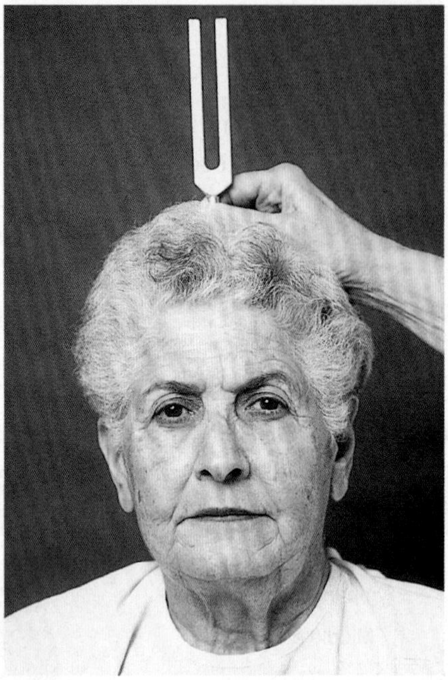

FIGURE 12-22 The Weber test.

In unilateral *sensorineural hearing loss*, sound is heard in the good ear.

- *Compare air conduction (AC) and bone conduction (BC) (Rinne test).* Place the base of a lightly vibrating tuning fork on the mastoid bone, behind the ear and level with the canal (Fig. 12-23A). When the patient can no longer hear the sound, quickly place the fork close to the ear canal and ask the patient if a vibration is heard (Fig. 12-23B). Here the "U" of the fork should face forward, which maximizes sound transmission for the patient. Normally the sound is heard longer through air than through bone (AC > BC).

In *conductive hearing loss*, sound is heard through bone as long as or longer than it is through air (BC = AC or BC > AC). In *sensorineural hearing loss*, sound is heard longer through air (AC > BC)—although both are decreased.

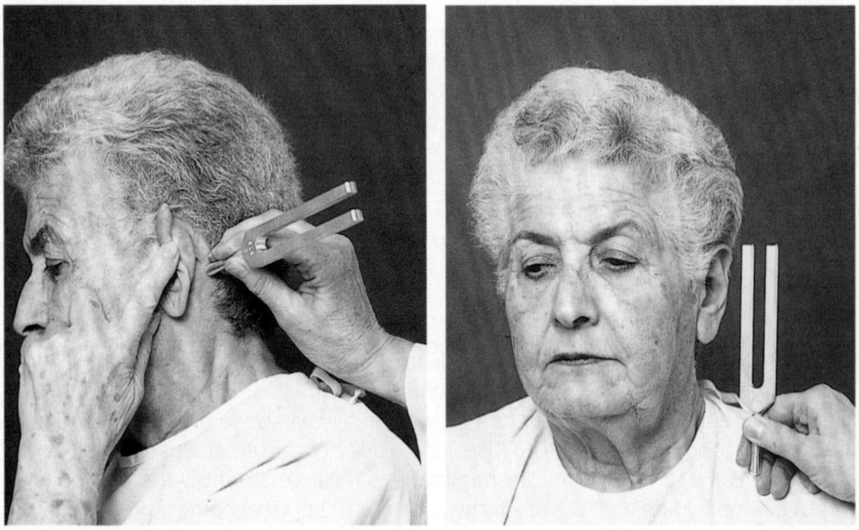

FIGURE 12-23 The Rinne test. **A.** Bone conduction. **B.** Palpating the maxillary sinuses.

PHYSICAL EXAMINATION OF THE NOSE

Equipment necessary for physical examination of the nose includes:

- Penlight
- Otoscope
- Nasal speculum or largest speculum available
- Gloves

Inspect the anterior and inferior surfaces of the nose. Gentle pressure on the tip of the nose with your thumb usually widens the nostrils. Use a penlight or otoscope light for a partial view of each nasal **vestibule** (opening of the nose) (Fig. 12-24). If the nasal tip is tender, be gentle and manipulate the nose as little as possible.

Tenderness of the nasal tip or alae suggests local infection such as a **furuncle**, especially if there is a small erythematous and/or swollen area.

Note any asymmetry or deformity of the nose.

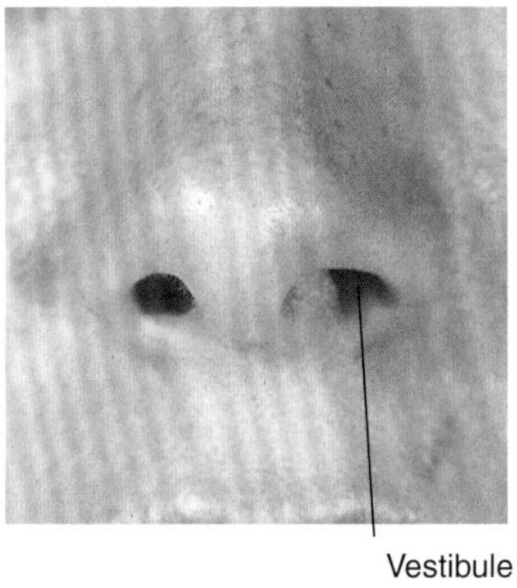

FIGURE 12-24 The vestibule of the nose.

Test for nasal obstruction, if indicated, by pressing on each ala nasi in turn and asking the patient to inhale.

Inspect the inside of the nose with a nasal speculum or with an otoscope and the largest ear speculum available (Fig. 12-25). Tilt the patient's head back slightly and insert the speculum gently into the vestibule of each nostril, avoiding contact with the sensitive nasal septum. Hold the otoscope handle to one side to avoid the patient's chin and improve your mobility. By directing the speculum posteriorly, then upward in small steps, try to see the inferior and middle turbinates, the nasal septum, and the narrow nasal

Deviation of the lower septum is common and may be easily visible, as illustrated in Figure 12-24. Deviation seldom obstructs air flow.

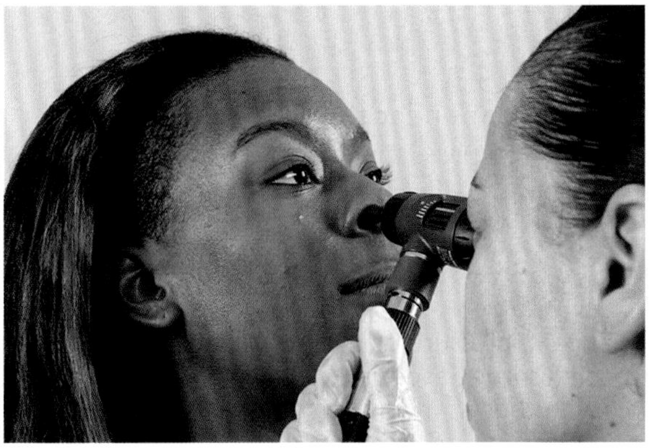

FIGURE 12-25 Inspecting the inside of the nose.

passage between them (Fig. 12-26). Some asymmetry of the two sides is normal.

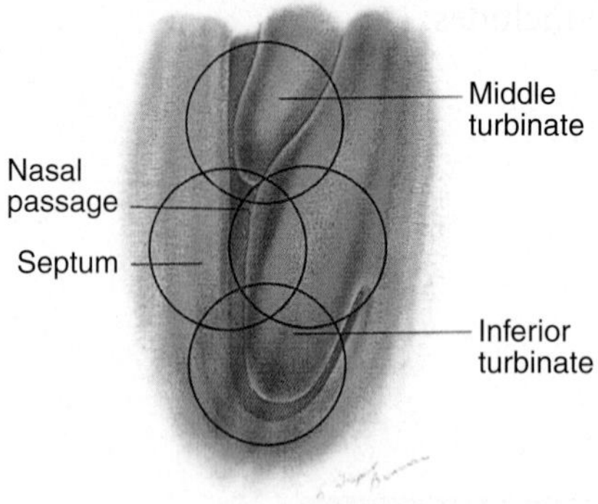

FIGURE 12-26 The turbinates of the nose.

Observe the nasal mucosa, the nasal septum, and any abnormalities:

- Inspect the *nasal mucosa* that covers the septum and turbinates. Note its color and any swelling, bleeding, or exudate. If exudate is present, note its character: clear, mucopurulent, or purulent. The nasal mucosa is normally somewhat redder than the oral mucosa.

In *viral rhinitis,* the mucosa is reddened and swollen; in *allergic rhinitis,* it may be pale, bluish, or red.

- Inspect the *nasal septum.* Note any deviation, inflammation, or perforation of the septum. The lower anterior portion of the septum (where the patient's finger can reach) is a common source of epistaxis.

Fresh blood or crusting may be present. Causes of septal perforation include trauma, surgery, and the intranasal use of cocaine or amphetamines, which can also cause septal ulceration.

- Note any *abnormalities* such as ulcers or polyps.

Nasal polyps are pale, semitranslucent sacs of inflamed tissue that can obstruct the airway.

Inspection of the nasal cavity through the anterior naris is usually limited to the vestibule, the anterior portion of the septum, and the lower and middle turbinates. Examination with a nasopharyngeal mirror is required for detection of posterior abnormalities. This technique is used by otorhinolaryngologists (ear, nose, and throat [ENT] specialists).

Dispose of all nasal and ear specula after use. (Check the policies of your institution.)

Palpate for sinus tenderness. Press up on the *frontal sinuses* from under the bony brows, avoiding pressure on the eyes (Fig. 12-27A). Then press up on the *maxillary sinuses* (Fig. 12-27B). Apply sufficient pressure to elicit pain or tenderness if present.

CLINICAL TIP

Local tenderness, together with symptoms such as facial pain, pressure or fullness, purulent nasal discharge, nasal obstructions, and smell disorder, especially when present for more than 7 days, suggest *acute bacterial rhinosinusitis* involving the frontal or maxillary sinuses (Cottrell et al., 2020).

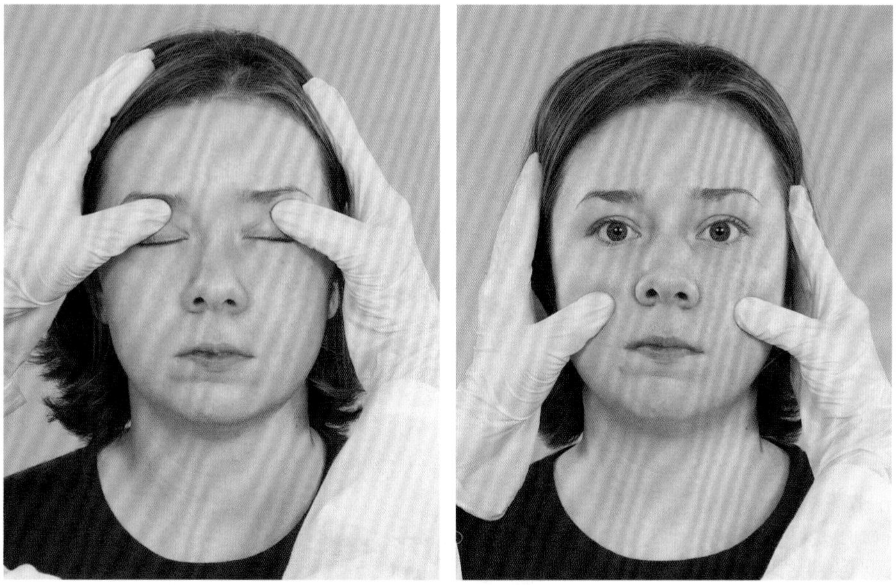

FIGURE 12-27 **A.** Palpating the frontal sinuses. **B.** Palpating the maxillary sinuses.

PHYSICAL EXAMINATION OF THE MOUTH AND THROAT

Equipment for examination of the mouth and throat includes:

- Penlight
- Tongue blade
- Gloves
- Gauze pad

Assess the teeth and dental hygiene. Take note if the teeth are real or if the patient wears dentures. Offer a paper towel and ask the patient to remove the dentures so that you can see the underlying mucosa. If you detect any suspicious ulcers or nodules, put on a glove and palpate any lesions, noting any thickening or infiltration of the tissues that might suggest malignancy.

CLINICAL TIP
Bright red edematous mucosa underneath a denture suggests *denture stomatitis* (denture sore mouth). There may be ulcers or papillary granulation tissue. Referral to a dentist is warranted.

The Lips

Observe the color and moisture of the lips, and note any lumps, ulcers, cracking, or scaling. See Table 12-5, "Abnormalities of the Lips."

Assess for central cyanosis or pallor from anemia.

TABLE 12-5 Abnormalities of the Lips

Angular Cheilitis

Angular cheilitis starts with softening of the skin at the angles of the mouth followed by fissuring. It may be due to nutritional deficiency or more commonly, to over-closure of the mouth, as in people with no teeth or with ill-fitting dentures. Saliva wets and macerates the infolded skin, often leading to secondary infection with *Candida*, as seen here.

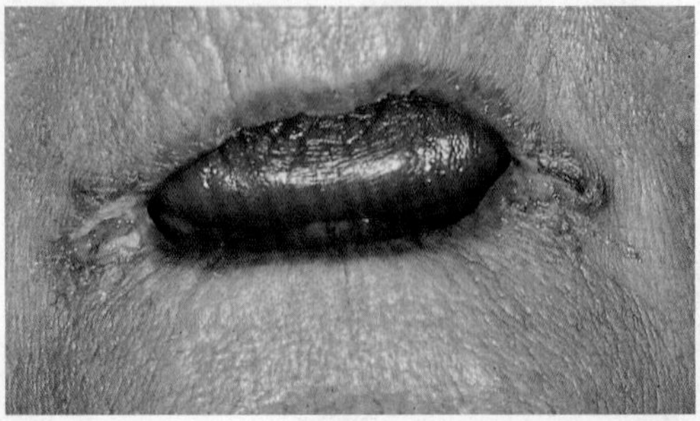

Actinic Cheilitis

Actinic cheilitis is a precancerous condition that results from excessive exposure to sunlight and affects primarily the lower lip. Fair-skinned men who work outdoors are most often affected. The lip loses its normal redness and may become scaly, somewhat thickened, and slightly everted. Because solar damage also predisposes to carcinoma of the lip, be alert to this possibility.

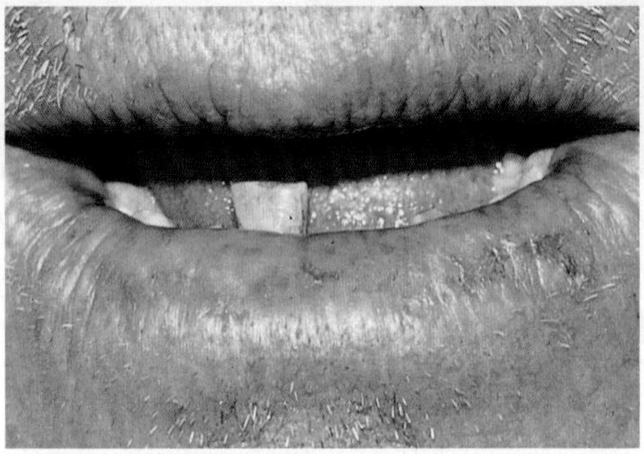

Herpes Simplex (*Cold Sore, Fever Blister*)

Herpes simplex virus (HSV) produces recurrent and painful vesicular eruptions of the lips and surrounding skin. A small cluster of vesicles first develops. As these break, yellow-brown crusts form; healing takes 10–14 days. Both new and erupted vesicles are visible here.

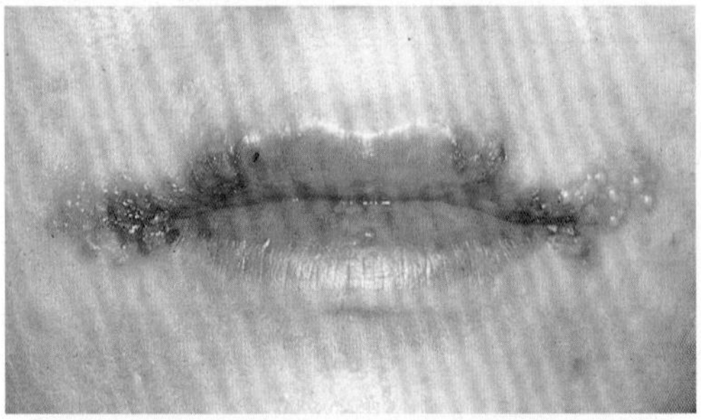

Angioedema

Angioedema is a localized subcutaneous or submucosal swelling caused by leakage of intravascular fluid into interstitial tissue. Two types are common. When vascular permeability is triggered by mast cells in allergic and NSAID reactions, look for associated urticaria and pruritus. These are uncommon in angioedema from bradykinin and complement-derived mediators, the mechanism in ACE inhibitor reactions. Angioedema is usually benign and resolves within 24–48 h. It can be life-threatening when it involves the larynx, tongue, or upper airway or develops into anaphylaxis.

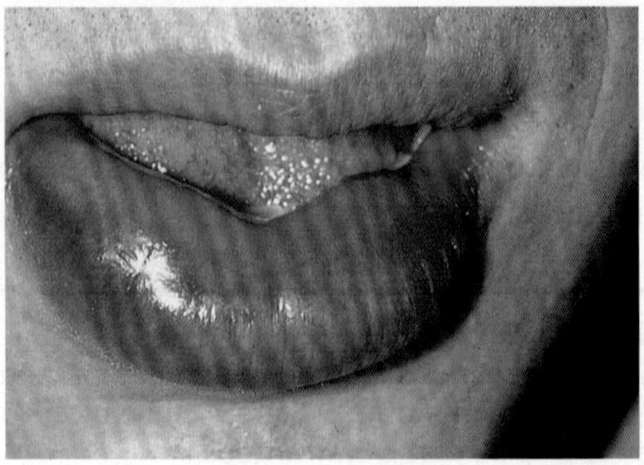

Hereditary Hemorrhagic Telangiectasia (Osler–Weber–Rendu Syndrome)

Multiple small red spots on the lips strongly suggest hereditary hemorrhagic telangiectasia, an autosomal dominant endothelial disorder causing vascular fragility and arteriovascular malformations (AVMs). Telangiectasias are also visible on the oral mucosa, nasal septal mucosa, and fingertips. Nosebleeds, gastrointestinal bleeding, and iron deficiency anemia are common. AVMs in the lungs and brain can cause life-threatening hemorrhage and embolic disease.

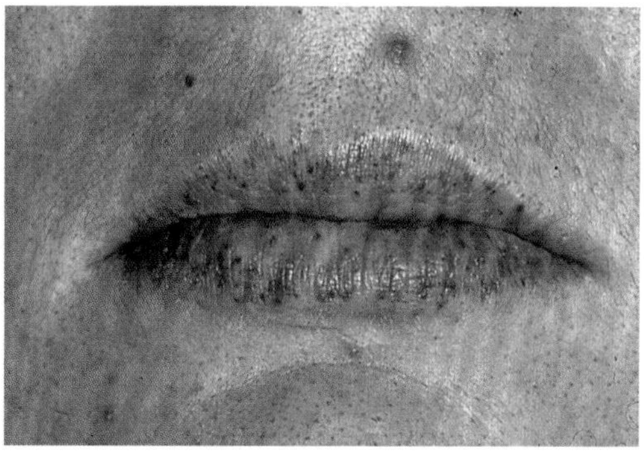

Peutz–Jeghers Syndrome

Look for prominent small brown pigmented spots in the dermal layer of the lips, buccal mucosa, and perioral area. These spots may also appear on the hands and feet. In this autosomal dominant syndrome, these characteristic skin changes accompany numerous intestinal polyps. The risk of gastrointestinal and other cancers ranges from 40–90%. Note that these spots rarely appear around the nose and mouth.

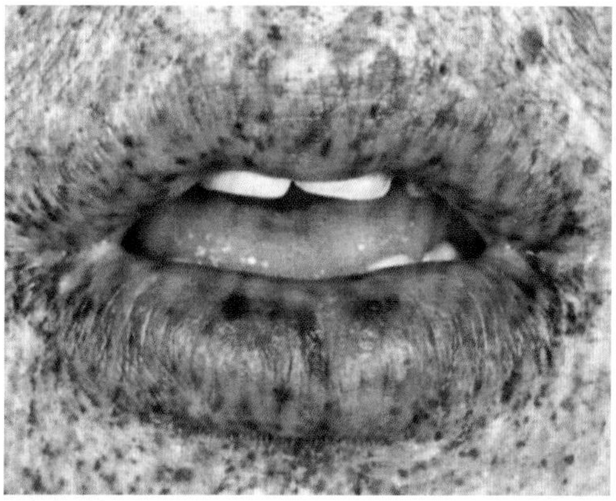

Chancre of Syphilis

This ulcerated papule with an indurated edge usually appears after 3–6 wk of incubating infection from the spirochete *Treponema pallidum*. These lesions may resemble a carcinoma or crusted cold sore. Similar primary lesions are common in the pharynx, anus, and vagina but may escape detection since they are painless, nonsuppurative, and usually heal spontaneously in 3–6 wk. Wear gloves during palpation since these chancres are infectious.

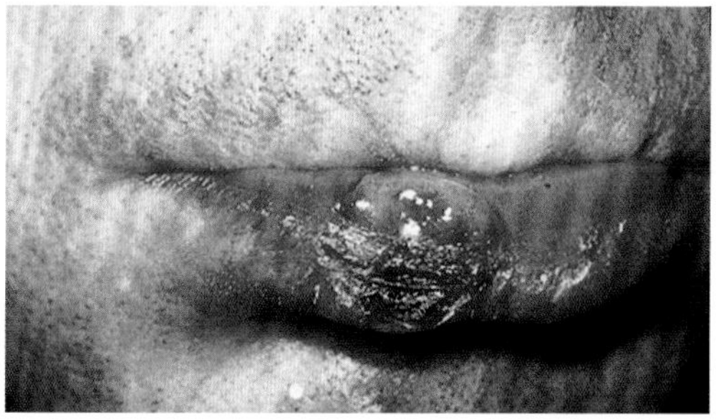

Carcinoma of the Lip

Like actinic cheilitis, *squamous cell carcinoma* usually affects the lower lip. It may appear as a scaly plaque, as an ulcer with or without a crust, or as a nodular lesion, as illustrated here. Fair skin and prolonged exposure to the sun are common risk factors.

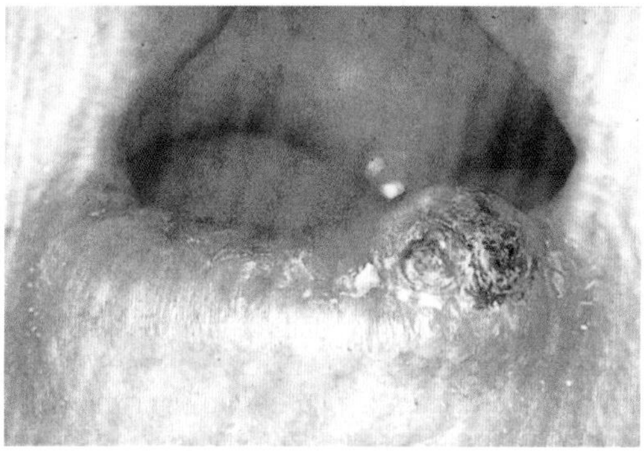

Sources of photos: *Angular Cheilitis, Herpes Simplex, Angioedema*—Neville, B. W., Damm, D. D., & White, D. K. (1991). *Color atlas of clinical oral pathology*. Lea & Febiger; Used with permission; *Actinic Cheilitis, Hereditary Hemorrhagic Telangiectasia*—Langlais, R. P., Miller, C. S. & Gehrig, J. S. (2017). *Color atlas of common oral diseases* (5th ed.). Wolters Kluwer; *Peutz–Jeghers Syndrome*—Robinson, H. B. G., & Miller, A. S. (1990). *Colby, Kerr, and Robinson's color atlas of oral pathology* (5th ed.). JB Lippincott; *Chancre of Syphilis*—Wisdom, A. A. (1989). *Colour atlas of sexually transmitted diseases* (2nd ed.). Wolfe Medical Publications; *Carcinoma of the Lip*—Tyldesley, W. R. (1991). *A colour atlas of orofacial diseases* (2nd ed.). Wolfe Medical Publications.

The Oral Mucosa

Look into the patient's mouth with a good light and the help of a tongue depressor. Inspect the oral mucosa for color, ulcers, white patches, and nodules.

Leukoedema is a grayish, blue-white coloring on the buccal mucosa (Fig. 12-28). This is commonly present more often in people with darker skin. This can develop where the upper and lower teeth meet and is irritated from sucking or chewing and is also more pronounced in smokers (Huang et al., 2020). Also look for **aphthous** ulcers (canker sores) as depicted in Figure 12-29. Table 12-6 outlines other findings possible in the pharynx, palate, and oral mucosa.

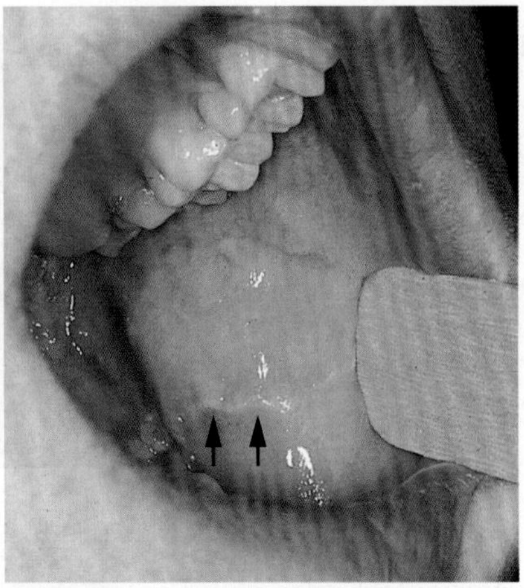

FIGURE 12-28 Leukoedema.

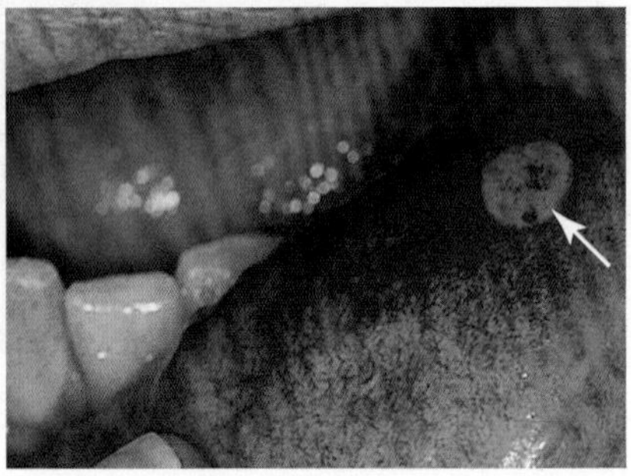

FIGURE 12-29 An aphthous ulcer.

TABLE 12-6 Findings in the Pharynx, Palate, and Oral Mucosa

Large Normal Tonsils

Normal tonsils may be large without being infected, especially in children. They may protrude medially beyond the pillars and even to the midline. Here they touch the sides of the uvula and obscure the pharynx. Their color is pink. The white marks are light reflections, not exudate.

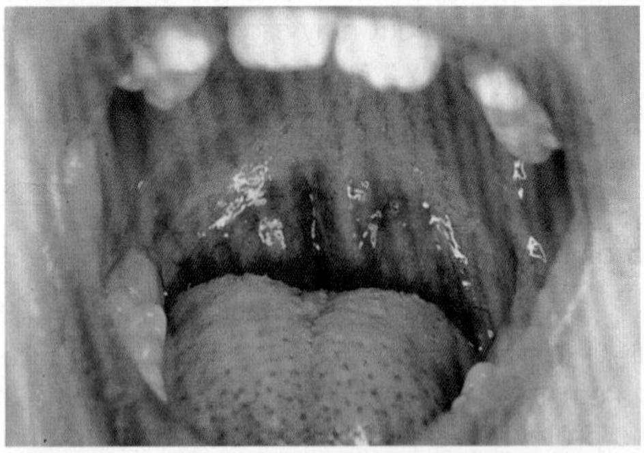

Exudative Tonsillitis

This red throat has a white exudate on the tonsils. This, together with fever and enlarged cervical nodes, increases the probability of *group A streptococcal infection* or *infectious mononucleosis*. Anterior cervical lymph nodes are usually enlarged in the former, posterior nodes in the latter.

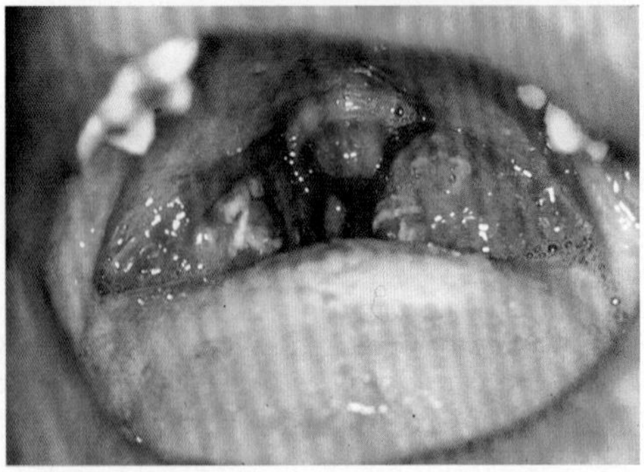

Pharyngitis

These two photos show reddened throats without exudate.

In **A**, redness and vascularity of the pillars and uvula are mild to moderate.

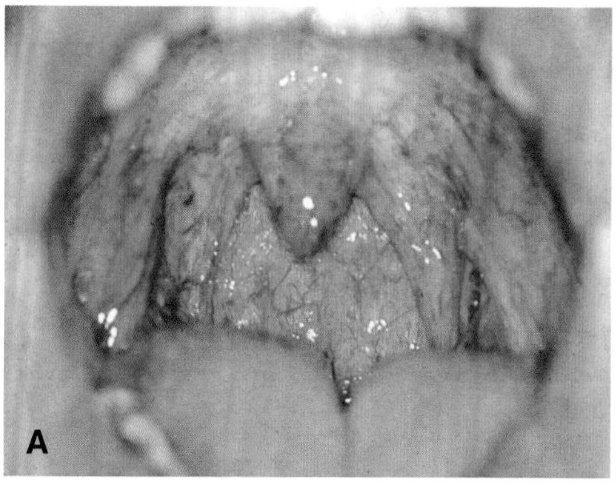

In **B**, redness is diffuse and intense. Each patient would probably complain of a sore throat, or at least a scratchy one. Possible causes include several kinds of viruses and bacteria. If the patient has no fever, exudate, or enlargement of cervical lymph nodes, the chances of infection by either of two common causes—*group A streptococci* and *Epstein-Barr virus* (infectious mononucleosis)—are reduced.

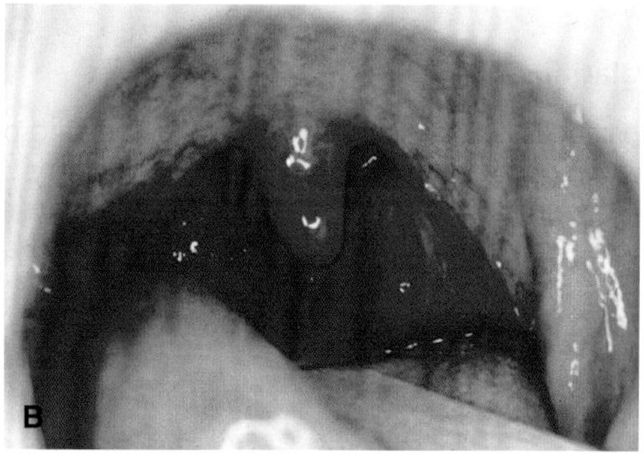

Diphtheria

Diphtheria, an acute infection caused by *Corynebacterium diphtheriae* is now rare but still important to be able to identify. The throat is dull red, and a gray exudate (pseudomembrane) is present on the uvula, pharynx, and tongue. The airway may become obstructed. Prompt diagnosis may lead to lifesaving treatment.

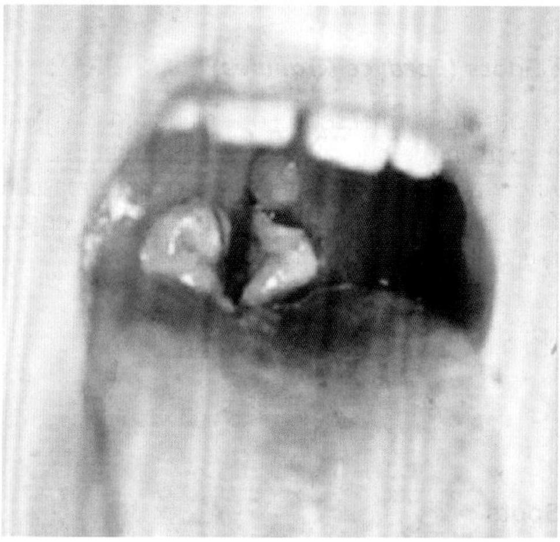

Thrush on the Palate (*Candidiasis*)

Thrush is a yeast infection due to *Candida*. Shown here on the palate, it may appear elsewhere in the mouth. Thick, white plaques are somewhat adherent to the underlying mucosa. Predisposing factors include (1) prolonged treatment with antibiotics or corticosteroids and (2) AIDS.

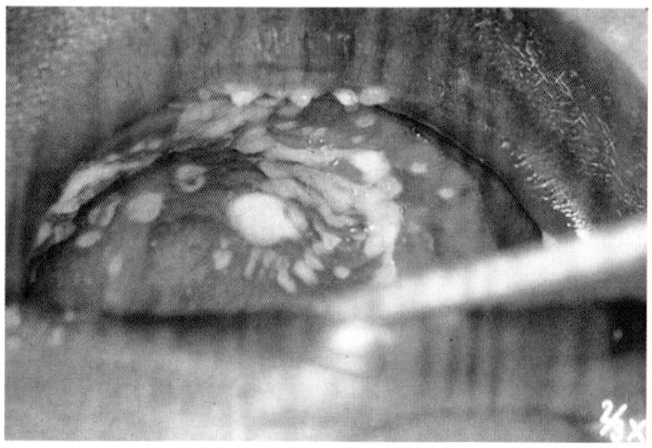

(continued)

TABLE 12-6 Findings in the Pharynx, Palate, and Oral Mucosa (*Continued*)

Kaposi Sarcoma in AIDS

The deep purple color of these lesions suggests Kaposi sarcoma, a low-grade vascular tumor associated with human herpesvirus 8. The lesions may be raised or flat. About a third of patients with Kaposi sarcoma have lesions in the oral cavity; other affected sites are the gastrointestinal tract and the lungs. Antiretroviral therapy has markedly reduced the prevalence of this disease.

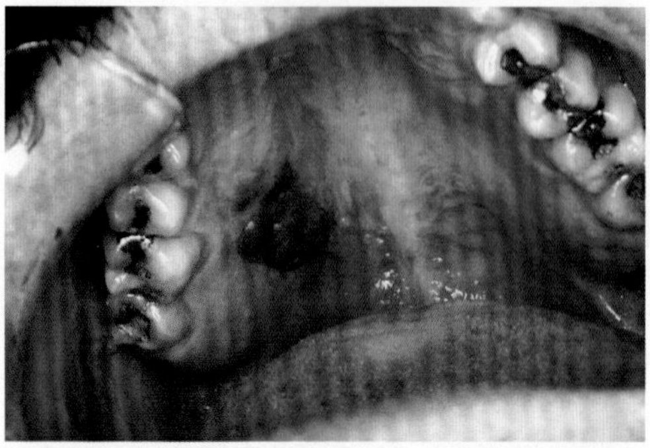

Torus Palatinus

A torus palatinus is a midline bony growth in the hard palate that is fairly common in adults. Its size and lobulation vary. Although alarming at first glance, it is harmless. In this example, an upper denture has been fitted around the torus.

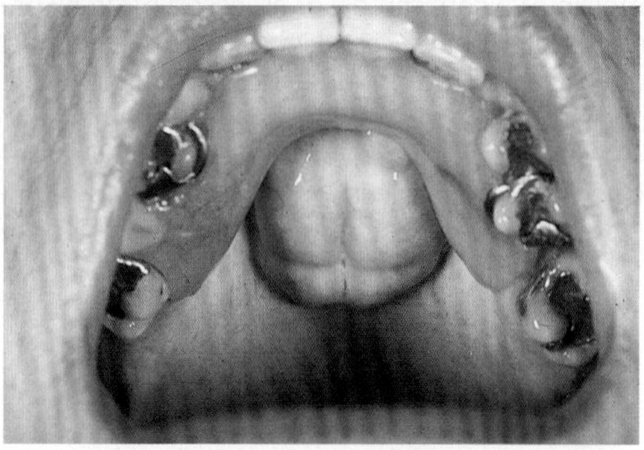

Fordyce Spots (*Fordyce Granules*)

Fordyce spots are normal sebaceous glands that appear as small yellowish spots in the buccal mucosa or on the lips. A worried person who has suddenly noticed them may be reassured. Here they are seen best anterior to the tongue and lower jaw. These spots are usually not so numerous.

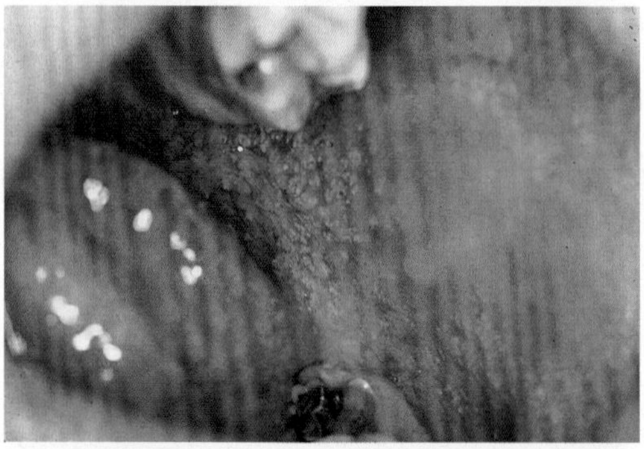

Koplik Spots

Koplik spots are an early sign of measles (rubeola). Search for small white specks that resemble grains of salt on a red background. They usually appear on the buccal mucosa near the first and second molars. In this photo, look also in the upper third of the mucosa. The rash of measles appears within a day.

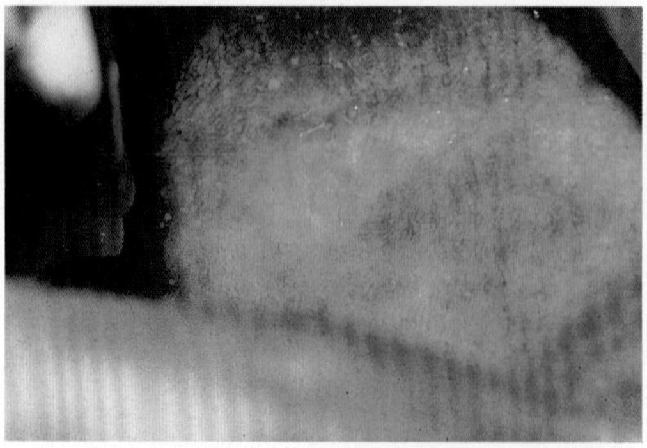

Petechiae

Petechiae are small red spots that result when blood escapes from capillaries into the tissues. Petechiae in the buccal mucosa, as shown, are often caused by accidentally biting the cheek. Oral petechiae may be due to infection or decreased platelets, as well as to trauma.

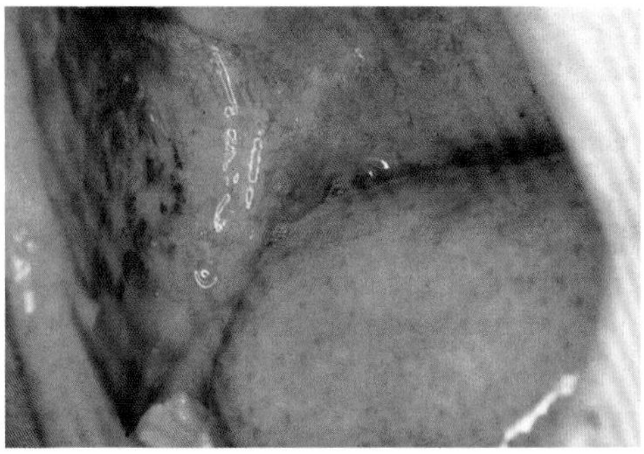

Leukoplakia

A thickened white patch (*leukoplakia*) may occur anywhere in the oral mucosa. The extensive example shown on this buccal mucosa resulted from frequent chewing of tobacco, a local irritant. This benign reactive process of the squamous epithelium may lead to cancer and should be biopsied. Another risk factor is human papillomavirus infection.

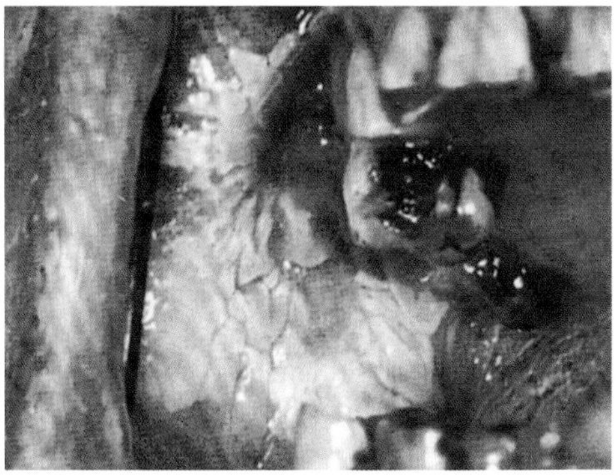

Sources of photos: *Large Normal Tonsils, Exudative Tonsillitis, Pharyngitis (**A** and **B**), Koplik Spots, Petechiae, Thrush on the Palate*—The Wellcome Trust, National Medical Slide Bank, London, UK; *Diphtheria*—Centers for Disease Control and Prevention; *Kaposi Sarcoma in AIDS*—CDC/ Sol Silverman, Jr., D. D. S., University of California, San Francisco; *Fordyce Spots*—Neville, B. W., Damm, D. D., & White, D. K. (1991). *Color atlas of clinical oral pathology*. Lea & Febiger; Used with permission; *Leukoplakia*—Robinson, H. B. G., & Miller, A. S. (1990). *Colby, Kerr, and Robinson's color atlas of oral pathology* (5th ed.). JB Lippincott.

The Gums and Teeth

Note the color of the gums which are normally pink. Patchy brownness may be present, especially but not exclusively in darker-skinned people.

Redness may indicate *gingivitis,* and a black line may indicate *lead poisoning.*

Inspect the gum margins and the interdental papillae for swelling or ulceration. Table 12-7 outlines other findings possible in the gums and teeth.

Swollen interdental papillae are present in *gingivitis*.

Inspect the teeth as they can provide information about development, hygiene, nutritional deficits, and cultural differences. Individuals with larger teeth may have protruding jaws, though this does not present a problem.

Assess for missing, discolored, misshapen, or abnormally positioned teeth. Note *malocclusion* of the teeth, and facial or jaw pain. Check for loose teeth with your gloved thumb and index finger. Loose-fitting dentures may contribute to ulcers in the mouth or tooth decay and ultimately cause halitosis (bad breath) (Kumbargere Nagraj et al., 2019).

Overall, White individuals have more decay and 51% have complete tooth loss compared to 39% in African Americans, though there is a higher prevalence of periodontal disease among African Americans (Andrews & Boyle, 2015).

CLINICAL TIP
Breath odor is indicative of many issues, such as diabetic ketoacidosis, renal failure, or mouth, nose, or pharynx infection (Kumbargere Nagraj et al., 2019).

TABLE 12-7 Findings in the Gums and Teeth

Marginal Gingivitis

Marginal gingivitis is common during adolescence, early adulthood, and pregnancy. The gingival margins are reddened and swollen, and the interdental papillae are blunted, swollen, and red. Brushing the teeth often makes the gums bleed. *Plaque*—the soft white film of salivary salts, protein, and bacteria that covers the teeth and leads to gingivitis—is not readily visible.

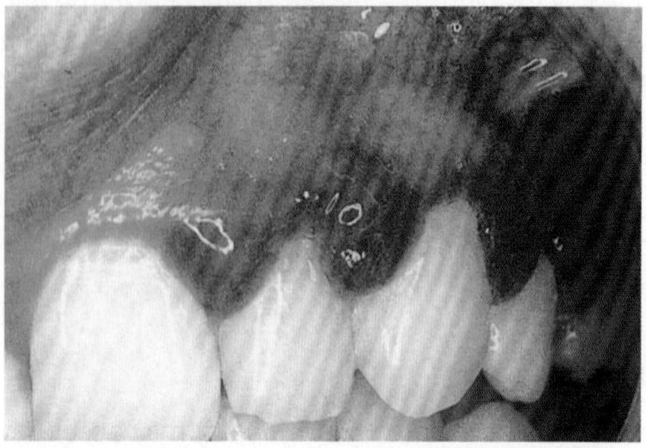

Acute Necrotizing Ulcerative Gingivitis

This uncommon form of gingivitis occurs suddenly in adolescents and young adults and is accompanied by fever, malaise, and enlarged lymph nodes. Ulcers develop in the interdental papillae. Then the destructive (necrotizing) process spreads along the gum margins, where a grayish pseudomembrane develops. The red, painful gums bleed easily; the breath is foul.

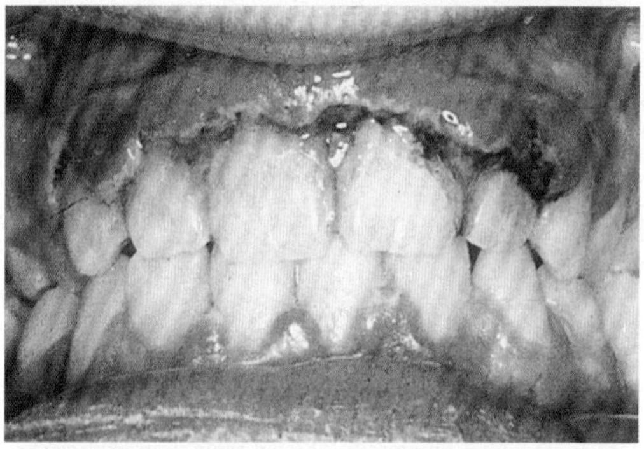

Gingival Hyperplasia

Gums enlarged by hyperplasia are swollen into heaped-up masses that may even cover the teeth. The redness of inflammation may coexist, as in this example. Causes include phenytoin (Dilantin) therapy (as in this case), puberty, pregnancy, and leukemia.

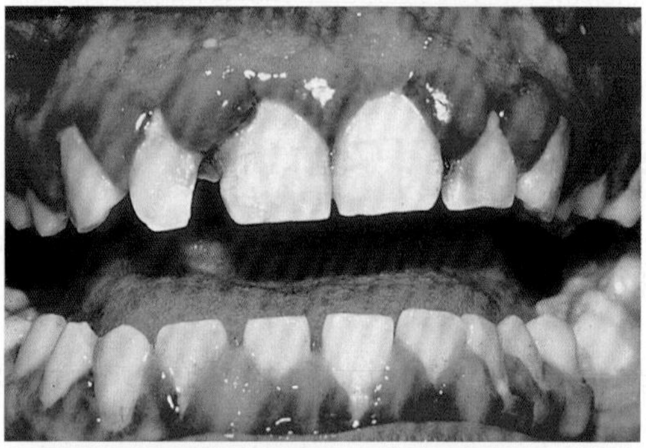

Pregnancy Tumor (*Pregnancy Epulis, Pyogenic Granuloma*)

Red purple papules of granulation tissue form in the gingival interdental papillae, in the nasal cavity, and sometimes on the fingers. They are red and soft and usually bleed easily. They occur in 1–5% of pregnancies and usually regress after delivery. Note the accompanying gingivitis in this example.

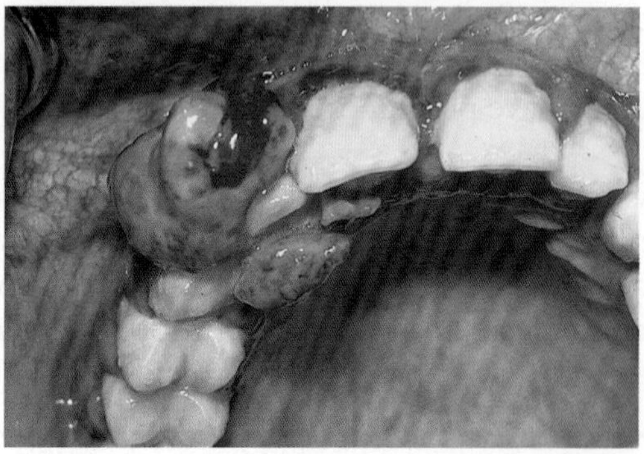

Attrition of Teeth; Recession of Gums

In many elderly people, the chewing surfaces of the teeth have been worn down by repetitive use so that the yellow-brown dentin becomes exposed—a process called *attrition*. Note the *recession of the gums*, which has exposed the roots of the teeth, giving a "long in the tooth" appearance.

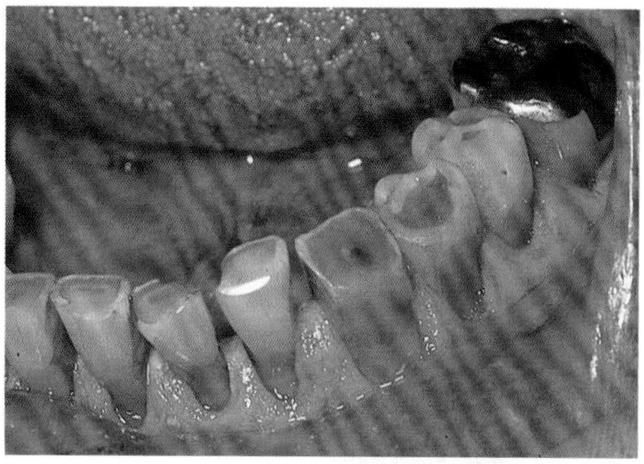

Erosion of Teeth

Teeth may be eroded by chemical action. Note here the erosion of the enamel from the lingual surfaces of the upper incisors, exposing the yellow-brown dentin. This results from recurrent regurgitation of stomach contents, as in bulimia.

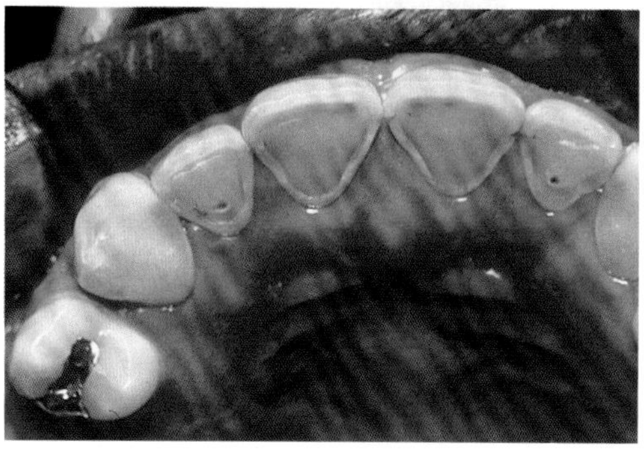

Abrasion of Teeth with Notching

The biting surface of the teeth may become abraded or notched by recurrent trauma, such as holding nails or opening bobby pins between the teeth. Unlike Hutchinson teeth, the sides of these teeth show normal contours; size and spacing of the teeth are unaffected.

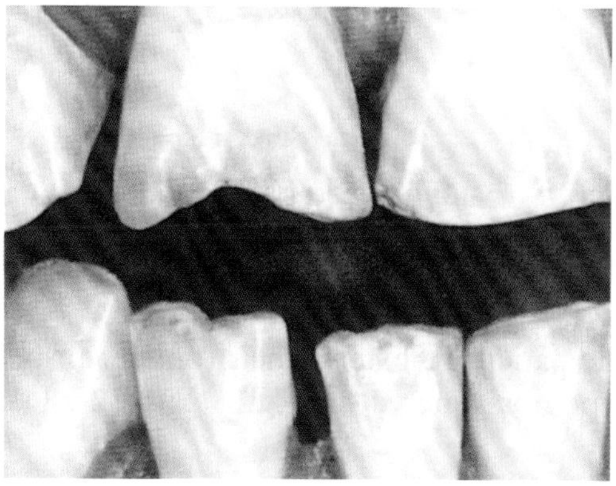

Hutchinson Teeth

Hutchinson teeth are smaller and more widely spaced than normal and are notched on their biting surfaces. The sides of the teeth taper toward the biting edges. The upper central incisors of the permanent (not the deciduous) teeth are most often affected. These teeth are a sign of congenital syphilis.

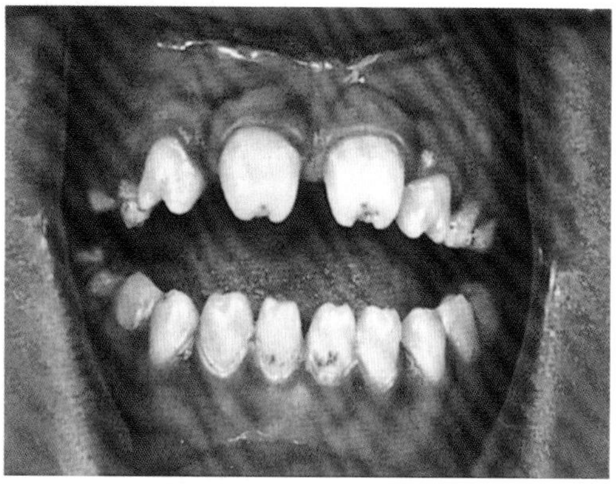

Sources of photos: *Marginal Gingivitis, Acute Necrotizing Ulcerative Gingivitis*—Tyldesley, W. R. (1991). *A Colour atlas of orofacial diseases* (2nd ed.). Wolfe Medical Publications; *Gingival Hyperplasia*—Courtesy of Dr. James Cottone; *Pregnancy Tumor, Attrition of Teeth, Erosion of Teeth*—Langlais, R. P., Miller, C. S., & Gehrig, J. S. (2017). *Color atlas of common oral diseases* (5th ed.). Wolters Kluwer, Used with permission; *Abrasion of Teeth, Hutchinson Teeth*—Robinson, H. B. G., & Miller, A. S. (1990). *Colby, Kerr, and Robinson's color atlas of oral pathology* (5th ed.). JB Lippincott.

The Roof of the Mouth

Inspect the color, architecture, and continuity of the hard palate.

Cleft lip is a separation or split of the upper lip, which can extend down from the base of the nose. *Cleft palate* is an opening or split of the roof of the mouth, involving the hard and/or the soft palate (Fig. 12-30).

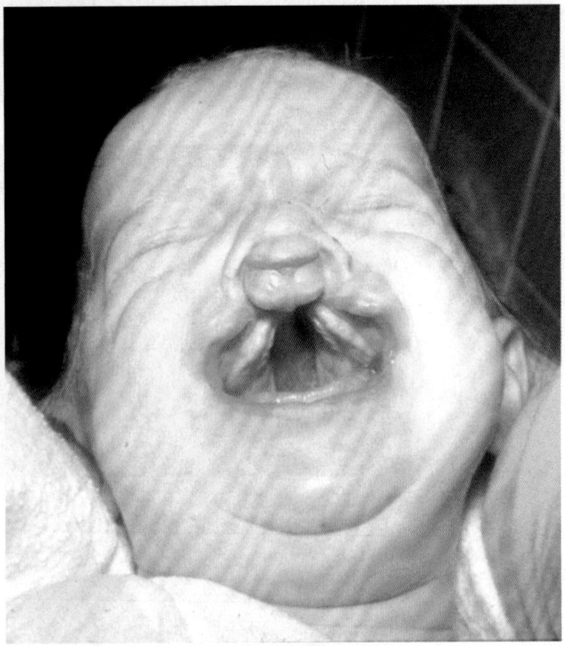

FIGURE 12-30 Bilateral cleft lip and cleft palate.

The Tongue and the Floor of the Mouth

Ask the patient to extend their tongue. Inspect it for symmetry—a test of the hypoglossal nerve (CN XII) (Fig. 12-31).

Torus mandibularis is a bony protrusion from the medial mandible near the surface close to the tongue. Torus palatinus is a bony growth in the middle of the hard palate.

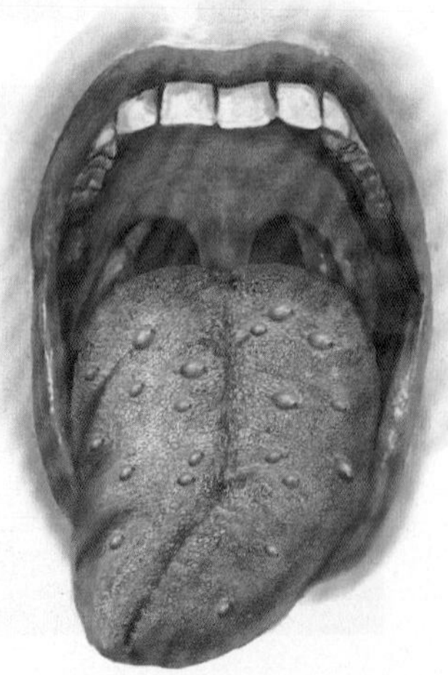

FIGURE 12-31 Asymmetric protrusion of the tongue suggests a lesion of CN XII with the tongue pointing "toward" the lesion.

Note the color and texture of the dorsum of the tongue. Inspect the entire oral cavity, especially the sides and undersurface of the tongue and the floor of the mouth (Fig. 12-32). These are the areas where cancer most often develops. Note any white or reddened areas, nodules, or ulcerations.

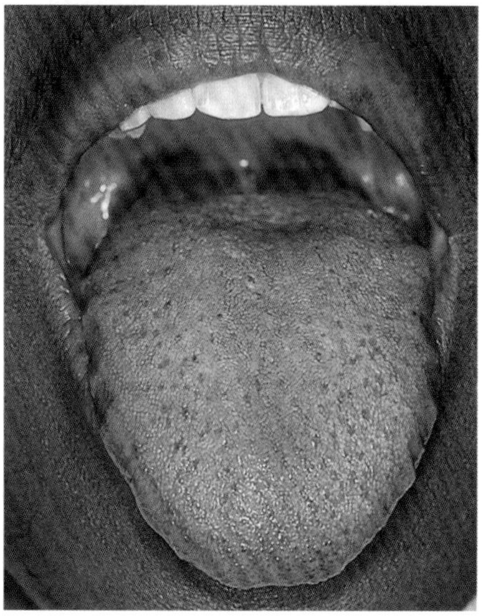

FIGURE 12-32 Inspecting the oral cavity.

Wearing gloves, palpate all lesions. Ask the patient to protrude the tongue. With your right hand, grasp the tip of the tongue with a square of gauze and gently pull it to the patient's left (Fig. 12-33). Inspect the side of the tongue, and then palpate it with your gloved left hand, feeling for any induration. Reverse the procedure for the right side. Table 12-8 outlines possible findings on or under the tongue.

Men older than 50 years, smokers, and heavy users of chewing tobacco and alcohol are at the highest risk for cancers of the tongue and oral cavity, usually *squamous cell carcinomas* on the side or base of the tongue (Liu et al., 2019). Any persistent nodule or ulcer, red or white, is suspect, especially if indurated. These discolored lesions represent *erythroplakia* (red, fiery patches) and *leukoplakia* (white patches) and should be biopsied (Myers et al., 2020).

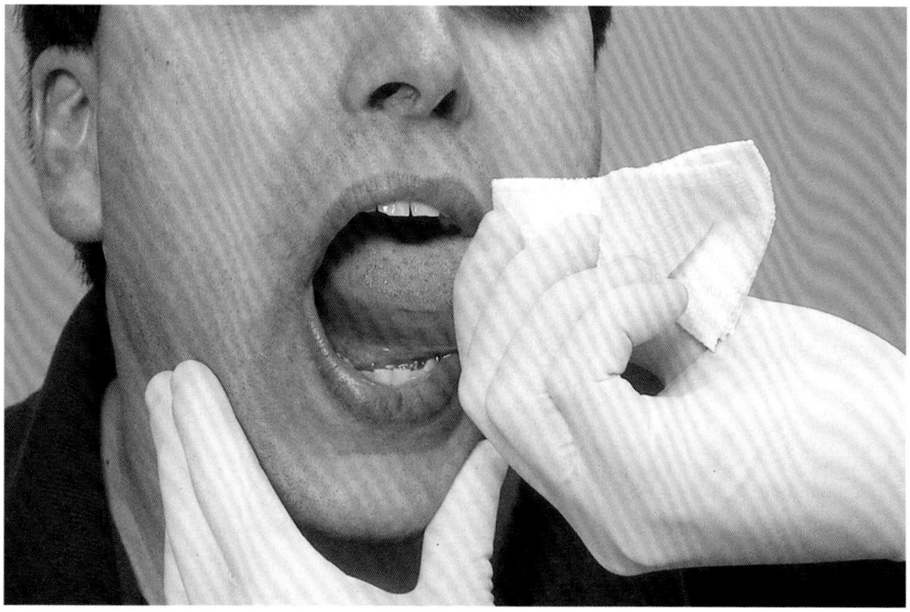

FIGURE 12-33 Inspection of the tongue.

TABLE 12-8 Findings on or Under the Tongue

Geographic Tongue

In this benign condition, the dorsum shows scattered smooth red areas denuded of papillae. Together with the normal rough and coated areas, they give a map-like pattern that changes over time.

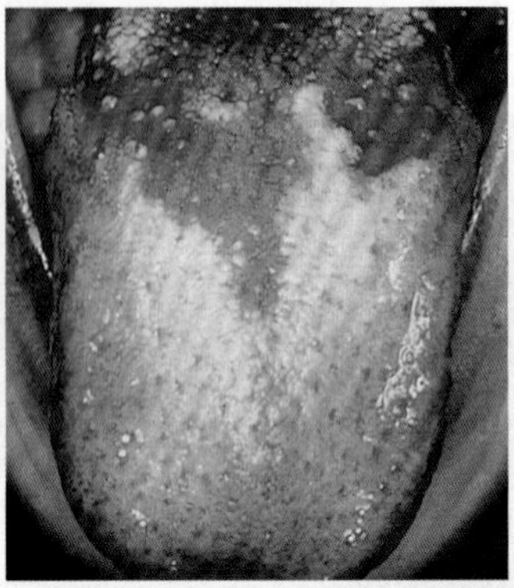

Hairy Tongue

Note the "hairy" yellowish to brown or black hypertrophied and elongated papillae on the tongue's dorsum. This benign condition is associated with *Candida* and bacterial overgrowth, antibiotic therapy, and poor dental hygiene. It may occur spontaneously.

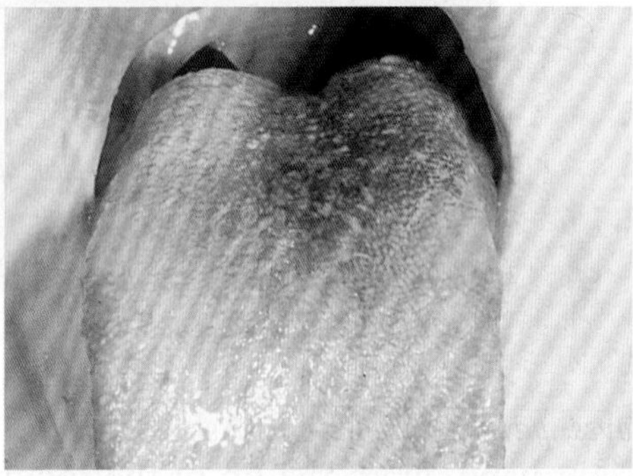

Fissured Tongue

Fissures appear with increasing age, sometimes termed *furrowed tongue*. Food debris may accumulate in the crevices and become irritating, but a fissured tongue is benign.

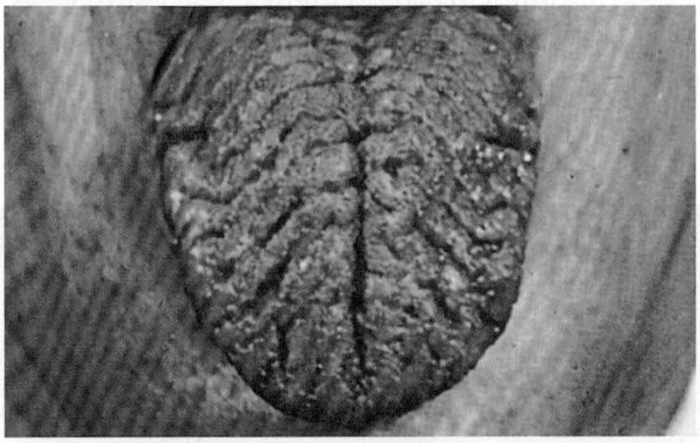

Smooth Tongue (*Atrophic Glossitis*)

A smooth and often sore tongue that has lost its papillae, sometimes just in patches, suggests a deficiency in riboflavin, niacin, folic acid, vitamin B_{12}, pyridoxine, or iron, or treatment with chemotherapy.

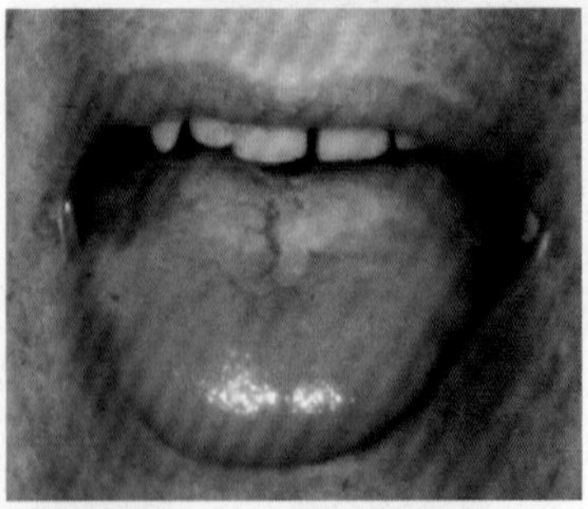

Candidiasis

Note the thick white coating from *Candida* infection. The raw red surface is where the coat was scraped off. Infection may also occur without the white coating. It is seen in immunosuppression from chemotherapy or prednisone therapy.

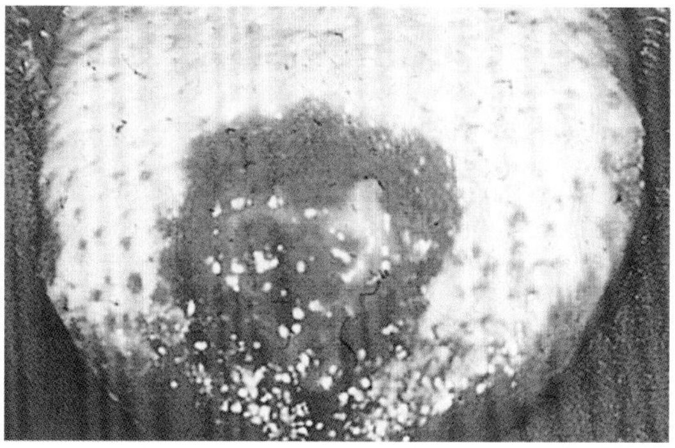

Hairy Leukoplakia

These whitish raised asymptomatic plaques with a feathery or corrugated pattern commonly occur on the sides of the tongue. Unlike candidiasis, these areas cannot be scraped off. This condition is caused by Epstein–Barr virus infection and is seen with HIV and AIDS.

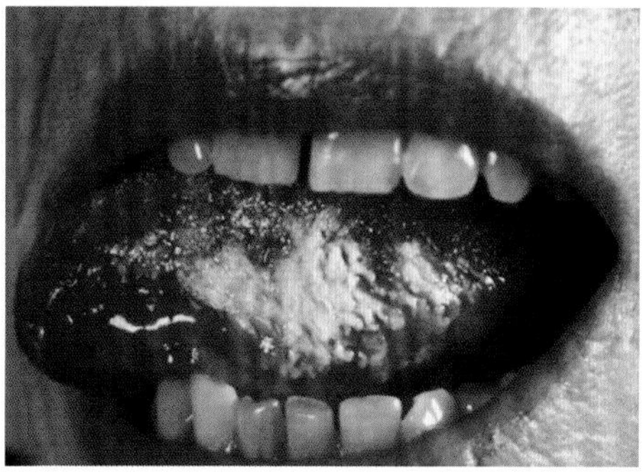

Varicose Veins

Small purplish or blue-black round swellings appear under the tongue with age. These dilatations of the lingual veins have no clinical significance.

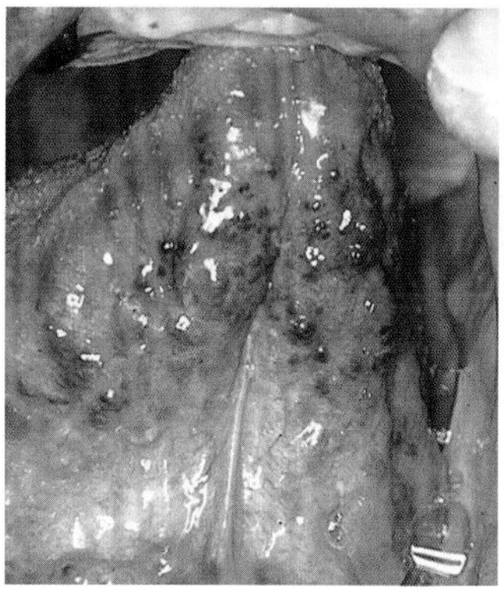

Aphthous Ulcer (*Canker Sore*)

A painful, round or oval shallow whitish-gray oval ulceration surrounded by a halo of reddened mucosa. It may be single or multiple and may also occur on the gingiva and oral mucosa. It heals in 7–10 days, but may recur, for example, in Behcet disease.

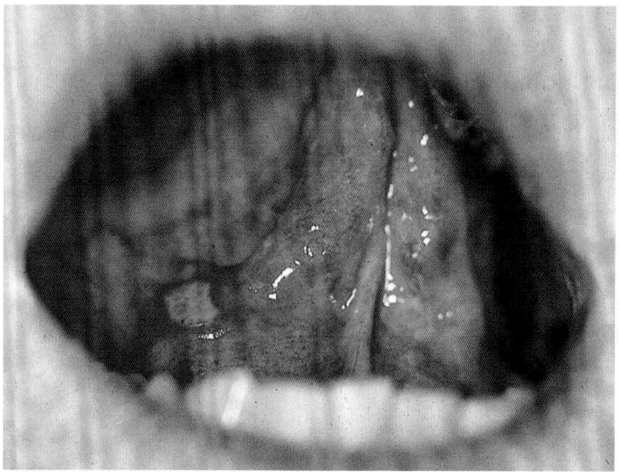

(continued)

TABLE 12-8 Findings on or Under the Tongue *(Continued)*

Mucous Patch of Syphilis

This painless lesion in the secondary stage of syphilis is highly infectious. It is slightly raised, oval, and covered by a grayish membrane. It may be multiple and occur elsewhere in the mouth.

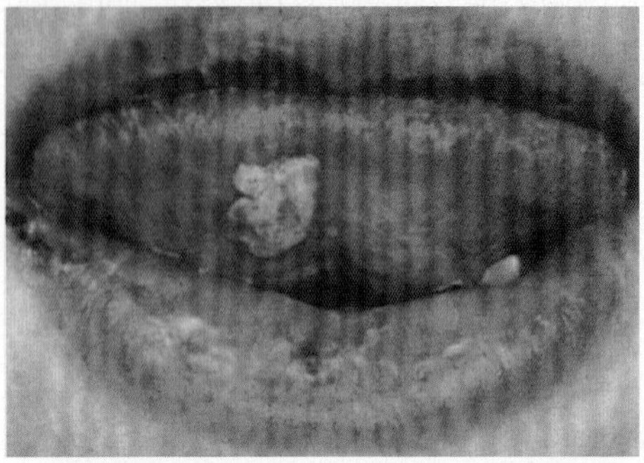

Leukoplakia

With this persisting painless white patch in the oral mucosa, the undersurface of the tongue appears painted white. Patches of any size raise the possibility of squamous cell carcinoma and require a biopsy.

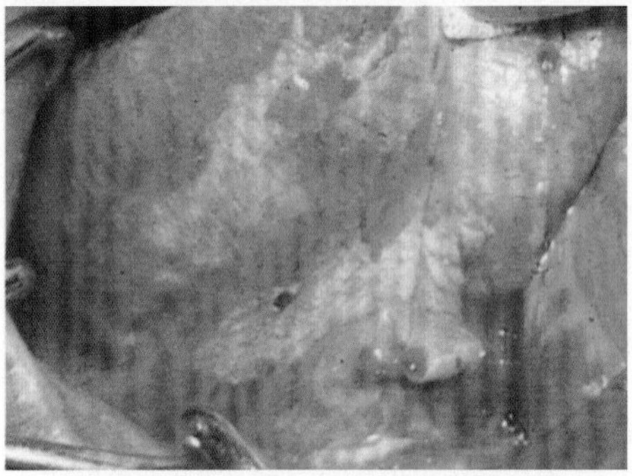

Tori Mandibulares

Rounded bony growths on the inner surfaces of the mandible are typically bilateral, asymptomatic, and harmless.

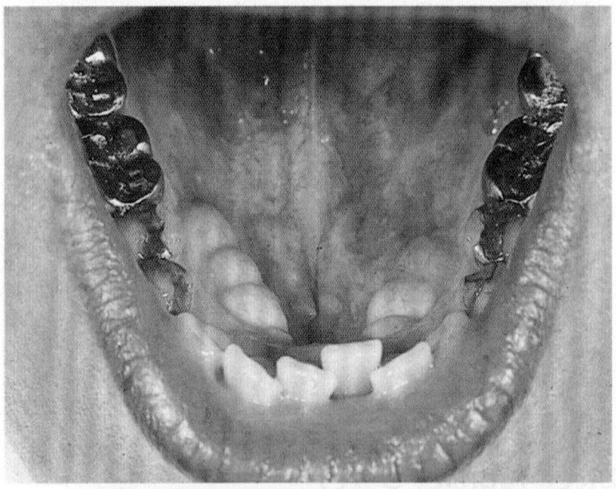

Carcinoma, Floor of the Mouth

This ulcerated lesion is in a common location for carcinoma. Medially, note the reddened area of mucosa, called *erythroplakia*, suggesting possible malignancy.

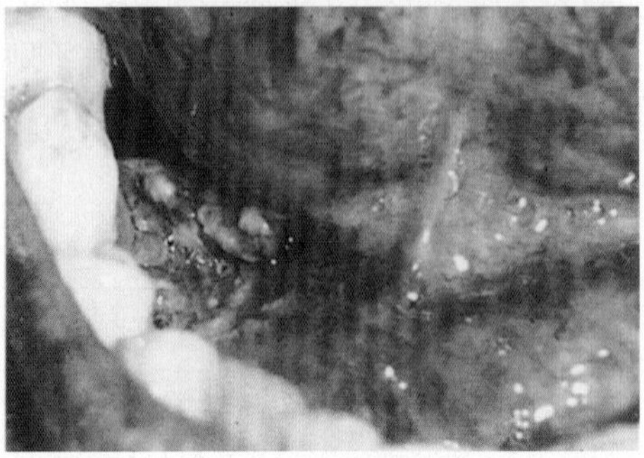

Sources of photos: *Fissured Tongue, Candidiasis, Mucous Patch, Leukoplakia, Carcinoma*—Robinson, H. B. G., & Miller, A. S. (1990). *Colby, Kerr, and Robinson's color atlas of oral pathology* (5th ed.). JB Lippincott; *Smooth Tongue*—Weksler, B. B., Schechter, J. P., & Ely, S. (2017). *Wintrobe's atlas of clinical hematology* (2nd ed.). Wolters Kluwer; *Geographic Tongue*—The Wellcome Trust, National Medical Slide Bank, London, UK; *Hairy Leukoplakia*—Goodheart, H. P., & Gonzalez, M. E. (2015). *Goodheart's photoguide to common pediatric and adult skin disorders* (4th ed.). Wolters Kluwer; *Varicose Veins*—Neville, B. W., Damm, D. D., & White, D. K. (1991). *Color atlas of clinical oral pathology*. Lea & Febiger; Used with permission.

The Pharynx

With the patient's mouth open but the tongue not protruded, ask the patient to say "ah" or yawn. This action helps you see the pharynx well. If you are not able to visualize the pharynx, press a tongue blade firmly down on the midpoint of the arched tongue—back far enough to see the pharynx but not so far that you cause gagging. Simultaneously, ask for an "ah" or a yawn. Note the rise of the soft palate and the uvula—a test of CN X (the vagal nerve). With CN X paralysis (Fig. 12-34), the soft palate fails to rise and the uvula deviates to the opposite side (points "away" from the lesion).

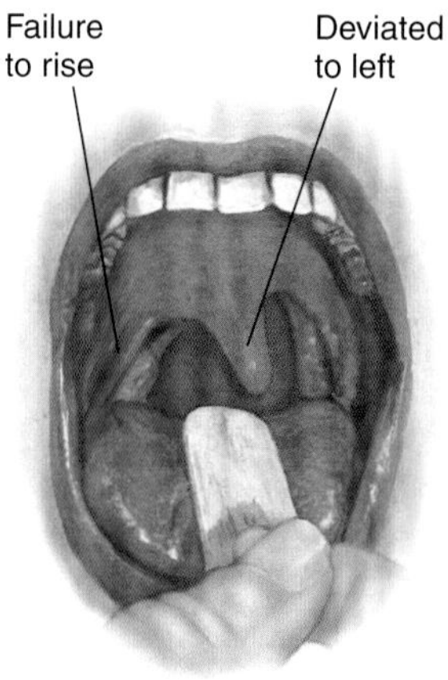

FIGURE 12-34 Deviation of the uvula indicative of CN X paralysis.

Inspect the soft palate, anterior and posterior pillars, uvula, tonsils, and pharynx. Note their color and symmetry and look for exudate, swelling, ulceration, or tonsillar enlargement. Tonsils have crypts, or deep folds of squamous epithelium where whitish spots of normal exfoliating epithelium may sometimes be seen.

Tonsils are graded based on size (Fig. 12-35):

- +1: Tonsils are visible.
- +2: Tonsils are between the tonsillar pillars and the uvula.
- +3: Tonsils are touching the uvula.
- +4: Tonsils are touching each other.

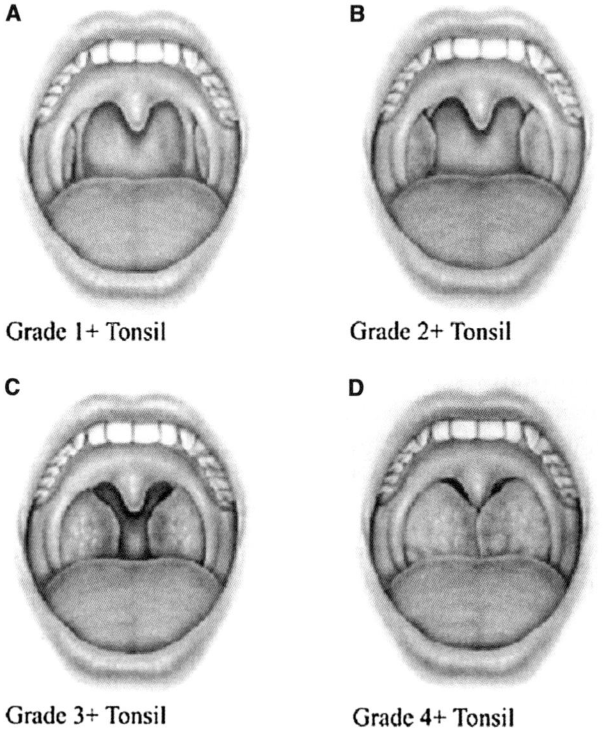

FIGURE 12-35 Grading of the tonsils. (Reprinted with permission from Johnson, J., & Rosen, C. A. (2013). *Bailey's head and neck surgery: Otolaryngology* (5th ed.). Wolters Kluwer.)

If possible, palpate any suspicious area for induration or tenderness.

See Table 12-6, "Findings in the Pharynx, Palate, and Oral Mucosa."

Discard your tongue blade and gloves after use and wash hands.

RECORDING YOUR FINDINGS

Box 12-5 includes examples of documentation of physical examination of the ears, nose, and mouth, and throat.

BOX 12-5 RECORDING THE PHYSICAL EXAMINATION—EARS, NOSE, AND THROAT

Ears—Acuity to whispered voice: L, "4-P-9"; R, "2-K-6." Tympanic membranes (TMs) intact, pearly gray, with cone of light at 7:00, L ear; 5:00, R ear. Weber midline. AC > BC. *Nose*—Nasal mucosa pink, septum midline; no sinus tenderness. *Mouth and throat*—Oral mucosa pink, dentition 32 teeth, white, visible decay, pharynx without exudates.

OR

Ears—Acuity diminished to whispered voice; intact to spoken voice, L decreased to "4-P-9," TMs intact, pearly gray. *Nose*—Mucosa swollen with erythema and clear drainage. Septum midline. Tender over maxillary sinuses. *Mouth and throat*—Oral mucosa pink, dental caries in lower molars, pharynx erythematous, no exudates.

HEALTH PROMOTION, DISEASE PREVENTION, AND EDUCATION: THE EARS

Important topics for health promotion of the ears include:

- Hearing screening
- Ear protection

Hearing is a critical sense for experiencing the world around us, and areas of importance are health promotion and disease prevention. Nursing education is vital in maintaining hearing and a healthy outlook for clients.

Hearing Screening

Universal screening for all newborns in the United States has been the standard of care since 2008. The Early Hearing Detection and Intervention (EHDI) program not only screens but includes evaluations to diagnose infants who do not pass the initial screening with interventions for those with hearing loss (Vos et al., 2019). This early detection will assist with early interventions in language and communication. Additional information can be obtained from the National Institute for Deafness and Communication Disorders at www.nidcd.nih.gov.

Hearing Loss

The World Health Organization has determined that close to 50% of people between the ages of 12 and 35 use personal devices at unsafe audible levels. Loss of hearing is a chronic condition and is two times more prevalent than cancer or diabetes (Blackwell et al., 2014). The National Health Interview Survey (NHIS) discovered that about 21% of individuals 18 years and older had trouble hearing when there was background noise, 11.2% had tinnitus, and 5.9% were sensitive to normal sounds (Zelaya et al., 2015).

Sound is measured in decibels. Sounds at or above 85 dB will cause hearing loss; even sounds less than 75 dB with repeated exposure are likely to cause loss. Normal conversation happens at 60 dB. Non-Hispanic White adults are more likely than other racial and ethnic groups to experience loss of hearing (CDC, 2020b). African Americans have a higher amount of melanin in the cochlea, and research indicates this may reduce hearing loss due to environmental noise (Andrews & Boyle, 2015). Prevention is key, and patients should be reminded to use ear protection when exposed to loud noises in their daily lives (e.g., lawnmowers, leaf blowers, chainsaws, concerts, train stations, battlefields, sirens) and to limit exposure (e.g., concerts, earbuds, cell phones). The key is to avoid noises that are too close, too loud, and/or too long.

More than 5% of the people in the world (about 466 million) have disabling hearing loss. The rate is projected to increase to over 900 million by 2050 (World Health Organization, 2020). Hearing loss in the later years is not only from noise exposure but also from **presbycusis** (age-associated hearing loss), which affects many older adults. One third of adults older than 65 years are affected by disabling hearing loss with the greatest prevalence in sub-Saharan Africa, Asia Pacific, and South Asia (World Health Organization, 2020). Hearing loss can contribute to emotional isolation and social withdrawal. Loss of hearing may go undetected if it is gradual since many do not realize hearing is decreasing. Unlike vision prerequisites for driving, there is no mandate for widespread testing of hearing, and many older adults avoid using hearing aids. Questionnaires and handheld audiometers work well for periodic screening. Less sensitive tests are the clinical "whisper test," rubbing fingers, or the use of the tuning fork.

HEALTH PROMOTION, DISEASE PREVENTION, AND EDUCATION: THE MOUTH AND THROAT

Important topics for health promotion regarding the mouth and throat include:

- Oral and dental screening
- Cancer prevention

Approximately 20% of children 5 to 11 years of age and 13% of teenagers 12 to 19 years of age have at least one untreated decayed primary tooth (CDC, 2020a). Children in low-income homes ages 5 to 19 years old are twice as likely to get cavities as children in higher-income homes (CDC,

2020a). This issue persists throughout life; those 50 to 69 years of age have higher rates of periodontal disease. The rate is highest for non-Hispanic Black individuals (31.2%), Mexican Americans (28.2%), and non-Hispanic White individuals (16.9%). As these groups age, the percentages rise to 47.1%, 32.0%, and 24.1%, respectively (Finnegan et al., 2016).

Nurses play an active role in promoting oral health. Health disparities regarding oral health are apparent among certain racial and ethnic groups. Overall non-Hispanic Black, Hispanic, Native American, and Alaskan Native individuals have poorer oral health. Untreated tooth decay and periodontal disease is three times as likely in adults 35 to 44 years of age with less than a high school education (Finnegan et al., 2016).

Effective screening begins with careful examination of the mouth. Inspect the oral cavity for decayed or loose teeth, inflammation of the gingiva, and signs of periodontal disease (bleeding, pus, recession of the gums, and bad breath). Inspect the mucous membranes, the palate, the oral floor, and the surfaces of the tongue for ulcers and leukoplakia, warning signs for oral cancer and HIV disease. Use of dental dams during oral sex will act as a barrier to bodily fluids and help reduce transmission of STIs such as herpes, genital warts, and HIV.

Concept Mastery Alert

Gingival Hyperplasia

While a finding of gingival hyperplasia may lead the novice nurse to consider a history of tobacco use, common causes also include phenytoin (Dilantin), puberty, pregnancy, and leukemia.

To improve oral health, counsel patients to adopt daily hygiene measures. Use of fluoride-containing toothpaste reduces tooth decay, and brushing and flossing daily delays periodontal disease by removing bacterial plaques. Urge patients to seek dental care at least annually to receive the benefits of more specialized preventive care such as scaling, planing (smoothing rough spots on tooth roots to prevent gum disease), and topical fluorides and sealants (CDC, 2020a).

Diet, tobacco and alcohol use, changes in salivary flow from medication, and proper use of dentures should also be addressed. As with children, adults should avoid excessive intake of foods high in refined sugars such as sucrose, which enhance attachment and colonization of cariogenic bacteria. Use of all tobacco products and excessive alcohol, the principal risk factors for oral cancers, should be avoided.

Saliva cleanses and lubricates the mouth. Many medications reduce salivary flow, increasing risk for tooth decay, mucositis, and gum disease from *xerostomia* (dryness of the mouth), especially for the elderly. For those wearing dentures, dental examinations should be scheduled annually, and patients should be counseled about the importance of removing and cleaning the dentures each night to reduce bacterial plaque and risk of malodor. Regular massage of the gums relieves soreness and pressure from dentures on the underlying soft tissue.

Bibliography

Alford, R. L., & Sutton, V. R. (2011). *Medical genetics in the clinical practice of ORL*. Karger.

Andrews, M. A., & Boyle, J. S. (2015). *Transcultural concepts in nursing care* (7th ed.). Lippincott Williams & Wilkins.

Babu, S., Schutt, C. A., & Bojrab, D. I. (2019). *Diagnosis and treatment of vestibular disorders*. Springer International Publishing.

Bagai, A., Thavendiranathan, P., & Detsky, A. S. (2006). Does this patient have hearing impairment? *JAMA, 295*(4), 416–428.

Blackwell, D. L., Lucas, J. W., & Clarke, T. C. (2014). Summary Health Statistics for US adults: National Health Interview Survey, 2012. *Vital and Health Statistics. Series 10, Data from the National Health Survey*, (260), 1–161.

Carrillo Muñoz, R., Ballve Moreno, J. L., Villar Balboa, I., Rando Matos, Y., Cunillera Puertolas, O., Almeda Ortega, J., Perez, E. R., Curto, X. M., Ripollès, C. R., Farres, N. M., Mendez, A. M., Nova, J. C. G., Santos, M. B., Miñano, J. J. V., Erazo, D. L. P., Sánchez, A. M. H., & Grupo de estudio del vértigo en atención primaria Florida. (2019). Disability perceived by primary care patients with posterior canal benign paroxysmal positional vertigo. *BMC Family Practice, 20*(1), 156. https://doi.org/10.1186/s12875-019-1035-3

Centers for Disease Control and Prevention (CDC). (2016). Pharyngitis (strep throat). Retrieved September 14, 2020, fromhttps://www.cdc.gov/groupastrep/diseases-hcp/strep-throat.html

Centers for Disease Control and Prevention. (2020a). Children's Oral Health. Retrieved September 14, 2020, from https://www.cdc.gov/oralhealth/basics/childrens-oral-health/index.html

Centers for Disease Control and Prevention. (2020b). Statistics about the Public Health Burden of Noise-Induced Hearing Loss. Retrieved September 14, 2020, from https://www.cdc.gov/nceh/hearing_loss/public_health_scientific_info.html

Cottrell, J., Yip, J., Chan, Y., Chin, C. J., Damji, A., de Almeida, J. R., Desrosiers, M., Eskander, A., Janjua, A., Kilty, S., Lee, J. M., Macdonald, K. I., Meen, E. K., Rudmik, L., Sommer, D. D., Sowerby, L., Tewfik, M. A., Thamboo, A., Vescan, A. D., … Monteiro, E. (2020). Quality indicators for the diagnosis and management of acute bacterial rhinosinusitis. *American Journal of Rhinology & Allergy, 34*(4), 519–531. https://doi.org/10.1177/1945892420912158

DeMuri, G. P., Gern, J. E., Eickhoff, J., Lynch, S. V., & Wald, E. R. (2018). Dynamics of bacterial colonization with Streptococcus pneumoniae, Haemophilus influenzae and Moraxella catarrhalis during symptomatic and asymptomatic viral upper respiratory infection. *Clinical Infectious Diseases, 66*(7), 1045–1053.

Eggermont, J. J. (2017). *Hearing loss: Causes, prevention, and treatment*. Elsevier.

Finnegan, D. A., Rainchuso, L., Jenkins, S., Kierce, E., & Rothman, A. (2016). Immigrant caregivers of young children: oral health beliefs, attitudes, and early childhood caries knowledge. *Journal of Community Health, 41*(2), 250–257. Retrieved September 14, 2020, from http://www.ncbi.nlm.nih.gov/pubmed/26370378

Harrison, E., & Cronin, M. (2016). Otalgia. *Australian Family Physician, 45*(7), 493–497.

Huang, B., Lin, C., Lee, Y., & Chiang, C. (2020). Differential diagnosis between leukoedema and white spongy nevus. *Journal of Dental Sciences, 15*(4), 554–555. https://doi.org/10.1016/j.jds.2020.05.018

Kim, S. H., Kim, T. H., Byun, J. Y., Park, M. S., & Yeo, S. G. (2015). Clinical differences in types of otalgia. *Journal of Audiology Otology, 19*(1), 34–38.

Kovacs, E., Wang, X., & Grill, E. (2019). Economic burden of vertigo: A systematic review. *Health Economics Review, 9*(1), 37–14. https://doi.org/10.1186/s13561-019-0258-2

Kumbargere Nagraj, S., Eachempati, P., Uma, E., Singh, V. P., Ismail, N. M., Varghese, E., & Kumbargere Nagraj, S. (2019). Interventions for managing halitosis. *Cochrane Database of Systematic Reviews*, 12(12), CD012213. https://doi.org/10.1002/14651858.CD012213.pub2

Liu, C., Tong, Z., Tan, J., & Xin, Z. (2019). Analysis of Treg/Th17 cells in patients with tongue squamous cell carcinoma. *Experimental and Therapeutic Medicine, 18*(3), 2187–2193.

Luo, R., Sickler, J., Vahidnia, F., Lee, Y.-C., Frogner, B., & Thompson, M. (2019). Diagnosis and Management of Group a Streptococcal Pharyngitis in the United States, 2011–2015. *BMC Infectious Diseases, 19*(1), 193.

McShefferty, D., Whitmer, W. M., Swan, I. R. C., & Akeroyd, M. A. (2013). The effect of experience on the sensitivity and specificity of the whispered voice test: a diagnostic accuracy study. *BMJ Open, 3*(4), e002394.

Murray, L. L. A. (2019). Vertigo. *Australasian Journal on Ageing, 38*(4), 291. https://doi.org/10.1111/ajag.12727

Myers, D., Allen, E., Essa, A., & Gbadamosi-Akindele, M. (2020). Rapidly growing squamous cell carcinoma of the tongue. *Cureus, 12*(3), e7164. https://doi.org/10.7759/cureus.7164

Prokop-Prigge, K. A., Mansfield, C. J., Parker, M. R., Thaler, E., Grice, E. A., Wysocki, C. J., & Preti, G. (2015). Ethnic/racial and genetic influences on cerumen odorant profiles. *Journal of Chemical Ecology, 41*(1), 67–74.

Shirai, N., & Preciado, D. (2019). Otitis media: What is new? *Current Opinion in Otolaryngology & Head and Neck Surgery, 27*(6), 495–498. https://doi.org/10.1097/MOO.0000000000000591

Stachler, R. J., Francis, D. O., Schwartz, S. R., Damask, C. C., Digoy, G. P., Krouse, H. J., McCoy, S. J., Ouellette, D. R., Patel, R. R., Reavis, C. C. W., Smith, L. J., Smith, M., Strode, S. W., Woo, P., & Nnacheta, L. C. (2018). Clinical practice guideline: Hoarseness (dysphonia) (update). *Otolaryngology Head and Neck Surgery, 158*(1_suppl), S1–S42.

Tiase, V. L., Tang, K., Vawdrey, D. K., Raso, R., Adelman, J. S., Yu, S. P., Applebaum, J. R., & Lalwani, A. K. (2020). Impact of hearing loss on patient falls in the inpatient setting. *American Journal of Preventive Medicine, 58*(6), 839–844. https://doi.org/10.1016/j.amepre.2020.01.019

Vos, B., Noll, D., Pigeon, M., Bagatto, M., & Fitzpatrick, E. M. (2019). Risk factors for hearing loss in children: A systematic literature review and meta-analysis protocol. *Systematic Reviews, 8*(1), 172–177. https://doi.org/10.1186/s13643-019-1073-x

Wald, E. R., & DeMuri, G. P. (2018). Antibiotic recommendations for acute otitis media and acute bacterial sinusitis: Conundrum no more. *Pediatric Infectious Disease Journal, 37*(12), 1255–1257. https://doi.org/10.1097/INF.0000000000002009

Wheatley, L. M., & Togias, A. (2015). Clinical practice. Allergic rhinitis. *New England Journal of Medicine, 372*(5), 456–463.

World Health Organization. (2020). Deafness and hearing loss. Retrieved September 14, 2020, from https://www.who.int/health-topics/hearing-loss#tab=tab_1

Zelaya, C. E., Lucas, J. W., & Hoffman, H. J. (2015). MAR Quick Stats: Percentage of adults with selected hearing problems, by type of problem and age group—National Health Interview Survey, United States, 2014. *MAR, 64*(37), 1058. https://www.cdc.gov/mmwr/preview/mmwrhtml/mm6437a8.htm

Zhang, M., Bi, Z., Fu, X., Wang, J., Ruan, Q., Zhao, C., Duan, J., Zeng, X., Zhou, D., Chen, J., & Bao, Z. (2019). A parsimonious approach for screening moderate-to-profound hearing loss in a community-dwelling geriatric population based on a decision tree analysis. *BMC Geriatrics, 19*(1), 214.

13 THE RESPIRATORY SYSTEM

KEY TERMS

adventitious sounds
bronchophony
cough
dyshemoglobinemia
dyspnea
egophony
fremitus
hemoptysis
hyperventilation
pneumothorax
pulmonary embolism
pulse oximetry
wheezes
whispered pectoriloquy

Learning Objectives

The student will:

1. Describe the structure and functions of the airways, alveoli, lungs, and pleura.
2. Identify the locations of each lung lobe using landmarks on the thorax.
3. Describe the mechanics of breathing.
4. Obtain a thorough history of the respiratory system.
5. Appropriately prepare and position the patient for the respiratory examination.
6. Identify the percussion and auscultation sites for assessment of the lungs.
7. Correctly inspect, palpate, percuss, and auscultate the thorax.
8. Describe the normal lung sounds and their locations.
9. Describe adventitious sounds and voice sounds and their origins.
10. Describe the equipment necessary to perform a respiratory examination, pulse oximetry, and peak flow assessment.
11. Discuss risk reduction and health promotion strategies to reduce respiratory disease.

ANATOMY AND PHYSIOLOGY

Review the *anatomy of the chest wall*, identifying the structures illustrated in Figure 13-1. Note that the intercostal space between two ribs has the same number as the rib above it.

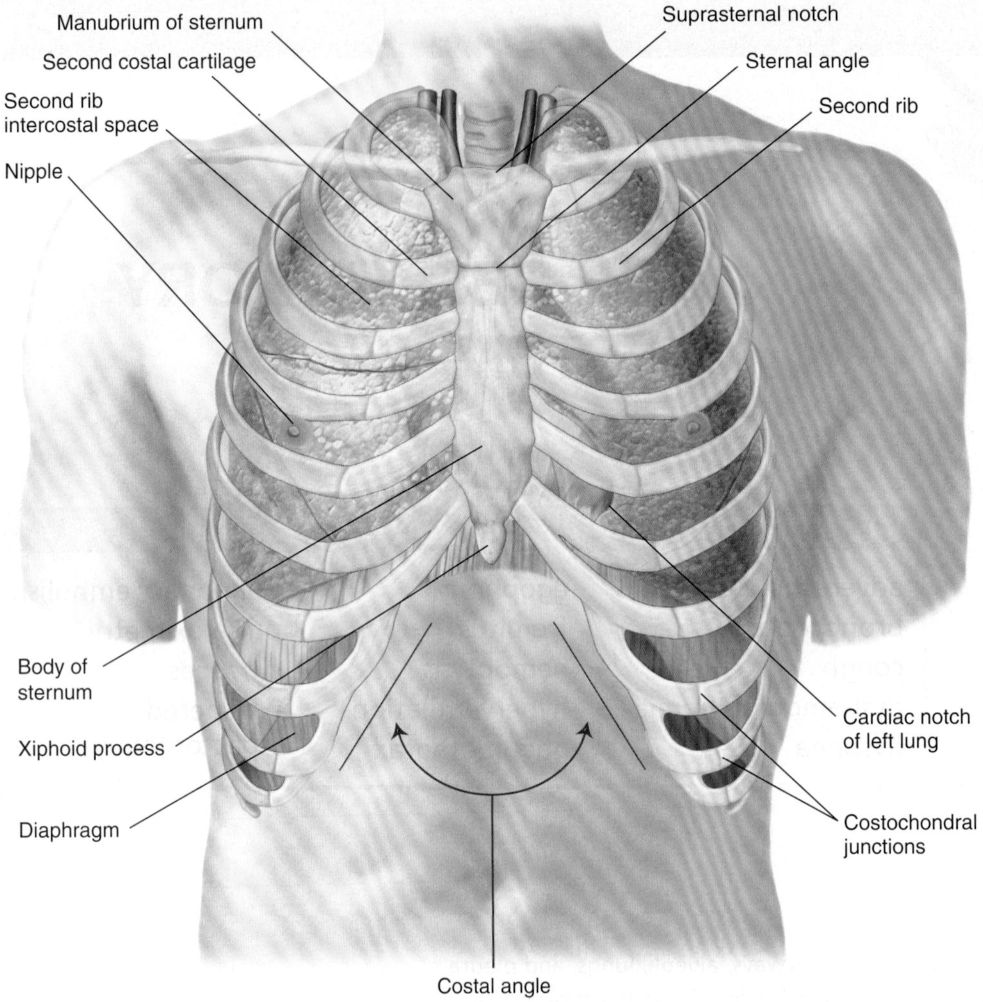

FIGURE 13-1 Anatomy of the chest wall.

Locating Findings on the Chest

The Vertical Axis

Chest findings are described in two dimensions: *along the vertical axis* and *around the circumference of the chest.*

To identify *vertical* locations, count the ribs and intercostal spaces. Begin by finding the *sternal angle*, also termed the angle of Louis. Place your finger in the hollow curve of the suprasternal notch, and then move your finger down approximately 5 cm to the horizontal bony ridge joining the manubrium to the body of the sternum. Then move your finger laterally and find the adjacent second rib. From here, using two fingers, "walk down" the intercostal spaces, one space at a time, on an oblique line, illustrated by the red numbers in Figure 13-2. It is easier to identify intercostal spaces in women when they lie down, as the supine position displaces breast tissue across the chest. Avoid pressing too hard on tender breast tissue.

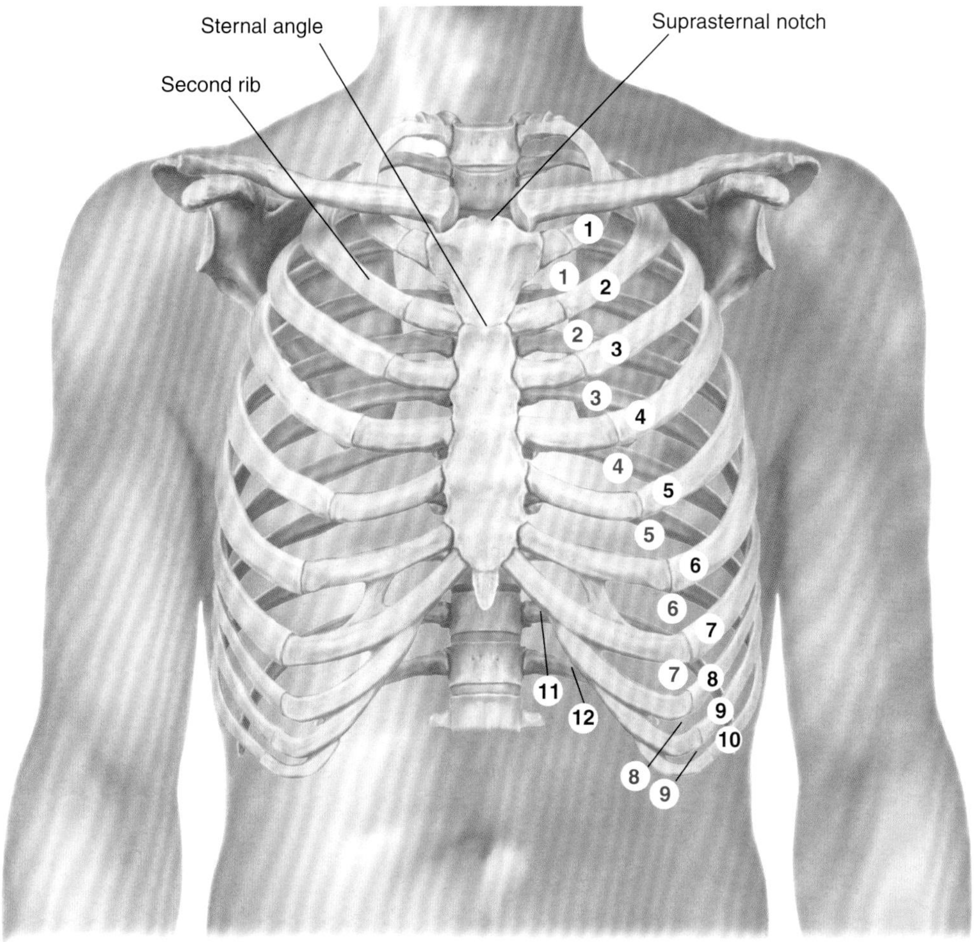

FIGURE 13-2 Vertical examination of the ribs and intercostal spaces.

The costal cartilages of the first seven ribs articulate with the sternum; the cartilages of the eighth, ninth, and 10th ribs articulate with the costal cartilages just above them. The 11th and 12th ribs, the "floating ribs," have no anterior attachments. The cartilaginous tip of the 11th rib can usually be felt laterally, and the 12th rib may be felt posteriorly. On palpation, costal cartilages and ribs feel identical.

Posteriorly, the 12th rib is another possible starting point for counting ribs and intercostal spaces; it helps locate findings on the lower posterior chest and provides an option when the anterior approach is unsatisfactory. With the fingers of one hand, press in and up against the lower border of the 12th rib, then "walk up" the intercostal spaces numbered in red in Figure 13-3, or follow a more oblique line up and around to the front of the chest.

The inferior tip of the scapula is another useful bony landmark—it usually lies at the level of the seventh rib or intercostal space.

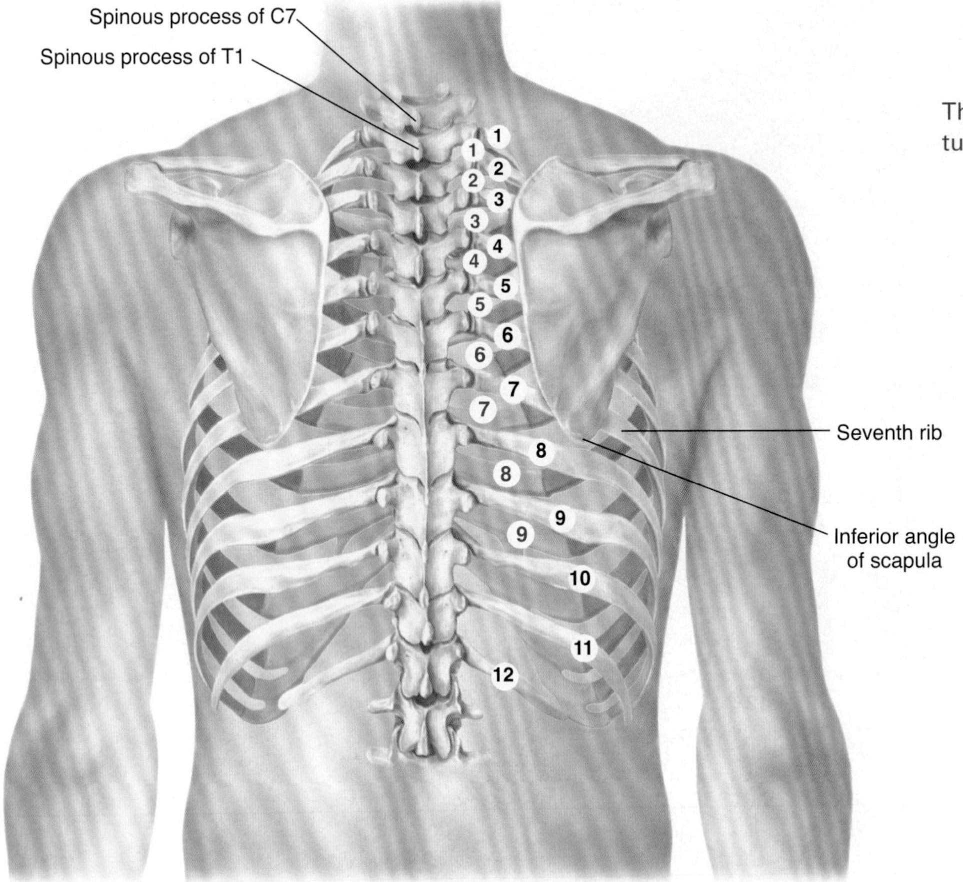

FIGURE 13-3 The ribs and intercostal spaces on the posterior chest.

The lower end of an endotracheal tube is usually at the level of T4.

The spinous processes of the vertebrae are also useful anatomic landmarks. When the neck is flexed forward, the most protruding process is usually the vertebra of C7, known as the vertebral prominens. If two processes are equally prominent, they are C7 and T1. You can often palpate and count the processes below them, especially when the spine is flexed.

Circumference of the Chest

To locate findings around the *circumference of the chest,* use a series of vertical lines, shown in the following figures. The *midsternal* and *vertebral lines* are easily seen. The others are estimated. The *midclavicular line* drops vertically from the midpoint of the clavicle (Fig. 13-4). To find it, identify both ends of the clavicle accurately (see Chapter 18, "The Musculoskeletal System").

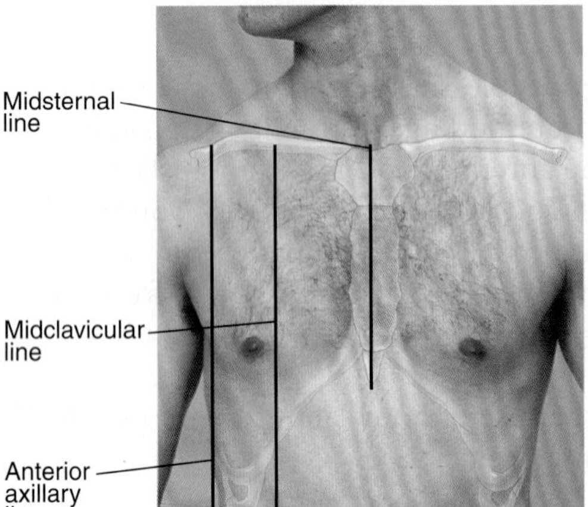

FIGURE 13-4 The vertical anterior chest lines.

The *anterior* and *posterior axillary lines* drop vertically from the anterior and posterior axillary folds, which are the muscle masses that border the axilla. The *midaxillary line* drops from the apex of the axilla. See Figure 13-5.

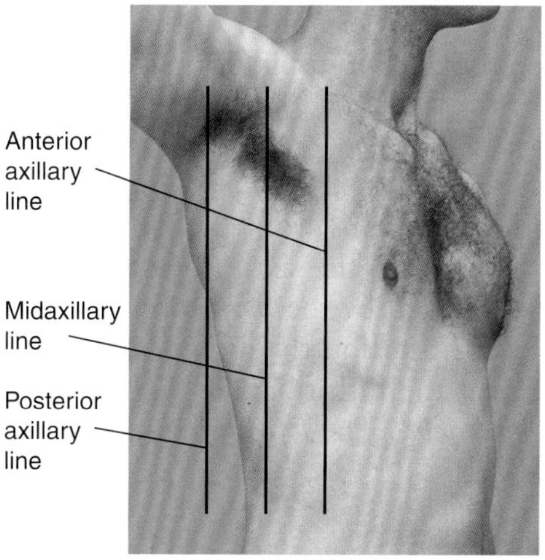

FIGURE 13-5 The axillary lines.

Posteriorly, the *vertebral line* overlies the spinous processes of the vertebrae. The scapular line drops from the inferior angle of the scapula. See Figure 13-6.

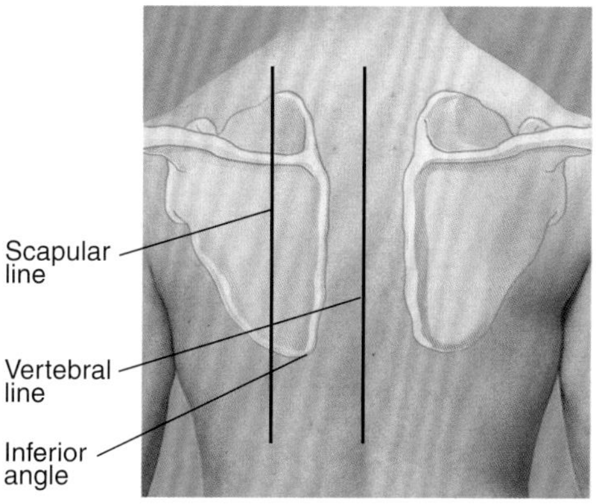

FIGURE 13-6 The posterior chest lines.

Lungs, Fissures, and Lobes

Using exterior landmarks, picture the lungs and their fissures and lobes on the chest. Anteriorly (Fig. 13-7A), the apex of each lung rises approximately 2 to 4 cm above the inner third of the clavicle. The lower border of the lung crosses the sixth rib at the midclavicular line and the eighth rib at the

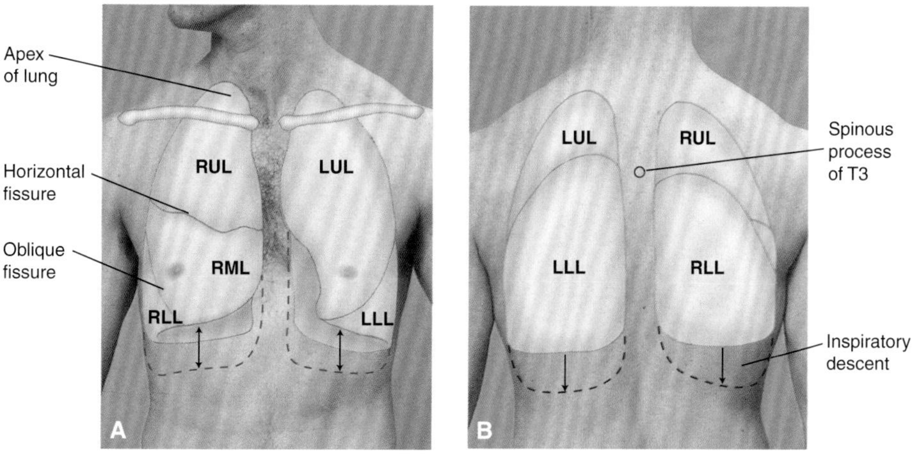

RUL: Right upper lobe
RML: Right middle lobe
RLL: Right lower lobe
LUL: Left upper lobe
LLL: Left lower lobe

FIGURE 13-7 The lobes of the lungs from the anterior (**A**) and posterior (**B**) views.

midaxillary line. Posteriorly (Fig. 13-7B), the lower border of the lung lies at about the level of the T10 spinous process. On inspiration, it descends farther.

Each lung is divided roughly in half by an *oblique (major) fissure.* This fissure may be approximated by a string that runs from the T3 spinous process obliquely down and around the chest to the sixth rib at the mid-clavicular line. The right lung is further divided by the *horizontal (minor) fissure.* Anteriorly, this fissure runs close to the fourth rib and meets the oblique fissure in the midaxillary line near the fifth rib. The *right lung* is thus divided into *upper*, *middle*, and *lower lobes.* The *left lung* has only *two lobes*, upper and lower. See Figure 13-8A,B.

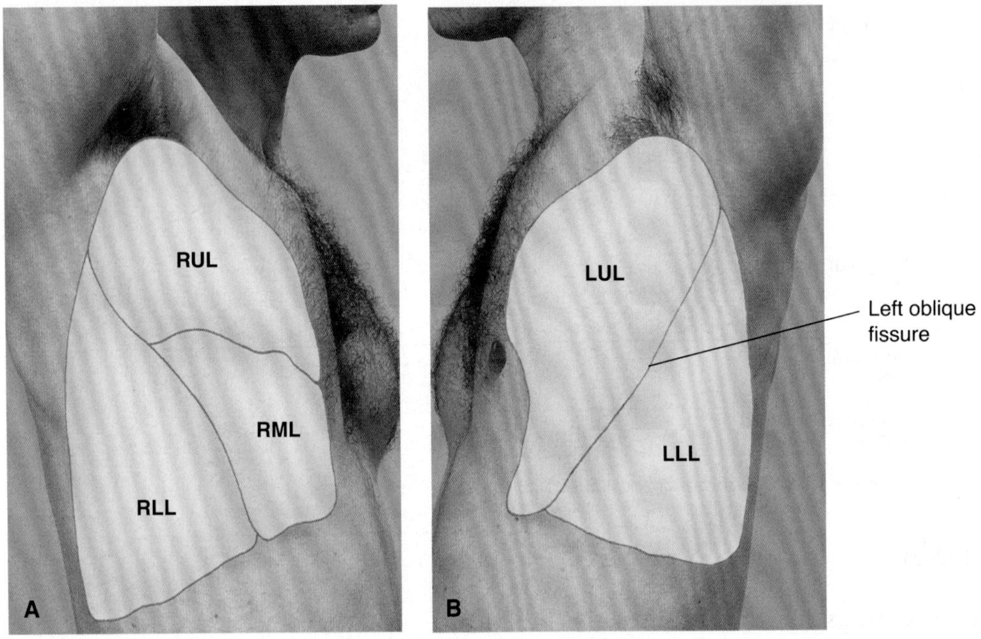

FIGURE 13-8 The lobes of the lungs from the right (**A**) and left (**B**) sides.

Locations on the Chest

Learn the general anatomic terms used to locate chest findings, such as:

- Supraclavicular—above the clavicles
- Infraclavicular—below the clavicles
- Interscapular—between the scapulae
- Infrascapular—below the scapulae
- Bases of the lungs—the lowermost portions
- Upper, middle, and lower lung fields

Usually, physical examination findings correlate with the underlying lobe. Signs in the right upper lung field, for example, almost certainly originate in the right upper lobe. Signs in the right middle lung field laterally, however, could come from any of three different lobes.

The Trachea and Major Bronchi

Breath sounds over the trachea and bronchi have a harsher quality than breath sounds over the lung parenchyma. Know the location of these structures (Fig. 13-9). The trachea bifurcates into its mainstem bronchi at the levels of the sternal angle anteriorly and the T4 spinous process posteriorly. The right main bronchus is wider, shorter, and more vertical than the left main bronchus, which extends more laterally.

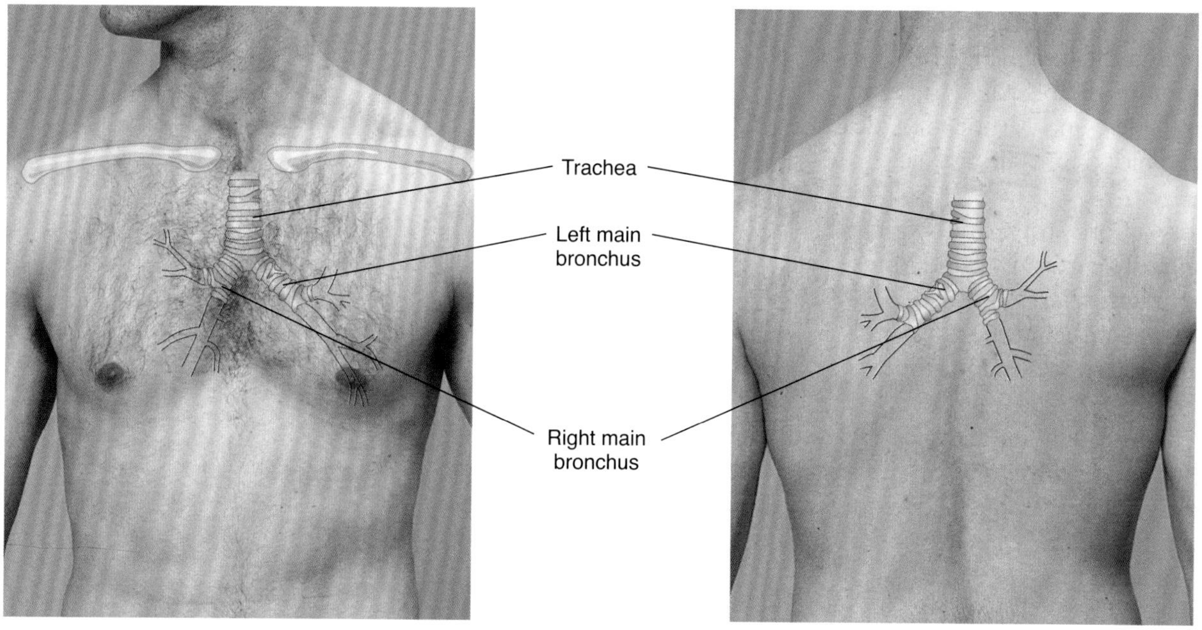

FIGURE 13-9 The trachea and major bronchi from the anterior and posterior views.

The Pleurae

The pleurae are two serous membranes that cover the outer surface of each lung. The *visceral pleura* lies next to the lung and the *parietal pleura* lines the inner rib cage and upper surface of the diaphragm. Their smooth opposing surfaces, lubricated by pleural fluid, allow the lungs to move easily within the rib cage during inspiration and expiration (Fig. 13-10). The *pleural space* is the *potential* space between visceral and parietal pleurae.

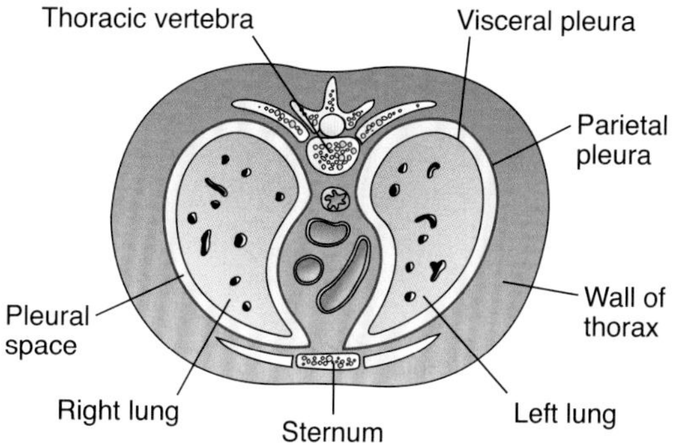

FIGURE 13-10 Cross-section of the chest showing the pleurae. (Modified from Cohen, B. J. (2007). *Medical terminology: An illustrated guide* (5th ed.). Lippincott Williams & Wilkins.)

Accumulation of fluid between the pleurae is called a *plural effusion.*

The visceral pleura lacks sensory nerves, but the parietal pleura is richly innervated by the intercostal and phrenic nerves. Inflammation of the parietal pleura produces pleuritic pain with deep inspiration, for example, in *pleurisy, pneumonia,* and *pulmonary embolism.*

Breathing

Breathing is largely an automatic act controlled by the respiratory center in the brainstem and mediated by the muscles of respiration. The *diaphragm* is the primary muscle of inspiration. When it contracts during inhalation, it descends in the chest and enlarges the thoracic cavity. At the same time, it compresses the abdominal contents, pushing the abdominal wall outward. The muscles in the rib cage and neck also expand the thorax during inspiration, especially the intercostal muscles, and the *scalenes*, which run from the cervical vertebrae to the first two ribs.

During inspiration, as these muscles contract, the thorax expands. Intrathoracic pressure decreases, drawing air through the tracheobronchial tree into the *alveoli*, or distal air sacs, and expanding the lungs (Fig. 13-11). Oxygen diffuses into the blood of adjacent pulmonary capillaries, and carbon dioxide diffuses from the blood into the alveoli.

After inspiratory effort stops, the expiratory phase begins. The chest wall and lungs recoil, the diaphragm relaxes and rises passively, air flows outward, and the chest and abdomen return to their resting positions.

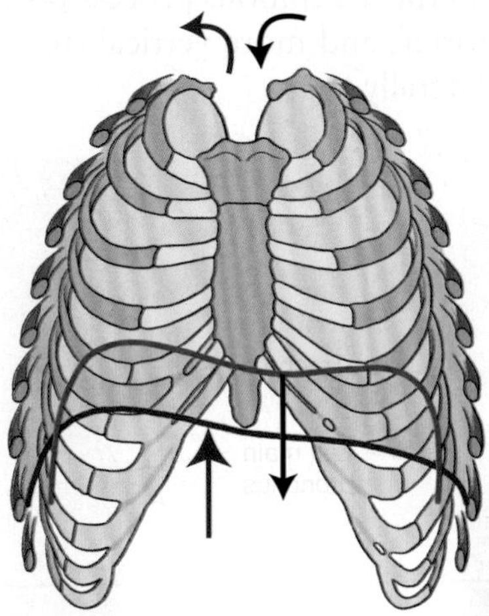

FIGURE 13-11 Diaphragmatic expansion.

Normal breathing is quiet and easy, barely audible near the open mouth as a faint whish. When a healthy person lies supine, the breathing movements of the thorax are relatively slight. In contrast, the abdominal movements are usually easy to see. In the sitting position, movements of the thorax become more prominent.

During exercise and in certain diseases, extra work is required to breathe, and accessory muscles join the inspiratory effort. The *sternocleidomastoids* are the most important of these (Fig. 13-12), and the *scalenes* may become visible. Abdominal muscles assist in expiration.

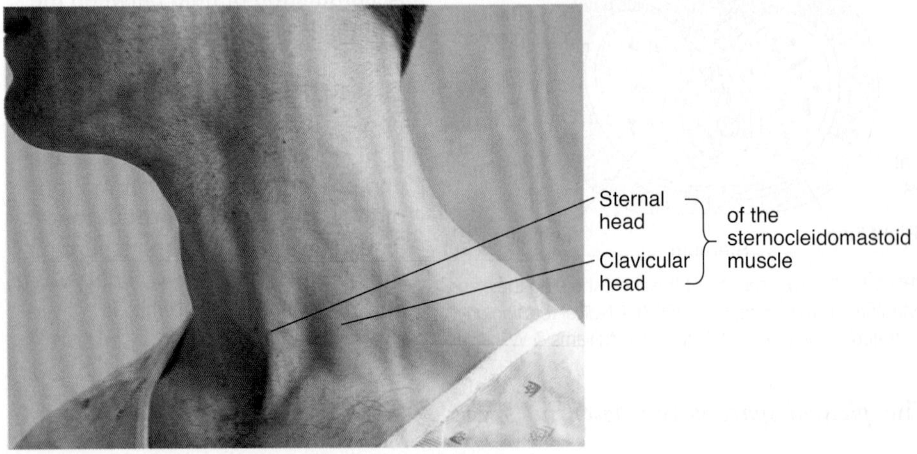

FIGURE 13-12 The sternocleidomastoid muscle.

Changes in the thorax and lungs due to age are described later in the textbook. The older adult changes are discussed in Chapter 24, "Assessing Older Adults" and the infant and child changes in Chapter 23, "Assessing Children: Infancy through Adolescence."

THE HEALTH HISTORY

Common or concerning symptoms identified in the respiratory system history are listed in Box 13-1.

BOX 13-1 COMMON OR CONCERNING SYMPTOMS

- Shortness of breath (dyspnea)
- Wheezing
- Cough
- Blood-streaked sputum (hemoptysis) or purulent sputum
- Chest pain

Sputum is a mixture of saliva and mucus coughed up from the respiratory tract.

The thorax houses several organs and structures, and the nurse must use astute questioning to ascertain the patient's problem. Dyspnea, wheezing, cough, and hemoptysis usually point to a respiratory problem; however, they may also indicate a cardiac condition. Chest pain may be caused by cardiac, respiratory, gastrointestinal, or musculoskeletal etiologies. The initial history questions should be as broad as possible.

Dyspnea is air hunger, a nonpainful but uncomfortable awareness of breathing that is inappropriate to the level of exertion, commonly termed "shortness of breath" (Table 13-1). This is a serious symptom that warrants a full explanation and assessment. It can result from pulmonary or cardiac disease.

To assess for dyspnea, the nurse should ask if the patient has experienced difficulty breathing and further explore it using "OLD CART."

- *Onset:* When did you first feel short of breath?
  Did anything bring on the shortness of breath (e.g., exposure to an allergen)?
- *Location:* Is the difficulty in your throat or neck area or your chest?
- *Duration:* Does this occur at a particular time of day?
  Did it come on suddenly or gradually?

CLINICAL TIP
Sudden onset may indicate anaphylaxis or pulmonary embolism (a blood clot in a lung artery) (both emergencies), spontaneous pneumothorax (the presence of air in the plural space, causing collapse of the lung), or anxiety.

  Is it continuous or intermittent?
  Does it occur at rest or with exertion or activity?
- *Characteristic symptoms:* Can you talk in full sentences or only short phrases?

Determine the severity of the dyspnea based on the patient's ability to talk and complete daily activities.

TABLE 13-1 Dyspnea

Problem	Process	Timing
Asthma (Kerlin, 2014; Panettieri, 2007)	Bronchial hyperresponsiveness involving release of inflammatory mediators, increased airway secretions, and bronchoconstriction	Acute episodes separated by symptom-free periods Nocturnal episodes common
Pneumonia (Neiderman, 2009)	Infection of lung parenchyma from the respiratory bronchioles to the alveoli	An acute illness, timing varies with the causative agent
Spontaneous Pneumothorax	Leakage of air into pleural space through blebs on visceral pleura, with resulting partial or complete collapse of the lung	Sudden onset of dyspnea
Acute Pulmonary Embolism (Agnelli & Becattini, 2010; Moore, 2019)	Sudden occlusion of part of the pulmonary arterial tree by a blood clot that usually originates in deep veins of legs or pelvis	Sudden onset of tachypnea, dyspnea
Chronic Bronchitis[a] (Wenzel & Fowler, 2006)	Excessive mucus production in bronchi followed by chronic obstruction of airways	Chronic productive cough followed by slowly progressive dyspnea
Chronic Obstructive Pulmonary Disease (COPD)[a] (Global Initiative for Chronic Obstructive Lung Disease, 2020; Littner, 2011; Neiwoehner, 2010)	Overdistention of air spaces distal to terminal bronchioles with destruction of alveolar septa and chronic obstruction of the airways	Slowly progressive dyspnea; relatively mild cough later
Diffuse Interstitial Lung Diseases *(such as sarcoidosis, widespread neoplasms, asbestosis, and idiopathic pulmonary fibrosis)*	Abnormal and widespread infiltration of cells, fluid, and collagen into interstitial spaces between alveoli Many causes	Progressive dyspnea, which varies in its rate of development with the cause
Left-Sided Heart Failure *(left ventricular failure or mitral stenosis)*	Elevated pressure in pulmonary capillary bed with movement of fluid into interstitial spaces and alveoli, decreased compliance (increased stiffness) of the lungs, increased work of breathing	Dyspnea may progress slowly or suddenly as in acute pulmonary edema
Anxiety with Hyperventilation	Overbreathing with resultant respiratory alkalosis and fall in the partial pressure of carbon dioxide in the blood	Episodic, often recurrent

[a]Chronic bronchitis and chronic obstructive pulmonary disease may coexist.

Source: Parshall, M. B., Schwartzstein, R. M., Adams, L., Banzett, R. B., Manning, H. L., Bourbeau, J., Calverley, P. M., Gift, A. G., Harver, A., Lareau, S. C., Mahler, D. A., Meek, P. M., & O'Donnell, D. E.; American Thoracic Society Committee on Dyspnea. (2012). An official American Thoracic Society statement: Update on the mechanisms, assessment, and management of dyspnea. *American Journal of Respiratory and Critical Care Medicine*, *185*(4), 435–452.

Factors that Aggravate	Factors that Relieve	Associated Symptoms	Setting
Variable, including allergens, irritants, respiratory infections, cold and exercise, and emotion	Separation from aggravating factors	Wheezing, cough, tightness in chest	Environmental conditions
Exertion, smoking	Rest, though dyspnea may become persistent	Pleuritic pain, cough, sputum, fever, though not necessarily always present	Varied
		Pleuritic pain, cough	Often a previously healthy young adult or adult with emphysema
Exertion	Rest, though dyspnea may become persistent	Often none Retrosternal oppressive pain if the occlusion is massive Pleuritic pain, cough, syncope and hemoptysis, and/or unilateral leg swelling and pain from an instigating deep vein thrombosis Anxiety (see "Anxiety with Hyperventilation")	Postpartum or postoperative periods; prolonged bed rest; congestive heart failure, chronic lung disease, and fractures of hip or leg; deep venous thrombosis (often not clinically apparent)
Exertion, inhaled irritants, respiratory infections	Expectoration; rest, though dyspnea may become persistent	Chronic productive cough, recurrent respiratory infections; possible wheezing	History of smoking, air pollutants, recurrent respiratory infections
Exertion	Rest, though dyspnea may become persistent	Cough, with scant mucoid sputum	History of smoking, air pollutants, sometimes a familial deficiency in α_1-antitrypsin
Exertion	Rest, though dyspnea may become persistent	Often weakness, fatigue Cough less common than in other lung diseases	Varied Exposure to one of many substances may be causative
Exertion, lying down	Rest, sitting up, though dyspnea may become persistent	Often cough, orthopnea, paroxysmal nocturnal dyspnea; sometimes wheezing	History of heart disease or its predisposing factors
More often occurs at rest than after exercise An upsetting event may not always be evident	Breathing in and out of a paper or plastic bag sometimes helps the associated symptoms	Sighing, lightheadedness, numbness or tingling of the hands and feet, palpitations, chest pain	Other manifestations of anxiety may be present

Is the shortness of breath worse when you are lying down or upright?
Has shortness of breath altered your lifestyle or daily activities? How many steps or flights of stairs can you climb before pausing for breath? Can you carry groceries, vacuum the floor, or make the bed without experiencing dyspnea?

- *Associated manifestations:* Are there any associated symptoms, such as wheezing or cough? Chest pain? Nausea?
- *Relieving factors:* Does anything make your dyspnea better?
- *Treatment:* Have you seen anyone or tried any medications or treatments?

Anxious patients may present a different picture. They may describe difficulty taking a breath that feels deep enough, or a smothering sensation with the inability to get enough air. If they are hyperventilating, they may report *paresthesias*, which are sensations of tingling or "pins and needles" around the lips or in the hands and feet.

Anxious patients may have episodic dyspnea during both rest and exercise, and **hyperventilation**, or rapid shallow breathing. At other times, they may sigh frequently.

Wheezes are musical respiratory sounds that may be audible to the patient and others. Wheezes are caused by partial obstruction of the lower airways. The airway may be narrowed by bronchoconstriction, edema, secretions as in asthma, or a foreign body.

Ask if the patient is experiencing wheezing, and if so, explore this with "OLD CART."

- *Onset:* When did you first notice the wheezing? Did anything precipitate it (e.g., exposure to an allergen, cold)?
- *Location:* Is it coming from your throat area or chest?
- *Duration:* Does the wheezing occur at a particular time of day?
  Did it come on suddenly or gradually?
  Is it continuous or intermittent?
  Does it occur at rest or with exercise or activity?
- *Characteristic symptoms:* Does the wheeze occur when you inhale, exhale, or both?
- *Associated manifestations:* Are there any associated symptoms, such as shortness of breath or cough?
- *Relieving factors:* Does anything make it better?
- *Treatment:* Have you seen anyone? Tried any medicines? Any treatments?

Cough is typically a reflex response to stimuli that irritate receptors in the larynx, trachea, or large bronchi (Table 13-2). These stimuli include mucus, pus, blood, dust, foreign bodies, and even extremely hot or cold air. Coughing may also be caused by inflammation of the respiratory mucosa or tension in the air passages from a tumor or enlarged peribronchial lymph nodes. Patients with asthma may experience a cough without wheezing. The narrowed airways trigger a cough on expiration as the patient tries to fully exhale the trapped air. Duration of a cough is important to document. An *acute cough* lasts less than 3 weeks, a *subacute cough* lasts 3 to 8 weeks, and a *chronic cough* lasts over 8 weeks.

TABLE 13-2 Cough and Hemoptysis

Problem	Cough and Sputum	Associated Symptoms and Setting
Acute Inflammation		
Laryngitis	Dry cough (without sputum), may become productive of variable amounts of sputum	An acute, fairly minor illness with hoarseness Often associated with viral nasopharyngitis
Acute Bronchitis (Wenzel & Fowler, 2006)	Cough may be dry or productive	An acute, often viral illness generally without fever or dyspnea; at times with burning retrosternal discomfort
Mycoplasma and Viral Pneumonias (Metlay et al., 1997)	Dry hacking cough, may become productive of mucoid sputum	An acute febrile illness, often with malaise, headache, and possibly dyspnea
Bacterial Pneumonias (Metlay et al., 1997)	Sputum is mucoid or purulent; may be blood streaked, diffusely pinkish, or rusty	An acute illness with chills, often high fever, dyspnea, and chest pain Commonly caused by *Streptococcus pneumoniae*, *Haemophilus influenzae*, *Moraxella catarrhalis*; *Klebsiella* in alcoholism, especially if there is underlying smoking, chronic bronchitis and COPD, cardiovascular disease, diabetes
Pertussis (*Bordetella pertussis*)	Cough comes in paroxysms; followed by a sudden forceful inhalation (*in children, a whooping sound is produced*.)	Begins with coryza (runny nose), sneezing, low-grade fever
Chronic Inflammation		
Postnasal Drip	Chronic cough; sputum mucoid or mucopurulent	Repeated attempts to clear the throat Postnasal discharge may be sensed by patient or seen in posterior pharynx Associated with chronic rhinitis, with or without sinusitis
Chronic Bronchitis (Wenzel & Fowler, 2006)	Chronic cough; sputum mucoid to purulent, may be blood-streaked or even bloody	Often with recurrent wheezing and dyspnea and prolonged history of tobacco abuse
Bronchiectasis (Barker, 2002)	Chronic cough; sputum purulent, often copious and foul-smelling; may be blood-streaked or bloody	Recurrent bronchopulmonary infections common; sinusitis may coexist
Pulmonary Tuberculosis (Escalante, 2009)	Cough dry or with mucoid or purulent sputum that is mucoid or purulent; may be blood-streaked or bloody	Early, no symptoms Later, anorexia, weight loss, fatigue, fever, and night sweats
Lung Abscess	Sputum purulent and foul-smelling; may be bloody	Usually from aspiration pneumonia with fever and infection from oral anaerobes and poor dental hygiene; often with dysphagia or episode of impaired consciousness

(*continued*)

TABLE 13-2 Cough and Hemoptysis (*Continued*)

Problem	Cough and Sputum	Associated Symptoms and Setting
Asthma (Kerlin, 2014; Panettieri, 2007)	Cough, at times with thick mucoid sputum, especially near end of an attack	Episodic wheezing and dyspnea but cough may occur alone Often with a history of allergies
Gastroesophageal Reflux	Chronic cough, especially at night or early in the morning	Wheezing, especially at night (often mistaken for asthma); early morning hoarseness; and repeated attempts to clear the throat Often with heartburn and regurgitation
Neoplasm		
Cancer of the Lung	Cough dry to productive; sputum may be blood-streaked or bloody	Commonly with dyspnea, weight loss, and tobacco use
Cardiovascular Disorders		
Left Ventricular Failure or Mitral Stenosis	Often dry, especially on exertion or at night; may progress to the pink, frothy sputum of pulmonary edema or to frank hemoptysis	Dyspnea, orthopnea, paroxysmal nocturnal dyspnea
Pulmonary Embolism (Agnelli & Becattini, 2010; Kerlin, 2010; Moore, 2019)	Dry to productive; may be dark, bright red, or mixed with blood	Dyspnea, anxiety, chest pain, fever; factors that predispose to deep venous thrombosis
Irritating Particles, Chemicals, or Gases		
	Variable There may be a latent period between exposure and symptoms	Exposure to irritants Eyes, nose, and throat may be affected

Source: Irwin, R. S., & Madison, J. M. (2000). The diagnosis and treatment of cough. *The New England Journal of Medicine*, *3432*(3), 1715–1721.

CLINICAL TIP

Cough may also be a symptom of *left-sided heart failure.* Viral upper respiratory infections are the most common cause of *acute cough*; other causes include acute bronchitis, pneumonia, asthma, pertussis, or foreign body.

Ask the patient if they have a cough, and if so, explore it with "OLD CART."

- *Onset:* When did you first notice the cough?
  Did anything precipitate the cough (e.g., a cold or respiratory infection)?
  Have you begun any new medicines recently?
- *Location:* Does your cough come from your throat or chest?
- *Duration:* Does this happen at a particular time of day?
  Did it come on suddenly or gradually?
  Does it come and go or last all the time?

Some medications such as angiotensin-converting enzyme (ACE) inhibitors produce a persistent dry cough as a side effect.

Does it occur at rest or with exercise or activity?
Does it wake you at night?

- *Characteristic symptoms:* Do you feel the urge to cough when you inhale or exhale?
- Does the cough come in spasms that make breathing difficult?'

Paroxysms (sudden uncontrollable attacks) of coughing followed by a "whooping" intake of breath occur with pertussis.

Do you cough up mucus or phlegm? If yes, what is the color? Odor? Consistency? Amount? How much mucus do you think you cough up in 24 hours—a teaspoon, tablespoon, quarter cup, half cup, or cupful?
Have you noticed blood in the mucus? Describe the color and amount of blood. Have you had any mouth injuries or nosebleeds recently? Any ulcers?

Mucoid sputum is translucent, white or grey; *purulent* sputum is yellowish or greenish. Foul-smelling sputum is seen in anaerobic lung abscess; tenacious sputum in cystic fibrosis. Large volumes of purulent sputum may occur in bronchiectasis or lung abscess.

CLINICAL TIP
Hemoptysis is coughing up of blood from the lungs; it may vary from blood-streaked phlegm to frank blood. Blood or blood-streaked material may originate in the mouth, pharynx, or gastrointestinal tract and is easily misidentified. Blood originating in the stomach is usually darker than blood from the respiratory tract, and food particles may be mixed into it. Hemoptysis is rare in infants, children, and adolescents, though common with cystic fibrosis.

If the patient is actively coughing, ask them to cough into a tissue in order to examine its characteristics.

- *Associated manifestations:* Do you have any other symptoms like shortness of breath or wheezing?
- *Relieving factors:* Does anything make your cough better?
- *Treatment:* Have you seen anyone or tried any medicines or treatments?

Chest pain may be caused by cardiac, respiratory, gastrointestinal, or musculoskeletal etiologies (Table 13-3). Lung tissue itself has no pain fibers. Pain in lung conditions, such as pneumonia or pulmonary infarction, usually arises from inflammation of the adjacent parietal pleura. Sources of chest pain are outlined in Table 13-4.

This chapter will focus on pulmonary complaints. See Chapter 14, "The Cardiovascular System," and Chapter 16, "The Gastrointestinal and Renal Systems" for history questions related to nonpulmonary chest pain. If the patient reports chest pain that is likely pulmonary in nature, ask more about it using "OLD CART."

- *Onset:* When did the pain begin?
  Have you experienced chest pain previously? When?
  Is this the same pain?
  Did you fall or have any chest injuries prior to the pain?
- *Location:* Where in your chest do you feel the pain?
- *Duration:* Does the pain occur with breathing? Does the pain come and go or last all the time?

TABLE 13-3 Chest Pain

Problem	Process	Location	Quality
Pulmonary			
Pleuritic Pain	Inflammation of the parietal pleura, as in pleurisy, pneumonia, pulmonary infarction, or neoplasm	Chest wall overlying the process	Sharp, knife-like
Cardiovascular			
Angina Pectoris	Temporary myocardial ischemia, usually secondary to coronary atherosclerosis	Retrosternal or across the anterior chest, often radiates to the shoulders, arms, neck, lower jaw, or upper abdomen	Pressing, squeezing, tight, heavy, occasionally burning
Myocardial Infarction	Prolonged myocardial ischemia resulting in irreversible muscle damage or necrosis	Same as in angina	Same as in angina
Pericarditis	Irritation of parietal pleura adjacent to the pericardium	Precordial, may radiate to the tip of the shoulder and to the neck	Sharp, knife-like Crushing
Dissecting Aortic Aneurysm	A splitting within the layers of the aortic wall, allowing passage of blood to dissect a channel	Anterior or posterior chest, radiating to the neck, back, or abdomen	Ripping, tearing
Gastrointestinal and Other			
Gastrointestinal Reflux Disease	Irritation or inflammation of the esophageal mucosa due to reflux of gastric acid from lowered esophageal sphincter tone	Retrosternal, may radiate to the back	Burning, may be squeezing
Diffuse Esophageal Spasm	Motor dysfunction of the esophageal muscle	Retrosternal, may radiate to the back, arms, and jaw	Usually squeezing
Chest Wall Pain, Costochondritis	Variable, including trauma, inflammation of costal cartilage	Often below the left breast or along the costal cartilages; also elsewhere	Stabbing, sticking, or dull, aching
Anxiety (Panic Disorder)	Unclear	Precordial, below the left breast, or across the anterior chest	Stabbing, sticking, or dull, aching

Note: Chest pain may be referred from extrathoracic structures such as the neck (arthritis) and abdomen (biliary colic, acute cholecystitis). Pleural pain may be from abdominal conditions such as subdiaphragmatic abscess.

Severity	Timing	Factors that Aggravate	Factors that Relieve	Associated Symptoms
Often severe	Persistent	Inspiration, coughing, movements of the trunk		Related to the underlying illness
Mild to moderate, sometimes perceived as discomfort rather than pain	Usually 1–3 min but up to 10 min Prolonged episodes up to 20 min	Often exertion, especially in the cold; meals; emotional stress May also occur at rest	Often but not always rest, nitroglycerin	Sometimes dyspnea, nausea, sweating
Often but not always severe pain	20 min to several hours	Not always triggered by exertion	Not relieved by rest	Nausea, vomiting, sweating, weakness
Often severe	Persistent	Breathing, changing position, coughing, lying down, sometimes swallowing	Sitting forward may relieve it	Related to the underlying illness
Very severe	Abrupt onset, early peak, persistent for hours or more	Hypertension		If in the thoracic aorta: hoarseness, dysphagia, also syncope, hemiplegia, paraplegia
Mild to severe	Variable	Large meal; bending over, lying down	Antacids, sometimes belching	Sometimes regurgitation, dysphagia
Mild to severe	Variable	Swallowing of food or cold liquid; emotional stress	Sometimes nitroglycerin	Dysphagia
Variable	Fleeting to hours or days	Coughing; movement of chest, trunk, arms	Often local tenderness	
Variable	Fleeting to hours or days	May follow effort, emotional stress	Breathlessness, palpitations, weakness, anxiety	

TABLE 13-4 Locations of Chest Pain and Related Causes

Location	Related Cause(s)
Trachea and large bronchi	Bronchitis
Parietal pleura	Pericarditis, pneumonia
Chest wall, including:	
• Musculoskeletal system	Costochondritis
• Skin	Herpes zoster
Myocardium	Angina pectoris, myocardial infarction
Pericardium	Pericarditis
Aorta	Dissecting aortic aneurysm
Esophagus	Gastric esophageal reflux disease, esophageal spasm
Extrathoracic structures:	
• Neck	Cervical arthritis
• Gallbladder	Biliary colic
• Stomach	Gastritis

Note: Anxiety may also result in chest pain, though the mechanism of pain is unclear.

- *Characteristic symptoms:* Describe your pain. Is your chest tender to touch? Rate the pain on a scale of 1 to 10.
- *Associated manifestations:* When you have the chest pain, does anything else happen, for example, loss of consciousness, nausea, numbness, or tingling?
- *Relieving factors:* Does anything make it better?
- *Treatment:* Have you seen anyone or tried any medicines or treatments?

Past History

Questions to ask about the patient's history may include:

- Have you had any prior lung problems, such as infections, COVID-19, asthma, bronchitis, emphysema, pneumonia, tuberculosis, collapsed lung (pneumothorax), or cystic fibrosis? If yes, ask about onset, duration, treatment, and sequelae.

- Have you had chest surgery, biopsy, or trauma to your chest? If yes, ask the purpose, date, and outcome of the event.

- Do you have any allergies that affect your breathing or respiratory system? If yes, ask the patient to describe their symptoms and treatment.

- Have you had tuberculosis skin testing (purified protein derivative [PPD]) or a chest x-ray? When? What were the results?

Ask patients born outside the United States if they received the bacillus Calmette-Guerin (BCG) vaccine. This vaccine is given in some countries to reduce the risk of contracting tuberculosis.

- Have you had any other lung function testing? When? What were the results?
- Have you had the flu vaccine? When?
- Have you had the Tdap version of the tetanus immunization?

Immunity to pertussis from the childhood (DPT) vaccine has been shown to be weakening. Vaccination with the Tdap vaccine is recommended.

- If the patient is over 65 years, ask, have you had the pneumonia (pneumococcal) vaccines? PCV13 (Prevnar 13), PPSV23 (Pneumovax 23)
- Have you traveled outside the United States within the last 6 months? If yes, where?

Family History

Questions to ask regarding the patient's family history may include:

- Does anyone in your family currently have a lung infection or disease?
- Has anyone had lung cancer, asthma, or cystic fibrosis?
- Did anyone smoke in your home when you were growing up?

Lifestyle and Personal Habits

Questions to ask regarding the patient's lifestyle and personal habits include:

- Do you smoke or have you ever smoked tobacco or marijuana?
  - How many cigarettes or packs per day do you smoke?
  - When did you start? How long have you smoked/did you smoke?
- Do you smoke e-cigarettes or vape?
  - What brands do you use?
  - How many times per day do you vape?
  - When did you start?
- Do you use or have you ever used snuff?

- Do you chew or have you ever chewed tobacco?
- Are you exposed to second-hand smoke?
    - Where are you exposed?
    - How many hours per day?
    - For how many years?
- Are you exposed to any environmental conditions at home or work that affect your breathing (e.g., mold, sawdust, asbestos, coal dust, insecticides, radon, paint, or pollution)?
- Are you taking any prescription, herbal, cannabidiol (CBD) or marijuana, and/or over-the-counter (OTC) medications for breathing or respiratory problems?
- Do you use oxygen or other treatments for breathing problems (e.g., nebulizer treatments)?

PHYSICAL EXAMINATION

For best results, examine the posterior and lateral thorax and lungs while the patient is sitting and the anterior thorax and lungs with the patient supine. Proceed in an orderly fashion: inspect, palpate, percuss, and auscultate the entire chest. Try to visualize the underlying lobes, and compare one side with the other, noting any asymmetrical findings. For men, arrange the patient's gown so that you can see the chest fully. For women, cover the anterior chest when you examine the back and sides. For the anterior examination, drape the gown over each half of the chest as you examine the other half.

With the patient sitting, examine the posterior and lateral thorax and lungs. The patient's arms should be folded across the chest with hands resting, if possible, on the opposite shoulders. This position moves the scapulae laterally and increases your access to the lung fields. Following the complete posterior and lateral thorax examination, ask the patient to lie down.

With the patient supine, examine the anterior thorax and lungs. The supine position makes it easier to examine women because the breasts can be gently displaced. Furthermore, wheezes, if present, are more likely to be heard. (Some clinicians examine both the back and the front of the chest with the patient sitting. This technique is also satisfactory.)

For patients who cannot sit up without aid, obtain assistance so that you can examine the posterior chest in the sitting position. If this is impossible, roll the patient to one side and then to the other. Percuss the upper lung, and auscultate both lungs in each position. Because ventilation is relatively greater in

Hospitalized or long-term care patients who cannot sit up for routine lung assessment every shift may be examined using this technique.

the dependent (i.e., lower) lung, your chances of hearing abnormal wheezes or crackles are greater on the dependent side (see the Table 13-8, "Characteristics of Breath Sounds").

Initial Survey of Respiration and the Thorax

Observe and document the rate, rhythm, depth, and effort of breathing. This may have been done already with the vital signs. A healthy adult breathes quietly and regularly about 12 to 20 times a minute. An occasional sigh is to be expected. Note whether expiration lasts longer than usual. Table 13-5 outlines abnormalities to assess for in the rate and rhythm of breathing.

See Chapter 7, "General Survey Including Vital Signs and Pain," for information on assessing respiratory rate and rhythm.

TABLE 13-5 Abnormalities in Rate and Rhythm of Breathing

When observing respiratory patterns, note the rate, depth, and regularity of the patient's breathing. Traditional terms, such as tachypnea, are given below so that you will understand them, but simple descriptions are recommended.

Normal

The respiratory rate is about 14–20 per min in normal adults and up to 44 per min in infants.

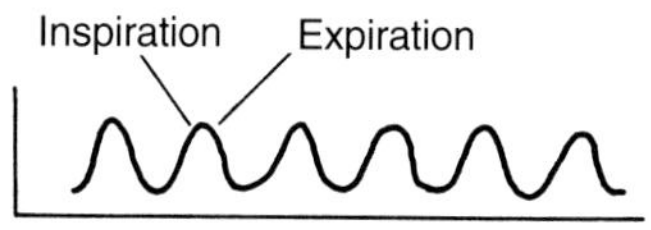

Slow Breathing (*Bradypnea*)

Slow breathing with or without an increase in tidal volume that maintains alveolar ventilation; abnormal alveolar hypoventilation without increased tidal volume can arise from uremia, drug-induced respiratory depression, and increased intracranial pressure.

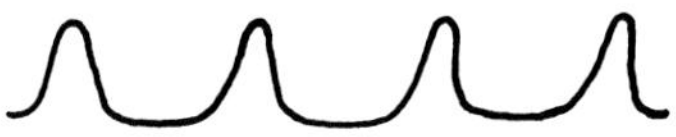

Sighing Respiration

Breathing punctuated by frequent sighs suggests hyperventilation syndrome, a common cause of dyspnea and dizziness. Occasional sighs are normal.

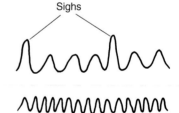

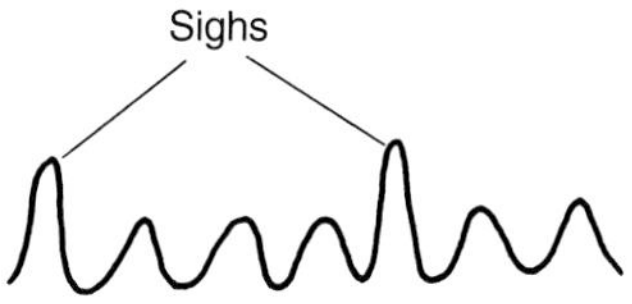

Rapid Shallow Breathing (*Tachypnea*)

Rapid shallow breathing has numerous causes, including salicylate intoxication, restrictive lung disease, pleuritic chest pain, and an elevated diaphragm.

Cheyne–Stokes Breathing

Periods of deep breathing alternate with periods of apnea (no breathing). This pattern is normal in children and older adults during sleep. Causes include heart failure, uremia, drug-induced respiratory depression, and brain injury (typically bihemispheric).

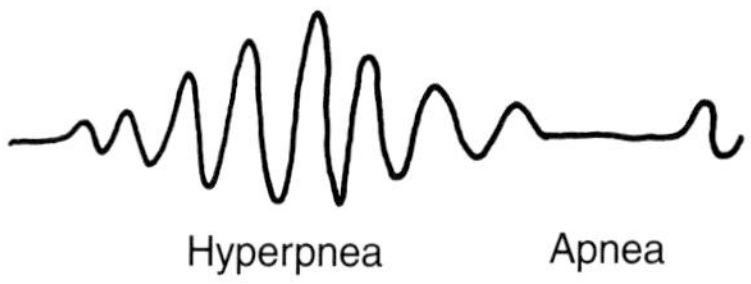

Obstructive Breathing

In obstructive lung disease, expiration is prolonged due to narrowed airways increasing the resistance to air flow. Causes include asthma, chronic bronchitis, and COPD.

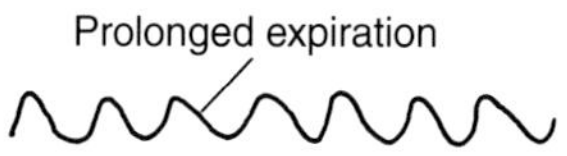

(*continued*)

TABLE 13-5 Abnormalities in Rate and Rhythm of Breathing (*Continued*)

Rapid Deep Breathing (*Hyperpnea, Hyperventilation*)

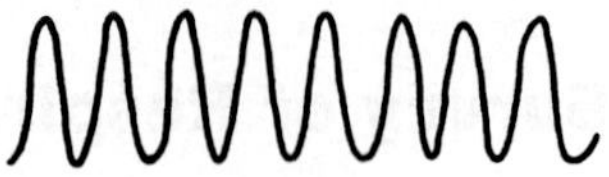

In hyperpnea, rapid deep breathing occurs in response to metabolic demand from causes such as exercise, high altitude, sepsis, and anemia. In hyperventilation, this pattern is independent of metabolic demand, except in respiratory acidosis. Lightheadedness and tingling may arise from decreased CO_2 concentration. In the comatose patient, consider hypoxia or hypoglycemia affecting the midbrain or pons. Kussmaul breathing is compensatory overbreathing due to systemic acidosis. The breathing rate may be fast, normal, or slow.

Ataxic Breathing (*Biot Breathing*)

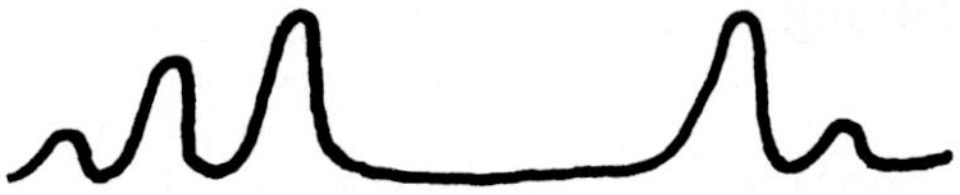

Breathing is irregular; periods of apnea alternate with regular deep breaths which stop suddenly for short intervals. Causes include meningitis, respiratory depression, and brain injury, typically at the medullary level.

Begin by inspecting the patient for signs of respiratory difficulty.

- *Observe the patient's facial expression*; it should be relaxed and calm.

Low oxygenation produces anxiety and restlessness.

- *Observe the patient's level of consciousness.*

A decreased level of consciousness indicates poor oxygenation to the brain and other disease processes.

- *Assess the patient's color* for cyanosis, especially in the face, mucous membranes, and nail beds (shown in the toes in Fig. 13-13; note the contrast with the normal fingers).

Cyanosis signals hypoxia. Clubbing of the nails (see Table 9-12, "Findings in or Near the Nails") may be present in *cystic fibrosis* or *congenital heart disease.*

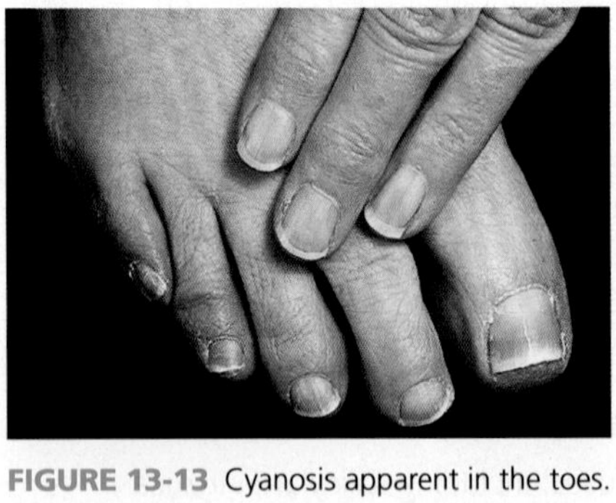

FIGURE 13-13 Cyanosis apparent in the toes.

- *Listen to the patient's breathing.* Are there any audible sounds (e.g., *wheezing* or *stridor*)? If so, do they occur during inhalation exhalation or both?

CLINICAL TIP
Audible stridor, a high-pitched inspiratory sound, is an ominous sign of airway obstruction in the larynx or trachea. Audible wheezing indicates severe asthma.

- *Inspect the neck.* During inspiration, is there contraction of the accessory muscles, namely, the sternocleidomastoid and scalene muscles, or supraclavicular retraction? Is the trachea midline?

Inspiratory contraction of the sternocleidomastoid and scalenes at rest signals severe difficulty in breathing. Lateral displacement of the trachea may be seen in *pneumothorax, pleural effusion*, or *atelectasis*.

- *Observe the shape of the chest.* Its anteroposterior (AP) diameter should be less than its lateral diameter. The normal ratio is usually 0.70 to 0.75 and increases with aging. The upper limit is approximately 0.9 (McGee, 2018).

The AP diameter also may increase in *chronic obstructive pulmonary disease* (COPD).

Examination of the Posterior Chest

Refer back to Chapter 6, "Physical Examination: Getting Started," for a description of how to perform the four assessment techniques.

Inspection

From a midline position behind the patient, note the *shape of the chest* and *how the chest moves,* including:

- Deformities or asymmetry (Table 13-6)

TABLE 13-6 Deformities of the Thorax

Normal Adult

The thorax in the normal adult is wider than it is deep. Its lateral diameter is larger than its anteroposterior diameter.

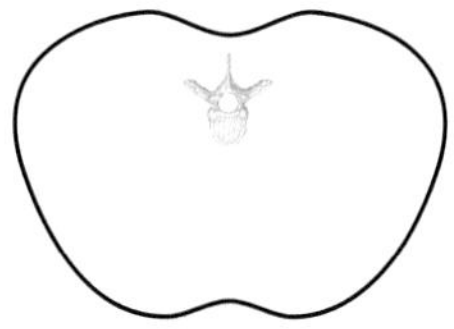

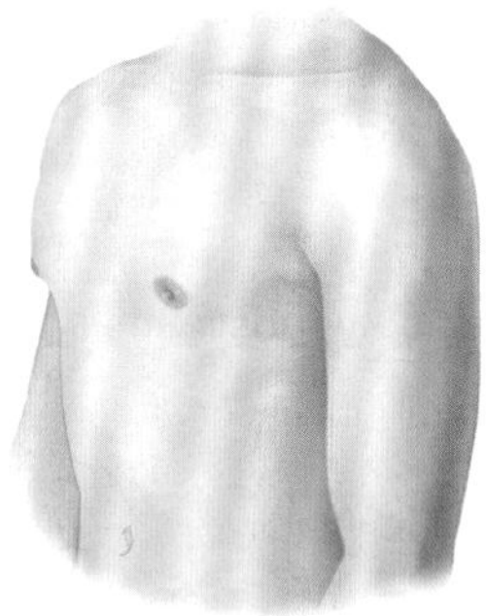

Funnel Chest (*Pectus Excavatum*)

Note depression in the lower portion of the sternum. Compression of the heart and great vessels may cause murmurs.

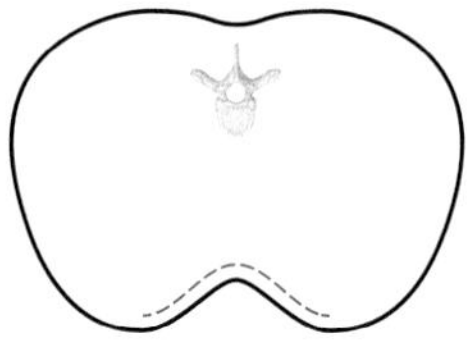

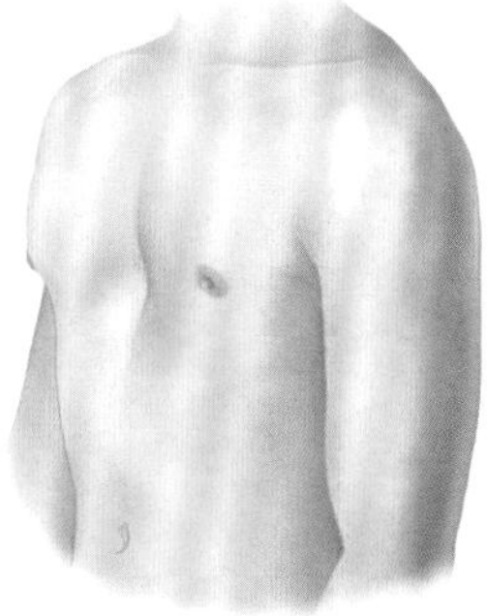

(continued)

TABLE 13-6 Deformities of the Thorax (*Continued*)

Barrel Chest

There is an increased anteroposterior diameter. This shape is normal during infancy and often accompanies aging and chronic obstructive pulmonary disease.

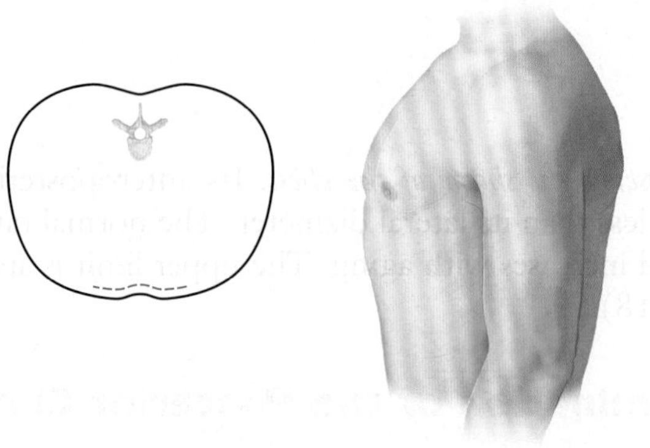

Pigeon Chest (*Pectus Carinatum*)

The sternum is displaced anteriorly, increasing the anteroposterior diameter. The costal cartilages adjacent to the protruding sternum are depressed.

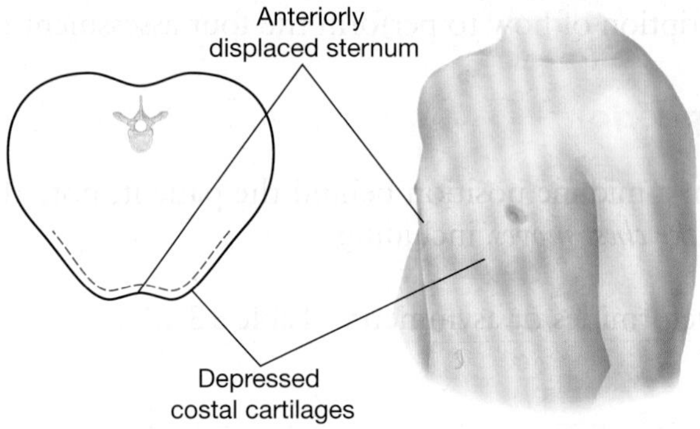

Traumatic Flail Chest

Multiple rib fractures may result in paradoxical movements of the thorax. As descent of the diaphragm decreases intrathoracic pressure, on inspiration the injured area caves inward; on expiration, it moves outward.

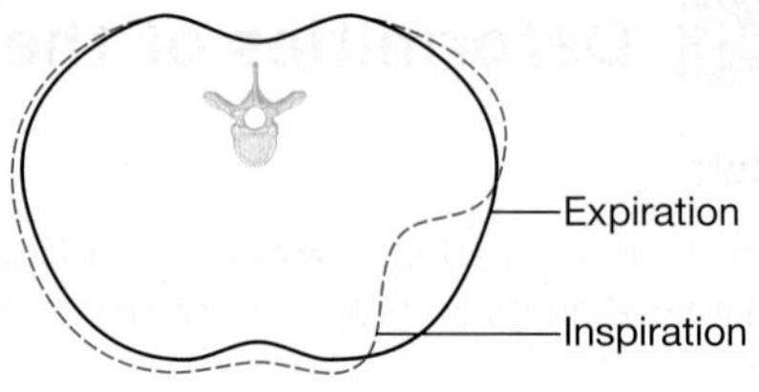

Thoracic Kyphoscoliosis

Abnormal spinal curvatures and vertebral rotation deform the chest. Distortion of the underlying lungs may make interpretation of lung findings difficult.

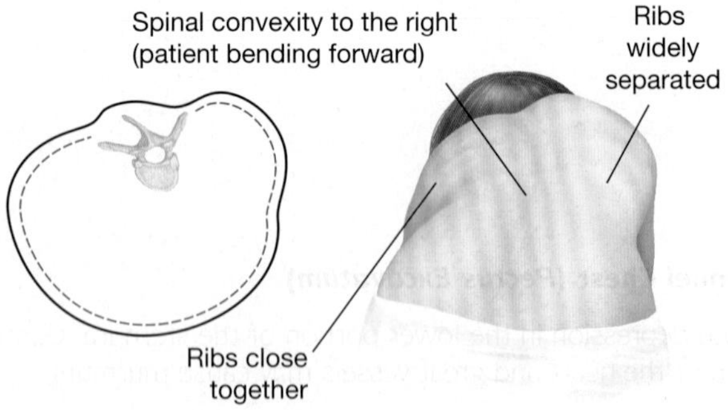

- Intercostal retractions during inspiration. Retractions are most apparent in the lower intercostal spaces.

CLINICAL TIP
Retraction is seen in severe *asthma*, *COPD*, or upper airway obstruction.

- Impaired respiratory movement on one or both sides or a unilateral lag (or delay) in movement

Unilateral impairment or lagging of respiratory movement suggests disease of the underlying lung or pleura.

Palpation

As you palpate the chest, focus on areas of tenderness and abnormalities in the overlying skin, muscles and ribs, respiratory expansion, and fremitus.

Intercostal tenderness may occur over inflamed pleura.

- *Identify tender areas.* Gently palpate any area where pain has been reported or where lesions or bruises are evident.

Bruises or tenderness may be apparent over a fractured rib.

- *Assess any observed abnormalities* such as masses.
- *Test chest expansion.* Place your thumbs at about the level of the 10th ribs with your fingers loosely grasping and parallel to the lateral rib cage. As you position your hands, slide them medially just enough to raise a loose fold of skin on each side between your thumb and the spine.

  Ask the patient to inhale deeply. Let your hands expand with the chest movement. Watch the distance between your thumbs as they move apart during inspiration, and feel for the range and symmetry of the rib cage as it expands and contracts (Fig. 13-14). Your thumbs should move equally apart.

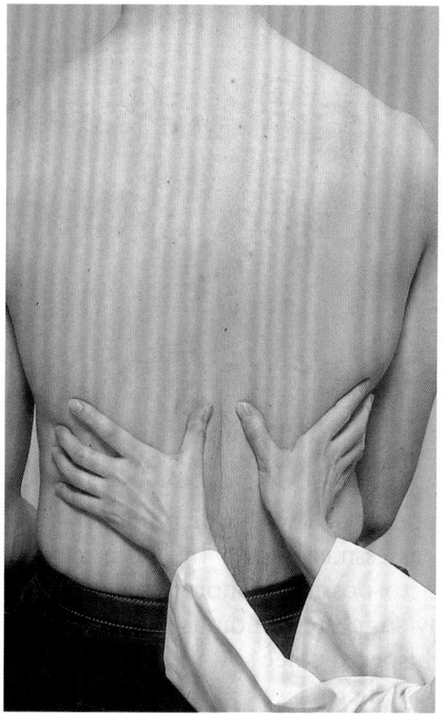

FIGURE 13-14 Testing chest expansion.

Causes of unilateral decrease or delay in chest expansion include *pleural effusion, lobar pneumonia,* pleural pain with associated splinting, unilateral bronchial obstruction, and *chronic fibrosis* of the underlying lung or pleura.

- *Feel for tactile fremitus.* **Fremitus** refers to the palpable vibrations transmitted through the bronchopulmonary tree to the chest wall as the patient is speaking. To detect fremitus, use either the ball (the bony part of the palm at the base of the fingers) or the ulnar surface of your hand to optimize the vibratory sensitivity of the bones in your hand. Ask the patient to repeat the words "ninety-nine" or "one-one-one." If fremitus is faint, ask the patient to speak more loudly or in a deeper voice. The simultaneous use of both hands to compare sides increases your speed and may facilitate detection of asymmetry (Fig. 13-15).

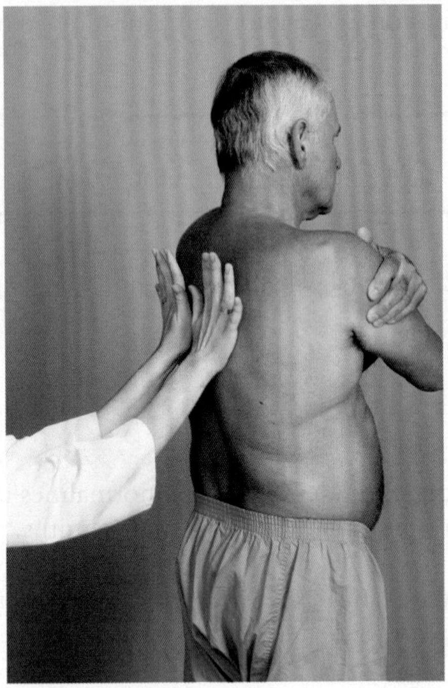

FIGURE 13-15 Using both hands to palpate fremitus. (Reprinted with permission from Lippincott Professional Development Collection, Wolters Kluwer, May 2013.)

Fremitus is decreased or absent when the voice is soft or when the transmission of vibrations from the larynx to the surface of the chest is impeded. Causes include a very thick chest wall; an obstructed bronchus; *COPD*; and pleural effusion, fibrosis (*pleural thickening*), air (*pneumothorax*), or an infiltrating tumor.

- *Palpate and compare symmetric areas* of the lungs in the pattern shown in Figure 13-16. Place your hands on the patient's back between the spine and scapula. Move your hands down the patient's back and around the scapula. Identify and locate any areas of increased, decreased, or absent fremitus. Fremitus is typically more prominent in the interscapular area than in the lower lung fields and sides. For the fourth location in Figure 13-16, place your hands on the lateral chest below the axillae. Fremitus is often more prominent on the right side than on the left. It disappears below the diaphragm. Tactile fremitus is a somewhat imprecise assessment tool, but as a scouting technique, it directs your attention to possible abnormalities. Later in the examination, you will check any suggested findings by listening for breath sounds, voice sounds, and whispered voice sounds. All these attributes tend to increase or decrease together.

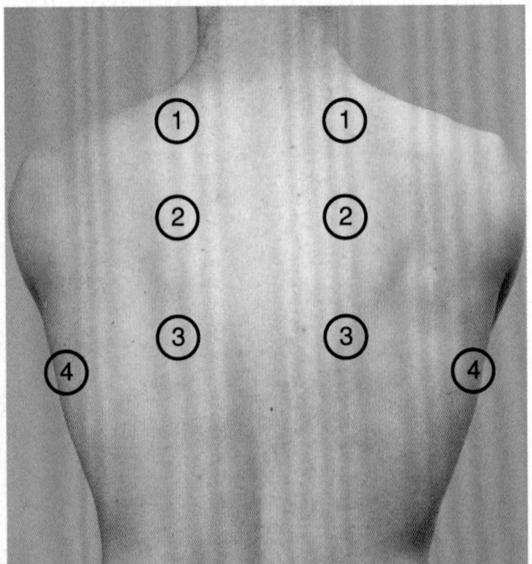

FIGURE 13-16 Locations for palpating fremitus.

Look for *asymmetric* fremitus: asymmetric *decreased* fremitus is seen in unilateral pleural effusion, pneumothorax, and neoplasm from decreased transmission of low-frequency sounds; asymmetric *increased* fremitus is seen in unilateral pneumonia from increased transmission (McGee, 2018).

Percussion

Percussion sets the chest wall and underlying tissues in motion, producing audible sound. Percussion helps establish whether the underlying tissues are air-filled, fluid-filled, or solid. It penetrates only 5 to 7 cm into the chest, however, and will not help detect deep-seated lesions.

The technique of percussion can be practiced on any surface. As you practice, listen for changes in percussion notes over different types of materials or different parts of the body. The key points for good technique, described for a right-handed person, are as follows:

- Hyperextend the middle finger of your left hand, known as the *pleximeter finger* (Fig. 13-17). Press its distal interphalangeal joint firmly on the surface to be percussed. *Avoid surface contact by any other part of the hand because this dampens out vibrations.* Note that the thumb and second, fourth, and fifth fingers are not touching the chest.

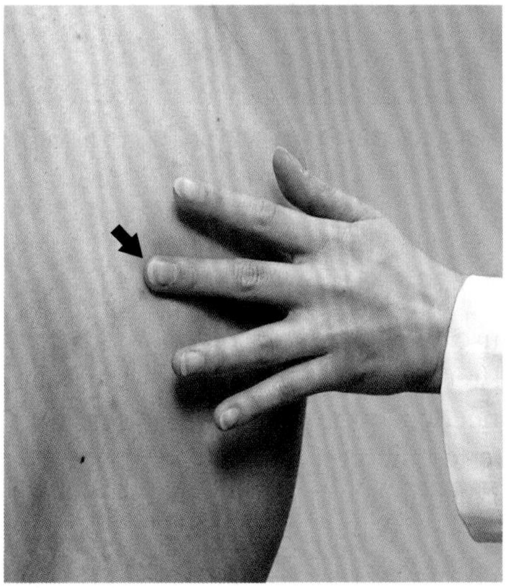

FIGURE 13-17 Using the pleximeter finger.

- Position your right forearm quite close to the surface, with the hand cocked upward. The middle finger is the *plexor finger*. It should be partially flexed, relaxed, and poised to strike (Fig. 13-18).

- With a *quick, sharp but relaxed wrist motion*, strike the pleximeter finger with the right middle finger, or plexor finger. Aim at your distal interphalangeal joint. You are trying to transmit vibrations through the bones of this joint to the underlying chest wall.

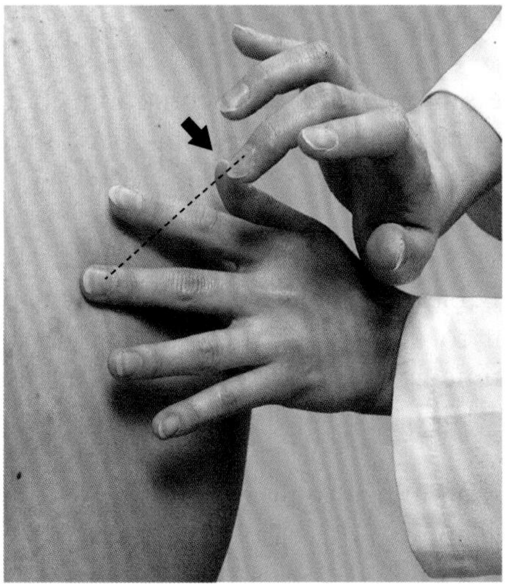

FIGURE 13-18 Preparing to strike with the plexor finger.

- Strike using the *tip of the plexor finger*, not the finger pad. Your finger should be almost at right angles to the pleximeter (Fig. 13-19). A short fingernail is recommended to avoid self-injury.

- Withdraw your striking finger quickly to avoid dampening the vibrations you have created.

In summary, the movement is at the wrist. It is directed, brisk yet relaxed, and slightly bouncy.

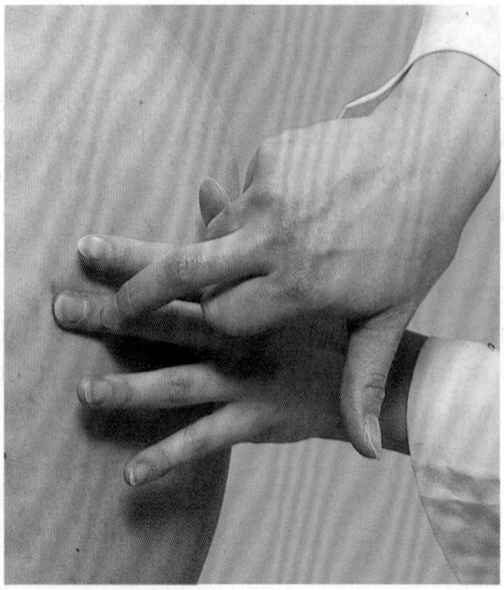

FIGURE 13-19 The plexor finger striking the pleximeter finger.

Left-handed individuals should reverse the hand positions and place the right middle finger on the chest and use the left middle finger as the plexor finger.

Concept Mastery Alert

Percussion of the Chest

Touching the patient's chest with only the pleximeter finger will help maximize resulting vibrations. Surface contact by any other part of the hand or arm when percussing will dampen vibrations.

Percussion Notes

With your plexor or tapping finger, use the lightest percussion that produces a clear note. A thick chest wall requires stronger percussion than a thin one. However, if a *louder* note is needed, apply more pressure with the *pleximeter* finger (this is more effective for increasing percussion note volume than tapping harder with the plexor finger). Consider the following:

- *When percussing the lower posterior chest*, stand somewhat to the side rather than directly behind the patient. This allows you to place your pleximeter finger more firmly on the chest and your plexor strike is more effective, making a better percussion note.

- *When comparing two areas*, use the same percussion technique in both areas. Percuss or strike twice in each location comparing percussion notes.

- *Learn to identify five percussion notes.* You can practice four of them on yourself. These notes differ in their basic qualities of sound: intensity, pitch, and duration. Train your ear to distinguish these differences by concentrating on one quality at a time as you percuss first in one location, then in another. Review Table 13-7. Healthy lungs are *resonant.*

While the patient keeps both arms crossed in front of the chest, percuss the thorax in symmetric locations from the apex to the base.

- *Alternate percussing one side of the chest and then the other at each level* in a ladder-like pattern, as shown in Figure 13-20. Begin above the scapula. Omit the areas over the scapulae; the thickness of muscle and bone alters the percussion notes of the lungs. The lateral numbers 6 and 7 should be percussed on the midaxillary line. Identify and locate the area and quality of any abnormal percussion note.

TABLE 13-7 Percussion Notes and Their Characteristics

	Relative Intensity	Relative Pitch	Relative Duration	Example of Location	Pathologic Examples
Flatness	Soft	High	Short	Thigh	Large pleural effusion
Dullness	Medium	Medium	Medium	Liver	Lobar pneumonia
Resonance	Loud	Low	Long	Healthy lung	Simple chronic bronchitis
Hyperresonance	Very loud	Lower	Longer	Usually none	COPD, pneumothorax
Tympany	Loud	High[a]	Longer	Gastric air bubble or puffed-out cheek	Large pneumothorax

[a]Distinguished mainly by its musical timbre.

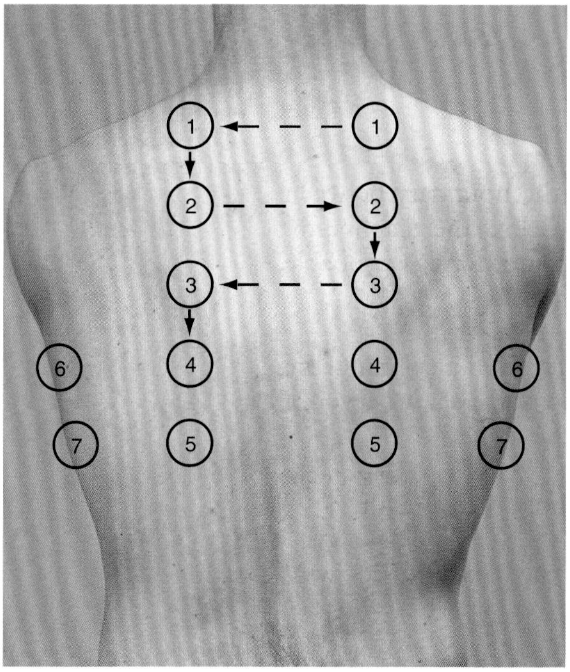

FIGURE 13-20 "Ladder" pattern for percussion and auscultation.

CLINICAL TIP

Dullness replaces resonance when fluid or solid tissue replaces air-containing lung or occupies the pleural space beneath your percussing fingers. Examples include *lobar pneumonia*, in which the alveoli are filled with fluid and blood cells; and pleural accumulations of serous fluid (*pleural effusion*), blood (*hemothorax*), pus (*empyema*), fibrous tissue, or tumor.

Generalized hyperresonance may be heard over the hyperinflated lungs of COPD or *asthma*, but this is not a reliable sign. *Unilateral hyperresonance* suggests a large pneumothorax or possibly a large air-filled bulla in the lung.

- *Identify the descent of the diaphragm*, or *diaphragmatic excursion* (Figs. 13-21 and 13-22). First, *determine the level of diaphragmatic dullness* during quiet respiration. Holding the pleximeter finger *above and parallel* to the expected level of dullness, percuss downward in progressive steps until dullness clearly replaces resonance. Confirm this level of change by percussion near the scapular line and more laterally.

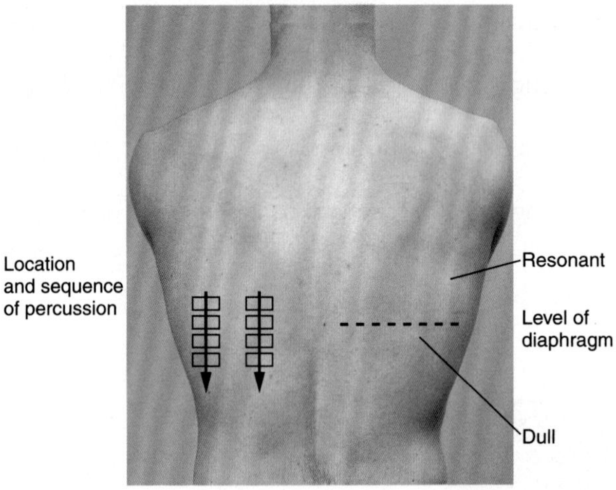

FIGURE 13-21 Diaphragmatic excursion.

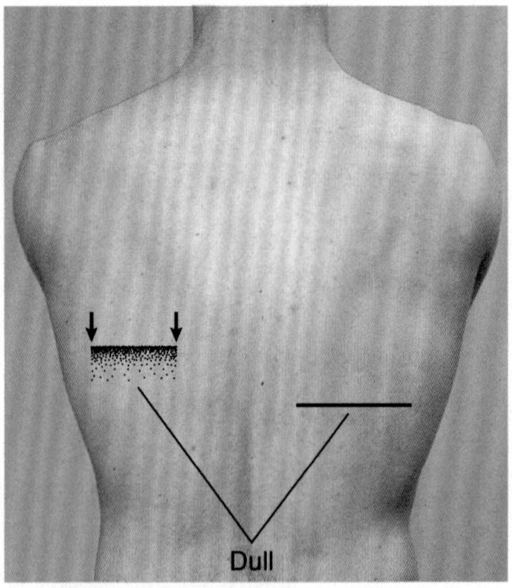

FIGURE 13-22 An abnormally high level suggests pleural effusion, or a high diaphragm as in atelectasis or diaphragmatic paralysis.

Note that with this technique, you are identifying the boundary between the resonant lung tissue and the duller structures below the diaphragm. You are not percussing the diaphragm itself. You can infer the probable location of the diaphragm from the level of dullness.

Now, *estimate the extent of diaphragmatic excursion* by determining the distance between the level of dullness on full expiration and the level of dullness on full inspiration, normally about 3 to 5 cm.

- Ask the patient to breathe in, then out fully and hold their breath.
- Percuss down to dullness and mark this point on the patient's back with a pen.
- Next ask the patient to breathe in fully and hold their breath, and continue percussing down until dullness is heard; mark this point.
- Repeat on the opposite side.
- Measure the distances; they should be equal through the right side though may be 1 cm higher due to the liver.

The diaphragmatic excursion should be 3 to 5 cm in adults, though in athletes it may be up to 7 to 8 cm.

Auscultation

Auscultation is the most important examination technique for assessing air flow through the tracheobronchial tree. Together with percussion, it also helps the nurse assess the condition of the surrounding lungs and pleural space. Auscultation involves (1) listening to the sounds generated by breathing, (2) listening for any **adventitious** (extra) sounds, and (3) if abnormalities are suspected, listening to the sounds of the patient's spoken or whispered voice as they are transmitted through the chest wall.

CLINICAL TIP
Sounds from bedclothes, paper gowns, and the chest itself can generate confusion in auscultation. Hair on the chest may cause crackling sounds. Either press harder or wet the hair. If the patient is cold or tense, you may hear muscle contraction sounds—muffled, low-pitched rumbling or roaring noises. A change in the patient's position may eliminate this noise. You can reproduce this sound on yourself by doing a Valsalva maneuver (straining down) as you listen to your own chest.

Breath Sounds (Lung Sounds)

Learn to identify patterns of breath sounds by their intensity, pitch, and the relative duration of their inspiratory and expiratory phases. Normal breath sounds (Fig. 13-23) are:

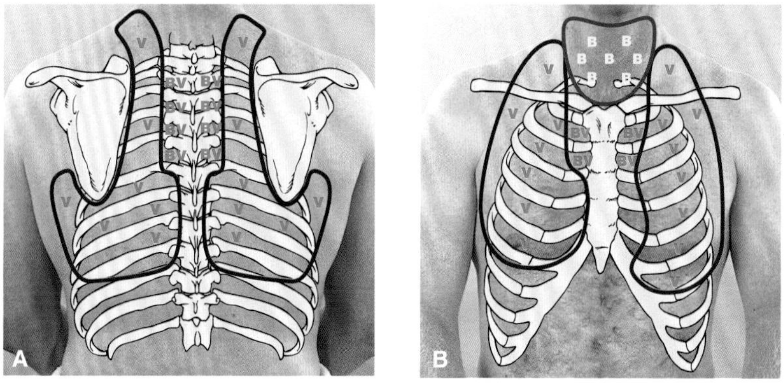

FIGURE 13-23 **A.** Location of vesicular sounds (V) and bronchovesicular sounds (BV) on the posterior thorax. (Reprinted with permission from Weber, J. R., & Kelley, J. H. (2017). *Health assessment in nursing* (6th ed.). Wolters Kluwer.) **B.** Location of the bronchial sounds (B), vesicular sounds, and bronchovesicular sounds on the anterior thorax. (Reprinted with permission from Weber, J. R., & Kelley, J. H. (2017). *Health assessment in nursing* (6th ed.). Wolters Kluwer.)

- *Vesicular*, or soft and low-pitched. They are heard throughout inspiration, continue without pause through expiration, and then fade away about one third of the way through expiration.
- *Bronchovesicular*, with inspiratory and expiratory sounds about equal in length, at times separated by a silent interval. Detecting differences in pitch and intensity is often easier during expiration.
- *Bronchial*, or louder and higher in pitch, with a short silence between inspiratory and expiratory sounds. Expiratory sounds last longer than inspiratory sounds.
- *Tracheal*, very loud, harsh sounds with inspiratory and expiratory sounds equal in length, over the trachea in the neck.

The characteristics of normal breath sounds are summarized in Table 13-8.

TABLE 13-8 Characteristics of Breath Sounds

	Duration of Sounds	Intensity of Expiratory Sound	Pitch of Expiratory Sound	Locations Where Normally Heard
Vesicular[a] 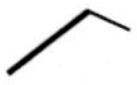	Inspiratory sounds last longer than expiratory ones.	Soft	Relatively low	Over most of both lungs
Bronchovesicular 	Inspiratory and expiratory sounds are about equal.	Intermediate	Intermediate	Often in the first and second intercostal spaces anteriorly and between the scapulae
Bronchial 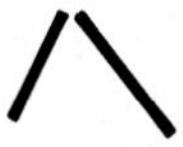	Expiratory sounds last longer than inspiratory ones.	Loud	Relatively high	Over the manubrium, if heard at all
Tracheal 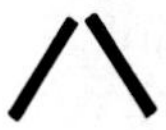	Inspiratory and expiratory sounds are about equal.	Very loud	Relatively high	Over the trachea in the neck

[a]The thickness of the bars indicates intensity; the steeper their incline, the higher the pitch.
Source: Bohadana, A., Izbicki, G., & Kraman, S. S. (2014). Fundamentals of lung auscultation. *The New England Journal of Medicine*, *370*(8), 744–751; and McGee, S. (2018). *Evidence-based physical diagnosis* (4th ed.). Saunders.

If bronchovesicular or bronchial breath sounds are heard in locations distant from those listed, suspect that air-filled lung has been replaced by fluid-filled or solid lung tissue.

Table 13-9 outlines normal and altered breath and voice sounds.

Listen to the breath sounds with the diaphragm of a stethoscope. Tell the patient to breathe deeply through an open mouth. Always place the stethoscope directly on the skin. Clothing may alter the quality of the breath sounds and introduce extra friction sounds. Use the pattern suggested for percussion, moving from one side to the other and comparing symmetric areas of the lungs. If you hear or suspect abnormal sounds, auscultate adjacent areas so that you can fully describe the extent of any abnormality. Listen to at least one full breath in each location. Be alert for patient discomfort resulting from hyperventilation (e.g., lightheadedness, faintness), and allow the patient to rest as needed.

Note the *intensity* of the breath sounds. Breath sounds are usually louder in the lower posterior lung fields and may also vary from area to area. If the breath sounds seem faint, ask the patient to breathe more deeply. You may then hear them easily. When patients do not breathe deeply enough or have a thick chest wall, as in obesity, breath sounds may remain diminished.

Breath sounds may be decreased when air flow is decreased (as in obstructive lung disease or muscular weakness) or when the transmission of sound is poor (as in *pleural effusion, pneumothorax,* or *COPD*).

TABLE 13-9 Normal and Altered Breath and Voice Sounds

The origins of breath sounds are still unclear (Bohadana et al., 2014). Turbulent air flow in the pharynx, glottis, and subglottic region produce tracheal breath sounds, which are similar to bronchial sounds. The inspiratory component of vesicular breath sounds seems to arise in the lobar and segmental airways; the expiratory component arises in the more central larger airways. Normally, tracheal and bronchial sounds may be heard over the trachea and mainstem bronchi; vesicular breath sounds predominate throughout most of the lungs.

Fluids and solids transmit sound and vibration waves better than air. When lung tissue loses its air, it transmits high-pitched sounds much better. If the tracheobronchial tree is open, bronchial breath sounds may replace the normal vesicular sounds over airless areas of the lung. This change is seen in lobar pneumonia when the alveoli fill with fluid, red cells, and white cells—a process called *consolidation*. Other causes include pulmonary edema or hemorrhage. Bronchial breath sounds usually correlate with an increase in tactile fremitus and transmitted voice sounds. These findings are summarized below.

	Normal Air-Filled Lung	Airless Lung, as in Lobar Pneumonia
	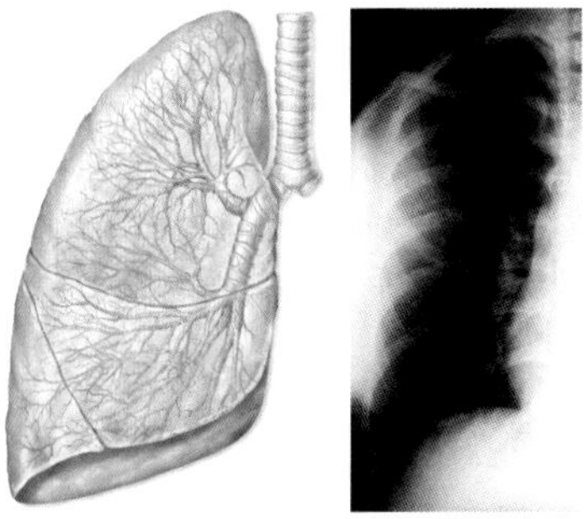	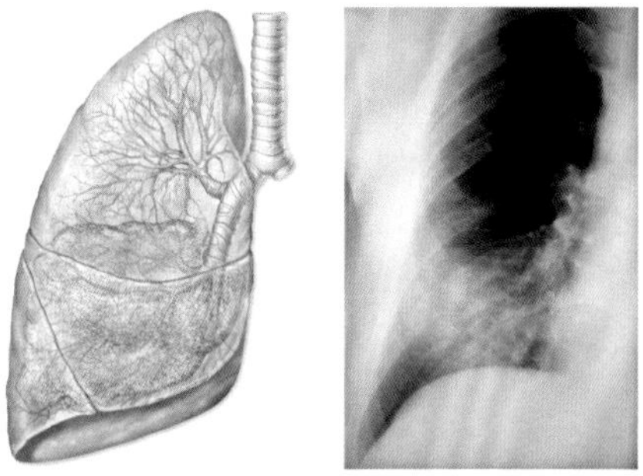
Breath Sounds	Predominantly vesicular	Bronchial or bronchovesicular over the involved area
Transmitted Voice Sounds	Spoken words muffled and indistinct Spoken "ee" heard as "ee" Whispered words faint and indistinct, if heard at all	Spoken words louder, clearer (*bronchophony*) Spoken "ee" heard as "ay" (*egophony*) Whispered words louder, clearer (*whispered pectoriloquy*)
Tactile Fremitus	Normal	Increased

Is there a *silent gap* between the inspiratory and expiratory sounds? A gap suggests bronchial breath sounds.

Listen for the *pitch, intensity, and duration of the expiratory and inspiratory sounds.* Are vesicular breath sounds distributed throughout the chest wall? Are there bronchovesicular or bronchial breath sounds in unexpected places? If so, where are they?

Adventitious (Extra) Sounds

Listen for any **adventitious sounds** (extra sounds) that are superimposed on the usual breath sounds. Detection of adventitious sounds—*crackles* (sometimes called *rales*), *wheezes,* and *rhonchi*—is an important part of your examination, often leading to diagnosis of cardiac and pulmonary conditions. The most common kinds of these sounds are outlined in Table 13-10.

TABLE 13-10 Adventitious Lung Sounds: Causes and Qualities

Crackles

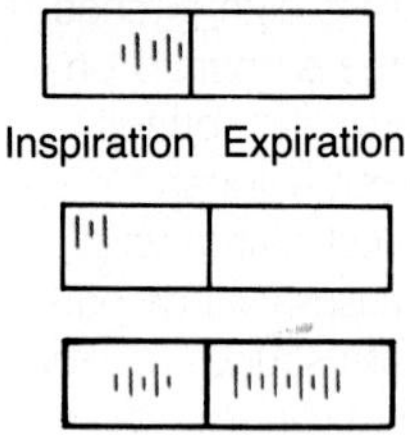

Crackles are discontinuous nonmusical sounds that can be early inspiratory (as in *COPD*), late inspiratory (as in *pulmonary fibrosis*), or biphasic (as in *pneumonia*). They are currently considered to result from a series of tiny explosions when small distal airways, deflated during expiration, pop open during inspiration. With few exceptions, recent acoustic studies indicate that the role of secretions as a cause of crackles to secretions is less likely.

- *Fine crackles* are soft, higher-pitched, and more frequent per breath than coarse crackles. They are heard from *mid to late inspiration*, especially in the dependent areas of the lung, and change according to body position. They have a shorter duration and higher frequency than coarse crackles. Fine crackles appear to be generated by the "sudden inspiratory opening of small airways held close by surface forces during the previous expiration."
  Examples include *pulmonary fibrosis* (known for "Velcro rales") and interstitial lung disease such as *interstitial fibrosis and interstitial pneumonitis heart failure*.
- *Coarse crackles* appear in early inspiration and last throughout expiration (*biphasic*), have a popping sound, are heard over any lung region, and do not vary with body position. They have a longer duration and lower frequency than fine crackles, change or disappear with coughing, and are transmitted to the mouth. Coarse crackles appear to result from "boluses of gas passing through airways as the open and close intermittently."
  Examples include *COPD*, *asthma*, and *bronchiectasis*; *pneumonia* (crackles may become finer and change from mid to late inspiratory during recovery); and *heart failure*.

Wheezes and Rhonchi

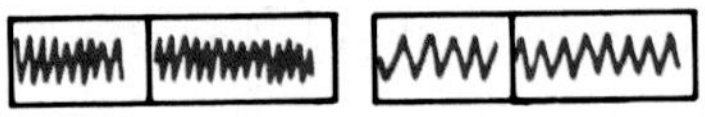

Wheezes are continuous musical sounds that occur during rapid airflow when bronchial airways are narrowed almost to the point of closure. Wheezes can be inspiratory, expiratory, or biphasic. They may be heard throughout the lung or localized due to a foreign body, mucous plug, or tumor. Although wheezes are typical of asthma, they can occur in a number of pulmonary diseases. Recent studies suggest that as the airways become more narrowed, wheezes become less audible, culminating finally in "the silent chest" of severe asthma that requires immediate intervention.

Rhonchi are now considered to be a variant of wheezes, arising from the same mechanism but lower in pitch. Unlike wheezes, rhonchi may disappear with coughing, so secretions may be involved.

Stridor

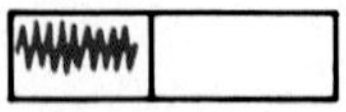

Stridor is a continuous high-frequency, high-pitched musical sound produced during airflow through a narrowing in the upper respiratory tract. Stridor is best heard over the neck during inspiration but can be biphasic. Causes of the underlying airway obstruction include tracheal stenosis from intubation, airway edema after device removal, croup, epiglottitis, foreign body, and anaphylaxis. Immediate intervention is warranted.

Pleural Friction Rub

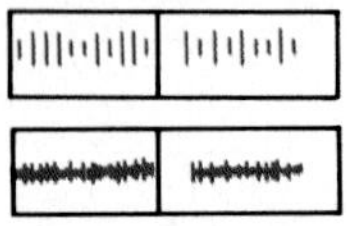

A *pleural friction rub* is a discontinuous, low-frequency, grating sound that arises from inflammation and roughening of the visceral pleura as it slides against the parietal pleura. This nonmusical sound is biphasic, heard during inspiration and expiration, and is often described as creaking or like two pieces of leather rubbing together. It is often best heard in the axilla and base of the lungs.

Mediastinal Crunch (*Hamman Sign*)

A *mediastinal crunch* is a series of precordial crackles synchronous with the heartbeat, not with respiration. Best heard in the left lateral position, it arises from air entry into the mediastinum causing mediastinal emphysema (*pneumomediastinum*). It usually produces severe central chest pain and may be spontaneous. It has been reported in cases of tracheobronchial injury, blunt trauma, pulmonary disease, use of recreational drugs, childbirth, and rapid ascent of scuba divers (Kouritas et al., 2015).

Source: Bohadana, A., Izbicki, G., & Kraman, S. S. (2014). Fundamentals of lung auscultation. *The New England Journal of Medicine*, *370*(8), 744–751; and McGee, S. (2018). *Evidence-based physical diagnosis* (4th ed.). Saunders.

If you hear *crackles*, especially those that do not clear after coughing, listen carefully for the following characteristics (Bohadana et al., 2014; McGee, 2018). These are clues to the underlying condition:

Crackles may be from abnormalities of the lungs (*pneumonia, fibrosis, early congestive heart failure*) or of the airways (*bronchitis, bronchiectasis*).

- Loudness, pitch, and duration (summarized as fine or coarse crackles)

Fine, late inspiratory crackles that persist from breath to breath suggest abnormal lung tissue.

- Number (few to many)
- Timing in the respiratory cycle
- Location on the chest wall
- Persistence of their pattern from breath to breath
- Any change after a cough or a change in the patient's position

Clearing of crackles, wheezes, or rhonchi after coughing or position change suggests thickened secretions, as in *bronchitis* or *atelectasis*.

In some healthy people, crackles may be heard at the lung bases anteriorly after maximal expiration. Crackles in dependent portions of the lungs may also occur after prolonged time lying flat (e.g., upon waking in the morning).

If you hear *wheezes* or *rhonchi*, note their timing (inspiratory, expiratory, or both) and location. Do they change with deep breathing or coughing?

Wheezes suggest narrowed airways as in *asthma, COPD,* or *bronchitis*. Ronchi suggest secretions in large airways. During a severe asthma exacerbation, wheezing may decrease or cease due to lack of air flow in the bronchial tree. This is a clinical emergency.

More information on these adventitious sounds as well as others are described in Table 13-11.

TABLE 13-11 Adventitious Breath Sounds

Crackles (or Rales)	Wheezes and Rhonchi
Discontinuous	**Continuous**
• Intermittent, nonmusical, and brief • Like dots in time • *Fine crackles:* soft, high-pitched, very brief (5–10 msec) • *Coarse crackles:* somewhat louder, lower in pitch, brief (20–30 msec)	• ≥250 msec, sinusoidal prolonged (but not necessarily persisting throughout the respiratory cycle) • Like dashes in time • *Wheezes:* musical, relatively high-pitched (≥400 Hz) with hissing or shrill quality • *Rhonchi:* relatively low-pitched (≤200 Hz) with snoring quality

Source: Bohadana, A., Izbicki, G., & Kraman, S. S. (2014). Fundamentals of lung auscultation. *The New England Journal of Medicine, 370*(8), 744–751; and McGee, S. (2018). *Evidence-based physical diagnosis* (4th ed.). Saunders.

Transmitted Voice Sounds

Sound waves travel better through consolidated tissue as when airways are blocked by inflammation and secretions. If you hear abnormally located bronchovesicular or bronchial breath sounds or adventitious sounds, assess transmitted voice sounds (see Table 13-9). With the diaphragm of the stethoscope, listen in symmetric areas over the chest wall as you:

- Ask the patient to say "ninety-nine." Normally the sounds transmitted through the chest wall are muffled and indistinct.

Louder, clearer voice sounds are called **bronchophony**.

- Ask the patient to say "ee." You will normally hear a muffled long E sound.

When "ee" is heard as "ay," an *E-to-A change* (**egophony**) is present, as in lobar consolidation from *pneumonia.* The quality sounds nasal.

- Ask the patient to whisper "ninety-nine" or "one-two-three." The whispered voice is normally heard faintly and indistinctly, if at all.

Louder, clearer whispered sounds are called **whispered pectoriloquy** and also indicate consolidation as in pneumonia.

Examination of the Anterior Chest

When examined in the supine position, the patient should lie comfortably with arms somewhat abducted. A patient who is having difficulty breathing should be examined in the sitting position or with the head of the bed elevated to a comfortable level.

Individuals with severe asthma or COPD may prefer to sit leaning forward, with lips pursed during exhalation and arms supported on their knees or a table. This is called the *tripod position* (Fig. 13-24).

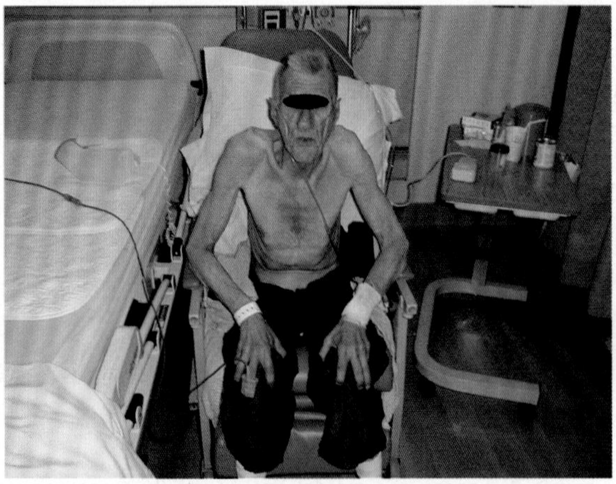

FIGURE 13-24 The tripod position.

Inspection

Observe *the shape of the patient's chest* and the *movement of the chest wall.* Note:

- Deformities or asymmetry of the thorax (see Table 13-6)

- Work of breathing: Intercostal, supraclavicular and/or substernal retractions during inspiration are seen in severe asthma, COPD, or upper airway obstruction.

- Unilateral lag or impaired respiratory movement in both sides which may indicate underlying disease of the lungs or pleura (e.g., asbestosis, nerve damage, or trauma)

- Bruising or other skin lesions

Palpation

Palpation has four potential uses:

- *Identification of tender areas.*

Tender pectoral muscles or costal cartilages corroborate but do not prove that chest pain has a musculoskeletal origin.

- *Assessment of observed abnormalities.*

- *Assessment of chest expansion.* Place your thumbs along each costal margin, your hands along the lateral rib cage (Fig. 13-25). As you position your hands, slide them medially a bit to raise loose skin folds between your thumbs. Ask the patient to inhale deeply (the thorax expands). Observe how far your thumbs diverge and feel for the extent and symmetry of respiratory movement.

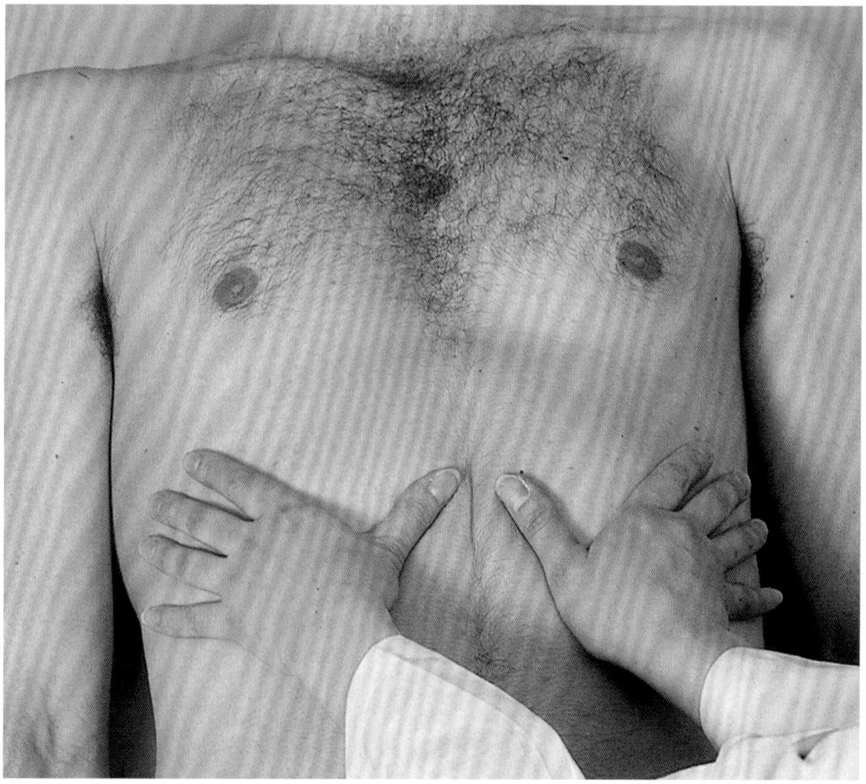

FIGURE 13-25 Chest expansion hand position.

- *Assessment of tactile fremitus* (Fig. 13-26). Compare both sides of the chest, using the ball or ulnar surface of your hand. Fremitus is usually decreased or absent over the precordium. When examining a woman, ask her to hold her breasts to the side or gently displace the breasts as necessary.

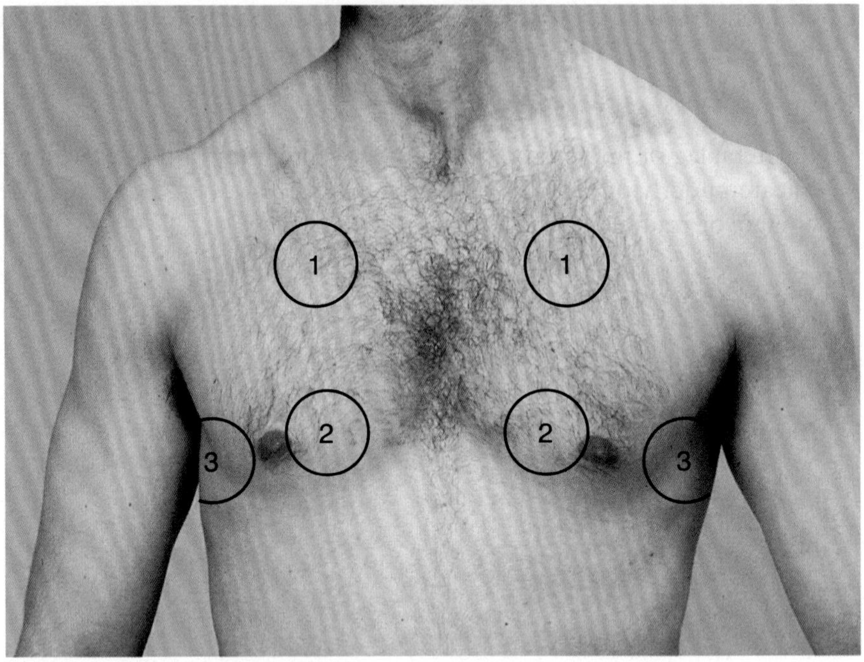

FIGURE 13-26 Locations for feeling fremitus.

Percussion

When percussing the anterior chest:

- Percuss the anterior and lateral chest, again comparing both sides (Fig. 13-27). The heart normally produces an area of dullness to the left of the sternum from the third to the fifth intercostal spaces. Percuss the left lung lateral to it. Identify and locate any area with an abnormal percussion note.

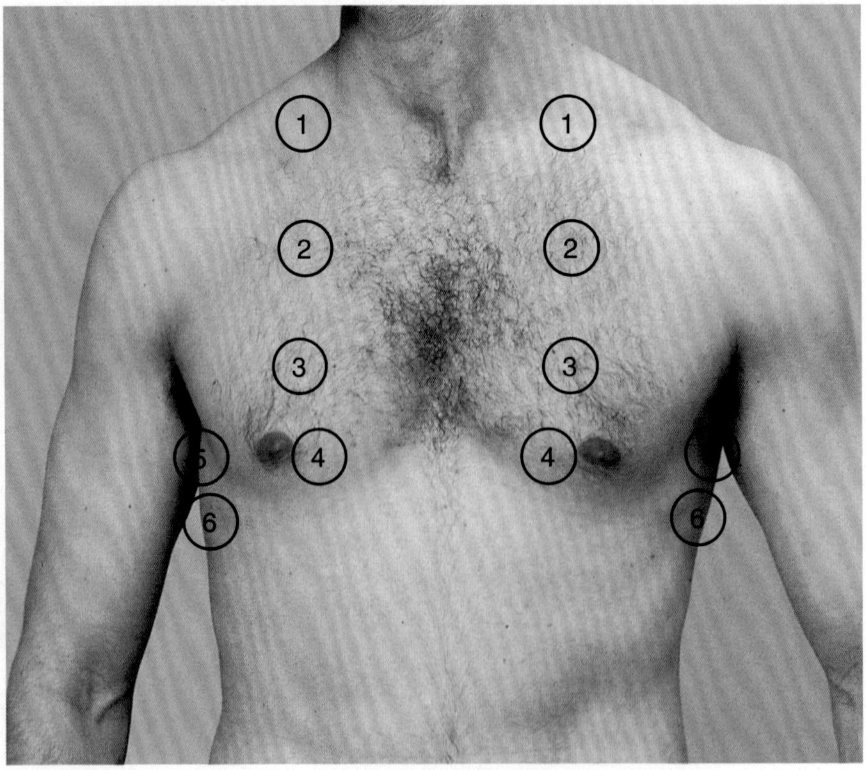

FIGURE 13-27 Percussing the anterior and lateral chest.

CLINICAL TIP

Dullness replaces resonance when fluid or solid tissue replaces air-containing lung or occupies the pleural space. Because pleural fluid usually sinks to the lowest part of the pleural space (posteriorly in a supine patient), only a very large effusion can be detected anteriorly.

The hyperresonance of *COPD* may totally replace cardiac dullness.

In a woman, to enhance percussion, ask her to hold her breast up and to the right. Alternatively, gently displace the breast with your left hand while percussing with the right.

The dullness of right middle lobe pneumonia typically occurs behind the right breast. Unless the breast is displaced, you may miss the abnormal percussion note.

- With your pleximeter finger above and parallel to the expected upper border of liver dullness, percuss in progressive steps downward in the right midclavicular line. Identify the upper border of liver dullness (Fig. 13-28). Later, during the abdominal examination, you will use this method to estimate the size of the liver. As you percuss down the chest on the left, the resonance of normal lung usually changes to the tympany of the gastric air bubble.

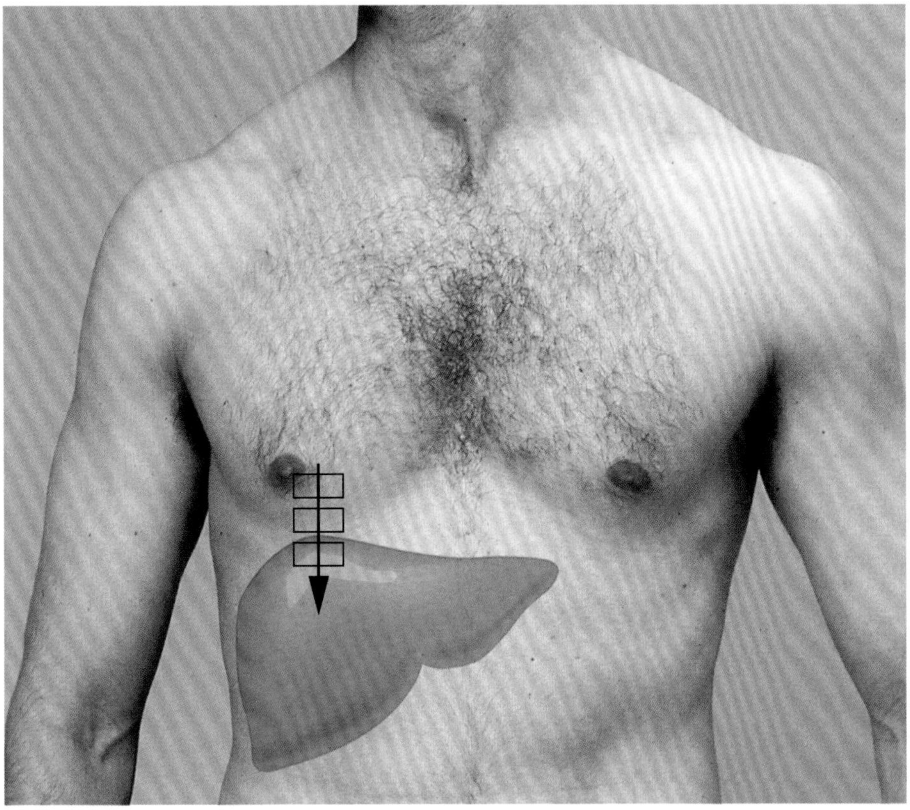

FIGURE 13-28 A lung affected by COPD often displaces the upper border of the liver downward. It also lowers the level of diaphragmatic dullness posteriorly.

Auscultation

Listen to the chest anteriorly and laterally as the patient breathes with the mouth open, more deeply than normal. Compare symmetric areas of the lungs, using the pattern suggested for percussion and extending it to adjacent areas as indicated.

- *Listen to the breath sounds*, noting their intensity and identifying any variations from normal vesicular breathing. Breath sounds are usually louder in the upper anterior lung fields. Bronchovesicular breath sounds may be heard over the large airways, especially on the right.
- *Identify any adventitious sounds*, time them in the respiratory cycle, and locate them on the chest wall. Do they clear with deep breathing?
- If indicated, *listen for transmitted voice sounds.*

Physical findings in additional select chest disorders are described in Table 13-12.

TABLE 13-12 Physical Findings in Select Chest Disorders

This table lists the typical changes seen in respiratory disorders. The changes described vary with the extent and severity of the disorder. Use the table for the direction of typical changes, not for absolute distinctions.

Condition	Percussion Note	Trachea	Breath Sounds	Adventitious Sounds	Tactile Fremitus and Transmitted Voice Sounds
Normal					
The tracheobronchial tree and alveoli are open. Pleurae are thin and close together. Mobility of the chest wall is unimpaired.	Resonant	Midline	Vesicular, except perhaps bronchovesicular and bronchial sounds over the large bronchi and trachea, respectively	None, except perhaps a few transient inspiratory crackles at the bases of the lungs	Normal
Chronic Bronchitis					
The bronchi are chronically inflamed and a productive cough is present. Airway obstruction may develop.	Resonant	Midline	Vesicular (normal)	None or scattered coarse crackles in early inspiration and perhaps expiration; or *wheezes* or *rhonchi*	Normal
Left-Sided Heart Failure (*Early*)					
Increased pressure in the pulmonary veins causes congestion and interstitial edema (around the alveoli); bronchial mucosa may become edematous.	Resonant	Midline	Vesicular	*Late inspiratory crackles* in the dependent portions of the lungs; possibly *wheezes*	Normal
Lobar Pneumonia					
Alveoli fill with fluid or blood cells, as in pneumonia pulmonary edema, or pulmonary hemorrhage.	Dull over the airless area	Midline	*Bronchial* over the involved area	*Late inspiratory crackles* over the involved area	*Increased over* the involved area with *bronchophony*, *egophony*, and *whispered pectoriloquy*

Condition	Percussion Note	Trachea	Breath Sounds	Adventitious Sounds	Tactile Fremitus and Transmitted Voice Sounds
Partial Lobar Obstruction (Atelectasis)					
When a plug in a mainstem bronchus (as from mucus or a foreign object) obstructs bronchial air flow, affected alveoli collapse and become airless.	Dull over the airless area	May be *shifted toward involved side*	*Usually absent* when bronchial plug persists Exceptions include right upper lobe atelectasis, where adjacent tracheal sounds may be transmitted	None	Usually absent when the bronchial plug persists In exceptions (e.g., right upper lobe atelectasis) may be increased
Pleural Effusion					
Fluid accumulates in the pleural space and separates air-filled lung from the chest wall, blocking the transmission breath sounds.	Dull to flat over the fluid	*Shifted toward the unaffected side* in a large effusion	*Decreased to absent*, but bronchial breath sounds may be heard near top of large effusion	None, except a *possible pleural* rub	*Decreased to absent, but may be increased* toward the top of a large effusion
Pneumothorax					
When air leaks into the pleural space, usually unilaterally, the lung recoils away from the chest wall. Pleural air blocks transmission of sound.	Hyperresonant or tympanitic over the pleural air	*Shifted toward the unaffected side, if it is a* tension pneumothorax	*Decreased to absent* over the pleural air	None, except a *possible pleural rub*	*Decreased to absent* over the pleural air
Chronic Obstructive Pulmonary Disease (COPD)					
Slowly progressive disorder in which the distal air spaces enlarge and lungs become hyperinflated. Chronic bronchitis may precede or follow the development of COPD.	Diffusely hyperresonant	Midline	*Decreased to absent with delayed expiration*	None, or the crackles, wheezes, and rhonchi of associated chronic bronchitis	Decreased
Asthma					
Widespread, usually reversible, airflow obstruction with bronchial hyperresponsiveness and underlying inflammation. During attacks, as air flow decreases, lungs hyperinflate.	Resonant to diffusely hyperresonant	Midline	*Often obscured by wheezes*	*Wheezes, possibly crackles*	Decreased

SPECIAL TECHNIQUES

Pulse Oximetry

Pulse oximetry measures the arterial oxygenation saturation, or SpO_2. A probe is placed on the patient's finger (Fig. 13-29) or earlobe. The toe is used for infants and young children. A diode emits light, and a detector on the opposite side of the probe measures the amount of light absorbed by oxyhemoglobin. The oximeter compares the amount of light emitted to the amount absorbed and calculates the percentage of oxygen saturation. A healthy person has an SpO_2 of 95% to 100%. Poor perfusion, hypotension, **dyshemoglobinemias** (disorders in which the hemoglobin molecule is functionally altered and prevented from carrying oxygen), dyes in some nail polishes, and excessive ambient light may cause inaccurate readings. Pulse oximetry is routinely used for respiratory diseases such as asthma, pneumonia, COPD, COVID-19, and lung cancer.

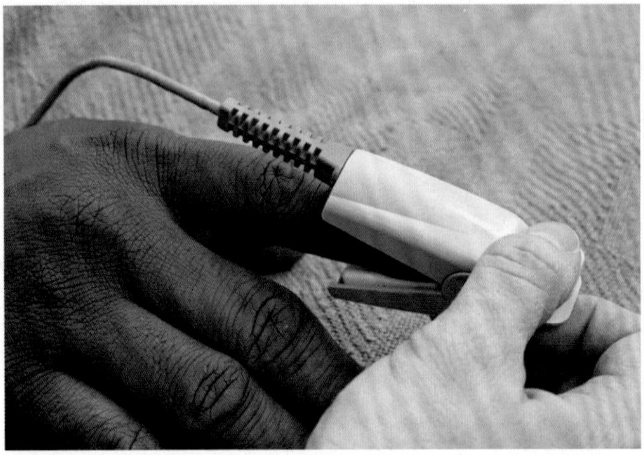

FIGURE 13-29 Pulse oximeter on the finger.

Peak Flow Assessment

A peak flow meter (Fig. 13-30) assesses the maximum volume of air expelled from the lungs during a vigorous exhalation. A decrease in peak

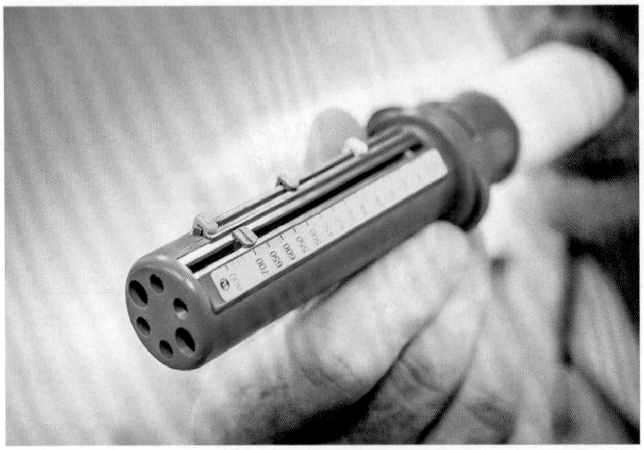

FIGURE 13-30 Patient using a peak flow meter. (Oxford Media Library/Shutterstock)

flow volume occurs in diseases that reduce outflow of air; for example, asthma. As peak flow decreases, the severity of an exacerbation increases. Regular monitoring of a patient's peak flow can evaluate the effectiveness of treatment for chronic asthma. Peak flow rate can be accurately performed by most people over 5 years of age.

To measure peak flow, move the marker on the meter to the bottom of the numbered scale and instruct the patient to:

- Stand up straight. Remove gum or candy from your mouth.
- Take a deep breath. Fill your lungs all the way.
- Hold your breath and place the mouthpiece in your mouth between your teeth. Close your lips around it. Do not put your tongue against or inside the hole.
- Blow out as hard and fast as you can in a single blow.

Note the number. Move the marker back to the bottom and have the patient repeat these steps two more times. The highest of the three numbers is recorded as the patient's peak flow.

The patient's first burst of air is the most important, so blowing for a longer time will not improve the result.

If the patient coughs, disregard that attempt and have the patient repeat the steps again.

Identification of a Fractured Rib

Local pain and tenderness of one or more ribs raise the question of fracture. By AP compression of the chest, you can help to distinguish a fracture from soft tissue injury. With one hand on the sternum and the other on the thoracic spine, squeeze the chest. Stop squeezing if patient complains of pain. Ask about the severity of the pain and its location. An increase in the local pain (distant from your hands) suggests rib fracture rather than a soft tissue injury.

Risk factors for rib fracture include:

- Weak bone density
- Heavy alcohol use
- Falls

Older women presenting with rib fractures should be evaluated for osteoporosis.

RECORDING YOUR FINDINGS

Box 13-2 includes examples of documentation of findings from physical examination of the thorax and lungs.

BOX 13-2 RECORDING THE PHYSICAL EXAMINATION—THE THORAX AND LUNGS

"Thorax is symmetric with equal expansion. Lungs resonant. Anterior and posterior breath sounds clear bilaterally. Diaphragm descends 4 cm bilaterally."

OR

"Thorax symmetric with moderate kyphosis and increased AP diameter, decreased expansion. Lungs are hyperresonant. Breath sounds distant with delayed expiratory phase and scattered expiratory wheezes. Fremitus decreased; no bronchophony, egophony, or whispered pectoriloquy. Diaphragm descends 2 cm bilaterally."

Suggests *COPD.*

HEALTH PROMOTION AND COUNSELING

Important topics for health promotion and counseling regarding the respiratory system include:

- Tobacco cessation
- Immunizations

Tobacco Cessation

According to the Centers for Disease Control and Prevention (CDC), tobacco use is the leading cause of preventable disease, disability, and death in the United States. Each year, nearly half a million Americans die prematurely of smoking or exposure to secondhand smoke. In 2018, an estimated 49.1 million U.S. adults (19.7%) reported currently using tobacco products, including cigarettes (13.7%), cigars (3.9%), e-cigarettes (3.2%), smokeless tobacco (2.4%), and pipes (regular, water pipe, or hookah) (1.0%). Of middle and high school students, 4.7 million reporting using at least one tobacco product, including e-cigarettes. Cigarette smoking remains higher among adults who are male, multiracial or Native American/Alaska Native, lesbian, gay, or bisexual, and those who have less education, live below the poverty line, and/or have a disability or serious psychological distress (CDC, 2020a).

Tobacco use and addiction often begin during middle school and high school years. Adolescence is a critical window for brain development, and nicotine use at this time might have lasting adverse consequences for brain development, cause addiction, and lead to continued tobacco use.

Recent increases in the use of e-cigarettes is driving increases in tobacco product use among youth. In 2019, about 12 of every 100 middle school students (12.5%) and about 31 of every 100 high school students (31.2%) reported current use of a tobacco product. In 2019, nearly one in every four middle school students (24.3%) and over half (53.3%) of high school students said they had tried a tobacco product (CDC, 2020f).

Overall, smoking is damaging to health in a number of ways (Table 13-13).

TABLE 13-13 Adverse Effects of Smoking on Health and Disease

Condition	Increased Risk Compared with Nonsmokers
Coronary artery disease	2–4 times higher
Stroke	2–4 times higher
COPD mortality	12–13 times higher
Lung cancer mortality	23 times higher in men 25.7 times higher in women

Source: Centers for Disease Control and Prevention (CDC). (2020a). Fact sheet: Smoking and tobacco use: Health effects of cigarette smoking. http://www.cdc.gov/tobacco/data_statistics/fact_sheets/health_effects/effects_cig_smoking/index.htm

In addition to respiratory tract cancers, smoking contributes to cancers of the bladder, cervix, colon and rectum, kidney, oropharynx, larynx, esophagus, stomach, liver, and pancreas, as well as acute myeloid leukemia (CDC, 2020e). Smoking increases risk of infertility, preterm birth, low birth weight, and sudden infant death syndrome. Smoking is associated with developing diabetes, cataracts, and rheumatoid arthritis. Nonsmokers exposed to smoke also have increased risk of lung cancer, ear and respiratory infections, asthma, and residential fires.

Cigarette smoking among U.S. adults has declined from 17.8% in 2013 to nearly 14% in 2018. Three in five adults who ever smoked cigarettes have quit. In addition, nearly 70% of adults who smoke say they want to quit, and just over half try to quit each year (CDC, 2020g). Nurses should focus on smoking prevention and cessation, especially in adolescents and pregnant women. Health care providers should advise smokers to quit during every visit. Use the "5 As" framework (Box 13-3) or the stages

BOX 13-3 ASSESSING READINESS TO QUIT SMOKING

The 5 As

1. *Ask* about tobacco use.
2. *Advise* the patient to quit through clear, personalized messages.
3. *Assess* willingness to quit.
4. *Assist* the patient with quitting.
5. *Arrange* follow-up and support.

Stages of Change Model

1. Precontemplation—"I don't want to quit."
2. Contemplation—"I am concerned but not ready to quit now."
3. Preparation—"I am ready to quit."
4. Action—"I just quit."
5. Maintenance—"I quit 6 months ago."

Source: Norcross, J. C., & Prochaska, J. O. (2002). Using the stages of change. *Harvard Mental Health Letter, 18*(11), 5–7; U.S. Preventive Services Task Force. (2020). Tobacco smoking cessation in adults, including pregnant persons: Interventions. Draft evidence review. Retrieved June 02, 2020, from https://www.uspreventiveservicestaskforce.org/uspstf/document/draft-evidence-review/tobacco-smoking-cessation-in-adults-including-pregnant-women-interventions

of change model (precontemplation, contemplation, preparation, action, maintenance) (Norcross & Prochaska, 2002) to assess readiness to quit.

Nicotine is highly addictive, comparable to heroin and cocaine, and quitting tobacco use is difficult. Cognitive therapy techniques will help patients recognize signs of withdrawal such as irritability, difficulty concentrating, anxiety, and depressed mood. Guide patients to better understand craving, triggers for smoking, strategies for managing withdrawal, coping with stress, and preventing relapse. Combining counseling with pharmacotherapy is more effective than either therapy alone. Three drugs have been shown to improve and sustain quitting rates: nicotine replacement therapies; bupropion, a norepinephrine and dopamine reuptake inhibitor and nicotinic receptor antagonist; and varenicline, a nicotinic receptor partial agonist that stimulates dopamine release, thought to relieve cravings (U.S. Food & Drug Administration, 2020).

Immunizations

Influenza Vaccine

Influenza can cause substantial morbidity and mortality, especially during the late fall and winter. The numbers of annual deaths related to influenza vary depending on the virus type and subtype, ranging from a few thousand to over 60,000 deaths per year. Because influenza viruses mutate from year to year, each vaccine contains three to four flu strains and is modified yearly. The CDC Advisory Committee on Immunization Practices (ACIP) updates its recommendations for vaccination annually, and these should be reviewed each year by health care providers (CDC, 2019).

Annual vaccination is recommended for all people aged 6 months and older, especially the following groups (CDC, 2019):

- Adults with chronic pulmonary conditions and chronic medical conditions
- Adults who are immunosuppressed or morbidly obese
- Adults 50 years of age or older
- Women who are or will be pregnant during influenza season
- Residents of nursing homes and chronic care facilities
- Native Americans and Alaska Natives
- Health care personnel
- Household contacts and caregivers of children 5 years of age or younger (especially infants aged 6 months or younger) and of adults 50 years of age or older with medical conditions placing them at higher risk for complications of influenza

Pneumococcal Vaccine

Pneumococcus (*Streptococcus pneumoniae*) is the most common cause of bacteremia (bloodstream infections), pneumonia, meningitis, and middle ear infections in young children. The CDC estimates that 150,000 hospitalizations from pneumococcal pneumonia occur annually in the United States. Pneumococci account for up to 30% of adult community-acquired pneumonia. Bacteremia occurs in up to 25% to 30% of patients with pneumococcal pneumonia. An estimated 5,000 cases of pneumococcal bacteremia (without pneumonia) occur each year. Pneumococci cause over 50% of all cases of bacterial meningitis in the United States (CDC, 2020c).

Two vaccines used in the United States help protect against pneumococcal disease (CDC, 2020d):

- Pneumococcal conjugate vaccine (PCV13)
- Pneumococcal polysaccharide vaccine (PPSV23)

The CDC recommends PCV13 for:

- all children younger than 2 years.
- people 2 years or older with certain medical conditions.
- some adults 65 and older; these individuals should discuss this with their health care providers.

The CDC recommends PPSV23 for:

- all adults 65 years or older.
- people aged 2 through 64 with certain medical conditions.
- adults aged 19 through 64 who smoke cigarettes.

Pertussis Vaccine

Pertussis (*Bordetella pertussis*) is an acute infectious respiratory illness that remains endemic in the United States despite routine childhood vaccination. Immunity to pertussis wanes approximately 5 to 10 years after completion of the childhood vaccination series, leaving adolescents and adults susceptible to it. Pertussis poses the highest risk to infants and young children. Therefore, to protect them, the CDC recommends (CDC, 2020b):

- Adults 19 years and older who have not received a dose of Tdap (*Tetanus, diphtheria, and acellular pertussis*) should get one as soon as possible, to protect themselves and infants. The Tdap booster can replace one of the 10-year Td booster vaccines.

- For adolescents 11 through 18 years of age, Tdap is routinely recommended as a single dose with preferred administration at 11 through 12 years of age.
- Infants should receive the five-dose series of DTaP (pediatric diphtheria, tetanus, and acellular pertussis) vaccine.
- Pregnant women should receive a dose of Tdap during each pregnancy, preferably during weeks 27 through 36. The mother's antibodies will transfer to the fetus providing protection to the newborn before the infant can receive the DTaP vaccine themselves.

COVID-19 Vaccines

Multiple COVID-19 vaccines became available toward the end of 2020, each with their own guidelines. Whichever vaccine manufacturer a patient receives, they should follow through with the associated guidelines. For example, one vaccine manufacturer (Pfizer) recommends two doses of the vaccine administered 3 weeks apart for people over 16 years of age, and another (Moderna) recommends two doses administered 4 weeks apart for individuals over 18 years of age. Yet another, (Johnson & Johnson) has a single dose vaccination. At the time of printing, vaccine development was underway with new information and guidelines coming out regularly for younger age groups, booster vaccinations, side effects and new manufacturers. The CDC website is a good resource for updated information.

BIBLIOGRAPHY

CITATIONS

Agnelli, G., & Becattini, C. (2010). Acute pulmonary embolism. *The New England Journal of Medicine*, *363*, 266–274.

Barker, A. (2002). Bronchiectasis. *The New England Journal of Medicine*, *346*(18), 1383–1393.

Bohadana, A., Izbicki, G., & Kraman, S. S. (2014). Fundamentals of lung auscultation. *The New England Journal of Medicine*, *370*(8), 744–751.

Centers for Disease Control and Prevention (CDC). (2019). Prevention and control of seasonal influenza with vaccines: Recommendations of the advisory committee on immunization practices—United States, 2019–20 influenza season. https://www.cdc.gov/mmwr/volumes/68/rr/rr6803a1.htm?s_cid=rr6803a1_w#influenzavaccinecompositionandavailableproducts

Centers for Disease Control and Prevention (CDC). (2020a). Fact sheet: Smoking and tobacco use: Health effects of cigarette smoking. http://www.cdc.gov/tobacco/data_statistics/fact_sheets/health_effects/effects_cig_smoking/index.htm

Centers for Disease Control and Prevention (CDC). (2020b). Pertussis: Summary of vaccine recommendations: For healthcare professionals. https://www.cdc.gov/vaccines/vpd/pertussis/recs-summary.html

Centers for Disease Control and Prevention (CDC). (2020c). Pneumococcal disease. Clinical features. https://www.cdc.gov/pneumococcal/clinicians/clinical-features.html

Centers for Disease Control and Prevention (CDC). (2020d). Pneumococcal disease. Pneumococcal vaccination. https://www.cdc.gov/pneumococcal/vaccination.html

Centers for Disease Control and Prevention (CDC). (2020e). Smoking and tobacco use. Current cigarette smoking among adults in the United States. Retrieved August 6, 2020, from https://www.cdc.gov/tobacco/data_statistics/fact_sheets/adult_data/cig_smoking/index.htm

Centers for Disease Control and Prevention (CDC). (2020f). Smoking and tobacco use. Youth and tobacco use. https://www.cdc.gov/tobacco/data_statistics/fact_sheets/youth_data/tobacco_use/index.htm

Centers for Disease Control and Prevention (CDC). (2020g). What you need to know about quitting smoking: Advice from the surgeon general. https://www.hhs.gov/sites/default/files/2020-cessation-sgr-consumer-guide.pdf

Escalante, P. (2009). In the clinic: Tuberculosis. *Annals of Internal Medicine*, *150*, ITC61–614.

Global Initiative for Chronic Obstructive Lung Disease. (2020). Global strategy for the diagnosis, management, and prevention of chronic obstructive pulmonary disease. Retrieved August 6, 2020, from https://goldcopd.org/wp-content/uploads/2019/12/GOLD-2020-FINAL-ver1.2-03Dec19_WMV.pdf

Irwin, R. S., & Madison, J. M. (2000). The diagnosis and treatment of cough. *The New England Journal of Medicine, 3432*(3), 1715–1721.

Kerlin, M. P. (2010). In the clinic: Acute pulmonary embolism. *The New England Journal of Medicine, 363*, 26.

Kerlin, M. P. (2014). In the clinic. Asthma. *Annals of Internal Medicine, 160*(5), ITC3-1.

Kouritas, V. K., Papagiannoupoulos, K., Lazaridis, G., et al. (2015). Pneumomediastinum. *Journal of Thoracic Disease, 7*(Suppl 1), S44–S49.

Littner, M. (2011). In the clinic: Chronic obstructive pulmonary disease. *Annals of Internal Medicine, 154*(7), ITC4-1–ITC4-15.

McGee, S. (2018). *Evidence-based physical diagnosis* (4th ed.). Saunders.

Metlay, J. P., Kapoor, W. N., & Fine, M. J. (1997). Does this patient have community-acquired pneumonia? Diagnosing pneumonia by history and physical examination. *JAMA, 278*(17), 1440–1445.

Moore, D. J. (2019). Sudden onset of shortness of breath: Consider pulmonary embolism. *American Nurse Today, 14*(3), 20–23.

Neiderman, M. (2009). In the clinic: Community-acquired pneumonia. *Annals of Internal Medicine, 151*, ITC4-1–ITC4-16.

Neiwoehner, D. R. (2010). Outpatient management of severe COPD. *The New England Journal of Medicine, 362*(15), 1407–1416.

Norcross, J. C., & Prochaska, J. O. (2002). Using the stages of change. *Harvard Mental Health Letter, 18*(11), 5–7.

Panettieri, R. A. (2007). In the clinic. Asthma. *Annals of Internal Medicine, 146*(11), ITC6-1–ITC6-14.

Parshall, M. B., Schwartzstein, R. M., Adams, L., Banzett, R. B., Manning, H. L., Bourbeau, J., Calverley, P. M., Gift, A. G., Harver, A., Lareau, S. C., Mahler, D. A., Meek, P. M., & O'Donnell, D. E.; American Thoracic Society Committee on Dyspnea. (2012). An official American Thoracic Society statement: Update on the mechanisms, assessment, and management of dyspnea. *American Journal of Respiratory and Critical Care Medicine, 185*(4), 435–452.

U.S. Food and Drug Administration. (2020). Want to quit smoking? FDA-approved products can help. Retrieved August 5, 2020, from https://www.fda.gov/consumers/consumer-updates/want-quit-smoking-fda-approved-products-can-help

U.S. Preventive Services Task Force. (2020). Tobacco smoking cessation in adults, including pregnant persons: Interventions. Draft evidence review. Retrieved June 02, 2020, from https://www.uspreventiveservicestaskforce.org/uspstf/document/draft-evidence-review/tobacco-smoking-cessation-in-adults-including-pregnant-women-interventions

Wenzel, R. P., & Fowler, A. A. (2006). Acute bronchitis. *The New England Journal of Medicine, 355*(20), 2125–2130.

ADDITIONAL REFERENCES

Centers for Disease Control and Prevention (CDC). (2019, November 21). Vaccines and preventable diseases: Pneumococcal vaccination. http://www.cdc.gov/vaccines/vpd-vac/pneumo/default.htm

Kendrick, K. R., Baxi, S. C., & Smith, R. M. (2000). Usefulness of the modified 0–10 Borg scale in assessing the degree of dyspnea in patients with COPD and asthma. *Journal of Emergency Nursing, 26*(3), 216–222.

14 THE CARDIOVASCULAR SYSTEM

KEY TERMS

amplitude	murmur	regurgitation
bruit	palpitations	stroke volume
cardiac cycle	point of maximal impulse	systole
diastole	precordium	tamponade
electrocardiogram	pulse contour	thrill
hypertension		

Learning Objectives

The student will:

1. Describe the structure and functions of the heart and great vessels.
2. Describe the two phases of the cardiac cycle.
3. Describe the normal heart sounds and their origin.
4. Identify the landmarks and key auscultation sites of the precordium.
5. Describe the electrical conduction system of the heart.
6. Explain the normal electrocardiogram waveform pattern.
7. Obtain an accurate history of the cardiovascular system.
8. Appropriately prepare and position the patient for the cardiovascular examination.
9. Describe the equipment necessary to perform a cardiovascular examination.
10. Examine the carotid arteries and jugular veins of the neck.
11. Inspect, palpate, and auscultate the precordium to evaluate the cardiovascular system.
12. Describe extra heart sounds and their origin.
13. Discuss risk reduction and health promotion strategies to reduce coronary heart disease.
14. Discuss risk factors for coronary heart disease.

The cardiovascular system is made up of the heart and blood vessels. The main functions of this system are delivering oxygen and nutrients to the cells of the body, removing waste products, and maintaining perfusion to the organs and tissues. The heart is the pump that drives circulation of the blood and the blood vessels are the pathways to and from the tissues. To assess a patient's cardiovascular health, the nurse gathers a thorough focused health history and uses this information to perform an appropriate physical examination of the patient's heart and blood vessels. This chapter will discuss the assessment of the heart and great vessels, aorta, pulmonary artery, venae cavae, and pulmonary veins. Chapter 15, "The Peripheral Vascular System and Lymphatic System," covers the assessment of the peripheral blood vessels and lymphatic system.

ANATOMY AND PHYSIOLOGY

In order to perform an accurate assessment of the cardiovascular system, the nurse must have a thorough understanding of the anatomy and physiology of the system, including the heart muscle, chambers, valves, great vessels, and conduction system; peripheral arteries and veins; the capillaries; and the lymph system.

Location of the Heart and Great Vessels

The heart is a hollow muscular organ a little larger than the patient's fist. It lies in the pericardial cavity in the mediastinum under the sternum and between the second and fifth intercostal spaces. About two thirds of the heart lies to the left of the midline of the sternum.

The area of the exterior chest that overlays the heart and great vessels is called the **precordium**. It is helpful to visualize the underlying structures of the heart as you examine the precordium. Note that the heart is rotated so that the *right ventricle* occupies most of the anterior cardiac surface (Fig. 14-1). This chamber and the pulmonary artery form a wedge-shaped structure behind and to the left of the sternum, outlined in Figure 14-1 in black.

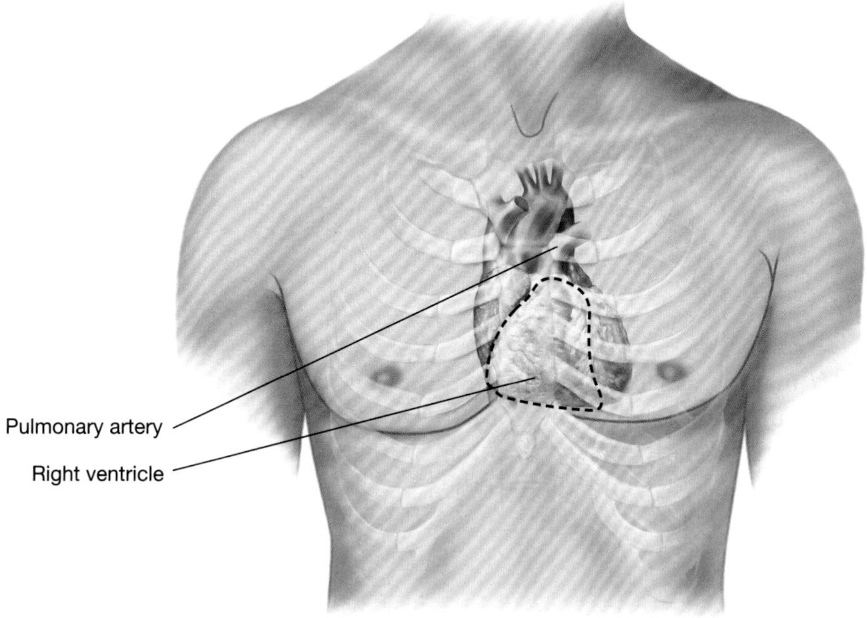

FIGURE 14-1 Location of the pulmonary artery and right ventricle.

The inferior border of the right ventricle lies at the junction of the sternum and the xiphoid process. The right ventricle narrows as it rises to meet the pulmonary artery just below the sternal angle. This is called the "*base of the heart*" and is located at the right and left second intercostal spaces next to the sternum.

The *left ventricle* lies behind the right ventricle and to the left, outlined in black in Figure 14-2. It forms the left margin of the heart. Its tapered inferior tip is often termed the *cardiac "apex."* It is clinically important because it produces the apical impulse, identified during palpation of the precordium as the **point of maximal impulse**, or PMI. This impulse locates the left border of the heart and is normally found in the fifth intercostal space 7 to 9 cm lateral to the midsternal line, at or just medial to the left midclavicular line. It is common to not be able to feel the PMI in a healthy patient with a normal heart.

The apical impulse is easily palpated in children and slender adults, but as the anteroposterior chest diameter increases, it becomes more difficult to feel. Obesity or a thick chest wall also makes palpation of the apical impulse difficult (McGee, 2018).

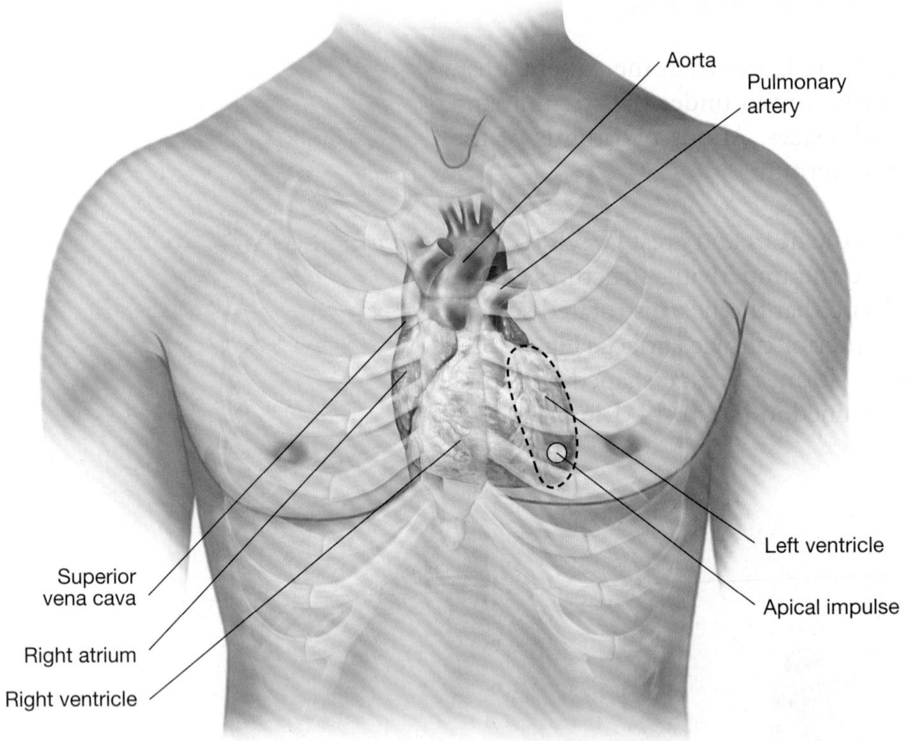

FIGURE 14-2 Structures of the heart in relation to the left ventricle.

In supine patients, the *diameter of the PMI* may be as large as a quarter, approximately 1 to 2.5 cm. A PMI greater than 2.5 cm is evidence of left ventricular hypertrophy (LVH), or enlargement. Similarly, *displacement of the PMI* lateral to the midclavicular line or greater than 10 cm lateral to the midsternal line also suggests LVH, or enlargement.

Note that in some patients, the most prominent precordial impulse may not be at the apex of the left ventricle. For example, in patients with chronic obstructive pulmonary disease, the most prominent palpable impulse or PMI may be in the xiphoid or epigastric area as a result of *right ventricular hypertrophy*.

Above the heart lie the *great vessels.* The *pulmonary artery*, which carries unoxygenated blood to the lungs, bifurcates quickly into its left and right branches. The *aorta* curves upward from the left ventricle to the level of the sternal angle, where it arches backward to the left and then downward. On the medial border, the *superior* and *inferior venae cavae* channel venous blood from the upper and lower portions of the body, respectively, into the right atrium.

The Heart Wall

The wall of the heart is composed of three layers. The *pericardium*, the outermost layer, is composed of two tough fibrous membranes that enclose and protect the heart. A few milliliters of serous fluid between the membranes provide lubrication for smooth movement of the heart. The *myocardium* is the heart muscle that does the pumping. The *endocardium* is a thin, smooth layer of endothelial tissue that lines the inner surface of the chambers and valves of the heart.

Cardiac Chambers, Valves, and Circulation

Circulation through the heart is shown in Figure 14-3, which illustrates the cardiac chambers, valves, and direction of blood flow. Blood from the body's organs and tissues returns to the heart via the superior and inferior venae cavae; empties into the right atrium; and travels through the tricuspid valve into the right ventricle, which pumps it through the pulmonary valve into the pulmonary artery. After passage through the lungs, the blood returns to the left atrium through the pulmonary veins and passes through the mitral valve into the left ventricle, where it is pumped through the aortic valve into the aorta for distribution of oxygenated blood throughout the body. Because of their positions, the *tricuspid* and *mitral valves* are often called *atrioventricular valves.* The *aortic* and *pulmonic valves* are called *semilunar valves* because each of their leaflets is shaped like a half moon. Although Figure 14-3 shows all the valves in an open position, they do not open simultaneously in the living heart.

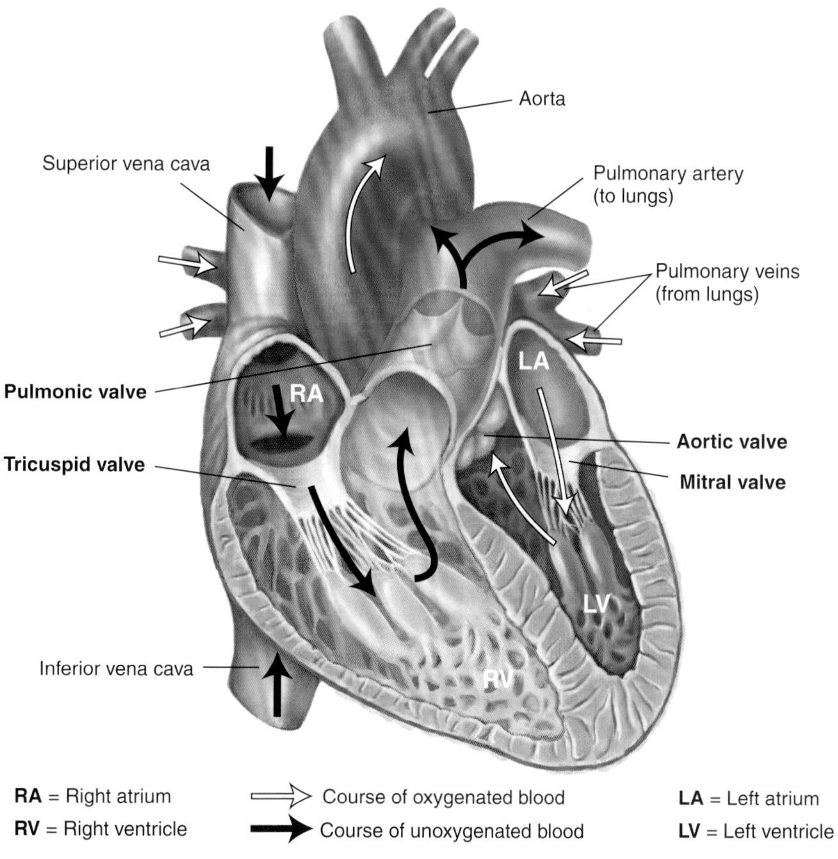

FIGURE 14-3 The cardiac chambers and valves and direction of blood flow.

As the heart valves close, the heart sounds arise from vibrations emanating from the leaflets, the adjacent cardiac structures, and the flow of blood. Carefully study the positions and movements of the valves in relation to events in the cardiac cycle in order to understand the heart sounds.

The Cardiac Cycle

Ventricular Pressures

The heart serves as a pump that generates varying pressures within its chambers as they contract and relax. **Systole** is the period of ventricular contraction. In Figure 14-4, pressure in the left ventricle rises from less than 5 mm Hg in its resting state to a normal peak of 120 mm Hg. After the ventricle ejects much of its blood into the aorta, the pressure levels off and starts to fall. **Diastole** is the period of ventricular relaxation. Ventricular pressure falls to below 5 mm Hg, and blood flows from atrium to ventricle. Late in diastole, ventricular pressure rises slightly during inflow of blood from atrial contraction. Systole and diastole make up the **cardiac cycle**.

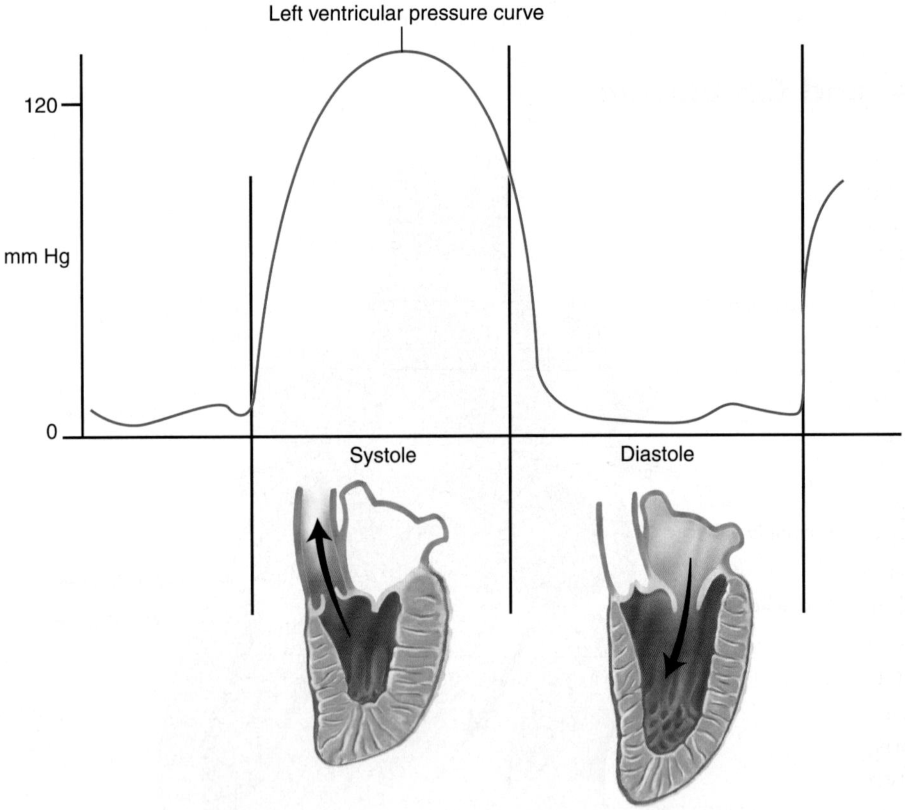

FIGURE 14-4 Ventricular pressure during systole and diastole.

Valve Openings and Closings

During *systole*, the aortic valve is open, allowing ejection of blood from the left ventricle into the aorta. The mitral valve is closed, preventing blood from **regurgitation** (leakage) back into the left atrium. In contrast, during *diastole*, the aortic valve is closed, preventing regurgitation of blood from the aorta back into the left ventricle. The mitral valve is open, allowing blood to flow from the left atrium into the relaxed left ventricle.

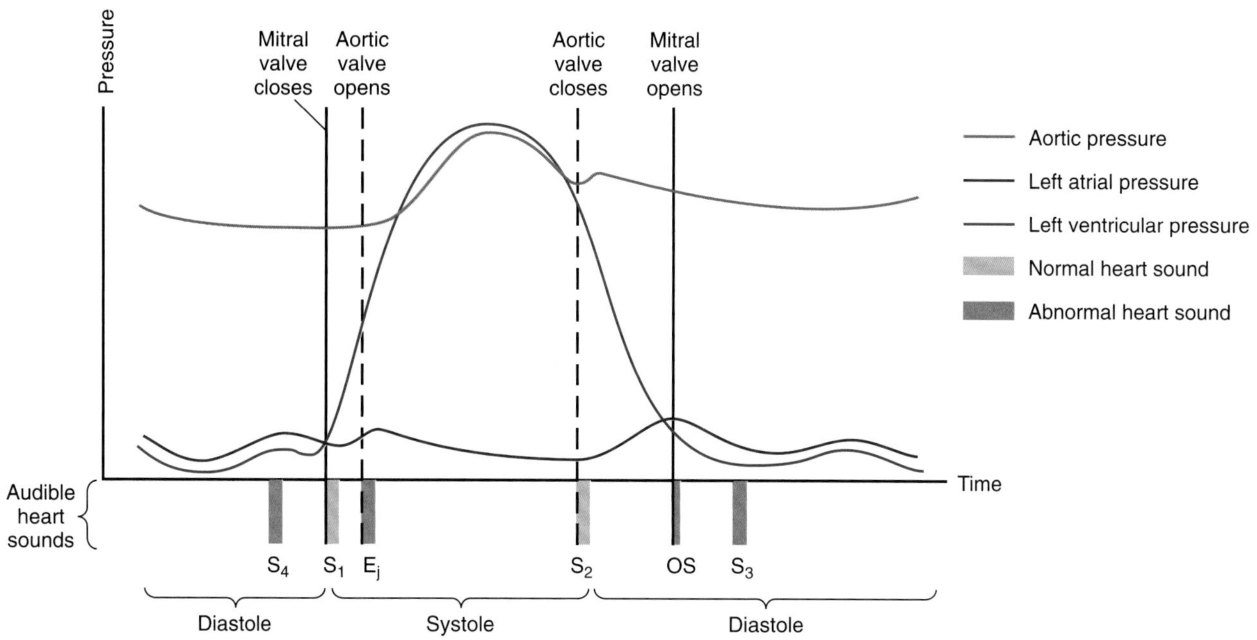

FIGURE 14-5 The cardiac cycle.

Understanding the interrelationships of the *pressures* in the left atrium, left ventricle, and aorta together with the position and movement of the valves is fundamental to understanding heart sounds. Trace these changing pressures and sounds through one cardiac cycle (Fig. 14-5). During auscultation, the first and second heart sounds define the duration of *systole* and *diastole*.

During *diastole*, pressure in the blood-filled left atrium slightly exceeds that in the relaxed left ventricle, and blood flows from left atrium to left ventricle across the open mitral valve. Just before the onset of ventricular systole, atrial contraction (*the "atrial kick"*) empties the atrium and produces a slight pressure rise in both chambers (Fig. 14-6).

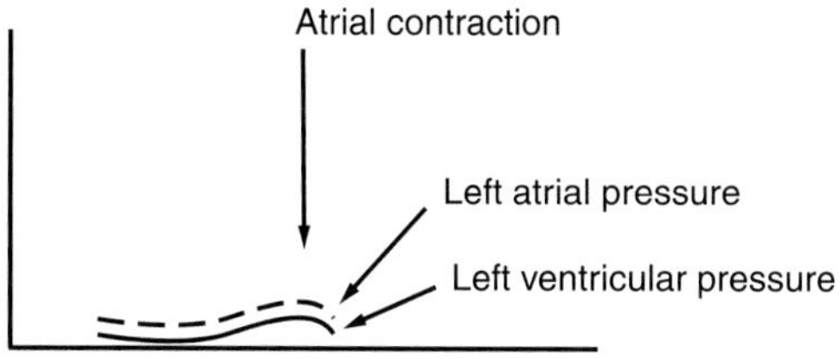

FIGURE 14-6 Atrial contraction slightly raises atrial and ventricular pressure.

During *systole*, the left ventricle starts to contract and ventricular pressure rapidly exceeds left atrial pressure, shutting the mitral valve (Fig. 14-7). *Closure of the mitral valve produces the first heart sound, S_1.*

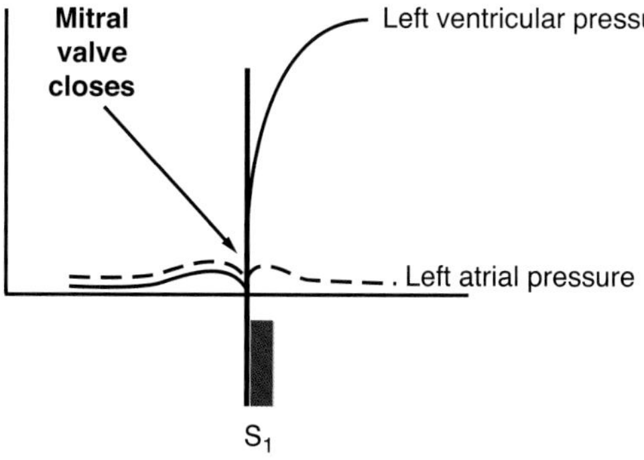

FIGURE 14-7 The mitral valve closes, causing S_1.

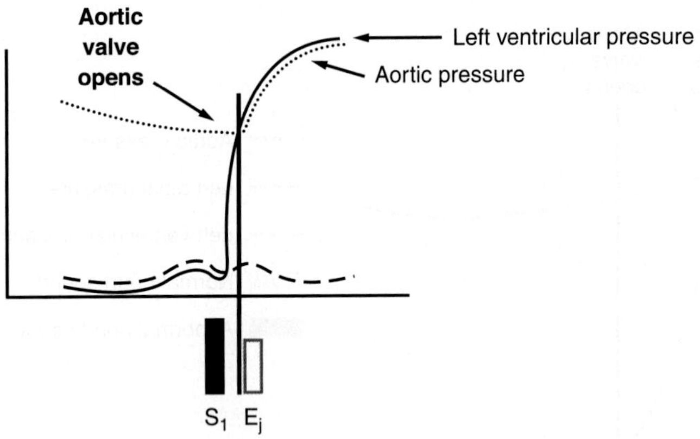

FIGURE 14-8 Rising left ventricular pressure causes the aortic valve to close.

As left ventricular pressure continues to rise, it quickly exceeds the pressure in the aorta and forces the aortic valve open (Fig. 14-8). *Normally, maximal left ventricular pressure corresponds to systolic blood pressure.*

In some pathologic conditions, an early systolic ejection sound (E_j) accompanies the opening of the aortic valve.

After the left ventricle ejects most of its blood, ventricular pressure begins to fall. When left ventricular pressure drops below aortic pressure, the aortic valve shuts (Fig. 14-9). *Aortic valve closure produces the second heart sound, S_2,* and another diastole begins.

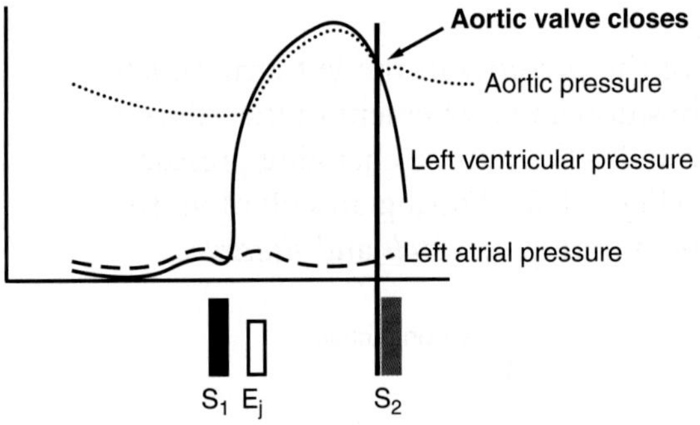

FIGURE 14-9 The aortic valve closes, producing S_2.

In *diastole*, left ventricular pressure continues to drop and falls below left atrial pressure. The mitral valve silently opens (Fig. 14-10).

An opening snap (OS) may be heard if valve leaflet motion is restricted, as in mitral stenosis.

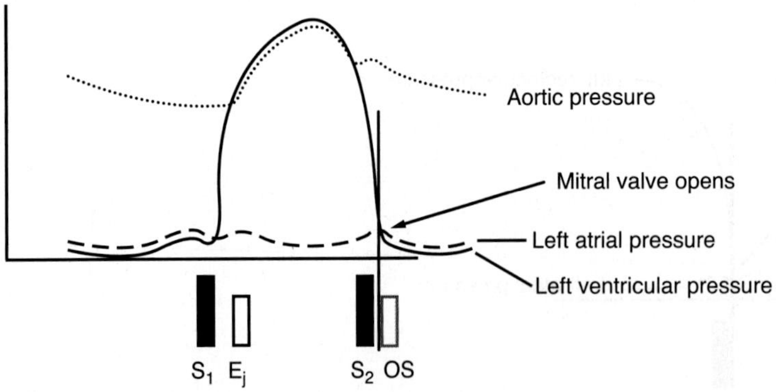

FIGURE 14-10 The mitral valve opens when left ventricular pressure drops below left atrial pressure.

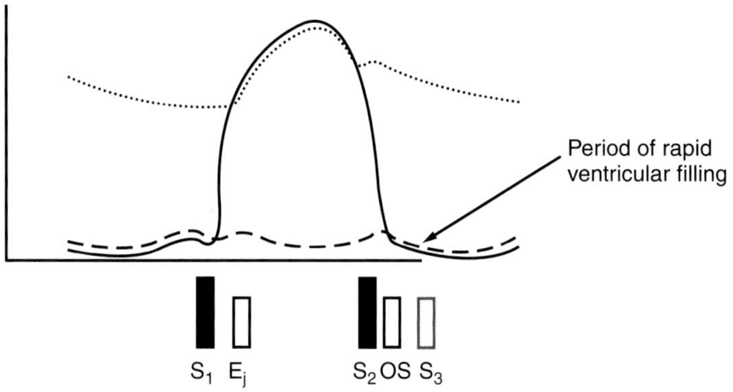

FIGURE 14-11 Blood flows early in diastole from the left atrium to the left ventricle.

After the mitral valve opens, there is a period of early rapid ventricular filling as blood flows early in diastole from the left atrium to the left ventricle (Fig. 14-11). In children and young adults, a third heart sound, S_3, may be heard and is caused by the rapid deceleration of the column of blood against the ventricular wall. In older adults, an S_3, sometimes termed "an S_3 gallop," usually indicates a pathologic change in ventricular compliance.

Finally, although not often heard in healthy adults, a fourth heart sound, S_4, marks atrial contraction (Fig. 14-12). It immediately precedes S_1 of the next beat and also reflects a pathologic change in ventricular compliance.

Compliance is the ease with which the heart muscle relaxes as it fills with blood. Poor compliance produces a stiff ventricle with reduced ability to expand as it receives blood.

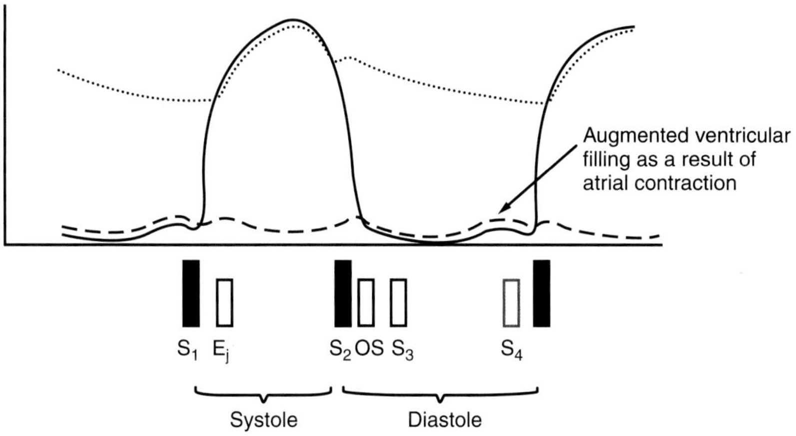

FIGURE 14-12 A fourth heart sound, not usually heard in healthy adults, indicates a pathologic change in ventricular compliance.

The Splitting of Heart Sounds

Split S_2

While these events are occurring on the left side of the heart, similar changes are occurring on the right involving the right atrium, right ventricle, tricuspid valve, pulmonic valve, and pulmonary artery. However, right ventricular and pulmonary arterial pressures are significantly lower than corresponding pressures on the left side.

Furthermore, right-sided events usually occur slightly later than those on the left. Instead of a single heart sound, two discernible sounds may be heard, the first from left-sided aortic valve closure, or A_2, and the second from right-sided closure of the pulmonic valve, or P_2.

S_2, and its two components, A_2 and P_2, are caused by the closure of the aortic and pulmonary valves, respectively. During inspiration, the filling time of the right heart increases, thereby increasing the *stroke volume* and lengthening the duration of right ventricle emptying compared to the left ventricle. This delays closure of the pulmonic valve, P_2, *splitting* S_2 into its two audible components (Fig. 14-13) (O'Gara & Loscalzo, 2018).

Stroke volume is the amount of blood ejected by the ventricle with each heartbeat.

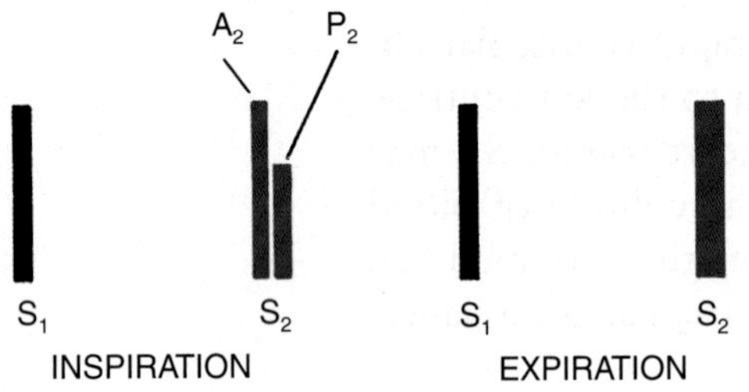

FIGURE 14-13 Split S_2.

During expiration, these two components fuse into a single sound, S_2.

The split S_2 may be difficult to hear in obese individuals or people with increased anteroposterior diameter chest walls.

Vein walls contain less muscle so they are more distensible than arteries and can store more blood. During inspiration, the pulmonary vascular bed has more capacity, which contributes to the increased filling time and delays closure of P_2.

Of the two components of the S_2, A_2 is normally louder, reflecting the high pressure in the aorta. It is heard throughout the precordium. P_2, in contrast, is relatively soft, reflecting the lower pressure in the pulmonary artery. It is heard best in its own area—the second and third left intercostal spaces close to the sternum. It is here that you should search for splitting of the S_2.

Split S_1

S_1 also has two components, an earlier mitral and a later tricuspid sound. The mitral sound, its principal component, is much louder, again reflecting the high pressures on the left side of the heart. It can be heard throughout the precordium and is loudest at the cardiac apex. The softer tricuspid component is heard best at the lower left sternal border, and it is here that you may hear a split S_1. The earlier, louder mitral component may mask the tricuspid sound, however, and splitting is not always detectable. Splitting of S_1 does not vary with respiration.

Heart Murmurs

Heart **murmurs** (Fig. 14-14) are distinguishable from heart sounds by their longer duration. They are attributed to turbulent blood flow and may be "innocent," as with flow murmurs of young adults, or diagnostic of valvular or congenital heart disease. A *stenotic valve* has an abnormally narrowed valvular orifice that obstructs blood flow, as in *aortic stenosis*, and causes a characteristic murmur. A valve that fails to fully close, as in *aortic regurgitation* or *insufficiency*, allows blood to leak backward in a retrograde direction and produces a *regurgitant* murmur.

"Stenosis" means narrowing; in this case, the aortic valve outlet is narrowed, producing turbulent blood flow.

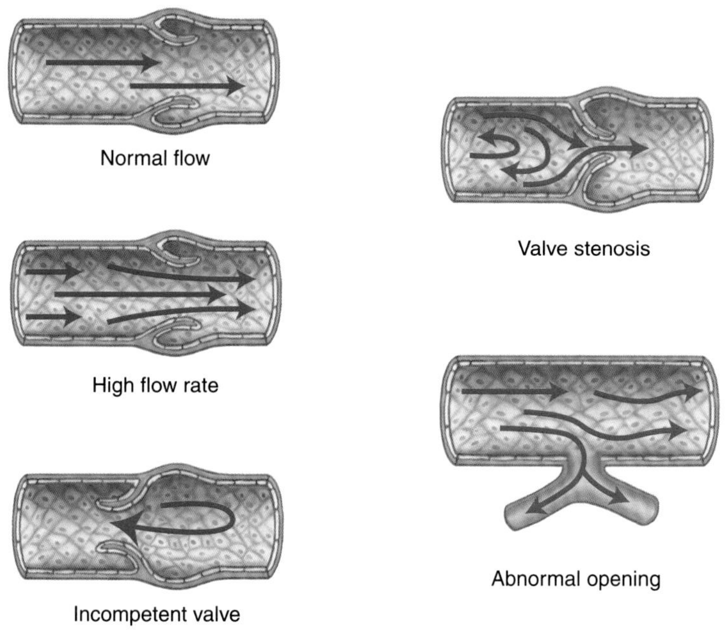

FIGURE 14-14 The mechanics of heart murmurs.

In the section on the cardiovascular physical examination, the characteristics of murmurs, including intensity, pitch, duration, and direction of radiation, will be discussed.

Relation of Auscultatory Findings to the Chest Wall

The locations on the chest wall where heart sounds and murmurs are heard help identify the valves or chambers where they originate. The sounds produced by the heart valves travel with the flow of blood. As you review the locations in Figure 14-15, picture the direction of blood flow between the upper and lower chambers and through the pulmonary artery and aorta. Sounds and murmurs arising from the mitral valve are usually heard best at and around the cardiac apex. Those originating in the tricuspid valve are heard best at or near the lower left sternal border. Murmurs arising from the pulmonic valve are usually heard best in the second and third left intercostal spaces close to the sternum but at times may also be heard at higher or lower levels. Murmurs originating in the aortic valve may be heard anywhere from the right second intercostal space to the apex. *These areas overlap*, as illustrated in Figure 14-15, and you will need

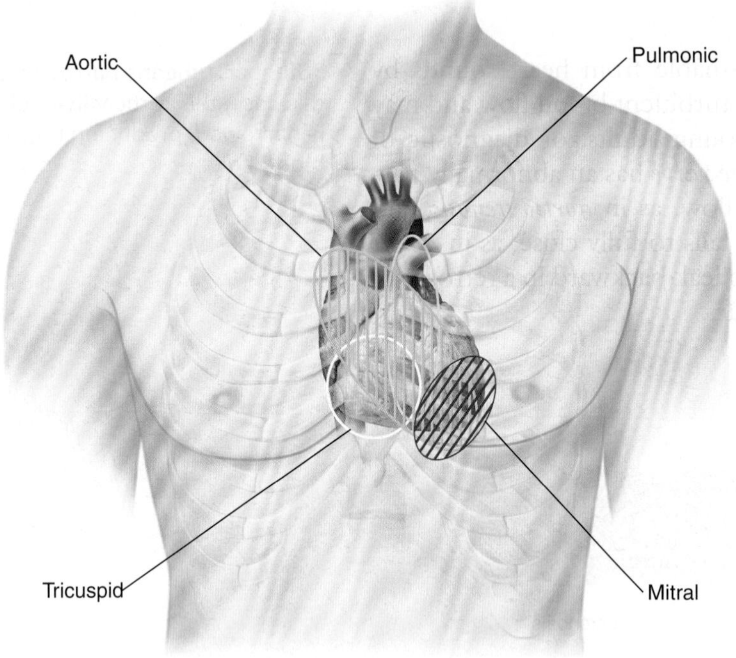

FIGURE 14-15 Locations of the origins of heart sounds.

to correlate auscultatory findings with other cardiac examination findings to identify sounds and murmurs accurately.

The Conduction System

An electrical conduction system stimulates and coordinates the contraction of cardiac muscle. Each electrical impulse is initiated in the *sinus node*, a group of specialized cardiac cells located in the right atrium near the junction of the vena cava. The sinus node acts as the cardiac pacemaker and automatically discharges an impulse about 60 to 100 times a minute. This impulse travels through both atria to the *atrioventricular node*, a specialized group of cells located low in the atrial septum. Here the impulse is delayed before passing down the bundle of His and its branches to the ventricular myocardium. Muscular contraction follows: first the atria, then the ventricles. The normal conduction pathway is diagrammed in Figure 14-16 in simplified form. The **electrocardiogram**, or ECG, records these events. Contraction of cardiac smooth muscle produces electrical activity, resulting in a series of waves on the ECG. The ECG consists of *six limb leads* in the *frontal plane* and *six chest or precordial leads* in the *transverse plane*.

- Electrical vectors (signals) approaching a lead cause a *positive, or upward, deflection.*
- Electrical vectors moving away from the lead cause a *negative, or downward, deflection.*
- When positive and negative vectors balance, they are *isoelectric*, appearing as a straight line.

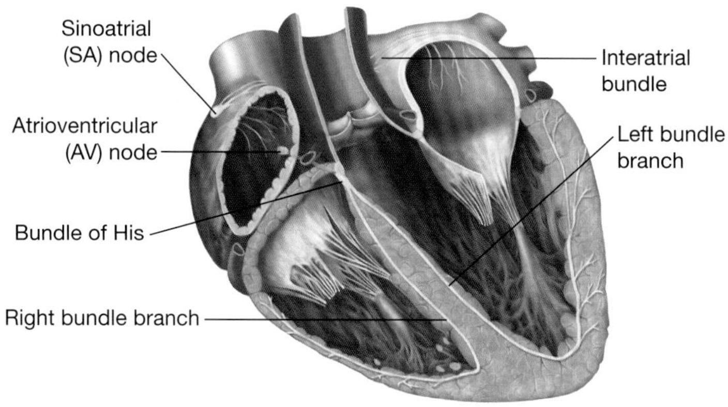

FIGURE 14-16 Electrical impulses travel through the heart's conduction system.

The components of the *normal ECG* and their duration are briefly summarized here and illustrated in Figure 14-17, but you will need further instruction and practice to interpret recordings from patients. The term "normal sinus rhythm" (NSR) is used to describe normal ECG transmission.

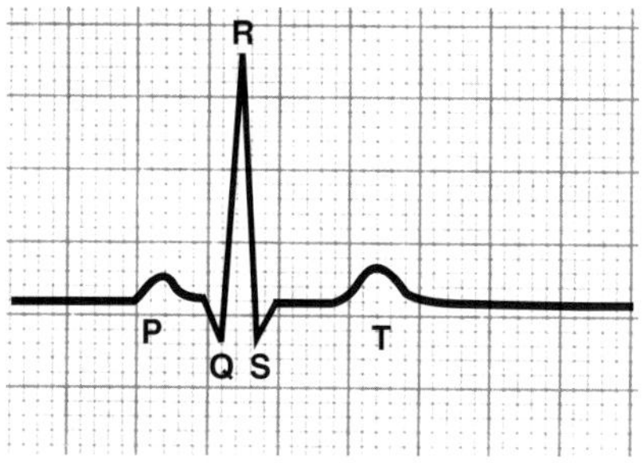

FIGURE 14-17 A normal electrocardiogram readout.

- The small *P wave* of atrial depolarization (duration up to 80 milliseconds; *PR interval* 120 to 200 milliseconds)
- The larger *QRS complex* of ventricular depolarization (up to 100 milliseconds), consisting of one or more of the following:
  - The *Q wave*, a downward deflection from septal depolarization
  - The *R wave*, an upward deflection from ventricular depolarization
  - The *S wave*, a downward deflection following an R wave
- A *T wave* of ventricular repolarization, or recovery (duration relates to QRS)

The electrical impulse slightly precedes the myocardial contraction that it stimulates. The relation of electrocardiographic waves to the cardiac cycle is shown in Figure 14-18.

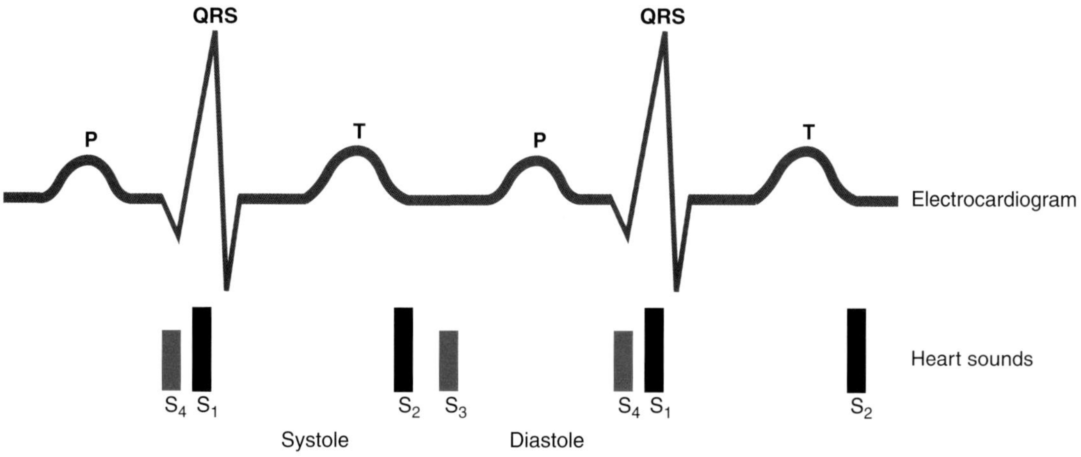

FIGURE 14-18 The relation of electrocardiographic waves to the cardiac cycle.

The Heart as a Pump

The left and right ventricles pump blood into the systemic and pulmonary arterial trees, respectively. *Cardiac output*, the volume of blood ejected from each ventricle over the course of 1 minute, is the product of *heart rate* and *stroke volume*. **Stroke volume** (the volume of blood ejected with each heartbeat) depends in turn on preload, myocardial contractility, and afterload.

- *Preload* refers to the load that stretches the cardiac muscle before contraction. The volume of blood in the right ventricle at the end of diastole then constitutes its preload for the next beat. Right ventricular preload is increased by increasing venous return to the right heart. Physiologic causes include inspiration and the increased volume of blood flow from exercising muscles. The increased blood volume in a dilated right ventricle of heart failure also increases preload. Causes of decreased right ventricular preload include exhalation, decreased left ventricular output, and pooling of blood in the capillary bed or the venous system.
- *Myocardial contractility* refers to the ability of the cardiac muscle, when given a load, to contract or shorten. Contractility increases when stimulated by the sympathetic nervous system and decreases when blood flow or oxygen delivery to the myocardium is impaired.
- *Afterload* refers to the degree of vascular resistance to ventricular contraction. Sources of resistance to left ventricular contraction include the tone in the walls of the aorta, the large arteries, and the peripheral vascular tree (primarily the small arteries and arterioles), as well as the volume of blood already in the aorta. Increased arterial blood pressure causes increased afterload.

Pathologic increases in preload and afterload, called *volume overload* and *pressure overload*, respectively, produce changes in ventricular function that may be clinically detectable. These changes include alterations in ventricular impulses, detectable by palpation, and in normal heart sounds. Pathologic heart sounds and murmurs may also develop.

The term *heart failure* is now preferred over "congestive heart failure" because not all patients have volume overload on initial presentation (Hunt et al., 2009).

Arterial Pulses and Blood Pressure

With each contraction, the left ventricle ejects a volume of blood into the aorta and on to the arterial tree. The ensuing pressure wave moves rapidly through the arterial system, where it is felt as the *arterial pulse*. Although the pressure wave travels quickly—many times faster than the blood itself—a palpable delay between ventricular contraction and peripheral pulses makes the pulses in the arms and legs unsuitable for timing events in the cardiac cycle.

Blood pressure in the arterial system varies during the cardiac cycle, peaking in systole and falling to its lowest trough in diastole (Fig. 14-19). These are the levels that are measured with the blood pressure cuff, or sphygmomanometer. The difference between systolic and diastolic pressures is known as the *pulse pressure*.

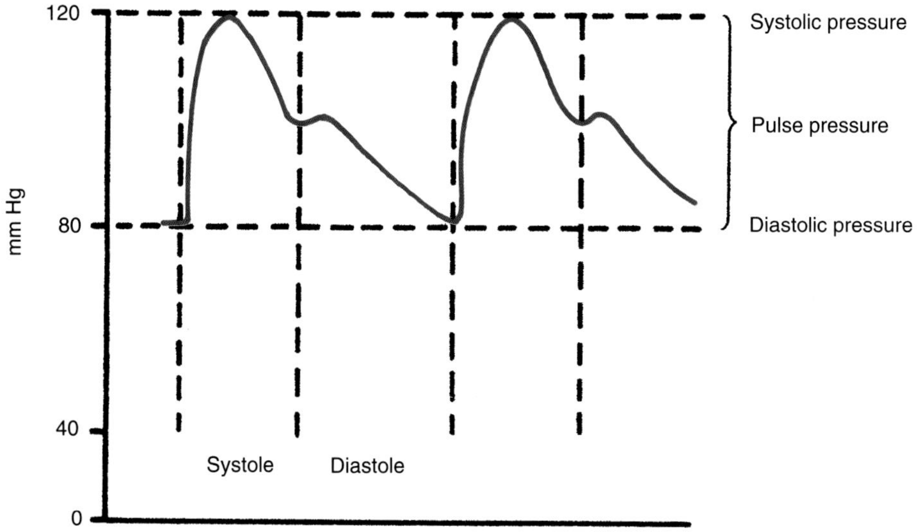

FIGURE 14-19 Blood pressure in the arterial system reaches its highest point during systole and its lowest during diastole.

Factors that influence arterial pressure are outlined in Box 14-1. Changes in any of these four factors alter systolic pressure, diastolic pressure, or both. Blood pressure levels fluctuate strikingly throughout any 24-hour period, varying with physical activity; emotional state; pain; noise; environmental temperature; use of coffee, tobacco, and other drugs; and even the time of day.

BOX 14-1 FACTORS INFLUENCING ARTERIAL PRESSURE

- Left ventricular stroke volume
- Distensibility of the aorta and the large arteries
- Peripheral vascular resistance, particularly at the arteriolar level
- Volume of blood in the arterial system

CLINICAL TIP

Hypertension is abnormally high arterial blood pressure. The heart must work harder to eject blood into the arteries. There are many causes of hypertension including smoking, being overweight or obese, age, genetics, kidney disease, adrenal disorders, sleep apnea, stress, lack of physical activity, excess dietary salt, and excess alcohol consumption (more than one to two drinks per day).

Jugular Vein Undulations

The oscillations visible in the internal jugular veins, and often in the external jugular veins, reflect changing pressures within the right atrium. Careful observation reveals that the undulating pulsations of the internal jugular veins, and sometimes the externals, are composed of two quick peaks (a and v) and two troughs (x and y) (Fig. 14-20).

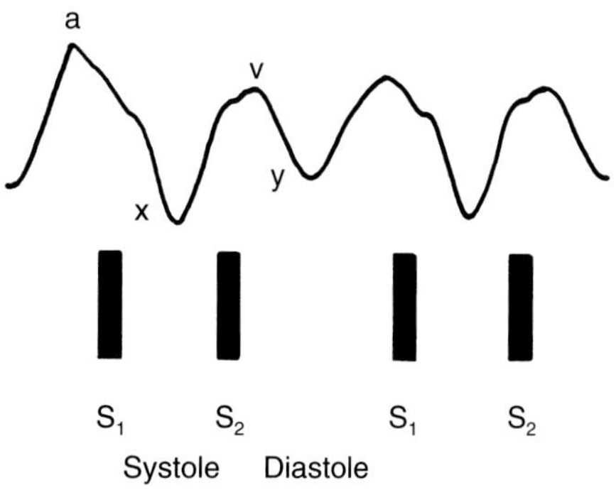

FIGURE 14-20 The jugular vein undulation pattern.

Jugular Venous Pressure

The jugular veins provide an important clinical index of right heart pressures and cardiac function. *Jugular venous pressure (JVP)* reflects right atrial pressure, which in turn equals *central venous pressure (CVP)* and right ventricular end-diastolic pressure. The JVP is best estimated from the *right internal jugular vein*, which has a more direct anatomic channel into the right atrium. Contrary to widely held views, a recent study has reaffirmed inspection of the *right external jugular vein* as a useful and accurate method for estimating CVP (Chua et al., 2013; Vinayak et al., 2006).

Pressure changes from right atrial filling, contraction, and emptying cause fluctuations in the JVP and its waveforms that are visible to the examiner. Careful observation of changes in these fluctuations yields clues about volume status, right and left ventricular function, patency of the tricuspid and pulmonary valves, pressures in the pericardium, and arrhythmias.

JVP falls with loss of blood and increases with right or left heart failure, pulmonary hypertension, tricuspid stenosis, and pericardial compression or **tamponade** (abnormal accumulation of fluid between the layers of the pericardium which places pressure on the heart; if severe it impairs cardiac pumping function).

The internal jugular veins (Fig. 14-21) lie under the sternocleidomastoid muscles in the neck and are not directly visible, so the nurse must learn to identify the *undulations* of the *internal jugular vein* or *external jugular vein* that are transmitted to the surface of the neck, making sure to carefully distinguish these venous undulations from the crisp pulsations of the carotid artery.

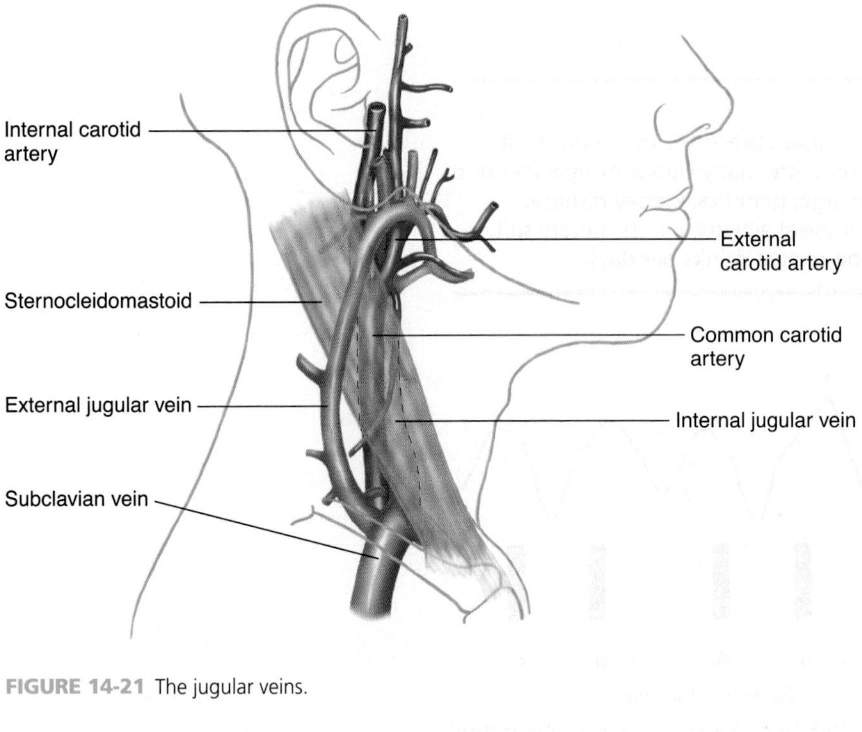

FIGURE 14-21 The jugular veins.

To estimate the level of the JVP, find the ***highest point of oscillation in the internal jugular vein*** or if necessary, the point above which the external jugular vein appears collapsed. The JVP is measured in vertical distance above the *sternal angle*, the bony ridge adjacent to the second rib where the manubrium joins the body of the sternum.

The visibility of the jugular veins varies by patient position due to gravity. Review Figure 14-22. In this patient, the pressure in the internal jugular vein is elevated.

- In *Position A*, the head of the bed is raised to 30 degrees, but the JVP cannot be measured because venous undulation is above the jaw and therefore not visible.
- In *Position B*, the head of the bed is raised to 60 degrees. The "top" of the internal jugular vein is now visible, so the vertical distance from the sternal angle or right atrium can be measured.
- In *Position C*, the patient is upright and the veins are barely discernible above the clavicle, making measurement impossible.

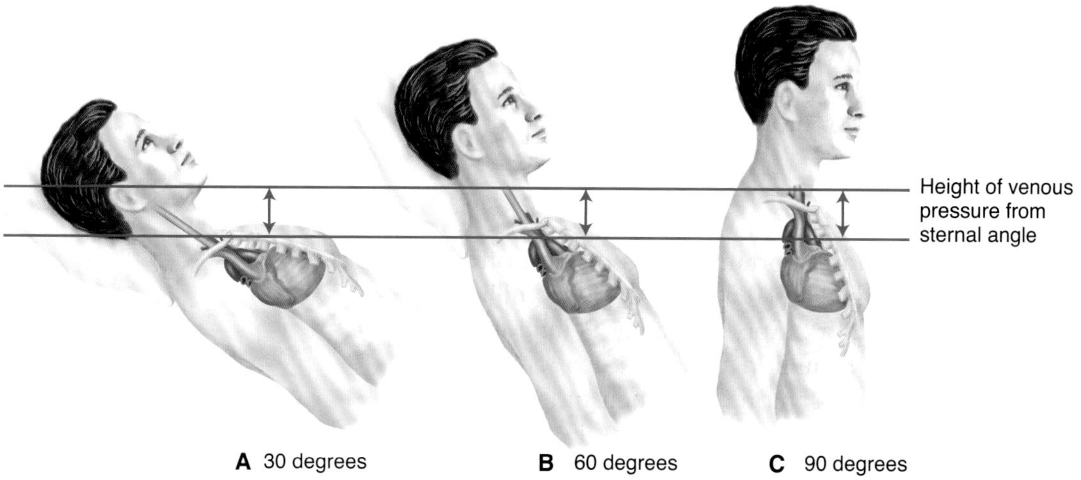

FIGURE 14-22 The height of venous pressure from the sternal angle facilitates measurement of the jugular venous pressure.

Note that the height of the venous pressure as measured from the sternal angle is the *same* in all three positions, but your ability to *measure* the height of the column of venous blood, or JVP, differs according to how you position the patient. The JVP measured at more than 4 cm above the sternal angle, or more than 9 cm above the right atrium, is considered abnormal. The techniques for measuring the JVP are fully described in the "Physical Examination" section.

THE HEALTH HISTORY

Common or concerning symptoms identified during the cardiovascular system history are listed in Box 14-2.

BOX 14-2 COMMON OR CONCERNING SYMPTOMS

- Chest pain or discomfort, pain or discomfort radiating to the neck, left shoulder or arm, and back
- Arrhythmias: skipped beats, palpitations
- Dyspnea
- Cough
- Edema
- Nocturia
- Fatigue
- Cyanosis or pallor

Assessing Cardiac Symptoms—Overview and Comparison with Baseline Activity Levels

Chest symptoms may be caused by cardiac, respiratory, gastrointestinal, or musculoskeletal etiologies. The nurse differentiates the cause of the symptoms through astute history questioning. This section focuses on chest symptoms from a cardiac standpoint. Cardiac symptoms reflect the heart's ability to function (i.e., to pump blood through the body and remove waste products).

Start the inquiry about the heart with broad open-ended questions. For each symptom, it is important to habitually ask the patient to quantify how it affects lifestyle or baseline level of activity. For example, in patients with chest pain, does the pain occur with walking? If yes, how far can you walk before the pain begins—50 ft, one block, or more?

Chest Pain

Chest pain is one of the most serious and important symptoms and often signals *coronary artery disease* (CAD), which currently affects 30.3 million people in the United States (CDC, 2021a). Approximately 9 million of these people have *angina pectoris*, and 8 million have had a *myocardial infarction*. CAD is the leading cause of death among both men and women, and it accounts for one in every four U.S. deaths (CDC, 2020a). Death rates are highest in African American men and women compared with other demographic groups (CDC, 2020a).

Classic pain on exertion, pressure, or discomfort in the chest, shoulder, back, neck, or arm in angina pectoris are seen in 50% of patients with acute myocardial infarction; atypical descriptors are also common, such as cramping, grinding, pricking; rarely, tooth or jaw pain is also reported (American Heart Association, n.d.).

CLINICAL TIP

Women experiencing myocardial infarctions frequently complain of different symptoms than men do. Rather than chest pain, they may experience upper body pain, for example, in one or both arms, the back, neck, jaw, or stomach. Dyspnea, cold sweats, nausea, indigestion, or lightheadedness may be the presenting symptom (American Heart Association, 2015, July 31).

Your initial questions should be broad: *Do you have any pain or discomfort in your chest?*

Acute coronary syndrome is used to refer to any of the clinical syndromes caused by acute myocardial ischemia, including unstable angina, non-ST elevation myocardial infarction, and ST elevation infarction.

Ask the patient to point to the pain and to describe its attributes.

Anterior chest pain, often tearing or ripping, radiating into the back or neck, may indicate *acute aortic dissection* (Creager & Loscalzo, 2018).

Move on to more specific questions, such as:

- Is the pain related to exertion?
- What kinds of activities bring on the pain?
- How intense is the pain on a scale of 1 to 10?
- Does it radiate into the neck, shoulder, or back or down your arm?
- Are there any associated symptoms such as shortness of breath, sweating, palpitations, or nausea?
- Does it ever wake you up at night?
- What do you do to make it better?

Palpitations

Palpitations involve an unpleasant awareness of the heartbeat. When describing palpitations, patients use terms such as skipping, racing, fluttering, pounding, or stopping of the heart.

Palpitations may result from an irregular heartbeat, from rapid acceleration or slowing of the heart, or from increased forcefulness of cardiac contraction. Such perceptions also depend on how patients respond to their own body sensations. Palpitations do not necessarily indicate heart disease. In contrast, the most serious dysrhythmias, such as ventricular tachycardia, often do not produce palpitations.

Ask the patient if they ever have palpitations. If the patient does not understand your question, reword it: Are you ever aware of your heartbeat? What is it like? How long did the palpitations last? Did they start and stop suddenly or come on gradually?

Shortness of Breath

Shortness of breath is a common patient concern and may represent *dyspnea*, *orthopnea*, or *paroxysmal nocturnal dyspnea*.

Dyspnea is an uncomfortable awareness of breathing that is inappropriate to a given level of exertion.

Ask do you ever have difficulty breathing or shortness of breath?

- When does it occur?
- What were you doing when you became short of breath?
- How many pillows do you use to sleep?

Orthopnea is dyspnea that occurs when the patient is lying down and improves when the patient sits up. Make sure, however, that the reason the patient uses extra pillows or sleeps upright is shortness of breath and no other causes.

- Have you ever awoken suddenly due to shortness of breath?

Paroxysmal nocturnal dyspnea, or PND, describes episodes of sudden dyspnea and orthopnea that awaken the patient from sleep, usually 1 or 2 hours after going to bed, prompting the patient to sit up, stand up, or go to a window for air. There may be associated wheezing and coughing. The episode usually subsides but may recur at about the same time on subsequent nights.

Cough

Cough can result from fluid leaking into the lungs.

CLINICAL TIP
Left-sided heart failure can cause fluid to leak into the lungs. Fine crackles or rales may be heard on auscultation.

Ask:

- Do you ever have a cough?
- Describe your cough.
- Do you cough up mucus? If yes, describe the mucus.
- When does it occur? Any particular time of day?

Edema

Edema refers to the accumulation of excessive fluid in the extravascular interstitial space. Focus your questions on the location, timing, and setting of the swelling, and on any associated symptoms.

Dependent edema appears in the lowest body parts: the feet and lower legs when sitting, or the sacrum when bedridden. Causes may be cardiac (*heart failure*), peripheral vascular disease, nutritional (*hypoalbuminemia*), or positional.

Ask:

- Have you had any swelling anywhere?
- Where? Anywhere else?
- When does it occur?
- Is it worse in the morning or at night?
- Do your shoes get tight?
- Are the rings tight on your fingers?
- Are your eyelids puffy or swollen in the morning?
- Have you had to let out your belt or waistband?

Nocturia

Nocturia is urination at night. It is dependent edema that is mobilized at night and returned to the kidneys for excretion during the night when the patient is reclining. Ask:

- Do you get up more than once during the night to urinate?
- How many times?

Fatigue

Fatigue is an overwhelming sustained sense of exhaustion. Ask:

CLINICAL TIP
Fatigue may signal that the heart is not adequately supplying the body with oxygen and nutrients.

- Do you feel more tired than previously?
- Are you able to perform your usual activities without resting?

Cyanosis or Pallor

Cyanosis or pallor indicates poor oxygenation of the body. Ask:

- Have you ever noticed your facial skin, lips, or fingers become blue or pale?
- How long did it last?

Cyanosis and pallor also may indicate that the heart is not adequately circulating blood.

Past History

Questions regarding the past history may include:

- Do you have a history of heart problems or heart disease?
- Do you have a history of:
  - Heart murmur?
  - Congenital heart disease?
  - Rheumatic fever?
  - High blood pressure? Do you know what the reading was?
  - Elevated cholesterol or triglycerides?
  - Peripheral arterial disease?
  - Cerebral arterial disease?
  - Diabetes?
- When was your last ECG? Cholesterol measurement? What were the results?
- Have you had any other heart tests? When? What were the results?

Family History

Ask the patient if there is any family history of CAD, hypertension, or sudden death at an age younger than 60. Is there a history of stroke? Diabetes? Obesity?

Family refers primarily to first-degree blood relatives (i.e., parent, sibling, child). However, information on grandparents, aunts, uncles, and first cousins can be useful as well.

Lifestyle Habits

Relative lifestyle habits to explore include:

- Nutrition—typical diet
- Smoking
- Alcohol use
- Exercise: Ask the patient to describe daily or weekly exercise and the type and amount
- Medications, prescribed and over-the-counter

PHYSICAL EXAMINATION

Preparation of the Patient

Appropriate preparation of the patient is essential for obtaining accurate findings during the cardiovascular examination. The patient should be comfortable and calm as anxiety may elevate the blood pressure or change the heart rate or rhythm. Review the examination procedure with the patient before putting on the examination gown. Explain why visualization of the anterior chest is important for data gathering. Have the patient put on the examination gown with the opening in the front, which enables the nurse to open the gown only as necessary during the examination. Assist the patient onto the examination table, if necessary, and immediately drape them with a sheet. Perform the examination from the patient's right side.

Equipment needed for a physical cardiovascular examination includes:

- Stethoscope with a bell and diaphragm
- Sphygmomanometer
- Two 15-cm rulers
- Watch with second hand
- Gooseneck lamp for tangential lighting

Blood Pressure and Heart Rate

As you begin the cardiovascular examination, review the blood pressure and heart rate recorded during the general survey and taking of vital signs at the start of the physical examination. If you need to repeat these measurements, or if they have not already been done, take the time to measure the blood pressure and heart rate using optimal technique (see Chapter 7, "General Survey Including Vital Signs and Pain").

The components of the cardiovascular examination include:

- Examination of the face
- Examination of the great vessels of the neck
- Inspection and palpation of the precordium
- Auscultation of heart sounds
- Inspection for peripheral edema

Face

As you are taking the patient's history inspect the face, noting its color and the presence of any orbital edema. Look for signs of anxiety. Pallor or cyanosis may indicate poor perfusion of oxygen, and orbital edema may indicate heart failure. Anxiety occurs during heart attacks.

CLINICAL TIP
Infants with cardiac disease may exhibit circumoral (around the mouth) cyanosis with feeding.

Great Vessels of the Neck

The Carotid Artery Pulse

The carotid pulse provides valuable information about cardiac function and is especially useful for detecting stenosis or insufficiency of the aortic valve. To compare regular and irregular rhythms, review Tables 14-1 and 14-2.

Amplitude and Contour

To assess **amplitude** (forcefulness) and contour of the carotid pulse, the patient should be lying down with the head of the bed elevated to about 30 degrees. First inspect the neck for carotid pulsations. These may be visible just medial to the sternocleidomastoid muscles. Then place your index and middle fingers on the right carotid artery in the lower third of the neck, press posteriorly, and feel for pulsations.

Pulse contour is the shape of the arterial pulse wave, which is an indicator of left ventricular stroke volume. A tortuous and kinked carotid artery may produce a unilateral pulsatile bulge.

Press just inside the medial border of a well-relaxed sternocleidomastoid muscle, roughly at the level of the cricoid cartilage (Fig. 14-23). Avoid pressing on the *carotid sinus*, which lies at the level of the top of the thyroid cartilage. For the left carotid artery, use your right fingers. Never press both carotids at the same time. This may decrease blood flow to the brain and induce syncope.

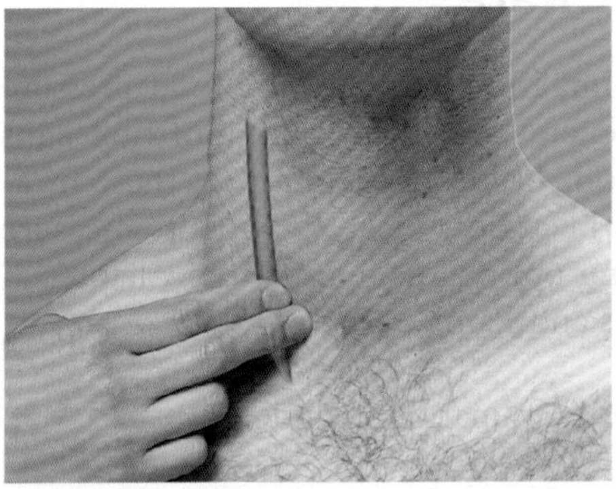

FIGURE 14-23 Palpating the carotid artery.

Causes of decreased pulsations include decreased stroke volume and local factors in the artery such as atherosclerotic narrowing or occlusion. Pressure on the carotid sinus may cause a reflex drop in pulse rate or blood pressure.

Slowly increase pressure until the maximal pulsation is felt, and then slowly decrease pressure until you best sense the arterial pressure and contour. Try to assess:

- The *amplitude of the pulse*. This correlates reasonably well with the pulse pressure.

Small, thready, or weak pulse occurs in *cardiogenic shock*; *bounding* pulse occurs in *aortic insufficiency* (see Table 15-5, "Abnormalities of the Arterial Pulse and Pressure Waves").

TABLE 14-1 Selected Heart Rates and Rhythms

Cardiac rhythms may be classified as *regular or irregular*. When rhythms are irregular or rates are fast or slow, an ECG should be obtained to identify the origin of the beats (sinus node, atrioventricular node, atrium, or ventricle) and the pattern of conduction. The range for normal sinus rhythm is reported at 50–90 beats/min (Spodick, 1996). Note that with AV (atrioventricular) block, arrhythmias may have a fast, normal, or slow ventricular rate.

IS THE RHYTHM REGULAR OR IRREGULAR?

Rhythm		ECG Pattern	Usual Resting Rate
REGULAR → WHAT IS THE RATE?	FAST (>100)	Sinus tachycardia	100–180
		Supraventricular (atrial or nodal) tachycardia	150–250
		Atrial flutter with a regular ventricular response	100–175
		Ventricular tachycardia	110–250
	OR		
	NORMAL (60–90)	Normal sinus rhythm	60–90
		Second-degree AV block	60–100
		Atrial flutter with a regular ventricular response	75–100
	OR		
	SLOW (<60)	Sinus bradycardia	<60
		Second-degree AV block	30–60
		Complete heart block	<40
IRREGULAR → WHAT IS THE PATTERN OF IRREGULARITY?	RHYTHMIC OR SPORADIC	With early beats, atrial or nodal (supraventricular) premature contraction OR ventricular premature contractions	See Table 14-2
		Sinus arrhythmia	See Table 14-2
	OR		
	TOTAL	Atrial fibrillation	See Table 14-2
		Atrial flutter with varying block	See Table 14-2

- The *contour of the pulse wave*, namely, the speed of the upstroke, the duration of its summit, and the speed of the downstroke. The normal upstroke is *brisk*. It is smooth and rapid and follows S_1 almost immediately. The summit is smooth, rounded, and roughly midsystolic. The downstroke is less abrupt than the upstroke.

CLINICAL TIP
Delayed carotid upstroke is seen in *aortic stenosis*.

TABLE 14-2 Selected Irregular Rhythms

Type of Rhythm	ECG Waves and Heart Sounds	
Atrial or Nodal Premature Contractions (*Supraventricular*)	**Rhythm.** A beat of atrial or nodal origin comes earlier than the next expected normal beat. A pause follows, and then the rhythm resumes. **Heart Sounds.** S_1 may differ in intensity from the S_1 of normal beats, and S_2 may be decreased.	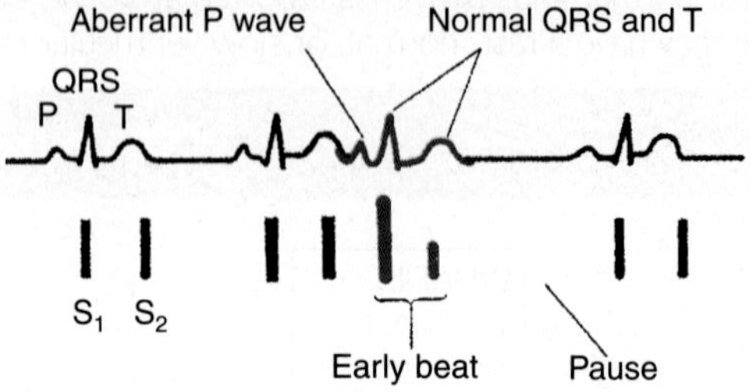
Ventricular Premature Contractions	**Rhythm.** A beat of ventricular origin comes earlier than the next expected normal beat. A pause follows, and the rhythm resumes. **Heart Sounds.** S_1 may differ in intensity from the S_1 of the normal beats, and S_2 may be decreased. Both sounds are likely to be split.	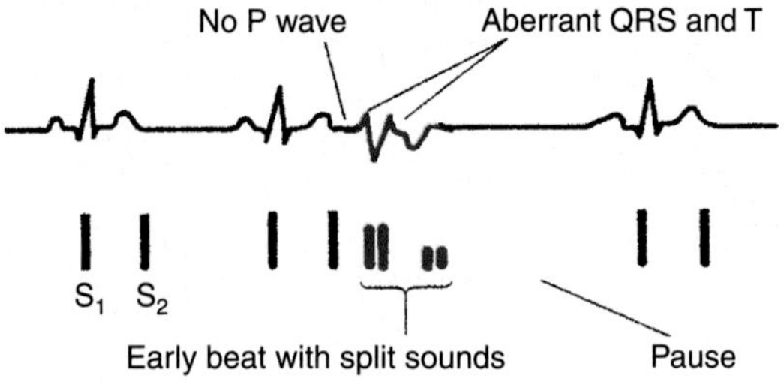
Sinus Arrhythmia	**Rhythm.** The heart varies cyclically, usually speeding up with inspiration and slowing down with expiration. **Heart Sounds.** Normal, though S_1 may vary with the heart rate.	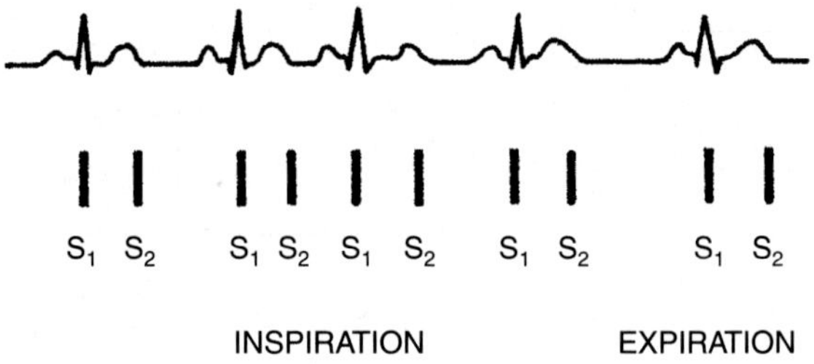
Atrial Fibrillation and Atrial Flutter with Varying AV Block	**Rhythm.** The ventricular rhythm is totally irregular, though short runs of the irregular ventricular rhythm may seem regular. **Heart Sounds.** S_1 varies in intensity.	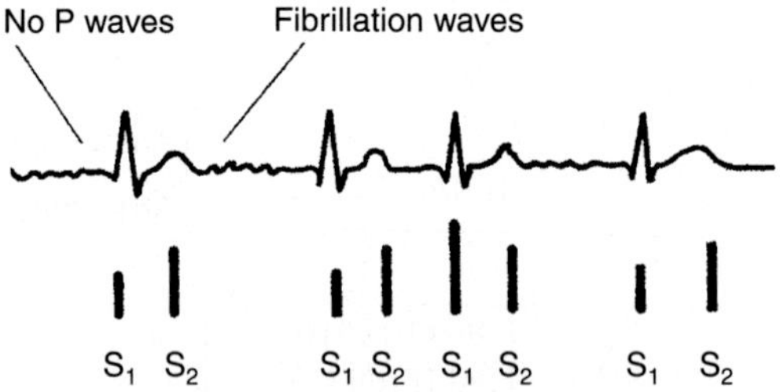

- Any *variations in amplitude*, either from beat to beat or with respiration.

Pulsus alternans (see Table 15-5, "Abnormalities of the Arterial Pulse and Pressure Waves"), bigeminal pulse (beat-to-beat variation); paradoxical pulse (respiratory variation).

- *The timing of the carotid upstroke in relation to S_1 and S_2.* Note that the normal carotid upstroke follows S_1 and precedes S_2. This relationship is helpful in correctly identifying S_1 and S_2, especially when the heart rate is increased and the duration of diastole, normally longer than systole, is shortened and approaches the duration of systole.

Thrills and Bruits

During palpation of the carotid artery, humming vibrations, or **thrills**, that feel like the throat of a purring cat may be detected. Routinely, but especially in the presence of a thrill, listen over both carotid arteries with the bell of the stethoscope for a **bruit**, a murmur-like sound of vascular rather than cardiac origin.

Note that an aortic valve murmur may radiate to the neck and sound like a carotid bruit.

Listen for carotid bruits if the patient is middle-aged or elderly or if cerebrovascular disease is suspected. Ask the patient to hold breathing for a moment so that breath sounds do not obscure the vascular sound, and then listen with the bell. Heart sounds alone do not constitute a bruit.

The prevalence of asymptomatic carotid bruits increases with age along with an increased risk of ischemic heart disease and stroke.

Further examination of arterial pulses is described in Chapter 15, "The Peripheral Vascular System and Lymphatic System."

The Brachial Artery

The carotid arteries reflect aortic pulsations more accurately, but in patients with carotid obstruction, kinking, or thrills, they are unsuitable. If so, assess the pulse in the *brachial artery*, applying the techniques described above for determining amplitude and contour.

Use the index and middle fingers to feel for the pulse just medial to the biceps tendon (Fig. 14-24). The patient's arm should rest with the elbow extended, palm up. With your free hand, you may need to flex the elbow to a varying degree to get optimal muscular relaxation.

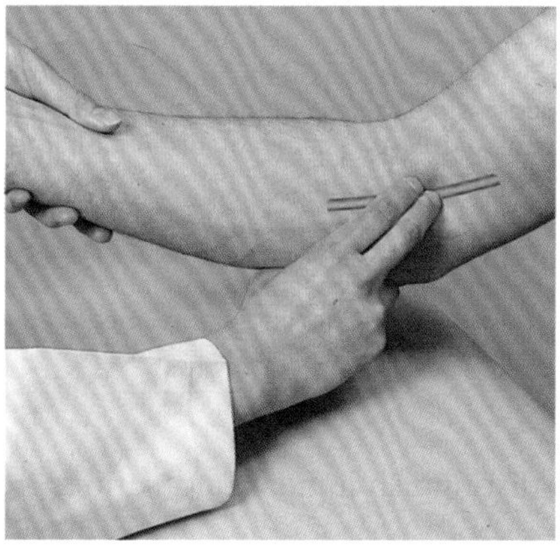

FIGURE 14-24 Palpating the brachial artery.

Jugular Venous Pressure

The JVP provides valuable information about the patient's volume status and cardiac function. The JVP reflects pressure in the right atrium, or CVP, and is best assessed from undulations in the right internal jugular vein (McGee, 2018).

Note, however, that the jugular veins are difficult to see in children younger than 12 years, so they are not useful for evaluating the cardiovascular system in this age group.

At the beginning of the assessment, consider the patient's volume status and how high the head of the bed or examining table needs to be elevated.

- The usual starting point for assessing the JVP is to elevate the head of the bed to 30 degrees. Identify the external jugular vein on each side, and then find the internal jugular venous undulations transmitted from deep in the neck to the overlying soft tissues. The JVP is the highest point of the jugular venous undulation that is usually evident in euvolemic patients.

A hypovolemic patient may have to lie flat before you see the neck veins. In contrast, when JVP is increased, an elevation up to 45 degrees, 60 degrees, or even 90 degrees may be required. Refer back to Figure 14-22.

- In patients who are *hypovolemic, the JVP may be low*, necessitating lowering *the head of the bed*, sometimes even to 0 degrees, to see the point of undulation best.
- Likewise, in volume-overloaded or *hypervolemic* patients, *the JVP may be high*, requiring raising *the head of the bed.*
- When documenting the JVP, record the height of the head of the bed, for example, JVP 2 cm from sternal angle with the head of the bed elevated 45 degrees.

Box 14-3 summarizes steps for assessing the JVP.

BOX 14-3 STEPS FOR ASSESSING THE JVP

- Make the patient comfortable. *Raise the head slightly on a pillow* to relax the sternocleidomastoid muscles.
- *Raise the head of the bed or examining table to about 30 degrees. Turn the patient's head slightly away from the side you are inspecting.*
- Use *tangential lighting* and examine both sides of the neck. Identify the external jugular vein on each side, and then find the internal jugular venous pulsations.
- *If necessary, raise or lower the head of the bed* until you can see the undulations of the internal jugular vein in the lower half of the neck.
- Focus on the *right internal jugular vein*. Look for undulations in the suprasternal notch between the attachments of the sternocleidomastoid muscle on the sternum and clavicle or just posterior to the sternocleidomastoid. Table 14-3 helps you distinguish internal jugular undulations from those of the carotid artery.
- *Identify the highest point of undulation in the right internal jugular vein.* Extend a ruler or card horizontally from this point and a second centimeter ruler vertically from the sternal angle, making an exact right angle. Measure the vertical distance in centimeters above the sternal angle where the horizontal object crosses the ruler. *This distance, measured in centimeters above the sternal angle or the right atrium, is the JVP* (see Fig. 14-25).

Table 14-3 outlines features that help distinguish jugular undulations from carotid artery pulsations.

TABLE 14-3 Distinguishing Jugular Undulations and Carotid Pulsations

Jugular Undulations	Carotid Pulsations
Rarely palpable	Palpable
Soft, biphasic, undulating quality usually with two elevations and two troughs per heartbeat	A more vigorous thrust with a *single outward component*
Undulations can be eliminated by light pressure on the vein(s) just above the sternal end of the clavicle	Pulsations not eliminated by this pressure
Height of undulations changes with position, dropping as the patient becomes more upright	Height of pulsations unchanged by position
Height of undulations usually falls with inspiration	Height of pulsations not affected by inspiration

Establishing the true vertical and horizontal lines to measure the JVP is difficult, much like the problem of hanging a picture straight when you are close to it. Place your ruler on the sternal angle and line it up with something in the room that you know to be vertical. Then place a card or rectangular object at an exact right angle to the ruler. This constitutes your horizontal line. Move it up or down—still horizontal—so that the lower edge rests at the top of the jugular pulsations, and read the vertical distance on the ruler (Fig. 14-25). Round your measurement off to the nearest centimeter.

Increased pressure suggests right-sided heart failure or less commonly, constrictive pericarditis, tricuspid stenosis, or superior vena cava obstruction (Aurigemma & Gasach, 2004; Lange & Hillis, 2004).

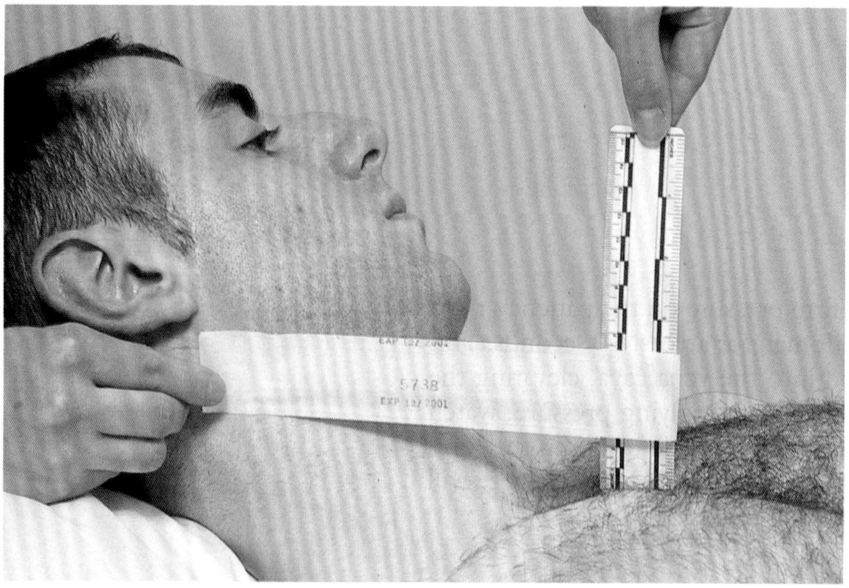

FIGURE 14-25 Establishing vertical and horizontal lines to measure the JVP.

Venous pressure measured at greater than 3 cm is considered *abnormal.*

An elevated JVP is 98% specific for an increased left ventricular end-diastolic pressure and low-left ventricular ejection fraction, although its role as a predictor of hospitalization and death from heart failure is less clear (Drazner et al., 2001; McGee, 2018).

If undulations in the internal jugular vein cannot be seen, look for them in the external jugular vein. If there is no undulation, use *the point above which the external jugular veins appear to collapse.* Make this observation on each side of the neck. Measure the vertical distance of this point from the sternal angle.

Local kinking or obstruction is the usual cause of unilateral distention of the external jugular vein.

The highest point of venous undulations may lie below the level of the sternal angle. Under these circumstances, venous pressure is not elevated and seldom needs to be measured.

Abdominojugular Test

If heart failure is suspected from the patient history or physical examination or if the JVP is elevated, perform the abdominojugular test. Position the patient supine with the head of the bed at the same angle used for the JVP

The abdominojugular test was formerly known as hepatojugular reflux. If heart failure is present, the JVP will remain elevated as long as the pressure is maintained.

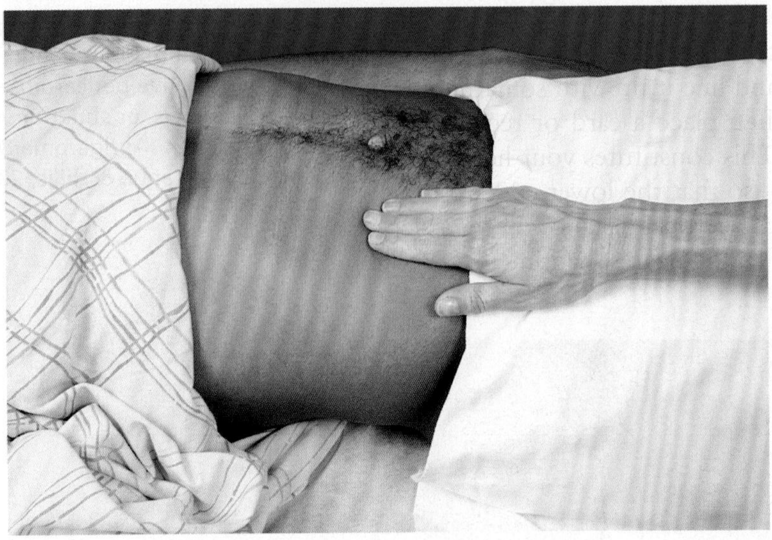

FIGURE 14-26 The abdominojugular test.

examination. With your right hand apply firm pressure on the patient's right upper quadrant (Fig. 14-26) or middle abdomen for at least 10 seconds. This maneuver forces the hepatic venous blood into the vena cava, elevating the venous blood volume and pressure. While you are applying pressure, watch the patient's jugular vein level. The healthy person is able to pump the extra blood through the heart within a few seconds. The jugular vein pressure will rise for a few seconds and then rapidly diminish to previous levels.

The Heart

For much of the cardiac examination, the patient should be *supine* with the upper body raised by elevating the head of the bed or table to about 30 degrees. Two other positions are also needed: (1) the left lateral decubitus position (the patient *lays on the left side*) and (2) *sitting and leaning forward*. These positions bring the ventricular apex and left ventricular outflow tract closer to the chest wall, enhancing detection of the PMI and aortic insufficiency. *The examiner should stand at the patient's right side.*

During the cardiac examination, remember to correlate the findings with the patient's JVP and carotid pulse. It is also important to document both the anatomic location of findings with their timing in the cardiac cycle.

Note the *anatomic locations* of sounds in terms of intercostal spaces and their distances from the midsternal or midclavicular lines. The midsternal line offers the most reliable zero point for measurement, but some feel that the midclavicular line accommodates the different sizes and shapes of patients.

Identify the *timing of impulses or sounds* in relation to the cardiac cycle. Timing of sounds is often possible through auscultation alone. In most people with normal or slow heart rates, it is easy to identify the paired heart sounds by listening through a stethoscope. S_1 is the first of these sounds,

S_2 is the second, and the relatively long diastolic interval separates one pair from the next (Fig. 14-27). The relative intensity of these sounds is also helpful. S_1 is usually louder than S_2 at the apex; S_2 is usually louder than S_1 at the base.

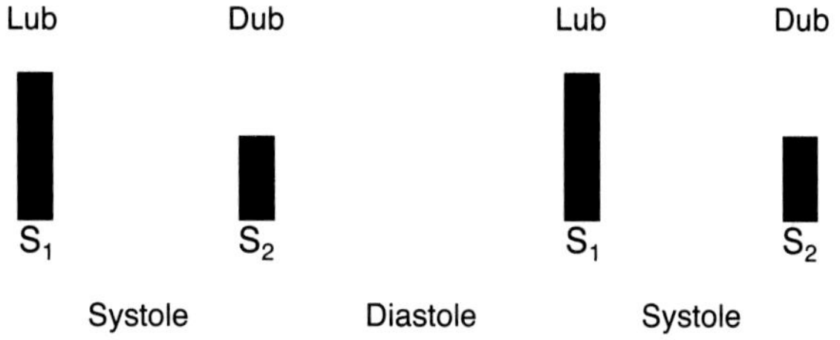

FIGURE 14-27 The timing of S_1 and S_2.

S_1 is sometimes called "lub" and S_2 "dub." Listen for the lub-dub sequence to distinguish the two sounds.

Even experienced nurses are sometimes uncertain about the timing of heart sounds, especially extra sounds and murmurs. "Inching" can then be helpful. Return to a place on the chest—most often the base—where it is easy to identify S_1 and S_2. Get their rhythm clearly in mind. Then inch your stethoscope down the chest in steps until you hear the new sound.

Auscultation alone, however, can be misleading. The intensities of S_1 and S_2, for example, may be abnormal. At rapid heart rates, diastole shortens, and at about a rate of 120, the durations of systole and diastole become indistinguishable. *Use palpation of the carotid pulse or of the apical impulse to help determine whether the sound or murmur is systolic or diastolic.* Because both the carotid upstroke and the apical impulse occur in systole, right after S_1, sounds or murmurs coinciding with them are systolic; sounds or murmurs occurring after the carotid upstroke or apical impulse are diastolic.

For example, S_1 is decreased in first-degree heart block, and S_2 is decreased in aortic stenosis.

Sequence of Cardiac Examination

Table 14-4 summarizes patient positions and a suggested sequence for the cardiac examination.

TABLE 14-4 Sequence of Cardiac Examination

Patient Position	Examination
Supine, with the head elevated 30 degrees	Inspect and palpate the precordium: the second right and left intercostal spaces; the right ventricle; and the left ventricle, including the apical impulse (diameter, location, amplitude, duration). Auscultate the second right and left intercostal spaces, along the left sternal border, down the left sternal border to the fourth and fifth interspaces, and across to the apex with the *diaphragm*.
Left lateral decubitus	Palpate the apical impulse if not previously detected. Auscultate the apex with the *bell* of the stethoscope.
Sitting, leaning forward, after full exhalation	Auscultate the right sternal border for tricuspid murmurs and sounds with the *bell*.

Low-pitched extra sounds such as an S_3, opening snap, diastolic rumble of *mitral stenosis*

Soft decrescendo diastolic murmur of *aortic insufficiency*

Inspection

Carefully *inspect* the anterior chest for the location of the *apical impulse* or *PMI* and heaves over the precordium, which indicate increased ventricular movement. Tangential light is useful for making this observation. Use *palpation* to confirm the characteristics of the apical impulse.

Palpation

Begin with general palpation of the chest wall. First palpate for *heaves (lifts)* using your *finger pads.* Hold them flat or obliquely on the body surface. Ventricular impulses may heave or lift your fingers.

Check for *thrills* formed by the turbulence of underlying murmurs by pressing the *ball of your hand* firmly on the chest. If subsequent auscultation reveals a loud murmur, go back to that area and check for thrills again.

Thrills may accompany loud, harsh, or rumbling murmurs as in *aortic stenosis, patent ductus arteriosus, ventricular septal defect,* and, less commonly, *mitral stenosis.* They are palpated more easily in patient positions that accentuate the murmur.

CLINICAL TIP

On rare occasions, a patient has *dextrocardia*—a heart situated on the right side. The apical impulse will then be found on the right. If you cannot find an apical impulse, percuss for the dullness of the heart and liver and for the tympany of the stomach. In *situs inversus*, all three of these structures are on opposite sides from normal. A right-sided heart with a normally placed liver and stomach is usually associated with congenital heart disease.

Be sure to assess the *right ventricle* by palpating the right ventricular area at the lower left sternal border and in the subxiphoid area, the pulmonary artery in the left second intercostal space, and the aortic area in the right second intercostal space (see Fig. 14-28 with palpation areas indicated).

Palpable pulsations of the right ventricle may indicate an enlarged right ventricle.

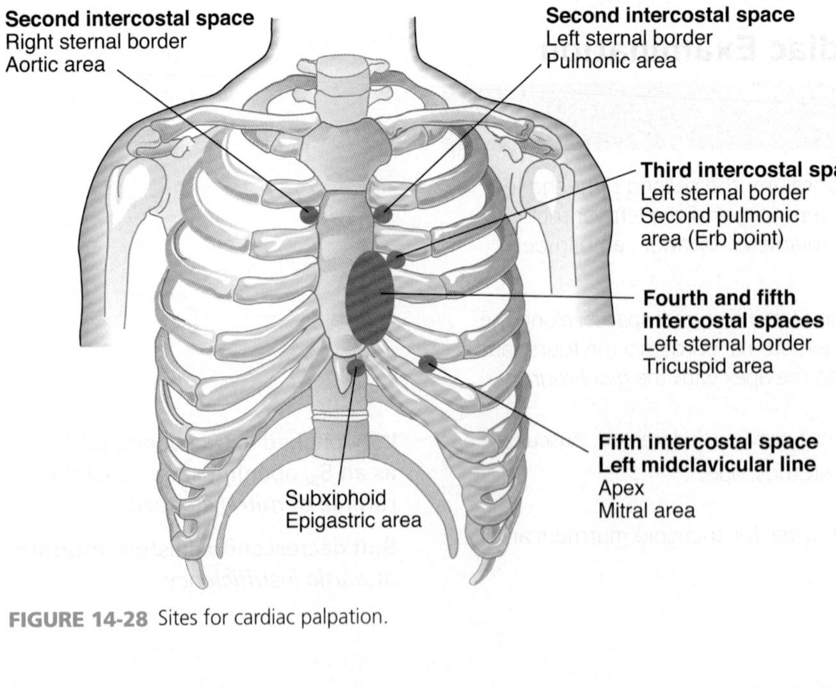

FIGURE 14-28 Sites for cardiac palpation.

The Apical Impulse or Point of Maximal Impulse

The apical impulse represents the brief early pulsation of the left ventricle as it moves anteriorly during contraction and touches the chest wall. Note that in most examinations the apical impulse is the PMI; however, some pathologic conditions may produce a pulsation that is more prominent than the apex beat, such as an enlarged right ventricle, a dilated pulmonary artery, or an aneurysm of the aorta.

If you cannot identify the apical impulse with the patient supine, ask the patient to roll partly onto the left side—this is the *left lateral decubitus* position. Palpate again, using the palmar surfaces of several fingers (Fig. 14-29). If you cannot find the apical impulse, ask the patient to exhale fully and stop breathing for a few seconds. When examining a woman, it may be helpful to displace the left breast upward or laterally as necessary; alternatively, ask her to do this for you.

The apex beat is palpable in only 25% to 40% of healthy adults in the supine position and in 50% of healthy adults in the left lateral decubitus position, especially those who are thin (McGee, 2018).

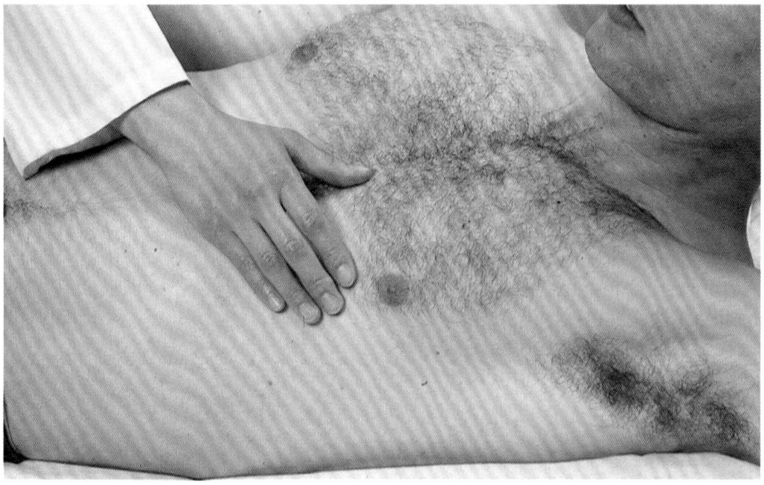

FIGURE 14-29 Palpating for the apical impulse with the patient in the left lateral decubitus position.

Once the apical impulse is found, make finer assessments with the fingertips, and then with one finger (Fig. 14-30).

Obesity, a very muscular chest wall, or an increased anteroposterior diameter of the chest, however, may make the apical impulse undetectable. Some hide behind the rib cage, despite positioning.

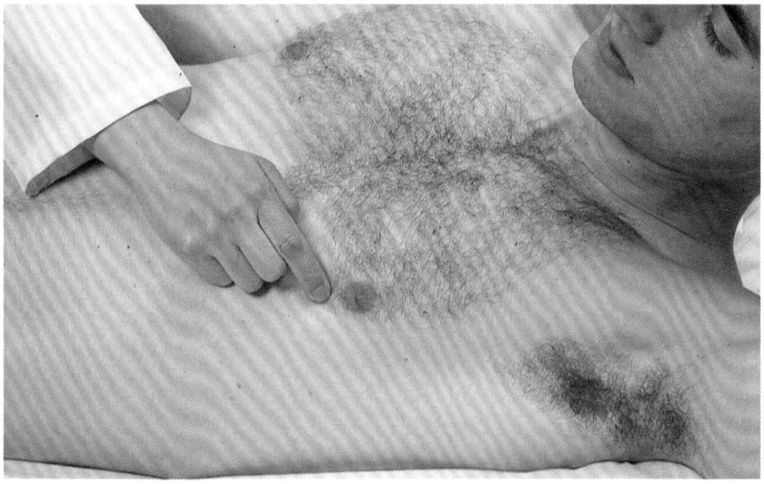

FIGURE 14-30 Making finer assessments once the apical impulse is found.

Now assess the location, diameter, amplitude, and duration of the apical impulse. You may wish to have the patient breathe out and briefly stop breathing to check your findings.

Review Table 14-5, "Variations and Abnormalities of the Apical Impulse."

TABLE 14-5 Variations and Abnormalities of the Apical Impulse

In the healthy heart, the apical impulse or *left ventricular impulse* is usually the *point of maximal impulse*, or *PMI*. This brief impulse is generated by the movement of the ventricular apex against the chest wall during contraction. The classical descriptors of the apical impulse are:

- *Location*: In the fourth or fifth intercostal space, ~7–10 cm lateral to the midsternal line depending on the diameter of the chest
- *Diameter*: *discrete*, or ≤2 cm
- *Amplitude*: *Brisk* and *tapping*
- *Duration*: ≤2/3 of systole

Careful examination of the apical impulse gives you important clues about underlying cardiovascular hemodynamics. The quality of the impulse changes as the left ventricle adapts to high-output states (anxiety, hyperthyroidism, and severe anemia) and to the more pathologic conditions of chronic pressure or volume overload. Note below the distinguishing features of the three types of apical impulses: the *hyperkinetic impulse* from transiently increased stroke volume (this change does not necessarily indicate heart disease); the *sustained* impulse of ventricular hypertrophy from chronic pressure load, known as *increased afterload*; and the *diffuse* impulse of ventricular dilation from chronic volume overload, or *increased preload*.

	Left Ventricular Impulse		
	Hyperkinetic	**Pressure Overload (Increased Afterload)**	**Volume Overload (Increased Preload)**
Examples of Causes	Anxiety, hyperthyroidism, severe anemia	Aortic stenosis, hypertension	Aortic or mitral regurgitation
Location	Normal	Normal	Displaced to the left and possibly downward
Diameter	2 cm, though increased amplitude may make it seem larger	>2 cm	>2 cm
Amplitude	More forceful tapping	More forceful tapping	*Diffuse*
Duration	<2/3 systole	*Sustained* (up to S_2)	Often slightly sustained

- *Location.* Try to assess location with the patient *supine* because the left lateral decubitus position displaces the apical impulse to the left. Locate two points: the intercostal spaces, usually the fifth or possibly the fourth, which give the vertical location; and the distance in centimeters from the *midsternal line*, which provides the horizontal location (Fig. 14-31).

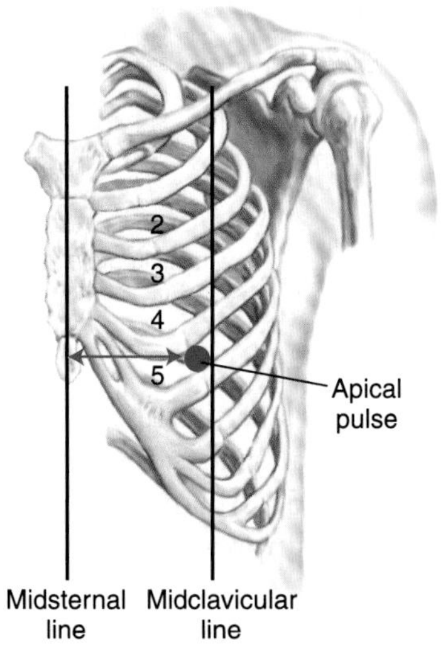

FIGURE 14-31 Locating the apical pulse in relation to the midsternal line.

Pregnancy or a high left diaphragm may displace the apical impulse upward and to the left.

Lateral displacement may occur with cardiac enlargement in *heart failure, cardiomyopathy, ischemic heart disease.* Displacement in deformities of the thorax and mediastinal shift, secondary to respiratory disease, may also occur. Lateral displacement outside the midclavicular line increases the likelihood of cardiac enlargement and a low-left ventricular ejection fraction.

- *Diameter.* Palpate the diameter of the apical impulse. In the supine patient, it usually measures less than 2.5 cm and occupies only one intercostal space. It may feel larger in the left lateral decubitus position.

In the left lateral decubitus position, a *diffuse* PMI with a diameter greater than 3 cm indicates left ventricular enlargement (McGee, 2018).

- *Amplitude.* Estimate the amplitude of the impulse. It is usually small and feels *brisk* and *tapping*. Some young people have an increased amplitude, or hyperkinetic impulse, especially when excited or after exercise; its duration, however, is normal (Fig. 14-32).

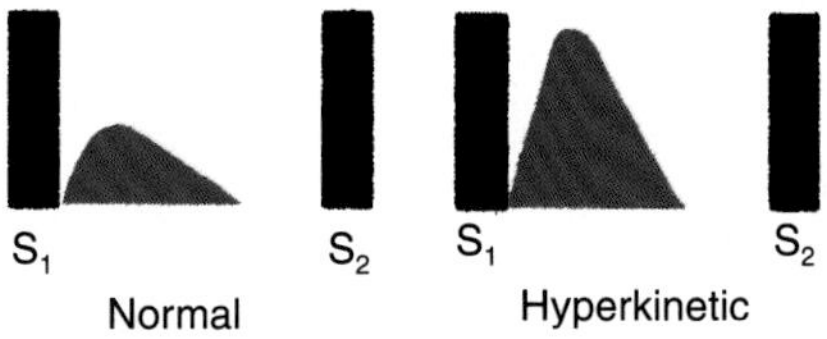

FIGURE 14-32 A normal amplitude and a hyperkinetic impulse.

CLINICAL TIP
Increased amplitude may also reflect *hyperthyroidism, severe anemia*, pressure overload of the left ventricle (as in *aortic stenosis*), or volume overload of the left ventricle (as in *mitral regurgitation*).

- *Duration.* Duration is the most useful characteristic of the apical impulse for identifying hypertrophy of the left ventricle. To assess duration, listen to the heart sounds as you feel the apical impulse, or watch the movement of your stethoscope as you listen at the apex. Estimate the proportion of systole occupied by the apical impulse. Normally it lasts through the first two thirds of systole, and often less, but does not continue to the second heart sound.

A *sustained*, high-amplitude impulse (Fig. 14-33) that is normally located suggests LVH from pressure overload (as in *hypertension*). If the impulse is also displaced laterally, it may indicate fluid volume overload.

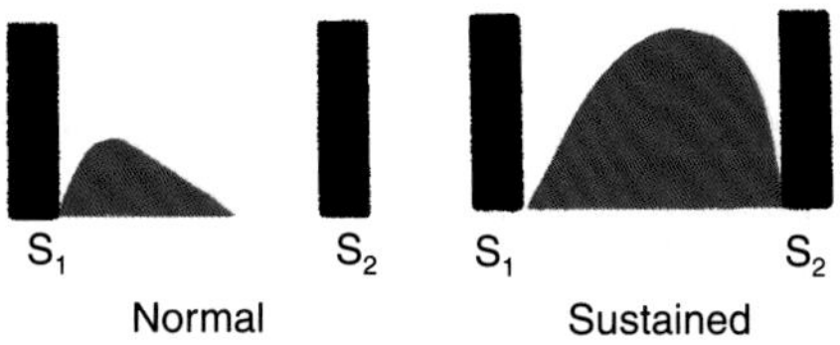

FIGURE 14-33 Normal duration of the apical impulse and sustained, high-amplitude apical impulse.

A sustained, low-amplitude (hypokinetic) impulse (Fig. 14-34) may result from *dilated cardiomyopathy*.

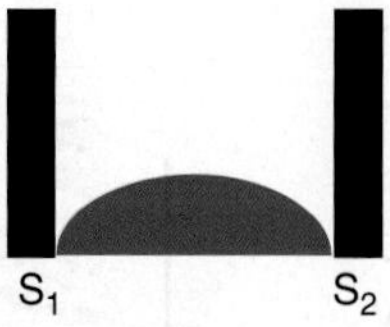

FIGURE 14-34 A hypokinetic apical impulse.

The Right Ventricular Area

The patient should rest supine at 30 degrees. Place the tips of your curved fingers in the third, fourth, and fifth intercostal spaces and try to feel the systolic impulse of the right ventricle (Fig. 14-35). Again, asking the patient to breathe out and then briefly stop breathing improves observation.

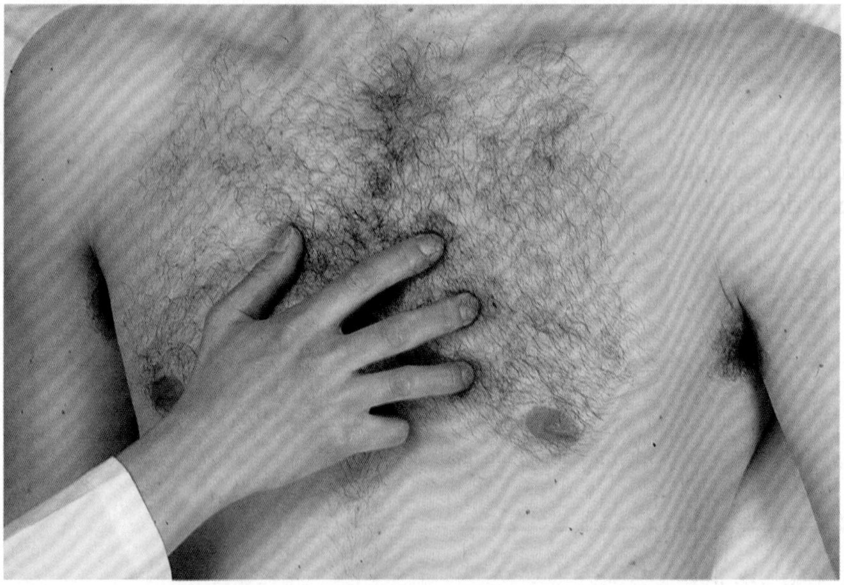

FIGURE 14-35 Palpating the right ventricular area at the third, fourth, and fifth intercostal spaces.

If an impulse or heave is palpable, assess its location, amplitude, and duration.

A marked increase in amplitude with little or no change in duration indicates chronic fluid volume overload of the right ventricle, as from an *atrial septal defect*. An impulse with increased amplitude and duration occurs with pressure overload of the right ventricle, as in *pulmonic stenosis* or *pulmonary hypertension*.

In patients with an increased anteroposterior (AP) diameter, palpation of the *right ventricle* in the *epigastric* or *subxiphoid area* is also useful (Fig. 14-36). With your hand flattened, press your index finger just under the rib cage and up toward the left shoulder and try to feel right ventricular pulsations.

In obstructive pulmonary disease, the hyperinflated lung may prevent palpation of an enlarged right ventricle in the left parasternal area. The impulse is felt easily, however, high in the epigastrium where heart sounds are also often heard best.

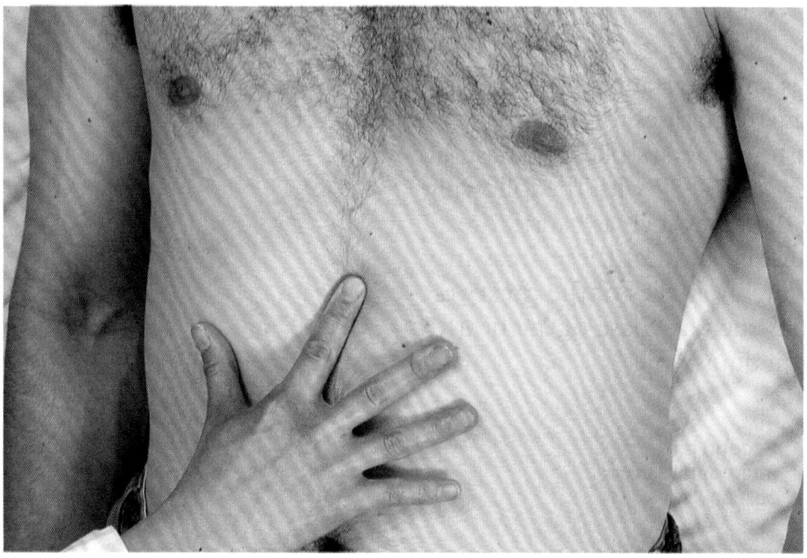

FIGURE 14-36 Palpation of the right ventricle at the epigastric area.

Asking the patient to inhale and briefly stop breathing is helpful. The inspiratory position moves your hand well away from the pulsations of the abdominal aorta, which might otherwise be confusing.

The Pulmonic Area

The left second intercostal space overlies the *pulmonary artery*. As the patient holds expiration, look and feel for an impulse and feel for possible heart sounds. In thin or shallow-chested patients, the pulsation of a pulmonary artery may sometimes be felt here, especially after exercise or with excitement.

A prominent pulsation here often accompanies dilatation or increased flow in the pulmonary artery. A palpable S_2 suggests increased pressure in the pulmonary artery (*pulmonary hypertension*).

The Aortic Area

The right second intercostal space overlies the aortic outflow tract. Search for pulsations and palpable heart sounds.

CLINICAL TIP
A palpable S_2 suggests *systemic hypertension*. A visible pulsation here suggests a *dilated or aneurysmal aorta*.

Percussion

Percussion is rarely used today to estimate cardiac size. X-rays, ECG, and echocardiography provide accurate measurement. Palpation of the apical impulse can provide a rough size estimate. When you cannot feel the apical impulse, however, percussion may be your only tool but may not be reliable. Starting well to the left on the chest, percuss from resonance toward cardiac dullness in the third, fourth, fifth, and possibly sixth intercostal spaces. It is especially difficult to obtain accurate findings in women. Ask the woman to lift her breast up and back before attempting percussion.

Auscultation

Auscultation of heart sounds and murmurs is an important skill of physical examination. In this section, you will learn the techniques for identifying S_1 and S_2, extra heart sounds in systole and diastole, and systolic and diastolic murmurs. Review the auscultatory areas in Figure 14-37 with the following caveats: (1) many authorities discourage use of names such as "aortic area," because murmurs may be loudest in other areas; and (2) these areas may not apply to patients with cardiac enlargement, anomalies of the great vessels, or dextrocardia. It is best to use locations such as "base of the heart," apex, or parasternal border to describe your findings.

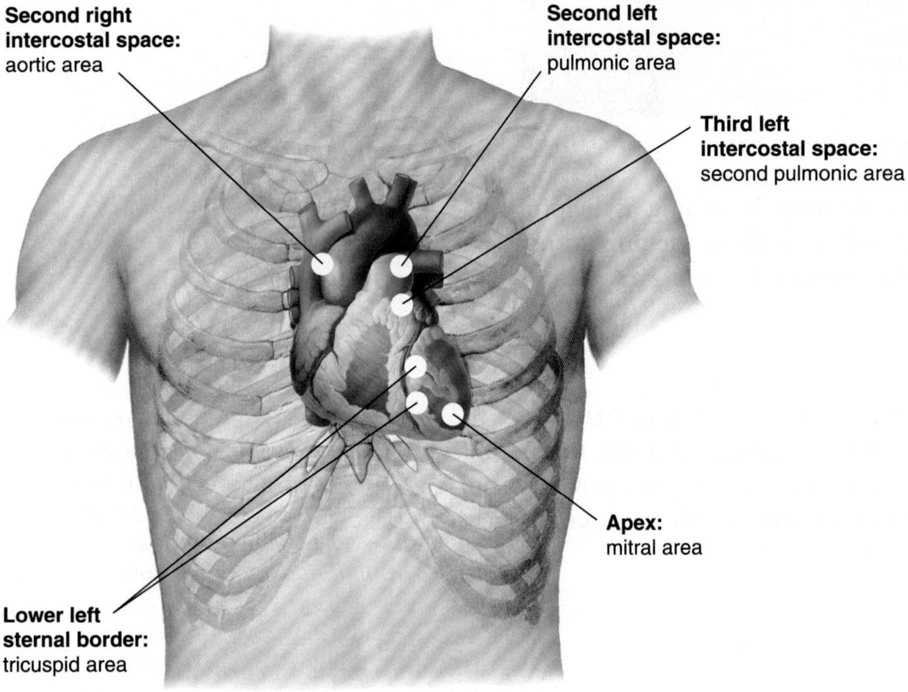

FIGURE 14-37 Sites for cardiac auscultation.

Know Your Stethoscope

The stethoscope has two sides, the diaphragm and the bell, which are acoustically different:

- *The diaphragm.* The diaphragm is better for picking up the relatively high-pitched sounds of S_1 and S_2, the murmurs of aortic and mitral regurgitation, and pericardial friction rubs. *Listen throughout the precordium* with the diaphragm, pressing it firmly against the chest.

- *The bell.* The bell is more sensitive to the low-pitched sounds of S_3 and S_4 and the murmur of mitral stenosis. Apply the bell lightly, with just enough pressure to produce an air seal with its full rim. *Use the bell at the apex, and then move medially along the lower sternal border.* Resting the heel of your hand on the chest like a fulcrum may help you maintain light pressure.

Pressing the bell firmly on the chest makes it function more like the diaphragm by stretching the underlying skin. Low-pitched sounds such as S_3 and S_4 may disappear with this technique—an observation that may help identify them. In contrast, high-pitched sounds such as a midsystolic click, an ejection sound, or an OS will persist or get louder.

There are three types of stethoscope heads. The simplest has only a diaphragm. This type is unsuitable for a full cardiac examination. The second type has a diaphragm on one side and a bell on the opposite side. The head of the stethoscope is rotated to open either the bell or the diaphragm. Lightly tapping on each side with the stethoscope in one's ears will reveal which side is open. The third type of head combines the diaphragm and bell on one side. The bell is activated by very light pressure (no ring should be seen on the skin when the stethoscope is removed) and with increased pressure it becomes a diaphragm. (A ring of blanched skin will remain for a few seconds.) This version comes as either a single-sided stethoscope (Fig. 14-38) or a double-sided stethoscope (Fig. 14-39) with a pediatric and adult side.

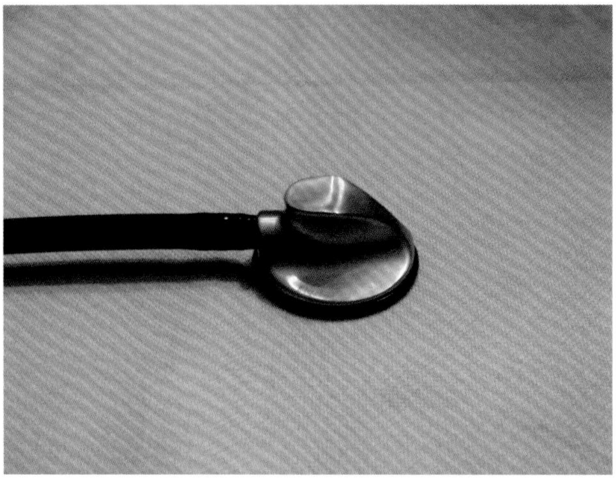

FIGURE 14-38 Single-sided stethoscope.

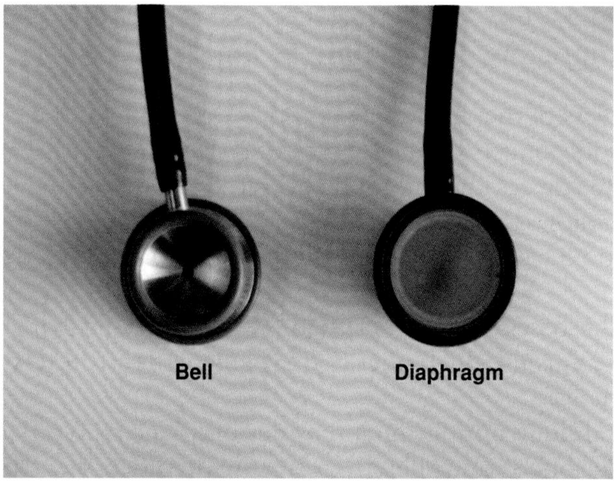

FIGURE 14-39 Double-sided stethoscope.

"Inching" Your Stethoscope

In a quiet room, listen to the heart with your stethoscope starting at either the base or apex. Either pattern is satisfactory:

- Some experts recommend *starting at the apex and inching to the base*: Move the stethoscope from the PMI medially to the left sternal border, superiorly to the second intercostal space, then across the sternum to the second intercostal space at the right sternal border.

- Alternatively, you can *start at the base and inch your stethoscope to the apex*: With your stethoscope in the right second intercostal space close to the sternum, move along the left sternal border in each intercostal space from the second through the fifth, and then to the apex.

Heart sounds and murmurs that originate in the four valves range widely as illustrated in Figure 14-40. Use anatomic location rather than valve area to describe where murmurs and sounds are best heard.

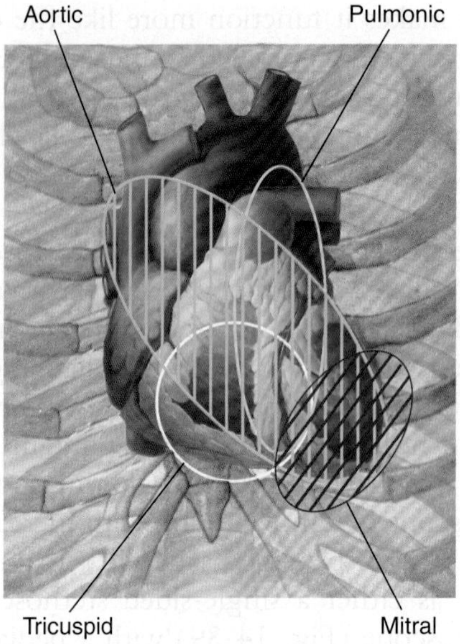

FIGURE 14-40 Anatomic locations of valve sounds.

The Importance of Timing S_1 and S_2

Regardless of the direction you move your stethoscope, keep your left index and middle fingers on the right carotid artery in the lower third of the neck to facilitate correct identification of S_1, just before the carotid upstroke, and S_2, which follows the carotid upstroke. Be sure to compare the relative intensities of S_1 and S_2 as you move your stethoscope through the listening areas:

- At the base, S_2 is louder than S_1 and may split with respiration. At the apex, S_1 is usually louder than S_2 unless the PR interval is prolonged.
- By carefully noting the intensities of S_1 and S_2, you will confirm each of these sounds and thereby correctly identify *systole*, the interval between S_1 and S_2, and *diastole*, the interval between S_2 and S_1.

When listening to the extra sounds of S_3 and S_4 and to murmurs, timing systole and diastole is an absolute prerequisite to the correct identification of these events in the cardiac cycle.

Listen to the entire precordium with the patient supine. For new patients and patients who need a complete cardiac examination, use two other positions to listen for S_3, S_4, and the murmurs of mitral stenosis and aortic regurgitation.

Use Important Maneuvers

Ask the patient to *roll partly onto the left side into the left lateral decubitus position*, bringing the left ventricle close to the chest wall. Place the bell of your stethoscope lightly on the apical impulse (Fig. 14-41).

This position accentuates or brings out a left-sided S_3 and S_4 and mitral murmurs, especially *mitral stenosis*. Otherwise, you may miss these important findings.

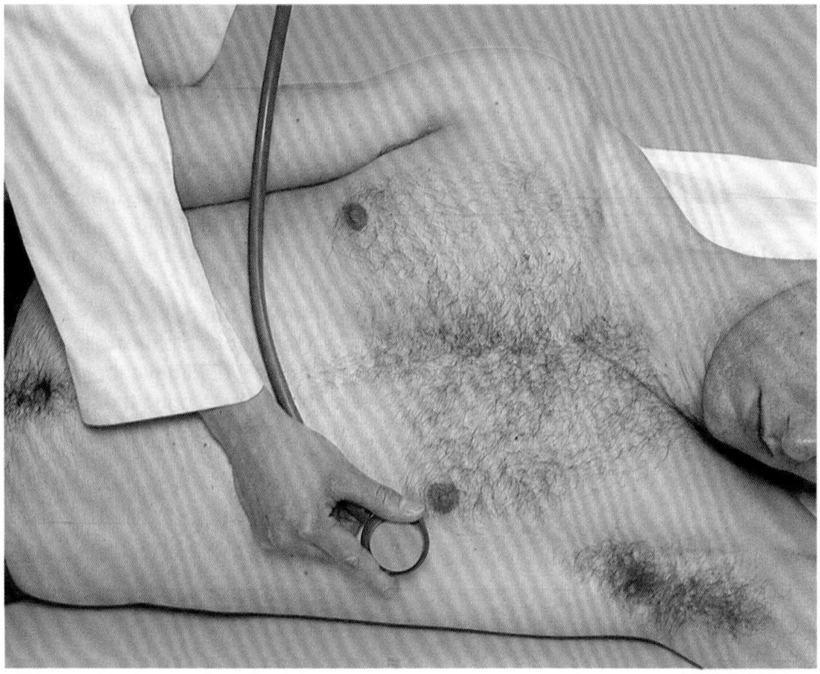

FIGURE 14-41 Auscultation in the left lateral decubitus position.

Next ask the patient to *sit up, lean forward, exhale completely, and stop breathing in expiration*. Pressing the diaphragm of your stethoscope on the chest (Fig. 14-42), listen along the left sternal border and at the apex, pausing periodically so the patient may breathe.

This position accentuates or brings out aortic murmurs. You may easily miss the soft diastolic murmur of *aortic regurgitation* unless you listen at this position.

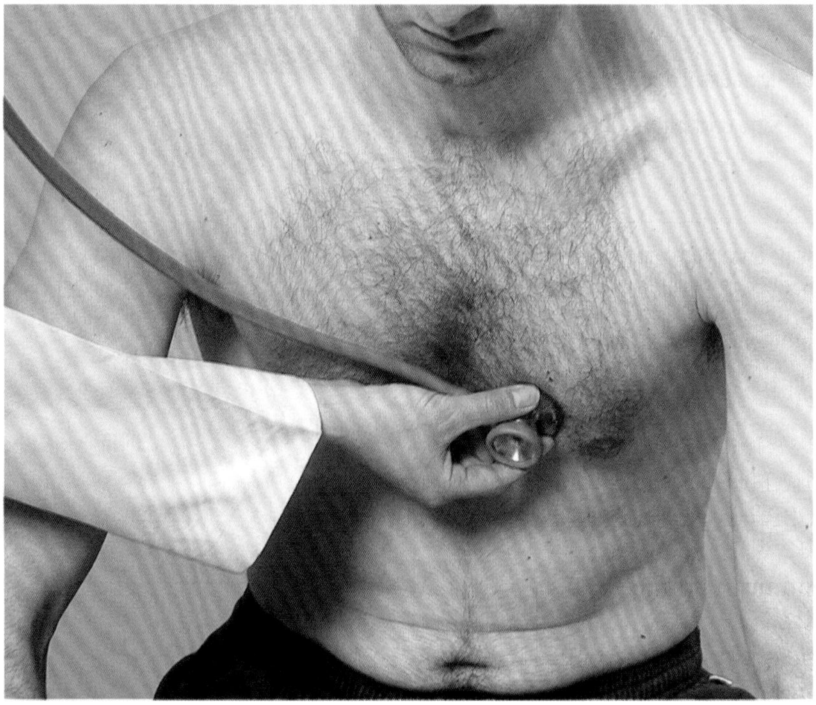

FIGURE 14-42 Auscultation with the patient sitting up and leaning forward.

Listening for Heart Sounds

Throughout your examination, take your time at each auscultatory area. Concentrate on each of the events in the cardiac cycle listed in Table 14-6 and sounds heard in systole and diastole.

Concept Mastery Alert

Auscultating Heart Sounds

Auscultating heart sounds can be challenging. To determine if an extra heart sound is heard after S_2, the nurse should observe the patient's respirations while listening to the heart. If the sound is a normal extra sound (split), then it will be heard on inspiration but not during expiration. To hear a possible diastolic murmur, the nurse would have the patient lean forward to bring the left ventricle closer to the chest wall.

TABLE 14-6 Auscultatory Sounds

Heart Sounds	Guides to Auscultation
S_1	Note its intensity and any splitting. Normal splitting is detectable along the lower left sternal border.
S_2	Note its intensity.
Split S_2	Listen for splitting of this sound in the second and third left intercostal spaces. Ask the patient to breathe quietly, and then slightly more deeply than normal. Does S_2 split into its two components, as it normally does? If not, ask the patient to (1) breathe a little more deeply or (2) sit up. Listen again. A thick chest wall may make the pulmonic component of S_1 inaudible. *Width of split.* How wide is the split? It is normally quite narrow. *Timing of split.* When in the respiratory cycle do you hear the split? It is normally heard late in inspiration. Does the split disappear as it should, during exhalation? If not, listen again with the patient sitting up. *Intensity of A_2 and P_2.* Compare the intensity of the two components, A_2 and P_2. A_2 is usually louder.
Extra Sounds in Systole	Such as ejection sounds or systolic clicks Note their location, timing, intensity, and pitch, and the effects of respiration on the sounds.
Extra Sounds in Diastole	Such as S_3, S_4, or an opening snap Note the location, timing, intensity, and pitch, and the effects of respiration on the sounds. (An S_3 or S_4 in athletes is a normal finding.)
Systolic and Diastolic Murmurs	Murmurs are differentiated from heart sounds by their longer duration.

Persistent splitting results from delayed closure of the pulmonic valve or early closure of the aortic valve.

Expiratory splitting suggests an abnormality.

A loud P_2 suggests *pulmonary hypertension.*

Review Table 14-7, "Variations in the First Heart Sound—S_1." Note that S_1 is louder at more rapid heart rates (and PR intervals are shorter).

Table 14-8 outlines variations in the second heart sound, S_2.

The systolic click of mitral valve prolapse is the most common of extra sounds in systole. See Table 14-9 for more information about extra heart sounds in systole. Table 14-10 outlines extra heart sounds in diastole.

TABLE 14-7 Variations in the First Heart Sound—S_1

Normal

S_1 is softer than S_2 at the *base* (right and left second intercostal spaces).

S_1 is often but not always louder than S_2 at the *apex*.

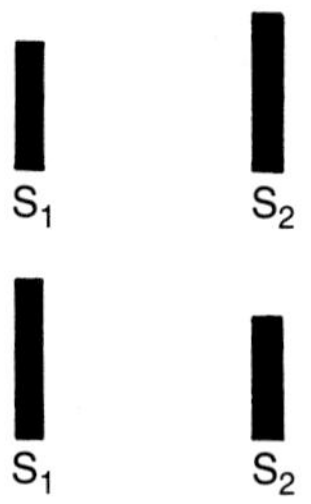

Accentuated S_1

S_1 is accentuated in (1) tachycardia, rhythms with a short PR interval, and high cardiac output states (e.g., exercise, anemia, hyperthyroidism) and (2) mitral stenosis. In these conditions, the mitral valve is still open wide at the onset of ventricular systole and then closes quickly.

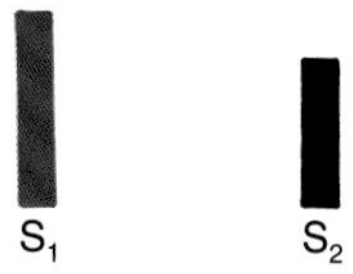

Diminished S_1

S_1 is diminished in first-degree heart block (delayed conduction from atria to ventricles). Here the mitral valve has had time after atrial contraction to float back into an almost closed position before ventricular contraction shuts it. It closes more quietly. S_1 is also diminished (1) when the mitral valve is calcified and relatively immobile, as in mitral regurgitation, and (2) when left ventricular contractility is markedly reduced, as in heart failure or coronary heart disease.

Varying S_1

S_1 varies in intensity (1) in complete heart block, when atria and ventricles are beating independently of each other, and (2) in any totally irregular rhythm (e.g., atrial fibrillation). In these situations, the mitral valve is in varying positions before being shut by ventricular contraction. Its closure sound, therefore, varies in loudness.

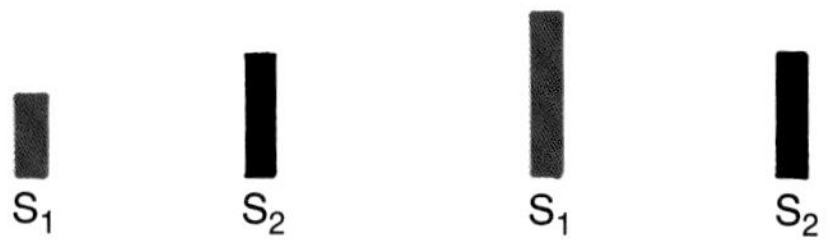

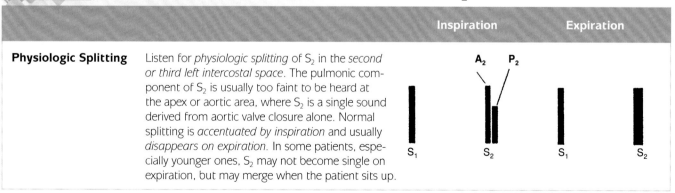

Split S_1

S_1 may be split normally along the lower left sternal border where the tricuspid component, often too faint to be heard, becomes audible. This split may sometimes be heard at the apex, but if heard, it should be differentiated from an S_4, an aortic ejection sound, or an early systolic click. Abnormal splitting of both heart sounds may be heard in right bundle branch block and in premature ventricular contractions.

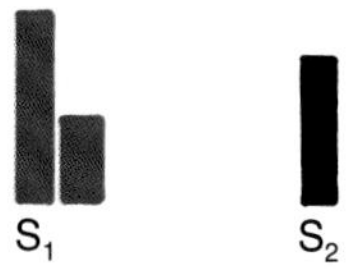

TABLE 14-8 Variations in the Second Heart Sound—S_2

		Inspiration	Expiration

Physiologic Splitting

Listen for *physiologic splitting* of S_2 in the *second or third left intercostal space*. The pulmonic component of S_2 is usually too faint to be heard at the apex or aortic area, where S_2 is a single sound derived from aortic valve closure alone. Normal splitting is *accentuated by inspiration* and usually *disappears on expiration*. In some patients, especially younger ones, S_2 may not become single on expiration, but may merge when the patient sits up.

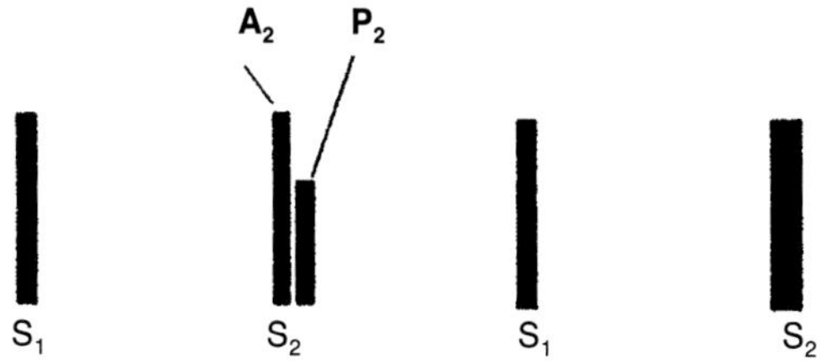

(continued)

TABLE 14-8 Variations in the Second Heart Sound—S_2 (*Continued*)

Inspiration **Expiration**

Pathologic Splitting
(involves splitting during expiration and suggests heart disease)

Wide splitting of S_2 refers to an increase in the usual splitting that persists throughout the respiratory cycle. Wide splitting can be caused by delayed closure of the pulmonic valve (as in pulmonic stenosis or right bundle branch block). As illustrated here, right bundle branch block also causes splitting of S_1 into its mitral and tricuspid components. Wide splitting can also be caused by early closure of the aortic valve as in mitral regurgitation.

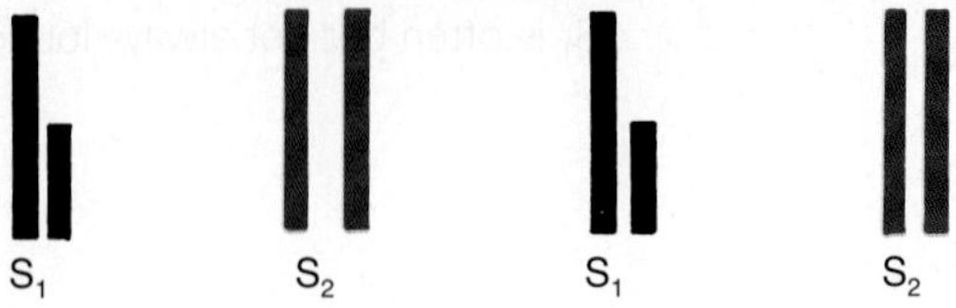

Fixed splitting refers to wide splitting that does not vary with respiration. It occurs in atrial septal defect and right ventricular failure.

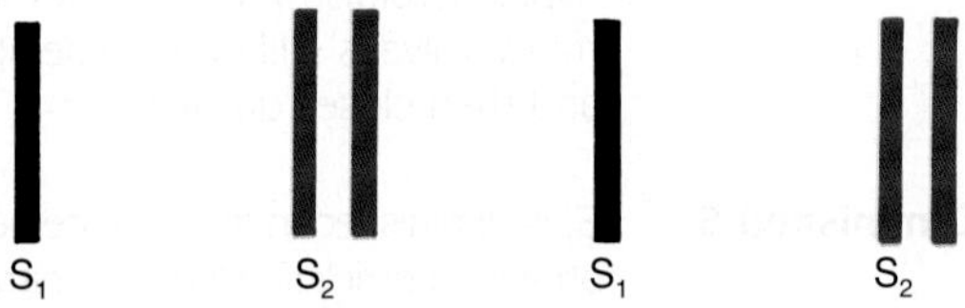

Paradoxical or reversed splitting refers to splitting that appears on expiration and disappears on inspiration. Closure of the aortic valve is abnormally delayed so that A_2 follows P_2 in expiration. Normal inspiratory delay of P_2 makes the split disappear. The most common cause of paradoxical splitting is left bundle branch block.

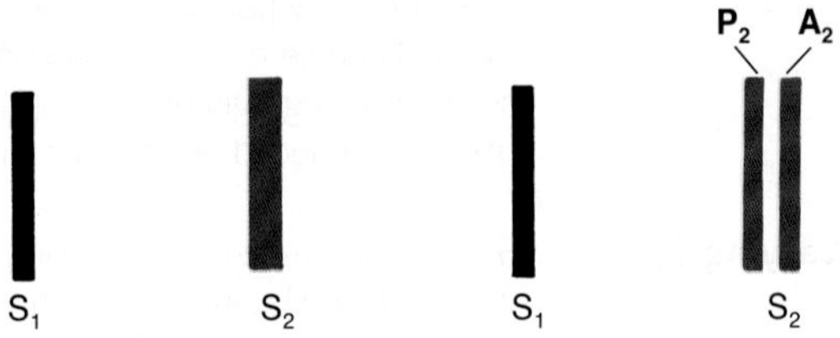

TABLE 14-9 Extra Heart Sounds in Systole

There are two kinds of extra heart sounds in systole: (1) early ejection sounds and (2) clicks, commonly heard in mid and late systole.

Early Systolic Ejection Sounds

Early systolic ejection sounds occur shortly after S_1, coincident with opening of the aortic and pulmonic valves (McGee, 2018). They are relatively high in pitch; have a sharp, clicking quality; and are heard better with the diaphragm of the stethoscope. An ejection sound indicates cardiovascular disease.

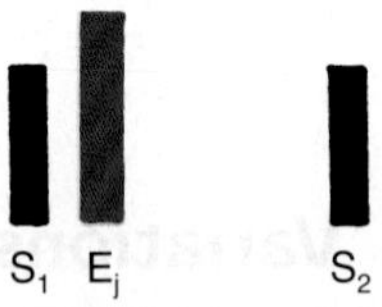

Listen for an *aortic ejection sound* at both the base and apex. It may be louder at the apex and usually does not vary with respiration. An aortic ejection sound may accompany a dilated aorta or aortic valve disease from congenital stenosis or a bicuspid valve (Kari et al., 2012; Siu & Silversides, 2010).

A *pulmonic ejection sound* is heard best in the second and third left intercostal spaces. When S_1, usually relatively soft in this area, appears to be loud, you may be hearing a pulmonic ejection sound. Its intensity often *decreases with inspiration*. Causes include dilatation of the pulmonary artery, pulmonary hypertension, and pulmonic stenosis.

Systolic Clicks

Systolic clicks are usually caused by *mitral valve prolapse*—an abnormal systolic ballooning of part of the mitral valve into the left atrium. The clicks are usually mid or late systolic. Prolapse of the mitral valve is a common cardiac condition, affecting about 2–3% of the general population. There is equal prevalence in men and women (Foster, 2010; Hayek et al., 2005; Topilsky et al., 2012).

The click is usually single, but you may hear more than one, usually *at or medial to the apex*, but also *at the lower left sternal border*. It is high-pitched, so listen with the diaphragm. The click is often followed by a late systolic murmur from mitral regurgitation—a flow of blood from the left ventricle to the left atrium. The murmur usually crescendos up to S_2. Auscultatory findings are notably variable. Most patients have only a click, some have only a murmur, and some have both. Systolic clicks may also be of extracardial or mediastinal origin.

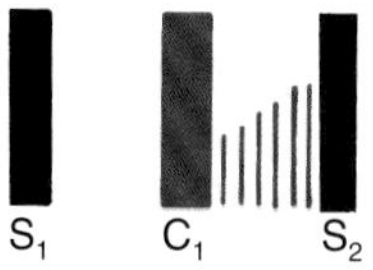

TABLE 14-10 Extra Heart Sounds in Diastole

Opening Snap

The *opening snap* is a very early diastolic sound usually produced by the opening of a *stenotic mitral valve*. It is heard best just medial to the apex and along the lower left sternal border. When it is loud, an opening snap radiates to the apex and to the pulmonic area, where it may be mistaken for the pulmonic component of a split S_2. Its high pitch and snapping quality help distinguish it from an S_2. It is heard better with the *diaphragm*.

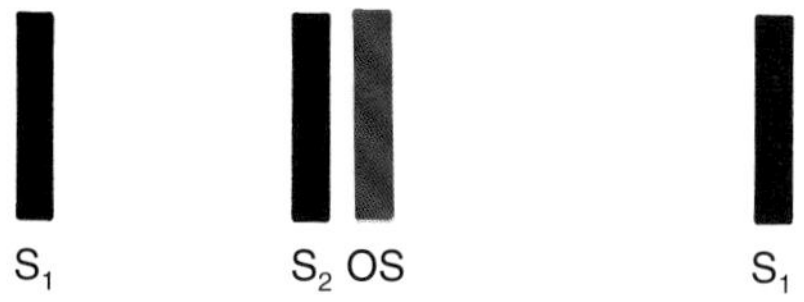

S_3

You will detect *physiologic* S_3 frequently in children and in young adults to the age of 35 or 40. It is common during the last trimester of pregnancy. Occurring early in diastole during rapid ventricular filling, it is later than an opening snap, dull and low in pitch, and heard best at the apex in the left lateral decubitus position. The *bell* of the stethoscope should be used with very light pressure.

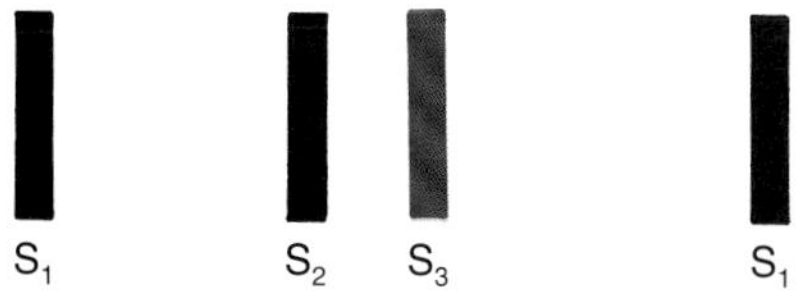

A *pathologic S_3* or *ventricular gallop* sounds just like a physiologic S_3. An S_3 in a person over age 40 (possibly a little older in women) is almost certainly pathologic, arising from altered left ventricular compliance at the end of the rapid filling phase of diastole (Shah & Michaels, 2006; Shah et al., 2008). Causes include decreased myocardial contractility, heart failure, and volume overloading of a ventricle, as in mitral or tricuspid regurgitation. A *left-sided S_3* is typically heard at the apex in the left lateral decubitus position. A *right-sided S_3* is usually heard along the lower left sternal border or below the xiphoid with the patient supine and is louder on inspiration. The term *gallop* comes from the cadence of three heart sounds, especially at rapid heart rates, and sounds like "Kentucky."

(*continued*)

TABLE 14-10 Extra Heart Sounds in Diastole *(Continued)*

S_4	An S_4 (*atrial sound* or *atrial gallop*) occurs just before S_1. It is dull, low in pitch, and heard better with the bell. Listen at the lower left sternal border for a right ventricular S_4. An S_4 is occasionally heard in an apparently normal person, especially in trained athletes and older age groups. More commonly, it is due to increased resistance to ventricular filling following atrial contraction. This increased resistance is related to decreased compliance (increased stiffness) of the ventricular myocardium (McGee, 2018; Shah et al., 2008). Causes of a left-sided S_4 include hypertensive heart disease, coronary artery disease, aortic stenosis, and cardiomyopathy. A *left-sided S_4* is heard best at the apex in the left lateral position; it may sound like "Tennessee." The less common *right-sided S_4* is heard along the lower left sternal border or below the xiphoid. It often gets louder with inspiration. Causes of a right-sided S_4 include pulmonary hypertension and pulmonic stenosis. An S_4 may also be associated with delayed conduction between the atria and ventricles. This delay separates the normally faint atrial sound from the louder S_1 and makes it audible. An S_4 is never heard in the absence of atrial contraction, which occurs with atrial fibrillation. Occasionally, a patient has both an S_3 and an S_4, producing a *quadruple rhythm* of four heart sounds. At rapid heart rates, the S_3 and S_4 may merge into one loud extra heart sound, called a *summation gallop*.	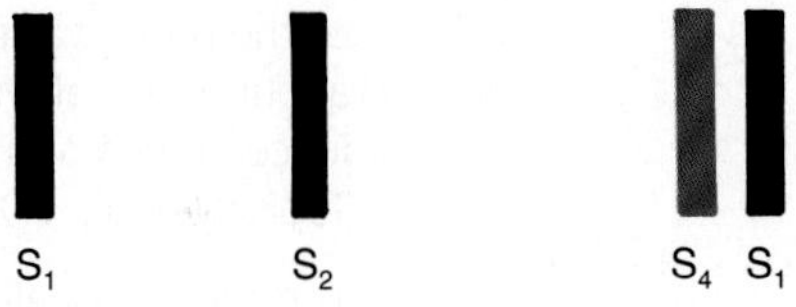

Correctly Identifying Heart Murmurs

Tables 14-11 to 14-13 discuss different types of heart murmurs. Tips for identifying heart murmurs are listed in Box 14-4.

BOX 14-4 TIPS FOR IDENTIFYING HEART MURMURS

- Time the murmur—does it occur in systole or diastole?
- Locate where the murmur is loudest on the precordium—at the base, along the sternal border, at the apex?
- Conduct any necessary maneuvers, such as having the patient lean forward and exhale or turn to the left lateral decubitus position.
- Determine the shape of the murmur—for example, is it crescendo (becomes louder) or decrescendo (becomes softer)? Is it pansystolic?
- Grade the intensity of the murmur from 1 to 6.
- Identify associated features such as the quality of S_1 and S_2; the presence of extra sounds such as S_3, S_4, or an OS; or the presence of additional murmurs.
- Be sure to listen in a quiet room.

Correctly identifying heart murmurs requires a logical and systematic approach, and a thorough understanding of cardiac anatomy and physiology.

TABLE 14-11 Pansystolic (Holosystolic) Murmurs

Pansystolic (holosystolic) murmurs are pathologic, arising from blood flow from a chamber with high pressure to one of lower pressure, through a valve or other structure that should be closed. The murmur begins immediately with S_1 and continues up to S_2.

	Mitral Regurgitation (Asgar et al., 2015; Bonow, 2013; Enriquez-Sarano et al., 2009)	Tricuspid Regurgitation (Irwin et al., 2010; McGee, 2018; Mutlak et al., 2009)	Ventricular Septal Defect
	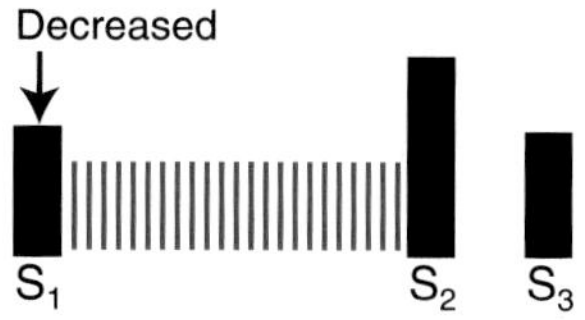	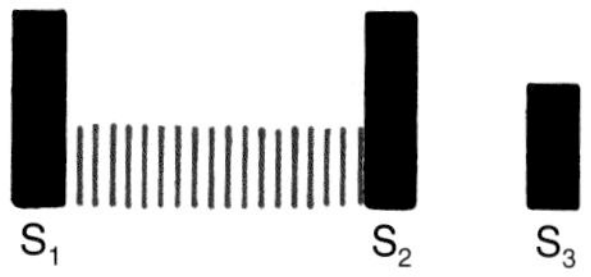	
Murmur			
Location	Apex	Lower left sternal border	Third, fourth, and fifth left intercostal spaces
Radiation	To the left axilla, less often to the left sternal border	To the right of the sternum, to the xiphoid area, and perhaps to the left midclavicular line, but not into the axilla	Often wide
Intensity	Soft to loud; if loud, associated with an apical thrill	Variable	Often very loud with a thrill
Pitch	Medium to high	Medium	High, holosystolic
Quality	Harsh, holosystolic	Blowing, holosystolic	Often harsh
Aids	Unlike tricuspid regurgitation, it does not become louder in inspiration.	Unlike mitral regurgitation, the intensity may increase slightly with inspiration.	
Associated Findings	S_1 normal (75%), loud (12%), soft (12%)	The right ventricular impulse is increased in amplitude and may be sustained.	S_2 may be obscured by the loud murmur.
	An apical S_3 reflects volume overload of the left ventricle. The apical impulse is increased in amplitude (diffuse), is laterally displaced, and may be sustained.	An S_3 may be audible along the lower left sternal border. The jugular venous pressure is often elevated, with large *v* waves in the jugular veins.	Findings vary with the severity of the defect and with associated lesions.
Mechanism	When the *mitral valve fails to close fully in systole*, blood regurgitates from the left ventricle to the left atrium, causing a murmur. This leakage creates volume overload on the left ventricle with subsequent dilatation.	When the *tricuspid valve fails to close fully in systole*, blood regurgitates from the right ventricle to the right atrium, producing a murmur. The most common cause is right ventricular failure and dilatation with resulting enlargement of the tricuspid orifice. Either pulmonary hypertension or left ventricular failure is the usual initiating cause.	A ventricular septal defect is a congenital abnormality in which *blood flows from the relatively high-pressure left ventricle into the low-pressure right ventricle through a hole*.

TABLE 14-12 Midsystolic Murmurs

Midsystolic ejection murmurs are the most common kind of heart murmur. They may be (1) *innocent*—without any detectable physiologic or structural abnormality; (2) *physiologic*—from physiologic changes in body metabolism; or (3) *pathologic*—arising from a structural abnormality in the heart or great vessels. Midsystolic murmurs tend to peak near midsystole and usually stop before S_2. The crescendo–decrescendo or "diamond" shape is not always audible, but the gap between the murmur and S_2 helps distinguish midsystolic from pansystolic murmurs.

	Innocent Murmurs	Physiologic Murmurs
	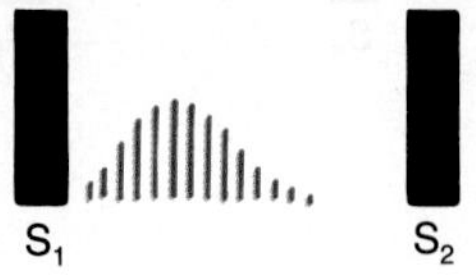	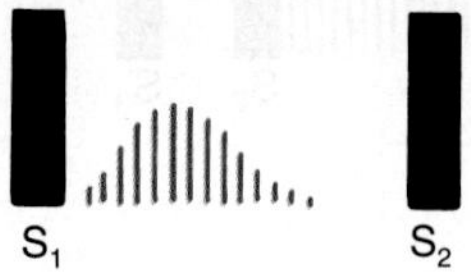
Murmur		
Location	Second to fourth left intercostal spaces between the left sternal border and the apex	Similar to innocent murmurs
Radiation	Little	
Intensity	Grades 1–2, possibly 3	
Pitch	Soft to medium	
Quality	Variable	
Aids	Usually decreases or disappears upon sitting	
Associated Findings	None: normal splitting, no ejection sounds, no diastolic murmurs, and no palpable evidence of ventricular enlargement Occasionally, both an innocent murmur and another kind of murmur are present.	Possible signs of a likely cause
Mechanism	Innocent murmurs result from turbulent blood flow, probably generated by ventricular ejection of blood into the aorta from the left and occasionally the right ventricle. Very common in children and young adults; may also be heard in older people There is no underlying cardiovascular disease.	Turbulence due to a temporary increase in blood flow in predisposing conditions such as anemia, pregnancy, fever, and hyperthyroidism

Pathologic Murmurs

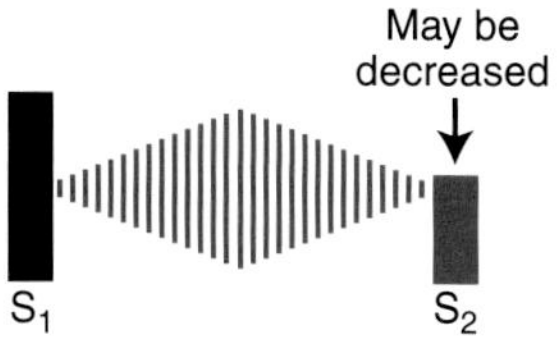

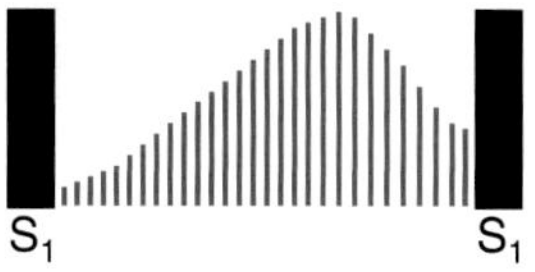

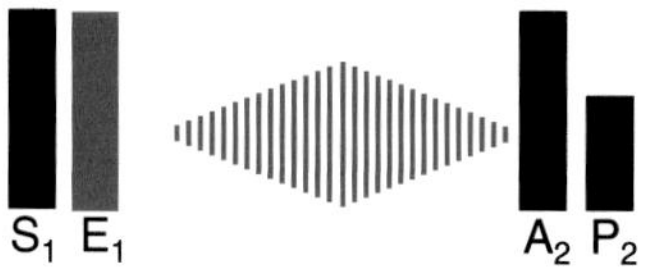

Aortic Stenosis (Otto & Prendergast, 2014)	Hypertrophic Cardiomyopathy (Ho, 2012)	Pulmonic Stenosis (Fitzgerald & Lim, 2011)
Right second intercostal space	Third and fourth left intercostal spaces	Second and third left intercostal spaces
Often to the carotids, down the left sternal border, even to the apex	Down the left sternal border to the apex, possibly to the base, but not to the neck	If loud, toward the left shoulder and neck
Sometimes soft but often loud, with a thrill	Variable	Soft to loud; if loud, associated with a thrill
Medium, harsh; crescendo–decrescendo may be higher at the apex	Medium	Medium; crescendo–decrescendo
Often harsh; may be more musical at the apex	Harsh	Often harsh
Heard best with the patient sitting and leaning forward	Decreases with squatting, increases with straining down from Valsalva maneuver and standing	
A_2 decreases as aortic stenosis worsens. A_2 may be delayed and merge with P_2 → single S_2 on expiration or paradoxical S_2 split. Carotid upstroke may be *delayed* with slow rise and small amplitude. Hypertrophied left ventricle may → *sustained* apical impulse and an S_4 from decreased compliance	S_3 may be present. An S_4 is often present at the apex (unlike mitral regurgitation). The apical impulse may be *sustained* and have two palpable components. The carotid pulse rises *quickly* unlike the pulse in aortic stenosis.	In severe stenosis, S_2 is widely split, and P_2 is diminished or inaudible. An early pulmonic ejection sound is common. May hear a right-sided S_4 Right ventricular impulse often increased in amplitude and *sustained*
Significant aortic valve stenosis impairs blood flow across the valve, causing turbulence, and increases left ventricular afterload. Causes are congenital, rheumatic, and degenerative; findings may differ with each cause. Other conditions mimic aortic stenosis without obstructing flow: *aortic sclerosis*, a stiffening of aortic valve leaflets associated with aging; a *bicuspid aortic valve*, a congenital condition that may not be recognized until adulthood; *a dilated aorta*, as in arteriosclerosis, syphilis, or Marfan syndrome; *pathologically increased flow across the aortic valve* during systole can accompany aortic regurgitation.	Massive ventricular hypertrophy is associated with unusually rapid ejection of blood from the left ventricle during systole. Outflow tract obstruction of flow may coexist. Accompanying distortion of the mitral valve may cause mitral regurgitation.	Pulmonic valve stenosis impairs flow across the valve, increasing right ventricular afterload. Congenital, usually found in children In an *atrial septal defect*, the systolic murmur from pathologically increased flow across the pulmonic valve may mimic pulmonic stenosis.

TABLE 14-13 Diastolic Murmurs

Diastolic murmurs almost always indicate heart disease. There are two basic types. *Early decrescendo diastolic murmurs* signify regurgitant flow through an incompetent semilunar valve, more commonly the aortic. *Rumbling diastolic murmurs in mid or late diastole* suggest stenosis of an atrioventricular valve, usually the mitral valve.

	Aortic Regurgitation (Babu et al., 2003; Enriquez-Sarano et al., 2009; Maganti et al., 2010; McGee, 2018)	Mitral Stenosis (Maganti et al., 2010; McGee, 2018)
	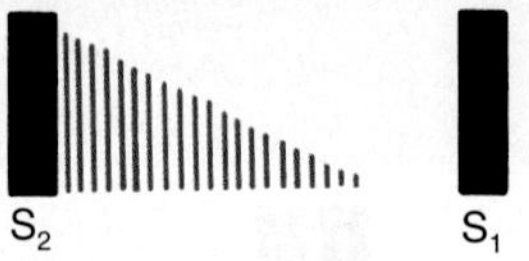	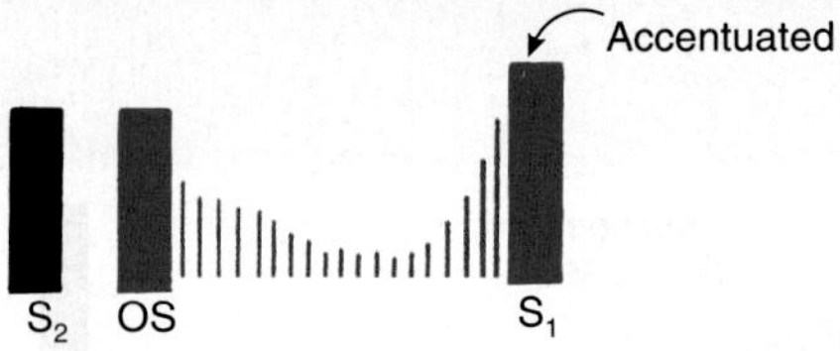
Murmur		
Location	Second to fourth left intercostal spaces	Usually limited to the apex
Radiation	If loud, to the apex, perhaps to the right sternal border	Little or none
Intensity	Grades 1–3	Grades 1–4
Pitch	High; *use the diaphragm*	High; *use the bell*
Quality	Blowing decrescendo; may be mistaken for breath sounds	Decrescendo rumble
Aids	The murmur is heard best with the *patient sitting, leaning forward*, with breath held after exhalation.	Placing the bell exactly on the apical impulse, turning the patient into a *left lateral position*, and mild exercise all help to make the murmur audible. It is heard better in exhalation.
Associated Findings	An ejection sound may be present. An S_3 or S_4, if present, suggests severe regurgitation. Progressive changes in the apical impulse include increased amplitude, displacement laterally and downward, widened diameter, and increased duration. The pulse pressure increases, and *arterial pulses are often large and bounding*. A midsystolic flow murmur or an Austin Flint murmur suggests large regurgitant flow.	S_1 is accentuated and may be palpable at the apex. An opening snap (OS) often follows S_2 and initiates the murmur. If pulmonary hypertension develops, P_2 is accentuated, and the right ventricular impulse becomes palpable. Mitral regurgitation and aortic valve disease may be associated with mitral stenosis.
Mechanism	The leaflets of the aortic valve fail to close completely during diastole, and blood regurgitates from the aorta back into the left ventricle. Volume overload on the left ventricle results. Two other murmurs may be associated: (1) a midsystolic murmur from the resulting increased forward flow across the aortic valve and (2) a mitral diastolic (*Austin Flint*) murmur, attributed to diastolic impingement of the regurgitant flow on the anterior leaflet of the mitral valve.	When the leaflets of the mitral valve thicken, stiffen, and become distorted from the effects of rheumatic fever, the *mitral valve fails to open sufficiently in diastole*. The resulting murmur has two components: (1) middiastolic (during rapid ventricular filling) and (2) presystolic (during atrial contraction). The latter disappears if atrial fibrillation develops, leaving only a middiastolic rumble.

Timing

First decide if you are hearing a *systolic murmur*, falling between S_1 and S_2, or a *diastolic murmur*, falling between S_2 and S_1. The S_1 or S_2 sounds may be hidden by a loud murmur. Palpating the carotid pulse as you listen can help you with timing. *Murmurs that coincide with the carotid upstroke are systolic.* Murmurs can be described as occurring *early, mid, late, or throughout (pan) systole or diastole.*

CLINICAL TIP
Diastolic murmurs usually indicate valvular heart disease. Systolic murmurs may indicate valvular disease but often occur when the heart valves are normal.

- Systolic murmurs are usually *midsystolic* or *pansystolic*. Late systolic murmurs may also be heard.

  - A *midsystolic murmur* (Fig. 14-43) begins after S_1 and stops before S_2. Brief gaps are audible between the murmur and the heart sounds. Listen carefully for the gap just before S_2. It is heard more easily and, if present, usually confirms the murmur as midsystolic, not pansystolic.

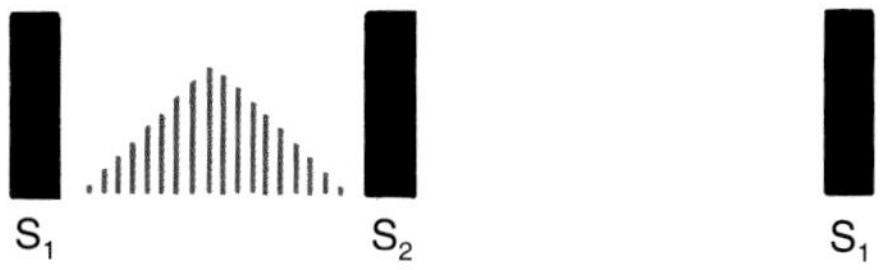

FIGURE 14-43 A midsystolic murmur.

Midsystolic murmurs typically arise from blood flow across the semilunar (aortic and pulmonic) valves. See Table 14-12, "Midsystolic Murmurs."

  - A *pansystolic (holosystolic) murmur* (Fig. 14-44) starts with S_1 and stops at S_2, without a gap between murmur and heart sounds.

FIGURE 14-44 A pansystolic (holosystolic) murmur.

Pansystolic murmurs often occur with regurgitant (backward) flow across the atrioventricular valves. See Table 14-11, "Pansystolic (Holosystolic) Murmurs."

  - A *late systolic murmur* (Fig. 14-45) usually starts in mid or late systole and persists up to S_2.

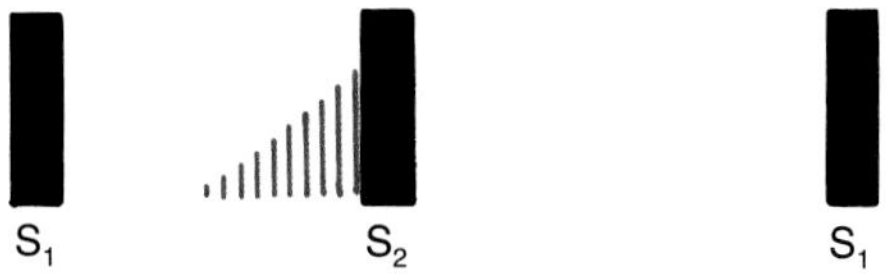

FIGURE 14-45 A late systolic murmur.

This is the murmur of mitral valve prolapse and is often but not always preceded by a systolic click.

- Diastolic murmurs may be early *diastolic*, *middiastolic*, or *late diastolic*.

  - An *early diastolic murmur* (Fig. 14-46) starts immediately after S_2 without a discernible gap and then usually fades into silence before the next S_1.

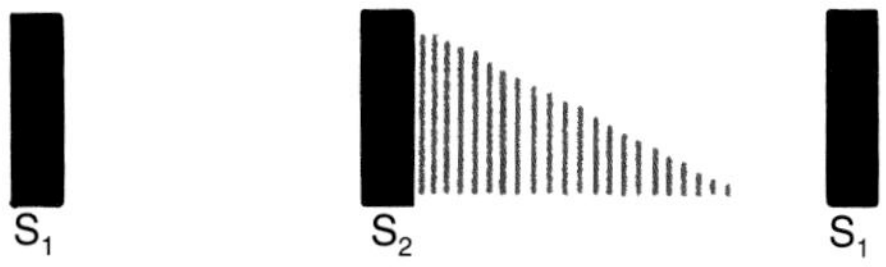

FIGURE 14-46 An early diastolic murmur.

Early diastolic murmurs typically accompany regurgitant flow across incompetent semilunar valves.

- A *middiastolic murmur* starts a short time after S_2. It may fade away in Figure 14-47, as illustrated, or merge into a late diastolic murmur.

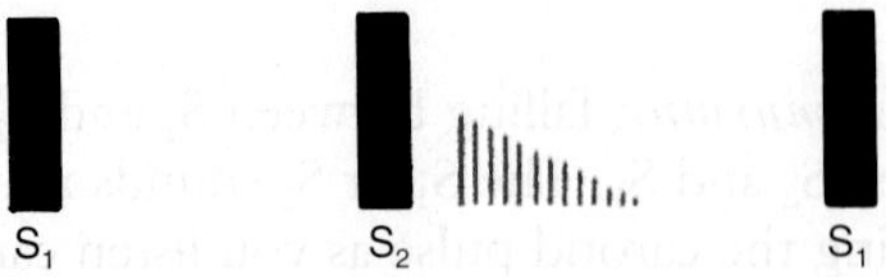

FIGURE 14-47 A middiastolic murmur.

Middiastolic and presystolic murmurs reflect turbulent flow across the atrioventricular valves. See Table 14-13, "Diastolic Murmurs."

- A *late diastolic (presystolic) murmur* (Fig. 14-48) starts late in diastole and typically continues up to S_1.

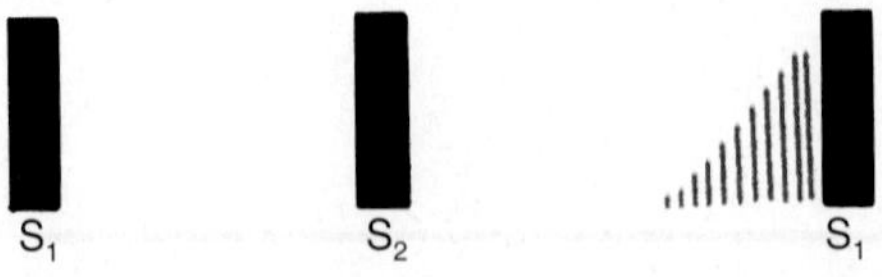

FIGURE 14-48 A late diastolic (presystolic) murmur.

The murmur of a patent ductus arteriosus starts in systole and continues into diastole without a pause, but not necessarily throughout diastole. It is called a *continuous murmur*. Other cardiovascular sounds, such as pericardial friction rubs or venous hums, have *both systolic and diastolic components* (Table 14-14). Observe and describe these sounds according to the characteristics used for systolic and diastolic murmurs.

TABLE 14-14 Cardiovascular Sounds with Both Systolic and Diastolic Components

Some cardiovascular sounds extend beyond one phase of the cardiac cycle. Three examples are: (1) a *venous hum*, a benign sound produced by turbulence of blood in the jugular veins—common in children; (2) a *pericardial friction rub*, produced by inflammation of the pericardial sac; and (3) *patent ductus arteriosus*, a congenital abnormality in which an open channel persists between the aorta and pulmonary artery. *Continuous murmurs* begin in systole and extend through S_2 into all or part of diastole, as in *patent ductus arteriosus*.

Venous Hum	Pericardial Friction Rub (Chizner, 2008; McGee, 2018)	Patent Ductus Arteriosus
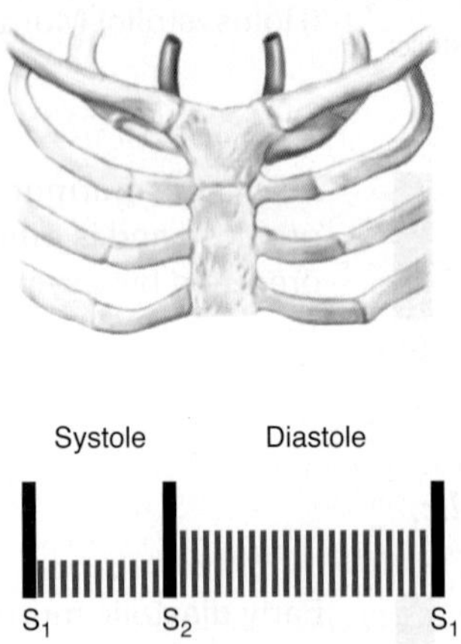	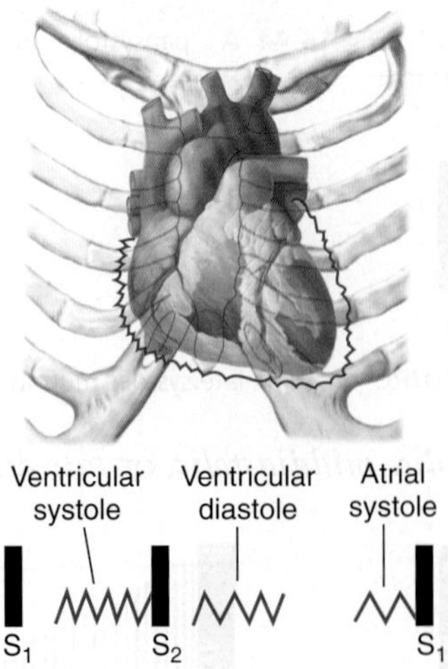	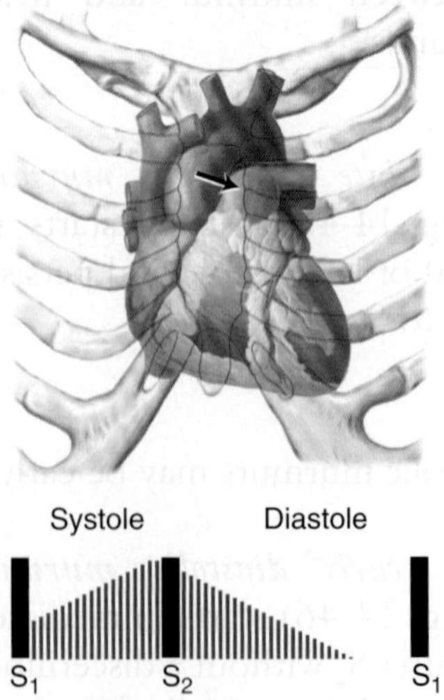

	Venous Hum	Pericardial Friction Rub (Chizner, 2008; McGee, 2018)	Patent Ductus Arteriosus
Timing	Continuous murmur without a silent interval Loudest in diastole	May have three short components, each associated with friction from cardiac movement in the pericardial sac: (1) atrial systole, (2) ventricular systole, and (3) ventricular diastole Usually the first two components are present; all three make diagnosis easy, and only one (usually the systolic) invites confusion with a murmur.	Continuous murmur in both systole and diastole, often with a silent interval late in diastole Loudest in late systole, obscures S_2, and fades in diastole
Location	Above the medial third of the clavicles, especially on the right	Variable, but usually heard best in the third interspace to the left of the sternum	Left second intercostal space
Radiation	First and second intercostal spaces	Little	Toward the left clavicle
Intensity	Soft to moderate Can be obliterated by pressure on the jugular veins	Variable May increase when the patient leans forward, exhales, and holds breath (in contrast to pleural rub)	Usually loud, sometimes associated with a thrill
Quality	Humming, roaring	Scratchy, scraping	Harsh, machinery-like
Pitch	Low (heard better with the *bell*)	High (heard better with the *diaphragm*)	Medium

Shape

The shape or configuration of a murmur is the most difficult for a novice to determine. Concentrate on learning the other characteristics of murmurs first. As your ears become attuned to listening, shape will become identifiable.

- A *crescendo murmur* grows louder (Fig. 14-49).

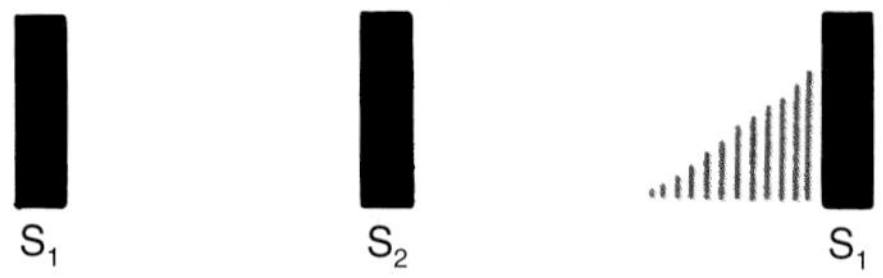

FIGURE 14-49 The late diastolic murmur of mitral stenosis in normal sinus rhythm.

- A *decrescendo murmur* grows softer (Fig. 14-50).

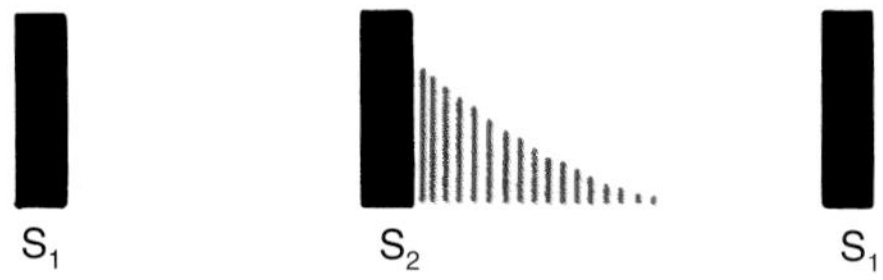

FIGURE 14-50 The early diastolic murmur of aortic regurgitation.

- A *crescendo–decrescendo murmur* (Fig. 14-51) first rises in intensity, then falls.

FIGURE 14-51 The midsystolic murmur of aortic stenosis and innocent flow murmurs.

- A *plateau murmur* has the same intensity throughout (Fig. 14-52).

FIGURE 14-52 The pansystolic murmur of mitral regurgitation.

Location of Maximal Intensity

Find the location where the murmur is heard in terms of the intercostal space and its relation to the sternum, the apex, or the midsternal, the midclavicular, or one of the axillary lines.

For example, a murmur best heard in the second right intercostal space often originates at or near the aortic valve.

Radiation or Transmission from the Point of Maximal Intensity

Radiation or transmission from the PMI reflects not only the site of origin but also the intensity of the murmur and the direction of blood flow. Explore the area around a murmur, and determine where else you can hear it.

A loud murmur of *aortic stenosis* often radiates into the neck (in the direction of arterial flow), especially on the right side.

Intensity

Intensity is usually graded on a 6-point scale and expressed as a fraction. The numerator describes the intensity of the murmur wherever it is loudest; the denominator indicates the scale you are using. Intensity is influenced by the thickness of the chest wall and the presence of intervening tissue.

An identical degree of turbulence would cause a louder murmur in a thin person than in a very muscular or obese person. Emphysematous lungs may diminish the intensity of murmurs.

Grade murmurs using the 6-point scale in Table 14-15. Note that Grades 4 through 6 require the added presence of a palpable thrill.

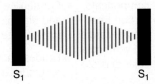

TABLE 14-15 Grades of Murmurs

Grade	Description
Grade 1	Very faint, heard only after listener has "tuned in"; may not be heard in all positions
Grade 2	Quiet, but heard immediately after placing the stethoscope on the chest
Grade 3	Moderately loud
Grade 4	Loud, with palpable thrill
Grade 5	Very loud, with thrill; may be heard when the stethoscope is partly off the chest
Grade 6	Very loud, with thrill; may be heard with stethoscope entirely off the chest

Pitch

Pitch is categorized as high, medium, or low.

Quality

Quality is described in terms such as blowing, harsh, rumbling, and musical.

A fully described murmur might be a "medium-pitched, grade 2/6, blowing decrescendo diastolic murmur, heard best in the fourth left intercostal space, with radiation to the apex" (aortic regurgitation).

Other Characteristics

Other characteristics of murmurs include variation with respiration or with the position of the patient. Document the position(s) of the patient or respiratory variation with the other characteristics.

Murmurs originating in the right side of the heart tend to vary with respiration more than left-sided murmurs.

Functional (innocent) murmurs are short, early, midsystolic murmurs that decrease in intensity with maneuvers that reduce left ventricular volume, such as standing, sitting up, and straining during the Valsalva maneuver.

Peripheral Edema

Inspect the patient's feet, ankles, and legs for edema. See Chapter 15, "The Peripheral Vascular System and Lymphatic System," for the examination techniques.

Peripheral edema may indicate heart failure.

Integrating Cardiovascular Assessment

Cardiovascular assessment requires more than careful examination. You need to correctly identify and interpret individual findings, fit them together in a logical pattern, and correlate your cardiac findings with the patient's blood pressure and heart rate, carotid upstroke and JVP, the arterial pulses, the remainder of your physical examination, and the patient's history.

For example, in a 60-year-old person with angina, you might hear a harsh 3/6 midsystolic crescendo–decrescendo murmur in the right second intercostal space radiating to the neck. These findings suggest aortic stenosis but could arise from aortic sclerosis (leaflets sclerotic but not stenotic), a dilated aorta, or increased flow across a normal valve. Assess any delay in the carotid upstroke and the intensity of A_2 for evidence of aortic stenosis. Check the apical impulse for LVH. Listen for aortic regurgitation as the patient leans forward and exhales.

Evaluating the common systolic murmur further illustrates this point. An asymptomatic teenager might have a grade 2/6 midsystolic murmur in the second and third left interspaces. Because this suggests a pulmonic murmur, you should assess the right ventricle for hypertrophy by carefully palpating the left parasternal area. Because pulmonic stenosis and atrial septal defects can cause this murmur, auscultate carefully for a split S_2, any ejection sounds, and variation with inspiration. Listen to the murmur after the patient sits up. Look for evidence of anemia, hyperthyroidism, or pregnancy that could cause such a murmur by increasing the flow across the aortic or the pulmonic valve. If all your findings are normal, your patient probably has a *functional murmur*—one with no pathologic significance.

Integrating this information allows you to generate a differential diagnosis about the origin of the murmur.

RECORDING YOUR FINDINGS

Box 14-5 includes examples of documentation that may be recorded for a cardiovascular examination.

BOX 14-5 RECORDING THE PHYSICAL EXAMINATION—THE CARDIOVASCULAR EXAMINATION

"Carotid upstrokes are brisk, without bruits. JVP is 3 cm above the sternal angle with the head of bed elevated to 30 degrees. Jugular venous distention diminishes rapidly with hepatojugular reflex. The apical impulse is 2 cm in diameter, 7 cm lateral to the midsternal line in the fifth intercostal space. S_1 and S_2 crisp with regular rhythm. At the base S_2 is $>S_1$ and at the apex S_1 is $>S_2$. No murmurs or extra sounds."

OR

"Carotid upstrokes are brisk; a bruit is heard over the left carotid artery. The JVP is 5 cm above the sternal angle with the head of bed elevated to 50 degrees. Venous distention diminishes over 10 seconds with hepatojugular reflux. The apical impulse is diffuse, 3 cm in diameter, palpated at the anterior axillary line in the fifth and sixth intercostal spaces. S_1 and S_2 are soft. S_3 presents at the apex. High-pitched harsh 2/6 holosystolic murmur best heard at the apex, radiating to the axilla."

Suggests heart failure with volume overload with partial left carotid occlusion and mitral regurgitation (Goldberg, 2010; Hunt et al., 2009; McMurray, 2010; Meyer et al., 2013).

HEALTH PROMOTION AND COUNSELING

Important topics for health promotion and counseling regarding the cardiovascular system include:

- Coronary heart disease (CHD) and stroke prevention
- Hypertension prevention and management
- Hyperlipidemia prevention and management

Key roles for the nurse in health promotion are:

- Screening patients for disease and risk factors
- Teaching patients the relationship of risk factors to diseases
- Educating patients on lifestyle changes to reduce risk factors
- Encouraging patients to adhere to healthy lifestyles and medical regimens to reduce the incidence of disease morbidity

Profile of Cardiovascular Disease

Cardiovascular disease (CVD) affects 85.6 million U.S. adults and includes hypertension, CHD, heart failure, stroke, peripheral vascular disease, and congenital cardiovascular defects. CHD remains the leading cause of death for both men and women, accounting for approximately one fourth of all U.S. deaths (CDC, 2020a).

According to the Centers for Disease Control and Prevention (CDC), hypertension is a prevalent condition, affecting 33.2% of the United States (CDC, 2021b). Uncontrolled hypertension is a risk factor for heart attack, stroke, and heart failure and a major contributing factor to cardiovascular and all-cause mortality in the United States (CDC, 2020b). Primary hypertension has no known cause and few symptoms, but it accounts for approximately 95% of adult hypertension. Box 14-6 outlines additional hypertension facts.

BOX 14-6 HYPERTENSION FACTS

- "Prevalence rates increase with age, from 7.3% in persons aged 18 to 39 years to 32.4% in those aged 40 to 59 years and to 65.0% in those aged 60 years or older. Non-Hispanic Black adults have the highest prevalence (42.1%) compared with White (28.0%), Hispanic (26.0%), and Asian Americans (24.7%)" and only 34% of those with hypertension have achieved blood pressure goals (CDC, 2019).
- For an adult 45 years of age without hypertension, the 40-year risk for developing hypertension is 93% for African Americans, 92% for Hispanic Americans, 86% for White Americans, and 84% for Chinese Americans (Whelton et al., 2018).
- Identifying and treating people with risk factors are not enough. The American Heart Association is expanding its focus beyond CVD prevention in adults to encouraging the development of healthy cardiovascular behaviors in childhood to lower the risk of developing cardiovascular disease later in adulthood (CDC, 2020a).

TABLE 14-16 Blood Pressure Classification for Adults

Category	Systolic (mm Hg)	Diastolic (mm Hg)	Recommendations
Normal blood pressure	<120	<80	Healthy lifestyle choices and yearly checks
Elevated blood pressure	120–129	<80	Healthy lifestyle changes, reassessed in 3–6 mo
High blood pressure, stage 1	130–139	80–89	10-y heart disease and stroke risk assessment; if less than 10% risk, lifestyle changes, reassessed in 3–6 mo. If higher, lifestyle changes and medication with monthly follow-ups until blood pressure is controlled.
High blood pressure, stage 2	≥140	≥90	Lifestyle changes and two different classes of medicine with monthly follow-ups until BP is controlled.
Hypertensive crisis	>180	>120	Consult Doctor immediately

Source: American Heart Association, Inc. Nearly half of U.S. adults could now be classified with high blood pressure, under new definitions. https://www.heart.org/en/news/2018/05/01/nearly-half-ofus-adults-could-now-be-classified-with-high-blood-pressure-under-new-definitions and Hypertensive crisis: When you should call 911 for high blood pressure. Retrieved May 17, 2021, from https://www.heart.org/en/health-topics/high-blood-pressure/understanding-blood-pressure-readings/hypertensive-crisis-when-you-should-call-911-for-high-blood-pressure.

Table 14-16 outlines the current blood pressure classifications for adults.

High serum cholesterol and related lipid disorders are correlated with an elevated risk for CVD in many of the world's populations (CDC, 2020c).

Diabetes and metabolic syndrome increase a person's risk for CVD. Metabolic syndrome is a group of lipid and nonlipid risk factors of metabolic origin that increases the risk of heart disease, stroke, and diabetes. It is closely linked to metabolic insulin resistance disorder (CDC, 2020c).

A client with three or more of these findings may have metabolic syndrome: (NIH, 2020)

- Large waist circumference (abdominal obesity)
  - Men: waist circumference of 40 in or more
  - Women: waist circumference of 35 in or more
- High blood pressure: 130 mm Hg or higher systolic or 85 mm Hg or higher diastolic or undergoing drug treatment
- High fasting blood sugar: Fasting glucose of 100 mg/dL or higher or being treated for high glucose
- High triglycerides: 150 mg/dL or higher or undergoing drug treatment for elevated triglycerides

- Low high-density lipoprotein (HDL; good) cholesterol or being treated with drugs
  - Men: <40 mg/dL
  - Women: <50 mg/dL

Risk Reduction

Identification of the patient's risk factors for CVD is a primary nursing function and a part of the history. The risks for cardiac disorders and hypertension overlap, as seen on the next page. The more risk factors an individual has, the greater is the chance of developing heart disease. Also, the greater the level of each risk factor, the greater is the risk (e.g., a low-density lipoprotein [LDL] cholesterol of 160 is a greater risk than a level of 135). Decreasing the number and severity of risk factors reduces the risk of developing heart disease.

Boxes 14-7 and 14-8 outline risk factors for coronary heart disease and hypertension, respectively.

BOX 14-7 CORONARY HEART DISEASE RISK FACTORS

Modifiable Risk Factors

- Diabetes
- Systolic and/or diastolic hypertension
- Elevated cholesterol and/or triglycerides
- Smoking
- Obesity
- Physical inactivity

Nonmodifiable Factors

- Increasing age
- History of cardiovascular disease
- Family history of early heart disease (younger than 55 years for men and 65 years for women)

BOX 14-8 HYPERTENSION RISK FACTORS

Modifiable Risk Factors

- Obesity
- Physical inactivity
- Smoking
- Microalbuminuria or a glomerular filtration rate of <60 mL/min
- Excess dietary sodium
- Insufficient intake of potassium
- Excess alcohol consumption

Nonmodifiable Factors

- Age
- Family history of hypertension or early CVD

Source: Centers for Disease Control and Prevention (CDC). (2020a). Heart disease facts. https://www.cdc.gov/heartdisease/facts.htm?CDC_AA_refVal=https%3A%2F%2Fwww.cdc.gov%2Fdhdsp%2Fdata_statistics%2Ffact_sheets%2Ffs_heart_disease.htm

The National Cholesterol Education Program (NCEP) wrote a report titled *Detection, Evaluation, and Treatment of High Cholesterol in Adults (Adult Treatment Panel III)* or *ATP III* that provides guidelines on how to prevent, detect, evaluate, and treat high blood cholesterol (Lipsy, 2003).

The *Eighth Report of the Joint National Committee on Prevention, Detection, Evaluation, and Treatment of High Blood Pressure (JNC-8)* describes how to prevent, detect, evaluate, and treat high blood pressure (James et al., 2014).

Risk assessment is a key element of the findings. Screening for adults should begin at 20 years, and the American Academy of Pediatrics recommends screening all children for cholesterol levels and hypertension. Adults 40 years and older should have their *10-year global risk* for heart disease estimated to help them keep their risk as low as possible (Box 14-9).

BOX 14-9 RISK FACTORS USED TO ASSESS THE 10-YEAR CORONARY HEART DISEASE RISK SCORE

- Age
- Gender
- Height, weight, waist circumference (or body mass index [BMI])
- Smoking
- History of CVD or diabetes
- Systolic and diastolic blood pressure
- Total cholesterol, LDL and HDL cholesterol
- Triglycerides
- Family history of early heart disease*

*Family is a blood-related parent, sibling, or child.
Source: Centers for Disease Control and Prevention (CDC). (2021b). National Center for Health Statistics: Hypertension. https://www.cdc.gov/nchs/fastats/hypertension.htm

CHD risk tools predict a patient's risk of suffering a heart attack or dying of heart disease over the next 10 years. For example, if the patient scores a 10% risk, it means in a group of 100 people with similar risk factors about 10 will have a heart attack or die from CHD in the next 10 years.

The American College of Cardiology and American Heart Association developed a risk tool based on the 2017 hypertension guidelines. It is available at http://www.cvriskcalculator.com/.

A more sensitive assessment tool called the Reynolds Risk Score was developed for women. This tool is based on data from both the Framingham Heart Study and the Women's Health Study from Harvard. The researchers added C-reactive protein to the risk analysis (Bassuk, 2008; Ridker et al., 2007). This tool can be found at www.reynoldsriskscore.org.

Screening for hypertension, CVD, hyperlipidemia, metabolic syndrome, and other risk factors should be carried out routinely. A suggested schedule can be found in Table 14-17; however, if a condition is present, more frequent screening is recommended. The nurse should encourage patients to obtain regular screenings (Prochaska & DiClemente, 1983).

TABLE 14-17 **Risk Factors and Screening Frequency for Adults Beginning at 20 Years**

Risk Factor	Frequency
Family history of CHD	Update regularly
Smoking status Diet Alcohol intake Physical activity	At each routine visit
Blood pressure BMI Waist circumference Pulse (to detect atrial fibrillation)	At each routine visit (at least every 2 y)
Fasting lipoprotein profile	Every 5 y if low risk; every 2 y if strong risk
Fasting glucose, HgA1C	If risk factors for hyperlipidemia or diabetes present

Source: American Heart Association. Heart health screenings. Retrieved August 23, 2020, from https://www.heart.org/en/health-topics/consumer-healthcare/what-is-cardiovascular-disease/heart-health-screenings#:~:text=An%20important%20aspect%20of%20lowering%20risk%20of%20cardiovascular,do%20you%20know%20which%20risk%20factors%20you%20have%3F

Healthy Lifestyles

Educating patients about healthy lifestyle choices and encouraging them to make changes is an important nursing role (Boxes 14-10 and 14-11). It is helpful to obtain a picture of the client's lifestyle before suggesting changes. Many patients will already include healthy choices in their lives. A nutrition history (see Chapter 8, "Nutrition and Hydration") and a "typical day" record can help the nurse identify good diet choices and where improvements can be made. Healthy choices should be affirmed. The nurse can then work with the patient to identify where further change is needed and create a mutually agreed upon change plan. The nurse can also supply resources that may help the patient achieve goals. For example, if the patient's goal is to stop smoking, the nurse can explain aids available to decrease the desire for nicotine. Prochaska and DiClemente's Stages of Change Model can be used during a patient assessment to help the nurse determine interventions appropriate to the patient's level (Prochaska & DiClemente, 1983).

BOX 14-10 LIFESTYLE MODIFICATIONS TO PREVENT OR MANAGE HYPERTENSION

- Maintenance of an optimal weight or BMI of 18.5 to 24.9
- Salt intake of <6 g of sodium chloride or 2,300 mg of sodium per day. However, individuals with hypertension, diabetes, or kidney disease, those 51 years or older or African American individuals should consume no more than 1,500 mg of sodium per day (*Healthy People 2030*).
- Regular aerobic exercise, such as brisk walking for at least 30 minutes per day most days of the week
- Moderate alcohol consumption per day of two drinks or fewer for men and one drink or fewer for women (two drinks = 1-oz ethanol, 24-oz beer, 10-oz wine, or 2- to 3-oz whiskey)
- Dietary intake of more than 3,500 mg of potassium
- Diet rich in fruits, vegetables, and low-fat dairy products with reduced content of saturated and total fat

Sources: Centers for Disease Control and Prevention (CDC). (2020, February 24). Prevent high blood pressure. https://www.CDC.gov/bloodpressure/prevent.htm; Whelton, P. K., Carey, R. M., Aronow, W. S., Casey, D. E., Collins, K. J., Himmelfarb, C. D., DePalma, S. M., Gidding, S., Jamerson, K. A., Jones, D. W., MacLaughlin, E. J., Muntner, P., Ovbiagele, B., Smith, S. C., Spencer, C. C., Stafford, R. S., Taler, S. J., Thomas, R. J., Williams, K. A., ... Wright, J. T. (2018). 2017 ACC/AHA/AAPA/ABC/ACPM/AGS/APhA/ASH/ASPC/NMA/PCNA Guideline for the Prevention, detection, evaluation, and management of high blood pressure in adults: A report of the American College of Cardiology/American Heart Association Task Force on Clinical Practice Guidelines. *Journal of the American College of Cardiology, 71*(19), e127–e248.

BOX 14-11 LIFESTYLE MODIFICATIONS TO PREVENT CARDIOVASCULAR DISEASE AND STROKE

- Complete cessation of smoking
- Optimal blood pressure control
- Healthy eating—see "Healthy Eating"
- Lipid management
- Regular aerobic exercise
- Optimal weight
- Diabetes management so that fasting glucose level is below 110 mg/dL and HgA1C is <7%
- Conversion of atrial fibrillation to normal sinus rhythm or, if chronic, anticoagulation

Sources: Hong, K. N., Fuster, V., Rosenson, R. S., Rosendorff, C., & Bhatt, D. L. (2017). How low to go with glucose, cholesterol, and blood pressure in primary prevention of CVD. *Journal of the American College of Cardiology, 70*(17), 2171–2185; Centers for Disease Control and Prevention (CDC). (2020, February 24). Prevent high blood pressure. https://www.CDC.gov/bloodpressure/prevent.htm

Healthy Eating

Begin with a nutrition history (see Chapter 8, "Nutrition and Hydration"), and then target low intake of cholesterol and total fat, especially less saturated and *trans* fats. Foods with monounsaturated fats, polyunsaturated fats, and omega-3 fatty acids in fish oils help lower blood cholesterol. Review the food sources of these healthy and unhealthy fats in Box 14-12.

BOX 14-12 FOOD SOURCES OF HEALTHY AND UNHEALTHY FATS

Healthy Fats

- *Foods high in monounsaturated fat*: nuts, such as almonds, pecans, and peanuts; sesame seeds; avocados; canola oil; olive and peanut oil; peanut butter
- *Foods high in polyunsaturated fat*: corn, safflower, cottonseed, and soybean oil; walnuts; pumpkin and sunflower seeds; soft (tub) margarine; mayonnaise; salad dressings
- *Foods high in omega-3 fatty acids*: albacore tuna, herring, mackerel, rainbow trout, salmon, sardines, anchovies, shrimp, flaxseed, walnuts

Unhealthy Fats

- *Foods high in trans fat*: snacks and baked goods with hydrogenated or partially hydrogenated oil, stick margarines, shortening, fried foods
- *Foods high in cholesterol*: dairy products, liver and organ meats, high-fat meat and poultry
- *Foods high in saturated fat*: high-fat dairy products—cream, cheese, ice cream, whole and 2% milk, butter, and sour cream; bacon; chocolate; lard and gravy from meat drippings; high-fat meats like ground beef, bologna, hot dogs, and sausage

Source: U.S. Department of Agriculture and U.S. Department of Health and Human Services. (2020, December). *Dietary Guidelines for Americans, 2020–2025* (9th ed.). Available at DietaryGuidelines.gov.

Counseling about Weight and Exercise

The 2020–2025 Dietary Guidelines for Americans reports that dietary factors are associated with CAD, hypertension, stroke, breast and colorectal cancer, diabetes, and osteoporosis. More than 74% of all Americans are now obese or overweight with a BMI of 25 or greater (U.S. Department of Agriculture and U.S. Department of Health & Human Services, 2020).

Counseling about weight has become an imperative role for nurses. Assess the patient's BMI as described in Chapter 8, "Nutrition and Hydration." Discuss the principles of healthy eating; patients who report high fat intake are more likely to accumulate body fat than are patients reporting high intake of protein and carbohydrate. Review the patient's eating habits and weight patterns within the family. Set realistic goals that will help the patient maintain healthy eating habits *for life*.

Exercise is a critical adjunct to weight control for maintaining health. *Healthy People 2030* notes only one in four adults and one in five adolescents in the United States meet physical activity guidelines for aerobic and muscle-strengthening activities. *Healthy People 2030* includes the objective, **"Increase the proportion of adults who meet the current minimum aerobic physical activity guideline needed for substantial health benefits"** (*Healthy People 2030*). To reduce the risk for CHD, counsel patients to perform aerobic exercise, or exercise that increases muscle oxygen uptake, for at least 30 minutes most days of the week. Spur motivation by emphasizing the immediate benefits to health and well-being. Deep breathing, sweating in cool temperatures, and pulse rates exceeding 60% of the maximum normal age-adjusted heart rate, or 220 minus the individual's age, are markers that help patients recognize onset of aerobic metabolism. Be sure to evaluate any cardiovascular, pulmonary, or musculoskeletal conditions that present risks before selecting an exercise regimen. The American Heart Association offers tips patients can use to incorporate exercise at www.heart.org/en/healthy-living/fitness.

Bibliography

CITATIONS

American Heart Association. (2015, July 31). Heart attack symptoms in a woman. Retrieved April 6, 2021, from https://www.heart.org/en/health-topics/heart-attack/warning-signs-of-a-heart-attack/heart-attack-symptoms-in-women

American Heart Association. (n.d.). Warning signs of a heart attack. Retrieved April 6, 2021, from https://www.heart.org/en/health-topics/heart-attack/warning-signs-of-a-heart-attack

Asgar, A. W., Mack, M. J., & Stone, G. W. (2015). Secondary mitral regurgitation in heart failure: Pathophysiology, prognosis, and therapeutic considerations. *Journal of the American College of Cardiology*, *65*, 1231.

Aurigemma, G. P., & Gasach, W. H. (2004). Diastolic heart failure. *New England Journal of Medicine*, *351*(11), 1097–1104.

Babu, A. N., Kymes, S. M., & Carpenter Fryer, S. M. (2003). Eponyms and the diagnosis of aortic regurgitation: What says the evidence? *Annals of Internal Medicine*, *138*(9), 736–742.

Bassuk, S. B. (2008). The Reynolds risk score—improving cardiovascular risk prediction in women. *AAOHN Journal*, *56*(4), 180.

Bonow, R. O. (2013). Chronic mitral regurgitation and aortic regurgitation: Have indications for surgery changed? *Journal of the American College of Cardiology*, *61*(7), 693–701.

Centers for Disease Control and Prevention (CDC). (2019). Hypertension cascade: Hypertension prevalence, treatment and control estimates among US adults aged 18 years and older applying the criteria from the American College of Cardiology and American Heart Association's 2017 Hypertension Guideline—NHANES 2013–2016. U.S. Department of Health and Human Services.

Centers for Disease Control and Prevention (CDC). (2020a). Heart disease facts. https://www.cdc.gov/heartdisease/facts.htm?CDC_AA_refVal=https%3A%2F%2Fwww.cdc.gov%2Fdhdsp%2Fdata_statistics%2Ffact_sheets%2Ffs_heart_disease.htm

Centers for Disease Control and Prevention (CDC). (2020b). High blood pressure. Know your risk for high blood pressure. Retrieved August 26, 2020, from https://www.cdc.gov/bloodpressure/risk_factors.htm

Centers for Disease Control and Prevention (CDC). (2020c). Know your risk for heart disease. Retrieved August 26, 2020, from https://www.cdc.gov/heartdisease/risk_factors.htm

Centers for Disease Control and Prevention (CDC). (2021a). National Center for Health Statistics: Heart disease. https://cdc.gov/nchs/fastats/heart-disease.htm

Centers for Disease Control and Prevention (CDC). (2021b). National Center for Health Statistics: Hypertension. https://www.cdc.gov/nchs/fastats/hypertension.htm

Chizner, M. A. (2008). Cardiac auscultation: Rediscovering the lost art. *Current Problems in Cardiology*, *33*(7), 326–408.

Chua, J., Parikh, N., & Fergusson, D. (2013). The jugular venous pressure revisited. *Cleveland Clinic Journal of Medicine*, *80*(10), 638–644.

Creager, M. A., & Loscalzo, J. (2018). Diseases of the aorta. In J. L. Jameson, et al. (Eds.), *Harrison's principles of internal medicine* (20th ed.). McGraw-Hill. Retrieved August 15, 2020, from https://accesspharmacy-mhmedical-com.uri.idm.oclc.org/content.aspx?sectionid=192030457&bookid=2129#192030487

Drazner, M. H., Rame, E., Stevenson, L. W., & Dries, D. L. (2001). Prognostic importance of elevated jugular venous pressure and a third heart sound in patients with heart failure. *New England Journal of Medicine*, *345*(8), 574–581.

Enriquez-Sarano, M., Akins, C. W., & Vahanian, A. (2009). Mitral regurgitation. *Lancet*, *373*(9672), 1382.

Fitzgerald, K. P., & Lim, M. J. (2011). The pulmonary valve. *Cardiology Clinics*, *29*, 223.

Foster, E. (2010). Mitral regurgitation due to degenerative mitral-valve disease. *New England Journal of Medicine*, *363*, 156.

Goldberg, L. R. (2010). In the clinic. Heart failure. *Annals of Internal Medicine*, *152*(11), ITC61–15.

Hayek, E., Gring, C. N., & Griffin, B. P. (2005). Mitral valve prolapse. *Lancet*, *365*, 507.

Healthy People 2030. 2030 Topics and objectives: Physical activity. U.S. Department of Health and Human Services. Retrieved January 9, 2021, from https://health.gov/healthypeople/objectives-and-data/browse-objectives/physical-activity

Ho, C. Y. (2012). Hypertrophic cardiomyopathy in 2012. *Circulation*, *125*, 1432.

Hunt, S. A., Abraham, W. T., Chin, M. H., Feldman, A. M., Francis, G. S., Ganiats, T. G., Jessup, M., Konstam, M. A., Mancini, D. M., Michl, K., Oates, J. A., Rahko, P. S., Silver, M. A., Stevenson, L. W., & Yancy, C. W. (2009). 2009 Focused guidelines for the diagnosis and management of heart failure in adults: A report of the American College of Cardiology Foundation/American Heart Association Task Force on Practice Guidelines: Developed in collaboration with the international society for heart and lung transplantation. *Circulation*, *119*(14), e391–e479.

Irwin, R. B., Luckie, M., & Khattar, R. S. (2010). Tricuspid regurgitation: Contemporary management of a neglected valvular lesion. *Postgraduate Medical Journal*, *86*(1021), 648–655.

James, P. A., Oparil, S., Carter, B. L., Cushman, W. C., Dennison-Himmelfarb, C., Handler, J., Lackland, D. T., LeFevre, M. L., MacKenzie, T. D., Ogedegbe, O., Smith, S. C. Jr, Svetkey, L. P., Taler, S. J., Townsend, R. R., Wright, J. T. Jr, Narva, A. S., & Ortiz, E. (2014). 2014 Evidence-based guideline for the management of high blood pressure in adults: Report from the panel members appointed to the Eighth Joint National Committee (JNC 8). *Journal of the American Medical Association*, *311*(5), 507.

Kari, F. A., Beyersdorf, F., & Siepe, M. (2012). Pathophysiological implications of different bicuspid aortic valve configurations. *Cardiology Research and Practice*, *2012*, 735–829.

Lange, R. A., & Hillis, L. D. (2004). Acute pericarditis. *New England Journal of Medicine*, *351*(21), 2195–2202.

Lipsy, R. J. (2003). The National Cholesterol Education Program Adult Treatment Panel III guidelines. *Journal of Managed Care Pharmacy*, *9*(1 Suppl), 2–5.

Maganti, K., Rigolin, V. H., Sarano, M. E., & Bonow, R. O. (2010). Valvular heart disease: Diagnosis and management. *Mayo Clinic Proceedings*, *85*(5), 483–500.

McGee, S. (2018). Palpation of the heart. In *Evidence-based physical diagnosis* (4th ed.). Saunders.

McMurray, J. J. (2010). Systolic heart failure. *New England Journal of Medicine*, *362*, 228–238.

Meyer, T., Shih, J., & Aurigemma, G. (2013). In the clinic. Heart failure with preserved ejection fraction (diastolic dysfunction). *Annals of Internal Medicine*, *158*(1), ITC5-1–ITC5-15.

Mutlak, D., Aronson, D., & Lessick, J., (2009). Functional tricuspid regurgitation in patients with pulmonary hypertension: is pulmonary artery pressure the only determinant of regurgitation severity? *Chest*, *135*(1), 115–121.

National Institutes of Health (NIH), National Heart, Lung and Blood Institute. (2020). Metabolic syndrome. Retrieved August 20, 2020, from https://www.nhlbi.nih.gov/health-topics/metabolic-syndrome

O'Gara, P. T., & Loscalzo, J. (2018). Physical examination of the cardiovascular system. In J. L. Jameson, et al. (Eds.), *Harrison's principles of internal medicine* (20th ed.). McGraw-Hill. Retrieved August 14, 2020, from https://accesspharmacy-mhmedical-com.uri.idm.oclc.org/content.aspx?bookid=2129&sectionid=186950064

Otto, C. M., & Prendergast, B. (2014). Aortic-valve stenosis-from patients at risk to severe valve obstruction. *New England Journal of Medicine*, *371*(8), 744–756.

Prochaska, J. O., & DiClemente, C. C. (1983). Stages and processes of self-change in smoking: Towards an integrative model of change. *Journal of Consulting and Clinical Psychology*, *51*(3), 390–395.

Ridker, P. M., Buring, J. E., Rifai, N., & Cook, N. R. (2007). Development and validation of improved algorithms for the assessment of global cardiovascular risk in women. *Journal of the American Medical Association*, *297*(6), 611–619.

Shah, S. J., Marcus, G. M., Gerber, I. L., McKeown, B. H., Vessey, J. C., Jordan, M. V., Huddleston, M., Foster, E., Chatterjee, K., & Michaels, A. D. (2008). Physiology of the third heart sound: Novel insights from tissue Doppler imaging. *Journal of the American Society of Echocardiography*, *21*(4), 394–400.

Shah, S. J., & Michaels, A. D. (2006). Hemodynamic correlates of the third heart sound and systolic time intervals. *Congest Heart Fail*, *12*(Suppl 1), 8–13.

Shah, S. J., Nakamura, K., Marcus, G. M., Gerber, I. L., McKeown, B. H., Jordan, M. V., Huddleston, M., Foster, E., & Michaels, A. D. (2008). Association of the fourth heart sound with increased left ventricular end-diastolic stiffness. *Journal of Cardiac Failure*, *14*(5), 431–436.

Siu, S. C., & Silversides, C. K. (2010). Bicuspid aortic valve disease. *Journal of the American College of Cardiology*, *55*, 2789.

Spodick, D. H. (1996). Normal sinus heart rate: Appropriate rate thresholds for sinus tachycardia and bradycardia. *Southern Medical Journal*, *89*, 666.

Topilsky, Y., Michelena, H., Bichara, V., Maalouf, J., Mahoney, D. W., & Enriquez-Sarano, M. (2012). Mitral valve prolapse with mid-late systolic mitral regurgitation: Pitfalls of evaluation and clinical outcome compared with holosystolic regurgitation. *Circulation*, *125*(13), 1643–1651.

U.S. Department of Agriculture and U.S. Department of Health and Human Services. (2020, December). *Dietary Guidelines for Americans, 2020–2025* (9th ed.). Available at DietaryGuidelines.gov.

Vinayak, A. G., Levitt, J., Gehlbach, B., Pohlman, A. S., Hall, J. B., & Kress, J. P. (2006). Usefulness of the external jugular vein examination in detecting abnormal central venous pressure in critically ill patients. *Archives of Internal Medicine*, *166*(19), 2132–2137.

Whelton, P. K., Carey, R. M., Aronow, W. S., Casey, D. E., Collins, K. J., Himmelfarb, C. D., DePalma, S. M., Gidding, S., Jamerson, K. A., Jones, D. W., MacLaughlin, E. J., Muntner, P., Ovbiagele, B., Smith, S. C., Spencer, C. C., Stafford, R. S., Taler, S. J., Thomas, R. J., Williams, K. A., ... Wright, J. T. (2018). 2017 ACC/AHA/AAPA/ABC/ACPM/AGS/APhA/ASH/ASPC/NMA/PCNA Guideline for the prevention, detection, evaluation, and management of high blood pressure in adults: A report of the American College of Cardiology/American Heart Association Task Force on Clinical Practice Guidelines. *Journal of the American College of Cardiology*, *71*(19), e127–e248.

ADDITIONAL REFERENCES

Bouthillet, K. (2020). Atypical presentation of myocardial infarction. *American Nurse Today*, *14*(7), 13.

Jameson, J. L., Fauci, A. S., Kasper, D. L., Hauser, S. L., Longo, D. L., & Loscalzo, J. (2018). *Harrison's principles of internal medicine* (20th ed.). McGraw-Hill Medical.

McSweeney, J., Cleves, M. A., Fischer, E. P., Moser, D. K., Wei, J., Pettey, C., Rojo, M. O., & Armbya, N. (2014). Predicting coronary heart disease events in women: A longitudinal cohort study. *Journal of Cardiovascular Nursing*, *29*(6), 482–492.

Ritchie, S. K., Murphy, E. C., Ice, C., Cottrell, L. A., Minor, V., Elliott, E., & Neal, W. (2010). Universal versus targeted blood cholesterol screening among youth: The CARDIAC project. *Pediatrics*, *126*(2), 260–265.

Wenger, N. K. (2012). Women and coronary heart disease: A century after Herrick: Understudied, underdiagnosed, and undertreated. *Circulation*, *126*(5), 604–611.

15 THE PERIPHERAL VASCULAR SYSTEM AND LYMPHATIC SYSTEM

KEY TERMS

atheroma	edema	pulmonary embolism (PE)
atherosclerosis	lymphadenopathy	venous insufficiency
claudication	lymphedema	venous thromboembolism (VTE)
deep vein thrombosis (DVT)	peripheral arterial disease (PAD)	

Learning Objectives

The student will:

1. Describe the structure and functions of arteries, veins, and lymph vessels and nodes.
2. Obtain a history of the peripheral vascular system.
3. Describe the equipment necessary to perform a peripheral vascular examination.
4. Appropriately prepare and position the patient for the peripheral vascular examination.
5. Identify the locations of and palpate the peripheral pulses for rate, rhythm, and amplitude.
6. Evaluate and interpret variations in pulse rhythm, rate, and amplitude.
7. Discuss risk reduction and health promotion strategies to prevent peripheral vascular disease.

Careful assessment of the peripheral vascular system is essential for detection of **peripheral arterial disease (PAD)**, which is the narrowing or blockage of the vessels that carry blood from the heart to the extremities. PAD is primarily caused by the buildup of fatty plaque in the arteries, which is called **atherosclerosis**. PAD can happen in any blood vessel, but it is more common in those of the legs than those of the arms.

In the United States, PAD affects roughly 8.5 million (7.2%) of the population over age 40 (Virani et al., 2020). Only about 10% of these individuals exhibited the classic symptom of intermittent **claudication**, a cramping pain that limits movement of the legs or arms during exercise. Approximately 40% do not report leg pain, and the remaining 50% have a variety of leg symptoms other than classic claudication. Prevalence increases with age, rising to 22.7% in American adults 80 years of age and older versus 1.6% among those 40 to 50 years of age (Virani et al., 2020). Detection is important because PAD is both a marker for cardiovascular morbidity and mortality, as well as a harbinger of functional decline. Risk of death from myocardial infarction and stroke triples in adults with PAD. PAD is defined by the American Heart Association as stenotic, occlusive, and aneurysmal disease of the aorta, its visceral arterial branches, and the arteries of the lower extremities, but not the coronary arteries.

Venous thromboembolism (VTE) is a disorder that includes deep vein thrombosis (DVT) and pulmonary embolism (PE). A **deep vein thrombosis (DVT)** occurs when a blood clot forms in a deep vein, accompanied by an inflammatory response in the vein wall. DVTs usually occur in the lower leg, thigh, or pelvis. Thrombi in the superficial veins are usually a response to vessel injury and rarely cause complications. DVTs in the upper extremities frequently reflect complications from the placement of central venous catheters, cardiac pacemakers, and defibrillators (Kucher, 2011). DVTs in the lower extremities put a patient at risk for **pulmonary embolism (PE)**, when a clot breaks loose and travels through the bloodstream to the lungs.

CLINICAL TIP

Dislodgement of the thrombus produces an *embolus* that can travel to the lungs, causing a pulmonary embolism, which blocks blood flow to the lungs, a life-threatening emergency because it impairs oxygenation.

Chronic **venous insufficiency** is caused by incompetent vein valves secondary to DVT or prolonged increased venous pressure as seen in prolonged standing or pregnancy. This can lead to varicose veins and skin changes.

ANATOMY AND PHYSIOLOGY

Arteries

Arteries contain three concentric layers of tissue: the *intima*, the *media*, and the *adventitia* (or the externa). The *internal elastic membrane* borders the intima and the media; the *external elastic membrane* separates the media from the adventitia (Fig. 15-1).

Atherosclerosis is a chronic inflammatory disease initiated by injury to vascular endothelial cells, provoking atheromatous plaque formation and the vascular lesions of hypertension.

The innermost layer of all blood vessels is the *intima*, a single continuous lining of the endothelial cells, which synthesize regulators of clotting, modulate blood flow through synthesis of vasoconstrictors and vasodilators, and regulate immune and inflammatory reactions.

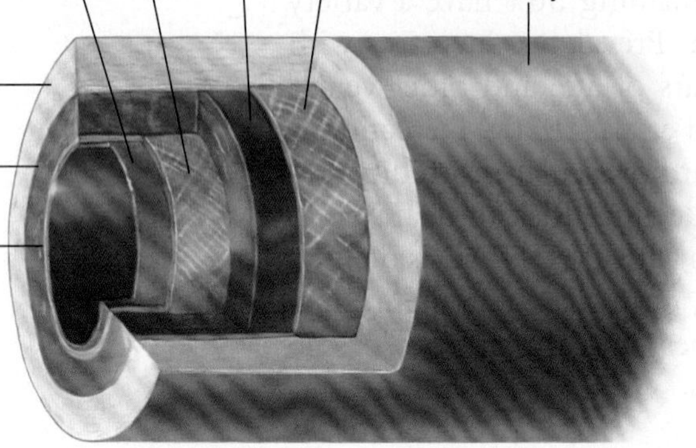

FIGURE 15-1 Anatomy of the artery.

An **atheroma** is a fatty thickening in the walls of arteries (Fig. 15-2). It begins in the intima as lipid-filled foam cells, then fatty streaks. Complex atheromas are thickened asymmetric plaques that narrow the lumen, reducing blood flow, and weaken the underlying media. They have a soft lipid core and a fibrous cap of smooth muscle cells and a collagen-rich matrix. Plaque rupture may precede thrombosis formation and lead to arterial occlusions in peripheral coronary or cerebral arteries (Mitchell, 2015).

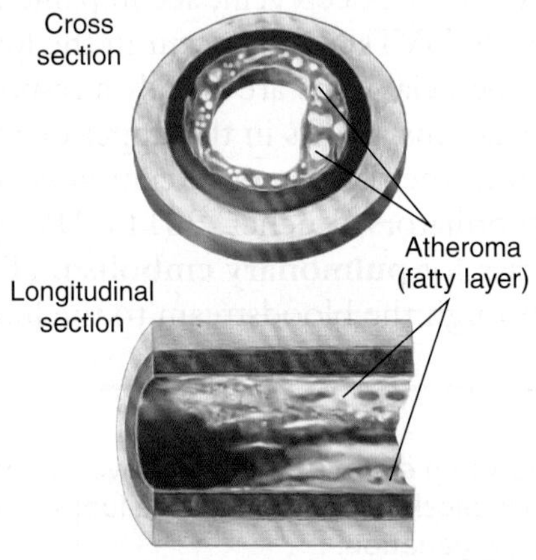

FIGURE 15-2 An atherosclerotic artery.

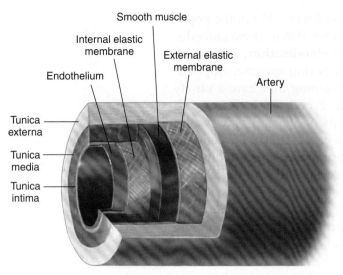

The *media* is composed of smooth muscle cells that dilate and constrict to accommodate blood pressure and flow. Its inner and outer boundaries are membranes of elastic fibers, or *elastin*, called *internal and external elastic laminae*. Small arterioles called the *vasa vasorum* perfuse the media. The outer layer of the artery is the *adventitia*, connective tissue containing nerve fibers and the vasa vasorum.

Arteries must respond to the variations that cardiac systole and diastole generate in cardiac output. Their anatomy and sizes vary according to their distance from the heart. The aorta and its immediate branches are large, highly elastic arteries such as the pulmonary, common carotid, and iliac arteries. These arteries course into *medium-sized muscular arteries* like the coronary and renal arteries. The elastic recoil and smooth muscle contraction and relaxation in the media of large and medium arteries propagate arterial pulsatile flow. Medium-sized arteries divide into *small arteries* less than 2 mm in diameter and even smaller *arterioles* with diameters from 20 to 100 micrometers (μm) or microns. Resistance to blood flow occurs primarily in the arterioles. Resistance is inversely proportional to the vessel radius. From the arterioles, blood flows into the vast network of *capillaries.* The diameter of each capillary is only 7 to 8 μm, the same diameter as a single red blood cell. Capillaries have an endothelial cell lining but no media, facilitating rapid diffusion of oxygen and carbon dioxide.

Arterial pulses are palpable in arteries lying close to the body surface. In the arms (Fig. 15-3), note pulsations in:

- the *brachial artery* at the bend of the elbow just medial to the biceps tendon.
- the *radial artery* on the lateral flexor surface.
- the *ulnar artery* on the medial flexor surface, though overlying tissues may obscure the ulnar artery.

Two vascular arches within the hand interconnect the radial and ulnar arteries, doubly protecting circulation to the hand and fingers against possible arterial occlusion.

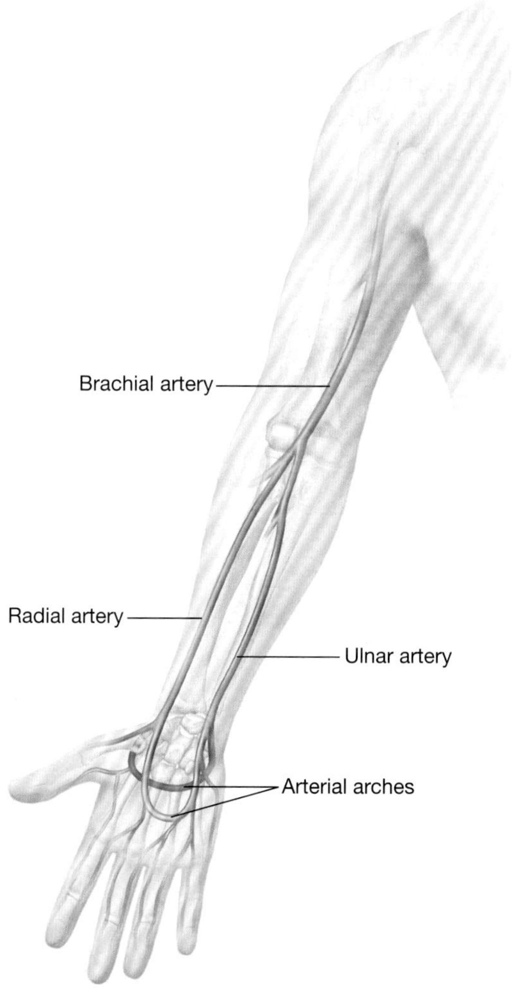

FIGURE 15-3 Arteries of the arm.

In the legs (Fig. 15-4), palpate pulsations in:

- the *femoral artery* just below the inguinal ligament, midway between the anterior superior iliac spine and the symphysis pubis.
- the *popliteal artery*, an extension of the femoral artery that passes medially behind the femur, palpable just behind the knee. The popliteal artery divides into the two arteries perfusing the lower leg and foot, namely:
  - The *dorsalis pedis artery* on the dorsum of the foot just lateral to the extensor tendon of the big toe.
  - The *posterior tibial artery* behind the medial malleolus of the ankle. An interconnecting arch between its two chief arterial branches protects circulation to the foot.

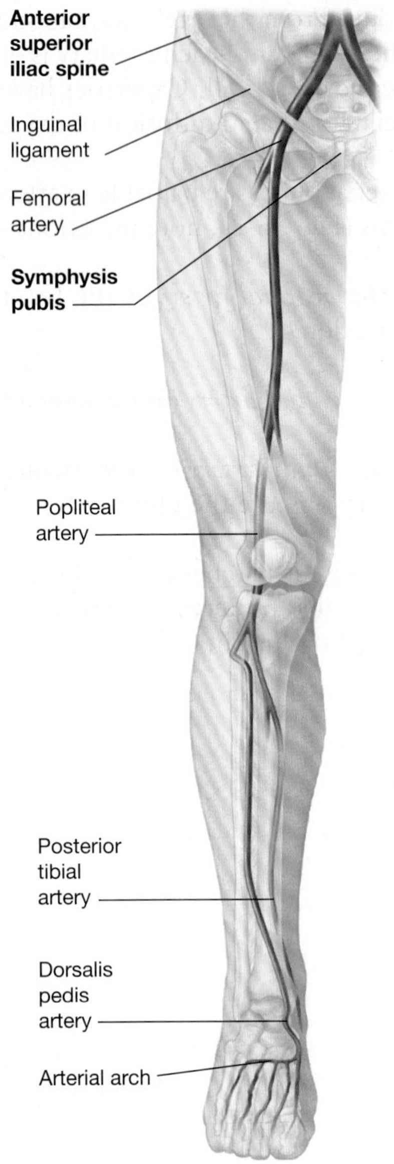

FIGURE 15-4 Arteries of the leg.

Veins

Unlike arteries, veins are thin-walled and highly distensible with a capacity for up to two thirds of circulating blood flow. The *venous intima* consists of nonthrombogenic endothelium. Protruding into the lumen are valves that promote unidirectional venous return to the heart. The *media* contains circumferential rings of elastic tissue and smooth muscle that change vein diameter in response to even minor changes in venous pressure (Mitchell, 2015). The smallest veins, or *venules*, drain capillary beds. Figure 15-5 illustrates differences between the structures of the artery and vein.

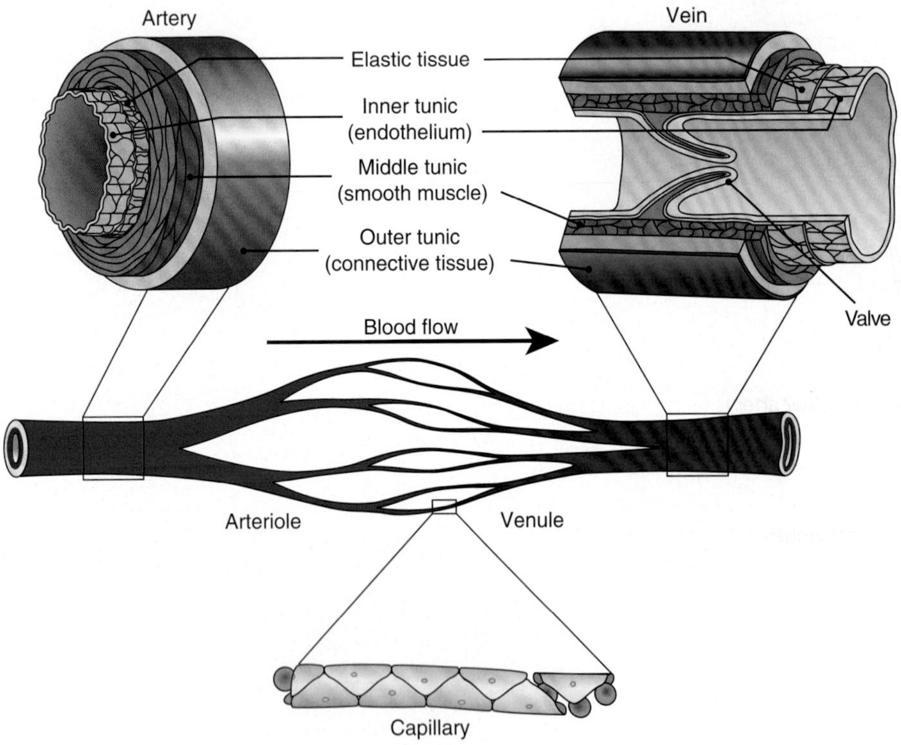

FIGURE 15-5 Differences in the structures of the artery and the vein.

Veins from the arms, upper trunk, and head and neck drain into the *superior vena cava*, which empties into the right atrium. Veins from the legs and lower trunk drain upward into the *inferior vena cava*. Because of their weaker wall structure, the leg veins are susceptible to irregular dilatation (varicosities), compression, ulceration, and invasion by tumors; they therefore warrant special attention.

The *deep veins* of the legs carry approximately 90% of the venous return from the lower extremities. They are well supported by surrounding tissues.

In contrast, the *superficial veins* (Fig. 15-6) are subcutaneous with relatively poor tissue support. They include:

- The *great saphenous vein,* which originates on the dorsum of the foot, passes just anterior to the medial malleolus, continues up the medial aspect of the leg, and joins the femoral vein of the deep venous system below the inguinal ligament
- The *small saphenous vein,* which begins at the side of the foot, passes upward along the posterior calf, and joins the deep venous system in the popliteal fossa

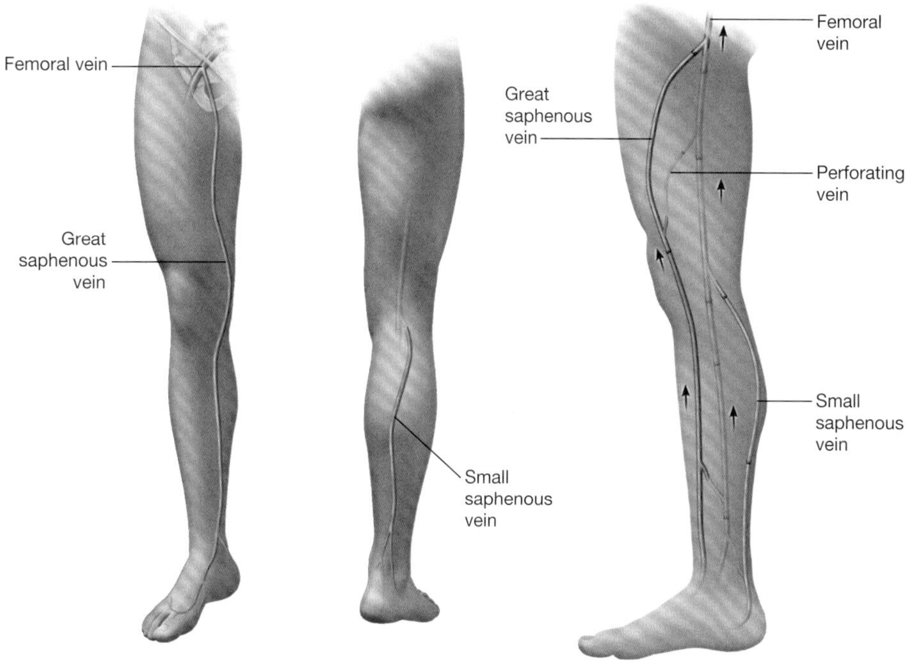

FIGURE 15-6 Veins of the leg from the front, back, and medial aspect.

Anastomotic veins connect the two saphenous veins that are readily visible when dilated. Bridging or *perforating* veins connect the superficial system with the deep system.

When competent, the one-way valves of the deep, superficial, and perforating veins propel blood toward the heart, preventing pooling, venous stasis, and backward flow. Contraction of the calf muscles during walking also serves as a venous pump, propelling blood upward against gravity.

The Lymphatic System and Lymph Nodes

The lymphatic system (Fig. 15-7) is an extensive vascular network that drains lymph fluid from body tissues and returns it to the venous circulation. The system starts peripherally as blind lymphatic capillaries; continues centrally as thin vascular channels, then collecting ducts; and empties into the major veins at the neck. The *right lymphatic duct* drains fluid from the

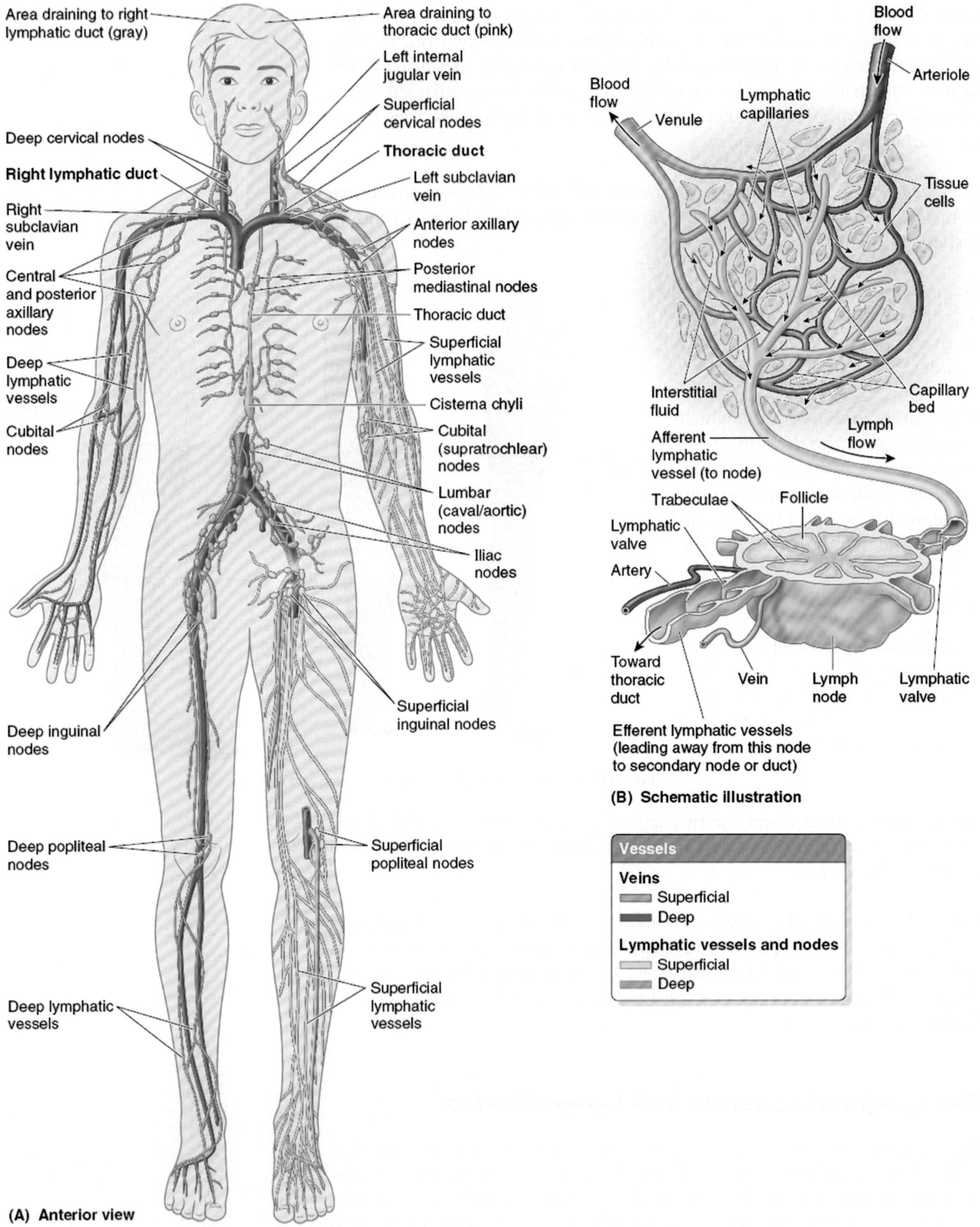

FIGURE 15-7 The lymphatic system and lymph nodes.

right side of the head, neck, thorax, and right upper limb and empties into the junction of the right internal jugular and the right subclavian veins. The *thoracic duct* collects lymph fluid from the rest of the body and empties into the junction of the left internal jugular and the left subclavian veins. Lymph fluid transported through these channels is filtered through lymph nodes interposed along the way.

Lymph nodes are round, oval, or bean-shaped structures that vary in size according to their location. Some lymph nodes, such as the preauricular nodes, if palpable at all, are typically very small. The inguinal nodes, in contrast, are relatively larger—often 1 cm in diameter and occasionally even 2 cm in an adult.

In addition to its vascular functions, the lymphatic system plays an important role in the body's immune system. Cells within the lymph nodes engulf cellular debris and bacteria and produce antibodies.

Only the superficial lymph nodes are accessible to physical examination. These include the head and cervical nodes (see Chapter 10), the clavicular nodes, the axillary nodes, and the epitrochlear and inguinal nodes.

The axillary lymph nodes drain most of the arm (Fig. 15-8). Lymphatics from the ulnar surface of the forearm and hand, the little and ring fingers, and the adjacent surface of the middle finger, however, drain first into the *epitrochlear nodes.* These are located on the medial surface of the arm approximately 3 cm above the elbow. Lymphatics from the rest of the arm drain mostly into the axillary nodes. A few may go directly to the infraclavicular nodes.

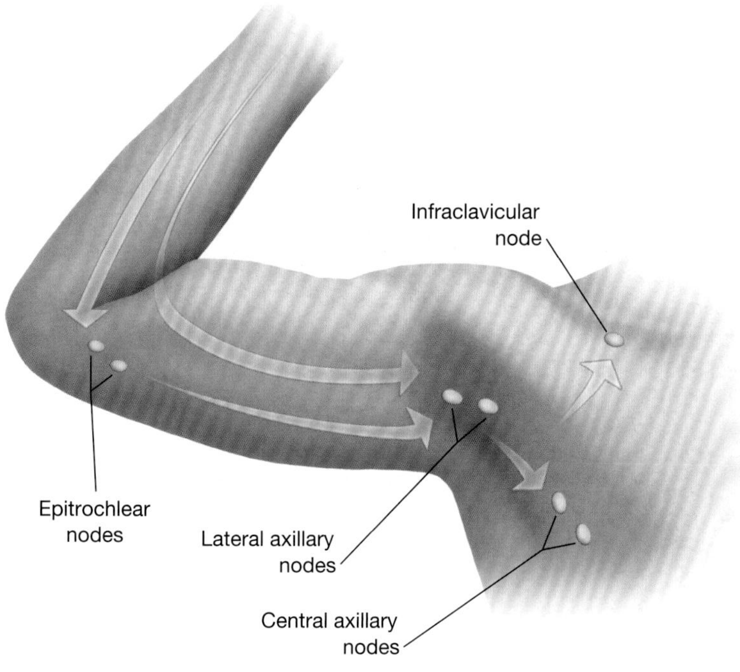

FIGURE 15-8 The lymph nodes of the arm.

The lymphatics of the lower limb follow the veins and consist of both deep and superficial systems. Only the superficial nodes are palpable. The *superficial inguinal nodes* include two groups (Fig. 15-9). The *horizontal group* lies in a chain high in the anterior thigh below the inguinal ligament. It drains the superficial portions of the lower abdomen and buttock, the external genitalia (but not the testes), the anal canal and perianal area, and the lower vagina. The *vertical group* clusters near the upper part of the saphenous vein and drains a corresponding region of the leg.

In contrast, lymphatics from the heel and outer aspect of the foot join the deep system at the level of the popliteal space. Lesions in this area, therefore, are not usually associated with palpable inguinal lymph nodes.

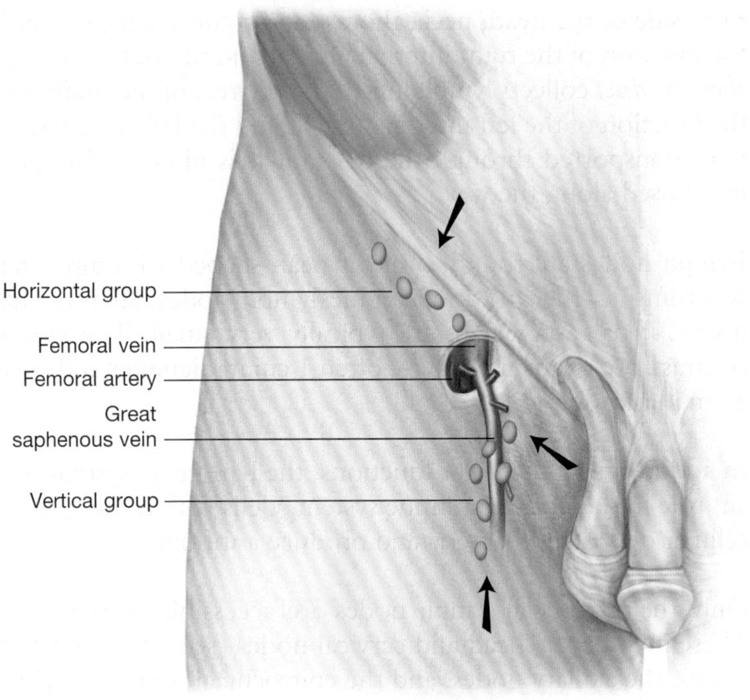

FIGURE 15-9 The superficial inguinal lymph nodes.

Fluid Exchange and the Capillary Bed

Blood circulates from arteries to veins through the capillary bed (Fig. 15-10). Here fluids diffuse across the capillary membrane, maintaining a dynamic equilibrium between the vascular and interstitial spaces. Most filtered fluid returns to the circulation not as fluid resorbed at the venous end of the capillaries, but as lymph through the lymphatic system (Braunwald & Loscalzo, 2018).

Lymphatic dysfunction or disturbances in capillary bed fluid exchange commonly result in **edema**, the presence of excess fluid in the interstitial spaces. Four mechanisms produce edema: (1) increased plasma volume from sodium retention; (2) increased capillary membrane permeability caused by burns, snake bites, angioedema, or allergic reactions; (3) low plasma protein levels (creating low colloid osmotic pressure) caused by renal disorders; and (4) blockage or inadequate removal of lymphatic fluid as seen in lymph node removal. This is termed as **lymphedema** and is usually nonpitting.

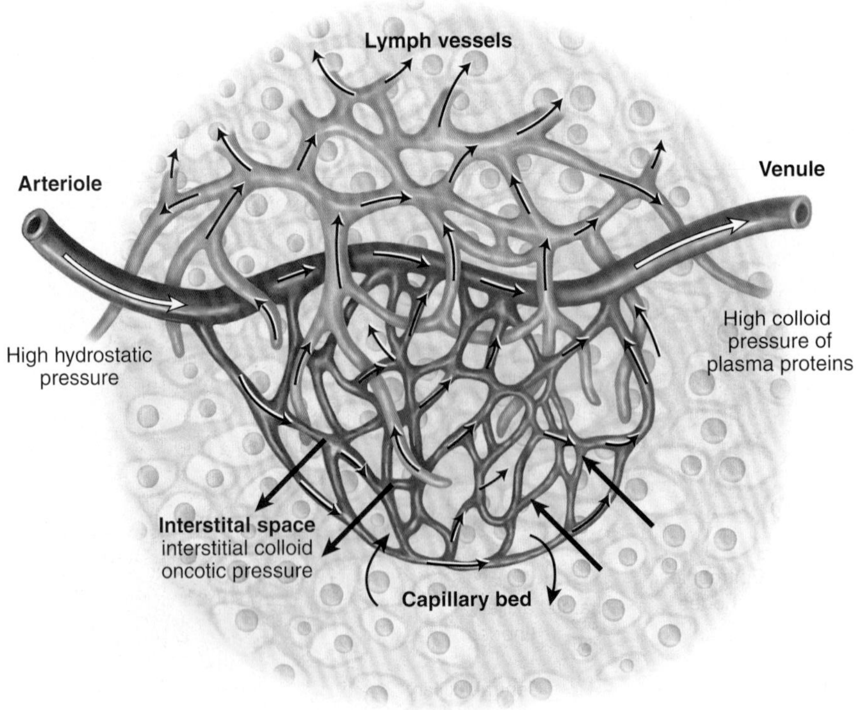

FIGURE 15-10 Capillary fluid exchange.

Edema may be pitting or nonpitting. In pitting edema, the interstitial water is mobile and can be translocated with the pressure exerted by a finger. A "pit," or depression, is left for 5 to 30 seconds. The degree of pitting is measured on a 1-to-4 scale (Table 15-1).

TABLE 15-1 Degree of Pitting Edema

Scale	Depression (mm)
1+	2
2+	4
3+	6
4+	8

Nonpitting edema reflects a condition in which serum proteins have accumulated in the interstitial space with the water and coagulated. This is frequently seen with local infection or trauma and is called brawny edema.

THE HEALTH HISTORY

The purpose of the history questions is to identify symptoms of peripheral arterial and venous disease. Common or concerning symptoms identified in the health history of the peripheral vascular system are listed in Box 15-1.

BOX 15-1 COMMON OR CONCERNING SYMPTOMS

- Pain in the arms or legs
- Intermittent claudication
- Cold, numbness, or pallor in the legs; hair loss
- Swelling in the calves, legs, or feet
- Swelling with redness or tenderness

Because most patients with peripheral vascular diseases report minimal symptoms, asking specifically about the symptoms that follow is recommended, especially in patients older than 50 and those with risk factors, like smoking, diabetes, hypertension, elevated cholesterol, and/or coronary artery disease (CAD). Questions may include:

- Do you have pain or cramping in your legs during walking or exertion? (This is termed *intermittent claudication.*)
  - Is it relieved by rest within 10 minutes?
  - Where is the pain felt? How far can you walk before the pain occurs?
- Do you have coldness or numbness in your legs or feet? Are your feet pale?
- Do you have hair on your shins?

These symptoms are caused by insufficient arterial supply to the legs, which may be caused by atherosclerosis.

- Do you have aching or pain at rest in the lower leg or foot? Is the pain alleviated by elevating the legs?
- Do you have fatigue or aching in the lower legs with prolonged standing?
- Do you have swelling of the feet or legs? If present, identify:

Edema, varicose veins, and aching in the legs are symptoms of venous stasis.

  - Where is the pain located?
  - What time of day it is present?
  - Is it bilateral or unilateral?
  - Does the swelling decrease after raising your legs?
  - Do you have any varicose veins?
    - Where are they located?
    - How long have they been present?
    - Do you have any discomfort from them?
- Do you have any wounds of the legs or feet that will not heal or heal very slowly?

Ulcers may be of venous or arterial origin.

  - Where is the wound located?
  - How long have you had the wound?
  - Did anything cause the wound (e.g., an injury)?
- Do your fingertips or toes change color in cold weather?

In Raynaud disease, the small arteries in the fingers and toes spasm in response to cold or stress causing them to become blue and numb. It is also known as Raynaud phenomenon or syndrome.

- Have you experienced erectile dysfunction?

Poor blood supply to the penile arteries can cause erectile dysfunction.

- Do you have abdominal pain after meals? Does it prevent you from eating?

Atherosclerosis of the mesenteric or celiac arteries can cause intestinal ischemia, producing abdominal pain and "food fear," where the patient is fearful of eating.

- Do you have tender or swollen lymph nodes (glands)?

Swollen nodes may indicate an infection or tumor.

Past History

When taking the patient's past history, explore the following topics:

- Medications, especially oral contraceptives or hormone replacement therapy

Estrogen use and pregnancy increase one's risk for blood clots.

- Pregnancy or recent childbirth
- Inflammatory diseases such as lupus, rheumatoid arthritis, or irritable bowel disease

Inflammation contributes to clot formation.

- Active cancer
- CAD

CAD and cerebral artery disease are also caused by atherosclerosis; an individual with either is at risk for PAD.

- Heart attack
- Congestive heart failure
- Stroke (cerebral arterial disease)
- Clotting disorders
- Hypertension
- Diabetes
- Problems in circulation, such as blood clots, leg ulcers, swelling, or poor healing of wounds
- Major surgery or fracture of a long bone in the last 4 weeks

Risk Factors

Risk factors to consider include:

- Obesity
- Smoking
- Hyperlipidemia
- Constrictive clothing
- Central venous lines

Family History

Topics for review of family history include:

- Peripheral vascular disease
- Varicose veins
- Abdominal aortic aneurysm (AAA)
- CAD
- Sudden death younger than 60 years of age
- Diabetes

Lifestyle or Health Patterns

Lifestyle and health patterns to discuss include:

- Prolonged standing or sitting (sedentary/stationary job, long-distance travel)
- Sedentary lifestyle
- Decreased mobility such as paralysis or cast

PHYSICAL EXAMINATION

Equipment needed for a physical examination of the peripheral vascular system include:

- Tape measure
- Doppler ultrasound device
- Tourniquet or blood pressure cuff

Important Areas of Examination

The upper and lower extremity areas of examination are outlined in Table 15-2.

TABLE 15-2 Areas of Examination

The Arms	The Legs
• Size, symmetry, skin color • Radial pulse, brachial • Epitrochlear lymph nodes	• Size, symmetry, skin color, tenderness • Femoral pulse and inguinal lymph nodes • Popliteal, dorsalis pedis, and posterior tibial pulses • Peripheral edema

The American College of Cardiology and the American Heart Association have urged close examination of the peripheral vascular system because PAD is often asymptomatic and underdiagnosed, leading to significant morbidity and mortality (Gerhard-Herman et al., 2017).

Arms

Inspection

Inspect both arms from the fingertips to the shoulders. Note:

1. Their size, symmetry, and any edema and lesions

Lymphedema of the arm and hand may follow axillary node dissection and radiation therapy.

2. The venous pattern

Prominent veins in an edematous arm suggest venous obstruction, such as a DVT.

3. The color of the skin and nail beds and the texture of the skin (Fig. 15-11)

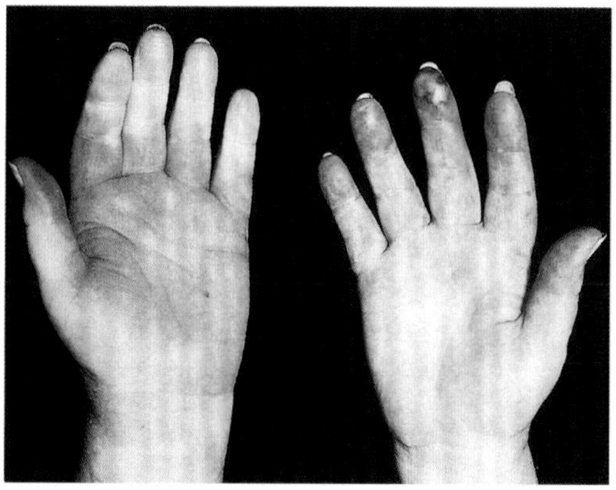

FIGURE 15-11 Skin color of the hands. (From Effeney, D. J., & Stoney, R. J. [1993]. *Wylie's atlas of vascular surgery: Disorders of the extremities.* Lippincott Williams & Wilkins.)

Palpation

Palpate the temperature of the arms and hands simultaneously with the backs of your fingers. Compare the temperature of the arms simultaneously.

Palpate the radial pulse with the pads of your fingers on the flexor surface of the wrist laterally (Fig. 15-12). Partially flexing the patient's wrist may help you feel this pulse. Compare the pulses in both arms. Pulses may be palpated simultaneously to facilitate comparison.

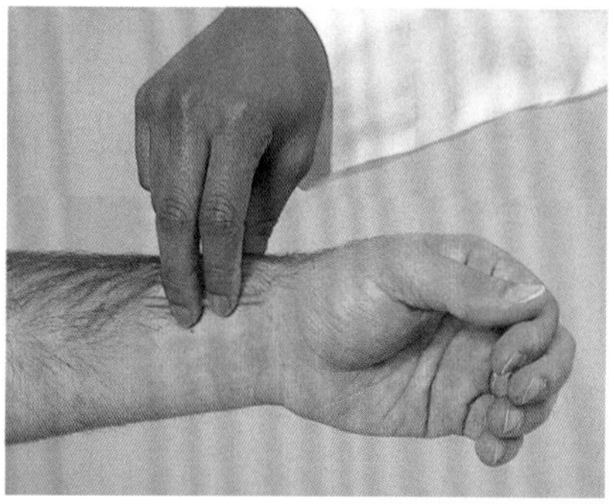

FIGURE 15-12 Palpating the radial pulse.

CLINICAL TIP

In Raynaud disease, wrist pulses are typically normal, but spasm of more distal arteries causes episodes of sharply demarcated pallor of the fingers (see Table 15-3, "Painful Peripheral Vascular Disorders and Their Mimics").

TABLE 15-3 Painful Peripheral Vascular Disorders and Their Mimics

Problem	Process	Location of Pain
Arterial Disorders		
Peripheral Arterial Disease	Atherosclerotic disease leading to obstruction of peripheral arteries causing exertional claudication (muscle pain relieved by rest) and atypical leg pain May progress to ischemic pain at rest	Usually calf muscles but also occurs in the buttock, hip, thigh, or foot, depending on the level of obstruction Rest pain may be distal in the toes or forefoot
Acute Arterial Occlusion	Embolism or thrombosis, possibly superimposed on arteriosclerosis obliterans	Distal pain, usually involving the foot and leg
Raynaud Phenomenon: Primary and Secondary (Varga, 2018)	*Raynaud phenomenon—primary:* Episodic reversible vasoconstriction in the fingers and toes, usually triggered by cold temperatures (capillaries are normal; no definable cause) *Raynaud phenomenon—secondary:* Symptoms/signs related to autoimmune diseases—scleroderma, lupus, mixed connective tissue disease, cryoglobulinemia, also to occupational vascular injury; drugs	Distal portions of one or more fingers. Pain is usually not prominent unless fingertip ulcers develop Numbness and tingling are common
Venous Disorders		
Superficial Phlebitis *Superficial Vein Thrombosis*	In the lower extremity: inflammation of a superficial vein A clot is confirmed by imaging	Pain and tenderness in a local area along the course of a superficial vein, most often in the saphenous system
Deep Venous Thrombosis (DVT)	DVT and PE are disorders of venous thromboembolic disease (VTE) DVTs are distal, limited to the deep calf veins, or proximal, in the popliteal, femoral, or iliac veins	Classically, painful calf swelling with erythema but can be painless; signs correlate poorly with site of thrombosis
Chronic Venous Insufficiency (Deep)	More severe form of chronic venous disease with chronic venous engorgement from venous occlusion or incompetency of venous valves	Diffuse aching of the leg(s)

Timing	Factors that Aggravate	Factors that Relieve	Associated Manifestations
May be brief if relieved by rest If there is *rest pain*, may be persistent and worse at night	Exercise such as walking If *rest pain*, leg elevation and bedrest	Rest usually stops the pain in 1–3 min *Rest pain* may be relieved by walking (increases perfusion), sitting with legs dependent	Local fatigue, numbness, progressing to cool, dry, hairless skin, trophic nail changes, diminished to absent pulses, pallor with elevation, ulceration, gangrene
Sudden onset Associated symptoms may occur without pain			Coldness, numbness, weakness, absent distal pulses
Relatively brief (minutes) but recurrent	Exposure to cold, emotional upset	Warm environment	*Primary RP:* distinct digital color changes of pallor, cyanosis, and hyperemia (redness); no necrosis *Secondary:* more severe, with ischemia, necrosis, and loss of digits; capillary loops are distorted
An acute episode lasting days or longer	Immobility, venous stasis and chronic venous disease, venous procedure, obesity	Supportive care, walking Measures prompted by further testing	Local induration, erythema If palpable nodules or cords, consider superficial or deep vein thrombosis, both associated with significant risk of DVT and PE
Often hard to determine due to lack of symptoms One third of untreated calf DVTs extend proximally	Immobilization or recent surgery, lower extremity trauma, pregnancy or postpartum state, hypercoagulable state (i.e., nephrotic syndrome, malignancy)	Antithrombotic and thrombolytic therapy	Asymmetric calf diameters more diagnostic than palpable cord or tenderness over femoral triangle Homan sign unreliable High risk of PE (50% with proximal DVT)
Chronic, increasing as the day wears on	Prolonged standing or sitting with legs dependent	Leg elevation, walking	Chronic edema, pigmentation, swelling, and possibly ulceration; especially if advanced age, pregnancy, increased weight, prior history or trauma

(*continued*)

TABLE 15-3 Painful Peripheral Vascular Disorders and Their Mimics (*Continued*)

Problem	Process	Location of Pain
Compartment Syndrome	Pressure builds from trauma or bleeding into one of the four major muscle compartments between the knee and ankle. Each compartment is enclosed by fascia that limits expansion and thus cannot expand to accommodate increasing pressure	Tight, bursting pain in calf muscles, usually in the anterior tibial compartment, sometimes with overlying dusky red skin
Acute Lymphangitis	Acute bacterial infection from *Streptococcus pyogenes* or *Staphylococcus aureus*, spreading up the lymphatic channels from a distal portal of entry such as a skin abrasion, dog bite or an ulcer	An arm or a leg
Mimics[a]		
Acute Cellulitis	Acute bacterial infection of the skin and subcutaneous tissues, most commonly from β-*hemolytic streptococci* (erysipelas) and *Staphylococcus aureus*	Arms, legs, or elsewhere

[a]Mistaken primarily for acute superficial thrombophlebitis.

Source: De Araujo, T., Valencia, I., Federman, D. G., & Kirsner, R. S. (2003). Managing the patient with venous ulcers. *Annals of Internal Medicine*, *138*(4), 326–334; and Gerhard-Herman, M. D., Gornik, H. L., Barrett, C., Barshes, N. R., Corriere, M. A., Drachman, D. E., Fleisher, L. A., Fowkes, F. G. R., Hamburg, N. M., Kinlay, S., Lookstein, R., Misra, S., Mureebe, L., Olin, J. W., Patel, R. A. G., Regensteiner, J. G., Schanzer, A., Shishehbor, M. H., Stewart, K. J., … Walsh, M. E. (2017). 2016 AHA/ACC guideline on the management of patients with lower extremity peripheral artery disease: executive summary: a report of the American College of Cardiology/American Heart Association Task Force on Clinical Practice Guidelines. *Circulation*, *135*(12), e686–e725.

The amplitude of the pulse is graded on a 3+ scale as outlined in Table 15-4.

A 0-to-4+ pulse amplitude scale is used by some institutions; record pulse findings per the institution's policy.

TABLE 15-4 Recommended Grading of Pulses

3+	Bounding
2+	Brisk, expected (normal)
1+	Diminished, weaker than expected
0	Absent, unable to palpate

Document pulse amplitude as a fraction with a denominator of 3. For example, a normal pulse would be recorded as "2+/3."

Bounding carotid, radial, and femoral pulses occur with aortic insufficiency; asymmetric diminished pulses occur with arterial occlusion from atherosclerosis or embolism.

Timing	Factors that Aggravate	Factors that Relieve	Associated Manifestations
Several hours if *acute* (pressure must be relieved to avert necrosis) During exercise if *chronic*	*Acute:* anabolic steroids; surgical complication; crush injury *Chronic:* occurs with exercise	*Acute:* surgical incision to relieve pressure *Chronic:* avoiding exercise; ice, elevation	Tingling, burning sensations in calf; muscles may feel tight, full, numbness, paralysis if unrelieved
An acute episode lasting days or longer			Red streak(s) on the skin with tenderness, enlarged, tender lymph nodes, and fever
An acute episode lasting days or longer			A local area of diffuse swelling, redness, and tenderness with enlarged, tender lymph nodes and fever; no palpable cord

If you cannot obtain the radial pulse, feel for the *brachial pulse* (Fig. 15-13). Flex the patient's elbow slightly, and palpate the artery just medial to the biceps tendon at the antecubital crease. The brachial artery can also be felt higher in the arm in the groove between the biceps and triceps muscles.

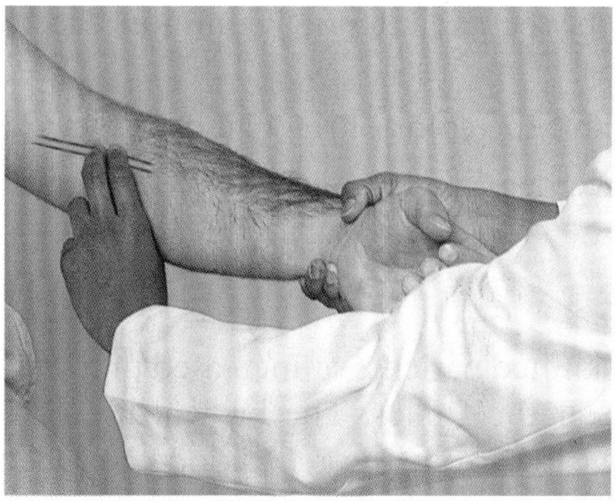

FIGURE 15-13 Palpating the brachial pulse.

Feel for the *epitrochlear nodes.* With the patient's elbow flexed to about 90 degrees and the forearm supported by your hand, reach around behind the arm and feel in the groove between the biceps and triceps muscles, about 3 cm above the medial epicondyle (Fig. 15-14). If a node is present, note its size, consistency, and tenderness.

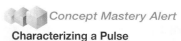

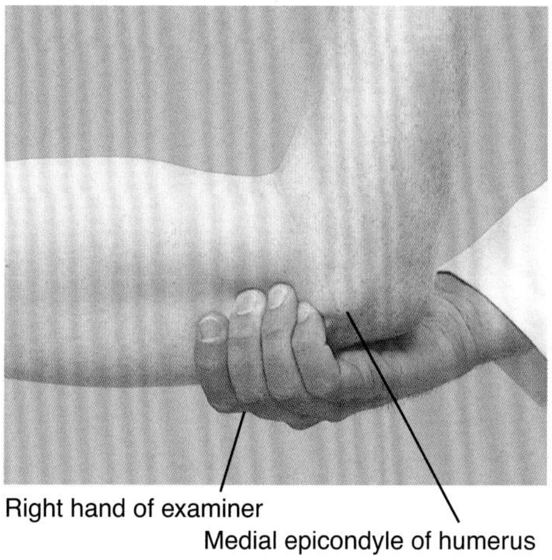

FIGURE 15-14 Palpating the epitrochlear nodes.

Concept Mastery Alert

Characterizing a Pulse

Identifying the characteristics of a pulse is important to determine if palpation reveals a normal finding, a finding associated with aging, or a problem. A bounding pulse may indicate decreased elasticity of the arterial walls, most commonly seen with aging. However, a bisferiens pulse, for example (one in which there is an increased arterial pulse with double systolic beats), suggests aortic stenosis.

CLINICAL TIP

An enlarged epitrochlear node may arise from local or distal infection or may be associated with generalized lymphadenopathy.

Epitrochlear nodes are nonpalpable in most normal people.

Legs

The patient should be lying down and draped so that the external genitalia are covered and the legs fully exposed. A good examination is impossible through stockings or socks.

Inspection

Inspect both legs from the groin and buttocks to the feet. Note:

1. Their size, symmetry, and edema. Measure leg circumferences in centimeters if discrepancy is suspected.
2. The venous pattern and any venous enlargement or varicosities; see Table 15-5, "Chronic Insufficiency of Arteries and Veins."
3. Pigmentation, rashes, scars, or ulcers; see Table 15-6, "Common Ulcers of the Ankles and Feet."
4. The color and texture of the skin and the color of the nail beds.
5. The distribution of hair on the lower legs, feet, and toes.

Tight socks may rub off the hair. If hair is absent, look for a clean demarcation where the top of the sock ends.

6. Look for brownish areas on light-skinned patients or increased pigmentation on dark-skinned patients near the ankles. The brown discoloration is caused by hemosiderin released from the red blood cells that seep into the skin with edema and break down.

Discoloration or ulcers just above the malleolus suggest chronic venous insufficiency.

7. Note the location, size, and depth of any ulcers in the skin. Note whether the edges of the wound are well demarcated or uneven and if there is bleeding.

TABLE 15-5 Chronic Insufficiency of Arteries and Veins

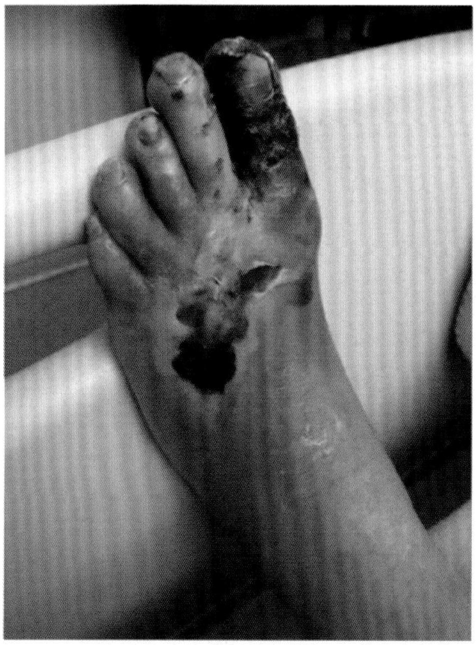

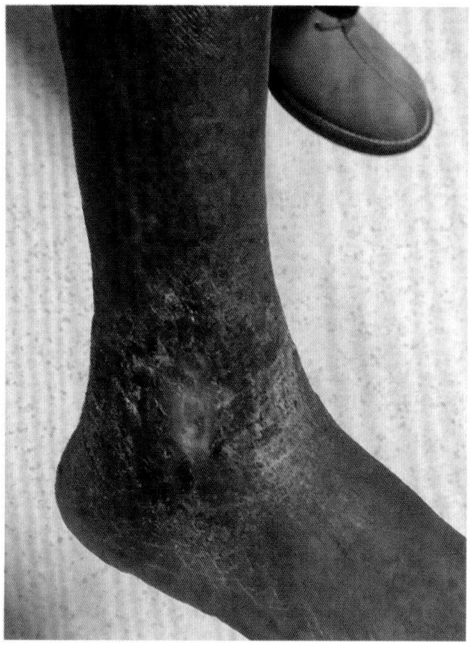

	Chronic Arterial Insufficiency (Advanced)	Chronic Venous Insufficiency (Advanced)
Pain	Intermittent claudication, progressing to pain at rest	Ulcer often painful (De Araujo et al., 2003); generalized leg aching, especially at end of day
Mechanism	Tissue ischemia	Venous stasis and hypertension
Pulses	Decreased or absent	Normal, though may be difficult to feel through edema
Color	Pale, especially on elevation; dusky red on dependency	Normal, or cyanotic on dependency Petechiae and then brown pigmentation appear with chronicity
Temperature	Cool	Normal
Edema	Absent or mild; may develop as the patient tries to relieve rest pain by lowering the leg	Present, often marked
Skin Changes	Trophic changes: thin, shiny, atrophic skin; loss of hair over the foot and toes; nails thickened and ridged	Often brown pigmentation around the ankle, stasis dermatitis, and possible thickening of the skin and narrowing of the leg as scarring develops
Ulceration	If present, involves toes or points of trauma on feet	If present, develops at sides of ankle, especially medially
Gangrene	May develop	Does not develop

Sources of photos: *Arterial Insufficiency*—Courtesy of Daniel Han, MD; *Venous Insufficiency*—Courtesy of Daniel Han, MD.

TABLE 15-6 Common Ulcers of the Ankles and Feet

Chronic Venous Insufficiency Ulcer

This condition usually appears over the medial and sometimes the lateral malleolus. The ulcer contains small, painful granulation tissue and fibrin; necrosis or exposed tendons are rare. Borders are irregular, flat, or slightly steep. Pain affects quality of life in 75% of patients. Associated findings include edema, reddish pigmentation and purpura, venous varicosities, the eczematous changes of stasis dermatitis (redness, scaling, and pruritus), and at times cyanosis of the foot when dependent. Gangrene is rare (De Araujo et al., 2003).

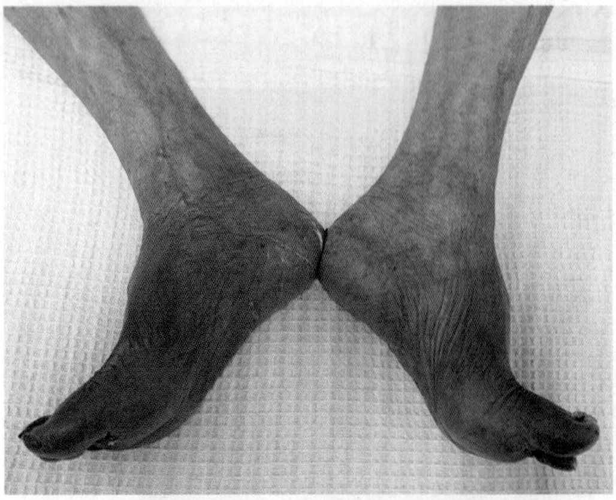

Arterial Insufficiency Ulcer

This condition occurs in the toes, feet, or possibly areas of trauma (e.g., the shins). Surrounding skin shows no callus or excess pigment, though it may be atrophic. Pain often is severe unless masked by neuropathy. Gangrene may occur, along with decreased pulses, trophic changes, foot pallor on elevation, and dusky rubor on dependency.

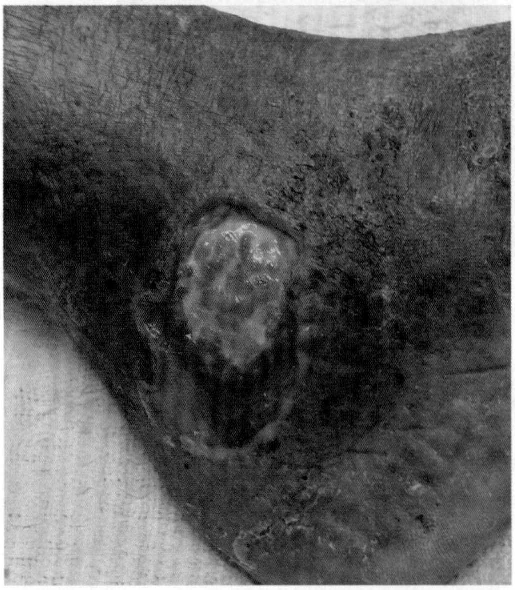

Neuropathic Ulcer

This condition develops in pressure points of areas with diminished sensation; seen in diabetic neuropathy, neurologic disorders, and Hansen disease. The surrounding skin is calloused. There is no pain, so the ulcer may go unnoticed. In uncomplicated cases, there is no gangrene. Associated signs include decreased sensation and absent ankle jerks.

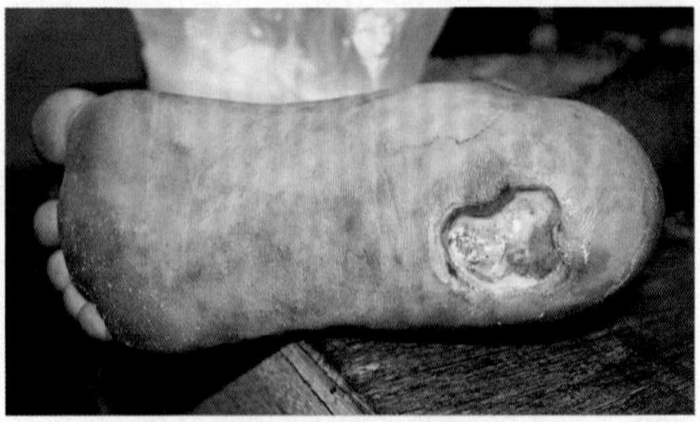

Source of photos: *Chronic Venous Insufficiency Ulcer*—Casa nayafana/Shutterstock; *Arterial Insufficiency Ulcer*—Alan Nissa/Shutterstock; *Neuropathic Ulcer*—Zay Nyi Nyi/Shutterstock.

Palpation

Palpate the temperature of both legs and feet simultaneously with the backs of your hands (Fig. 15-15). Compare the temperature of the legs. Bilateral coolness may be caused by a cold environment or anxiety.

Coldness, especially when unilateral or associated with other signs, suggests arterial insufficiency from inadequate arterial circulation.

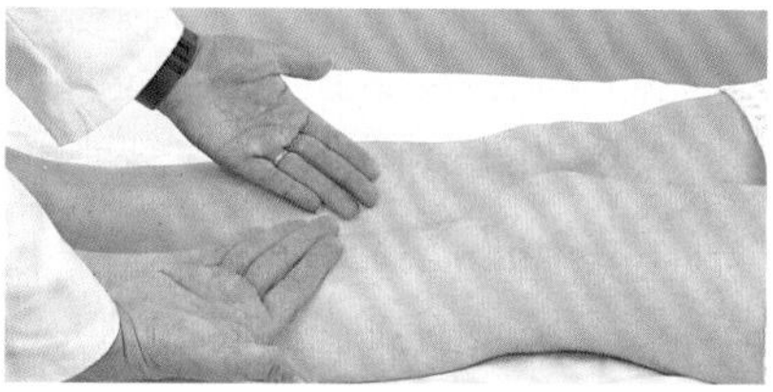

FIGURE 15-15 Palpating leg temperature.

Palpate for edema. Compare one foot and leg with the other, noting their relative size and the prominence of veins, tendons, and bones (Fig. 15-16).

Palpate for pitting edema. Press firmly but gently with your thumb for at least 5 seconds (1) over the dorsum of each foot (Fig. 15-17A); (2) behind each medial malleolus; and (3) over the shins. Look for *pitting*—a depression caused by pressure from your thumb (Fig. 15-17B). Normally, pitting edema is not present. If found, the severity of edema is graded on a 4-point scale (see Table 15-1).

Table 15-7 outlines peripheral causes of edema.

A

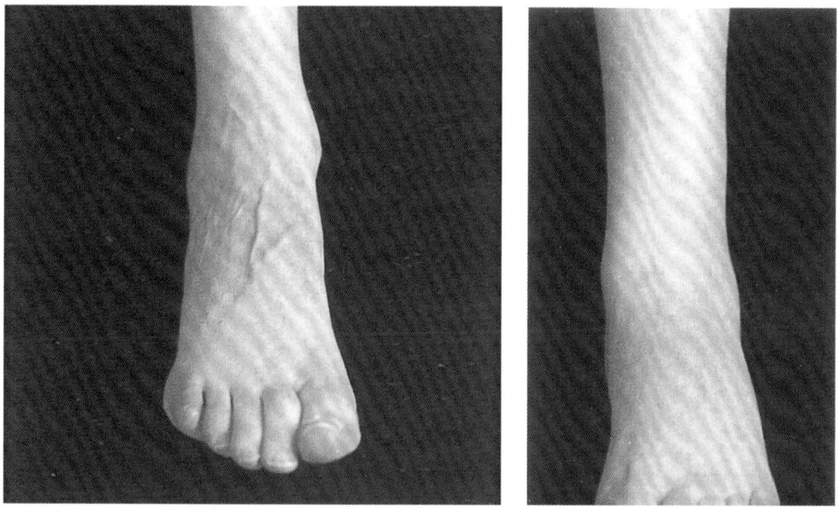

B

FIGURE 15-16 **A.** A normal foot. **B.** A foot in which edema has obscured the veins, tendons, and bony prominences.

A

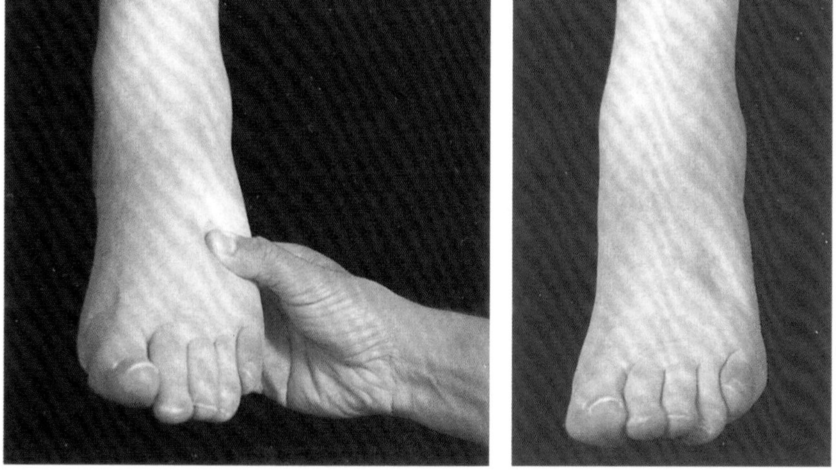

B

FIGURE 15-17 **A.** Palpating for pitting edema. **B.** A foot with 3+ pitting edema.

TABLE 15-7 Some Peripheral Causes of Edema

Approximately one third of total body water is extracellular. Approximately 25% of extracellular fluid is plasma; the remainder is interstitial fluid. Normally, fluid diffuses out of the capillaries, where most of it is returned to the vascular system by lymphatic drainage. Several clinical conditions disrupt this balance, resulting in *edema*, or a clinically evident accumulation of interstitial fluid. Pitting characteristics reflect the viscosity of the edema fluid, based primarily on its protein concentration (Grada & Phillips, 2017; McGee, 2018). When protein concentration is low, as in heart failure, pitting and recovery occur within a few seconds. In lymphedema, protein levels are higher and nonpitting is more typical. Not depicted below is *capillary leak syndrome,* in which protein leaks into the interstitial space, seen in burns, angioedema, snake bites, and allergic reactions.

Pitting Edema

Edema is a soft bilateral palpable swelling from increased interstitial fluid volume and retention of salt and water, demonstrated by pitting upon pressure, on the anterior tibiae and feet. There is no skin thickening, ulceration, or pigmentation. Pitting edema occurs in several conditions: when legs are dependent from prolonged standing or sitting, which leads to increased hydrostatic pressure in the veins and capillaries; congestive heart failure leading to decreased cardiac output; nephrotic syndrome, cirrhosis, or malnutrition leading to low albumin and decreased intravascular colloid oncotic pressure; and drug use.

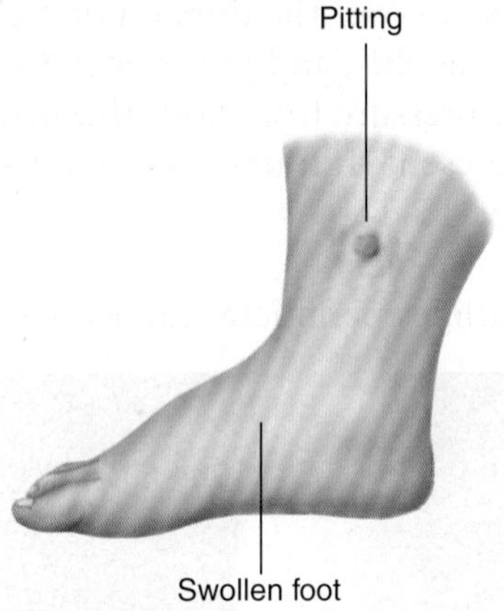

Chronic Venous Insufficiency

Edema is soft, with pitting upon pressure, and occasionally bilateral. Look for brawny changes and skin thickening, especially near the ankle. Ulceration, brownish pigmentation, and edema in the feet are common. Arises from chronic obstruction and from incompetent valves in the deep venous system.

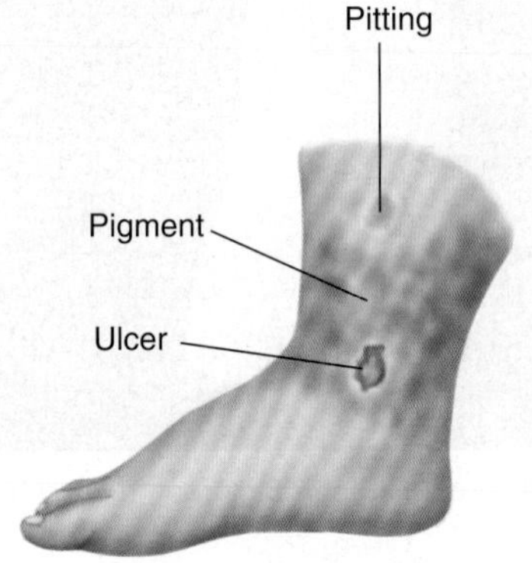

Lymphedema

Edema is initially soft and pitting, then becomes indurated, hard, and nonpitting. Skin is markedly thickened; ulceration is rare. There is no pigmentation. Edema often occurs bilaterally in the feet and toes. Lymphedema arises from interstitial accumulation of protein-rich fluid when lymph channels are infiltrated or obstructed by tumor, fibrosis, or inflammation, or disrupted by axillary node dissection and/or radiation.

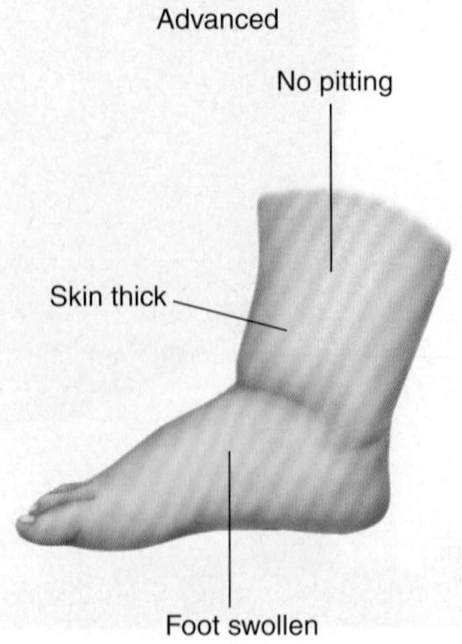

If you suspect edema, *measure the legs* to identify the edema and to follow its course. With a flexible tape, measure (1) the forefoot; (2) the smallest possible circumference above the ankle; (3) the largest circumference at the calf; and (4) the midthigh with the knee extended. Compare one side with the other. A difference of more than 1 cm just above the ankle or 2 cm at the calf is unusual and suggests edema.

If edema is present, look for possible causes in the peripheral vascular system. These include (1) recent DVT; (2) chronic venous insufficiency from previous DVT or incompetence of the venous valves; and (3) lymphedema. Note the extent of the swelling and how far up the leg it goes.

In *DVT*, the extent of edema suggests the location of the occlusion; the popliteal vein may be the location when the lower leg or the ankle is swollen, and the iliofemoral vein may be the location when the entire leg is swollen.

Is the swelling unilateral or bilateral?

Unilateral calf and ankle swelling and edema suggest DVT, chronic venous insufficiency from prior DVT, or incompetent venous valves; lymphedema may be another cause.

Bilateral edema is present in *heart failure*, *cirrhosis*, and *nephrotic syndrome*.

Venous distention suggests a venous cause of edema.

If risk factors for DVT are present, try to identify any venous tenderness that may accompany DVT. Very gently palpate the groin just medial to the femoral pulse for tenderness of the femoral vein. Next, with the patient's leg flexed at the knee and relaxed, palpate the calf by very gently compressing the calf muscles against the tibia with your finger pads. Search for any tenderness or cords. DVT may have no demonstrable signs, and diagnosis often depends on high clinical suspicion and other testing. *Firm palpation or massage over a DVT should be avoided as it may dislodge the clot, causing a PE or death.*

A painful, pale swollen leg, together with tenderness in the groin over the femoral vein, suggests deep *iliofemoral thrombosis*. Only half of patients with *DVT* in the calf have tenderness and cords deep in the calf. Calf tenderness is nonspecific and may be present without thrombosis.

Feel the thickness of the skin.

Thickened brawny skin suggests lymphedema and advanced venous insufficiency.

Palpate areas of local redness, noting the skin temperature, and then gently palpate for the firm cord of a thrombosed vein in the area. The calf is most often involved.

Local swelling, redness, warmth, and a subcutaneous cord suggest *superficial thrombophlebitis*.

A diminished or absent pulse indicates partial or complete occlusion proximally; for example, at the popliteal level, the dorsalis pedis and posterior tibial pulses are typically affected. Chronic arterial occlusion, usually from atherosclerosis, causes *intermittent claudication*.

Palpate the pulses to assess the arterial circulation:

- *The femoral pulse.* Press deeply below the inguinal ligament and about midway between the anterior superior iliac spine and the symphysis pubis (Fig. 15-18). As in deep abdominal palpation, the use of two hands, one on top of the other, may facilitate this examination, especially in obese patients.

An exaggerated, widened femoral pulse suggests a *femoral aneurysm,* a pathologic dilatation of the artery.

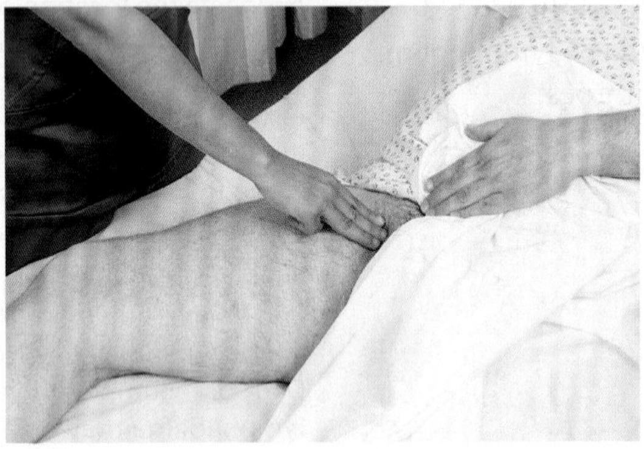

FIGURE 15-18 Palpating the femoral pulse.

- *The popliteal pulse.* The patient's knee should be somewhat flexed with the leg relaxed. Place the fingertips of both hands so that they meet in the midline behind the knee and press deeply into the popliteal fossa (Fig. 15-19). The popliteal pulse is often more difficult to find than other pulses. It is deeper and feels more diffuse.

An exaggerated, widened popliteal pulse suggests an aneurysm of the popliteal artery. Popliteal and femoral aneurysms are not common. They are usually caused by atherosclerosis and occur primarily in men older than 50.

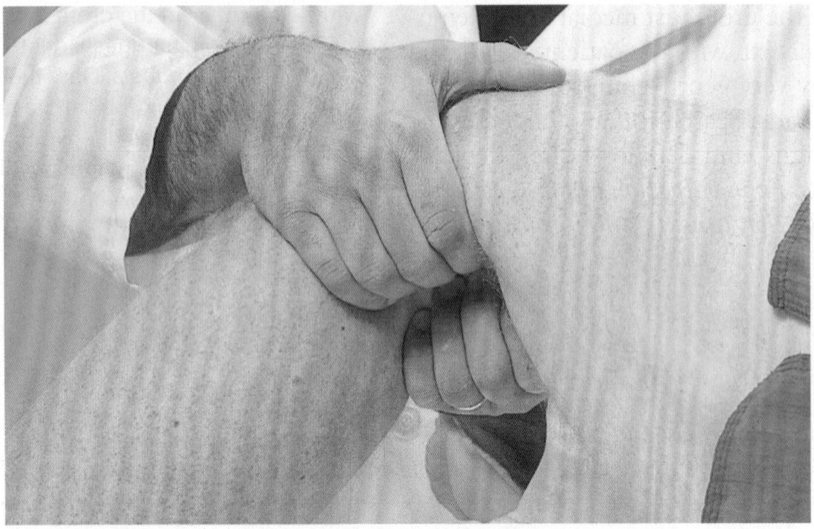

FIGURE 15-19 Palpating the popliteal pulse with the patient supine.

If you cannot palpate the popliteal pulse with this approach, try palpating it with the patient prone (Fig. 15-20). Flex the patient's knee to about 90 degrees, let the lower leg relax against your shoulder or upper arm, and press your two thumbs deeply into the popliteal fossa.

Atherosclerosis (arteriosclerosis obliterans) most commonly obstructs arterial circulation in the thigh. The femoral pulse is then normal, the popliteal decreased or absent.

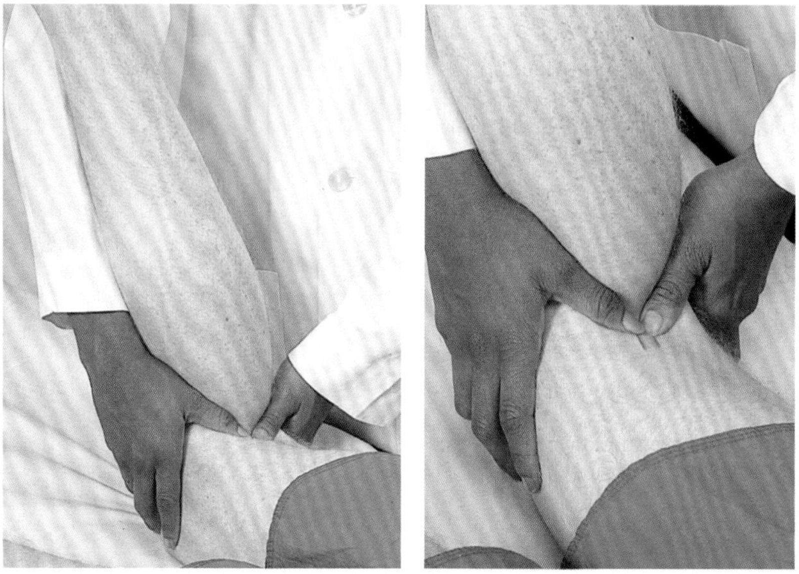

FIGURE 15-20 Palpating the popliteal pulse with the patient prone.

- *The dorsalis pedis pulse.* Palpate the dorsum of the foot (not the ankle) just lateral to the extensor tendon of the great toe (Fig. 15-21). If you cannot feel a pulse, explore the dorsum of the foot more laterally.

The dorsalis pedis artery may be congenitally absent or may branch higher in the ankle.

Decreased or absent pedal pulses (assuming a warm environment) with normal femoral and popliteal pulses suggest occlusive disease in the lower popliteal artery or its branches, often seen in *diabetes mellitus.*

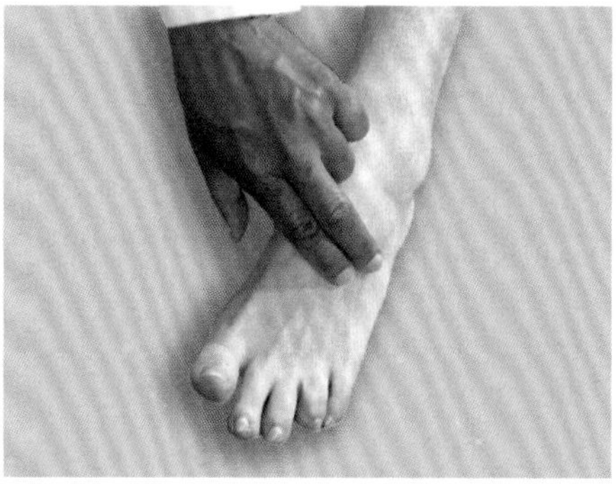

FIGURE 15-21 Palpating the dorsalis pedis pulse.

- *The posterior tibial pulse.* Curve your fingers behind and slightly below the medial malleolus of the ankle (Fig. 15-22). (This pulse may be hard to feel in an ankle that is enlarged due to fat deposits or edema.)

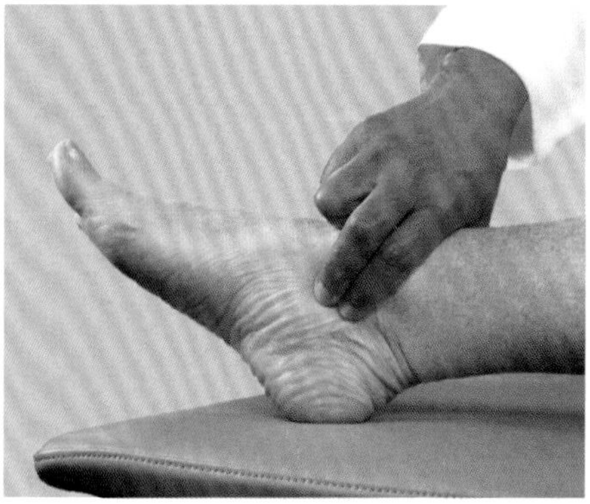

FIGURE 15-22 Palpating the posterior tibial pulse.

CLINICAL TIP

Sudden arterial occlusion from embolism or thrombosis causes pain and numbness or tingling. The limb distal to the occlusion becomes cold, pale, and pulseless. Emergency treatment is required. If collateral circulation is good, only numbness and coolness may result.

Tips for feeling difficult pulses are outlined in Box 15-2.

BOX 15-2 TIPS FOR FEELING DIFFICULT PULSES

1. Position your body and examining hand comfortably; awkward positions decrease your tactile sensitivity.
2. Once your hand is positioned properly, linger and vary the pressure of your fingers to pick up a weak pulsation. If unsuccessful, then gently explore the area more deliberately.
3. Do not confuse the patient's pulse with your own pulsating fingertips. If you are unsure, count your own heart rate and compare it with the patient's. The rates are usually different. Your carotid pulse is convenient for this comparison.

Palpate the *superficial inguinal nodes*, including both the horizontal and the vertical groups. Note their size, consistency, and discreteness, and note any tenderness. Nontender, discrete inguinal nodes up to 1 cm or even 2 cm in diameter are frequently palpable in healthy people.

Lymphadenopathy refers to enlargement of the nodes with or without tenderness.

At the end of the examination, ask the patient to stand, and *inspect the saphenous system for varicosities*. The standing posture allows any varicosities to fill with blood and makes them visible (Fig. 15-23). You can easily miss them when the patient is in a supine position. Feel for any varicosities, noting any signs of thrombophlebitis.

Varicose veins are dilated and tortuous. Their walls may feel somewhat thickened. Many varicose veins can be seen in the leg in Figure 15-23.

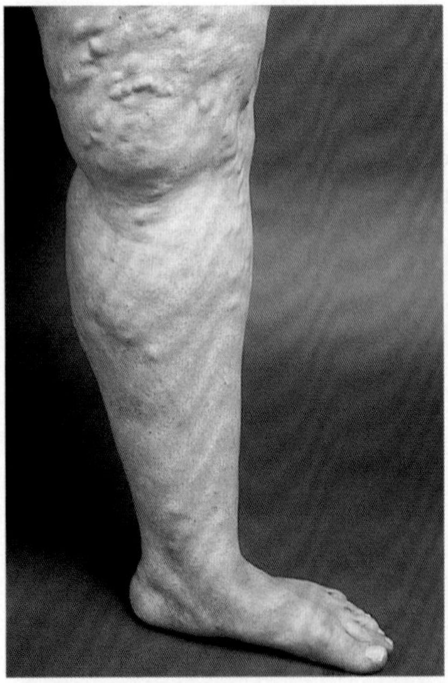

FIGURE 15-23 Varicosities visible upon standing.

RECORDING YOUR FINDINGS

Box 15-3 contains examples of documentation taken during the examination of the peripheral vascular system.

BOX 15-3 RECORDING THE PHYSICAL EXAMINATION—THE PERIPHERAL VASCULAR SYSTEM

"Extremities are warm without edema. No varicosities or stasis changes. Calves are supple and nontender. No femoral or abdominal bruits. Brachial, radial, femoral, popliteal, dorsalis pedis (DP), and posterior tibial (PT) pulses are 2+ and symmetric."

OR

"Extremities are pale below the midcalf, with notable hair loss. Rubor noted when legs are dependent but no edema or ulceration. Bilateral femoral bruits; no abdominal bruits heard. Brachial and radial pulses 2+; femoral, popliteal, DP, and PT pulses 1+ bilaterally." (Alternatively, pulses can be recorded as below.)

Suggests atherosclerotic *peripheral arterial disease*

	Radial	Brachial	Femoral	Popliteal	Dorsalis Pedis	Posterior Tibial
RT	2+	2+	1+	1+	1+	1+
LT	2+	2+	1+	1+	1+	1+

OR

"Bilateral pitting edema 2+ and brownish pigmentation present to midcalf bilaterally. 2-cm × 1-cm shallow ulcer with irregular edges and moderate exudate on right leg superior to medial malleolus. Granulation tissue visible in ulcer. Varicose veins present on posterior upper legs bilaterally."

Suggests venous ulcer

Recall that the written description of lymph nodes appears in Chapter 10, "The Head and Neck." Likewise, assessment of the carotid pulse is recorded in Chapter 14, "The Cardiovascular System."

SPECIAL TECHNIQUES

Evaluating the Arterial Supply to the Hand

To assess for arterial insufficiency in the arm or hand, try to palpate the *ulnar pulse* as well as the radial and brachial pulses. Press deeply on the flexor surface of the medial wrist (Fig. 15-24). Partially flexing the patient's wrist may help you. The pulse of a normal ulnar artery, however, may not be palpable.

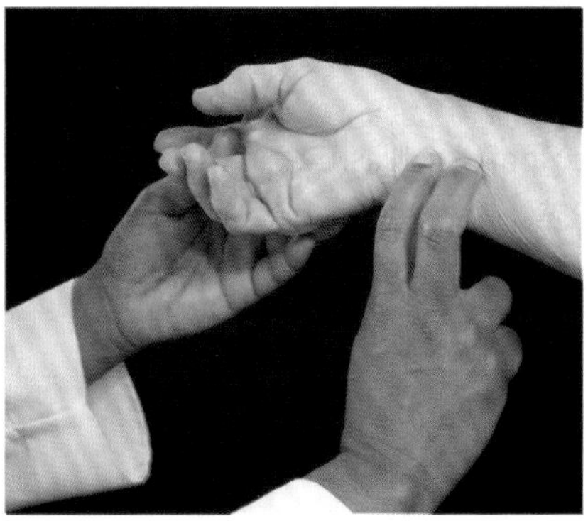

FIGURE 15-24 Palpating the ulnar pulse.

CLINICAL TIP
Arterial occlusive disease is much less common in the arms than in the legs. Absent or diminished pulses at the wrist occur in acute embolic occlusion and in Buerger disease, or thromboangiitis obliterans (a recurring progressive inflammation and thrombosis of small and medium arteries and veins of the hands and feet). It is strongly associated with use of tobacco products.

Allen Test

The *Allen test* compares patency of the ulnar and radial arteries. It also ensures the patency of the ulnar artery before puncturing the radial artery for blood samples or arterial lines. The patient should rest with the hands in lap, palms up.

Ask the patient to make a tight fist with one hand; then compress both radial and ulnar arteries firmly between your thumbs and fingers (Fig. 15-25).

Next, ask the patient to open the hand into a relaxed, slightly flexed position. The palm is pale (Fig. 15-26).

Extending the hand fully may cause pallor and a falsely positive test.

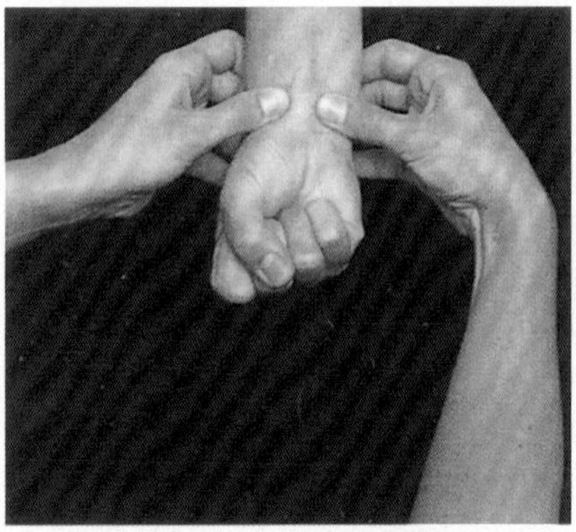

FIGURE 15-25 In the first step of the Allen test, the patient makes a tight fist, and the nurse compresses the radial and ulnar arteries.

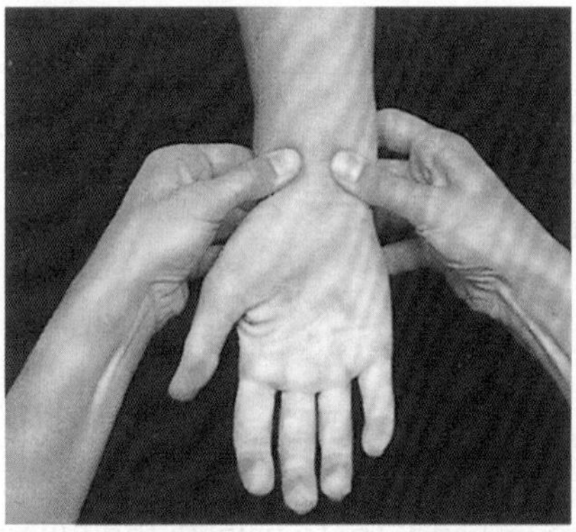

FIGURE 15-26 In the second step of the Allen test, the patient opens the hand, and the palm is pale.

Release pressure over the ulnar artery. If the ulnar artery is patent, the palm flushes within 3 to 5 seconds (Fig. 15-27).

Persisting pallor indicates occlusion of the ulnar artery or its distal branches.

Patency of the radial artery may be tested by repeating the test and releasing the radial artery while still compressing the ulnar artery (Fig. 15-28).

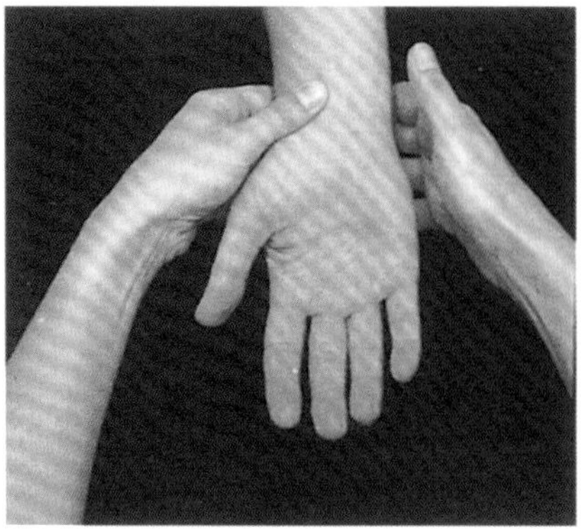

FIGURE 15-27 In the third step of the Allen test, the nurse releases pressure, and if the ulnar artery is patent, the palm flushes within seconds.

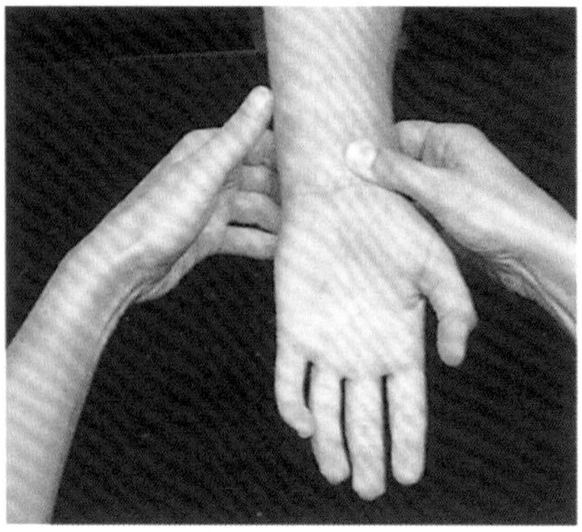

FIGURE 15-28 The nurse can test patency of the radial artery by repeating the test with the ulnar artery compressed and pressure on the radial artery released.

Evaluating Arterial Supply to the Legs

If pain or diminished pulses suggest arterial insufficiency, look for postural color changes. With the patient lying down, raise both legs to about 60 degrees until maximal pallor of the feet develops—usually within a minute. Have the patient flex the ankles up and down to drain venous blood. In light-skinned persons, either maintenance of normal color, or slight pallor is normal. In dark-skinned persons, evaluate the soles of the feet or nail beds for pallor.

Then ask the patient to sit up and dangle the legs over the side of the examination table. Compare both feet, noting the time required for:

- return of pinkness to the skin, normally about 10 seconds or less.
- filling of the veins of the feet and ankles, normally about 15 seconds.

These normal responses suggest an adequate circulation. However, if the return of color and filling of the veins take longer, the patient may have inadequate arterial supply to the legs.

Look for any unusual *rubor* (dusky redness) to replace the pallor of the dependent foot. Rubor may take a minute or more to appear.

Persistent dependent rubor suggests arterial insufficiency. If the patient's veins are incompetent, dependent rubor and the timing of color return and venous filling are not reliable tests of arterial insufficiency.

Normal responses accompanied by diminished arterial pulses suggest that a good collateral circulation has developed around an arterial occlusion.

If the patient has risk factors for peripheral artery disease, an ankle-brachial index (ABI) screening should be performed (Box 15-4). ABI is a noninvasive method to assess lower extremity arterial blood flow by comparing systolic blood pressure in the ankle to arm systolic pressure.

BOX 15-4 ANKLE-BRACHIAL INDEX SCREENING

Equipment

- Doppler device with 8-MHz probe (for obese individuals, a 4-MHz probe may be necessary)
- Doppler gel
- Blood pressure cuffs for arm and leg; cuffs should be 40% of limb circumference (or 20% of the limb diameter)

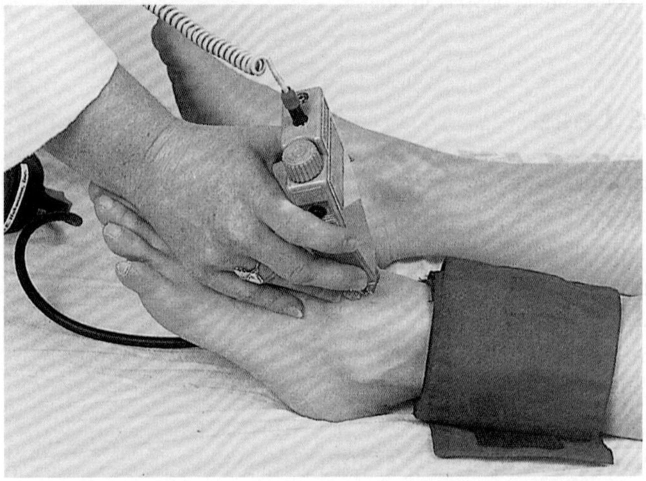

Procedure

1. Advise patients to avoid caffeine, tobacco, and heavy activity for at least 1 hour prior to the procedure.
2. Perform the ABI in a quiet, warm environment to prevent vasoconstriction.
3. Have patient empty the bladder and remove tight or restrictive clothing, shoes, and socks.
4. Explain the procedure to the patient and position them in the supine position. The patient should rest supine for 10 to 20 minutes before the procedure.
5. Apply the blood pressure cuff to the patient's arm and palpate the brachial pulse.
6. Apply a small mound of gel over the pulse; turn on the Doppler.
7. Place the tip of the Doppler probe in the gel at a 45-degree angle and listen for the "whooshing" sound, indicating the pulse. (The probe may be adjusted between 30 and 60 degrees to maximize the sound.)
8. Inflate the blood pressure cuff until the sound is no longer heard, and then inflate it 20 to 30 mm Hg above that point.
9. Deflate the cuff at a rate of 2 to 3 mm Hg/sec until the sound returns. This is the systolic blood pressure. Repeat the procedure in the other arm.
10. Place the ankle blood pressure cuff just above the malleoli. Locate the posterior tibial pulse with the Doppler and inflate the cuff 20 to 30 mm Hg above the number at which the pulse is last heard. Slowly release the pressure until the pulse is heard. This is the systolic pressure. Repeat the procedure using the dorsalis pedis pulse.
11. Obtain the systolic pressure for both pulses on the opposite ankle.

NOTE: The ankle blood pressure cuff must be of appropriate size in order to obtain accurate readings. Artery pressure is measured at the site of the cuff; if the cuff is placed higher on the leg, a false high systolic reading will be obtained.

BOX 15-4 ANKLE-BRACHIAL INDEX SCREENING (*Continued*)

Calculation

Divide the higher systolic pressure from each leg by the higher brachial systolic pressure to obtain the ABI for each leg.

Documentation

Describe the patient's tolerance of the procedure and any problems encountered during the test. Document all brachial and ankle pressures, the ABI value, and the interpretation of perfusion status.

Interpretation

<table>
<tr><th>ABI Value</th><th>Interpretation</th><th>Recommendation</th></tr>
<tr><td>>1.4</td><td>Calcification/Artery hardening</td><td>Refer to vascular specialist.</td></tr>
<tr><td>1.0–1.4</td><td>Normal</td><td rowspan="2">None.</td></tr>
<tr><td>0.9–1.0</td><td>Acceptable</td></tr>
<tr><td>0.8–0.9</td><td>Some arterial disease</td><td>Treat risk factors.</td></tr>
<tr><td>0.5–0.8</td><td>Moderate arterial disease</td><td>Refer to vascular specialist.</td></tr>
<tr><td><0.5</td><td>Severe arterial disease</td><td>Refer to vascular specialist.</td></tr>
</table>

Stanford Medicine 25. *Measuring and understanding the ankle brachial index (ABI).* Retrieved September 12, 2020, from https://stanfordmedicine25.stanford.edu/the25/ankle-brachial-index.html

Evaluating the Competency of Venous Valves

By the *retrograde filling (Trendelenburg) test*, you can assess the valvular competency in both the penetrating veins and the saphenous system:

- With the patient supine, elevate one leg to about 90 degrees to empty it of venous blood.
- Occlude the great saphenous vein in the upper thigh by manual compression or tourniquet, using enough pressure to occlude this vein but not the deeper vessels.
- Ask the patient to stand. While you keep the vein occluded, watch for venous filling in the leg. Normally the saphenous vein fills from below, taking about 35 seconds as blood flows through the capillary bed into the venous system.

Rapid filling of the superficial veins during occlusion of the saphenous vein indicates incompetent valves in the penetrating veins, which allows rapid retrograde flow from the deep to the saphenous system.

- After the patient stands for 20 seconds, release the compression and look for sudden additional venous filling. Normally slow venous filling continues since competent valves in the saphenous vein block retrograde flow.

Sudden additional filling of superficial veins after release of compression indicates incompetent valves in the saphenous vein.

When both steps of this test are normal, the response is termed negative-negative. Negative-positive and positive-negative responses may also occur. When both steps are abnormal, the test is positive-positive.

Pulsus Alternans

In *pulsus alternans*, the rhythm of the pulse remains regular, but the *force* of the arterial pulse alternates because of alternating strong and weak ventricular contractions. *Pulsus alternans* almost always indicates severe left-sided heart failure and is usually best felt by applying light pressure on the radial or femoral arteries. Use a blood pressure cuff to confirm your finding. After raising the cuff pressure, lower it slowly to the systolic level—the initial Korotkoff sounds are the strong beats. As you lower the cuff, you will hear the softer sounds of the alternating weak beats. See Table 15-8, "Abnormalities of the Arterial Pulse and Pressure Waves."

Alternately loud and soft Korotkoff sounds or a sudden doubling of the apparent heart rate as the cuff pressure declines indicates a pulsus alternans. The alternation may be more noticeable with the patient in an upright position.

TABLE 15-8 Abnormalities of the Arterial Pulse and Pressure Waves

Normal

The pulse pressure is approximately 30–40 mm Hg. The pulse contour is smooth and rounded. (The notch on the descending slope of the pulse wave is not palpable.)

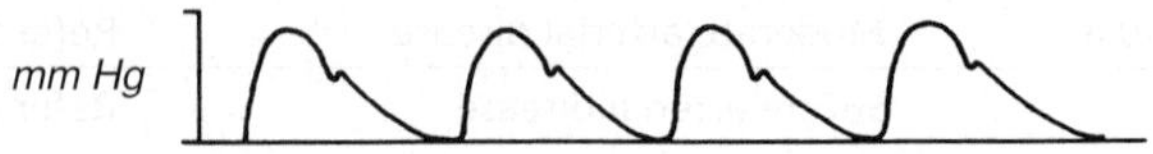

Weak

The pulse pressure is diminished, and the pulse feels weak and small. The upstroke may feel slowed, the peak prolonged. Causes include (1) decreased stroke volume, as in heart failure, hypovolemia, and severe aortic stenosis, and (2) increased peripheral resistance, as in exposure to cold and severe congestive heart failure.

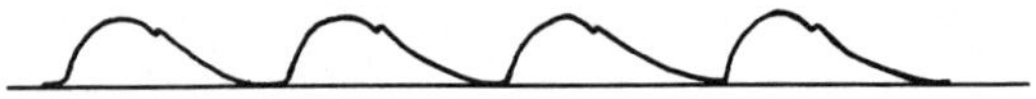

Bounding

The pulse pressure is increased, and the pulse feels strong and bounding. The rise and fall may feel rapid, the peak brief. Causes include (1) increased stroke volume, decreased peripheral resistance, or both, as in fever, anemia, hyperthyroidism, aortic regurgitation, arteriovenous fistulas, and patent ductus arteriosus; (2) increased stroke volume because of slow heart rates, as in bradycardia and complete heart block; and (3) decreased compliance (increased stiffness) of the aortic walls, as in aging or atherosclerosis.

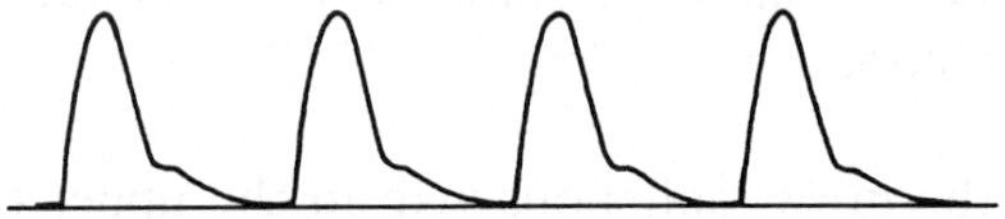

Bisferiens

A bisferiens pulse is an increased arterial pulse with a double systolic peak. Causes include pure aortic regurgitation and aortic stenosis with regurgitation.

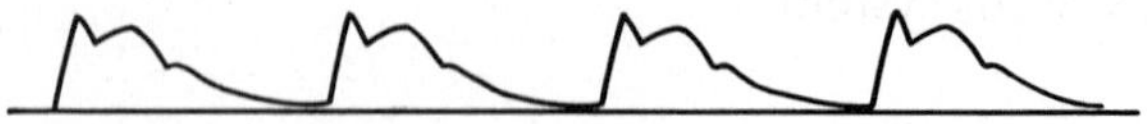

Pulsus Alternans

The pulse alternates in amplitude from beat to beat even though the rhythm is regular. When the difference between stronger and weaker beats is slight, it can be detected only by sphygmomanometry. Pulsus alternans indicates left ventricular failure and is usually accompanied by a left-sided S3.

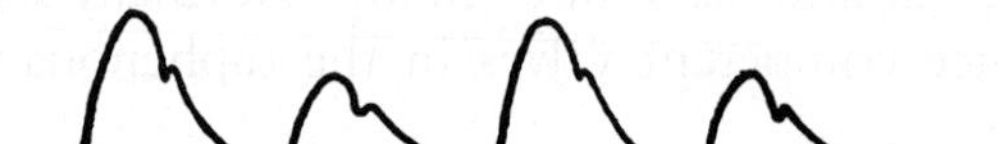

Bigeminal Pulse

This disorder of rhythm may mimic pulsus alternans. A bigeminal pulse is caused by a normal beat alternating with a premature contraction. The stroke volume of the premature beat is diminished in relation to that of the normal beats, and the pulse varies in amplitude accordingly.

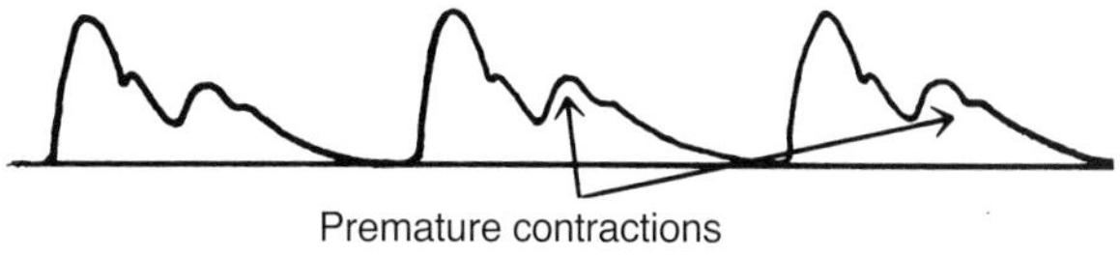

Paradoxical Pulse

A paradoxical pulse is a palpable decrease in the pulse's amplitude with quiet inspiration. A blood pressure cuff may be needed to detect the difference in amplitude. Systolic pressure decreases by more than 10 mm Hg during inspiration. A paradoxical pulse is found in pericardial tamponade, constrictive pericarditis (though less commonly), and obstructive lung disease.

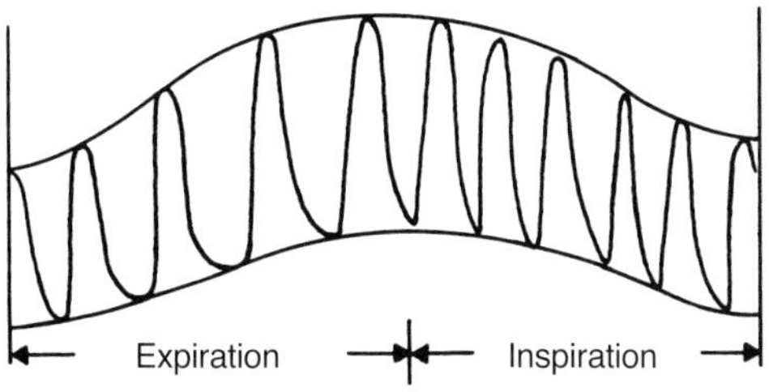

Paradoxical Pulse

Paradoxical pulse means the pulse beat amplitude is weaker during inspiration and stronger during expiration. This is due to a greater-than-normal drop in systolic blood pressure during inspiration. Normally, systolic blood pressure decreases slightly during inspiration, less than 10 mm Hg. In the presence of certain diseases, for example, cardiac tamponade, pericarditis, or obstructive airway disease, the fall in systolic pressure is greater than 10 mm Hg due to decreased left ventricular volume producing decreased left ventricular output and systolic pressure. The *paradox* in *pulsus paradoxus* is that on clinical examination, you can detect beats on cardiac auscultation during inspiration that cannot be palpated at the radial pulse.

CLINICAL TIP

The level identified by first hearing Korotkoff sounds is the highest systolic pressure during the respiratory cycle. The level identified by hearing sounds throughout the cycle is the lowest systolic pressure. A difference between these levels of more than 10 mm Hg indicates a paradoxical pulse.

To test for a paradoxical pulse:

- Inflate the blood pressure cuff above the patient's usual systolic pressure.
- As the patient breathes, lower the cuff pressure slowly to the systolic level. Note the pressure level at which the first sounds can be heard.
- Drop the pressure slowly until sounds can be heard throughout the respiratory cycle. Again, note the pressure level. The difference between these two levels is normally no greater than 3 or 4 mm Hg.

See Table 15-8, "Abnormalities of the Arterial Pulse and Pressure Waves."

HEALTH PROMOTION AND COUNSELING

Important Topics for Health Promotion and Counseling

Important topics for health promotion and counseling regarding arterial disease include:

- Smoking cessation
- Weight control
- Exercise program
- Hypertension control
- Hyperlipidemia control
- Diabetes management
- Limiting alcohol intake
- Foot care

Important topics for health promotion and counseling regarding venous disease include:

- Avoidance of prolonged sitting and standing
- Avoidance of constrictive clothing, including girdles and tight hose
- Exercise program
- Weight control
- Foot care
- Dehydration prevention

Diseases of the peripheral vascular system, peripheral arterial disease, venous stasis, and thromboembolic disorders can severely affect the lifestyle and quality of life of patients. Identifying modifiable risk factors and providing health promotion counseling can prevent or delay long-term complications, such as decreased mobility and amputation. Helping the patient understand the effects of smoking, obesity, hypertension, hyperlipidemia, and diabetes and the need for exercise encourages the patient to institute lifestyle changes that promote peripheral and cardiovascular health.

PAD has the same underlying pathology as CAD and is a common manifestation of atherosclerosis. Approximately 8.5 million people aged 40 or older in the United States have PAD. Men and women are equally affected by PAD; however, Black race/ethnicity is associated with an increased risk of PAD. People of Hispanic origin may have similar to slightly higher rates of PAD compared to non-Hispanic White people (Virani et al., 2020). The presence of PAD significantly increases the risk for cardiovascular events. Controlling risk factors will help prevent or decrease the complications of both diseases.

Early identification of peripheral vascular diseases and modification of risk factors are important nursing functions. Careful and thorough history taking is essential to identifying early peripheral vascular disease, especially in patients older than 60 years of age. Identification of risk factors should be performed with every patient. The nurse can use the ABI to assess peripheral arterial disease. Serial ABI testing will document any progression of the disease.

Since atherosclerotic renal arterial disease and AAA often accompany peripheral vascular disease, patients with risk factors should be referred to their physicians for screening of these diseases. Patients with worsening hypertension despite medication or new worsening of renal function should be evaluated. AAAs are rarely symptomatic, and the mortality rate for ruptured aneurysms is high. Risk factors for AAA include a history of having smoked or currently smoking, family history, PAD, CAD, hypertension, elevated cholesterol, and age older than 65.

Prevention and early identification of DVT are critical nursing responsibilities, especially in the care of hospitalized patients and patients with reduced mobility. The Virchow triad—venous stasis, hypercoagulability, and vessel wall damage—set the stage for the development of a DVT. Blood stasis, which usually occurs within the pockets of vein valves, is commonly a result of immobility, compression of the vein, and increased blood viscosity (as seen with dehydration). The Homan sign, with the patient's knee flexed and the ankle forcibly dorsiflexed, was considered the classic assessment maneuver to detect DVT; however, it should not be used because research has found this test to be unreliable, yielding many false positives and negatives (McGee, 2018). Almost every hospitalized patient is at risk for DVT. DVT risk assessment tools for hospitalized patients have been developed. The tools identify and rank risk factors and become part of the patient chart. Prevention strategies can then be initiated.

Patients should be educated about the risk of DVT outside the hospital as well. Conditions that produce dehydration, cramped positioning, or immobility, such as long plane travel, can cause a DVT to form. Patients with sedentary jobs should be advised to walk or flex their legs at their desks at least every hour. Ergonomic furniture may reduce the effects of prolonged flexion of the legs.

Bibliography

CITATIONS

Braunwald, E., & Loscalzo, J. (2018). Edema. In J. Jameson, A. S. Fauci, D. L. Kasper, S. L. Hauser, D. L. Longo, & J. Loscalzo (Eds.), *Harrison's principles of internal medicine* (20th ed.). McGraw Hill.

Centers for Disease Control and Prevention (CDC). (2020, September 8). Peripheral arterial disease (PAD). https://www.cdc.gov/heartdisease/pad.htm?CDC_AA_refVal=https%3A%2F%2Fwww.cdc.gov%2Fdhdsp%2Fdata_statistics%2Ffact_sheets%2Ffs_pad.htm

De Araujo, T., Valencia, I., Federman, D. G., & Kirsner, R. S. (2003). Managing the patient with venous ulcers. *Annals of Internal Medicine, 138*(4), 326–334.

Gerhard-Herman, M. D., Gornik, H. L., Barrett, C., Barshes, N. R., Corriere, M. A., Drachman, D. E., Fleisher, L. A., Fowkes, F. G. R., Hamburg, N. M., Kinlay, S., Lookstein, R., Misra, S., Mureebe, L., Olin, J. W., Patel, R. A. G., Regensteiner, J. G., Schanzer, A., Shishehbor, M. H., Stewart, K. J., ... Walsh, M. E. (2017). 2016 AHA/ACC guideline on the management of patients with lower extremity peripheral artery disease: executive summary: a report of the American College of Cardiology/American Heart Association Task Force on Clinical Practice Guidelines. *Circulation, 135*(12), e686–e725.

Grada, A. A., & Phillips, T. J. (2017). Lymphedema: diagnostic workup and management. *Journal of the American Academy Dermartology, 77*(6), 995–1006.

Kucher, N. (2011). Clinical practice. Deep-vein thrombosis of the upper extremities. *The New England Journal of Medicine, 364*(9), 861–869.

McGee, S. (2018). Chapter 54: Peripheral vascular disease. In *Evidence-based physical diagnosis* (4th ed.). Elsevier.

Mitchell, R. N. (2015). Chapter 11: Blood vessels. In: V. K. Kumar, A. K. Abbas, & J. C. Aster (Eds.). *Robbins and Cotran pathologic basis of disease* (9th ed.). Saunders/Elsevier.

Varga, J. (2018). Chapter 353: Systemic sclerosis (scleroderma) and related disorders. In J. Jameson, A. S. Fauci, D. L. Kasper, S. L. Hauser, D. L. Longo, & J. Loscalzo (Eds.). *Harrison's principles of internal medicine* (20th ed.).

Virani, S. S., Alonso, A., Benjamin, E. J., Bittencourt, M. S., Callaway, C. W., Carson, A. P., Chamberlain, A. M., Chang, A. R., Cheng, S., Delling, F. N., Djousse, L., Elkind, M. S. V., Ferguson, J. F., Fornage, M., Khan, S. S., Kissela, B. M., Knutson, K. L., Kwan, T. W., Lackland, D. T., ... American Heart Association Council on Epidemiology and Prevention Statistics Committee and Stroke Statistics Subcommittee. (2020). Heart disease and stroke statistics—2020 update: A report from the American Heart Association. *Circulation, 141*(9), e139–e596.

ADDITIONAL REFERENCES

Centers for Disease Control and Prevention (CDC). (2020). Venous thromboembolism (blood clots). Preventing healthcare-associated venous thromboembolism (VTE): A public health and patient safety challenge. Retrieved September 9, 2020, from https://www.cdc.gov/ncbddd/dvt/features/keyfinding-pba-vte.html

Creager, M. A., & Loscalzo, J. (2018). Arterial diseases of the extremities. In: J. Jameson, A. S. Fauci, D. L. Kasper, S. L. Hauser, D. L. Longo, & J. Loscalzo (Eds.). *Harrison's principles of internal medicine* (20th ed.). McGraw-Hill. https://accesspharmacy-mhmedical-com.uri.idm.oclc.org/content.aspx?bookid=2129&sectionid=192030522

National Institutes of Health (NIH). (2020a). Heart, Lung and Blood Institute. Peripheral artery disease (PAD). Retrieved September 9, 2020, from https://www.nhlbi.nih.gov/health-topics/peripheral-artery-disease

National Institutes of Health (NIH). (2020b). Heart, Lung and Blood Institute. Venous thromboembolism. Retrieved September 9, 2020, from https://www.nhlbi.nih.gov/health-topics/venous-thromboembolism

Ostomy, W., & Society, C. N. (2012). Ankle brachial index: Quick reference guide for clinicians. *Journal of Wound, Ostomy, and Continence Nursing, 39*(25), S21–S29.

16 THE GASTROINTESTINAL AND RENAL SYSTEMS

KEY TERMS

anorexia
ascites
cholecystitis
constipation
diarrhea
dyspepsia
dysphagia
functional (nonulcer) dyspepsia
functional incontinence
gastroesophageal reflux disease (GERD)
heartburn
hematemesis
hematuria
incisional hernias
mixed incontinence
nocturia
odynophagia
overflow incontinence
peritonitis
polyuria
pyelonephritis
splenomegaly
umbilical hernia
urge incontinence
urinary frequency
urinary incontinence
ventral hernia

Learning Objectives

The student will:

1. Identify the structures and function of the gastrointestinal and renal systems.
2. Identify the four quadrants and the organs in each quadrant.
3. Collect a health history of the gastrointestinal and renal systems.
4. Describe the physical examination techniques and the order performed to evaluate the gastrointestinal and renal systems.
5. Describe the techniques for assessing ascites, appendicitis, acute cholecystitis, hernias, and masses in the abdominal wall.
6. Document a complete gastrointestinal and renal system assessment utilizing information from the health history and the physical examination.
7. Determine the health promotion and counseling measures related to alcohol abuse, hepatitis, colorectal cancer, and urinary incontinence.

ANATOMY AND PHYSIOLOGY

The gastrointestinal and renal systems encompass many organs of the body. It is important to be familiar with the sites and functions of each organ and in which quadrant of the abdomen each organ is located for the assessment. The landmarks of the abdominal wall and pelvis are illustrated in Figure 16-1. The rectus abdominis muscles become more prominent when the patient raises the head and shoulders from the supine position.

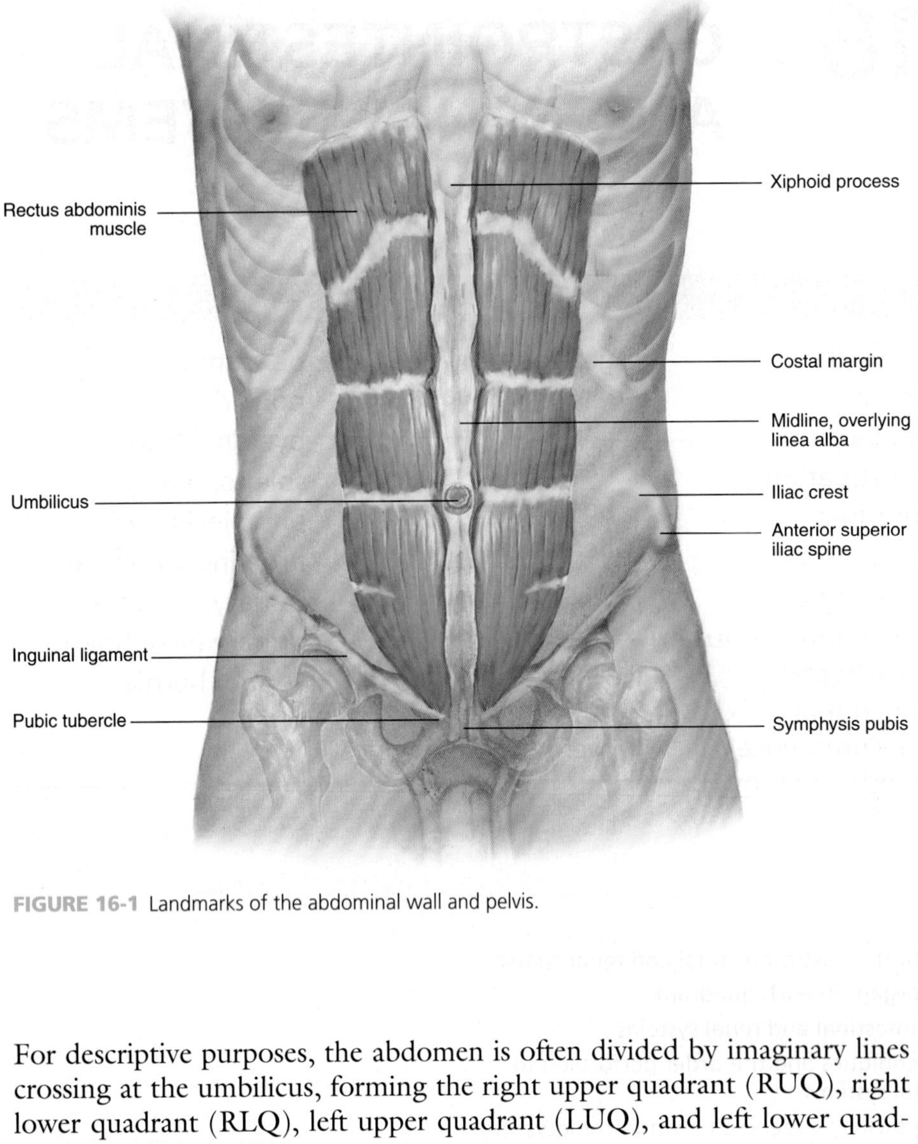

FIGURE 16-1 Landmarks of the abdominal wall and pelvis.

For descriptive purposes, the abdomen is often divided by imaginary lines crossing at the umbilicus, forming the right upper quadrant (RUQ), right lower quadrant (RLQ), left upper quadrant (LUQ), and left lower quadrant (LLQ) (Fig. 16-2).

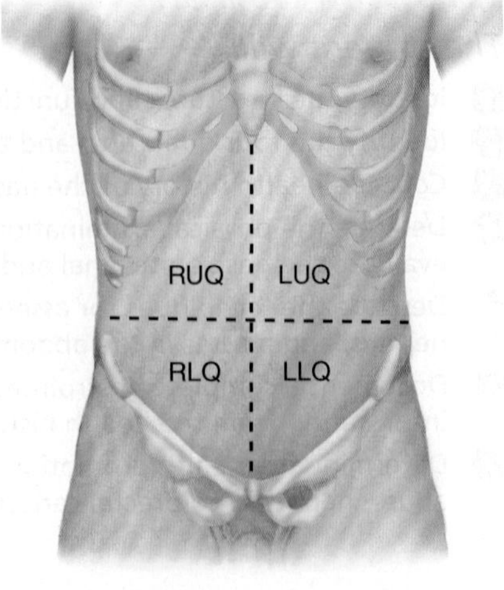

FIGURE 16-2 The four quadrants of the abdomen.

Examine the abdomen, moving in a clockwise rotation beginning in the RLQ. Several organs are often palpable with the exception of the stomach and much of the liver and spleen (Fig. 16-3). These lie high in the abdominal cavity close to the diaphragm, where they are protected by the thoracic ribs, beyond the reach of the palpating hand. The dome of the diaphragm lies at approximately the fifth anterior intercostal space.

In the *RUQ*, the soft consistency of the *liver* makes it difficult to palpate through the abdominal wall. The lower margin of the liver, the liver edge, is often palpable at the right costal margin. The *gallbladder*, which rests against the inferior surface of the liver, and the more deeply lying *duodenum* are generally not palpable. Moving medially, the examiner encounters the rib cage with its xiphoid process, which protects the stomach. The *abdominal aorta* often has visible pulsations and is usually palpable in the upper abdomen. At a deeper level, the *lower pole of the right kidney* may be felt, especially in children or a thinner person with relaxed abdominal muscles.

In the *LUQ*, the *spleen* is lateral to and behind the stomach, just above the left kidney in the left midaxillary line. Its upper margin rests against the dome of the diaphragm. The ninth, 10th, and 11th ribs protect most of the spleen. The tip of the spleen may be palpable below the left costal margin in a small percentage of adults. In healthy people, the *pancreas* cannot be detected. In the *LLQ*, the firm, narrow, tubular sigmoid *colon* is often felt, and portions of the transverse and descending colon may also be palpable, especially if stool is present.

In the lower midline, the *bladder* may be palpated and in women, the *uterus* and *ovaries* are palpable as well. In the *RLQ* are bowel loops and the *appendix* at the base of the cecum near the junction of the small and large intestines. In healthy people, these are not palpable.

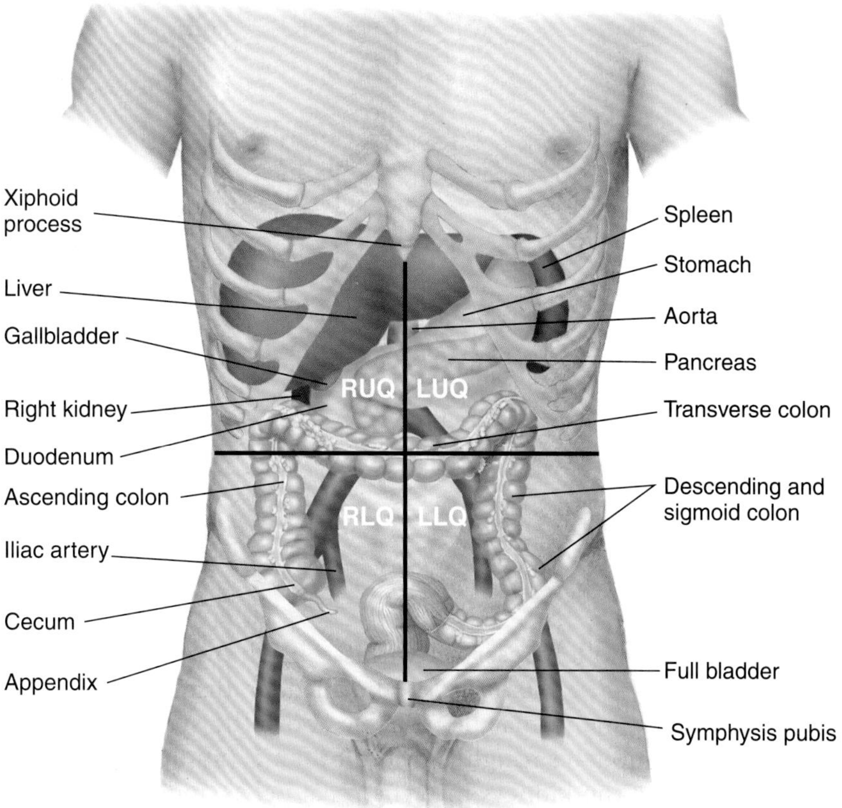

Right Upper Quadrant (RUQ)	Left Upper Quadrant (LUQ)
Ascending colon Duodenum Gallbladder Right kidney Liver Pancreas (head) Transverse colon Ureter (right)	Descending colon Left kidney Pancreas (body and tail) Spleen Stomach Transverse colon Ureter (left)
Right Lower Quadrant (RLQ)	**Left Lower Quadrant (LLQ)**
Appendix Ascending colon Bladder Cecum Rectum Ovary, uterus and fallopian tube (female) Prostate and spermatic cord (male) Small intestine Ureter (right)	Bladder Descending colon Ovary, uterus, fallopian tube (female) Prostate and spermatic cord (male) Small intestine Sigmoid colon Ureter (left)

FIGURE 16-3 Abdominal quadrants with organ locations.

The *kidneys* are retroperitoneal organs. They are not suspended by the mesentery and remain behind the parietal peritoneum. The ribs protect their upper portions. The *costovertebral angle* is formed by the lower border of the 12th rib and the transverse processes of the upper lumbar vertebrae (Fig. 16-4). This defines the region to assess for kidney tenderness, called costovertebral angle tenderness (CVAT).

The *mesentery* is the membrane that attaches the intestines to the wall of the abdomen, maintaining their position in the abdominal cavity and supplying them with blood vessels, nerves, and lymphatics.

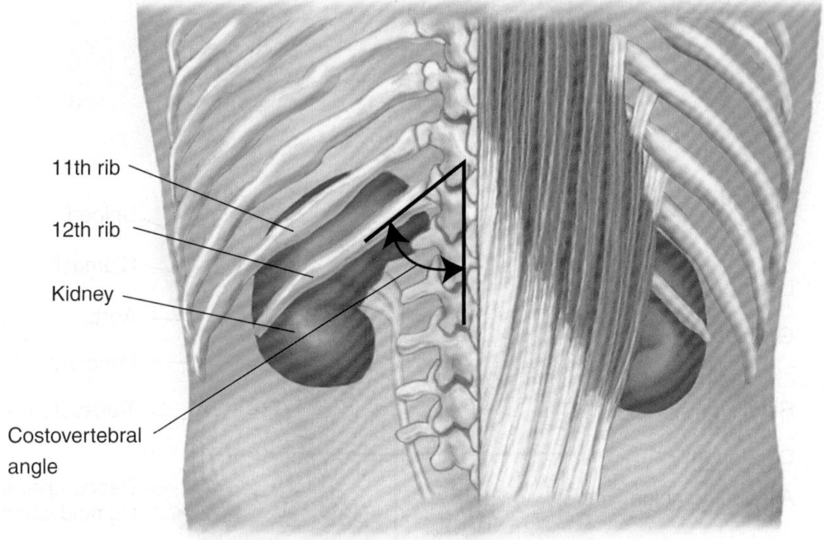

FIGURE 16-4 A posterior view of the costovertebral angle.

The *bladder* is a hollow reservoir with strong smooth muscle walls composed chiefly of *detrusor muscle.* The bladder distends as it fills with urine, at which time, it may be palpable above the symphysis pubis. The bladder accommodates roughly 400 to 500 mL (about 1.5 to 2 cups) of urine filtered by the kidneys into the renal pelvis and the ureters. Bladder expansion stimulates parasympathetic innervation at relatively low pressures, resulting in detrusor contraction and inhibition (relaxation) of the *internal urethral sphincter*, also under autonomic control. Voiding further requires relaxation of the *external urethral sphincter*, composed of striated muscle under voluntary control. Rising pressure triggers the conscious urge to void. Increased *intraurethral* pressure can overcome rising pressures in the bladder and prevent incontinence. Intraurethral pressure is related to factors such as smooth muscle tone in the internal urethral sphincter, the thickness of the urethral mucosa, and in women, sufficient support to the bladder and proximal urethra from pelvic muscles and ligaments to maintain proper anatomic relationships. Striated muscle around the urethra can also contract voluntarily to interrupt voiding (Holcomb, 2008).

Neuroregulatory control of the bladder functions at several levels. In infants, the bladder empties by reflex mechanisms in the sacral spinal cord. Voluntary control of the bladder depends on higher centers in the brain and on motor and sensory pathways connecting the brain and the reflex arcs of the sacral spinal cord. When voiding is inconvenient, higher centers in the brain can inhibit detrusor contractions until the capacity of the bladder, approximately 400 to 500 mL, is exceeded. The integrity of the sacral nerves that innervate the bladder can be tested by assessing perirectal and perineal sensation in the S2, S3, and S4 dermatomes (see dermatome maps in Chapter 20, "The Nervous System").

BOX 16-1 COMMON OR CONCERNING SYMPTOMS

Gastrointestinal

- Abdominal pain, acute and chronic
- Indigestion, nausea, vomiting including blood (*hematemesis*), loss of appetite, early satiety
- Difficulty swallowing (*dysphagia*)
- Painful swallowing (*odynophagia*)
- Food intolerance
- Unintentional weight loss or gain
- Change in bowel function
- Diarrhea, constipation
- Jaundice

Urinary and Renal

- Suprapubic pain
- Difficulty urinating (*dysuria*), urgency, or frequency
- Hesitancy, decreased stream in males
- Excessive urination (*polyuria*) or excess urination at night (*nocturia*)
- Urinary incontinence
- Blood in the urine (*hematuria*)
- Flank pain and ureteral colic

THE HEALTH HISTORY

Common or concerning symptoms identified during gastrointestinal and renal histories are listed in Box 16-1.

Gastrointestinal complaints rank high among reasons for office and emergency room visits. Patients complain of a wide variety of upper gastrointestinal symptoms, including abdominal pain, heartburn, nausea and vomiting, difficulty or pain with swallowing, vomiting of stomach contents or blood, loss of appetite, and jaundice. Lower gastrointestinal complaints are also common and may include diarrhea, constipation, change in bowel habits, and blood in the stool, often described as either bright red or dark and tarry.

Numerous symptoms also originate in the *genitourinary tract*: difficulty urinating, urgency and frequency, hesitancy and decreased stream in men, high urine volume, urinating at night, incontinence, blood in the urine, and flank pain and colic from renal stones or infection. These are often accompanied by gastrointestinal symptoms such as abdominal pain, nausea, and vomiting.

Often you will need to cluster several findings from both the patient's story and your examination as you sort through various explanations for the patient's symptoms. Your skills in history taking and examination are needed for sound clinical reasoning. Review Chapter 8, "Nutrition and Hydration," for important assessment points that correlate with the gastrointestinal and renal systems.

Patterns and Mechanisms of Abdominal Pain

Before exploring gastrointestinal and genitourinary symptoms, review the mechanisms and clinical patterns of abdominal pain (Table 16-1). Be familiar with the three broad categories of abdominal pain:

TABLE 16-1 Abdominal Pain

Problem	Process	Location	Quality
Gastroesophageal reflux disease (GERD) (American Gastroenterological Association, 2018; Davis-Yadley et al., 2016; DeVault & Castell, 2005; Shaheen et al., 2012; Spechler et al., 2019; Yadlapati & Pandolfino, 2020)	Prolonged exposure of esophagus to gastric acid due to impaired esophageal motility or excess relaxations of the lower esophageal sphincter *Helicobacter pylori* may be present	Chest or epigastric	Heartburn, regurgitation
Peptic ulcer and dyspepsia (American Gastroenterological Association, 2018; Tack & Talley, 2013)	Mucosal ulcer in stomach or duodenum >5 mm	Epigastric, may radiate straight to the back	Variable: epigastric gnawing or burning (dyspepsia); may also be boring, aching, or hunger-like No symptoms in up to 20% of cases
Acute appendicitis (D'Souza & Nugent, 2016; Evans & Curtin, 2014; Youatou Towo et al., 2012)	Acute inflammation of the appendix with distention or obstruction	Poorly localized *periumbilical pain*, usually migrates to the right lower quadrant	Mild but increasing, possibly cramping Steady and more severe
Acute cholecystitis (Friedman et al., 2011)	Inflammation of the gallbladder, usually from obstruction of the cystic duct by a gallstone in 90% of cases	Right upper quadrant or epigastrium; may radiate to the right shoulder of interscapular area	Steady, aching
Biliary colic (Tagliaferri et al., 2017)	Sudden obstruction of the cystic duct or common bile duct by a gallstone	Epigastric or right upper quadrant; may radiate to the right scapula and shoulder	Steady, aching; *not* colicky Usually lasts longer than 3 h
Acute bowel obstruction (Elliott et al., 2019)	Obstruction of the bowel lumen, commonly caused by (1) adhesions or hernias (small bowel) or (2) cancer or diverticulitis (colon)	*Small bowel:* periumbilical or upper abdominal *Colon:* lower abdominal or generalized	*Small bowel:* Cramping *Colon:* Cramping
Acute pancreatitis (Ahmed Ali et al., 2016; Sankaran et al., 2015)	Intrapancreatic trypsinogen activation to trypsin and other enzymes, resulting in autodigestion and inflammation of the pancreas	Epigastric, may radiate straight to the back or other areas of the abdomen; 20% of cases with severe sequelae of organ failure	Usually steady

Timing	Factors that May Aggravate	Factors that May Relieve	Associated Symptoms and Setting
After meals, especially spicy foods	Lying down, bending over Physical activity Diseases such as scleroderma, gastroparesis Drugs like nicotine that relax the lower esophageal sphincter	Antacids; proton pump inhibition Avoiding alcohol, smoking, fatty meals, chocolate, selected drugs such as theophylline, and calcium channel blockers	Wheezing, chronic cough, shortness of breath, hoarseness, choking sensation, dysphagia, regurgitation, halitosis, sore throat Increases risk of Barrett esophagus and esophageal cancer
Intermittent Duodenal ulcer is more likely than gastric ulcer or dyspepsia to cause pain that (1) wakes the patient at night and (2) occurs intermittently over a few weeks, then disappears for months, and then recurs	Variable	Food and antacids may bring relief	Nausea, vomiting, belching, bloating Heartburn (more common in duodenal ulcer) Weight loss (more common in gastric ulcer) Dyspepsia is more common among younger patients (20–29 y), gastric ulcer in those over 50 y, and duodenal ulcer in those 30–60 y
Lasts roughly 4–6 h depending on intervention	Movement or cough		Anorexia, nausea, possibly vomiting, which typically follow the onset of pain; low fever
Gradual onset; course longer than in biliary colic	Jarring, deep breathing		Anorexia, nausea, vomiting, fever No jaundice
Rapid onset over a few minutes, lasts 1 to several hours and subsides gradually Often recurrent	Fatty meals but also fasting Often precedes cholecystitis, cholangitis, pancreatitis		Anorexia, nausea, vomiting, restlessness
Small bowel: Paroxysmal; may decrease as bowel mobility is impaired *Colon:* Paroxysmal, though typically milder	Ingestion of food or liquids		Vomiting of bile and mucus (high obstruction) or fecal material (low obstruction) Obstipation develops Obstipation early Vomiting late if at all Prior symptoms of underlying cause
Acute onset, persistent pain	Lying supine Dyspnea if pleural effusions from capillary leak syndrome Selected medications, high triglycerides may exacerbate	Leaning forward with trunk flexed	Nausea, vomiting, abdominal distention, fever Often recurrent; 80% of cases with a history of previous attacks and alcohol abuse or gallstones

(*continued*)

TABLE 16-1 Abdominal Pain *(Continued)*

Problem	Process	Location	Quality
Chronic pancreatitis (Ahmed Ali et al., 2016; Sankaran et al., 2015)	Irreversible destruction of the pancreatic parenchyma from recurrent inflammation of either large ducts or small ducts	Epigastric, radiating through to the back	Severe, persistent, deep
Pancreatic cancer (American Cancer Society, 2020)	Predominantly adenocarcinoma (95%), 9% have 5-y survival	Epigastric in either upper quadrant; often radiates to the back	Steady, deep
Gastric cancer	Adenocarcinoma in 90–95% of cases, either intestinal (older adults) or diffuse (younger adults, worse prognosis)	Increasingly in "cardia" and GE junction; also in distal stomach	Variable
Acute diverticulitis (Mulligan, 2015)	Acute inflammation of a colonic diverticula, outpouching a 5–10 mm in diameter, usually in sigmoid or descending colon	Left lower quadrant	May be cramping at first, then becomes steady
Mesenteric ischemia (American Cancer Society, 2018)	Occlusion of blood flow to small bowel from arterial or venous thrombosis (especially superior mesenteric artery), cardiac embolus, or hypoperfusion Can be colonic	May be periumbilical at first, then diffuse May be postprandial, classically inducing "food fear"	Cramping at first, then steady Pain disproportionate to examination findings

- *Visceral pain* occurs when hollow abdominal organs such as the intestine or biliary tree contract unusually forcefully or are distended or stretched. Solid organs such as the liver can also become painful when their capsules are stretched. Visceral pain may be difficult to localize. It is typically palpable near the midline at levels that vary according to the structure involved, as illustrated in Figure 16-5. Visceral pain varies in quality and may be gnawing, burning, cramping, or aching. When it becomes severe, it may be associated with sweating, pallor, nausea, vomiting, and restlessness.

The *biliary tree* is a vessel system directing digestive juice secretions from the pancreas, gall bladder, and liver through the ducts into the duodenum. Visceral pain in the RUQ suggests liver distention against its capsule from various causes of hepatitis, such as *alcoholic hepatitis.* Visceral periumbilical pain suggests early *acute appendicitis* from distention of an inflamed appendix. It gradually changes to parietal pain in the RLQ from inflammation of the adjacent parietal peritoneum.

- *Parietal pain* originates from inflammation in the parietal peritoneum, also known as *peritonitis.* It is a steady, aching pain that is usually more severe than visceral pain and more precisely localized over the involved structure. It is typically aggravated by movement or coughing. Patients with parietal pain usually prefer to lie still.

Pain of duodenal or pancreatic origin may be referred to the back; pain from the biliary tree, to the right scapular region or the right posterior thorax. Pain from *pleurisy* or inferior wall myocardial infarction may be referred to the epigastric area.

Timing	Factors that May Aggravate	Factors that May Relieve	Associated Symptoms and Setting
Chronic or recurrent course	Alcohol, heavy or fatty meals	Possibly leaning forward with trunk flexed; often intractable	Symptoms of decreased pancreatic function may appear: diarrhea with fatty stools (*steatorrhea*) and diabetes mellitus
Persistent pain; relentlessly progressive illness	Smoking, chronic pancreatitis		Painless jaundice, anorexia, weight loss Glucose intolerance, depression
Pain is persistent, slowly progressive Duration of pain is typically shorter than in peptic ulcer.	Food *H. pylori* infection	Not relieved by food or antacids	Anorexia, nausea, early satiety, weight loss, and sometimes bleeding Most common in ages 50–70
Often a gradual onset	Smoking, use of NSAIDs, obesity, insufficient dietary fiber intake	Weight control, smoking cessation, high-fiber diet	Fever, constipation Nausea, vomiting, abdominal mass with rebound tenderness
Usually abrupt in onset, then persistent	Underlying cardiac disease		Vomiting, bloody stool, soft distended abdomen with peritoneal signs, shock; age >50

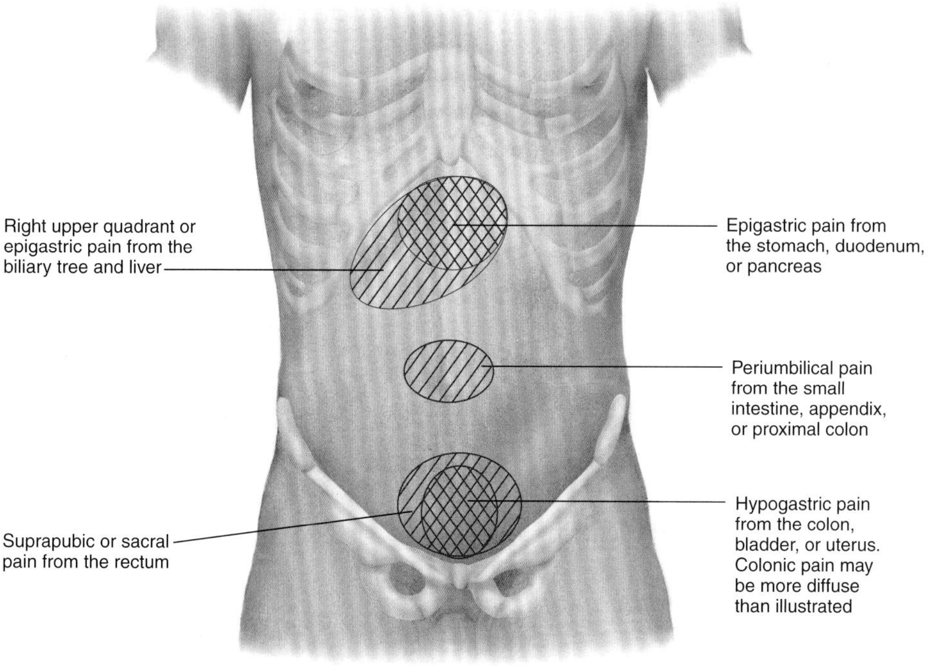
Right upper quadrant or epigastric pain from the biliary tree and liver
Epigastric pain from the stomach, duodenum, or pancreas
Periumbilical pain from the small intestine, appendix, or proximal colon
Hypogastric pain from the colon, bladder, or uterus. Colonic pain may be more diffuse than illustrated
Suprapubic or sacral pain from the rectum

FIGURE 16-5 The location of visceral pain can indicate the organ that may be the cause of the underlying problem.

- *Referred pain* is felt in more distant sites, which are innervated at approximately the same spinal levels as the inflamed structures. Referred pain often develops as the initial pain becomes more intense and thus seems to radiate or travel from the initial site. It may be palpated superficially or deeply but is usually well localized. Pain may also be referred to the abdomen from the chest, spine, or pelvis, and complicate the assessment of abdominal pain.

The Gastrointestinal Tract

Upper Abdominal Pain, Discomfort, and Heartburn

Over 40 million people in the United States were seen on an outpatient basis for gastrointestinal complaints in 2018 (Peery et al., 2019). Close to 22 million of these visits were for abdominal pain, 5.6 million for reflux disease, 4.7 million for vomiting, and 3.4 million for diarrhea (Peery et al., 2019). Gastrointestinal complaints are common.

Acute Upper Abdominal Pain or Discomfort

For patients with abdominal pain, causes range from benign to life-threatening, so take the time to conduct a careful history. Ask the patient to describe the pain in their own words and use "OLD CART" to fill in areas the patient did not mention or to clarify details for accuracy.

- *Onset:* Determine the *timing of the pain.* Is it *acute or chronic*? Acute abdominal pain has many patterns. Did the pain start suddenly or gradually? When did it begin?

Abdominal pain is seen in 4% to 5% of emergency department patients, usually for appendicitis, intestinal obstruction, or cholecystitis (Saccomano & Ferrara, 2013).

- *Location:* Ask the patient to *point to the pain.* Patients are not always able to clearly articulate their pain, especially when it is intense or radiates. The quadrant where the pain is located helps identify which of the underlying organs are involved. If clothing interferes with the person's ability to point to the pain, repeat the question during the physical examination.

Epigastric pain occurs with gastritis, gastroesophageal reflux disease (GERD), pancreatitis and perforated ulcers. RUQ pain occurs with cholecystitis, duodenal ulcer, or hepatitis (Cervellin et al., 2016).

- *Duration:* How long does the pain last?

  What is the pattern over a 24-hour period? Over weeks or months?

  Is the pain constant?

  Does the pain come and go?

  Are you dealing with an acute illness or a chronic and recurring one?

- *Characteristic symptoms:* Ask the patient to *describe the pain in their own words.* Pursue important details:

  - Where does the pain start?

- Does it radiate or travel anywhere?
- What is the pain like?
- If the patient has trouble describing the pain, try offering several choices: Is it aching?, burning?, gnawing?

  Ask the patient to rank the *severity of the pain* on a scale of 1 to 10. Note that severity does not always help identify the cause. Sensitivity to abdominal pain varies widely and tends to diminish in older adults, masking acute abdominal conditions. Pain threshold varies for each individual, and how patients accommodate to pain during daily activities also affects ratings of severity.

Doubling over with cramping, colicky pain may signal a *renal stone.* Sudden knife-like epigastric pain can occur with *pancreatitis* (Gougol et al., 2019; Kidney Stones, 2012).

- *Associated manifestations:* Ask the patient if they are experiencing any other symptoms (e.g., nausea, vomiting, indigestion, constipation, diarrhea, gastrointestinal bleeding, or fever).
- *Relieving factors:* As you explore factors that aggravate or relieve the pain, pay special attention to nonverbal cues, including body position and movement, changes in eating patterns, alcohol, medications (including antacids, aspirin and aspirin-like drugs, or over-the-counter medications), stress, and change in defecation or urinary patterns. Ask if indigestion or discomfort is related to exertion and relieved by rest.

Note that angina from inferior wall coronary artery disease may present as "indigestion," but is typically precipitated by exertion and relieved by rest. See Chapter 13, "The Respiratory System."

- *Treatment:* Determine what remedies the patient has tried and the results of each.

Chronic Upper Abdominal Discomfort or Pain

Dyspepsia is a chronic or recurrent discomfort or pain centered in the upper abdomen which is characterized by postprandial fullness, early satiety, and epigastric pain or burning (Tack & Talley, 2013). *Discomfort* is defined as a subjective negative feeling that is nonpainful. It can include various symptoms such as bloating, nausea, upper abdominal fullness, and heartburn.

Bloating, nausea, or belching can occur alone or be associated with other disorders. When they occur alone, they do not meet the criteria for dyspepsia.

Bloating may occur with inflammatory bowel disease, lactose intolerance, or ovarian cancer. Belching results from aerophagia or swallowing air.

Many patients with upper abdominal discomfort or pain will have **functional (nonulcer) dyspepsia**, defined as a 3-month history of nonspecific upper abdominal discomfort or nausea not attributable to structural abnormalities or peptic ulcer disease. Symptoms are usually recurring and typically present for more than 6 months (Tack & Talley, 2013).

Multifactorial causes of functional dyspepsia include delayed gastric emptying (20% to 40%), gastritis from *Helicobacter pylori (H. pylori)* (20% to 60%), peptic ulcer disease (up to 15% if *H. pylori* is present), *irritable bowel disease,* and psychosocial factors (Saccomano & Ferrara, 2013).

Many patients with chronic upper abdominal discomfort or pain complain of *heartburn*, *dysphagia*, or *regurgitation*. Heartburn and regurgitation reported together more than once a week usually receive a diagnosis of **gastroesophageal reflux disease (GERD)**. Approximately 20% of adults have symptoms of GERD (Spechler et al., 2019; Yadlapati & Pandolfino, 2020). These symptoms or mucosal damage on endoscopy are the diagnostic criteria for GERD. Risk factors include reduced salivary flow, which prolongs acid clearance by damping action of the bicarbonate buffer; delayed gastric emptying; selected medications; obesity; and hiatal hernia.

Heartburn is a rising retrosternal burning pain or discomfort occurring weekly or more often. It is typically aggravated by foods like alcohol, chocolate, citrus fruits, coffee, onions, and peppermint; or positions like bending over, exercising, lifting, or lying supine.

Note that angina from inferior wall coronary ischemia along the diaphragm may present as heartburn. See Chapter 13, "The Respiratory System."

Some patients with GERD have *atypical respiratory symptoms* such as chest pain, cough, wheezing, asthma, or aspiration pneumonia. Others complain of *pharyngeal symptoms*, such as hoarseness and chronic sore throat (American Gastroenterological Association, 2018).

Some patients may have "*alarm symptoms*," such as difficulty swallowing (**dysphagia**), pain with swallowing (**odynophagia**), frequent burping, recurrent vomiting, evidence of gastrointestinal bleeding, weight loss, anemia, or risk factors for gastric cancer or painless jaundice.

Patients with GERD who do not respond to empiric therapy, patients older than 55 years, and those with "alarm symptoms" warrant endoscopy to detect *esophagitis*, peptic strictures, *Barrett esophagus*, or esophageal cancer (Davis-Yadley et al., 2016). Approximately 50% to 85% of those with suspected GERD have no disease on endoscopy (American Gastroenterological Association, 2018; Davis-Yadley et al., 2016; Shaheen et al., 2012; Spechler et al., 2019). Approximately 10% of patients with chronic heartburn have Barrett esophagus, a metaplastic change in the esophageal lining from normal squamous to columnar epithelium. In those affected, dysplasia on endoscopy increases the risk of esophageal cancer from 0.1% to 0.5% (no dysplasia) to 6% to 19% per patient year (high-grade dysplasia) (Spechler & Souza, 2014).

Lower Abdominal Pain and Discomfort

Lower abdominal pain and discomfort may be acute or chronic. Asking the patient to point to the pain and characterize all its features, combined with findings on physical examination, will help identify possible causes. Some acute pain, especially in the suprapubic area or radiating from the flank, originates in the genitourinary tract.

Acute Lower Abdominal Pain

Patients may complain of *acute pain* localized to the *RLQ*. Find out if it is sharp and continuous or intermittent and cramping, causing them to double over.

RLQ pain or pain that migrates from the periumbilical region, combined with abdominal wall rigidity on palpation, is suspicious for appendicitis. In women, consider causes such as *pelvic inflammatory disease*, *ruptured ovarian follicle*, and *ectopic pregnancy* (Bao et al., 2013; Saccomano & Ferrara, 2013). Cramping pain radiating to the RLQ, LLQ, or groin could signify a renal stone.

When patients report acute pain in the LLQ or diffuse abdominal pain, investigate associated symptoms such as fever and loss of appetite.

LLQ pain, especially with a palpable mass, signals *diverticulitis*. Diffuse abdominal pain with abdominal distention, hyperactive high-pitched bowel sounds, and tenderness on palpation may indicate *small or large bowel obstruction*. Pain with absent bowel sounds, rigidity, percussion tenderness, and guarding points to *peritonitis*.

See Table 16-1, "Abdominal Pain."

Chronic Lower Abdominal Pain

If there is *chronic pain* in the quadrants of the lower abdomen, ask about changes in bowel habits and alternating diarrhea and constipation.

Change in bowel habits with a mass lesion indicates the possibility of *colon cancer*. Intermittent pain for 12 weeks of the preceding 12 months with relief from defecation, change in frequency of bowel movements, or change in form of stool (loose, watery, pellet-like) without structural or biochemical abnormalities are symptoms of *irritable bowel syndrome* (Kaplan, 2015; Ludlow, 2019; Ng et al., 2018).

Abdominal Pain Associated with Gastrointestinal Symptoms

Patients often experience abdominal pain in conjunction with other symptoms. Ask questions that relate, beginning with "How is your appetite?" This may lead to other symptoms such as *indigestion*, *nausea*, *vomiting*, and/or *anorexia*. *Indigestion* is a general term for distress associated with eating that can have many meanings. Urge your patient to be more specific.

Anorexia, nausea, and vomiting accompany many gastrointestinal disorders; including pregnancy, diabetic ketoacidosis, adrenal insufficiency, hypercalcemia, uremia, liver disease, emotional distress, and adverse drug reactions. Induced vomiting without nausea is more indicative of anorexia or bulimia.

Nausea, often described as "feeling sick to my stomach," may progress to retching and vomiting. *Retching* describes involuntary spasm of the stomach, diaphragm, and esophagus that precedes and culminates in *vomiting*, the forceful expulsion of gastric contents out of the mouth. Some patients may not actually vomit but raise esophageal or gastric contents without nausea or retching, called *regurgitation*.

Regurgitation occurs in GERD, esophageal stricture, and esophageal cancer.

Ask about any vomitus or regurgitated material and inspect it, if possible. Note the color, odor and quantity. Assist the patient with estimating the amount: A teaspoon? Two teaspoons? A cupful?

Vomiting and pain indicate small bowel obstruction. Fecal odor occurs with small bowel obstruction and gastrocolic fistula.

Ask specifically if the vomitus contains any blood and quantify the amount. Gastric juice is clear and mucoid. Small amounts of yellowish or greenish bile are common and have no special significance. Brownish or blackish vomitus with a coffee-grounds appearance suggests blood altered by gastric acid. Coffee-grounds emesis or red blood is termed **hematemesis**.

CLINICAL TIP
Hematemesis may accompany esophageal or gastric varices, gastritis, or peptic ulcer disease.

Is there any dehydration or electrolyte imbalance from prolonged vomiting or significant blood loss? Do the patient's symptoms suggest any complications of vomiting, such as aspiration into the lungs, seen in debilitated, obtunded, or elderly patients?

CLINICAL TIP
Symptoms of blood loss such as lightheadedness or syncope depend on the rate and volume of bleeding and are rare until blood loss exceeds 500 mL.

Anorexia is loss or lack of appetite. Find out if it arises from intolerance to certain foods, distortion of self-image, abdominal discomfort (real or perceived), or a fear of food (*cibophobia*). Check for associated symptoms of nausea, vomiting, or excessive exercise.

"Food fear" with abdominal pain and a slightly distended, soft, nontender abdomen are hallmarks of *mesenteric ischemia*, which is poor circulation in the vessels supplying blood flow to the mesenteric organs (i.e., stomach, liver, colon, and intestines). Patients may complain of unpleasant *abdominal fullness* after light or moderate meals, or *early satiety*, the inability to eat a full meal. A dietary assessment or recall may be warranted (see Chapter 8, "Nutrition and Hydration").

If a person has fullness or early satiety, consider *diabetic gastroparesis* (weakness in the muscles of the stomach), anticholinergic medications, *gastric outlet obstruction, gastric cancer*, and *hepatitis*.

Other Gastrointestinal Symptoms

Difficulty Swallowing and/or Painful Swallowing

Less commonly, patients may report difficulty swallowing from impaired passage of solid foods or liquids from the mouth to the stomach, or *dysphagia* (Table 16-2). Food seems to stick, or "not go down right," suggesting motility disorders or structural anomalies. The sensation of a lump or foreign body in the throat unrelated to swallowing, called a *globus* sensation, is not true dysphagia.

Indicators of *oropharyngeal dysphagia* include drooling, nasopharyngeal regurgitation, and cough from aspiration. Gurgling or regurgitation of undigested food occurs in GERD, motility disorders, and structural

TABLE 16-2 Dysphagia

Process and Problem	Timing	Factors that Aggravate	Factors that Relieve	Associated Symptoms and Conditions
Oropharyngeal dysphagia (due to motor disorders affecting the pharyngeal muscles)	Acute or gradual onset and a variable course, depending on the underlying disorder	Attempts to start the swallowing process		Aspiration into the lungs or regurgitation into the nose with attempts to swallow Neurologic evidence of stroke, bulbar palsy, or other neuromuscular conditions
Esophageal Dysphagia				
Due to Mechanical Narrowing				
Mucosal rings and webs	Intermittent	Solid foods	Regurgitation of the bolus of food	Usually none
Esophageal stricture	Intermittent; may become slowly progressive	Solid foods	Regurgitation of the bolus of food	A long history of heartburn and regurgitation
Esophageal cancer	May be intermittent at first; progressive over months	Solid foods, with progression to liquids	Regurgitation of the bolus of food	Pain in the chest and back and weight loss, especially late in the course of illness
Due to Motor Disorders				
Diffuse esophageal spasm	Intermittent	Solids or liquids	Maneuvers described below; sometimes nitroglycerin	Chest pain that mimics angina pectoris or myocardial infarction and lasts minutes to hours; possibly heartburn
Scleroderma or achalasia	Intermittent; may progress slowly	Solids or liquids	Repeated swallowing; movements such as straightening the back, raising the arms, or a Valsalva maneuver (straining down against a closed glottis)	Heartburn; other manifestations of scleroderma Regurgitation, often at night when lying down with nocturnal cough; possibly chest pain precipitated by eating

disorders like *esophageal stricture* and *Zenker diverticulum*. Causes are generally mechanical/obstructive in younger adults and neurologic/muscular in older adults (stroke, Parkinson disease) (Giraldo-Cadavid et al., 2017).

The nurse should ask the patient if they have any difficulty or pain swallowing (*odynophagia*). Ask the patient to point to where the dysphagia occurs. Pointing to below the sternoclavicular notch indicates *esophageal dysphagia*.

Pursue which types of foods provoke symptoms—solid foods or solids and liquids? Establish the timing. When does the dysphagia start? Is it intermittent or persistent? Is it progressing? If so, over what time period? Are there associated symptoms and medical conditions?

CLINICAL TIP

If solid foods trigger symptoms, consider structural esophageal causes such as *esophageal stricture*, webbing or *Schatzki ring*, and neoplasm; if both solids and liquids are triggers, a motility disorder, such as *achalasia* (a condition in which the muscles of the lower part of the esophagus fail to relax), is more likely.

Is there *odynophagia,* or pain on swallowing?

May be due to esophageal ulceration from ingestion of aspirin or nonsteroidal antiinflammatory drugs (NSAIDs), caustic ingestion, radiation, or infection from *Candida, cytomegalovirus, herpes simplex,* or *HIV*.

Change in Bowel Function

To assess *bowel function,* start with open-ended questions: "Have you noticed any change in your bowel movements?" "How often do they occur?" "Have you noticed any change in stool appearance?" The range of normal bowel movements varies from a few a day to only a few per week depending on the individual. Some patients may complain of passing excessive gas, or *flatus,* normally about 600 mL per day.

Causes may include *aerophagia,* eating gas-producing foods (e.g., legumes, *intestinal lactase deficiency,* or *irritable bowel syndrome*).

Diarrhea and Constipation

Patients vary widely in their views of diarrhea and constipation (Tables 16-3 and 16-4). Increased water content of the stool results in **diarrhea**, or stool volume greater than 200 g in 24 hours. Patients, however, usually focus on the change to loose, watery stools or increased frequency during 75% or more of defecations (Riddle et al., 2016; World Health Organization, 2020).

TABLE 16-3 Constipation

Problem	Process	Associated Symptoms and Setting
Life Activities and Habits		
Inadequate time or setting for the defecation reflex	Ignoring the sensation of a full rectum inhibits the defecation reflex	Hectic schedules, unfamiliar surroundings, bed rest
False expectations of bowel habits	Expectations of "regularity" or more frequent stools than a person's norm	Beliefs, treatments, and advertisements that promote the use of laxatives
Diet deficient in fiber	Decreased fecal bulk	Other factors such as debilitation and constipating drugs may contribute

Problem	Process	Associated Symptoms and Setting
Irritable Bowel Syndrome (Newman, 2019)		
	Functional change in frequency or form of bowel movement without known pathology; possibly from change in intestinal bacteria	Three patterns: diarrhea-predominant, constipation-predominant, or mixed. Symptoms present 6 mo or longer and abdominal pain for 3 mo or longer plus at least two of three features (improvement with defecation; onset with change in stool frequency; onset with change in stool form and appearance)
Mechanical Obstruction		
Cancer of the rectum or sigmoid colon	Progressive narrowing of the bowel lumen	Change in bowel habits; often diarrhea, abdominal pain, and bleeding In rectal cancer, tenesmus and pencil-shaped stools
Fecal impaction	A large, firm, immovable fecal mass, most often in the rectum	Rectal fullness, abdominal pain, and diarrhea around the impaction Common in debilitated, bedridden, and elderly patients
Other obstructing lesions (such as diverticulitis, volvulus, intussusception, or hernia)	Narrowing or complete obstruction of the bowel	Colicky abdominal pain, abdominal distention, and with intussusception, often "currant jelly" stools (red blood and mucus)
Painful Anal Lesions		
	Pain may cause spasm of the external sphincter and voluntary inhibition of the defecation reflex	Anal fissures, painful hemorrhoids, perirectal abscesses
Drugs		
	A variety of mechanisms	Opiates, anticholinergics, antacids containing calcium or aluminum, and many others
Depression		
	A disorder of mood	Fatigue, anhedonia, sleep disturbance, weight loss
Neurologic Disorders		
	Interference with the autonomic innervation of the bowel	Spinal cord injuries, multiple sclerosis, Hirschsprung disease, and other conditions
Metabolic Conditions		
	Interference with bowel motility	Pregnancy, hypothyroidism, hypercalcemia

TABLE 16-4 Diarrhea

Problem	Process	Characteristics of Stool	Timing	Associated Symptoms	Setting, Persons at Risk
Acute Diarrhea (Riddle et al., 2016)					
Secretory infection (noninflammatory)	Infection by viruses, preformed bacterial toxins (such as *Staphylococcus aureus*, *Clostridium perfringens*, toxigenic *Escherichia coli*, *Vibrio cholerae*), cryptosporidium, *Giardia lamblia*, rotavirus	Watery, without blood, pus, or mucus	Duration of a few days, possibly longer Lactase deficiency may lead to a longer course	Nausea, vomiting, periumbilical cramping pain Temperature normal or slightly elevated	Often travel, a common food source, or an epidemic
Inflammatory infection	Colonization or invasion of intestinal mucosa (nontyphoid *Salmonella*, *Shigella*, *Yersinia*, *Campylobacter*, enteropathic *E. coli*, *Entamoeba histolytica*, *C. difficile*)	Loose to watery, often with blood, pus, or mucus	An acute illness of varying duration	Lower abdominal cramping pain and often rectal urgency, tenesmus; fever	Travel, contaminated food or water. Frequent anal intercourse
Drug-Induced Diarrhea					
	Action of many drugs, such as magnesium-containing antacids, antibiotics, antineoplastic agents, and laxatives	Loose to watery	Acute, recurrent, or chronic	Possibly nausea; usually little if any pain	Prescribed or over-the-counter medications
Chronic Diarrhea (Arasaradnam et al., 2018)					
Diarrheal syndrome/irritable bowel syndrome (Newman, 2019)	Change in frequency and form of bowel movements without chemical or structural abnormality	Loose; ~50% with mucus; small to moderate volume Small, hard stools with constipation May be mixed pattern	Worse in the morning; rarely at night	Cramping lower abdominal pain, abdominal distention, flatulence, nausea Urgency, pain relieved with defecation	Young and middle-aged adults, especially women
Cancer of the sigmoid colon	Partial obstruction by a malignant neoplasm	May be blood-streaked	Variable	Change in usual bowel habits, cramping lower abdominal pain, constipation	

Problem	Process	Characteristics of Stool	Timing	Associated Symptoms	Setting, Persons at Risk
Inflammatory Bowel Disease					
Ulcerative colitis	Mucosal inflammation typically extending proximally from the rectum (*proctitis*) to varying lengths of the colon (*colitis* to *pancolitis*), with microulcerations and if chronic, inflammatory polyps	Frequent, watery, often containing blood	Abrupt Often recurrent, persisting, and may awaken at night	Cramping with urgency, tenesmus Fever, fatigue, weakness Abdominal pain if complicated by toxic megacolon May include episcleritis, uveitis, arthritis, erythema nodosum	Often young adults, Ashkenazi Jewish descendants Linked to altered CD4+ T-cell Th2 response Increases risk of colon cancer
Crohn disease of the small bowel (*regional enteritis*) or colon (*granulomatous colitis*)	Chronic transmural inflammation of the bowel wall with skip pattern involving the terminal ileum and/or proximal colon (and rectal sparing) May cause strictures	Small, soft to loose or watery with bleeding if *colitis*, obstructive symptoms if *enteritis*	Insidious onset; chronic or recurrent	Cramping periumbilical or right lower quadrant (*enteritis*) or diffuse (*colitis*) pain, with weight loss Perianal or perirectal abscesses and fistulas May cause small or large bowel obstruction	Often late teens or young adults More common in Ashkenazi Jewish descendants Increases risk of colon cancer
Voluminous Diarrhea					
Malabsorption syndrome	Defective membrane transport or absorption of intestinal epithelium (*Crohn, celiac disease, surgical resection*); impaired luminal digestion (*pancreatic insufficiency*); epithelial defects at brush border (*lactose intolerance*)	Typically bulky, soft, light yellow to gray, mushy, greasy or oily, and sometimes frothy; particularly foul-smelling; usually floats in the toilet (*steatorrhea)*	Onset of illness typically insidious	Anorexia, weight loss, fatigue, abdominal distention, often cramping lower abdominal pain Symptoms of nutritional deficiencies such as bleeding (vitamin K), bone pain and fractures (vitamin D), glossitis (vitamin B), and edema (protein)	Variable, depending on cause
Secretory diarrhea	Variable: from bacterial infection, secreting villous adenoma, fat or bile salt malabsorption, hormone-mediated conditions (gastrin in Zollinger–Ellison syndrome, vasoactive intestinal peptide)	Watery diarrhea of large volume	Variable	Weight loss, dehydration, nausea, vomiting, and cramping abdominal pain	Variable depending on cause

(*continued*)

TABLE 16-4 Diarrhea (*Continued*)

Problem	Process	Characteristics of Stool	Timing	Associated Symptoms	Setting, Persons at Risk
Osmotic Diarrhea					
Lactose intolerance	Intestinal lactase deficiency	Watery diarrhea of large volume	Follows the ingestion of milk and milk products; relieved by fasting	Cramping abdominal pain, abdominal distention, flatulence	In >50% of African Americans, Asians, Native Americans, Hispanic Americans; in 5–20% of Caucasians
Abuse of osmotic purgatives	Laxative habit, often surreptitious	Watery diarrhea of large volume	Variable	Often none	Persons with anorexia nervosa or bulimia nervosa

Ask about the duration:

- *Acute diarrhea* lasts 2 weeks or less.
- *Persistent diarrhea* lasts more than 14 days and less than 30 days.
- *Chronic diarrhea* is defined as lasting 4 weeks or more.

CLINICAL TIP
Acute diarrhea is usually caused by infection (Riddle et al., 2016); chronic diarrhea is typically noninfectious in origin, as in *Crohn disease* and *ulcerative colitis.*

Ask about the characteristics of the diarrhea, including volume, frequency, and consistency. Is there mucus, pus, or blood? Is there associated *tenesmus* (a constant urge to defecate) accompanied by pain, cramping, and involuntary straining?

High-volume, frequent watery stools are usually from the small intestine; small-volume stools with *tenesmus*, or diarrhea with mucus, pus, or blood occurs in rectal inflammatory conditions.

Does diarrhea occur at night? Nocturnal diarrhea usually has pathologic significance; it may indicate systemic disease, dietary changes, or alcohol-related factors (Arasaradnam et al., 2018).

Are the stools greasy or oily? Frothy? Foul-smelling? Floating on the surface because of excessive gas?

CLINICAL TIP
Oily residue, sometimes frothy or floating, occurs with *steatorrhea,* or fatty diarrheal stools, from malabsorption in *celiac sprue, pancreatic insufficiency, cystic fibrosis,* or *small-bowel bacterial overgrowth.*

Associated features should be considered when identifying possible causes. These include current and/or alternative medications, especially antibiotics or excessive use of laxatives (*factitious diarrhea*), recent travel, dietary patterns, baseline bowel habits, and risk factors for immunocompromise.

CLINICAL TIP

Diarrhea is common with the use of penicillin and macrolides, magnesium-based antacids, metformin, and herbal and alternative medicines. Also, consider *Clostridioides* (formerly *Clostridium*) *difficile* infection if there has been recent health care exposure or antibiotic use (Riddle et al., 2016).

Another common symptom is **constipation**. Recent criteria stipulate that constipation should be present for at least 12 weeks of the prior 6 months with at least two of the following conditions: fewer than three bowel movements per week; 25% or more defecations with either straining or sensation of incomplete evacuation; lumpy or hard stools; or need for manual facilitation (Herrington, 2018; Trads et al., 2018).

Ask about frequency of bowel movements, passage of hard or painful stools, straining, and a sense of incomplete rectal emptying or pressure. Types of primary or functional constipation are normal transit, slow transit, impaired expulsion (from pelvic floor disorders), and constipation-predominant irritable bowel syndrome. Secondary causes include medications and conditions like amyloidosis, diabetes, and central nervous system (CNS) disorders (Herrington, 2018; Shah et al., 2015; Trads et al., 2018).

Check if the patient actually looks at the stool and can describe its color and bulk.

Thin, pencil-like stool occurs in an obstructing "apple core" lesion of the sigmoid colon.

What remedies has the patient tried? Do medications or stress play a role? Are there associated systemic disorders? Causes of constipation may include medications such as anticholinergic agents, calcium channel blockers, iron supplements, and opiates. Constipation also occurs with *diabetes*, *hypothyroidism*, *hypercalcemia*, *multiple sclerosis*, *Parkinson disease*, and *systemic sclerosis.*

Occasionally, there is no passage of either feces or gas, or *obstipation*. Obstipation may signify intestinal obstruction.

Inquire about the color of stools. Is there *melena*, or black tarry stools, or *hematochezia* (stools that are red or maroon-colored) (Table 16-5)? Pursue such important details as quantity and frequency of any blood.

Melena may appear with as little as 100 mL of *upper gastrointestinal bleeding*, and *hematochezia*, is usually from *lower gastrointestinal bleeding*, but may occur with brisk upper gastrointestinal bleeding.

Is the blood mixed in with the stool or on the surface? Does it appear as streaks on the toilet paper or is it more copious? Blood on the surface or on toilet paper may occur with *hemorrhoids.*

TABLE 16-5 Black and Bloody Stools

Problem	Selected Causes	Associated Symptoms and Setting
Melena		
Refers to passage of black, tarry stools Fecal blood tests are positive Involves ≥60 mL of blood into the gastrointestinal tract (less in children), usually from the esophagus, stomach, or duodenum with transit time of 7–14 h Less commonly, if slow transit, blood loss originates in the jejunum, ileum, or ascending colon In infants, melena may result from swallowing blood during the birth process	Gastritis, GERD, peptic ulcer (gastric or duodenal)	Usually epigastric discomfort from heartburn, dysmotility; if peptic ulcer, pain after meals (delay of 2–3 h if duodenal ulcer). May be asymptomatic
	Gastritis or stress ulcers	Recent ingestion of alcohol, aspirin, or other antiinflammatory drugs; recent body trauma, severe burns, surgery, or increased intracranial pressure
	Esophageal or gastric varices	Cirrhosis of the liver or other cause of portal hypertension
	Reflux esophagitis Mallory–Weiss tear, a mucosal tear in the esophagus due to retching and vomiting	Retching, vomiting, often recent ingestion of alcohol
Black Stool		
Black stool from other causes with negative fecal blood tests Stool change has no pathologic significance	Ingestion of iron, bismuth salts, licorice, or even chocolate cookies	Asymptomatic
Stool with Red Blood (*Hematochezia*)		
Usually originates in the colon, rectum, or anus, and much less frequently in the jejunum or ileum Upper gastrointestinal hemorrhage may also cause red stool, usually with large blood loss ≥1 L Rapid transit time through the intestinal tract leaves insufficient time for the blood to turn black.	Colon cancer	Often a change in bowel habits, weight loss
	Hyperplasia or adenomatous polyps	Often no other symptoms
	Diverticula of the colon	Often no other symptoms unless inflammation causes diverticulitis
	Inflammatory conditions of the colon and rectum:	
	• Ulcerative colitis, Crohn disease	See Table 16-3.
	• Infectious diarrhea	See Table 16-3.
	• Proctitis (various causes) from frequent anal intercourse	Rectal urgency, tenesmus
	Ischemic colitis	Lower abdominal pain, sometimes fever or shock in older adults; abdomen typically soft to palpation
	Hemorrhoids	Blood on the toilet paper, on the surface of the stool, or dripping into the toilet
	Anal fissure	Blood on the toilet paper or on the surface of the stool; anal pain
Reddish but Nonbloody Stools	Ingestion of beets	Pink urine, which usually precedes the reddish stool: from poor metabolism of betacyanin

Jaundice

In some patients, you will find jaundice (icterus), the yellowish discoloration of the skin, mucous membranes and sclerae from increased levels of bilirubin (a bile pigment derived chiefly from the breakdown of hemoglobin) (Fargo et al., 2017). Normally the hepatocytes conjugate (combine), unconjugated bilirubin with other substances, making the bile water-soluble, and then excrete the conjugated bilirubin into the bile. The bile passes through the cystic duct into the common bile duct, which also drains the extrahepatic ducts from the liver. More distally, the common bile duct and the pancreatic ducts empty into the duodenum at the ampulla of Vater (hepatopancreatic duct) (Fargo et al., 2017). Box 16-2 outlines the mechanisms of jaundice.

BOX 16-2 MECHANISMS OF JAUNDICE

- Increased production of bilirubin
- Decreased uptake of bilirubin by the hepatocytes
- Decreased ability of the liver to conjugate bilirubin
- Decreased excretion of bilirubin into the bile, resulting in absorption of *conjugated* bilirubin back into the blood

Predominantly, unconjugated bilirubin occurs from the first three mechanisms, as in *hemolytic anemia* (increased destruction) and *Gilbert syndrome* (a common, harmless liver condition in which the liver doesn't properly process bilirubin). Impaired excretion of conjugated bilirubin occurs with *viral hepatitis*, *cirrhosis*, *primary biliary cirrhosis*, and drug-induced cholestasis from medications such as oral contraceptives, methyl testosterone, and chlorpromazine.

Intrahepatic jaundice can be *hepatocellular*, from damage to the hepatocytes, or *cholestatic*, from impaired excretion as a result of damaged hepatocytes or intrahepatic bile ducts. *Extrahepatic* jaundice arises from obstruction of the extrahepatic bile ducts, most commonly the cystic and common bile ducts.

CLINICAL TIP

Gallstones or pancreatic, cholangio, or duodenal carcinoma may obstruct the common bile duct.

As the patient with jaundice is assessed, pay special attention to the associated symptoms and the setting in which the illness occurred. What was the *color of the urine* as the patient became ill? When the level of conjugated bilirubin increases in the blood, it may be excreted into the urine, turning the urine a dark yellowish brown or tea color. Unconjugated bilirubin is not water-soluble, so it is not excreted into urine. Is there any associated pain?

Dark urine from bilirubin indicates impaired excretion of bilirubin into the gastrointestinal tract. Painless jaundice points to malignant obstruction of the bile ducts, seen in *duodenal* or *pancreatic carcinoma*; painful jaundice is commonly infectious in origin, as in *hepatitis A* and *cholangitis*.

Ask also about the *color of the stools*. When excretion of bile into the intestine is completely obstructed, the stools become gray or light-colored (*acholic*) without bile.

Acholic stools may occur briefly in *viral hepatitis*; they are common in obstructive jaundice.

Does the skin itch without other obvious explanation? Is there associated pain? What is its pattern? Has it been recurrent in the past?

CLINICAL TIP
Itching indicates cholestatic or obstructive jaundice; pain may signify a distended liver capsule, biliary cholic, or pancreatic cancer.

With a finding of jaundice, liver disease must be considered (Box 16-3).

BOX 16-3 LIVER DISEASE AND JAUNDICE

The nurse must ask the patient about risk factors for:

- *Hepatitis*: Travel or meals in areas of poor sanitation, which could result in ingestion of contaminated water or food (hepatitis A); parenteral or mucous membrane exposure to infectious body fluids such as blood, serum, semen, and vaginal fluid, especially through sexual contact with an infected partner or use of shared needles for injection drug use (hepatitis B); sharing of needles of infected persons or tainted blood transfusions (hepatitis C)
- *Alcoholic hepatitis* or *alcoholic cirrhosis*: Screen the patient carefully about alcohol use with, for example, the AUDIT questionnaire (see Chapter 4, "The Health History")
- *Toxic liver damage* from medications, industrial solvents, or environmental toxins
- *Gallbladder disease* or *surgery* that may result in extrahepatic biliary obstruction
- *Hereditary disorders* present in the family history

The Renal System

General questions for a urinary history include:

- Do you have any difficulty passing your urine?
- How often do you go (Table 16-6)?
- Do you have to get up at night? How often?
- How much urine do you pass at a time?
- Is there any pain or burning?
- Do you ever feel rushed getting to the toilet in time?
- Do you ever leak any urine or wet yourself unintentionally?
- Can you sense when your bladder is full and when voiding occurs?

Involuntary voiding or lack of awareness suggests cognitive or neurosensory deficits.

TABLE 16-6 Frequency, Nocturia, and Polyuria

Problem	Mechanisms	Selected Causes	Associated Symptoms
Frequency	Decreased bladder capacity		
	• Increased bladder sensitivity to stretch because of inflammation	*Infection,* stones, tumor, or foreign body in the bladder	Burning on urination, urinary urgency, sometimes gross hematuria
	• Decreased elasticity of the bladder wall	Infiltration by scar tissue or tumor	Symptoms of associated inflammation (see above) are common
	• Decreased cortical inhibition of bladder contractions	Motor disorders of the central nervous system, such as a stroke	Urinary urgency; neurologic symptoms such as weakness and paralysis
	Impaired bladder emptying with residual urine in the bladder:		
	• Partial mechanical obstruction of the bladder neck or proximal urethra	Most commonly, benign prostatic hyperplasia; urethral stricture and other obstructive lesions of the bladder or prostate	Prior obstructive symptoms: hesitancy in starting the urinary stream, straining to void, reduced size and force of the stream, and dribbling during or at the end of urination
	• Loss of S2–4 innervation to the bladder	Neurologic disease affecting the sacral nerves or nerve roots (e.g., diabetic neuropathy)	Weakness or sensory defects
Nocturia			
With high volumes	Most types of polyuria		
	Decreased concentrating ability of the kidney with loss of the normal decrease in nocturnal urinary output	Chronic renal insufficiency due to a number of diseases	Possibly other symptoms of renal insufficiency
	Excessive fluid intake before bedtime	Habit, especially involving alcohol and coffee	
	Fluid-retaining, edematous states; daytime accumulation of dependent edema that is excreted at night when the patient is supine	Heart failure, nephrotic syndrome, hepatic cirrhosis with ascites, chronic venous insufficiency	Edema and other symptoms of the underlying disorder; urinary output during the day may be reduced as fluid accumulates in the body
With low volumes	Urinary frequency; voiding while up at night without a real urge, a "pseudo-frequency"	Insomnia	Variable
Polyuria	Deficiency of antidiuretic hormone (diabetes insipidus)	A disorder of the posterior pituitary and hypothalamus	Thirst and polydipsia, often severe and persistent; nocturia
	Renal unresponsiveness to antidiuretic hormone (nephrogenic diabetes insipidus)	A number of kidney diseases, including hypercalcemic and hypokalemic nephropathy; drug toxicity (e.g., from lithium)	
	Solute diuresis:		
	• Electrolytes, such as sodium salts	Large saline infusions, potent diuretics, certain kidney diseases	Variable
	• Nonelectrolytes, such as glucose	Uncontrolled diabetes mellitus	Thirst, polydipsia, and nocturia
	Excessive water intake	Primary polydipsia	Polydipsia tends to be episodic. Thirst may not be present. Nocturia is usually absent

Ask women if sudden coughing, sneezing, or laughing cause loss of urine. Occasional leakage is not necessarily significant. *Stress incontinence* arises from decreased intraurethral pressure (Table 16-7)

Ask men:

- Do you have trouble starting your stream?
- Do you have to stand close to the toilet to void?

TABLE 16-7 Urinary Incontinence[a]

Problem	Mechanisms	Symptoms	Physical Signs
Stress Incontinence			
The urethral sphincter is weakened so that transient increases in intra-abdominal pressure raise the bladder pressure to levels that exceed urethral resistance.	In women, pelvic floor weakness and inadequate muscular and ligamentous support of the bladder and proximal urethra change in the angle between the bladder and the urethra. Causes include childbirth and surgery. Local conditions affecting the internal urethral sphincter, such as postmenopausal atrophy of the mucosa and urethral infection, may also contribute In men, stress incontinence may follow prostatic surgery	Momentary leakage of small amounts of urine with coughing, laughing, and sneezing while the person is in an upright position Urine loss is unrelated to a conscious urge to urinate	Stress incontinence may be demonstrable, especially if the patient is examined before voiding and in a standing position Atrophic vaginitis may be evident. Bladder distention is absent
Urge Incontinence			
Detrusor contractions are stronger than normal and overcome the normal urethral resistance. The bladder is typically *small*.	Decreased cortical inhibition of detrusor contractions from strokes, brain tumors, dementia, and lesions of the spinal cord above the sacral level Hyperexcitability of sensory pathways, as in bladder infections, tumors, and fecal impaction Deconditioning of voiding reflexes, as in frequent voluntary voiding at low bladder volumes	Involuntary urine loss preceded by an urge to void The volume tends to be moderate Urgency Frequency and nocturia with small to moderate volumes If acute inflammation is present, pain on urination Possibly "pseudo-stress incontinence"—voiding 10–20 sec after stresses such as a change of position, going up or down stairs, and possibly coughing, laughing, or sneezing	The small bladder is not detectable on abdominal examination When cortical inhibition is decreased, mental deficits or motor signs of central nervous system disease are often present When sensory pathways are hyperexcitable, signs of local pelvic problems or a fecal impaction may be present

Problem	Mechanisms	Symptoms	Physical Signs
Overflow Incontinence			
Detrusor contractions are insufficient to overcome urethral resistance, causing urinary retention. The bladder is typically flaccid and *large*, even after an effort to void.	Obstruction of the bladder outlet, as in *benign prostatic hyperplasia* or tumor Weakness of the detrusor muscle associated with peripheral nerve disease at S2–4 level Impaired bladder sensation that interrupts the reflex arc, as in diabetic neuropathy	When intravesicular pressure overcomes urethral resistance, continuous dripping or dribbling incontinence ensues Decreased force of the urinary stream Prior symptoms of partial urinary obstruction or other symptoms of peripheral nerve disease may be present	Examination often reveals an enlarged, sometimes tender bladder. Other signs include prostate enlargement, motor signs of peripheral nerve disease, a decrease in sensation (including perineal sensation), and diminished to absent reflexes
Functional Incontinence			
This is a functional inability to get to the toilet in time because of impaired health or environmental conditions.	Problems in mobility resulting from weakness, arthritis, poor vision, or other conditions Environmental factors such as an unfamiliar setting, distant bathroom facilities, bed rails, or physical restraints	Incontinence on the way to the toilet or only in the early morning	The bladder is not detectable on physical examination. Look for physical or environmental clues to the likely cause
Incontinence Secondary to Medications			
Drugs may contribute to any type of incontinence listed.	Sedatives, tranquilizers, anticholinergics, sympathetic blockers, and potent diuretics	Variable A careful history and chart review are important	Variable

[a]Patients may have more than one kind of incontinence.

Source: Junqueira, J. B., & Santos, V. L. C. G. (2018). Urinary incontinence in hospital patients: Prevalence and associated factors. *Revista Latino-Americana De Enfermagem*, *25*, e2970. Published 2018 January 8. https://doi.org/10.1590/1518-8345.2139.2970; and Newman, D., Burgio, K., Markland, A., & Goode, P. (2014). Urinary incontinence: Nonsurgical treatments. *Geriatric Urology*, 141–168. https://doi.org/10.1007/978-1-4614-9047-0_11

- Is there a change in the force or size of your stream, or do you begin straining to void?
- Do you hesitate or stop in the middle of voiding?
- Is there dribbling when you are finished?

These findings are common in men with partial bladder outlet obstruction from *benign prostatic hyperplasia* or *urethral stricture.*

Suprapubic Pain

Disorders in the urinary tract may cause pain in either the abdomen or the back. Bladder disorders may cause *suprapubic pain.* With a *bladder infection*, pain in the lower abdomen is typically dull and pressure-like. In sudden overdistention of the bladder, pain is often agonizing; in contrast, chronic bladder distention is usually painless.

Pain from sudden overdistention accompanies acute urinary retention.

Dysuria, Urgency, or Frequency

Infection or irritation of either the bladder or urethra often leads to *pain on urination*, usually felt as a burning sensation. Some clinicians refer to this as *dysuria*, while others reserve this term for difficulty voiding. Women may report internal urethral discomfort, sometimes described as a pressure or an external burning from the flow of urine across irritated or inflamed labia. Men typically feel a burning sensation proximal to the glans penis. In contrast, *prostatic pain* is felt in the perineum and occasionally in the rectum.

Painful urination accompanies cystitis (bladder infection), *urethritis* and *urinary tract infections,* bladder stones, tumors, and in men, acute *prostatitis.* Women report that internal burning occurs with *urethritis* and external burning with *vulvovaginitis.*

Other commonly associated urinary symptoms are *urgency* and *frequency.* Urgency is an unusually intense and immediate desire to void, sometimes leading to involuntary voiding or urge incontinence. Frequency is abnormally frequent voiding. Ask about any related fever or chills, blood in the urine, or any pain in the abdomen, flank, or back (Fig. 16-6). Men with partial obstruction to urinary outflow often report *hesitancy* in starting the urine stream, straining to void, reduced caliber and force of the urinary stream, or dribbling as voiding is completed (Kinjo et al., 2020; Liu et al., 2019).

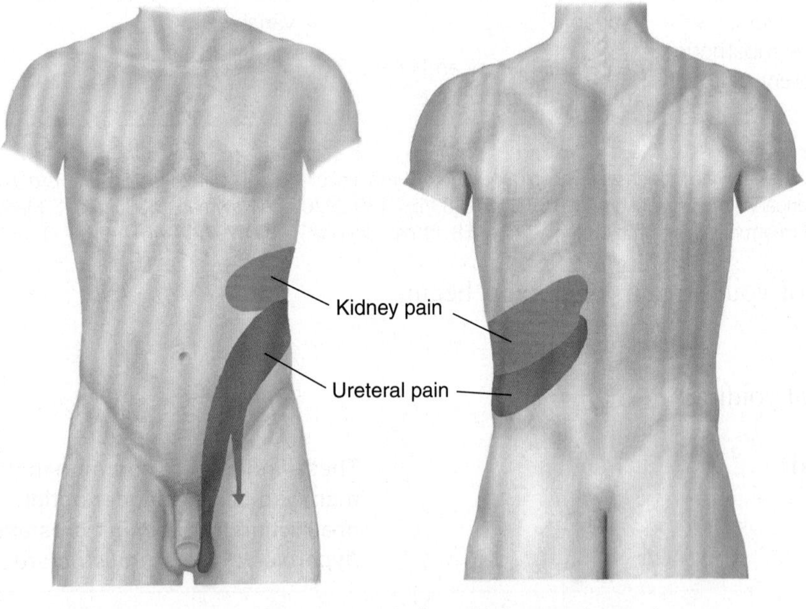

FIGURE 16-6 The location of the pain may indicate if it is ureteral or renal.

Urgency suggests urinary tract infection or irritation from possible urinary calculi. Frequency is common with *urinary tract infection* and *bladder neck obstruction.* In men, painful urination without frequency or urgency suggests *urethritis.* Associated flank or back pain suggests **pyelonephritis** (kidney infection) (Johnson & Russo, 2018).

Polyuria or Nocturia

Additional terms are used to describe important alterations in the pattern of urination. **Polyuria** refers to a significant increase in 24-hour urine volume, roughly defined as exceeding 3 L. It should be distinguished from **urinary frequency**, which can involve voiding in high amounts, seen in polyuria, or in small amounts, as in infection. **Nocturia** refers to urinary frequency at night, sometimes defined as awakening the patient more than once; urine volumes may be large or small. Clarify the patient's daily total fluid intake. Note any change in nocturnal voiding patterns and the number of trips to the bathroom to void.

Causes of polyuria include the high fluid intake of *psychogenic polydipsia* and poorly controlled *diabetes*, the decreased secretion of antidiuretic hormone (ADH) of *central diabetes insipidus*, and the decreased renal sensitivity to ADH of *nephrogenic diabetes insipidus*.

Urinary Incontinence

Urinary incontinence is an involuntary loss of urine that can be socially limiting or cause problems with hygiene. The prevalence rate of incontinence for women is 28% and 16% for men (Junqueira & Santos, 2018). If the patient reports incontinence, ask questions to ascertain when this occurs and how often. Refer back to Table 16-7.

Bladder control involves complex neuroregulatory and motor mechanisms. Several central or peripheral nerve lesions affecting S2 to S4 can affect normal voiding. Does the patient sense when the bladder is full? And when voiding occurs? There are five broad categories of incontinence, including *stress*, *urge*, *overflow*, *functional*, and *mixed incontinence*.

Stress incontinence with increased intra-abdominal pressure suggests decreased contractility of urethral sphincter or poor support of bladder neck. **Urge incontinence**, if unable to hold the urine, suggests detrusor overactivity. **Overflow incontinence** may indicate neurologic disorders or anatomic obstruction from pelvic organs or the prostate, limiting bladder emptying until the bladder becomes overdistended (Newman et al., 2014).

To determine the type of incontinence, the nurse should ask:

- Do you leak small amounts of urine with increased intra-abdominal pressure from coughing, sneezing, laughing, or lifting?
- Is it difficult to hold the urine once there is an urge to void?
- Is a large amount of urine lost?
- Is there a sensation of bladder fullness? Frequent leakage?
- Do you void small amounts of urine but have difficulty emptying the bladder?

In addition, the patient's functional status may significantly affect voiding behaviors even when the urinary tract is intact. Is the patient mobile? Alert?

Able to respond to voiding cues and reach the bathroom? Is alertness or voiding affected by medications?

Functional incontinence may arise from impaired cognition, musculoskeletal problems, or immobility. **Mixed incontinence** is a combination of the other types of incontinence.

Hematuria

Blood in the urine, or **hematuria**, is an important cause for concern. When visible to the naked eye, it is called *gross hematuria*. The urine may appear frankly bloody. Alternately, blood may be detected only during microscopic urinalysis, known as *microscopic hematuria*. Smaller amounts of blood may tinge the urine with a pinkish or brownish cast. In women, be sure to distinguish menstrual blood from hematuria. If the urine is reddish, ask about ingestion of beets or medications that might discolor the urine. Test the urine with a dipstick and microscopic examination before you settle on recording the term *hematuria*.

Kidney or Flank Pain; Ureteral Colic

Disorders of the urinary tract may also cause *kidney pain*, often reported as *flank pain*, at or below the posterior costal margin near the costovertebral angle. It may radiate anteriorly toward the umbilicus (see Fig. 16-6). Kidney pain is a visceral pain usually produced by distention of the renal capsule, and it is typically dull, aching, and steady. *Ureteral colic* is dramatically different, severe, colicky pain originating at the costovertebral angle and radiating around the trunk into the lower quadrant of the abdomen and groin, or possibly into the upper thigh, testicle, or labium. Ureteral pain results from sudden distention of the ureter and associated distention of the renal pelvis. Ask about any associated fever, chills, or hematuria.

CLINICAL TIP
Flank pain, fever, and chills suggest *acute pyelonephritis.* Renal or ureteral colic is caused by sudden obstruction of a ureter, for example, from urinary stones or blood clots.

PHYSICAL EXAMINATION

Equipment needed for a physical examination of the abdomen include:

- Tangential lighting
- Stethoscope
- Tape measure with centimeter markings

For the abdominal examination (Box 16-4), the patient should be relaxed and have an empty bladder. Explain the steps of the examination and

BOX 16-4 TIPS FOR EXAMINING THE ABDOMEN

- Ensure the patient is comfortable in the supine position with a pillow under the head and perhaps another under the knees. Slide your hand under the low back to see if the patient is relaxed and lying flat on the table.
- Ask the patient to keep the arms at the sides or folded across the chest. When the arms are above the head, the abdominal wall stretches and tightens, which hinders palpation.
- To expose the abdomen when draping the patient, place the drape or sheet at the level of the symphysis pubis, then raise the gown to below the nipple line just above the xiphoid process. The groin should be visible, but the genitalia should remain covered. The abdominal muscles should be relaxed to enhance all aspects of the examination, especially palpation.
- Before you begin palpation, ask the patient to point to any areas of pain so you can examine these areas last.
- Warm your hands and stethoscope. To warm your hands, rub them together or place them under warm water. Approach the patient calmly and avoid quick, unexpected movements. Avoid having long fingernails which could inadvertently scratch the patient.
- Stand at the patient's *right side* and proceed in a systematic fashion with inspection, auscultation, percussion, and palpation. Visualize each organ in the region you are examining. Watch the patient's face for any signs of pain or discomfort.
- If necessary, distract the patient with conversation or questions. If the patient is frightened or ticklish, begin palpation with the patient's hand under yours. After a few moments, slip your hand underneath to palpate directly.

An arched back thrusts the abdomen forward and tightens the abdominal muscles.

optimize lighting for the examination. The patient should be draped, with exposure of the abdomen.

The Abdomen

Inspection

First observe the general appearance of the patient. Are they lying quietly or walking guarding the abdomen? Are they gripping the handrail, clenching their fists at their sides, or do you notice other nonverbal cues that suggest abdominal pain or discomfort?

Starting from the usual standing position at the patient's right side, inspect the surface, contours, and movements of the abdomen. Watch for peristalsis or bulges. It may be helpful to sit or bend down to view the abdomen tangentially.

During the *skin* assessment, note:

- *Scars.* Describe or diagram their locations.
- *Striae.* Old silver striae or stretch marks are normal (Fig. 16-7).
- *Dilated veins.* A few small veins may be visible normally.

Pink–purple striae are found in *Cushing syndrome.*

CLINICAL TIP
Dilated veins suggest portal hypertension from *hepatic cirrhosis* or *inferior vena cava obstruction.*

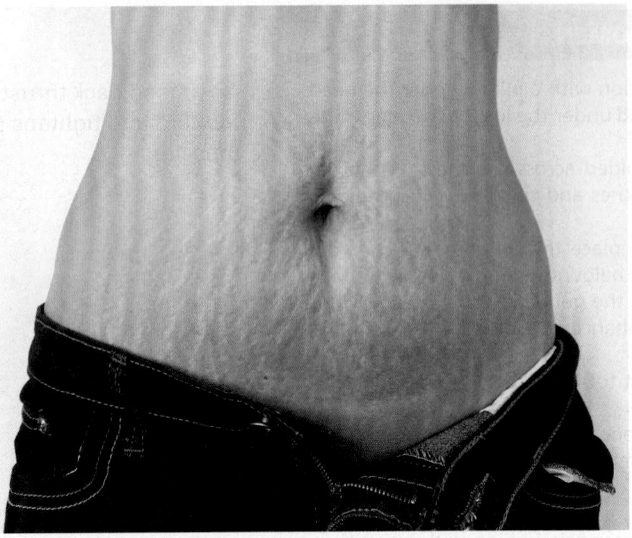

FIGURE 16-7 Striae on the abdomen.

- *Rashes and lesions.* Describe and/or diagram these.
- *Ecchymosis.* Describe the color of the discoloration and location. This is leakage of blood from a vessel into the surrounding tissue.

CLINICAL TIP
Ecchymosis of the abdominal wall is seen with intraperitoneal or retroperitoneal hemorrhage.

- *The umbilicus.* Observe its contour and location and any inflammation or bulges suggesting a hernia (Table 16-8).

TABLE 16-8 Localized Bulges in the Abdominal Wall

Localized bulges in the abdominal wall include *ventral hernias* (defects in the wall through which tissue protrudes) and subcutaneous tumors such as *lipomas.* The more common ventral hernias are umbilical, incisional, and epigastric. Hernias and a diastasis rectus usually become more evident when the patient is supine and raises the head and shoulders.

Umbilical Hernia

A protrusion through a defective umbilical ring is most common in infants but also occurs in adults. In infants, but not in adults, it usually closes spontaneously within 1–2 y.

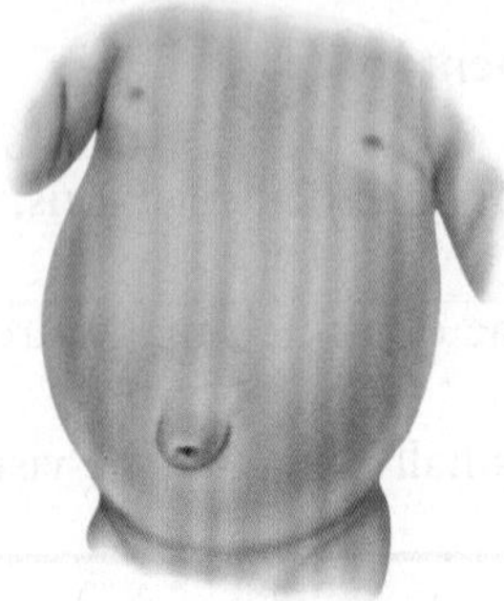

Diastasis Recti

Separation of the two rectus abdominis muscles through which abdominal contents form a midline ridge typically extending from the xiphoid to the umbilicus and seen only when the patient raises the head and shoulders. Often present in patients with repeat pregnancies, obesity, and chronic lung disease. It is clinically benign.

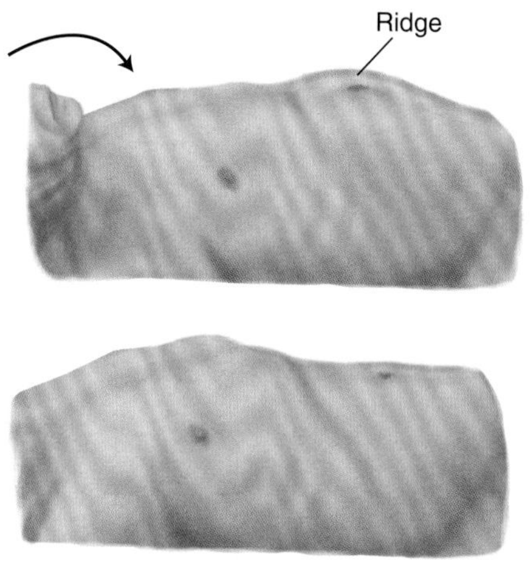

Incisional Hernia

This is a protrusion through an operative scar. Palpate to detect the length and width of the defect in the abdominal wall. A small defect through which a large hernia has passed has a greater risk for complications than a large defect.

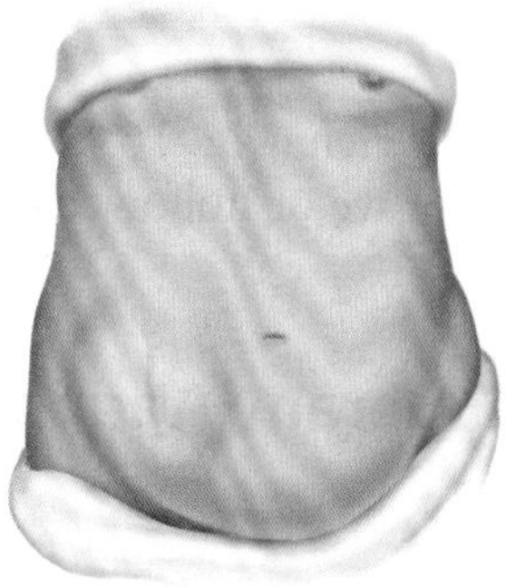

Epigastric Hernia

A small midline protrusion through a defect in the linea alba occurs between the xiphoid process and the umbilicus. With the patient coughing or performing a Valsalva maneuver, palpate by running your finger pad down the linea alba to feel it.

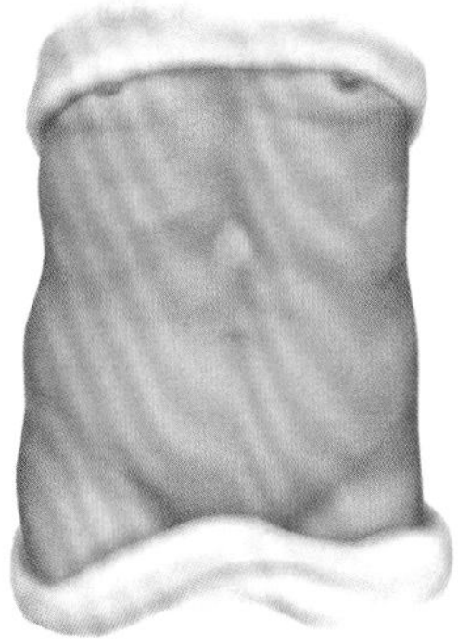

Lipoma

Common, benign, fatty tumors usually in the subcutaneous tissues almost anywhere in the body, including the abdominal wall. Small or large, they are usually soft and often lobulated. Press your finger down on the edge of a lipoma. The tumor typically slips out from under your finger and is well demarcated, nonreducible, and usually nontender.

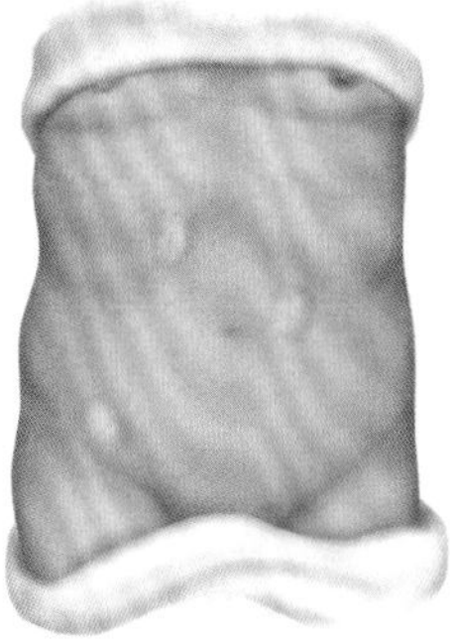

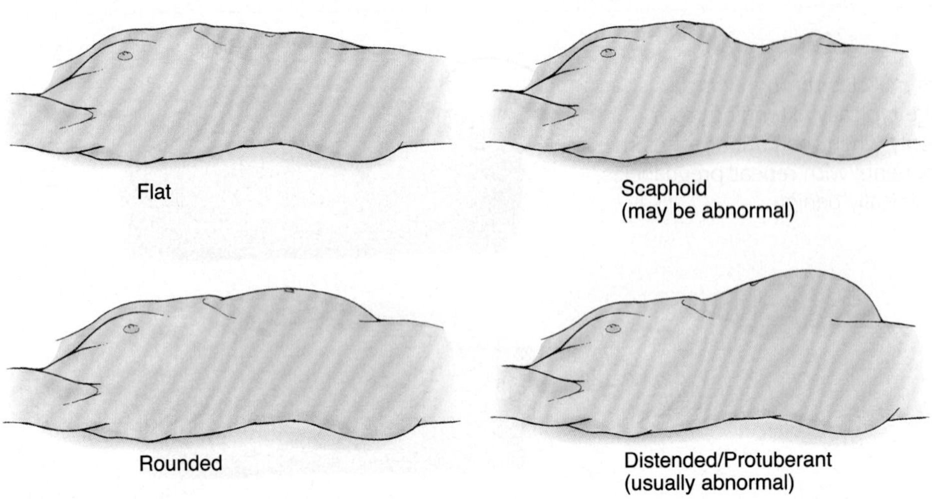

FIGURE 16-8 Examine the contour of the abdomen.

- The contour of the abdomen (Fig. 16-8): Is the abdomen flat, rounded, scaphoid (markedly concave or hollowed), or protuberant (Table 16-9).

TABLE 16-9 Protuberant Abdomen

Fat

Fat is the most common cause of a protuberant abdomen. Fat thickens the abdominal wall, the mesentery, and omentum. The umbilicus may appear sunken. A *pannus,* or apron of fatty tissue, may extend below the inguinal ligaments. Lift it to look for inflammation in the skin folds or even for a hidden hernia.

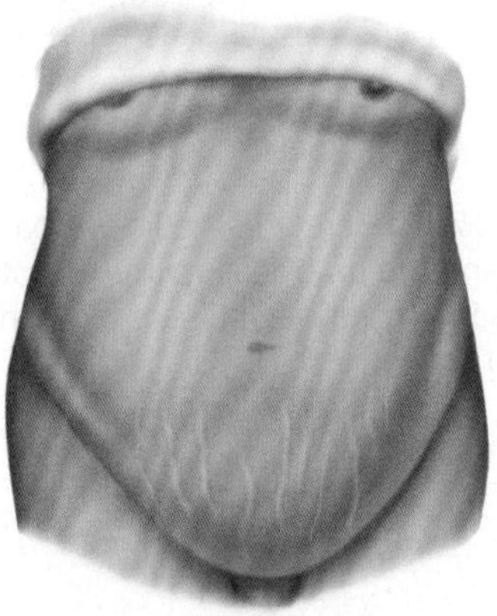

Gas

Gaseous distention may be localized or generalized. It causes a tympanitic percussion note. Select foods may cause mild distention from increased intestinal gas production. More serious are intestinal obstruction and adynamic (paralytic) ileus. Note the location of the distention. Distention becomes more marked in obstruction in the colon than in the small bowel.

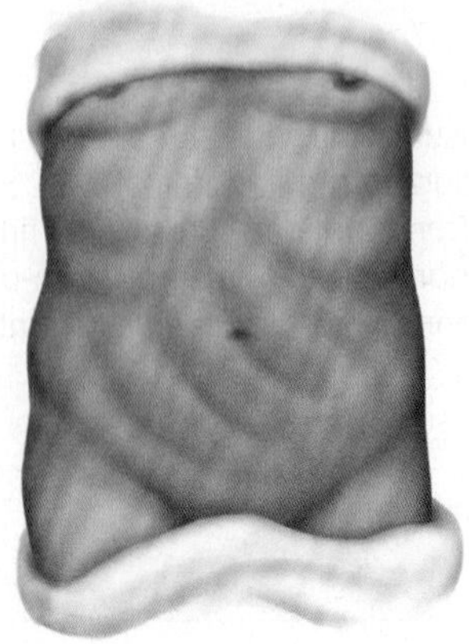

Tumor

A large, solid tumor, usually rising out of the pelvis, is dull to percussion. Air-filled bowel is displaced to the periphery. Causes include ovarian tumors and uterine fibroids. Occasionally, a markedly distended bladder may be mistaken for such a tumor.

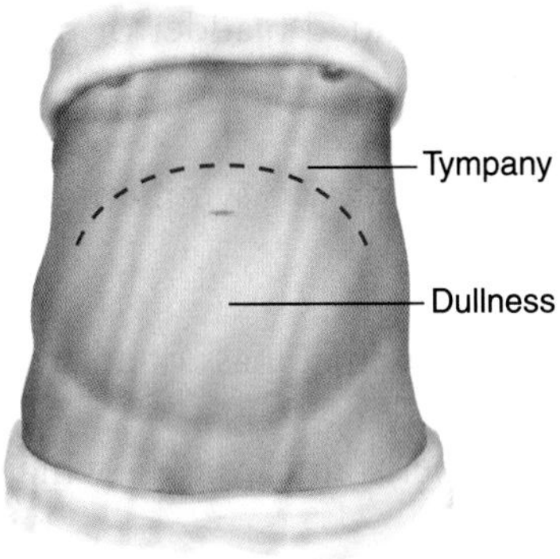

Pregnancy

Pregnancy is a common cause of a pelvic "mass." Listen for the fetal heart.

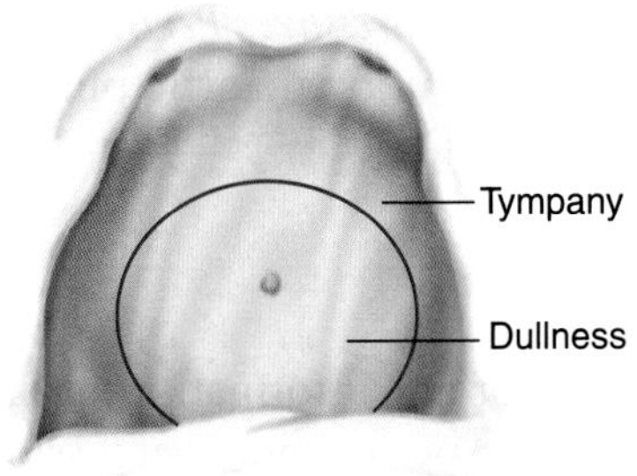

Ascitic Fluid

Ascitic fluid seeks the lowest point in the abdomen, producing bulging flanks that are dull to percussion. The umbilicus may protrude. Turn the patient onto one side to detect the shift in position of the fluid level (shifting dullness).

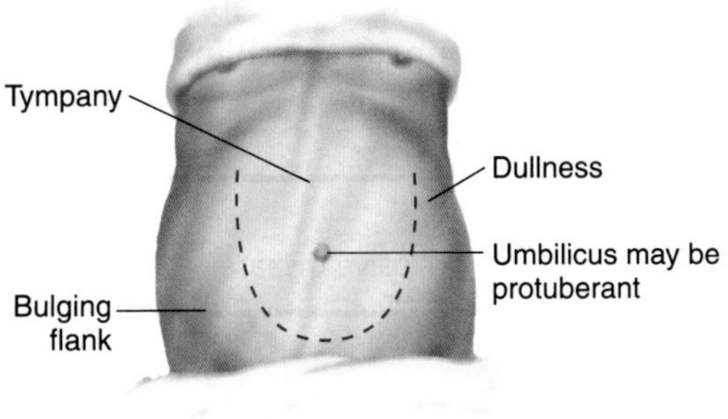

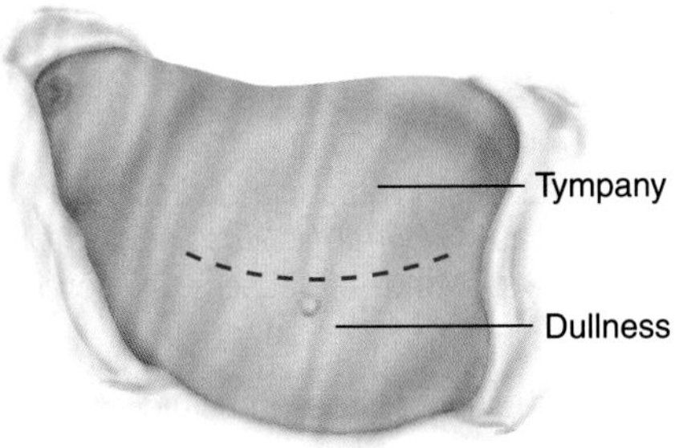

- Observe for the bulging flanks of **ascites** (the accumulation of fluid); the suprapubic bulge of a distended bladder or pregnant uterus; or femoral, umbilical, or inguinal hernias.
- Inspect for *abdominal symmetry*. Asymmetry suggests a hernia, enlarged organ, or mass.
- Inspect for the lower abdominal mass of an ovarian or uterine tumor.
- Inspect for increased peristaltic waves which suggest an *intestinal obstruction*.
- Inspect for the increased pulsations of an *abdominal aortic aneurysm (AAA)* or of *increased pulse pressure*. *Peristalsis* may be visible normally in very thin people and the normal aortic pulsation is frequently visible in the epigastrium.

Auscultation

Auscultation provides important information about bowel motility. Auscultate the abdomen before performing percussion or palpation because these maneuvers may alter the frequency of bowel sounds. Learn to identify variations in normal bowel sounds and to detect changes suggestive of peritoneal inflammation or obstruction (Table 16-10). Auscultation may also reveal bruits, or vascular sounds resembling heart murmurs, over the aorta or other arteries in the abdomen.

CLINICAL TIP
Bruits suggest vascular occlusive disease.

TABLE 16-10 Sounds in the Abdomen

Bowel Sounds

Bowel sounds may be:

- Increased, as in diarrhea or early intestinal obstruction
- *Decreased*, then absent, as in *adynamic ileus* and *peritonitis*; before deciding that bowel sounds are absent, sit down and listen where shown for 2 min or even longer

High-pitched tinkling sounds suggest intestinal fluid and air under tension in a dilated bowel. *Rushes of high-pitched sounds* coinciding with an abdominal cramp indicate intestinal obstruction.

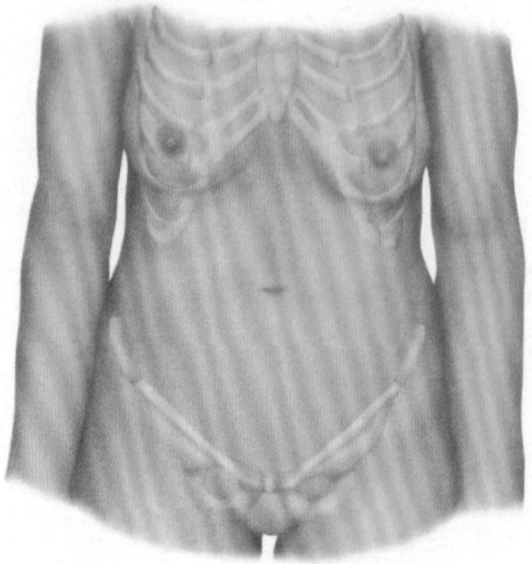

Bruits

A *hepatic bruit* suggests carcinoma of the liver or cirrhosis. *Arterial bruits* with both systolic and diastolic components suggest partial occlusion of the aorta or large arteries. Such bruits in the epigastrium are suspicious for *renal artery stenosis* or *renovascular hypertension*.

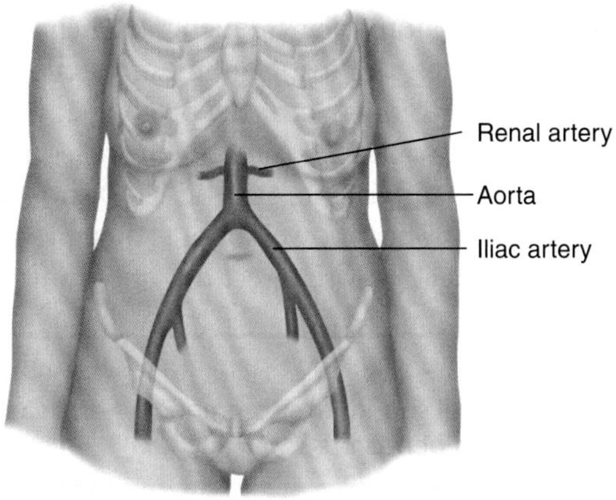

Venous Hum

A venous hum is rare. It is a soft humming noise with both systolic and diastolic components. It indicates increased collateral circulation between portal and systemic venous systems, as in *hepatic cirrhosis*.

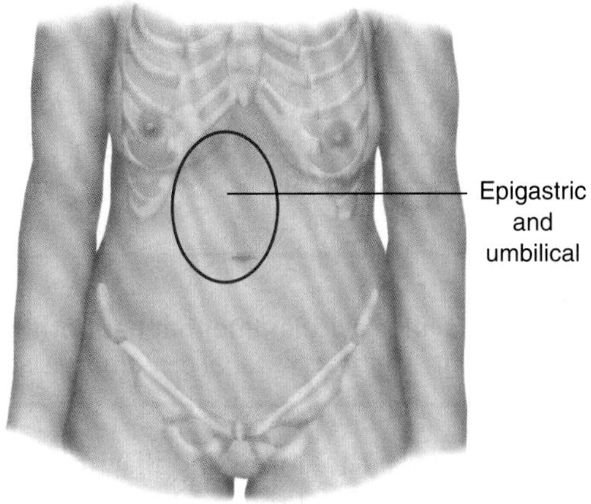

Friction Rubs

Friction rubs are rare. They are grating sounds with respiratory variation. They indicate inflammation of the peritoneal surface of an organ, as in liver cancer, chlamydial or gonococcal perihepatitis, recent liver biopsy, or splenic infarct. When a systolic bruit accompanies a hepatic friction rub, suspect carcinoma of the liver.

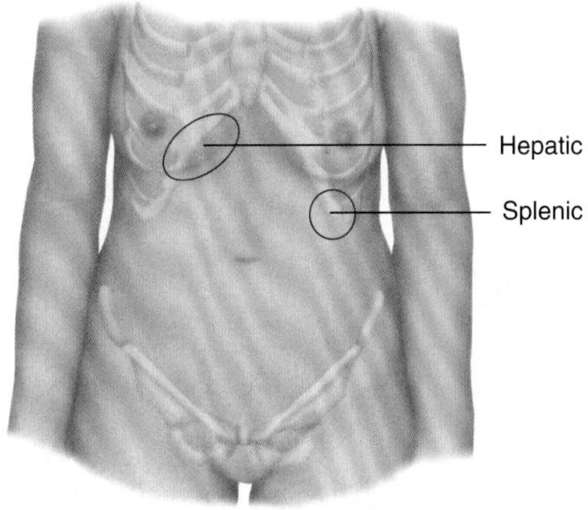

Place the diaphragm of your stethoscope gently on the abdomen. Listen for bowel sounds and note their frequency and character. Normal sounds consist of clicks and gurgles, occurring at an estimated frequency of 5 to 34 per minute. Occasionally, you may hear the prolonged gurgles of hyperperistalsis from stomach growling, called *borborygmi*. Bowel sounds are transmitted throughout the abdomen and listening in the RLQ should be sufficient to hear bowel sounds. If unable to hear bowel sounds, then proceed to listen in all four quadrants, moving in a clockwise direction, questioning why this alteration exists.

CLINICAL TIP
Altered bowel sounds are common in diarrhea, intestinal obstruction, *paralytic ileus*, and *peritonitis*.

Abdominal Bruits and Friction Rubs

If the patient has high blood pressure, listen in the epigastrium and in each upper quadrant for *bruits*. Later in the examination, when the patient sits up, listen also in the costovertebral angles. Epigastric bruits confined to systole may be heard normally.

CLINICAL TIP
A bruit in the midclavicular line that has both systolic and diastolic components strongly suggests *renal artery stenosis* as the cause of hypertension.

Listen for bruits over the aorta, the iliac arteries, and the femoral arteries (Fig. 16-9). Bruits confined to systole are relatively common, however, and do not necessarily signify occlusive disease.

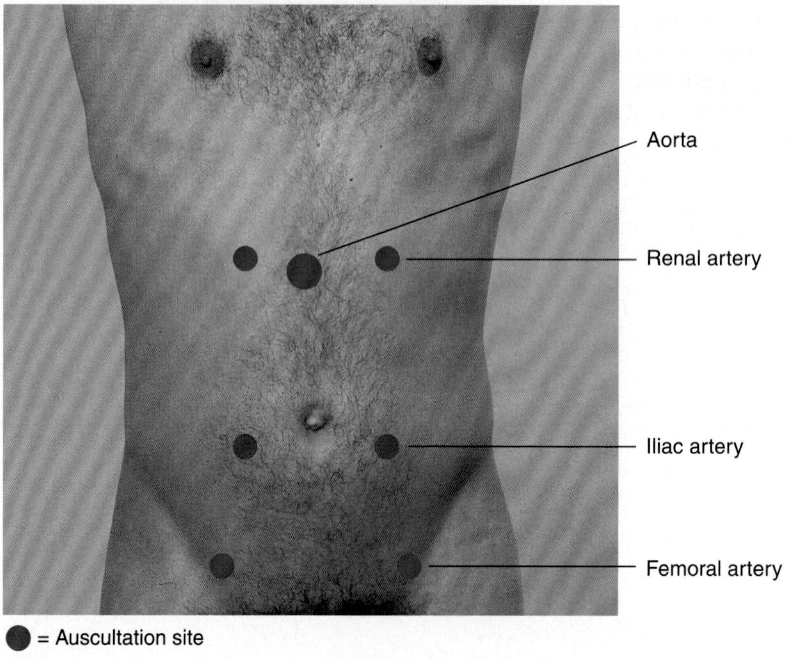

FIGURE 16-9 Locations of bruits may indicate more information about potential occlusive disease.

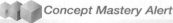

Concept Mastery Alert

Auscultating Bowel Sounds

When evaluating a patient for a possible intestinal obstruction, the nurse needs to assess the patient's bowel sounds, auscultating in each abdominal quadrant for 5 minutes. This time frame is necessary before determining whether a patient has bowel sounds. Typically, in a patient with an intestinal obstruction, the nurse would auscultate a change in pitch or rushes of high-pitched sounds.

CLINICAL TIP

Bruits with both systolic and diastolic components suggest the turbulent blood flow of partial arterial occlusion or arterial insufficiency. If a bruit is heard over the aorta, follow up to determine if this is indicative of an abdominal aortic aneurysm.

Listen over the liver and spleen (Fig. 16-10) for *friction rubs*, which have a grating sound (see Table 16-10).

Friction rubs are present with hepatoma, gonococcal infection around the liver, splenic infarction, and pancreatic carcinoma.

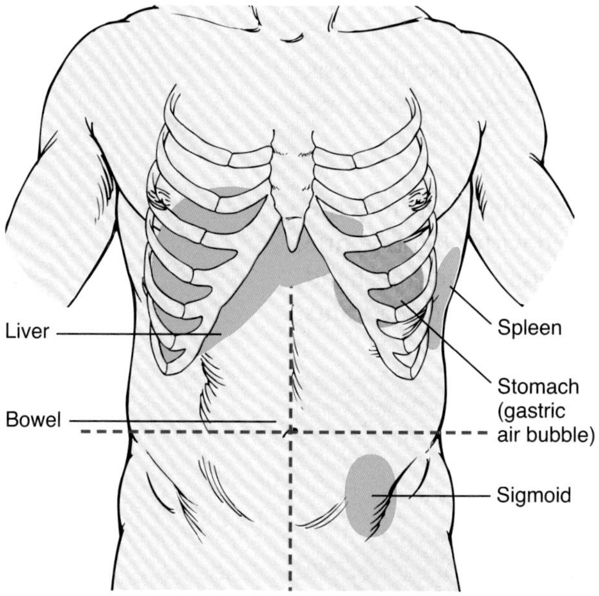

FIGURE 16-10 The nurse assesses tympany and dullness with abdominal percussion. Dullness (*blue*) indicates fluid or feces; tympany (*orange*) indicates gas.

Percussion

Percussion helps you assess the amount and distribution of gas in the abdomen, viscera, masses that are solid or fluid-filled, and the sizes of the liver and spleen.

Percuss the abdomen lightly in all four quadrants to assess the distribution of *tympany* and *dullness* (Fig. 16-10). Tympany usually predominates because of gas in the gastrointestinal tract, but scattered areas of dullness from fluid and feces are also common.

A protuberant abdomen that is tympanic throughout suggests *intestinal obstruction* or *paralytic ileus.* Refer back to Table 16-9, "Protuberant Abdomens."

Note any large dull areas that might indicate an underlying mass or enlarged organ. This observation will guide palpation.

Dull areas are heard over a pregnant uterus, ovarian tumor, distended bladder, or large liver or spleen.

On each side of a protuberant abdomen, note any changes in sound. You may hear the abdominal tympany change to dullness over the solid posterior structures.

CLINICAL TIP
Dullness in both flanks prompts further assessment for ascites.

Briefly percuss the lower anterior chest between the lungs above and costal margins. On the right, you will usually find the dullness of the liver; on the left, the tympany that overlies the gastric air bubble and the splenic flexure of the colon.

In the rare condition of situs inversus, organs are reversed: the air bubble will be on the right with liver dullness on the left.

Palpation

Light Palpation

Gentle palpation aids detection of abdominal tenderness, muscular resistance, and some superficial organs and masses. It also serves to reassure and relax the patient.

Keeping your hand and forearm on a horizontal plane, with fingers together and flat on the abdominal surface, palpate the abdomen with a light, gentle, dipping motion, approximately 1 cm (Fig. 16-11). As you move your hand, raise it just off the skin and glide smoothly, palpating in all four quadrants.

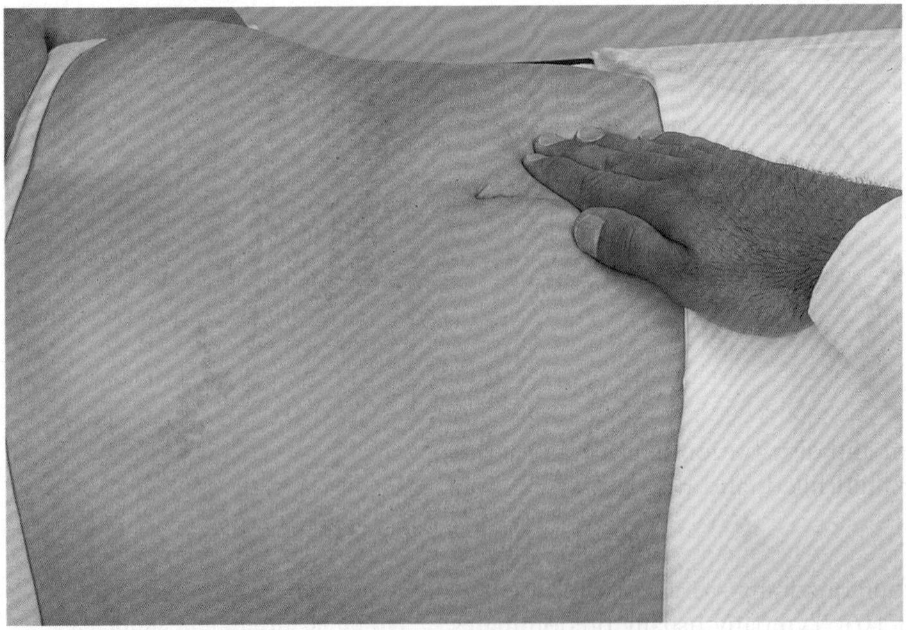

FIGURE 16-11 Light palpation.

Identify any superficial organs or masses and any area of tenderness or increased resistance to palpation. If resistance is present, try to distinguish voluntary guarding from involuntary muscular spasm. Voluntary guarding usually decreases with the following techniques.

Involuntary rigidity (muscular spasm) typically persists despite these maneuvers, suggesting *peritoneal inflammation.*

Use methods described earlier to assist the patient relax. Also ask the patient to exhale and then palpate to aid in the relaxation of abdominal muscles. Ask the patient to mouth-breathe with the jaw wide open.

Deep Palpation

Deep palpation is usually required to delineate the liver edge, the kidneys, and abdominal masses. Again, using the palmar surfaces of your fingers, press down about 5 to 8 cm (2 to 3 in) in all four quadrants (Fig. 16-12). Identify any masses and note their locations, sizes, shapes, consistencies, tenderness, pulsations, and any mobility with respiration or with the examining hand. Correlate your findings from palpation with the percussion notes.

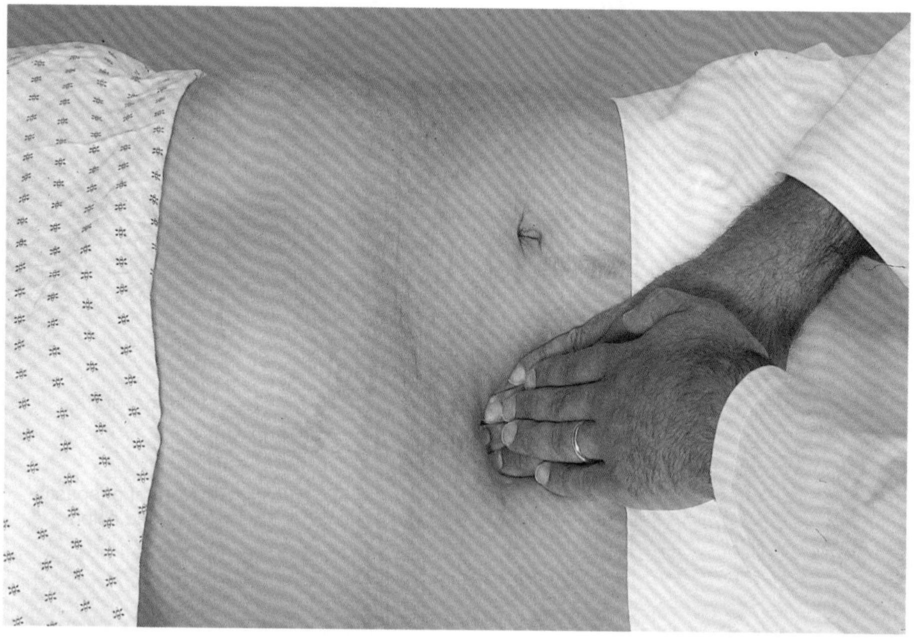

FIGURE 16-12 Two-handed deep palpitation.

CLINICAL TIP
Abdominal masses may be categorized in several ways: physiologic (pregnant uterus); inflammatory (diverticulitis of the colon); vascular (an AAA); neoplastic (carcinoma of the colon); or obstructive (a distended bladder or dilated loop of bowel).

Assessment for Peritoneal Inflammation

Abdominal pain and tenderness, especially when associated with muscular spasm, suggest inflammation of the parietal peritoneum, or **peritonitis**. Signs of peritonitis include a positive cough test, guarding, rigidity, rebound tenderness (Table 16-11), and percussion tenderness (Box 16-5). Even before palpation, ask the patient to cough and determine where the cough produces pain. Then, palpate gently with one finger to localize the area of pain. Pain produced by light percussion has similar localizing value. These maneuvers may establish the area of peritoneal inflammation.

TABLE 16-11 Tender Abdomen

Abdominal Wall Tenderness

Tenderness may originate in the abdominal wall. When the patient raises the head and shoulders, this tenderness persists, whereas tenderness from a deeper lesion (protected by the tightened muscles) decreases.

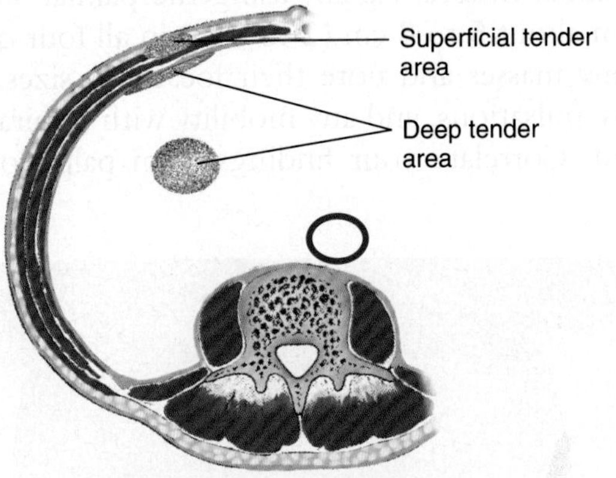

Visceral Tenderness

The structures shown may be tender to deep palpation. Usually the discomfort is dull with no muscular rigidity or rebound tenderness. A reassuring explanation to the patient may prove helpful.

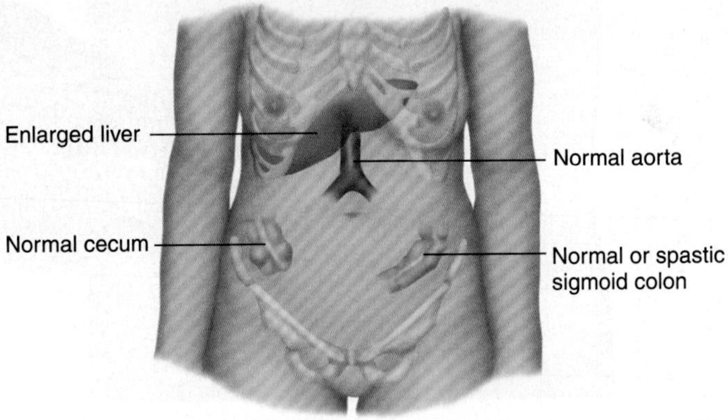

Tenderness from Disease in the Chest and Pelvis

Acute Pleurisy

Abdominal pain and tenderness may result from acute pleural inflammation. When unilateral, it may mimic *acute cholecystitis* or *appendicitis*. Rebound tenderness and rigidity are less common; chest signs are usually present.

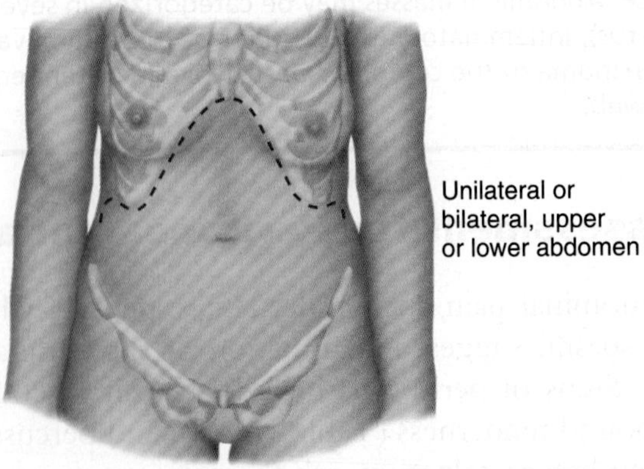

Acute Salpingitis

Frequently bilateral, the tenderness of acute salpingitis (inflammation of the fallopian tubes) is usually maximal just above the inguinal ligaments. Rebound tenderness and rigidity may be present. On pelvic examination, motion of the cervix and uterus causes pain.

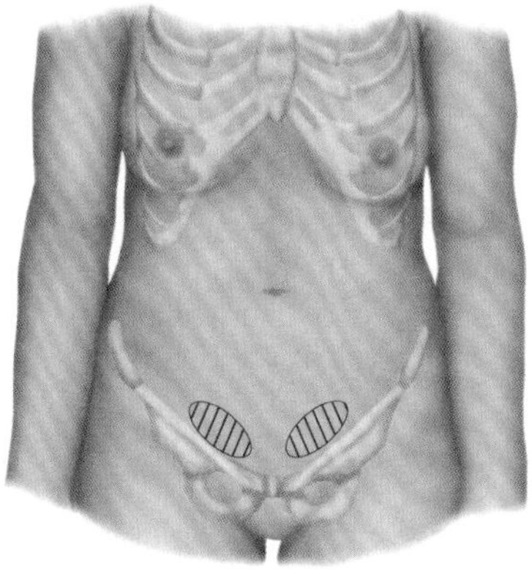

Tenderness of Peritoneal Inflammation

Tenderness associated with peritoneal inflammation is more severe than visceral tenderness. Muscular rigidity and rebound tenderness are frequently but not necessarily present. Generalized peritonitis causes exquisite tenderness throughout the abdomen, together with board-like muscular rigidity. These signs on palpation, especially abdominal rigidity, double the likelihood of peritonitis (Junqueira & Santos, 2018). Local causes of peritoneal inflammation include:

Acute Cholecystitis (Friedman et al., 2011)

Signs are maximal in the right upper quadrant. Check for the Murphy sign.

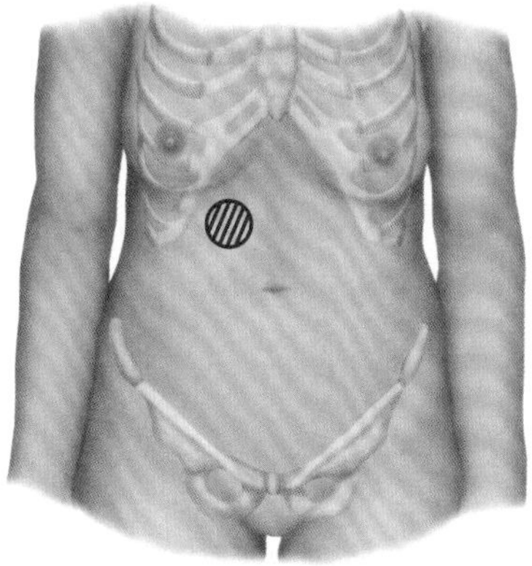

Acute Pancreatitis (Ahmed Ali et al., 2016; Sankaran et al., 2015)

In acute pancreatitis, epigastric tenderness and rebound tenderness are usually present, but the abdominal wall may be soft.

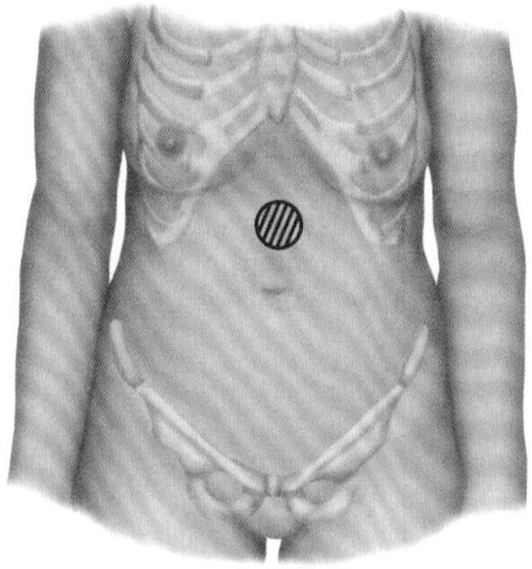

(continued)

TABLE 16-11 Tender Abdomen (*Continued*)

Acute Appendicitis (D'Souza & Nugent, 2016; Evans & Curtin, 2014; Saccomano & Ferrara, 2013)

Right lower quadrant signs are typical of acute appendicitis but may be absent early in the course. The typical area of tenderness, McBurney point, is illustrated. Examine other areas of the right lower quadrant as well as the right flank.

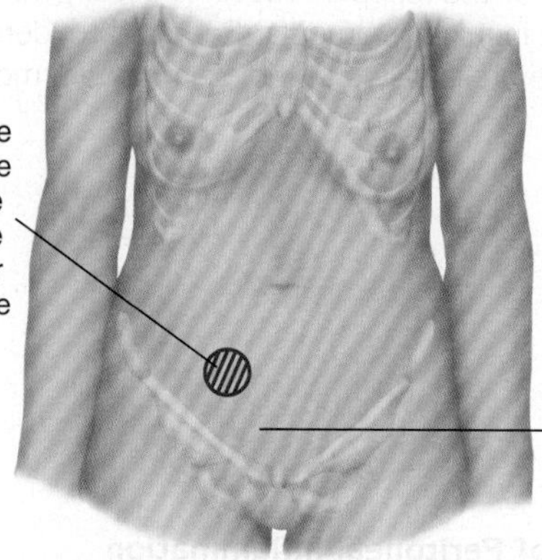

Acute Diverticulitis (Mulligan, 2015)

Acute diverticulitis is a confined inflammatory process, usually in the left lower quadrant that involves the sigmoid colon. If the sigmoid colon is redundant, there may be suprapubic or right-sided pain. Look for localized peritoneal signs and a tender underlying mass. Microperforation, abscess, and obstruction may ensue.

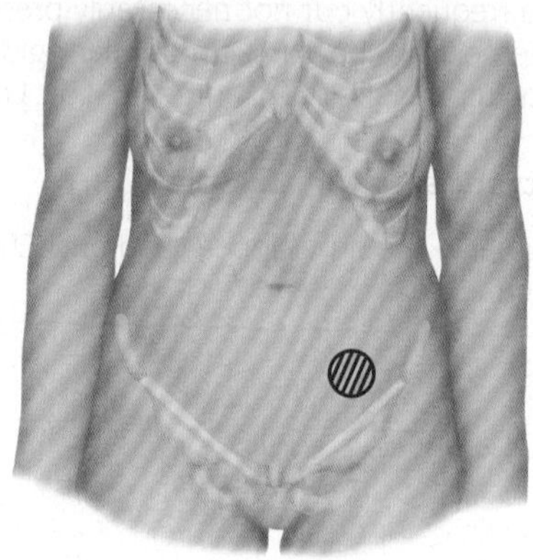

BOX 16-5 SIGNS OF PERITONITIS

Guarding is a voluntary contraction of the abdominal wall, often accompanied by a grimace that may diminish when the patient is distracted.

Rigidity is an involuntary reflex contraction of the abdominal wall from peritoneal inflammation that persists over several examinations.

Rebound tenderness refers to pain expressed by the patient after the examiner presses down on an area of tenderness and suddenly removes the hand. To assess rebound tenderness, ask the patient "Which hurts more, when I press or let go?" Press down with your fingers firmly and slowly, then withdraw your hand quickly. The maneuver is positive if withdrawal produces pain. Percuss gently to check for percussion tenderness.

When positive, these signs roughly double the likelihood of *peritonitis*; rigidity makes peritonitis almost four times more likely (Ross et al., 2018). Causes include *appendicitis*, *cholecystitis*, and a perforation of the bowel wall (Evans & Curtin, 2014).

The Liver

The rib cage shelters most of the liver and can make assessment difficult. Liver size and shape can be estimated by percussion and palpation. Liver consistency and tenderness is examined by palpation.

Percussion

Measure the vertical span of liver dullness in the right midclavicular line. First, locate the midclavicular line carefully to improve accurate measurement. Use a light to moderate percussion stroke, because a heavier stroke can underestimate liver size (Loloi et al., 2018). Starting at a level below the umbilicus (in an area of tympany, not dullness), percuss upward toward the liver. Identify the *lower border of dullness* in the midclavicular line.

Next, identify the *upper border of liver dullness* in the midclavicular line. Starting at the nipple line, percuss downward in the midclavicular line until lung resonance shifts to liver dullness (Fig. 16-13). Gently displace a woman's breast as necessary to be sure to start in a resonant area. The course of percussion is shown in the picture below.

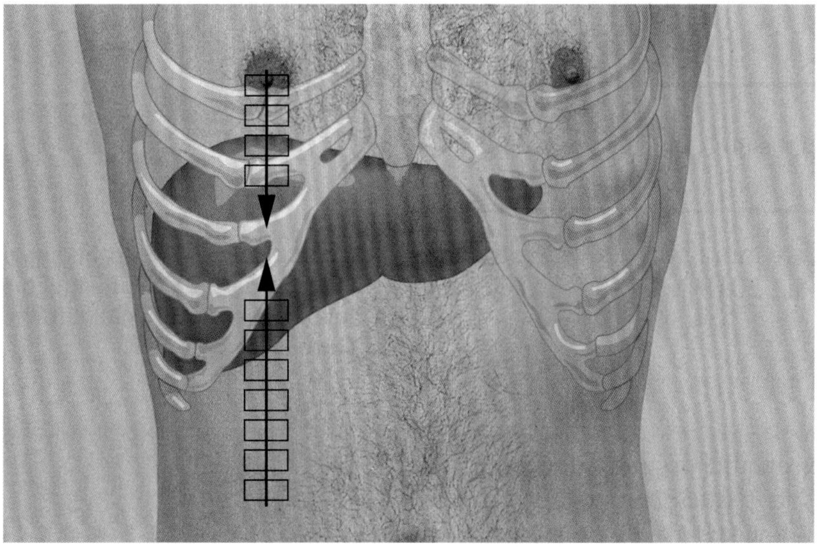

FIGURE 16-13 Percuss downward from the nipple line until lung resonance shifts to liver dullness.

CLINICAL TIP

The span of liver dullness is *increased* when the liver is enlarged. The span of liver dullness is *decreased* when the liver is small, or when free air is present below the diaphragm, as from a *perforated bowel or hollow viscus (organ)*. Liver span may decrease with resolution of *hepatitis* or *congestive heart failure* or less commonly, with progression of *fulminant hepatitis*. Liver dullness may be displaced downward by the low diaphragm of *chronic obstructive pulmonary disease*. Span, however, remains normal.

Now measure in centimeters the distance between the two points—the vertical span of liver dullness. Normal liver span (Fig. 16-14) is generally greater in men than in women and greater in taller than shorter people. If the liver seems to be enlarged, outline the lower edge by percussing medially and laterally.

Dullness of a right pleural effusion or consolidated lung, if adjacent to liver dullness, may falsely *increase* estimated liver size.

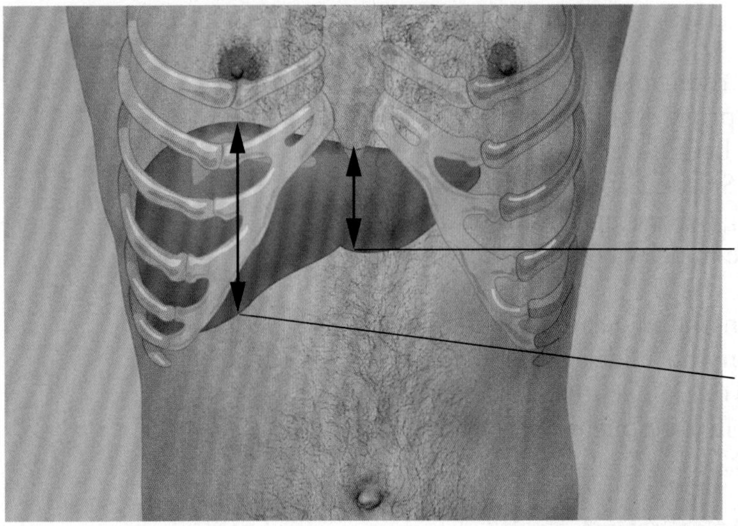

FIGURE 16-14 Normal liver spans.

CLINICAL TIP
Gas in the colon may produce tympany in the RUQ, obscure liver dullness, and falsely *decrease* estimated liver size.

Measurements of liver span by percussion are more accurate when the liver is enlarged with a palpable edge (Loloi et al., 2018).

In *chronic liver disease*, finding an enlarged palpable liver edge roughly doubles the likelihood of *cirrhosis* (Ueda & Ishida, 2015).

Palpation

Place your left hand behind the patient, parallel to and supporting the right 11th and 12th ribs and adjacent soft tissues below (Fig. 16-15). Remind the patient to relax on your hand if necessary. By pressing the left

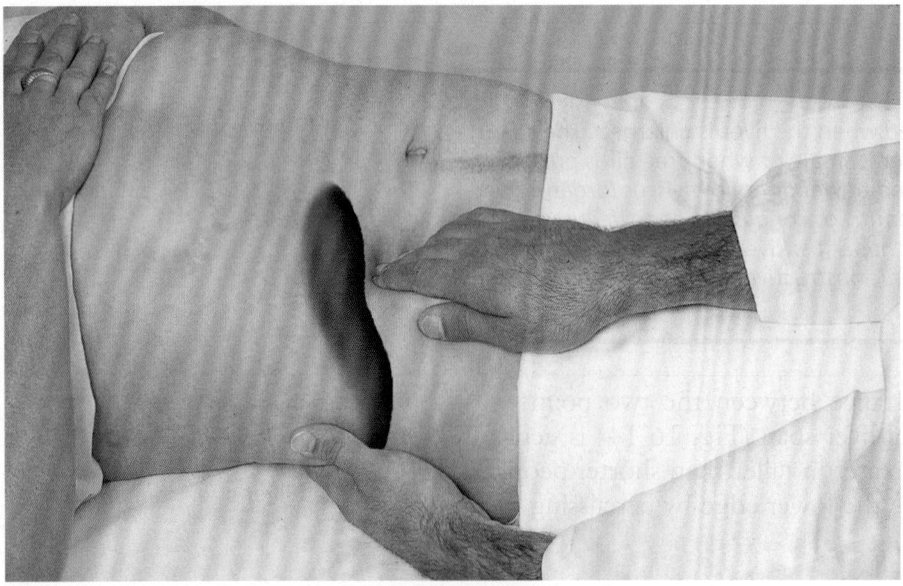

FIGURE 16-15 The hand supporting the ribs can make the liver more easily palpated.

hand forward, the patient's liver may be felt more easily by the examining hand.

Place your right hand on the patient's right abdomen lateral to the rectus muscle, with the fingertips well below the lower border of liver dullness. Some examiners point their fingers up toward the patient's head, whereas others prefer a somewhat more oblique position. In either case, press gently in and up.

Ask the patient to take a deep breath. Try to feel the liver edge as it slides down to meet the fingertips. When palpable, the normal liver edge is soft, sharp, and regular with a smooth surface. If you feel the edge, slightly lighten the pressure of the palpating hand so that the liver can slip under the finger pads and you can feel its anterior surface. Note any tenderness. The normal liver may be slightly tender.

CLINICAL TIP

Firmness or hardness of the liver, bluntness or rounding of its edge, and surface irregularity are suspicious for liver disease.

On inspiration, the liver is palpable about 3 cm below the right costal margin in the midclavicular line (Fig. 16-16). Some people breathe more with the chest than with the diaphragm. It may be helpful to train such a patient to "breathe with the abdomen," which brings the liver, as well as the spleen and kidneys, into a palpable position during inspiration.

An obstructed, distended gallbladder may merge with the liver, forming a firm oval mass below the liver's edge that is dull to percussion.

Palpate the liver edge, altering the examining pressure according to the thickness and resistance of the abdominal wall. If you cannot feel the edge, move your palpating hand closer to the costal margin and try again.

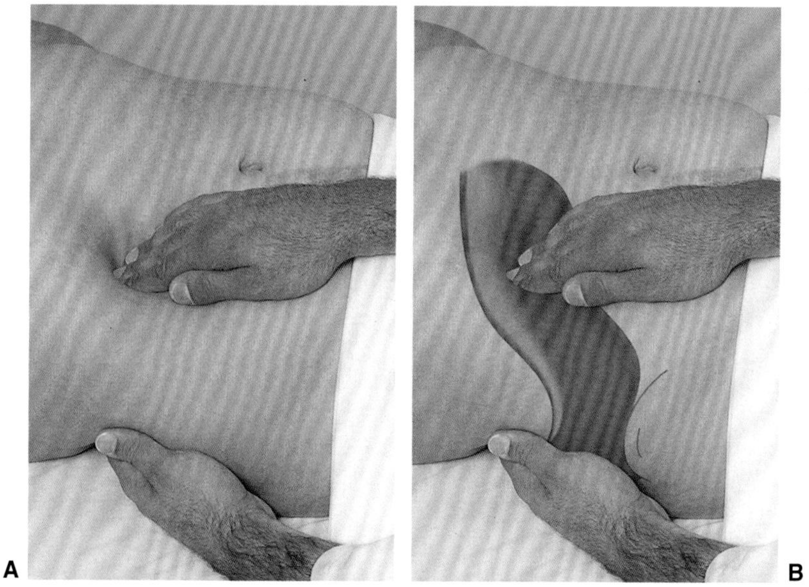

FIGURE 16-16 **A.** Palpate the abdomen about 3 cm below the right costal margin. **B.** The liver will descend to your fingertips when the patient inhales.

Try to trace the liver edge both laterally and medially. Palpation through the rectus muscles can be difficult. A palpable liver edge does not reliably indicate hepatomegaly. See Table 16-12 to learn to distinguish between apparent and real liver enlargement.

TABLE 16-12 Liver Enlargement: Apparent and Real

A palpable liver does not necessarily indicate hepatomegaly (an enlarged liver), but more often results from a change in consistency—from the normal softness to an abnormal firmness or hardness, as in cirrhosis. Clinical estimates of liver size should be based on both percussion and palpation, although even these techniques are imperfect compared to ultrasound.

Downward Displacement of the Liver by a Low Diaphragm

This finding is common when the diaphragm is flattened and low, as in chronic obstructive pulmonary disease. The liver edge may be palpable well below the costal margin. Percussion, however, reveals a low upper edge also, and the vertical span of the liver is normal.

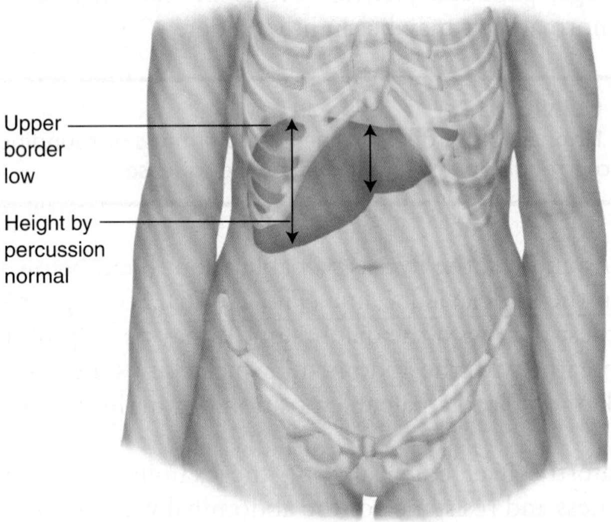

Normal Variations in Liver Shape

In some individuals, the right lobe of the liver may be elongated and easily palpable as it projects downward toward the iliac crest. Such an elongation, sometimes called *Riedel lobe*, represents a variation in shape, not an increase in liver volume or size.

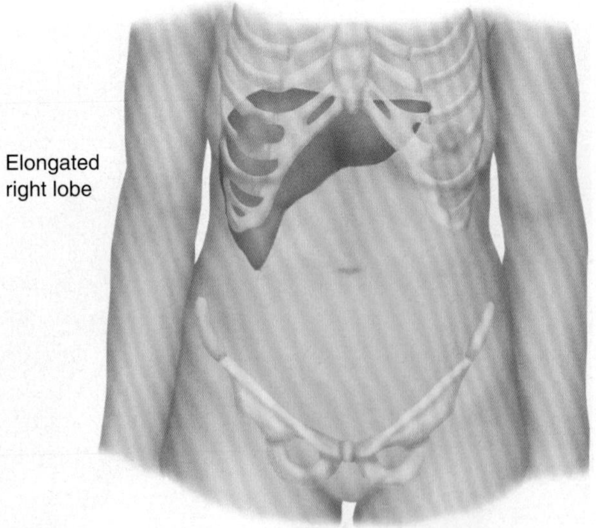

Smooth Large Liver

Cirrhosis may produce an enlarged liver with a firm, *nontender* edge. The cirrhotic liver may also be scarred and contracted. Many other diseases may produce similar findings such as hemochromatosis, amyloidosis, and lymphoma. An enlarged liver with a smooth, *tender* edge suggests inflammation, as in hepatitis, or venous congestion, as in right-sided heart failure.

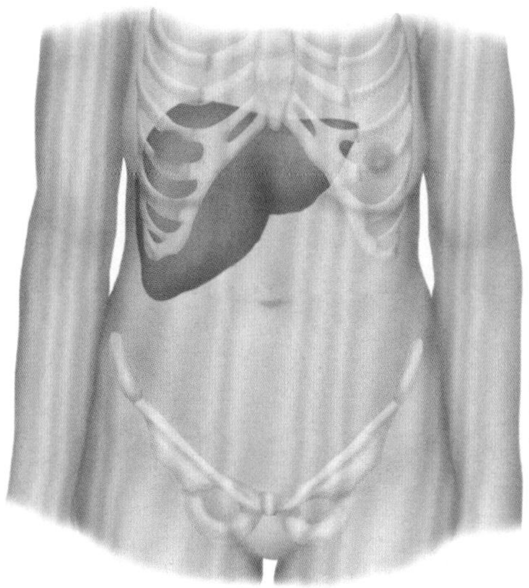

Irregular Large Liver

An enlarged liver that is firm or hard with an irregular edge or surface suggests *hepatocellular carcinoma*. There may be one or more nodules. The liver may or may not be tender.

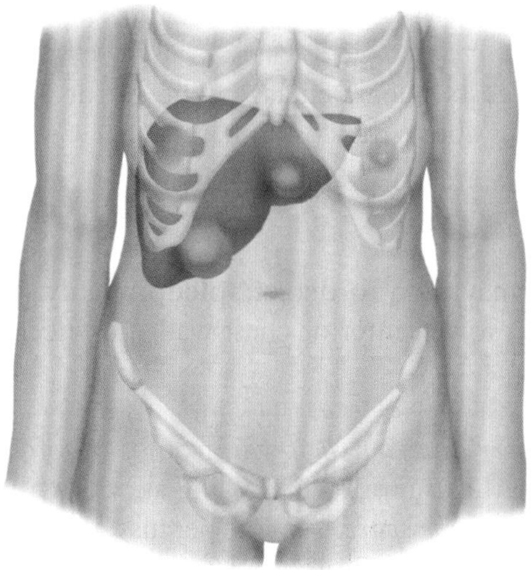

The "*hooking technique*" may be helpful, especially when the patient is obese. Stand to the right of the patient's chest. Place both hands, side by side, on the right abdomen below the border of liver dullness. Press in with your fingers and up toward the costal margin (Fig. 16-17A). Ask the patient to take a deep breath. The liver edge is palpable with the finger pads of both hands (Fig. 16-17B).

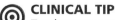

CLINICAL TIP
Tenderness over the liver suggests inflammation found in *hepatitis* or congestion from *heart failure*.

The Spleen

When a spleen enlarges, it expands anteriorly, downward, and medially, often replacing the tympany of the stomach and colon with the dullness of a solid organ. It then becomes palpable below the costal margin. Dullness

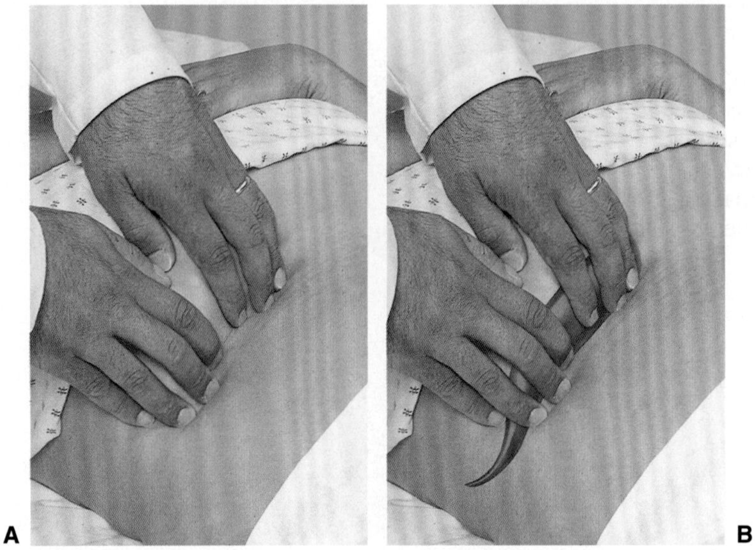

FIGURE 16-17 **A.** Pressing in and up toward the costal margin is the "hooking technique." **B.** This helps find the liver edge.

to percussion suggests splenic enlargement, but it may be absent when an enlarged spleen lies above the costal margin.

Percussion

Two techniques may help to detect **splenomegaly**, an enlarged spleen—percussing the left lower anterior chest wall and checking for a splenic percussion sign.

Percuss the left lower anterior chest wall from the border of cardiac dullness at the sixth rib to the anterior axillary line and down the costal margin, an area termed the *Traube space.* As you percuss along the routes shown by the arrows in Figure 16-18, note the lateral extent of tympany. Percussion is moderately accurate in detecting splenomegaly (sensitivity, 60% to 80%; specificity, 72% to 94%) (Loloi et al., 2018).

If percussion dullness is present, palpation correctly detects splenomegaly more than 80% of the time (Grover, 1993).

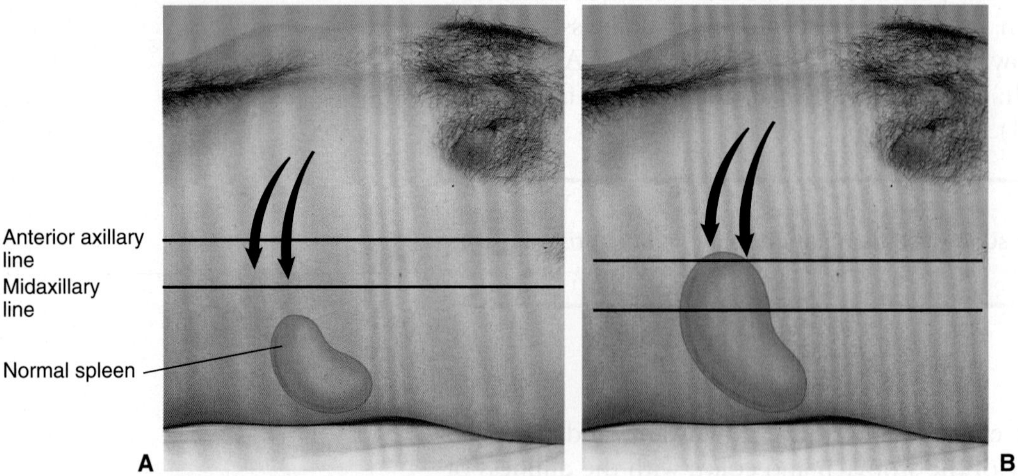

FIGURE 16-18 **A.** Location of a normal spleen. **B.** Location of an enlarged spleen.

If tympany is prominent, especially laterally, splenomegaly is not likely. The dullness of a normal spleen is usually hidden within the dullness of other posterior tissues.

Fluid or solids in the stomach or colon may also cause dullness in the Traube space.

Check for a splenic percussion sign. Percuss the lowest intercostal space in the left anterior axillary line (Fig. 16-19). This area is usually tympanic. Then ask the patient to take a deep breath, and percuss again. When spleen size is normal, the percussion note usually remains tympanic.

If either or both of these tests are positive, pay extra attention to palpation of the spleen.

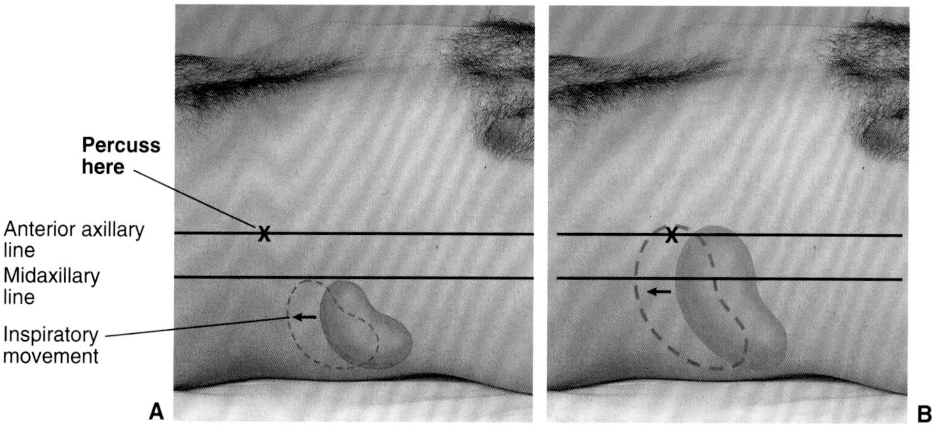

FIGURE 16-19 A. Negative splenic percussion sign. **B.** Positive splenic percussion sign.

CLINICAL TIP
A change in percussion note from tympany to dullness on inspiration is a *positive splenic enlargement*; however, this is only moderately useful in detecting splenomegaly.

Palpation

To enhance relaxation of the abdominal wall, the patient should keep the arms at the sides and flex the neck and legs for comfort, as necessary. With your left hand, reach over and around the patient to support and press forward the lower left rib cage and adjacent soft tissue (Fig. 16-20). With your right hand below the left costal margin, press in toward the spleen. Begin palpation low enough so that you can detect an enlarged spleen. If your hand is too close to the costal margin, you will not be able to reach under the rib cage.

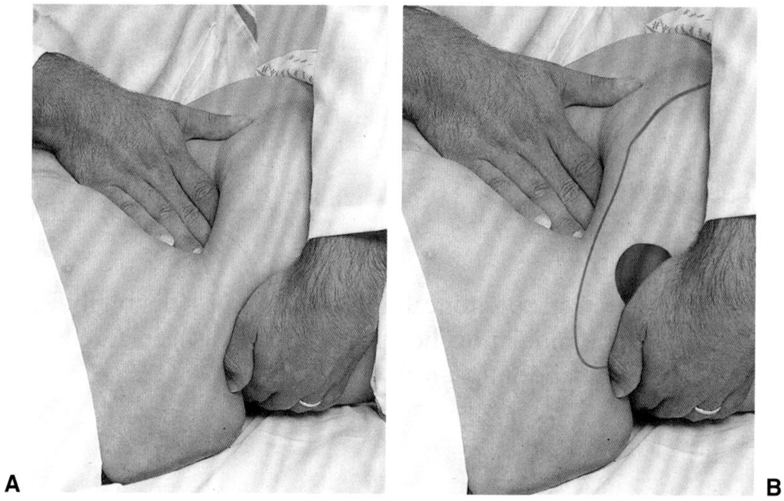

FIGURE 16-20 A. To palpate for splenomegaly, support the patient with one hand and press below the left costal margin with the other. **B.** If palpable, the enlarged spleen tip (purple) is deep to the left costal margin on deep inspiration.

CLINICAL TIP
An enlarged spleen may be missed if the examiner starts palpation too high in the abdomen to feel the lower edge.

Ask the patient to take a deep breath. Try to feel the tip or edge of the spleen as it comes down to meet your fingertips. Note any tenderness, assess the splenic contour, and measure the distance between the spleen's lowest point and the left costal margin. Approximately 5% of normal adults have a palpable spleen tip.

Splenomegaly is eight times more likely when the spleen is palpable. The types of pathologic conditions underlying splenomegaly are vast and categorized into the following categories: congestive, hematologic, inflammatory, infectious, infiltrative, and neoplastic (Sjoberg et al., 2018). Examples of associated conditions include portal hypertension, hematologic malignancies, HIV infection, and splenic infarct or hematoma.

Repeat with the patient lying on the right side with legs somewhat flexed at hips and knees (Fig. 16-21). In this position, gravity may bring the spleen forward and to the right into a palpable location.

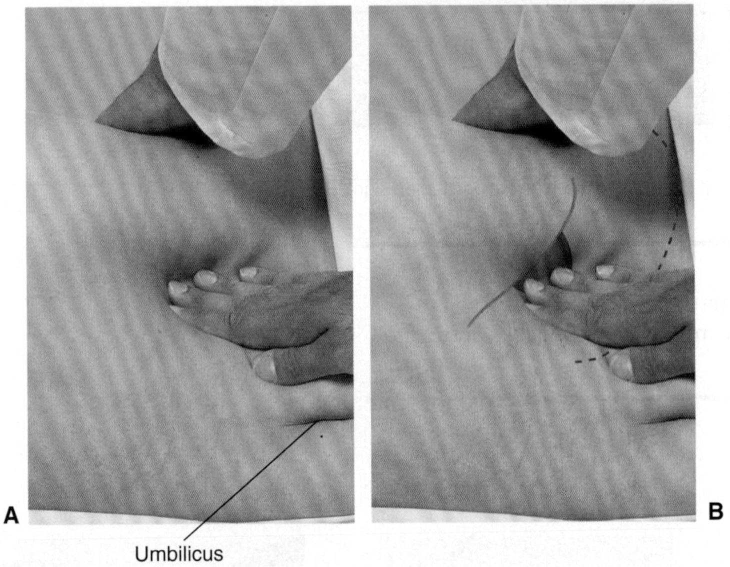

FIGURE 16-21 **A.** Palpating the spleen with the patient lying on their right side. **B.** The enlarged spleen is palpable about 2 cm below the left costal margin on deep inspiration.

The Kidneys

Palpation

The kidneys are retroperitoneal and usually not palpable but learning the techniques for examination helps you distinguish enlarged kidneys from other organs and abdominal masses.

A left flank mass may represent either *splenomegaly* or an enlarged left kidney. Suspect *splenomegaly* if there is a palpable notch on the medial border, the edge extends beyond the midline, percussion is dull, and the fingers can probe deep to the medial and lateral borders but *not* between the mass and the costal margin. Confirm the findings with further evaluation.

Palpation of the Left Kidney

Move to the patient's *left side*. Place your right hand behind the patient, just below and parallel to the 12th rib with your fingertips just reaching the costovertebral angle. Lift, trying to displace the kidney anteriorly. Place the left hand gently in the LUQ, lateral and parallel to the rectus muscle. Ask the patient to take a deep breath. At the peak of inspiration, press your left hand firmly and deeply into the LUQ, just below the costal margin, and try to "capture" the kidney between your two hands. Ask the patient to breathe out and then to stop breathing briefly. Slowly release the pressure of your left hand, feeling at the same time for the kidney to slide back into its expiratory position. If the kidney is palpable, document its size, contour, and any tenderness.

Alternatively, try to palpate for the left kidney using the deep palpation technique similar to feeling for the spleen. Standing to the patient's right side, with your left hand, reach over and around the patient to lift up beneath the left kidney, and with your right hand, feel deep in the LUQ. Ask the patient to take a deep breath, and feel for a mass. A normal left kidney is rarely palpable.

Suspect an enlarged kidney if there is normal tympany in the LUQ, and you can probe with your fingers between the mass and the costal margin but not deep to its medial and lower borders.

Palpation of the Right Kidney

A normal right kidney may be palpable especially when the patient is thin and the abdominal muscles are relaxed. To capture the right kidney, return to the patient's right side. Use your left hand to lift up from the back, and your right hand to feel deep in the LUQ (Fig. 16-22). Proceed as before. The kidney may be slightly tender. The patient is usually aware of a capture and release. Occasionally, a right kidney is more anterior and must be distinguished from the liver. The lower pole of the kidney is rounded, and the liver edge, if palpable, tends to be sharper and extend farther medially and laterally. It cannot be captured.

Causes of kidney enlargement include hydronephrosis, cysts, and tumors. Bilateral enlargement suggests *polycystic kidney disease.* Hydronephrosis is visible on ultrasound and is indicative of ureteral stones.

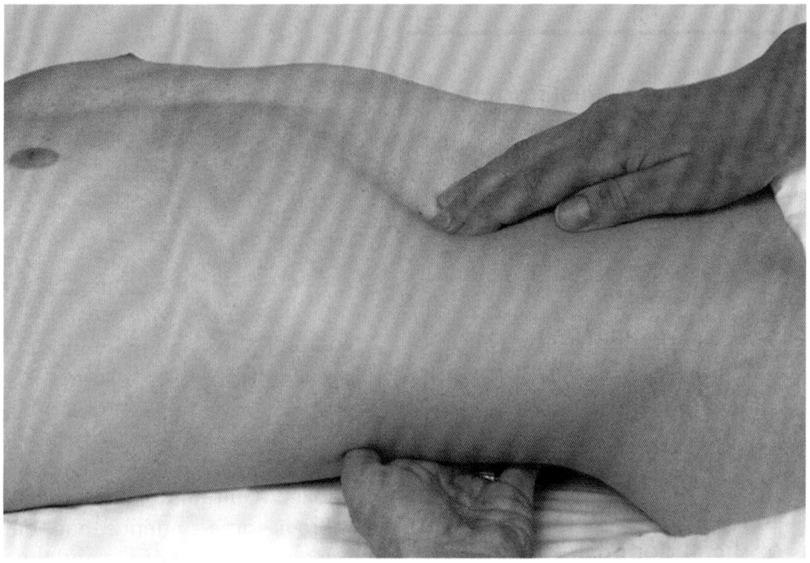

FIGURE 16-22 Palpating the right kidney.

Assessing Percussion Tenderness of the Kidneys

Assess percussion tenderness over the costovertebral angles. Pressure from your fingertips may be enough to elicit tenderness; if not, use fist percussion. Place the ball of one hand in the costovertebral angle and strike it with the ulnar surface of your fist (Fig. 16-23). Use enough force to cause a perceptible but painless jar or thud.

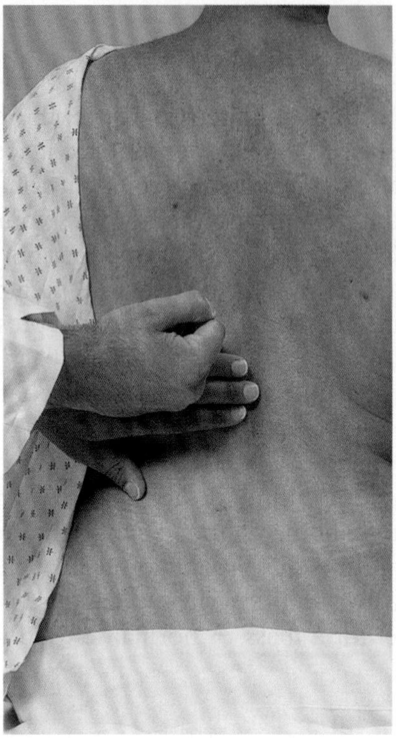

FIGURE 16-23 Fist percussion to elicit costovertebral angle tenderness.

CLINICAL TIP
Pain with pressure or fist percussion suggests *pyelonephritis* associated with fever and dysuria but may also be musculoskeletal.

To save the patient from needless exertion and repositioning, integrate this assessment into your examination of the posterior lungs or back.

The Bladder

The bladder cannot normally be palpated unless it is distended above the symphysis pubis. Percuss to check for dullness and to determine the height of the bladder above the symphysis pubis. Bladder volume must be 400 to 600 mL before dullness becomes apparent (McGee, 2018). On palpation, the dome of the distended bladder feels smooth and round. Check for tenderness.

CLINICAL TIP
Bladder distention from outlet obstruction is caused by *urethral stricture, prostatic hyperplasia,* medication side effects, and neurologic disorders such as *stroke* or *multiple sclerosis.* Suprapubic tenderness may be assessed with *bladder infection.*

The Aorta

Press firmly deep in the upper abdomen, slightly to the left of the midline, and identify the aortic pulsations. In people older than age 50, assess the width of the aorta by pressing deeply in the upper abdomen with one hand on each side of the aorta (Fig. 16-24). In this age group, a normal aorta is not more than 3.0 cm wide (average, 2.5 cm). This measurement does not include the thickness of the abdominal wall. The ease of feeling aortic pulsations varies greatly with the thickness of the abdominal wall and with

Note that the U.S. Preventive Services Task Force (USPSTF) gives a "B" rating recommendation for ultrasound screening for men over 65 to 75 years who have ever smoked (Guirguis-Blake et al., 2019). There is some evidence that health outcomes may improve and the benefits outweigh the harm.

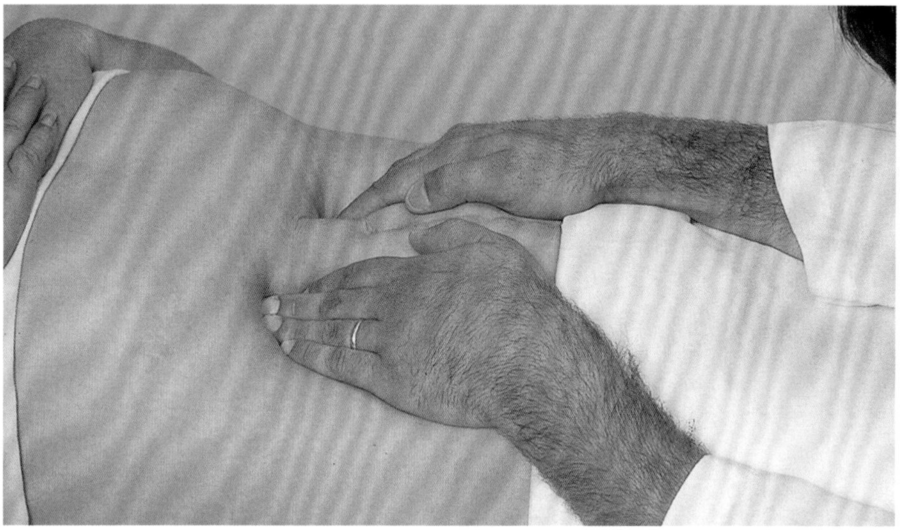

FIGURE 16-24 Press deeply into the upper abdomen with one hand on each side of the aorta to assess its width.

the anteroposterior diameter of the abdomen (Fig. 16-25). Risk factors for AAA are age 65 years or older, history of smoking, male gender, having a first-degree relative with a history of AAA repair, coronary and peripheral artery disease, hypertension, and previous myocardial infarction (Keisler & Carter, 2015). A periumbilical or upper abdominal mass with expansile pulsations that is 3.0 cm or larger suggests an AAA. Sensitivity of palpation increases as AAAs enlarge: for widths of 3.0 to 3.9 cm, 29%; 4.0 to 4.9 cm, 50%; 5.0 cm or greater, 76% (Kent, 2014). Screening by palpation followed by ultrasound decreases mortality, especially in male smokers older than 65 years of age. Pain may signal rupture. Rupture is 15 times more likely in AAAs that are larger than 4 cm than it is in smaller aneurysms, and it carries an 85% to 90% mortality rate (Alix, 2016). The prevalence has decreased over the past 20 years and is seen in 1.2% to 3.3% of men older than 60 years of age (Guirguis-Blake et al., 2019).

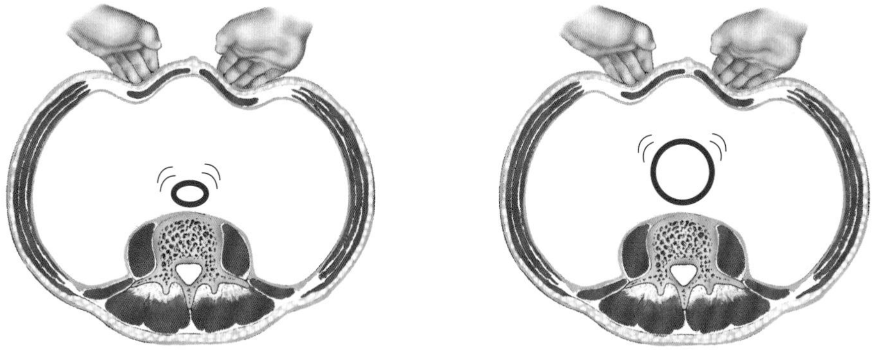

FIGURE 16-25 Palpation of aortic pulsations varies with the thickness of the abdominal wall and the anteroposterior diameter of the abdomen.

SPECIAL TECHNIQUES

Special techniques during examination of the abdomen can assess for:

- Ascites
- Appendicitis
- Acute cholecystitis
- A ventral hernia
- A mass in abdominal wall

Assessing Possible Ascites

A protuberant abdomen with bulging flanks is suspicious for ascites, the most common complication of cirrhosis (Tan et al., 2017). Because ascitic fluid characteristically sinks with gravity, whereas gas-filled loops of bowel rise, dullness appears in the dependent areas of the abdomen. Percuss for dullness outward in several directions from the central area of tympany. Map the border between tympany and dullness (Fig. 16-26).

Ascites can be a clue to *increased hydrostatic pressure* in cirrhosis (most common), heart failure, constrictive pericarditis, or inferior vena cava or hepatic vein obstruction. This may be from decreased osmotic pressure in nephrotic syndrome, malnutrition, or ovarian cancer.

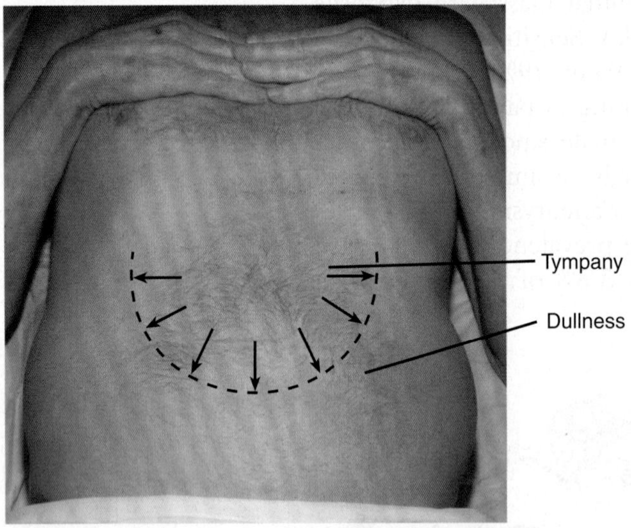

FIGURE 16-26 Mapping the border between tympany and dullness to assess for ascites.

Two additional techniques help to confirm ascites, although both signs may be misleading.

Test for shifting dullness. Percuss the border of tympany and dullness with the patient supine, then ask the patient to roll onto one side (Fig. 16-27). Percuss and mark the borders again. In a person without ascites, the borders between tympany and dullness usually stay relatively constant.

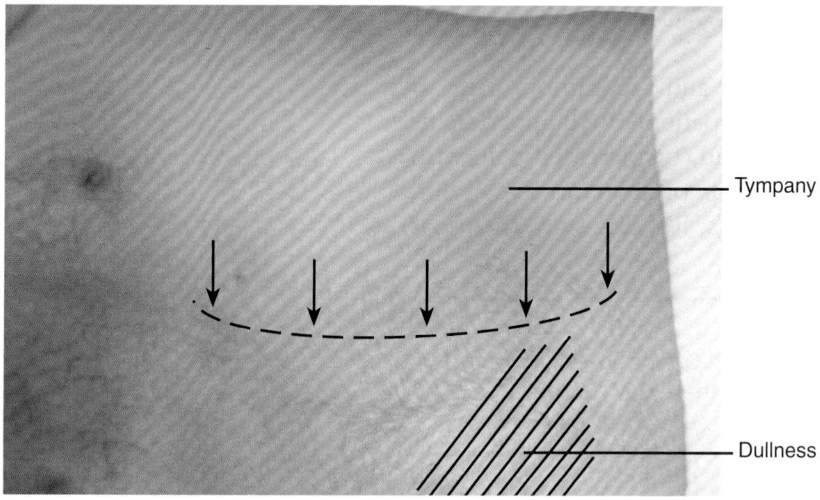

FIGURE 16-27 Assess for shifting dullness to help confirm ascites. Here, dullness is present at the left abdominal border toward the right with the patient on the right side.

Test for a fluid wave. Ask the patient or an assistant to press the edges of both hands firmly down the midline of the abdomen. This pressure helps stop the transmission of a wave through fat. While you tap one flank sharply with your fingertips, feel on the opposite flank for an impulse transmitted through the fluid, as shown in Figure 16-28. Unfortunately, this sign is often negative until ascites is obvious, and it is sometimes positive in people without ascites.

In ascites, dullness shifts to the more dependent side, whereas tympany shifts to the top.

An easily palpable impulse suggests ascites. A positive fluid wave, shifting dullness, and peripheral edema make the diagnosis of ascites three to six times more likely (Hou & Sanyal, 2009).

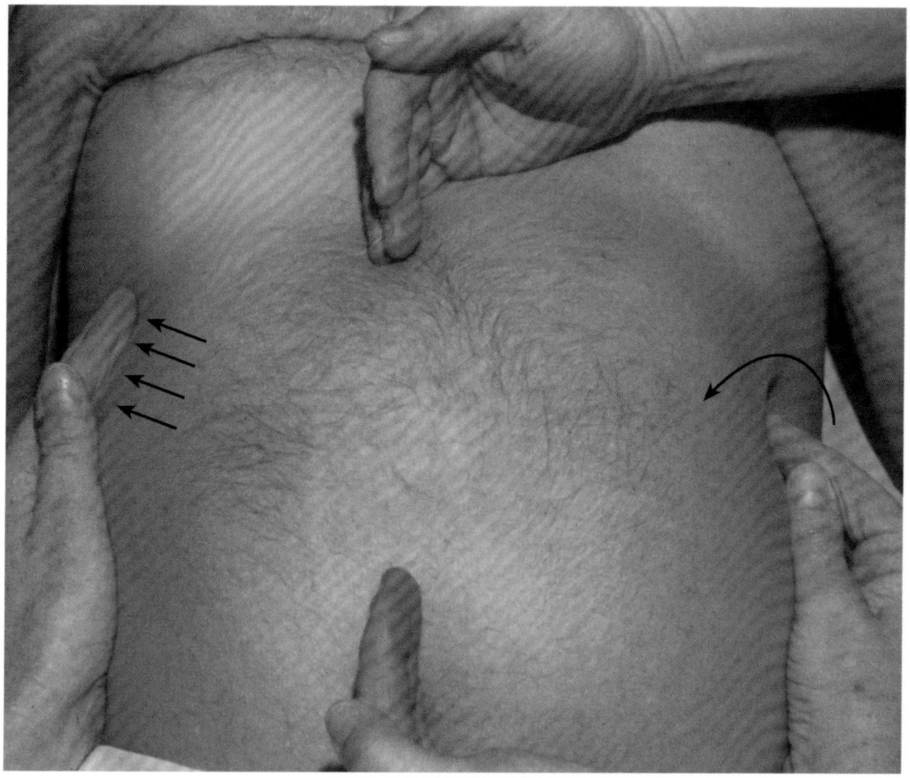

FIGURE 16-28 Test for a fluid wave by tapping one flank sharply with the fingertips while feeling the opposite flank for an impulse transmitted through fluid.

Assessing Possible Appendicitis

Appendicitis is an inflammation of the appendix and a common cause of acute abdominal pain. In addition to acute pain, patients with appendicitis may also present with nausea, vomiting, fever, and/or increased pain with coughing. Assess carefully for the peritoneal signs of acute abdomen and the additional signs of McBurney point tenderness, Rovsing sign, the psoas sign, and the obturator sign.

CLINICAL TIP

Appendicitis is twice as likely in the presence of RLQ tenderness, Rovsing sign, and the psoas sign; it is three times more likely if there is McBurney point tenderness (D'Souza & Nugent, 2016).

The pain of *appendicitis* classically begins near the umbilicus, then migrates to the RLQ. Older adults are less likely to report this pattern.

Ask the patient to point to where the pain began and where it is now. Ask the patient to cough and determine where pain occurs.

Palpate carefully for an area of local tenderness. *McBurney point* lies 2 in from the anterior superior spinous process of ilium on a line drawn from that process to the umbilicus (Youatou Towo et al., 2012).

Localized tenderness anywhere in the RLQ, even in the right flank, suggests *appendicitis*.

Palpate the tender area for guarding, muscular rigidity, and rebound tenderness.

Early voluntary guarding may be replaced by involuntary muscular rigidity and signs of peritoneal inflammation. There may also be RLQ pain on quick withdrawal or deferred rebound tenderness.

Palpate for the *Rovsing sign* and for referred rebound tenderness. Press deeply and evenly in the *left* lower quadrant. Then quickly withdraw your fingers. Pain in the RLQ during *left-sided* pressure is a positive Rovsing sign. Pain in the RLQ when pressure is released from the LLQ is referred rebound tenderness.

Assess for a *psoas sign*. Place your hand just above the patient's right knee and ask the patient to raise that thigh against your hand. Alternatively, ask the patient to turn onto the left side. Then extend the patient's right leg at the hip. Flexion of the leg at the hip makes the psoas muscle contract; extension stretches it. Increased abdominal pain on either maneuver is a positive psoas sign, suggesting irritation of the psoas muscle by an inflamed appendix.

Assess for the *obturator sign* (though this sign has very low sensitivity). Flex the patient's right thigh at the hip with the knee bent and rotate the leg internally at the hip. This maneuver stretches the internal obturator muscle. Right hypogastric pain is a positive obturator sign, suggesting irritation of the obturator muscle by an inflamed appendix.

Localized pain with this maneuver in all or part of the RLQ may accompany appendicitis.

A physician or nurse practitioner may perform a rectal examination and in women, a pelvic examination. These maneuvers have low sensitivity and specificity, but they may help identify an inflamed appendix atypically located within the pelvic cavity. They may also suggest other causes of the abdominal pain.

Right-sided rectal tenderness may also be caused by inflammation of an organ nearby, such as an inflamed seminal vesicle.

Assessing Possible Acute Cholecystitis

When RUQ pain and tenderness suggest acute **cholecystitis**, which is inflammation of the gallbladder, assess *Murphy sign*. Hook your left thumb or the fingers of your right hand under the costal margin at the point where the lateral border of the rectus muscle intersects with the costal margin. Alternatively, palpate the RUQ with the fingers of your right hand near the costal margin. If the liver is enlarged, hook your thumb or fingers under the liver edge at a comparable point below. Ask the patient to take a deep breath, which forces the liver and gall bladder down toward the examining fingers. Watch the patient's breathing and note the degree of tenderness.

CLINICAL TIP

A sharp increase in tenderness with inspiratory effort is a positive Murphy sign. When positive, Murphy sign triples the likelihood of *acute cholecystitis* (Friedman et al., 2011).

Assessing Ventral Hernias

Ventral hernias occur when the muscles of the abdominal wall are weak and abdominal tissue or a loop of intestine bulge out. These are also known as **incisional hernias**, typically seen at the scar site from a previous surgery. Approximately one third of patients with open abdominal surgery will develop a ventral hernia at an incision site.

During assessment, ask the patient to raise both head and shoulders off the table. The bulge of a hernia will usually appear with this action, but it should not be confused with *diastasis recti*, which is a benign 2- to 3-cm gap in the rectus muscles often seen in obese and postpartum patients.

Umbilical hernias are caused by a weakness in the abdominal wall at the umbilicus and are usually present at birth.

Inguinal and femoral hernias are discussed in Chapter 21, "Reproductive System." They can give rise to important abdominal problems and should not be overlooked.

The cause of intestinal obstruction or peritonitis may be missed by overlooking a strangulated femoral or inguinal hernia.

Assessing a Mass in the Abdominal Wall

Occasionally, there is a mass in the abdominal wall rather than inside the abdominal cavity. To distinguish an abdominal mass from a mass in the abdominal wall, ask the patient either to raise the head and shoulders or to strain down, thus tightening the abdominal muscles. Feel for the mass again.

CLINICAL TIP
A mass in the abdominal wall remains palpable; an intra-abdominal mass is obscured by muscular contraction.

RECORDING YOUR FINDINGS

Box 16-6 includes examples of documentation of abdominal assessment findings.

BOX 16-6 RECORDING THE PHYSICAL EXAMINATION—THE ABDOMEN

"Abdomen protuberant with active bowel sounds. Soft, nontender; no palpable masses or hepatosplenomegaly. Liver span 7 cm in right midclavicular line; edge smooth and palpable 1 cm below the right costal margin. Spleen and kidneys not palpable. No costovertebral angle tenderness."

OR

"Abdomen flat. No bowel sounds. Firm, board-like, increased tenderness, guarding, and rebound tenderness in the right mid-quadrant. Liver percusses 7 cm in the right MCL; edge not felt. Spleen and kidneys not palpable. No palpable masses. No CVA tenderness."

Suggests peritonitis from possible *appendicitis*.

HEALTH PROMOTION

Important topics for health promotion and counseling regarding the gastrointestinal and renal systems include:

- Screening for alcohol use and misuse
- Risk factors for hepatitis A, B, and C
- Screening for colon cancer
- Prevention of urinary incontinence

Screening for Alcohol Misuse

According to the National Institute on Alcohol Abuse and Alcoholism, in 2018, 86.4% of people over age 18 reported drinking in their lifetimes (Samhsa.gov, 2020a). Binge drinking was reported by 26.9% in the past year, and 7% of participants reported heavy drinking in the past month (Samhsa.gov, 2020b).

Approximately 15.1 million adults in the United States have an *alcohol use disorder* (AUD) with only 6.7% receiving treatment (National Institute on

Alcohol Abuse and Alcoholism, 2020a). Addictions are increasingly viewed as chronic relapsing behavioral disorders with substance-induced alterations of brain neurotransmitters resulting in tolerance, physical dependence, sensitization, craving, and relapse.

Alert clinicians often notice clues of unhealthy alcohol use from social patterns and behavioral problems that emerge during the history. The patient may report past episodes of substance use, unstable relationships, difficulty holding jobs, or legal problems related to violent behaviors or driving under the influence (Mitchell et al., 2020). Excessive alcohol use has numerous short-term health risks, including injuries, violence (e.g., homicide, suicide, sexual assault, intimate partner violence), alcohol poisoning, and adverse effects on reproductive health (risky sexual behaviors, miscarriage, and fetal alcohol disorders). Medical issues are often associated with chronic alcohol use such as cirrhosis, pancreatitis or cancer, other gastrointestinal or cardiovascular diseases, neurologic disorders, nutritional deficiencies, or additional mental health problems. Examination of the abdomen may reveal classic findings of liver disease such as hepatosplenomegaly, ascites, or even *caput medusa* (dilated abdominal vein).

Other classic findings include jaundice, spider angiomas, palmar erythema, and gynecomastia.

See Chapter 19, "Mental Status and Mental Health Assessment" for more about alcohol misuse.

Because early detection of at-risk behaviors may be difficult to identify, knowledge of basic alcohol screening criteria is critical. The USPSTF recommends screening and behavioral counseling interventions for adolescents and adults in primary care settings, including pregnant women (O'Connor et al., 2018). Learn the best approach to identify problem drinking. If your patient reports drinking alcoholic beverages, ask the initial screening question about heavy drinking (Box 16-7) and follow-up with a well-validated screening tool—the Alcohol Use Disorders Identification Test (AUDIT) or the shorter AUDIT-C questionnaire (Babor et al., 2020; Madson et al., 2018). Keep in mind cutoffs for problem drinking. See Box 16-7.

See Chapter 4, "The Health History."

BOX 16-7 SCREENING FOR PROBLEM DRINKING

Standard Drink Equivalents: One standard drink is equivalent to 12 oz of regular beer or wine cooler, 8 oz of malt liquor, 5 oz of wine, or 1.5 oz of 80-proof spirits

Initial Screening Question: "How many times in the past year have you had four or more drinks a day (women)/five or more drinks a day (men)?"

National Institute of Alcohol Abuse and Alcoholism: Definitions of Drinking and Levels for Adults (National Institute on Alcohol Abuse & Alcoholism [NIAAA], 2020b)

	Women	Men
Moderate drinking	≤1 drink/day	≤2 drinks/day
Unsafe drinking levels (increased risk for developing an alcohol use disorder)	>3 drinks/day and >7 drinks/wk[a]	>4 drinks/day and >14 drinks/wk
Binge drinking[b]	≥4 drinks on one occasion	≥5 drinks on one occasion

[a]Pregnant women and those with health problems that could be worsened by drinking should not drink any alcohol.
[b]Brings blood alcohol level to 0.08%, usually within 2 hours.

Tailor your recommendations to the severity of the drinking problem, ranging from brief behavioral counseling interventions to inpatient detoxification and/or long-term rehabilitation.

Prevention: Hepatitis A, B, and C

The best strategy for protection and prevention of transmission and infection of hepatitis A and B is adherence to the vaccination guidelines. Education about how the hepatitis viruses spread, behavioral strategies to reduce the risk of infection, and the benefits of vaccination for groups at risk is important.

Hepatitis A

Transmission of the hepatitis A virus (HAV) is the fecal–oral route. Fecal shedding followed by inadequate hand washing can contaminate water and food. Those at highest risk include those who have traveled to or live in countries where hepatitis A is common, and those who have had sex with infected individuals, use recreational drugs, eat raw or undercooked shellfish from contaminated waters, have clotting disorders, or live with or care for a person with hepatitis A. Infected children are often asymptomatic and play a key role in spreading infection. For immediate protection and prophylaxis for household contacts and travel and to reduce transmission, advise hand washing with soap and water after bathroom use or changing diapers, and before preparing or eating food (CDC, 2019). HAV infection is rarely fatal, is an acute illness lasting approximately 2 months, and does not cause chronic hepatitis (CDC, 2019). Box 16-8 outlines the Centers for Disease Control and Prevention recommendations for hepatitis A vaccination.

BOX 16-8 CDC RECOMMENDATIONS FOR HEPATITIS A VACCINATION

- All children ages 12 to 23 months
- Children 2 to 18 years old who are unvaccinated
- Infants 6 to 12 months old who will be traveling to places where hepatitis A vaccination is recommended
- Healthy individuals 1 to 40 years old traveling to counties with intermediate to high endemicity of hepatitis A
- People who are homeless
- Individuals with chronic liver disease or HIV
- Men who have sex with men
- Illicit drug use
- Individuals working with HAV-infected animals or work with HAV in research setting
- Individuals in close contact with a person who has HAV (postexposure prophylaxis)
- Individuals who anticipate close contact with a person from endemic region (e.g., adoptee)
- Anybody who wants protection

Source: Doshani, M., Weng, M., Moore, K. L., Romero, J. R., & Nelson, N. P. (2019). Recommendations of the advisory committee on immunization practices for use of hepatitis a vaccine for persons experiencing homelessness. *MMWR. Morbidity and Mortality Weekly Report, 68*(6), 153–156. Published 2019 February 15. https://doi.org/10.15585/mmwr.mm6806a6

Postexposure Prophylaxis

Healthy unvaccinated individuals should receive either a hepatitis A vaccine or a single dose of *immune globulin* (preferred for those aged 40 and over) within 2 weeks of being exposed to HAV. These recommendations apply to close personal contacts of individuals with confirmed HAV, coworkers of infected food handlers, and staff and attendees (and their household members) of child care centers where HAV has been diagnosed in children, staff, or households of attendees.

Hepatitis B

Hepatitis B virus (HBV) poses a more serious (Box 16-9) threat than infection with HAV, however, it is preventable with a vaccine. Exposure to HBV is via infected blood, semen, or other body fluids from an infected individual to a noninfected person. The virus can occur during sexual contact, while sharing syringes, or during childbirth. It is not contracted through food or water. Approximately 95% of infections in healthy adults are self-limited with elimination of the virus from blood and development of immunity (CDC, 2020a).

BOX 16-9 CDC RECOMMENDATIONS FOR HEPATITIS B VACCINATION

- All infants and children younger than 19 years old who are not vaccinated
- Sexual contacts, including sex partners of individuals who test positive for hepatitis B surface antigens, people with more than one sex partner in the prior 6 months, people seeking evaluation and treatment for sexually transmitted infections (STIs), and men who have sex with men
- People with percutaneous (through the skin) or mucosal exposure to blood, including injection drug use
- Household contacts of individuals who are antigen-positive
- Residents and staff of facilities for the developmentally disabled
- Health care workers with exposure to blood or other potentially infectious body fluids
- People on dialysis
- People with diabetes who are 19 to 59 years old, and per direction of the individual's health care provider if 60 or older
- Travelers to endemic areas
- People with hepatitis C infection, chronic liver disease, or HIV infection
- People seeking protection from hepatitis B infection
- All adults in high-risk settings, such as STI clinics, HIV testing and treatment programs, drug abuse treatment programs and programs for injection drug users, correctional facilities, programs for men having sex with men, chronic hemodialysis facilities and end-stage renal disease programs, and facilities for people with developmental disabilities.

Source: Schillie, S., Vellozzi, C., Reingold, A., Harris, A., Haber, P., Ward, J. W., & Nelson, N. P. (2018). Prevention of hepatitis B virus infection in the United States: Recommendations of the advisory committee on immunization practices. *MMWR. Recommendations and Reports*, *67*(1), 1–31. Published 2018 January 12. https://doi.org/10.15585/mmwr.rr6701a1

Hepatitis C

There is no vaccination for hepatitis C, so prevention targets counseling to avoid risk factors. Screening should be recommended for high-risk groups.

Hepatitis C virus (HCV) is primarily transmitted by percutaneous exposure to blood, usually via exposure to contaminated needles or syringes or receiving blood or blood products that have not been checked for HCV. Anti-HVC antibody is present in approximately 2% of U.S. adults. However, prevalence increases significantly in groups at high risk, particularly injection drug users who share needles (CDC, 2020b). Additional risk factors for HCV infection include those who sustain needle stick injuries or mucosal exposure to HCV-positive blood, HIV infection, and birth from an HCV positive mother. *Sexual transmission is rare.* Hepatitis C becomes a chronic disease in over 50% of those infected and is a major risk factor for cirrhosis, hepatocellular carcinoma, and the need for liver transplant for end-stage liver disease (CDC, 2020b).

The majority of people with chronic HCV are unaware of being infected. Response to antiviral therapy ranges from 40% to over 90% depending on the viral genotype and the combination of drugs used for treatment. The CDC recommends screening for hepatitis C infection in all pregnant women during each pregnancy and for drug use via injection (Schillie et al., 2020).

Screening for Colorectal Cancer

Colorectal cancer is the third most common type of cancer and cause of cancer death in both men and women (Lin et al., 2016). Most cases of colorectal cancer occur in individuals 50 or older. Colorectal cancer cases are seen most often after the age of 50 with the overall risk during a lifetime at 1 in 25 for females and 1 in 23 for males (U.S. Cancer Statistics Working Group, 2020). Evidence supports screening guidelines by multisociety task forces, including the American Cancer Society and the USPSTF placing emphasis on risk stratification and endorsement of colorectal cancer screening (U.S. Cancer Statistics Working Group, 2020).

Risk Factors

Modifiable risk factors for colorectal cancer include diets high in red meat, processed meat, overweight stature, lack of exercise, smoking, and increased alcohol intake. Nonmodifiable risk factors for colorectal cancer are age 50 and older, personal history of colorectal cancer, adenomatous polyps, long-standing inflammatory bowel disease, family history of colorectal neoplasia, a hereditary colorectal cancer syndrome (e.g., Lynch syndrome), type 2 diabetes, and African American and Ashkenazi Jewish descent (American Cancer Society, 2017).

Prevention

The most effective prevention strategy is to screen for and remove precancerous adenomatous polyps. Screening programs using fecal blood testing or flexible sigmoidoscopy have been shown in randomized trials to reduce the risk of developing colorectal cancer by about 15% to 20% (CDC, 2020b; Schillie et al., 2020). Physical activity, dietary increase of fruits and vegetables, aspirin and NSAIDs, and postmenopausal combined hormone replacement therapy (estrogen and progestin) are also associated with a decreased risk of colorectal cancer (American Cancer Society, 2017). However, the USPSTF recommends against routinely using aspirin and NSAIDs for prevention in average-risk persons because the potential harms, including gastrointestinal bleeding, hemorrhagic stroke, and renal impairment, outweigh the benefits (American Cancer Society, 2017). Furthermore, while hormone replacement therapy may decrease the risk of colorectal cancer, it can significantly increase the risk of breast cancer.

Screening Tests

Screening tests include stool tests that detect occult fecal blood, such as fecal immunochemical tests, high-sensitivity guaiac-based tests, and tests that detect abnormal DNA. Endoscopic tests are also used for screening, including colonoscopy, which visualizes the entire colon and can remove polyps, and flexible sigmoidoscopy, which visualizes the distal 60 cm of the bowel. Imaging tests include the double-contrast barium enema and computerized tomography (CT) colonography. Any abnormal finding on a stool test, imaging study, or flexible sigmoidoscopy warrants further evaluation with colonoscopy. Screening programs using fecal blood testing or flexible sigmoidoscopy have been shown in randomized trials to reduce the risk colorectal cancer death by about 15% to 30% (Singal et al., 2017; White et al., 2017). Although colonoscopy is the gold standard diagnostic test for screening, there is no direct evidence from randomized trials that screening with colonoscopy reduces colorectal cancer incidence or mortality. Complications of colonoscopy include perforation and bleeding (Singal et al., 2017). Patients are usually sedated during the procedure but extensive bowel preparation is required beginning the day before the procedure. The USPSTF screening recommendations for colorectal cancer are outlined in Box 16-10.

BOX 16-10 **U.S. PREVENTIVE SERVICES TASK FORCE SCREENING RECOMMENDATIONS FOR COLORECTAL CANCER**

- Adults aged 50 to 75 have a high certainty and benefit of screening
- Adults aged 45–49, moderate certainty and benefit of screening
- Adults aged 76 to 85 do not need to be screened routinely; providers should take into consideration overall health and ability to withstand treatment and existence of comorbid conditions

Source: U.S. Preventive Services Task Force (USPSTF). (2021). Final Recommendation: Colorectal cancer: Screening. https://www.uspreventiveservicestaskforce.org/uspstf/recommendation/colorectal-cancer-screening.

The American Cancer Society (2018) recommends beginning screening at 45 years of age.

Urinary Incontinence

Urinary incontinence is the involuntary loss of bladder control. Incontinence is inconvenient and a disruption to daily activities can be physically uncomfortable, and can cause embarrassment and be socially isolating (Scemons, 2013).

Women experience urinary incontinence more often than men do. Those at higher risk for urinary incontinence include women who are postpartum and women between the ages of 60 and 80 years. Men experience urinary incontinence more frequently after prostate surgery. Many patients believe incontinence is normal, but it is not. Information needs to be disseminated more widely for patients to be aware that urinary incontinence is reversible. Nurses play an integral part during the health history in screening for patients who are experiencing urinary incontinence (Newman et al., 2014). The Sandvik scale, also known as the bladder incontinence severity index (ISI), is based on two questions: How often do you experience urine leakage? How much urine do you lose each time you are incontinent? (Sandvik et al., 2006). See Box 16-11.

BOX 16-11 BLADDER INCONTINENCE SEVERITY INDEX (ISI)

1. How often do you experience urine leakage (incontinence)?
   0—never
   1—less than once a month
   2—one or several times a month
   3—one or several times a week
   4—every day/night
2. How much urine do you lose each time?
   1—drops/little
   2—more
3. Total score (multiply question 1 by question 2).
   0—dry
   1 to 2—slight incontinence
   3 to 5—moderate incontinence
   6 to 8—severe incontinence

Source: Hensley, D., Driscoll, A., & Bradway, C. (2013). *Urologic nursing: Scope and standards of practice* (2nd ed.). Jannetti; and Scemons, D. (2013). Urinary incontinence in adults. *Nursing, 43*(11), 52–60. https://doi.org/10.1097/01.NURSE.0000435202.96023.d6

Identification and education of patients with urinary incontinence is key. Teaching pelvic floor muscle exercises to strengthen the pelvic muscles can be life-changing for many who deal with incontinence. Other modalities include behavioral changes, use of a pessary, or biofeedback to reduce and/or eliminate urinary incontinence (Johannessen et al., 2017). This will promote healthy lifestyles and improved quality of life for these individuals.

BIBLIOGRAPHY

CITATIONS

Ahmed Ali, U., Issa, Y., Hagenaars, J. C., Bakker, O. J., van Goor, H., Nieuwenhuijs, V. B., Bollen, T. L., van Ramshorst, B., Witteman, B. J., Brink, M. A., Schaapherder, A. F., Dejong, C. H., Spanier, B. W., Heisterkamp, J., van der Harst, E., van Eijck, C. H., Besselink, M. G., Gooszen, H. G., van Santvoort, H. C., ... Dutch Pancreatitis Study Group. (2016). Risk of recurrent pancreatitis and progression to chronic pancreatitis after a first episode of acute pancreatitis. *Clinical Gastroenterology and Hepatology, 14*(5), 738–746. https://doi.org/10.1016/j.cgh.2015.12.040

Alix, K. (2016). Endovascular repair of the juxtarenal AAA: The future of endovascular nursing. *Journal of Vascular Nursing, 34*(2), 69. https://doi.org/10.1016/j.jvn.2016.04.027

American Cancer Society (ACS). (2017). *Colorectal cancer facts & figures 2017–2019.* https://www.cancer.org/content/dam/cancer-org/research/cancer-facts-and-statistics/colorectal-cancer-facts-and-figures/colorectal-cancer-facts-and-figures-2017-2019.pdf

American Cancer Society (ACS). (2020). *Cancer facts & figures 2020.* American Cancer Society. https://www.cancer.org/content/dam/cancer-org/research/cancer-facts-and-statistics/annual-cancer-facts-and-figures/2020/cancer-facts-and-figures-2020.pdf.

American Gastroenterological Association. (2018). Clinical gastroenterology and hepatology, *16*(5), A27. https://doi.org/10.1016/j.cgh.2018.02.014

Arasaradnam, R. P., Brown, S., Forbes, A., Fox, M. R., Hungin, P., Kelman, L., Major, G., O'Connor, M., Sanders, D. S., Sinha, R., Smith, S. C., Thomas, P., & Walters, J. R. F. (2018). Guidelines for the investigation of chronic diarrhoea in adults: British Society of Gastroenterology, 3rd edition. *Gut, 67*(8), 1380–1399. https://doi.org/10.1136/gutjnl-2017-315909

Babor, T., Higgins-Biddle, J., Saunders, J., & Monteiro, M. (2020). *AUDIT: The alcohol use disorders identification test: Guidelines for use in primary care* (2nd ed.). World Health Organization. https://apps.who.int/iris/bitstream/handle/10665/67205/WHO_MSD_MSB_01.6a.pdf;jsessionid=5FA678733BFE16C3A978CD9EB23D79B7?sequence=1

Bao, J., Lopez, J. A., & Huerta, S. (2013). Acute abdominal pain and abnormal CT findings. *JAMA, 310*(8), 848–849. https://doi.org/10.1001/jama.2013.276158

Centers for Disease Control and Prevention (CDC). (2019). Commentary portion of U.S. 2017 surveillance data for viral hepatitis. https://www.cdc.gov/hepatitis/statistics/2017surveillance/index.htm

Centers for Disease Control and Prevention (CDC). (2020a). *Hepatitis B information. Division of viral hepatitis.* Retrieved July 8, 2020, from https://www.cdc.gov/hepatitis/hbv/index.htm

Centers for Disease Control and Prevention (CDC). (2020b). *Hepatitis C information. Division of viral hepatitis.* Retrieved July 8, 2020, from https://www.cdc.gov/hepatitis/hcv/index.htm

Centers for Disease Control and Prevention (CDC). (2021, January 14). *Deaths from excessive alcohol use.* https://www.cdc.gov/alcohol/features/excessive-alcohol-deaths.html

Cervellin, G., Mora, R., Ticinesi, A., Meschi, T., Comelli, I., Catena, F., & Lippi, G. (2016). Epidemiology and outcomes of acute abdominal pain in a large urban emergency department: Retrospective analysis of 5,340 cases. *Annals of Translational Medicine*, *4*(19), 362. https://doi.org/10.21037/atm.2016.09.10

Davis-Yadley, A. H., Neill, K. G., Malafa, M. P., & Pena, L. R. (2016). Advances in the endoscopic diagnosis of Barrett esophagus. *Cancer Control*, *23*(1), 67–77. https://doi.org/10.1177/107327481602300112

DeVault, K. R., & Castell, D. O.; American College of Gastroenterology. (2005). Updated guidelines for the diagnosis and treatment of gastroesophageal reflux disease. *American Journal of Gastroenterology*, *100*(1), 190–200. https://doi.org/10.1111/j.1572-0241.2005.41217.x

Doshani, M., Weng, M., Moore, K. L., Romero, J. R., & Nelson, N. P. (2019). Recommendations of the advisory committee on immunization practices for use of hepatitis a vaccine for persons experiencing homelessness. *MMWR. Morbidity and Mortality Weekly Report*, *68*(6), 153–156. Published 2019 February 15. https://doi.org/10.15585/mmwr.mm6806a6

D'Souza, N., & Nugent, K. (2016). Appendicitis. *American Family Physician*, *93*(2), 142–143.

Elliott, K. R., Dunn, M. J., Krueger, T. D., & Steele, D. A. (2019). Utilization of point-of-care ultrasonography (POCUS) for small bowel obstruction. *Advanced Emergency Nursing Journal*, *41*(2), 107–110. https://doi.org/10.1097/TME.0000000000000237

Evans, M. M., & Curtin, M. (2014). Acute appendicitis: A case study describing standards of care. *Medsurg Nursing*, *23*(6), 3–15.

Fargo, M. V., Grogan, S. P., & Saguil, A. (2017). Evaluation of jaundice in adults. *American Family Physician*, *95*(3), 164–168.

Friedman, A., Mukerji, P., Buadu, A., & Grandone, C. (2011). Sonography of acute cholecystitis: Murphy's sign or Murphy's Law? *Ultrasound in Medicine & Biology*, *37*(8), S87. https://doi.org/10.1016/j.ultrasmedbio.2011.05.390

Giraldo-Cadavid, L. F., Leal-Leaño, L. R., Leon-Basantes, G. A., Bastidas, A. R., Garcia, R., Ovalle, S., & Abondano-Garavito, J. E. (2017). Accuracy of endoscopic and videofluoroscopic evaluations of swallowing for oropharyngeal dysphagia. *Laryngoscope*, *127*(9), 2002–2010. https://doi.org/10.1002/lary.26419

Gougol, A., Machicado, J. D., Matta, B., Paragomi, P., Pothoulakis, I., Slivka, A., Whitcomb, D. C., Yadav, D., & Papachristou, G. I. (2019). Prevalence and associated factors of abdominal pain and disability at 1-year follow-up after an attack of acute pancreatitis [Erratum in *Pancreas.* 2020 March; 49(3):e25]. *Pancreas*, *48*(10), 1348–1353. https://doi.org/10.1097/MPA.0000000000001434

Grover, S. (1993). Does this patient have splenomegaly? *JAMA*, *270*(18), 2218. https://doi.org/10.1001/jama.1993.03510180088040

Guirguis-Blake, J. M., Beil, T. L., Senger, C. A., & Coppola, E. L. (2019). Primary care screening for abdominal aortic aneurysm: Updated evidence report and systematic review for the US Preventive Services Task Force. *JAMA*, *322*(22), 2219–2238. https://doi.org/10.1001/jama.2019.17021

Hensley, D., Driscoll, A., & Bradway, C. (2013). *Urologic nursing: Scope and standards of practice* (2nd ed.). Jannetti.

Herrington, H. (2018). Constipation. *Clinical Gastroenterology and Hepatology*, *16*(2), A22. https://doi.org/10.1016/j.cgh.2017.11.043

Holcomb, S. (2008). Acute abdomen: What a pain! *Nursing*, *38*(9), 34–40. https://doi.org/10.1097/01.nurse.0000334644.51961.47

Hou, W., & Sanyal, A. (2009). Ascites: Diagnosis and management. *Medical Clinics of North America*, *93*(4), 801–817. https://doi.org/10.1016/j.mcna.2009.03.007

Johannessen, H. H., Wibe, A., Stordahl, A., Sandvik, L., & Mørkved, S. (2017). Do pelvic floor muscle exercises reduce postpartum anal incontinence? A randomised controlled trial. *BJOG*, *124*(4), 686–694. https://doi.org/10.1111/1471-0528.14145

Johnson, J. R., & Russo, T. A. (2018). Acute pyelonephritis in adults [Erratum in N Engl J Med. 2018 March 15;378(11):1069]. *New England Journal of Medicine*, *378*(1), 48–59. https://doi.org/10.1056/nejmcp1702758

Junqueira, J. B., & Santos, V. L. C. G. (2018). Urinary incontinence in hospital patients: Prevalence and associated factors. *Revista Latino-Americana De Enfermagem*, *25*, e2970. Published 2018 January 8. https://doi.org/10.1590/1518-8345.2139.2970

Kaplan, G. G. (2015). The global burden of IBD: From 2015 to 2025. *Nature Reviews, Gastroenterology & Hepatology*, *12*(12), 720–727. https://doi.org/10.1038/nrgastro.2015.150

Kidney stones. *Nursing*, 2012, *42*(12), 29. https://doi.org/10.1097/01.nurse.0000422643.21501.3f

Keisler, B., & Carter, C. (2015). Abdominal aortic aneurysm. *American Family Physician*, *91*(8), 538–543.

Kent, K. C. (2014). Clinical practice. Abdominal aortic aneurysms. *New England Journal of Medicine*, *371*(22), 2101–2108. https://doi.org/10.1056/NEJMcp1401430

Kinjo, M., Nakamura, Y., Taguchi, S., Yamaguchi, T., Tambo, M., Okegawa, T., & Fukuhara, H. (2020). Sex differences in prevalence and patient behavior regarding lower urinary tract symptoms among Japanese medical checkup examinees. [published online ahead of print, 2020 June 12]. *Urology*, *S0090-4295*(20), 30672–30675. https://doi.org/10.1016/j.urology.2020.05.065

Lin, J. S., Piper, M., & Perdue, L. A. (2016). *Screening for colorectal cancer: A systematic review for the U.S. Preventive Services Task Force.* Evidence Synthesis No. 135. AHRQ Publication No. 14-05203-EF-1. Agency for Healthcare Research and Quality.

Liu, G., Andreev, V. P., Helmuth, M. E., Yang, C. C., Lai, H. H., Smith, A. R., Wiseman, J. B., Merion, R. M., Erickson, B. A., Cella, D., Griffith, J. W., Gore, J. L., DeLancey, J. O. L., & Kirkali, Z.; LURN Study Group. (2019). Symptom based clustering of men in the LURN observational cohort study. *Journal of Urology*, *202*(6), 1230–1239. https://doi.org/10.1097/JU.0000000000000354

Loloi, J., Patel, A., & Riley, T. (2018). Do physical exam and ultrasound liver size findings correlate? Teaching the abdominal examination through reflective practice 936. *American Journal of Gastroenterology*, *113*(Supplement), S523–S524. https://doi.org/10.14309/00000434-201810001-00936

Ludlow, H. (2019). Clinical assessment. In: A. Strum & L. White (Eds.), *Inflammatory bowel disease nursing manual.* Springer. https://doi-org.proxy.library.upenn.edu/10.1007/978-3-319-75022-4_4

Madson, M. B., Schutts, J. W., Jordan, H. R., Villarosa-Hurlocker, M. C., Whitley, R. B., & Mohn, R. S. (2018). Identifying at-risk college student drinkers with the AUDIT-US: A receiver operating characteristic curve analysis. [published online ahead of print, 2018 August 1]. *Assessment*, 1073191118792091. https://doi.org/10.1177/1073191118792091

McGee, S. (2018). *Evidence-based physical diagnosis.* Elsevier.

Mesenteric ischemia. *Gastroenterology Nursing.* 2018, *41*(4), E1–E2. https://doi.org/10.1097/sga.0000000000000412

Mitchell, A. M., Mahmoud, K. F., Finnell, D., Savage, C. L., Weber, M., & Bacidore, V. (2020). The essentials competencies: A framework for substance use-related curricula. *Nurse Educator*, *45*(4), 225–228. https://doi.org/10.1097/NNE.0000000000000753

Mulligan, C. (2015). Update on diverticular disease and implications for primary care. *The Journal for Nurse Practitioners*, *11*(9), 883–888. https://doi.org/10.1016/j.nurpra.2015.07.010

National Institute on Alcohol Abuse and Alcoholism (NIAAA). (2020a). Alcohol facts and statistics. Retrieved April 17, 2021, from https://pubs.niaaa.nih.gov/publications/AlcoholFacts%26Stats/AlcoholFacts%26Stats.htm

National Institute on Alcohol Abuse and Alcoholism (NIAAA). (2020b). Helping patients who drink too much: A clinician's guide. Retrieved June 29, 2020, from https://pubs.niaaa.nih.gov/publications/practitioner/cliniciansguide2005/guide.pdf

Newman, D. K. (2019). Prompted voiding for individuals with urinary incontinence. *Journal of Gerontological Nursing*, *45*(2), 14–26.

Newman, D., Burgio, K., Markland, A., & Goode, P. (2014). Urinary incontinence: Nonsurgical treatments. *Geriatric Urology*, 141–168. https://doi.org/10.1007/978-1-4614-9047-0_11

Ng, S. C., Shi, H. Y., Hamidi, N., Underwood, F. E., Tang, W., Benchimol, E. I., Panaccione, R., Ghosh, S., Wu, J. C. Y., Chan, F. K. L., Sung, J. J. Y., & Kaplan, G. G. (2018). Worldwide incidence and prevalence of inflammatory bowel disease in the 21st century: A systematic review of population-based studies. *Lancet*, *390*(10114), 2769–2778. https://doi.org/10.1016/S0140-6736(17)32448-0

O'Connor, E. A., Perdue, L. A., Senger, C. A., Rushkin, M., Patnode, C. D., Bean, S. I., & Jonas, D. E. (2018). Screening and behavioral counseling interventions to reduce unhealthy alcohol use in adolescents and adults: Updated evidence report and systematic review for the US Preventive Services Task Force. *JAMA*, *320*(18), 1910–1928. https://doi.org/10.1001/jama.2018.12086

Peery, A. F., Crockett, S. D., Murphy, C. C., Lund, J. L., Dellon, E. S., Williams, J. L., Jensen, E. T., Shaheen, N. J., Barritt, A. S., Lieber, S. R., Kochar, B., Barnes, E. L., Fan, Y. C., Pate, V., Galanko, J., Baron, T. H., & Sandler, R. S. (2019). Burden and cost of gastrointestinal, liver, and pancreatic diseases in the United States: Update 2018 [Erratum in *Gastroenterology.* 2019 May;156(6):1936]. *Gastroenterology*, *156*(1), 254–272.e11. https://doi.org/10.1053/j.gastro.2018.08.063

Riddle, M. S., DuPont, H. L., & Connor, B. A. (2016). ACG clinical guideline: Diagnosis, treatment, and prevention of acute diarrheal infections in adults. *American Journal of Gastroenterology*, *111*(5), 602–622. https://doi.org/10.1038/ajg.2016.126

Ross, J. T., Matthay, M. A., & Harris, H. W. (2018). Secondary peritonitis: Principles of diagnosis and intervention. *BMJ (Clinical Research Ed.)*, *361*, k1407. Published 2018 June 18. https://doi.org/10.1136/bmj.k1407

Saccomano, S., & Ferrara, L. (2013). Evaluation of acute abdominal pain. *Nurse Practitioner*, *38*(11), 46–53. https://doi.org/10.1097/01.npr.0000433077.14775.f1

Samhsa.gov. (2020a). Section 2 PE Tables—Results from the 2018 National Survey on Drug Use and Health: Detailed Tables, Sections 1–3, SAMHSA, CBHSQ. Retrieved June 29, 2020, from https://www.samhsa.gov/data/sites/default/files/cbhsq-reports/NSDUHDetailedTabs2018R2/NSDUHDetTabsSect2pe2018.htm#tab2-1b.

Samhsa.gov. (2020b). Section 5 PE Tables—Results from the 2018 National Survey on Drug Use and Health: Detailed Tables, Sections 1–3, SAMHSA, CBHSQ. Retrieved June 29, 2020, from https://www.samhsa.gov/data/sites/default/files/cbhsq-reports/NSDUHDetailedTabs2018R2/NSDUHDetTabsSect5pe2018.htm#tab5-4b

Sandvik, H., Espuna, M., & Hunskaar, S. (2006). Validity of the incontinence severity index: Comparison with pad-weighing tests. *International Urogynecology Journal and Pelvic Floor Dysfunction*, *17*(5), 520–524. https://doi.org/10.1007/s00192-005-0060-z

Sankaran, S. J., Xiao, A. Y., Wu, L. M., Windsor, J. A., Forsmark, C. E., & Petrov, M. S. (2015). Frequency of progression from acute to chronic pancreatitis and risk factors: A meta-analysis. *Gastroenterology*, *149*(6), 1490–1500.e1. https://doi.org/10.1053/j.gastro.2015.07.066

Scemons, D. (2013). Urinary incontinence in adults. *Nursing*, *43*(11), 52–60. https://doi.org/10.1097/01.NURSE.0000435202.96023.d6

Schillie, S., Vellozzi, C., Reingold, A., Harris, A., Haber, P., Ward, J. W., & Nelson, N. P. (2018). Prevention of hepatitis B virus infection in the United States: Recommendations of the advisory committee on immunization practices. *MMWR. Recommendations and Reports*, *67*(1), 1–31. Published 2018 January 12. https://doi.org/10.15585/mmwr.rr6701a1

Schillie, S., Wester, C., Osborne, M., Wesolowski, L., & Ryerson, A. B. (2020). CDC recommendations for hepatitis C screening among adults—United States, 2020. *MMWR Recommendations and Reports*, *69*(2), 1–17. Published 2020 April 10. https://doi.org/10.15585/mmwr.rr6902a1

Shah, B. J., Rughwani, N., & Rose, S. (2015). In the clinic. Constipation. *Annals of Internal Medicine*, *162*(7), ITC1. https://doi.org/10.7326/AITC201504070

Shaheen, N. J., Weinberg, D. S., Denberg, T. D., Chou, R., Qaseem, A., & Shekelle, P.; Clinical Guidelines Committee of the American College of Physicians. (2012). Upper endoscopy for gastroesophageal reflux disease: Best practice advice from the clinical guidelines committee of the American College of Physicians. *Annals of Internal Medicine*, *157*(11), 808–816. https://doi.org/10.7326/0003-4819-157-11-201212040-00008

Singal, A. G., Gupta, S., Skinner, C. S., Ahn, C., Santini, N. O., Agrawal, D., Mayorga, C. A., Murphy, C., Tiro, J. A., McCallister, K., Sanders, J. M., Bishop, W. P., Loewen, A. C., & Halm, E. A. (2017). Effect of colonoscopy outreach vs fecal immunochemical test outreach on colorectal cancer screening completion: A randomized clinical trial. *JAMA*, *318*(9), 806–815. https://doi.org/10.1001/jama.2017.11389

Sjoberg, B. P., Menias, C. O., Lubner, M. G., Mellnick, V. M., & Pickhardt, P. J. (2018). Splenomegaly: A combined clinical and radiologic approach to the differential diagnosis. *Gastroenterology Clinics of North America*, *47*(3), 643–666. https://doi.org/10.1016/j.gtc.2018.04.009

Spechler, S. J., Hunter, J. G., Jones, K. M., Lee, R., Smith, B. R., Mashimo, H., Sanchez, V. M., Dunbar, K. B., Pham, T. H., Murthy, U. K., Kim, T., Jackson, C. S., Wallen, J. M., von Rosenvinge, E. C., Pearl, J. P., Laine, L., Kim, A. W., Kaz, A. M., Tatum, R. P., ... Huang, G. D. (2019). Randomized trial of medical versus surgical treatment for refractory heartburn. *New England Journal of Medicine*, *381*(16), 1513–1523. https://doi.org/10.1056/NEJMoa1811424

Spechler, S. J., & Souza, R. F. (2014). Barrett's esophagus. *New England Journal of Medicine*, *371*(9), 836–845. https://doi.org/10.1056/NEJMra1314704

Tack, J., & Talley, N. J. (2013). Functional dyspepsia–symptoms, definitions and validity of the Rome III criteria. *Nature Reviews. Gastroenterology & Hepatology*, *10*(3), 134–141. https://doi.org/10.1038/nrgastro.2013.14

Tagliaferri, E., Bergmann, H., Hammans, S., Shiraz, A., Stüber, E., & Seidlmayer, C. (2017). Agenesis of the gallbladder: Role of clinical suspicion and magnetic resonance to avoid unnecessary surgery. *Case Reports in Gastroenterology*, *10*(3), 819–825. Published 2017 January 6. https://doi.org/10.1159/000453656

Tan, M., Menon, S., & Black, D. (2017). The impact on patients of a nurse-led clinical service in gastroenterology. *British Journal of Nursing*, *26*(13), 734–738. https://doi.org/10.12968/bjon.2017.26.13.734

Trads, M., Deutch, S. R., & Pedersen, P. U. (2018). Supporting patients in reducing postoperative constipation: Fundamental nursing care—a quasi-experimental study. *Scandinavian Journal of Caring Sciences*, *32*(2), 824–832. https://doi.org/10.1111/scs.12513

U.S. Cancer Statistics Working Group. (2020). *U.S. cancer statistics data visualizations tool based on 2019 submission data (1999–2017)*. https://www.cdc.gov/cancer/uscs/dataviz/index.htm

Ueda, T., & Ishida, E. (2015). Indirect fist percussion of the liver is a more sensitive technique for detecting hepatobiliary infections than Murphy's sign. *Current Gerontology and Geriatrics Research*, *2015*, 431638. https://doi.org/10.1155/2015/431638

U.S. Preventive Services Task Force (USPSTF). (2021). Final Recommendation: Colorectal cancer: Screening. https://www.uspreventiveservicestaskforce.org/uspstf/recommendation/colorectal-cancer-screening

White, A., Thompson, T. D., White, M. C., Sabatino, S. A., de Moor, J., Doria-Rose, P. V., Geiger, A. M., & Richardson, L. C. (2017). Cancer screening test use—United States, 2015. *MMWR Morbidity and Mortality Weekly Report*, *66*(8), 201–206. Published 2017 March 3. https://doi.org/10.15585/mmwr.mm6608a1

World Health Organization (WHO). (2020). Top 10 causes of death, Global health observatory data. Retrieved June 25, 2020, from http://www.who.int/gho/mortality_burden_disease/causes_death/top_10/en/. Published 2020.

Yadlapati, R., & Pandolfino, J. E. (2020). Medical versus surgical treatment for refractory heartburn. *The New England Journal of Medicine*, *382*(3), 296–297. https://doi.org/10.1056/NEJMc1915309

Youatou Towo, P., Ramadan, A. S., Ngatchou, W., Djiélé, J. N., Etienne, A., Capelluto, E., & Mols, P. P. (2012). Predictors of early outcome after acute appendicitis: Is delaying surgery for acute appendicitis an option? A retrospective study. *European Journal of Trauma and Emergency Surgery*, *38*(6), 641–646. https://doi.org/10.1007/s00068-012-0208-8

17 THE BREASTS AND AXILLAE

KEY TERMS

areola	hidradenitis	mammogram
BRCA genes	lactation	mastitis
galactorrhea	lactiferous	supernumerary
gynecomastia	lymphadenopathy	

Learning Objectives

The student will:

1. Identify the structures and functions of the breasts and axillae.
2. Elicit a health history of the breasts and axillae.
3. Describe the physical examination techniques performed to evaluate the breasts and axillae.
4. Demonstrate how to perform a clinical breast examination.
5. Document a complete breast and axilla assessment using information from the health history and the physical examination.
6. Describe the measures for prevention or early detection of breast cancer.

Hormonal changes at puberty in women cause the breast tissue to enlarge, preparing the ductal system for **lactation**, the production of milk. Until puberty, the male and female breasts are similar.

ANATOMY AND PHYSIOLOGY

The Female Breast

The female breast lies against the anterior thoracic wall, extending from the second rib down to the sixth rib, and from the sternum across to the midaxillary line (Fig. 17-1). Its surface area is generally rectangular rather than round. The breast overlies the pectoralis major and at its inferior margin, the serratus anterior.

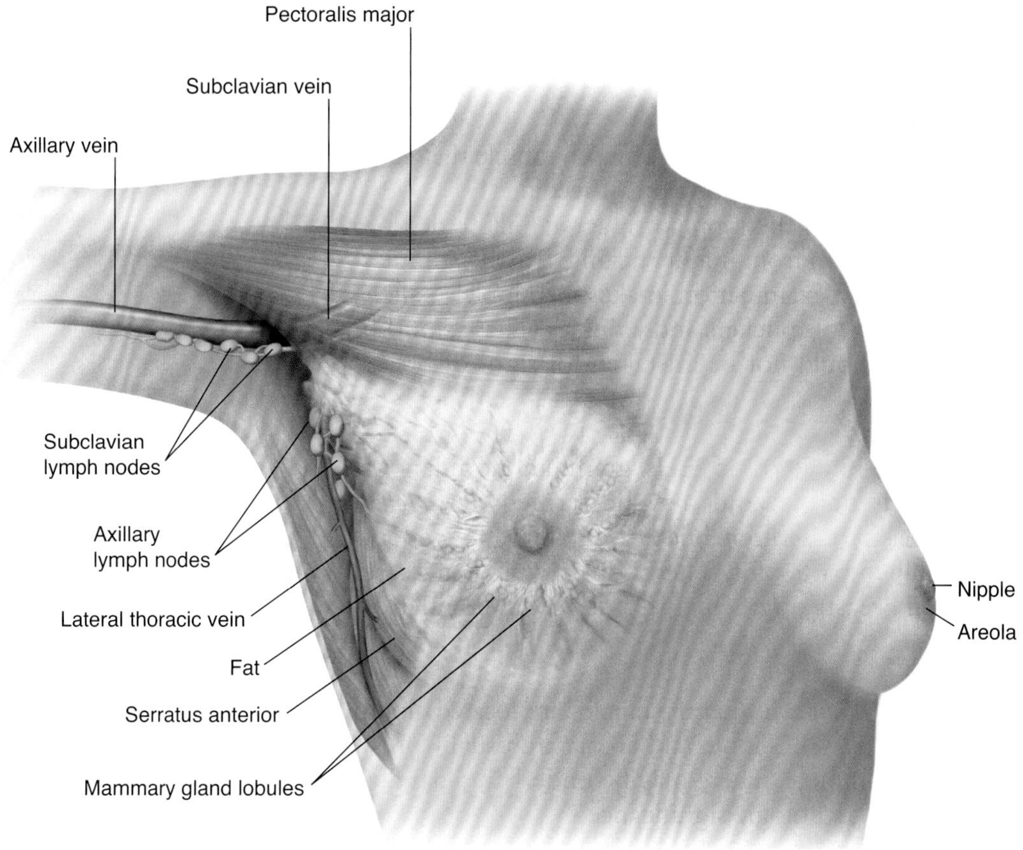

FIGURE 17-1 Anatomy of the breast.

The breast is hormonally sensitive tissue, responsive to the changes of monthly menstrual cycles and aging. At the tip of the breast is an area called the **areola** and at the center is the nipple. About 15 to 20 **lactiferous** (milk producing) ducts empty into a depression at the top of the nipple (Fig. 17-2). Each duct leads from the alveoli within the breast called lobules, where the milk is secreted. Along their length, the duct widens into areas that form reservoirs where milk can be stored. These ducts and lobules form the *glandular tissue. Fibrous connective tissue* provides structural support in the form of fibrous bands or suspensory ligaments connected to both the skin and the underlying fascia. *Adipose tissue*, or fat, surrounds the breast, predominantly in the superficial and peripheral areas. After menopause, there are fewer lobules noted, and glandular tissue atrophies and is replaced with fat. The proportions of these components vary with age, the general state of nutrition, pregnancy, exogenous hormone use, and other factors.

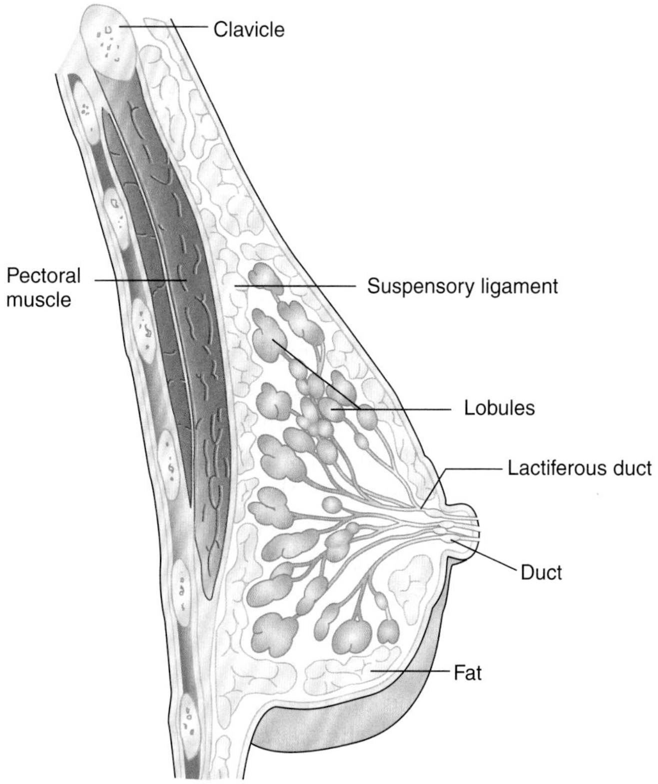

FIGURE 17-2 Structures of the breast from the sagittal view.

The surface of the areola has small, rounded elevations formed by sebaceous glands, sweat glands, and accessory areolar glands. A few hairs are often seen on the areola.

Both the nipple and the areola are well supplied with smooth muscle that contracts to express milk from the ductal system during breast-feeding (Fig. 17-3). Rich sensory innervation, especially in the nipple, triggers "milk letdown" following neurohormonal stimulation from infant sucking. Tactile stimulation of the area, including the breast examination, makes the nipple smaller, firmer, and more erect while the areola puckers and wrinkles. These smooth muscle reflexes are normal and should not be mistaken for signs of breast disease.

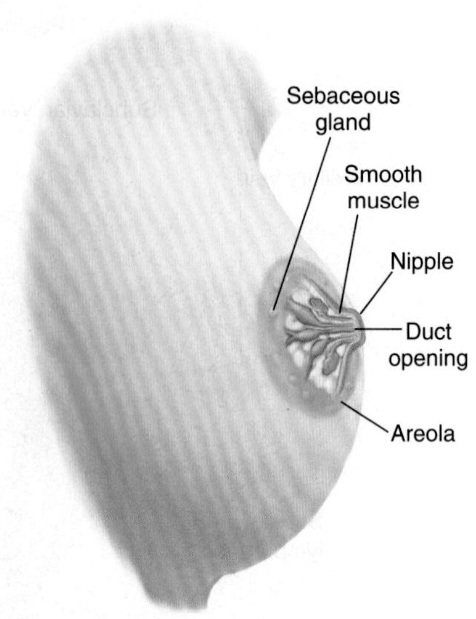

FIGURE 17-3 Anatomy of the nipple and areola.

The adult breast may be soft, but it often feels granular, nodular, or lumpy. This uneven texture is normal and may be termed *physiologic nodularity* or fibrocystic breast. It is often bilateral. It may be evident throughout the breast or only in parts of it. The nodularity may increase before menses—a time when breasts often enlarge and become tender or even painful.

Occasionally, one or more extra or **supernumerary** nipples are located along the "milk line" (Fig. 17-4). Only a small nipple and areola are usually present, often mistaken for a common mole. There may be underlying glandular tissue. An extra nipple has no pathologic significance.

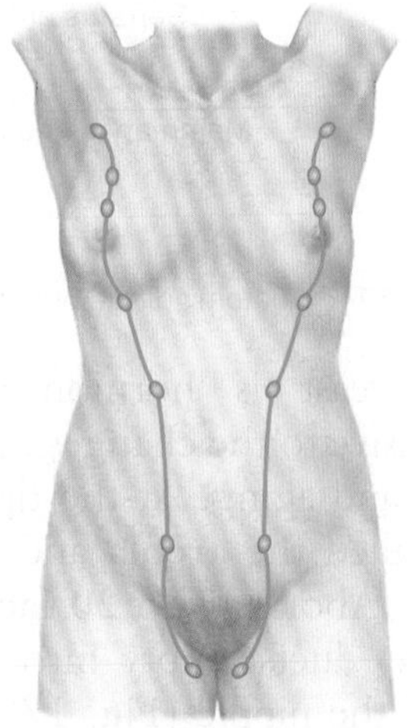

FIGURE 17-4 The "milk line."

The Male Breast

The male breast consists chiefly of a small nipple and areola. These overlie a thin disc of undeveloped breast tissue consisting primarily of ducts. There is a lack of estrogen and progesterone stimulation, ductal branching and the development of lobules is minimal (Harris et al., 2014). It may be difficult to distinguish male breast tissue from the surrounding muscles of the chest wall. A firm button of breast tissue, 2 cm or more in diameter, has been described in roughly one of three adult men.

Lymphatics

Lymphatics from most of the breast drain toward the axilla (Fig. 17-5). Of the axillary lymph nodes, the *central nodes* are palpable most frequently. They lie along the chest wall, usually high in the axilla and midway between the anterior and posterior axillary folds. Channels from three

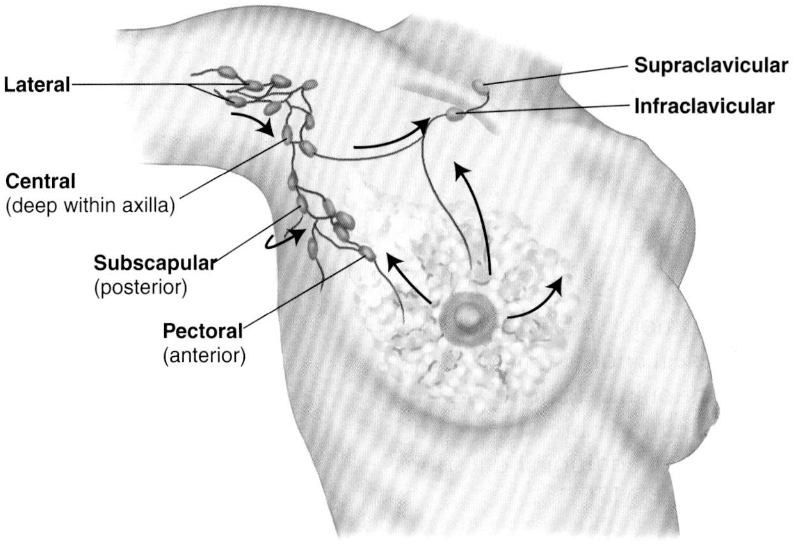

FIGURE 17-5 The axillary lymph nodes.

other groups of lymph nodes drain into them and are seldom palpable. They include:

- *Pectoral nodes—anterior*, located along the lower border of the pectoralis major inside the anterior axillary fold. These nodes drain the anterior chest wall and much of the breast.
- *Subscapular nodes—posterior*, located along the lateral border of the scapula; palpated deep in the posterior axillary fold. They drain the posterior chest wall and a portion of the arm.
- *Lateral nodes*—located *along the upper humerus.* They drain most of the arm.

Lymph drains from the central axillary nodes to the *infraclavicular* and *supraclavicular* nodes.

Not all the lymphatics of the breast drain into the axilla. Malignant cells from a breast cancer may spread directly to the infraclavicular nodes or into deep channels within the chest.

THE HEALTH HISTORY

Common or concerning symptoms identified during a breast and axilla history are listed in Box 17-1.

During the breast examination, remember to consider the client's cultural background, sexual orientation, and gender identity elicited during the general health history. Once a rapport has developed, begin with an open-ended question, such as, "Have you noticed any changes in your breasts?"

BOX 17-1 COMMON OR CONCERNING SYMPTOMS IN FEMALES OR MALES

- Breast lump or mass
- Breast pain or discomfort
- Change in shape
- Nipple discharge
- Edema
- Rashes
- Scaling
- Dimpling
- Retraction
- Gynecomastia (males)

If the patient does not have any comments, then more specific questions are necessary as they may trigger a memory and reveal another area that the patient thought was "nothing" or not worth mentioning. Patients may be too embarrassed to ask or answer questions regarding their breasts. In addition, if the patient does have a positive response, then additional questions should be asked related to the finding, using "OLD CART."

Lump or Mass

Ask the patient, "Have you ever felt a lump in your breast or under your arm?" If the answer is yes, use "OLD CART" to further explore this issue.

- *Onset:* When did you first notice the lump?
- *Location:* In which breast is the lump? Where on the breast?
- *Duration:* Does the lump remain at all times, or does it come and go?
  If it comes and goes, when is it present and when does it disappear?
- *Characteristic symptoms:* What does the lump feel like?
  Are there multiple lumps or one distinct lump?
- *Associated manifestations:* What else happens when the lump is present?
  Is there pain or discharge?
  Can you only feel it during menstruation?
- *Relieving factors:* Does anything make it go away?
  What relieves the lump? What relieves the pain?
- *Treatment:* Have you done anything about the lump to try to make it disappear?
  Have you spoken to a health care provider?

Lumps may be physiologic or pathologic, ranging from cysts and fibroadenomas (benign tumors found commonly, consist of connective tissue and glandular breast tissue) to breast cancer. See Table 17-1, "Common Breast Masses" and Table 17-2, "Visible Signs of Breast Cancer."

Pain or Discomfort

If the patient reports pain or discomfort, ask:

- *Onset:* Do you ever have breast pain or discomfort?
  When do you have pain or discomfort?
- *Location:* Where do you have pain or discomfort?
- *Duration:* Does the pain or discomfort come and go, or is it constant?
- *Characteristic symptoms:* Describe the pain or discomfort.

Concept Mastery Alert

Physiologic versus Pathologic Breast Lumps

When collecting the health history of a patient who reports a lump or swelling in the breast, the nurse must gather additional information to evaluate whether the lump is physiologic or pathologic. The priority question would be to first determine if the lumps change in size during the menstrual cycle. Women with fibrocystic breasts will often have lumpy areas in the breast that increase in size in the 2 weeks prior to the menstrual period and then decrease in size during the period and for the first 2 weeks after the period. Pain is often associated with these lumps, so a report of pain from the patient does not provide specific information about whether lump is physiologic or pathologic.

- *Associated manifestations:* What else happens with the pain or discomfort?
- *Relieving factors:* What have you done to make the pain or discomfort feel better?
- *Treatment:* Have you done anything to treat the pain?

There are many other questions related to the breast, and the "OLD CART" mnemonic ensures all areas of questioning are covered. Additional examples of questions for a variety of findings related to the breast and axilla continue in the following sections.

Change in Shape

Ask the patient, "Have you noticed any change in the *shape* of your breast?" If the answer is yes, ask:

- When did you notice the change in shape?
- Where is the change? Which breast?
- When did this occur?
- Did anything else happen at this time?
- Can you associate anything else with this?
- How are you coping with the treatment?

Discharge

Ask, "Have you ever had *nipple discharge*?" If the answer is yes, ask:

- When does the discharge occur?
- In which breast does it occur? Is it unilateral or bilateral?
- How long does the discharge last?
- Can you describe the discharge? Color? Consistency? Amount? Odor?
- What is associated with the discharge?
- How do you deal with the discharge?

CLINICAL TIP
Galactorrhea, or the inappropriate discharge of milk-containing fluid, is abnormal if it occurs 6 or more months after childbirth or the cessation of breast feeding.

TABLE 17-1 Common Breast Masses

The three most common kinds of breast masses are *fibroadenomas* (benign tumors), *cysts*, and *breast cancer*. The clinical characteristics of these masses are listed below. However, any breast mass should be carefully evaluated and usually warrants further investigation by ultrasound, aspiration, mammography, or biopsy. The masses depicted below are large for purposes of illustration. Ideally, breast cancer should be identified early, when the mass is small. *Fibrocystic changes*, not illustrated, are also commonly palpable as nodular, rope-like densities in women aged 25–50. They may be tender or painful. They are considered benign and are not viewed as a risk factor for breast cancer.

	Fibroadenoma	Cysts	Cancer
Illustration	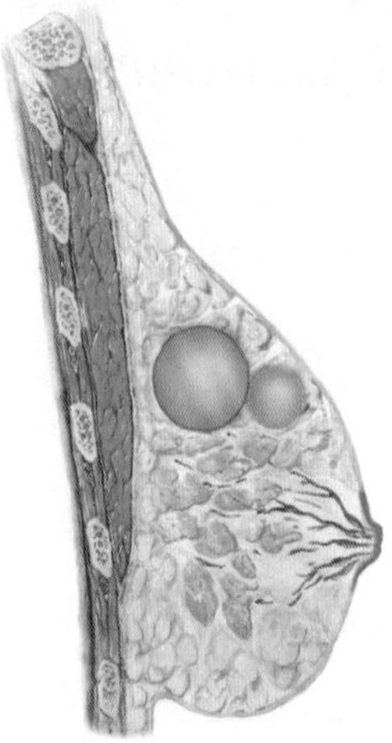	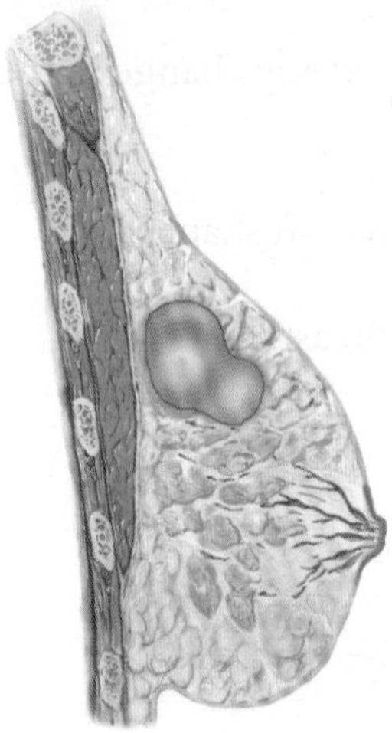	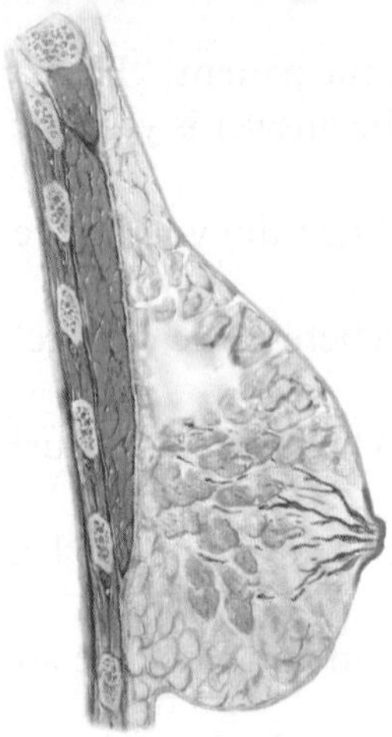
Usual Age	15–25, usually puberty and young adulthood, but up to age 55	30–50, regress after menopause except with estrogen therapy	30–90, most common over age 50
Number	Usually single, may be multiple	Single or multiple	Usually single, though may coexist with other nodules
Shape	Round, disc-like, or lobular	Round	Irregular or stellate
Consistency	May be soft, usually firm	Soft to firm, usually elastic	Firm or hard
Delineation	Well delineated	Well delineated	Not clearly delineated from surrounding tissues
Mobility	Very mobile	Mobile	May be fixed to skin or underlying tissues
Tenderness	Usually nontender	Often tender	Usually nontender
Retraction Signs	Absent	Absent	May be present

TABLE 17-2 Visible Signs of Breast Cancer

Retraction Signs

As breast cancer advances, it causes fibrosis (scar tissue). Shortening of this tissue produces *dimpling*, *changes in contour*, and *retraction or deviation of the nipple*. Other causes of retraction include fat necrosis and mammary duct ectasia.

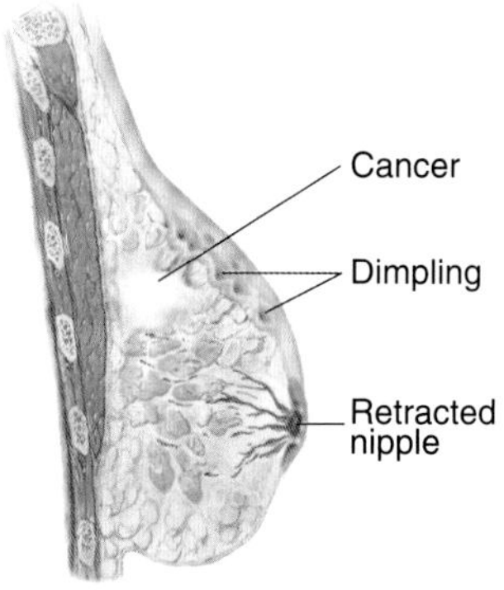

Nipple Retraction and Deviation
A retracted nipple is flattened or pulled inward, as illustrated here. It may also be broadened and feels thickened. When involvement is radially asymmetric, the nipple may deviate or point in a different direction from its normal counterpart, typically toward the underlying cancer.

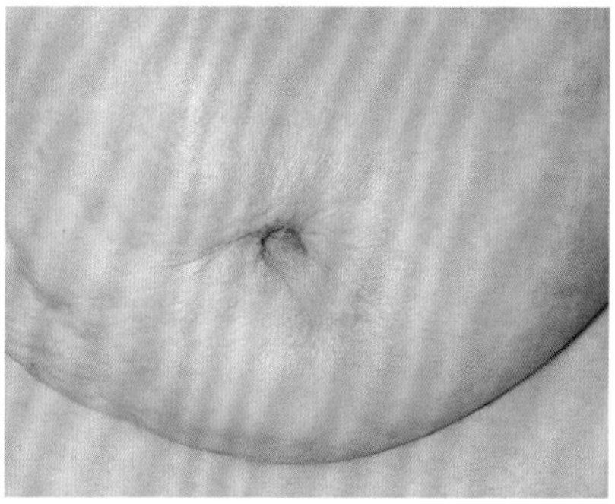

Skin Dimpling
Look for this sign with the patient's arm at rest, during special positioning, and on moving or compressing the breast, as illustrated here.

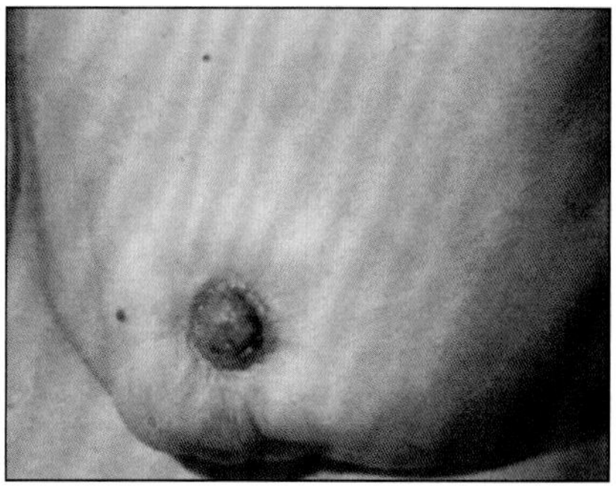

Abnormal Contours
Look for any variation in the normal convexity of each breast, and compare one side with the other. Special positioning may be useful. Shown here is marked flattening of the lower outer quadrant of the left breast.

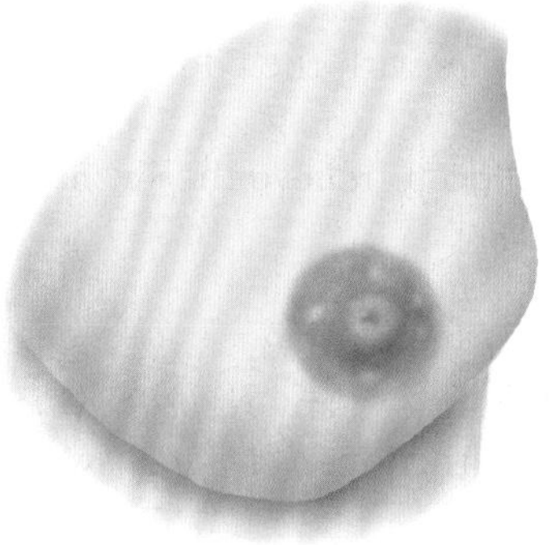

(continued)

TABLE 17-2 Visible Signs of Breast Cancer *(Continued)*

Edema of the Skin

Edema of the skin is produced by lymphatic blockade. It appears as thickened skin with enlarged pores—the so-called *peau d'orange* (orange peel) *sign*. It is often seen first in the lower portion of the breast or areola.

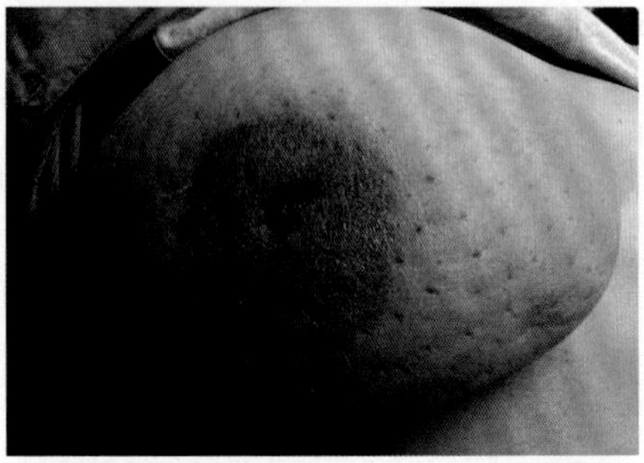

Paget Disease of the Nipple

This uncommon form of breast cancer usually starts as a scaly, eczema-like lesion that may weep, crust, or erode. A breast mass may be present. Suspect Paget disease in any persisting dermatitis of the nipple and areola. Can present with invasive breast cancer or ductal carcinoma in situ (National Comprehensive Cancer Network, n.d.).

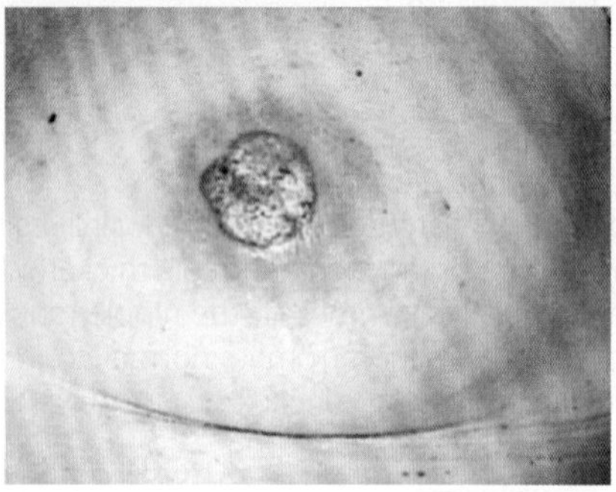

Edema

Ask, "Have you noticed any breast *edema* (swelling)?" If the answer is yes, ask:

- When does the edema occur?
- Where does it occur? Which breast? Which quadrant?
- How long does it last?
- Is it painful?
- What is the color of the breast?
- What else occurs with the edema?
- What do you do to relieve the swelling?

Rashes or Scaling

Ask, "Have you noticed any *rashes*? *Scaling*?" (Scaling consists of thin flakes of keratinized epithelium.) If the answer to either of these is yes, ask:

- When did this begin?
- Where did this begin?

- How long has it been going on?
- Besides the rash or scaling of the skin, what else is happening?
- Does it hurt?
- What do you do to relieve the rash or scaling?

Dimpling

Ask, "Have you noticed *dimpling* (small indents) of the breast tissue?" If the answer is yes, ask:

- When did this begin?
- In which breast did this begin?
- How long has it been going on? Is it constant?
- Are there any other symptoms occurring at this time?
- Do you associate anything with this?
- Are you treating this?

Retraction

Ask, "Have you ever had nipple *retraction*?" If the answer is yes, ask:

- When did the retraction occur?
- Which nipple is retracted?
- How long does it last? Does it evert at any time? When?
- What happens when the nipple retracts?
- Does anything else occur during the retraction?
- Do you do anything to protract the nipple?

CLINICAL TIP

Nipple retraction is when the nipple is pulled inward. This is not an issue if the breast has had an inverted nipple since birth; however, it is noteworthy if this is a change as it could be an indicator of breast cancer or adhesions below the skin surface (see Table 17-2).

Past History

Additional relevant questions to ask while taking the history include:

- What medications (hormone replacement therapy [HRT], oral contraceptives [OCs]) are you currently taking?
  - When did you begin taking the medication?
  - What is the medication name and dosage?
  - Are you having any side effects?
- What other medications have you taken in the past?
  - When did you take them?
  - For how long did you take them?
  - Why did you stop?
  - Were there any side effects?
- Have you ever been pregnant?
  - When?
  - How many live births? Abortions? Miscarriages?
  - How old were you when your first baby was delivered? Was the birth at full term?
  - Did you breast-feed your child(ren)? For how long?
- Menstrual history
  - How old were you at menarche (first menses)?
  - How old were you at menopause?
  - How many days in your cycle?
- Previous history of breast cancer and/or reproductive cancer (e.g., ovarian)
  - When did you have breast cancer and/or reproductive cancer?
  - In which breast did you have cancer or where was the reproductive cancer?
  - How did you find the cancer? Was there a lump?
  - How was it treated?
  - Who was on your health care team?
- Have you ever had a breast biopsy?
  - If yes, when? Where?
  - What were the results?
- Breast self-examination (BSE)
  - How often do you perform a BSE?
  - When do you perform BSEs?
  - What technique do you use?
  - Have you ever palpated a lump or found any changes?
- Clinical breast examination (CBE)
  - When was your last examination by a health care provider?
  - What were the results?

- **Mammogram** (x-ray of the breast) or magnetic resonance imaging (MRI)
  When was your last mammogram or MRI?
  What were the results?
  What testing site do you use?
  Has the site changed? Did you transfer previous mammograms or MRI results to this site?

Family History

Questions regarding family history include:

- Do you have a family history of breast cancer? Was any genetic information found or testing done?
- Do you have a family history of reproductive cancer?
- If yes, who in the family has had either type of cancer (e.g., sisters, mother, daughters, maternal aunts, maternal grandmother)?
- Have you had **BRCA gene** (breast cancer gene) testing done?

Lifestyle Habits

Ask about relevant lifestyle habits:

- How much alcohol do you drink each day/week?
- What do you do for physical activity?

PHYSICAL EXAMINATION

The Female Breast

When clinicians perform a CBE, it is advisable to adopt a standardized approach, especially for palpation, and to use a systemic up and down search pattern, varying palpation pressure, and a circular motion with the finger pads.

CLINICAL TIP
The most significant risk factors for breast cancer are age, BRCA status, and breast density on mammogram. Personal history of breast cancer, family history, and reproductive factors affecting duration of uninterrupted estrogen exposure are also important (Centers for Disease Control and Prevention [CDC], 2020). For additional risk factors, see the "Assessing the Risk of Breast Cancer" section.

As you begin the examination, adopt a courteous and gentle approach. Let the patient know that you are about to examine the breasts. This may be a good time to ask if the individual has noticed any lumps or other problems and to enhance any awareness of screening guidelines. Because breasts tend to swell and become more nodular before menses from increasing estrogen stimulation, the best time for examination is 5 to 7 days *after* the onset of menstruation. Nodules appearing prior to menstruation should be reevaluated at this later time. Adequate inspection initially requires full exposure of the chest, but later in the examination, drape one breast while you are palpating the other.

Inspection

Inspect the breasts and nipples with the patient in the sitting position, disrobed to the waist. A thorough examination of the breast includes careful inspection for skin changes, symmetry, contours, and retraction in four views—arms at the sides, arms over the head, arms pressed against the hips, and leaning forward. When examining an adolescent girl, assess her breast development according to the Tanner Sexual Maturity Ratings described in Chapter 23, "Assessing Children: Infancy Through Adolescence."

Arms at the Sides

Note the clinical features as follows.

- The appearance of the skin, including:
  - Color

Redness in a light complexion or deeper pigmentation in a dark skin woman may be from local infection or inflammatory carcinoma.

- Thickening of the skin and unusually prominent pores, which may accompany lymphatic obstruction

Thickening and prominent pores suggest breast cancer.

- The *size and symmetry of the breasts.* Some difference in the size of the breasts, including the areolae, is common and is usually normal, as shown in Figure 17-6.

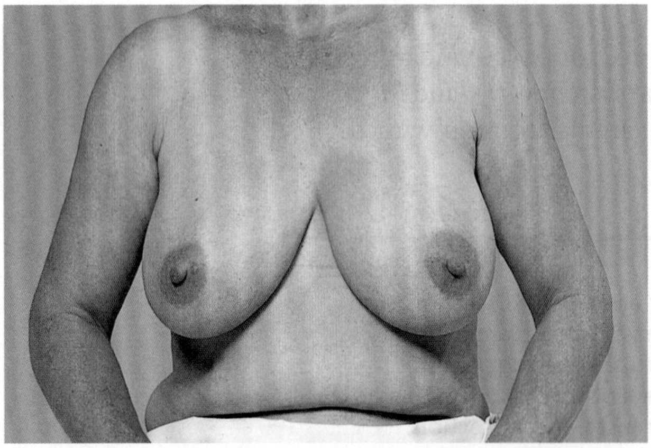

FIGURE 17-6 Some asymmetry between the sizes of the breasts and areolae is common.

- The *contour of the breasts.* Look for changes such as masses, dimpling, or flattening. Compare one side with the other.

Flattening of the normally convex breast suggests cancer. See Table 17-2, "Visible Signs of Breast Cancer."

- The *characteristics of the nipples*, including *size and shape*, *direction* in which they point, any *rashes or ulceration*, or any *discharge*.

Asymmetry of directions in which nipples point suggests an underlying cancer. Rashes or ulceration may indicate Paget disease of the breast (Lakhera et al., 2020) (see Table 17-2).

Occasionally, the shape of the nipple is *inverted*, or depressed below the areolar surface (Fig. 17-7). It may be enveloped by folds of areolar skin, as illustrated. Longstanding inversion is usually a normal variant of no clinical consequence, except for possible difficulty when breast-feeding.

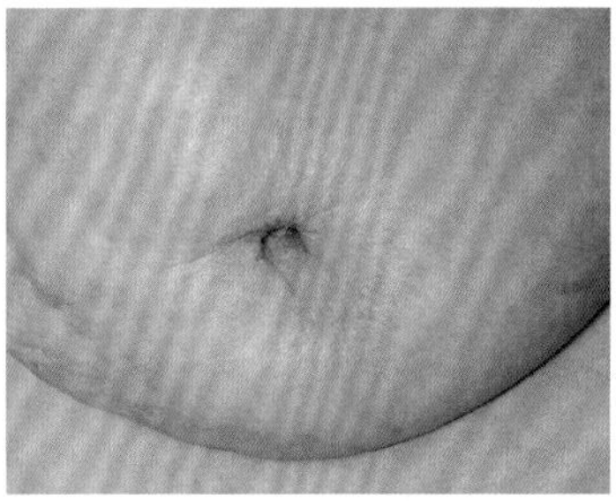

FIGURE 17-7 An inverted nipple.

Recent or fixed flattening or depression of the nipple suggests nipple retraction. A retracted nipple may also be broadened and thickened, suggesting an underlying cancer.

Arms over the Head; Hands Pressed against the Hips; Leaning Forward

To bring out dimpling or retraction that may otherwise be invisible, ask the patient to raise the arms over the head (Fig. 17-8), and then press the hands against the hips to contract the pectoral muscles (Fig. 17-9). Inspect the

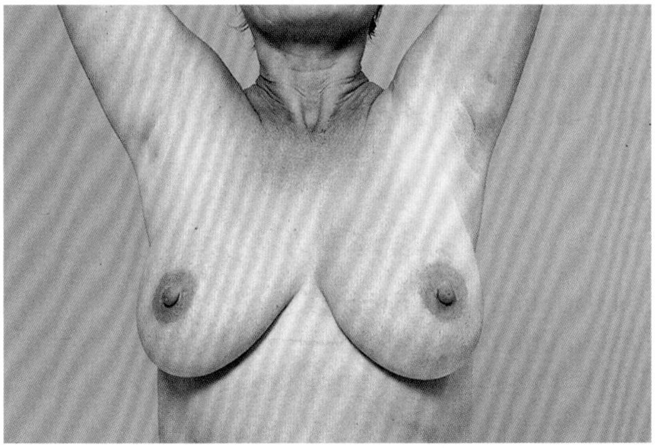

FIGURE 17-8 The arms over the head for breast inspection.

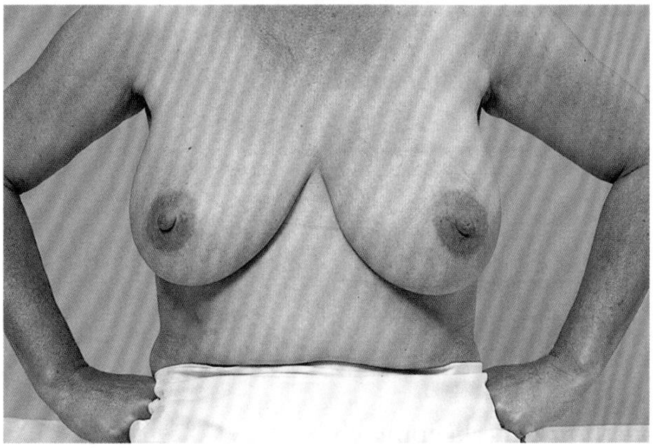

FIGURE 17-9 Hands pressed against the hips for breast inspection.

breast contours carefully in each position. If the breasts are large or pendulous, it may be useful to have the patient stand and lean forward, supported by the back of the chair (Fig. 17-10).

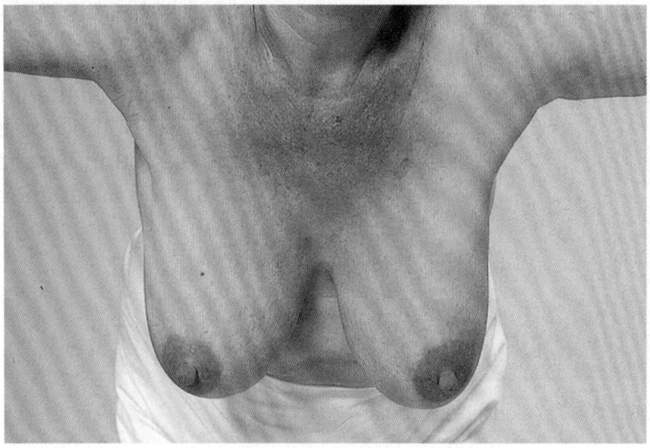

FIGURE 17-10 Leaning forward for breast inspection.

> **CLINICAL TIP**
> Dimpling or retraction of the breasts in these positions suggests an underlying cancer. When a cancer or its associated fibrous strands are attached to both the skin and the fascia overlying the pectoral muscles, pectoral contraction can draw the skin inward, causing dimpling.

Leaning forward may reveal an asymmetry of the breast or nipple not otherwise visible. Retraction of the nipple and areola suggests an underlying cancer (see Table 17-2).

Occasionally, these signs may be associated with benign lesions such as posttraumatic fat necrosis or mammary duct ectasia (distension of hollow tissue), but they must always be evaluated.

Palpation

Palpation is best performed when the breast tissue is flattened. The patient should be supine. Plan to palpate a rectangular area extending from the clavicle to the inframammary fold or lower bra line, and from the midsternal line to the posterior axillary line and well into the axilla for the tail of the breast.

A thorough examination will take time and focus.

> **CLINICAL TIP**
> When pressing deeply on the breast, you may mistake a normal rib for a hard breast mass.

Palpation should take place as follows:

- While lying supine, have the patient reach behind their head with their right hand when the right breast is examined. Placing the hand behind the head will displace the breast tissue for easier palpation.
- Use the finger pads of the second, third, and fourth fingers, keeping the fingers slightly flexed.

- The vertical stripe pattern is currently the best validated technique for detecting breast masses. It is important to be systematic.

- Palpate in small, dime-size, concentric circles at each examining point; if possible, apply light, medium, and deep pressure. You will need to press more firmly to reach the deeper tissues of a large breast.

- Continue in vertical overlapping strips until your examination covers the entire breast, including the periphery, tail, and axilla (Fig. 17-11).

- When you have completed all areas on the right breast, have the patient switch arms, placing the left hand behind the head to complete the assessment on the left side. Pay special attention to the upper outer quadrant and axilla, as 50% of breast lumps are found in the upper outer quadrant.

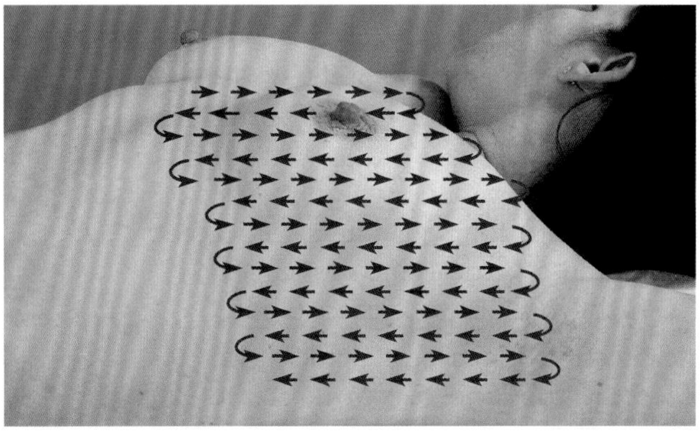

FIGURE 17-11 Palpation pattern for the clinical breast exam.

Examine the breast tissue carefully for:

- *Consistency* of the tissues. Normal consistency varies widely depending in part on the relative proportions of firmer glandular tissue and soft fat. Physiologic nodularity may be present, increasing before menses. There may be a firm transverse ridge of compressed tissue along the lower margin of the breast, especially in large breasts. This is the normal inframammary ridge, not a tumor.

A lump near a clogged nipple may suggest *mammary duct ectasia*, a benign but sometimes painful condition of dilated ducts with surrounding inflammation, sometimes with associated masses.

- *Tenderness.* This may be premenstrual fullness.

- *Nodules.* Palpate carefully for any lump or mass that is different from the rest of the breast tissue. This is sometimes called a dominant mass and may reflect a pathologic change that requires evaluation by mammogram, MRI, aspiration, or biopsy.

See Table 17-1, "Common Breast Masses."

Document the characteristics of any nodule:

- *Location*—which breast, the quadrant or clock site, centimeters from the nipple

- *Size*—in centimeters

- *Shape*—round or cystic, disc-like, or irregular in contour

- *Consistency*—soft, firm, or hard

- *Delineation*—well circumscribed or not

Hard, irregular, poorly circumscribed nodules, fixed to the skin or underlying tissues, strongly suggest breast cancer.

- *Tenderness*—tender or nontender

Cysts, inflamed areas, and some cancers may be tender.

- *Mobility*—assess in relation to the skin, pectoral fascia, and chest wall. Gently move the breast near the mass, and watch for dimpling

A mobile mass that becomes fixed when the arm relaxes is attached to the ribs and intercostal muscles; if fixed when the hand is pressed against the hip, it is attached to the pectoral fascia.

Next, try to move the mass itself while the patient relaxes the arm and then while pressing the hands into the hips.

If a lump is detected, documentation of the breast assessment is acceptable in either of two forms (Fig. 17-12):

1. Divide the breast into four quadrants with a horizontal line and a vertical line crossing at the nipple, which would be the center point.
2. Look at the breast as the face of a clock with 12 o'clock at the top, and 6 o'clock at the bottom.

If an area needs to be specifically identified (e.g., to determine the exact site of a lump), the distance in centimeters from the nipple in the respective quadrant is charted. The area that extends laterally across the exterior fold is called the tail of Spence.

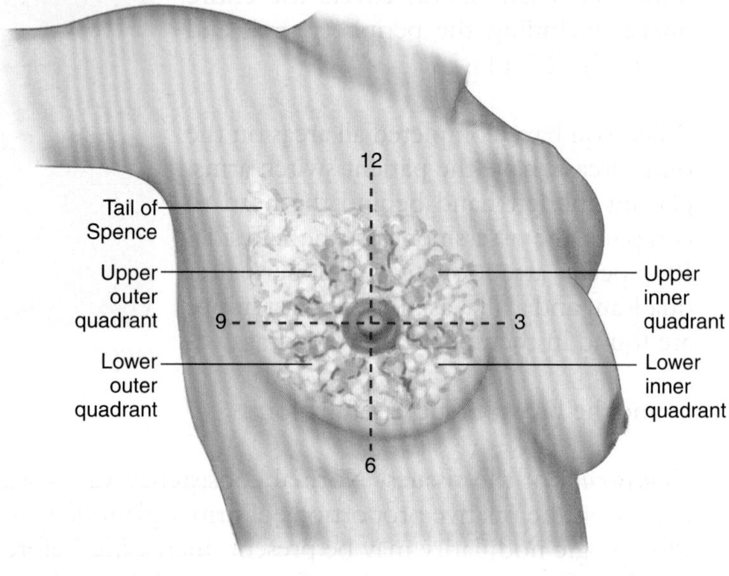

FIGURE 17-12 Document the location of a lump by either dividing the breast into quadrants or envisioning the face of a clock.

The Male Breast

Examination of the male breast may be brief, but it is important. *Inspect the nipple and areola* for nodules, swelling, or ulceration. *Palpate the areola and breast tissue* for nodules. If the breast appears enlarged, distinguish between the soft fatty enlargement of obesity and the firm disc of glandular enlargement caused by an imbalance of estrogen and testosterone, called **gynecomastia** (Fig. 17-13). This can occur in one or both breasts, and in newborns, adolescents, or older men due to changes in hormone levels. In addition, certain diseases or medications, including anabolic steroids for athletic enhancement, can contribute to the swollen breast tissue or tenderness. Gynecomastia usually resolves without treatment (Sansone et al., 2017; Yilmaz et al., 2018).

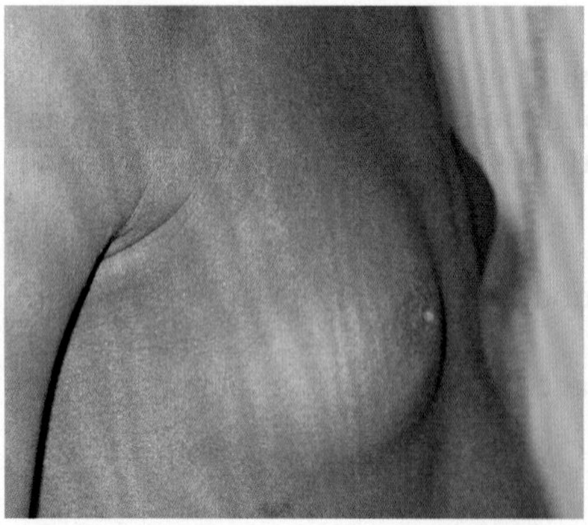

FIGURE 17-13 Gynecomastia.

CLINICAL TIP

A hard, irregular, eccentric, or ulcerating nodule suggests breast cancer. Male breast cancer constitutes only 1% of breast cancer cases (Katiyar et al., 2017; Yilmaz et al., 2018).

Breast cancer risk may increase for transgender men who are on testosterone (Susan, 2016).

The Axillae

Although the axillae may be examined with the patient lying down, a sitting position is preferable.

Inspection

Inspect the skin of each axilla, noting evidence of:

- Rash

Assess if rash is related to change in deodorant, lotions, or laundry detergent.

- Infection

The sweat glands may become infected (**hidradenitis suppurativa**).

- Nodules
- Unusual pigmentation

Deeply pigmented, velvety axillary skin suggests *acanthosis nigricans*; which has been associated with insulin resistance, hormonal disorders, and internal malignancy.

Palpation

To examine the left axilla, ask the patient to relax with the left arm down. Help by supporting the left wrist or hand with your left hand. Wearing a glove, cup together the fingers of your right hand and reach as high as you can toward the apex of the axilla (Fig. 17-14). Warn the patient that this may feel uncomfortable. Your fingers should lie directly behind the pectoral muscles, pointing toward the midclavicle. Now press your fingers in toward the chest wall and slide them downward, trying to feel the central lymph nodes against the chest wall. These nodes are often the most palpable of the axillary nodes. One or more soft, small (smaller than 1 cm), nontender nodes are frequently felt.

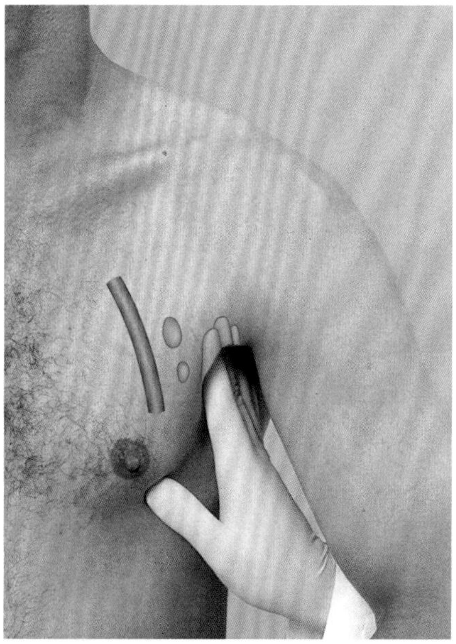

FIGURE 17-14 When palpating the axilla, reach as high as you can toward the apex.

Nodes that are large (1 cm or bigger) and firm or hard, matted together, or fixed to the skin or to underlying tissues suggest malignant involvement.

CLINICAL TIP
Enlarged axillary lymph nodes can occur from an infection of the hand or arm, recent immunizations or skin tests in the arm, or part of a generalized **lymphadenopathy** (an enlargement of one or more lymph nodes). Check the epitrochlear nodes and other groups of lymph nodes.

Use your gloved hand to examine the nodes of the axilla:

- *Central nodes*—Palpate in the base of the axilla. The central nodes receive lymph from the pectoral, lateral, and subscapular lymph nodes and drain into the apical lymph nodes. If the central nodes feel large, hard, or tender, or if there is a suspicious lesion in the drainage areas of the axillary nodes, palpate the other three groups of axillary lymph nodes.
- *Pectoral nodes*—Grasp the anterior axillary fold between your thumb and fingers; and with your fingers, palpate inside the border of the pectoral muscle (Fig. 17-15).
- *Lateral nodes*—From high in the axilla, feel along the upper humerus.
- *Subscapular nodes*—Step behind the patient, and with your fingers, feel inside the muscle of the posterior axillary fold (Fig. 17-16).

Also feel for infraclavicular nodes and reexamine the supraclavicular nodes.

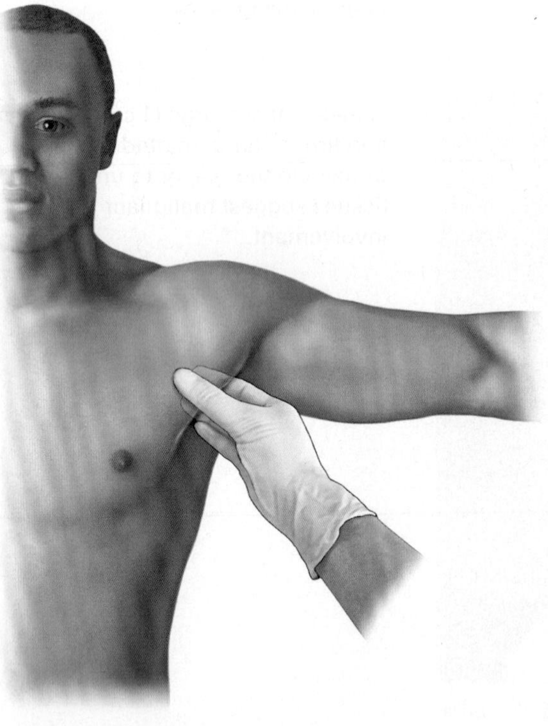

FIGURE 17-15 Palpating the pectoral nodes.

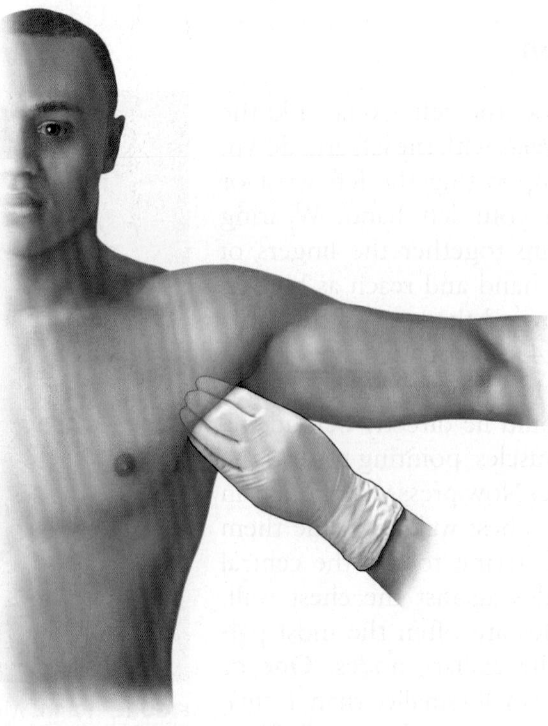

FIGURE 17-16 Palpating the subscapular nodes.

SPECIAL TECHNIQUES

Assessment of Nipple Discharge

If there is a history of spontaneous nipple discharge, try to determine its origin by compressing the areola with your index finger, placed in radial positions around the nipple (Fig. 17-17). Watch for discharge appearing through one of the duct openings on the nipple's surface. Note the color, consistency, and quantity of any discharge and the exact location where it appears. Discharge from the nipple is usually bilateral and the fluid is released when stimulated or compressed. The color alone is not indicative of the cause of the discharge.

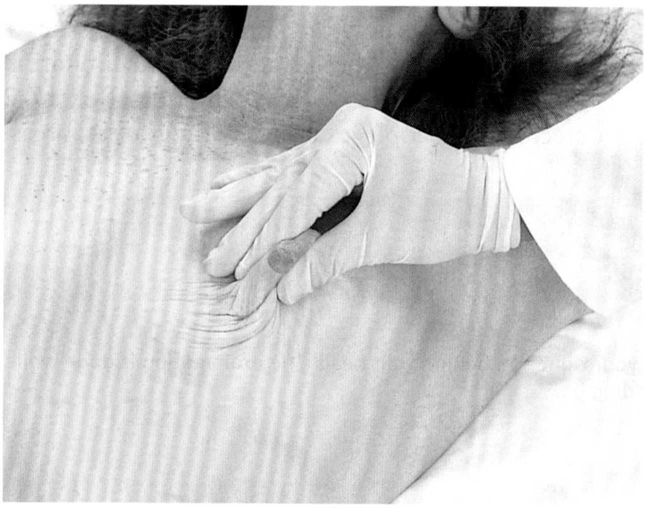

FIGURE 17-17 Compress the areola to assess nipple discharge.

CLINICAL TIP

Some findings include a milky discharge unrelated to a prior pregnancy and lactation, known as *nonpuerperal galactorrhea*. Causes include *hypothyroidism*, pituitary *prolactinoma*, and drugs that are dopamine agonists, including many psychotropic agents and phenothiazines.

Spontaneous unilateral bloody discharge from one or two ducts warrants further evaluation for intraductal *papilloma*, as shown in Figure 17-17; ductal carcinoma in situ (DCIS); or Paget disease of the breast (Sansone et al., 2017).

Examination of the Mastectomy or Breast Augmentation Patient

The woman with a mastectomy warrants special care on examination. Inspect the mastectomy scar and axilla carefully for any masses or unusual nodularity. Note any change in color or signs of inflammation. Lymphedema may be present in the axilla and upper arm from impaired lymph drainage after surgery. Palpate gently along the scar—these tissues may be more sensitive. Use a circular motion with two or three fingers. Note any enlargement of the lymph nodes or signs of inflammation or infection.

CLINICAL TIP

Masses, nodularity, and change in color or inflammation, especially in the incision line, suggest recurrence of breast cancer.

It is especially important to carefully palpate the breast tissue and incision lines or edges of the implant of women with breast augmentation or reconstruction.

Self-Awareness and Instructions for the Breast Self-Examination

Self-awareness and individual care is important for any part of the body. If a patient wants more information on how to monitor breast tissue and chooses to perform BSE after reviewing the advantages and limitations, the nurse should take the opportunity to teach this technique (Box 17-2). Breast masses can be detected by people examining their own breasts.

BOX 17-2 BREAST AWARENESS AND SELF-EXAMINATION INSTRUCTIONS

Lying Supine

- Lie down and place your right arm behind your head. The examination is done while lying down, not standing up.

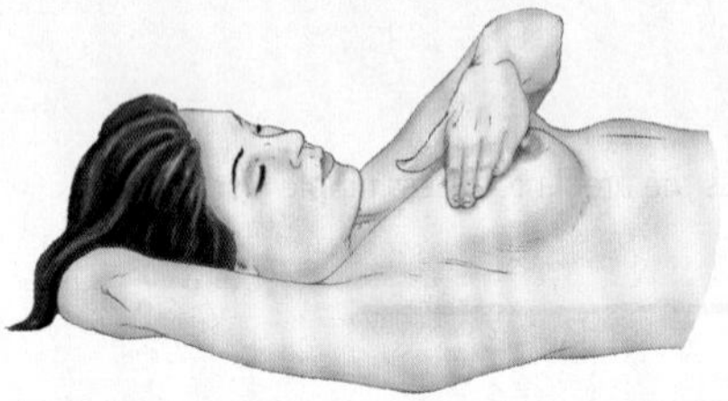

- Use the finger pads of the three middle fingers on your left hand to feel for lumps in the right breast. Use overlapping dime-sized circular motions of the finger pads to feel the breast tissue.

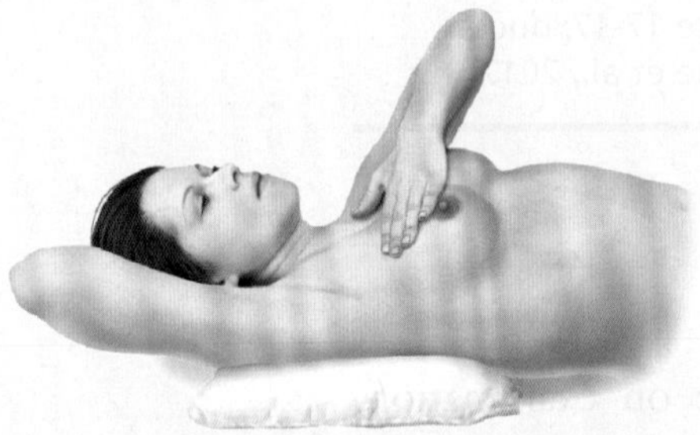

- Use three different levels of pressure to feel all the breast tissue. Light pressure is needed to feel the tissue closest to the skin; medium pressure to feel a little deeper; and firm pressure to feel the tissue closest to the chest and ribs. If you are not sure how hard to press, talk with your health care provider.
- Move in an up and down pattern. Be sure to check the entire breast.

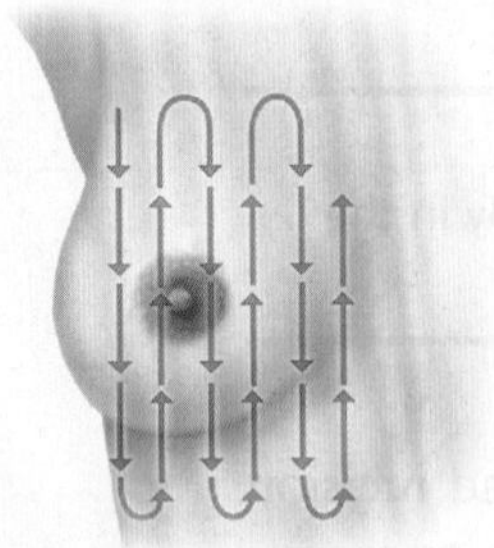

BOX 17-2 **BREAST AWARENESS AND SELF-EXAMINATION INSTRUCTIONS (*Continued*)**

- Repeat the examination on your left breast, putting your left arm behind your head and using the finger pads of your right hand to do the examination.

Standing

- Stand in front of a mirror with your hands pressing firmly on your hips. Look for any changes of size, shape, contour, dimpling, redness, or scaliness of the nipple or breast skin.

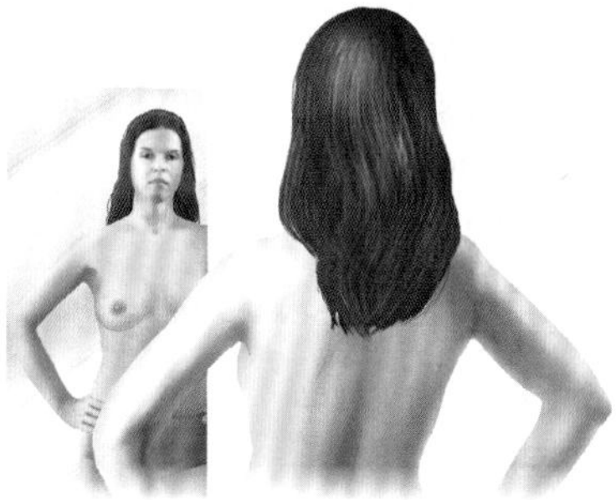

- Examine each underarm while sitting up or standing and with your arm only slightly raised so you can easily feel in this area.

Although BSE has not been shown to reduce breast cancer mortality, BSE is inexpensive and may promote stronger health awareness and more active self-care. For early detection of breast cancer, the BSE is an option that is most useful when coupled with regular breast examination by an experienced clinician and mammography or MRI. The BSE is an individual choice as research has shown that many lumps are randomly found though not during a monthly self-examination. If an individual chooses to practice BSE, it is best timed 5 to 7 days after the start of menses, when hormonal stimulation and breast tenderness is lower.

RECORDING YOUR FINDINGS

Box 17-3 illustrates examples of documentation of breast and axilla.

BOX 17-3 **RECORDING THE PHYSICAL EXAMINATION—BREASTS AND AXILLAE**

"Breasts symmetric, color tan without pigment changes and smooth bilaterally; no masses, dimpling, lumps, edema, thickening, rashes, or ulcerations; nipples everted, equal in size, point outward; no discharge, no axillary adenopathy detected."

OR

"Breasts pendulous with diffuse fibrocystic changes. Single firm 1 × 1 cm mass, mobile and nontender, with overlying *peau d'orange* (orange peel/thick and pitting) appearance in right breast, upper outer quadrant at 11 o'clock, 2 cm from the nipple, nipples everted, no discharge, no axillary adenopathy."

The second part of the recording suggests possible breast cancer.

HEALTH PROMOTION AND COUNSELING

Important topics for health promotion and counseling regarding the breast and axilla include:

- Palpable masses of the breast
- Assessing risk of breast cancer
- Breast cancer screening

Women may experience a wide range of changes in breast tissue and sensation, from cyclic swelling and nodularity to a distinct lump or mass. The examination of the breast provides a meaningful opportunity for the nurse to explore what to do if a lump or mass is detected, risk factors for breast cancer, and screening measures such as breast self-awareness, CBEs, mammography, and MRIs. Men can also be diagnosed with breast cancer. If any noted changes or lumps are detected, men should also see their health care providers. Inclusive care and attention of the breast for transgender patients are also crucial to promote.

Trans women have a high prevalence of dense breasts.

Palpable Masses of the Breast and Breast Symptoms

Invasive breast cancer occurs in approximately one in eight women (13%), and one in 39 women (3%) will die from breast cancer (American Cancer Society [ACS], 2019). Breast masses show marked variation in etiology, from fibroadenomas and cysts seen in younger patients to abscess or **mastitis** (inflammation of breast tissue) to primary breast cancer. On initial assessment, the individual's age and physical characteristics of the mass provide clues about its etiology. All breast masses require careful assessment. Nurses are patient advocates and help navigate the complex health care system. Nurses assist patients with following up on all breast irregularities for accurate diagnosis and treatment.

Assessing the Risk of Breast Cancer

Patients who have breasts are increasingly interested in information about breast cancer. Nurses and the health care team should be familiar with the literature detailing the epidemiology of and risk factors for breast cancer that supports recommendations for screening. Key facts and figures are presented here, but further reading will enhance counseling of patients.

Breast cancer continues to be the leading cancer diagnosis among women today with the exception of skin cancer (CDC, 2020). Early detection has increased recently. When diagnosed with breast cancer, 64% of patients have detected the breast cancer early and disease is localized; 27% have regional disease; and 6% have distant or metastatic disease (ACS, 2019). In recent years, ductal cancer has decreased 2.1% per year, and invasive cancer has risen 0.3% per year (ACS, 2019). The increase of invasive cancer is considered to be in part due to increasing body mass index (BMI) and decreased number of births, both of which are risk factors for breast cancer (Pfeiffer et al., 2018).

Non-Hispanic White women are more likely to be diagnosed with breast cancer than non-Hispanic Black women (ACS, 2019). However, death from breast cancer in non-Hispanic Black women surpasses all other racial/ethnic groups in breast cancer death rates. American Indian/Alaska Native and Hispanic women are the next lowest group. Asian/Pacific Islander women have both the lowest incidence and lowest death rate from breast cancer (ACS, 2019).

Health disparities are evident in the mortality rates associated with breast cancer. Factors that may contribute to these disparities include later diagnosis, decreased access to care and mammograms, longer intervals between mammograms, presence of comorbidities, and decreased follow-up with care providers. In addition, data also suggest that the tumors may be more aggressive in Black women (ACS, 2019). Nurses and the health care team should advocate for access to care, educate marginalized populations on the importance of screening mammograms, and give prompt attention and follow-up to any breast changes or lumps.

Men are more likely to be diagnosed with late-stage breast cancer (51%) than women (36%). This is likely due to later detection resulting from decreased awareness (ACS, 2019).

Both *modifiable* and *nonmodifiable risk factors* contribute to breast cancer. Many risk factors cannot be readily altered (nonmodifiable), such as gender, age, family history, race, genetics, personal history of breast cancer, age at first full-term pregnancy, early menarche, late menopause, and breast density (ACS, 2019). Others can be modified, though these tend to confer lower relative risk: postmenopausal obesity, use of estrogen-progesterone combination HRT, alcohol use, and physical inactivity. Not having children or having them later in life also puts individuals at a higher risk for breast cancer.

Health risks for breast cancer in transgender individuals are a concern, and finding a health care provider who is responsive is important. Ensuring early detection and timely care is a priority as many trans patients may have less access to providers and therefore may be diagnosed later. Assessing the individual risks and necessary screening tools is instrumental based on the needs of each person.

Selected Risk Factors that Affect Screening Decisions

BRCA1 and 2 Mutations

Begin evaluating a woman's risk for breast cancer as early as her 20s. Women of all ages should be asked if there is a family history of breast, ovarian, tubal, or peritoneal cancer on either the maternal or paternal side. Approximately 5% to 10% of women have genetic risk of BRCA1 or BRCA2 gene mutation (ACS, 2019). These genes are autosomal-dominant. The U.S. Preventative Services Task Force (USPSTF) recommends screening women to determine if there is a high risk of a mutation of BRCA1 or BRCA2 gene. The screening should be considered for women with positive family histories and at least a 5% to 10% chance of a gene mutation. Those with positive results from the screening should receive genetic counseling. BRCA testing should not be done routinely but instead based on the presence of risk factors. There are models available to determine risk. Each of these identifies different areas and may have variable results. The Gail model focuses primarily on nonfamilial risk factors while the Claus model highlights familial risk factors (Alvarado et al., 2016; Wang et al., 2018). The Tyrer-Cuzick model takes into account family history, length of time of estrogen exposure, and atypical hyperplasia which addresses issues of other models. Research using the Tyrer-Cuzick model also takes into consideration mammography breast density to increase the prediction of those at risk for breast cancer (Kurian et al., 2020; Rainey et al., 2020).

Benign Breast Conditions

Mammograms result in an increased number of breast biopsies, and clinicians should understand the effects of benign breast disease on risk for later breast cancer. Breast lesions are believed to evolve in somewhat linear fashion. This occurs in ductal hyperplasia, unfolded lobules, atypical hyperplasia, the pathologic stages of DCIS, and invasive cancer. These disorders are classified by degree of cellular proliferation on biopsy and degree of risk for breast cancer (Table 17-3). Women with atypia are more likely to have strong family history of breast cancer. Their risk increases when atypia is diagnosed at younger ages.

TABLE 17-3 Categories of Benign Breast Lesions

Nonproliferative changes
No increased risk
Changes include: Overgrowth of breast tissue, cysts (fibrocystic changes), fibrosis, mild hyperplasia
Proliferative without atypia
Small increased risk
Changes include: Ductal hyperplasia, fibroadenoma
Proliferative with atypia
Moderate increased risk
Changes include: Atypical ductal hyperplasia, atypical lobular hyperplasia

Source: Dyrstad, S. W., Yan, Y., Fowler, A. M., & Colditz, G. A. (2015). Breast cancer risk associated with benign breast disease: Systematic review and meta-analysis. *Breast Cancer Research and Treatment*, *149*(3), 569–575. https://doi.org/10.1007/s10549-014-3254-6

Breast Density

Mammographic breast density is a strong independent risk factor even after adjusting for the effects of other risk factors (Kiyang et al., 2015). Stromal and epithelial tissues appear radiologically light and dense, reflecting higher proportions of stromal and glandular tissue and increased ductal and atypical ductal hyperplasia. A proposed mechanism is proliferation of breast epithelial cells and stromal fibrosis in response to growth factors induced by circulating sex hormones.

An analysis of studies quantifying breast density found that women with radiologic density in more than 60% to 75% of the breast are at four to six times greater risk of breast cancer than women with lower breast density (Ripping et al., 2016). Breast density may account for up to 30% of the risk for breast cancer and has a strong inherited component (ACS, 2019).

Breast density affects the sensitivity and specificity of mammograms, dropping from 88% and 96% in women with predominantly fatty breast tissue to 62% and 89% in women with breasts that are extremely dense, respectively (Ripping et al., 2016). With approximately 36% of women 40 to 74 years of age having dense breasts and 7% with extremely dense breasts, the Food and Drug Administration (FDA) has proposed that mammograms should report breast density. There are no current guidelines about referring women with dense breasts for additional ultrasounds or MRIs (ACS, 2019).

Recommendations for Breast Cancer Screening and Chemoprevention

Mammography

Mammography is the most common screening modality, but recommendations from professional groups vary about when to start screening and intervals. The ACS supports screening mammograms for women between ages 40 and 44 if they choose to begin or have risk factors. For women aged 45 to 54, yearly mammograms are recommended, and at 55 and older mammograms are recommended every 2 years unless personal reasons indicate yearly screening. Mammograms continue every other year until the individual is no longer in good health or will not live beyond 10 years (ACS, 2019). The USPSTF suggests women aged 40 to 49 choose if they want a mammogram and recommend mammograms biennially for those aged 50 to 74. The USPSTF does not support women over 75 getting mammograms based on inadequate evidence. The use of CBE for people without symptoms or family histories of breast cancer have been shown to have low yield rates for detecting breast cancer. Neither CBEs nor BSEs are endorsed by any of the aforementioned organizations, though breast self-awareness is warranted if changes are noted. The World Health Organization does recommend CBE in low-resource settings only (National Comprehensive Cancer Network, n.d.; Oeffinger et al., 2015; Qaseem et al., 2019).

The evidence and rationale for decisions about age to begin screening bears thoughtful review of the balance of benefits and risks. For mammography, experts commonly raise concerns about *overdiagnosis*, defined as detection of lesions on mammogram that would not otherwise be detected and are not pathologic during a woman's lifetime (Løberg et al., 2015). Changes in the recommended guidelines underscore the need for clinicians to be well informed as they counsel individual patients, particularly as more evidence emerges to guide risk-based screening (ACS, 2019).

Digital Breast Tomosynthesis

Digital breast tomosynthesis is an imaging modality that uses 2D images to create a 3D image of the breast. This modality has been approved by the FDA for screening, though it is currently unavailable in many areas. Additionally, many insurance plans do not currently cover this type of screening.

Magnetic Resonance Imaging

Studies have investigated the use of screening MRI in people with a high risk for breast cancer of greater than 20% based on the risk assessment tools available (Gail, Claus, or Tyrer-Cuzick models); presence of a BRCA1 or BRCA2 gene mutation or a first-degree relative with a gene mutation; and having had chest radiation between the ages of 10 and 30 years. In these groups, breast MRI has helped improve detection of multicentric or contralateral breast cancer prior to management decisions about breast-conserving strategies or initiation of treatment regimens (ACS, 2019). However, cost is high, and specificity is 77%, resulting in more false positives, recalls, and biopsies (Saslow et al., 2007). Expertise in reading MRIs and MRI-guided biopsy is an important component for accuracy. Currently, the ACS recommends breast MRI for people at a high lifetime risk, or a risk of 20% or more (ACS, 2019). Women at moderately increased lifetime risk, or a risk of 15% to 20%, are encouraged to discuss benefits and drawbacks with their providers. MRI should not be done in isolation but rather in conjunction with a mammogram. Each test may pick up cancers that the other could miss.

Chemoprevention

The USPSTF recommends discussion of chemoprevention with estrogen-receptor modulators in people at high risk for breast cancer and at low risk for adverse effects, but it recommends against routine use for primary prevention in people at low or average risk. The USPSTF found substantial evidence that these modulators reduce the incidence of estrogen-receptor–positive breast cancer (Nelson et al., 2019). Clinicians are urged to review the literature on risks and benefits of these agents for people at high risk for developing breast cancer within 5 years.

Counseling about Breast Cancer

The Challenges of Communicating Risks and Benefits

As breast cancer screening and prevention options become more complex, nurses should consider how best to express statistics on risks and benefits in terms that patients can easily understand. Framing, or the effect of presenting the same information in terms of either increased benefit or decreased harm, is one of several ways of presenting data that can compromise informed consent. Nurse navigators can assist patients and families as they figure out the best options for them. The nurse can answer questions and coordinate the plan of care in consultation with the patient, family, and health care team.

Websites for Breast Cancer Information

Encourage patients to pursue breast cancer-related information from recommended reputable sources to help make informed choices during shared decision making. Box 17-4 lists some credible resources.

BOX 17-4 BREAST CANCER WEBSITES

Calculation of the risk of a breast cancer diagnosis and death at the level of individual women:

http://bcra.nci.nih.gov/brc/start.htm (Gail model)
https://www.cancer.gov/types/breast

Randomized Clinical Trials of New Modalities in Breast Cancer Screening:
http://www.clinicaltrials.gov

Support:
http://www.cancer.org/Treatment/SupportProgramsServices/

Susan G. Komen: www.komen.org

The Mautner Project of Whitman-Walker Health:
https://www.whitman-walker.org/care-program/cancer-navigation

National LGBT Cancer Network: www.cancer-network.org

Kelly Rooney Foundation: https://www.breastcancer.org/about_us/donate/rooney

BIBLIOGRAPHY

CITATIONS

Alvarado, M., Tiller, G., Kershberg, H., Solomon, S., Mullineaux, L., & Haque, R. (2016). Women without significant Claus model breast cancer risks may warrant breast MRI when pathogenic/likely-pathogenic variant (PV/LPV) is detected in a hereditary cancer moderate risk gene. *Cancer Research*. https://doi.org/10.1158/1538-7445.SABCS15-P2-09-26

American Cancer Society (ACS). (2019). Breast cancer facts & figures 2019–2020 [Ebook]. Retrieved October 3, 2020, from https://www.cancer.org/content/dam/cancer-org/research/cancer-facts-and-statistics/breast-cancer-facts-and-figures/breast-cancer-facts-and-figures-2019-2020.pdf

Centers for Disease Control and Prevention (CDC). (2020). What is breast cancer screening? Retrieved September 27, 2020, from https://www.cdc.gov/cancer/breast/basic_info/screening.htm

Dyrstad, S. W., Yan, Y., Fowler, A. M., & Colditz, G. A. (2015). Breast cancer risk associated with benign breast disease: Systematic review and meta-analysis. *Breast Cancer Research and Treatment, 149*(3), 569–575. https://doi.org/10.1007/s10549-014-3254-6

Harris, J. R., Morrow, M. M., Lippman, M. E., & Osborne, C. K. (2014). *Diseases of the breast* (5th ed.). Wolters Kluwer.

Katiyar, R., Patne, S. C., Kumar, S., & Khanna, R. (2017). Invasive papillary carcinoma of the male breast misdiagnosed as fibroadenoma on FNAB. *Journal of Clinical and Diagnostic Research: JCDR, 11*(2), ED06–ED07. https://doi.org/10.7860/JCDR/2017/24832.9211

Kiyang, L. N., Labrecque, M., Doualla-Bell, F., Turcotte, S., Farley, C., Cionti Bas, M., Blais, J., & Légaré, F. (2015). Family physicians' intention to support women in making informed decisions about breast cancer screening with mammography: A cross-sectional survey. *BMC Research Notes*, *8*, 663. https://doi.org/10.1186/s13104-015-1608-8

Kurian, A., Hughes, E., Bernhisel, R., Probst, B., Lanchbury, J., & Wagner, S. (2020). Performance of the IBIS/Tyrer-Cuzick (TC) model by race/ethnicity in the Women's Health Initiative. *Journal of Clinical Oncology*, *38*(15 suppl), 1503–1503. https://doi.org/10.1200/jco.2020.38.15_suppl.1503

Lakhera, K. K., Patni, S., Patni, N., & Jindal, R. (2020). Practical approach to extensive cutaneous spread without any underlying malignancy: A rare presentation of Paget's disease of breast. *BMJ Case Reports*, *13*(4), e233600. https://doi.org/10.1136/bcr-2019-233600

Løberg, M., Lousdal, M. L., Bretthauer, M., & Kalager, M. (2015). Benefits and harms of mammography screening. *Breast Cancer Research: BCR*, *17*(1), 63. https://doi.org/10.1186/s13058-015-0525-z

National Comprehensive Cancer Network. (n.d.). *Clinical practice guidelines in oncology. Breast cancer screening and diagnosis. National Comprehensive Cancer Network diagnosis.* Retrieved September 27, 2020, from https://www.nccn.org/professionals/physician_gls/pdf/breast-screening.pdf

Nelson, H. D., Fu, R., Zakher, B., Pappas, M., & McDonagh, M. (2019). Medication use for the risk reduction of primary breast cancer in women: Updated evidence report and systematic review for the US Preventive Services Task Force. *JAMA*, *322*(9), 868–886. https://doi.org/10.1001/jama.2019.5780

Oeffinger, K. C., Fontham, E. T., Etzioni, R., Herzig, A., Michaelson, J. S., Shih, Y. C., Walter, L. C., Church, T. R., Flowers, C. R., LaMonte, S. J., Wolf, A. M., DeSantis, C., Lortet-Tieulent, J., Andrews, K., Manassaram-Baptiste, D., Saslow, D., Smith, R. A., Brawley, O. W., Wender, R., & American Cancer Society. (2015). Breast cancer screening for women at average risk: 2015 guideline update from the American Cancer Society. *JAMA*, *314*(15), 1599–1614. https://doi.org/10.1001/jama.2015.12783

Pfeiffer, R. M., Webb-Vargas, Y., Wheeler, W., & Gail, M. H. (2018). Proportion of U.S. trends in breast cancer incidence attributable to long-term changes in risk factor distributions. *Cancer Epidemiology, Biomarkers & Prevention*, *27*(10), 1214–1222. https://doi.org/10.1158/1055-9965.EPI-18-0098

Qaseem, A., Lin, J. S., Mustafa, R. A., Horwitch, C. A., Wilt, T. J., & Clinical Guidelines Committee of the American College of Physicians. (2019). Screening for breast cancer in average-risk women: A guidance statement from the American College of Physicians. *Annals of Internal Medicine*, *170*(8), 547–560. https://doi.org/10.7326/M18-2147

Rainey, L., Eriksson, M., Trinh, T., Czene, K., Broeders, M., van der Waal, D., & Hall, P. (2020). The impact of alcohol consumption and physical activity on breast cancer: The role of breast cancer risk. *International Journal of Cancer*, *147*(4), 931–939. https://doi.org/10.1002/ijc.32846

Ripping, T. M., Hubbard, R. A., Otten, J. D., den Heeten, G. J., Verbeek, A. L., & Broeders, M. J. (2016). Towards personalized screening: Cumulative risk of breast cancer screening outcomes in women with and without a first-degree relative with a history of breast cancer. *International Journal of Cancer*, *138*(7), 1619–1625. https://doi.org/10.1002/ijc.29912

Sansone, A., Romanelli, F., Sansone, M., Lenzi, A., & Di Luigi, L. (2017). Gynecomastia and hormones. *Endocrine*, *55*(1), 37–44. https://doi.org/10.1007/s12020-016-0975-9

Saslow, D., Boetes, C., Burke, W., Harms, S., Leach, M. O., Lehman, C. D., Morris, E., Pisano, E., Schnall, M., Sener, S., Smith, R. A., Warner, E., Yaffe, M., Andrews, K. S., Russell, C. A., & American Cancer Society Breast Cancer Advisory Group. (2007). American Cancer Society guidelines for breast screening with MRI as an adjunct to mammography. *CA: A Cancer Journal for Clinicians*, *57*(2), 75–89. https://doi.org/10.3322/canjclin.57.2.75

Susan G. Komen Puget Sound. (2016). Breast *h*ealth *t*oolkit for the LGBTQ *c*ommunity [Ebook]. Retrieved October 1, 2020, from https://komenpugetsound.org/wp-content/uploads/2018/04/LGBTQ-Breast-Health-Toolkit-final.pdf

Wang, X., Huang, Y., Li, L., Dai, H., Song, F., & Chen, K. (2018). Assessment of performance of the Gail model for predicting breast cancer risk: A systematic review and meta-analysis with trial sequential analysis. *Breast Cancer Research: BCR*, *20*(1), 18. https://doi.org/10.1186/s13058-018-0947-5

Yilmaz, R., Cömert, R. G., Aliyev, S., Toktaş, Y., Önder, S., Emirikçi, S., & Özmen, V. (2018). Encapsulated papillary carcinoma in a man with gynecomastia: Ultrasonography, mammography and magnetic resonance imaging features with pathologic correlation. *European Journal of Breast Health*, *14*(2), 127–131. https://doi.org/10.5152/ejbh.2018.3761

18 THE MUSCULOSKELETAL SYSTEM

KEY TERMS

abduction
active range of motion
adduction
arthralgias
circumduction
condyles
crepitus
effusion
extension
fibrosis
flexion
hemiparesis
hemiplegia
muscle tone
myalgias
paraplegia
paresis
passive range of motion
plegia
quadriplegia
range of motion
rotation
shoulder girdle
synovium

Learning Objectives

The student will:

1. Describe the structure and functions of the bones, muscles, and joints.
2. Identify the key landmarks of each joint.
3. Obtain a history of the musculoskeletal system.
4. Identify the equipment necessary to perform a musculoskeletal examination.
5. Assess muscle strength using the muscle strength grading scale.
6. Inspect and palpate the joints, bones, and muscles.
7. Assess the range of motion of the major joints.
8. Document the findings of the musculoskeletal assessment.
9. Discuss risk reduction and health promotion strategies to reduce musculoskeletal injuries and disease.
10. Discuss risk factors for falls.
11. Discuss risk factors for osteoporosis.

ASSESSING THE MUSCULOSKELETAL SYSTEM

Musculoskeletal complaints and disorders are leading causes of health care visits in clinical practice. Since the musculoskeletal system is innervated by the neurologic system, examinations of the two systems are closely aligned. Indeed, these systems may be examined at the same time. Careful questioning during the history and acute observations will help the nurse distinguish the cause of the patient's symptoms.

Because of the nature of the musculoskeletal assessment, the organization of this chapter is different from the other body system chapters. Examination of joints requires both visualization and knowledge of surface landmarks and underlying anatomy. Therefore, to help students pair their knowledge of joint structure and function with methods of examination, the anatomy and physiology and physical examination for specific joints are combined.

Joint Structure and Function

Begin by reviewing basic anatomic terminology related to the joints.

- *Articular structures* include the joint capsule and articular cartilage, the **synovium** (a membrane in the joint that produces fluid to lubricate the joint and supply nutrients to the cartilage) and synovial fluid, intra-articular ligaments, and juxta-articular bone.

Articular disease typically involves swelling and tenderness of the entire joint and limits both active and **passive range of motion**, the full movement potential of a joint, usually its range of flexion and extension.

- *Extra-articular structures* include periarticular ligaments, tendons, bursae, muscle, fascia, bone, nerve, and overlying skin.
- *Ligaments* are rope-like bundles of collagen fibrils that connect bone to bone.
- *Tendons* are collagen fibers connecting muscle to bone.
- *Cartilage,* another form of collagen, overlies the articular surfaces of the bone ends and facilitates smooth painless movement of the joint.
- *Bursae* are pouches of synovial fluid that cushion the movement of tendons and muscles over bone or other joint structures.

Types of Joint Articulation

There are three types of joint articulation—synovial, cartilaginous, and fibrous—allowing varying degrees of joint movement (Table 18-1).

TABLE 18-1 Joints

Type of Joint	Extent of Movement	Example
Synovial	Freely movable	Knee, shoulder
Cartilaginous	Slightly movable	Vertebral bodies of the spine
Fibrous	Immovable	Skull sutures

Synovial Joints

The bones of synovial joints (Fig. 18-1) do not touch each other, and the joint articulations are *freely movable*. The bone ends are covered by *articular cartilage* and separated by a *synovial cavity* that cushions joint movement. The *synovial membrane* lines the synovial cavity and secretes a small amount of viscous lubricating fluid—the *synovial fluid*. The membrane is attached at the margins of the articular cartilage and pouched to allow joint movement. Surrounding the synovial membrane is a fibrous *joint capsule*, which is strengthened by ligaments extending from bone to bone.

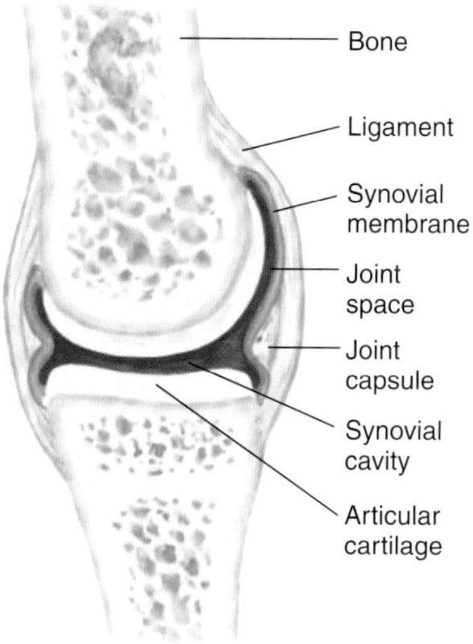

FIGURE 18-1 A synovial joint.

Cartilaginous Joints

Cartilaginous joints (Fig. 18-2), such as those between vertebrae and the symphysis pubis, are *slightly movable*. Fibrocartilaginous discs separate the bony surfaces. At the center of each disc is the *nucleus pulposus*, fibrocartilaginous material that serves as a cushion or shock absorber between bony surfaces.

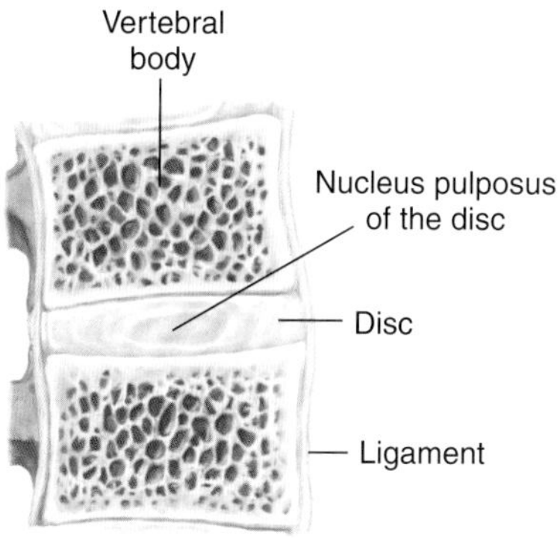

FIGURE 18-2 A cartilaginous joint.

Fibrous Joints

In fibrous joints (Fig. 18-3), such as the sutures of the skull, intervening layers of fibrous tissue or cartilage hold the bones together. The bones are almost in direct contact, which allows *no appreciable movement*.

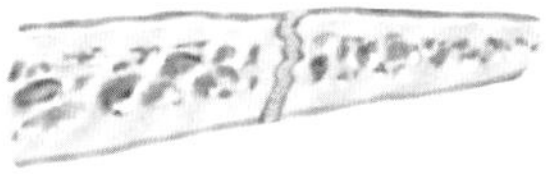

FIGURE 18-3 A fibrous joint.

Structure of Synovial Joints

Many of the joints examined are *synovial*, or movable, *joints*. The shape of the articulating surfaces of synovial joints determines the direction and extent of joint motion (Table 18-2).

TABLE 18-2 Synovial Joints

Type of Joint	Articular Shape	Movement	Example
Spheroidal (ball-and-socket)	Convex surface in concave cavity	Wide-ranging flexion, extension, abduction, adduction, rotation, circumduction	Shoulder, hip
Hinge	Flat, planar	Motion in one plane; flexion, extension	Interphalangeal joints of hand and foot; elbow
Condylar	Convex or concave articulating surfaces	Movement of two articulating surfaces	Knee; temporo-mandibular joint

- *Spheroidal joints* (Fig. 18-4) have a ball-and-socket configuration—a rounded, convex surface articulating with a cup-like cavity, allowing a wide range of rotatory movement, as in the shoulder and hip.

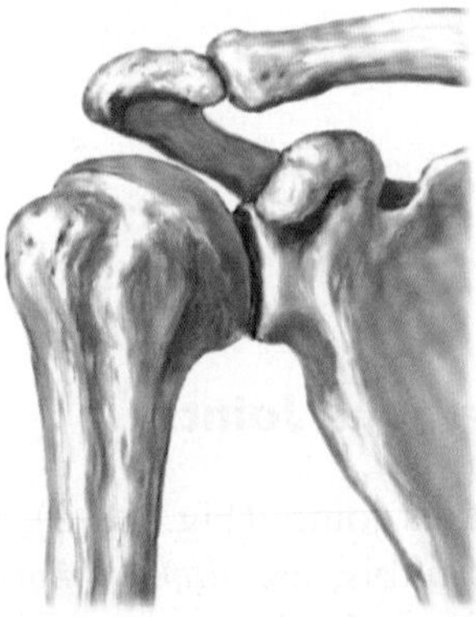

FIGURE 18-4 A spheroidal (ball-and-socket) joint.

- *Hinge joints* (Fig. 18-5) are flat, planar, or slightly curved, allowing only a gliding motion in a single plane, as in flexion and extension of the digits.

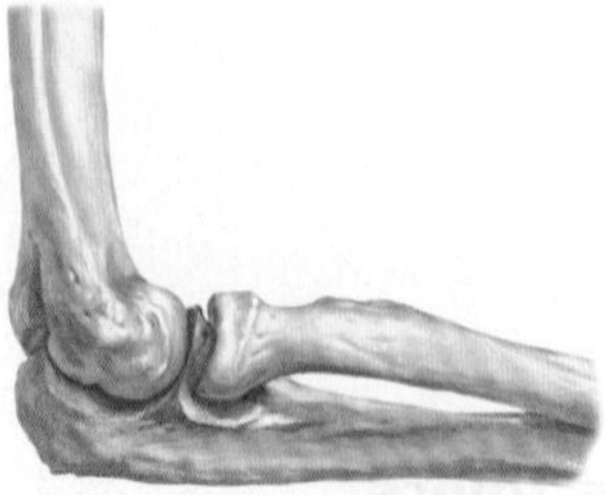

FIGURE 18-5 A hinge joint.

- In *condylar joints* (Fig. 18-6), such as the knee, the articulating surfaces are convex or concave, termed **condyles**. One articulating surface is convex and the matching surface is concave.

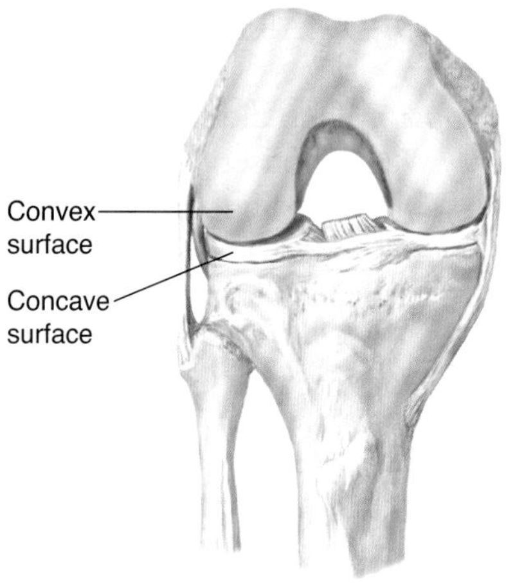

FIGURE 18-6 A condylar joint.

Easing joint action are *bursae*, disc-shaped synovial sacs that allow adjacent muscles or muscles and tendons to glide over each other during movement. They lie between the skin and the convex surface of a bone or joint (as in the prepatellar bursa of the knee, or in areas where tendons or muscles rub against bone, ligaments, or other tendons or muscles [as in the subacromial bursa of the shoulder]).

THE HEALTH HISTORY

Common or concerning symptoms identified during the health history of the musculoskeletal system are listed in Box 18-1.

BOX 18-1 COMMON OR CONCERNING SYMPTOMS

- Joint pain
- Joint pain associated with systemic symptoms, such as fever, chills, rash, weakness, and weight loss
- Low back pain
- Neck pain
- Bone pain
- Muscle pain or cramps
- Muscle weakness

Begin the history with a broad, open-ended question like, "Do you have any pain in your joints, bones, or muscles?"

Joint pain is a leading complaint of patients seeking health care. Joint pain may also be *extra-articular*, involving bones, muscles, and tissues around the joint such as tendons, ligaments, bursae, or overlying skin.

CLINICAL TIP
Pain may be due to sprains from stretching or tearing of ligaments, muscle or tendon strain, bursitis, or tendinitis.

Generalized "aches and pains" are called **myalgias** if they occur in muscles, and **arthralgias** if there is pain in a joint without evidence of arthritis.

The "OLD CART" mnemonic may be used to obtain more information:

- *Onset:* When did the pain begin?
  Was the onset rapid or slow?
  Did the pain follow an injury? Describe the injury.
- *Location:* Where is the pain located? Point to the site.
  Is the pain in one joint or multiple joints (or multiple muscles)?

Pain in one joint suggests trauma, monoarticular arthritis, possible tendinitis, or bursitis. Lateral hip pain near the greater trochanter suggests *trochanteric bursitis.*

  Does the pain migrate from joint to joint?
  Does the pain radiate (e.g., down a limb)?
- *Duration:* How long have you had the pain?
  Does the pain come and go or is it constant?
  Is it worse at a particular time of day or night?

A migratory pattern of joint pain occurs in *rheumatic fever*; progressive and symmetric joint involvement occurs in *rheumatoid arthritis.*

- *Characteristic symptoms:* Describe the pain. Is it sharp, dull, achy, or shooting? Use an appropriate pain scale to have the patient rate the pain.
- *Associated manifestations:* Do you have any other symptoms such as bruising, warmth, swelling, stiffness, deformity such as nodules, fever, chills, rash, muscle weakness, numbness, tingling, or burning?
  Do you have pain with weight bearing?
  Is your motion limited?
  Does the limitation affect activities, such as walking, rising from a chair, holding objects, or other activities of daily living?
- *Relieving/Exacerbating factors:* Does anything relieve the pain or make it worse, such as a heating pad or cool compress?
- *Treatment:* Have you taken any medication or tried other treatments to relieve the pain?

Extra-articular pain is present with inflammation of bursae (*bursitis*), tendons (*tendinitis*), or tendon sheaths (*tenosynovitis*) as well as *sprains* from stretching or tearing of ligaments.

Low Back Pain

Low back pain (Table 18-3) is the second most common reason for health care visits. Using open-ended questions gives a clearer picture of the problem, especially the location of the pain.

Low back pain has a lifetime prevalence of nearly 80% in the United States (Chou, 2014).

Determine if the pain is *on the midline*, over the vertebrae, or *off the midline.*

Midline back pain suggests a musculoligamentous injury, disc herniation, vertebra collapse, or spinal cord metastases. *Pain off the midline* suggests sacroiliitis, trochanteric bursitis, sciatica, or hip arthritis.

Is there radiation into the leg? If yes, is there any associated numbness or paresthesias?

CLINICAL TIP
Radiation of pain is seen in sciatica. Leg pain that resolves with rest and/or lumbar forward flexion suggests *spinal stenosis.*

Ask also about associated bladder or bowel dysfunction.

TABLE 18-3 Low Back Pain

Patterns	Possible Causes	Physical Signs
Mechanical Low Back Pain (Chou, 2014; Chou & Shekelle, 2010; Ropper & Zafonte, 2015; Rozenberg et al., 2012)		
Aching pain in the lumbosacral area; may radiate into lower leg, especially along L5 (lateral leg) or S1 (posterior leg) dermatomes. Refers to anatomic or functional abnormality in the absence of neoplastic, infectious, or inflammatory disease. Usually acute (<3 mo), idiopathic, benign, and self-limiting; represents 97% of symptomatic low back pain. Commonly work-related and occurring in patients 30–50 y. Risk factors include heavy lifting, poor conditioning, and obesity.	Often arises from muscle and ligament injuries (~70%) or age-related intervertebral disc or facet disease (~4%). (McGee, 2018c) Causes also include herniated disc (~4%), spinal stenosis (~3%), compression fractures (~4%), and spondylolisthesis (2%).	Paraspinal muscle or facet tenderness, pain with back movement, loss of normal lumbar lordosis, but no motor or sensory loss or reflex abnormalities. In osteoporosis, check for thoracic kyphosis, percussion tenderness over a spinous process, or fractures in the thoracic spine or hip (Golub & Laya, 2015).
Sciatica (Radicular Low Back Pain) (Chou, 2014; Ropper & Zafonte, 2015)		
Shooting pain below the knee, commonly into the lateral leg (L5) or posterior calf (S1); typically accompanies low back pain. Patients report associated paresthesias and weakness. Bending, sneezing, coughing, straining during bowel movements often worsen pain.	Sciatic pain very sensitive, ~95%, and specific, ~88%, for disc herniation. Usually from herniated intervertebral disc with compression or traction of nerve root(s) in people 50 y or older. Involves L5 and S1 roots in ~95% of disc herniations. Root or spinal cord compression from neoplastic conditions in fewer than 1% of cases. Tumor or midline disc herniation in bowel or bladder dysfunction, leg weakness from cauda equina syndrome (S2–S4).	Disc herniation most likely if calf wasting, weak ankle dorsiflexion, absent ankle jerk, positive crossed straight-leg raise (pain in affected leg when healthy leg tested); negative straight-leg raise makes diagnosis highly unlikely. Ipsilateral straight-leg raise sensitive, ~65–98%, but not specific, ~10–60%.
Chronic Back Stiffness (Assassi et al., 2014; Raychaudhuri & Deodhar, 2014)		
	Ankylosing spondylitis, an inflammatory polyarthritis, most common in men younger than 40 y. *Diffuse idiopathic skeletal hyperostosis (DISH)* affects men more than women, usually age ≥50 y.	
Pain Referred from the Abdomen or Pelvis		
Usually a deep, aching pain; the level varies with the source. Accounts for approximately 1% of low back pain.	Peptic ulcer, pancreatitis, pancreatic cancer, chronic prostatitis, endometriosis, dissecting aortic aneurysm, retroperitoneal tumor, and other causes.	Variable with the source. Local vertebral tenderness may be present. Spinal movements are not painful and range of motion is not affected. Look for signs of the primary disorder.

Neck Pain

Neck pain (Table 18-4) is also common. Although usually self-limited, it is important to ask about radiation into the arm, arm or leg weakness or paresthesias, and any changes in bladder or bowel function. Persisting pain after blunt trauma or a motor vehicle accident warrants referral to a specialist.

Radicular pain (radiating along a dermatome) may be from spinal nerve compression, most commonly C7 followed by C6.

TABLE 18-4 Pains in the Neck

Patterns	Possible Causes	Physical Signs
Mechanical Neck Pain		
Aching pain in the cervical paraspinal muscles and ligaments with associated muscle spasm and associated stiffness and tightness in the upper back and shoulder lasting up to 6 wk. No associated radiation, paresthesias, or weakness. Headache may be present.	Mechanism poorly understood, possibly sustained muscle contraction. Associated with poor posture, stress, poor sleep, poor head position during activities such as computer use, watching television, driving.	Local muscle tenderness, pain on movement. No neurologic deficits. Possible trigger points in *fibromyalgia*. *Torticollis* if prolonged abnormal neck posture and muscle spasm.
Mechanical Neck Pain—Whiplash		
Also mechanical neck pain with aching paracervical pain and stiffness, often beginning the day after injury. Occipital headache, dizziness, malaise, and fatigue may be present. Chronic whiplash syndrome if symptoms last more than 6 mo, present in 20–40% of injuries.	Musculoligamental sprain or strain from forced hyperflexion–hyperextension injury to the neck, as in rear-end collisions.	Localized paracervical tenderness, decreased neck range of motion, perceived weakness of the upper extremities. Causes of cervical cord compression such as fracture, herniation, head injury, or altered consciousness are excluded.
Cervical Radiculopathy—from Nerve Root Compression		
Sharp burning or tingling pain in the neck and one arm with associated paresthesias and weakness. Sensory symptoms often in myotomal pattern, deep in muscle, rather than dermatomal pattern.	Dysfunction of cervical spinal nerve, nerve roots, or both from foraminal encroachment of the spinal nerve (~75%), herniated cervical disc (~25%). Rarely from tumor, syrinx, or multiple sclerosis. Mechanisms may involve hypoxia of the nerve root and dorsal ganglion, release of inflammatory mediators.	C7 nerve root affected most often (45–60%), with weakness in triceps and finger flexors and extensors. C6 nerve root involvement also common with weakness in biceps, brachioradialis, and wrist extensors.
Cervical Myelopathy—from Cervical Cord Compression		
Neck pain with bilateral weakness and paresthesias in both upper and lower extremities, often with urinary frequency. Hand clumsiness, palmar paresthesias, and gait changes may be subtle. Neck flexion often exacerbates symptoms.	Usually from cervical *spondylosis*, defined as cervical degenerative disc disease from spurs, protrusion of ligamentum flavum, and/or disc herniation (~80%); also from cervical stenosis from osteophytes, ossification of ligamentum flavum. Large central or paracentral disc herniation may also compress cord.	Hyperreflexia; clonus at the wrist, knee, or ankle; extensor plantar reflexes (positive Babinski signs); and gait disturbances. May also see *Lhermitte sign:* neck flexion with resulting sensation of electrical shock radiating down the spine. Confirmation of cervical myelopathy warrants neck immobilization and neurosurgical evaluation.

Source: Bono, C. M., Ghiselli, G., Gilbert, T. J., Kreiner, D. S., Reitman, C., Summers, J. T., Baisden, J. L., Easa, J., Fernand, R., Lamer, T., Matz, P. G., Mazanec, D. J., Resnick, D. K., Shaffer, W. O., Sharma, A. K., Timmons, R. B., & Toton, J. F.; North American Spine Society. (2011). North American Spine Society. An evidence-based clinical guideline for the diagnosis and treatment of cervical radiculopathy from degenerative disorders. *The Spine Journal, 11*, 64–72; and Onks, C. A., & Billy, G. (2013). Evaluation and treatment of cervical radiculopathy. *Primary Care, 40*, 837–848.

EXAMINATION OF THE JOINTS

Important areas of examination for each of the major joints include:

- Inspect joint symmetry, alignment, and any bony deformities.
- Inspect and palpate surrounding tissues for skin changes, nodules, muscle atrophy, and crepitus.
- Perform range-of-motion maneuvers to test joint function and stability.
- Assess for signs of inflammation, swelling, warmth, tenderness, and redness.
- Assess muscle strength.

During the history, the patient's ability to carry out normal activities of daily living can be assessed. Keep these abilities in mind during the physical examination.

The detail needed for examination of the musculoskeletal system varies widely. This section presents examination techniques for both comprehensive and targeted assessment of joint function. Patients with extensive or severe musculoskeletal problems will require more time.

In the general survey of the patient, general appearance, body proportions, and ease of movement are assessed. The musculoskeletal examination should be systematic. It should include inspection and palpation of the bones and joints, assessment of range of motion and muscle strength. There are two phases to **range of motion**: *active* (by the patient) and *passive* (by the examiner).

Equipment needed for a physical examination of the musculoskeletal system includes:

- Tape measure
- Goniometer
- Skin marking pen

Tips for examining the musculoskeletal system are outlined in Box 18-2.

Examination of the muscles includes assessing muscle bulk, muscle tone, and muscle strength.

BOX 18-2 TIPS FOR SUCCESSFUL EXAMINATION OF THE MUSCULOSKELETAL SYSTEM

- During inspection, look for *symmetry.* Is there a symmetric change in joints on both sides of the body or only on one side? Is the change only in one or two joints?

Acute involvement of only one joint suggests trauma, septic arthritis, or gout. *Rheumatoid arthritis* typically involves several joints symmetrically distributed.

- Note any *joint deformities* or *malalignment of bones.*

This may indicate *Dupuytren contracture*, bowlegs, or knock knees.

- Use inspection and palpation to assess the *surrounding tissues,* note skin changes, subcutaneous nodules, and muscle atrophy. Assess for crepitus, an audible or palpable crunching during movement of tendons or ligaments over bone.

Look for subcutaneous nodules in *rheumatoid arthritis* or *rheumatic fever;* effusions in trauma; and crepitus over inflamed joints, in *osteoarthritis,* or in inflamed tendon sheaths.

- Test range of motion and maneuvers (described for each joint) to demonstrate *limitations in range of motion* or joint instability from excess mobility of joint ligaments, called *ligamentous laxity.* During range-of-motion evaluation, the angle of the joint can be measured with a *goniometer* (Fig. 18-7). This is useful for documenting the degree of limitation.

Decreased range of motion occurs in arthritis, inflammation of tissues around a joint, **fibrosis** (the development of fibrous connective tissue as a **reparative response to injury or damage** in or around a joint), or bony fixation (*ankylosis*). Ligamentous laxity of the anterior cruciate ligament (ACL) occurs in knee trauma.

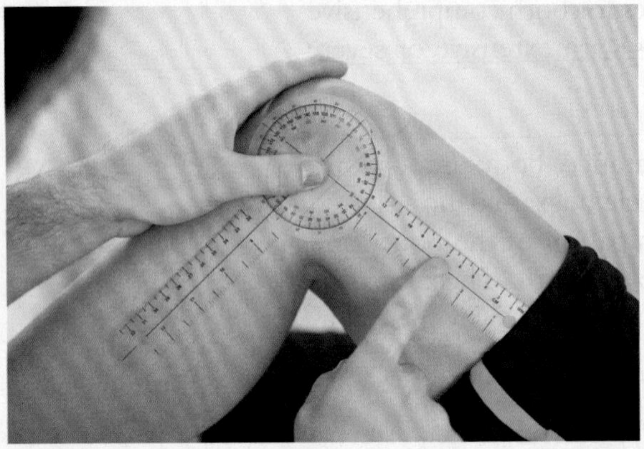

FIGURE 18-7 Using a goniometer to assess range of motion. (ESB Professional/Shutterstock.)

- Finally, test *muscle strength.*

Muscle atrophy or weakness occurs in *rheumatoid arthritis.*

Assess the four signs of inflammation:

- *Swelling.* Palpable swelling may involve (1) the synovial membrane, which can feel boggy or doughy; (2) effusion from excess synovial fluid within the joint space; or (3) soft-tissue structures such as bursae, tendons, and tendon sheaths.
- *Warmth.* Use the backs of your fingers to compare the involved joint with its unaffected contralateral joint, or with nearby tissues if both joints are involved.

Seen in arthritis, tendinitis, bursitis, and *osteomyelitis.*

- *Tenderness.* Try to identify the specific anatomic structure that is tender. Trauma may also cause tenderness.

Tenderness and warmth over a thickened synovium suggest arthritis or infection.

- *Redness.* Redness of the overlying skin is the *least* common sign of inflammation near the joints.

Redness over a tender joint suggests septic or gouty arthritis or possibly *rheumatoid arthritis.*

EXAMINATION OF THE MUSCLES

Muscle Bulk

Begin the examination by inspecting the size and contours of muscles. Do the muscles look shrunken, flat or concave, suggesting atrophy? If so, is the atrophy unilateral or bilateral? Is it proximal or distal?

Muscular *atrophy* refers to a loss of muscle bulk, or wasting. It results from diseases of the peripheral nervous system such as diabetic neuropathy as well as diseases of the muscles themselves. *Hypertrophy* is an increase in bulk with proportionate strength, whereas increased bulk with diminished strength is called *pseudohypertrophy* (seen in the *Duchenne form of muscular dystrophy*).

Flattening of the thenar and hypothenar eminences and furrowing between the metacarpals suggest atrophy. Localized atrophy of the thenar and hypothenar eminences occur in median and ulnar nerve damage, respectively.

When looking for atrophy, pay particular attention to the hands, shoulders, and thighs. The thenar and hypothenar eminences should be full and convex, and the spaces between the metacarpals, where the dorsal interosseous muscles lie, should be full or only slightly depressed. Atrophy of hand muscles may occur with normal aging, however, as in Figure 18-8.

Other causes of muscular atrophy include motor neuron diseases and rheumatoid arthritis.

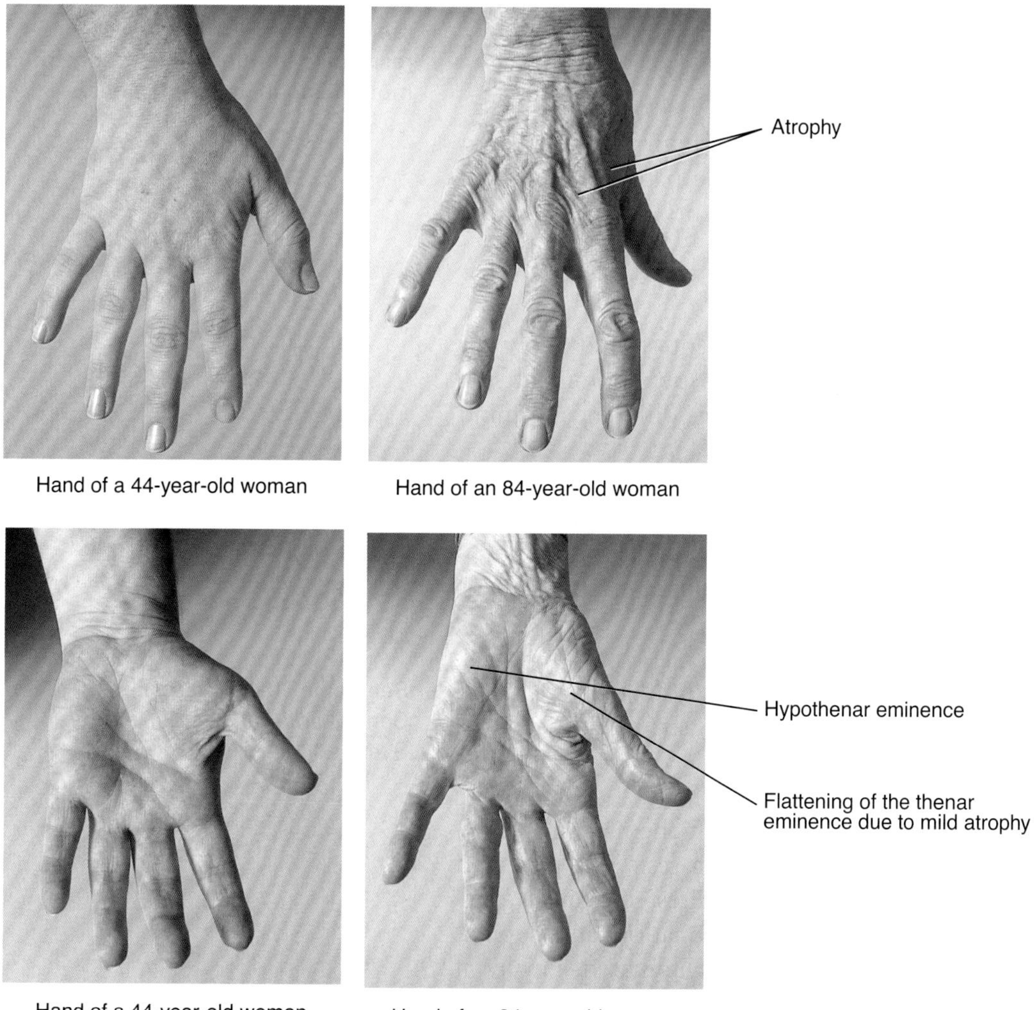

FIGURE 18-8 Muscular atrophy due to aging.

Look for fasciculations (fine tremors of the muscles), in atrophic muscles.

Fasciculations with atrophy and muscle weakness suggest disease of the peripheral motor unit.

Muscle Tone

When a normal muscle with an intact nerve supply is relaxed voluntarily, it maintains a slight residual tension known as **muscle tone**. This can best be assessed by feeling the muscle's resistance to passive stretch. Persuade the patient to relax. Take one hand with yours and while supporting the elbow, flex and extend the patient's fingers, wrist, and elbow, and put the shoulder through a moderate range of motion. With practice, these actions can be combined into a single smooth movement. On each side, note muscle tone and the resistance offered to your movements. Tense patients may show increased resistance. The feel of normal resistance is learned with repeated practice.

Decreased resistance occurs with diseases of the peripheral nervous system, cerebellar disease, or the acute stages of spinal cord injury. See Table 20-9, "Disorders of Muscle Tone."

If you suspect decreased resistance, hold the forearm and shake the hand loosely back and forth. Normally the hand moves back and forth freely but is not completely floppy.

Marked floppiness indicates muscle *hypotonia* or *flaccidity*, usually from a disorder of the peripheral motor system.

If resistance is increased, determine whether it varies as you move the limb or whether it persists throughout the range of motion and in both directions, for example, during both flexion and extension. Feel for any jerkiness in the resistance.

Spasticity is the increased resistance that worsens at the extremes of range. *Rigidity* is the increased resistance throughout the range of motion and in both directions.

To assess muscle tone in the legs, support the patient's thigh with one hand, grasp the foot with the other, and flex and extend the patient's knee and ankle on each side. Note the resistance to your movements.

Muscle Strength

People vary widely in their strength, and the assessment should allow for such variables as age, sex, and muscular training. A person's dominant side is usually slightly stronger than the other side. Keep this difference in mind when comparing sides.

Impaired strength is called weakness, or **paresis**. Absence of strength is called *paralysis*, or **plegia**. **Hemiparesis** refers to weakness of one half of the body; **hemiplegia** it is paralysis of one half of the body. **Paraplegia** means paralysis of the legs; **quadriplegia** is paralysis of all four limbs.

Test muscle strength by asking the patient to flex and extend actively against your resistance or to resist your movement. A muscle is strongest when it is shortest and weakest when longest.

See Table 20-11, "Disorders of the Central and Peripheral Nervous Systems."

If the muscles are too weak to overcome resistance, test them against gravity alone or with gravity eliminated. When the forearm rests in a pronated position, for example, dorsiflexion at the wrist can be tested against gravity alone. When the forearm is midway between pronation and supination, extension at the wrist can be tested with gravity eliminated. Finally, if the patient fails to move the body part, watch or feel for weak muscular contraction.

When documenting muscle strength, indicate the scale used (e.g., muscle strength 3 out of 5 or 3/5). See Box 18-3.

BOX 18-3 SCALE FOR GRADING MUSCLE STRENGTH

Muscle strength is graded on a 0 to 5 scale:

0—No muscular contraction detected
1—A barely detectable flicker or trace of contraction
2—Active movement of the body part with gravity eliminated
3—Active movement against gravity
4—Active movement against gravity and some resistance
5—Active movement against full resistance without evident fatigue; this is normal muscle strength

Methods for testing the major muscle groups are described in the next sections.

If the person has painful joints, move the person gently. Patients may move more comfortably by themselves. Let them show you how they manage movement. If joint trauma is present, ask the nurse practitioner or physician about an x-ray before attempting movement.

TEMPOROMANDIBULAR JOINT

Overview—Bony Structures and Joints

The temporomandibular joint (TMJ) is the most active joint in the body, opening and closing up to 2,000 times a day. It is formed by the fossa and articular tubercle of the temporal bone and the condyle of the mandible. It lies midway between the external acoustic meatus and the zygomatic arch (Fig. 18-9).

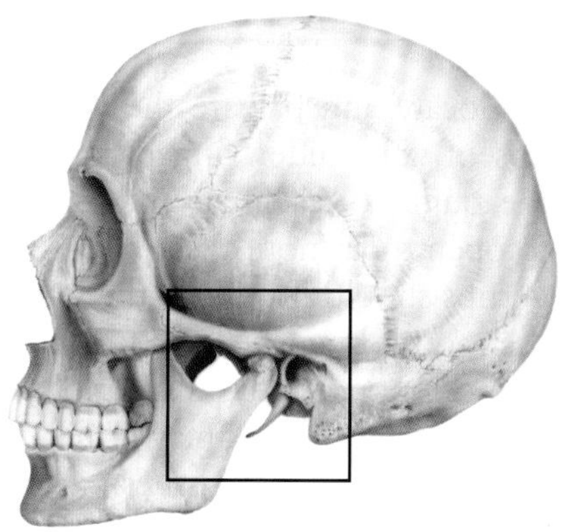

FIGURE 18-9 Location of the temporomandibular joint.

A fibrocartilaginous disc cushions the action of the condyle of the mandible against the synovial membrane and capsule of the articulating surfaces of the temporal bone (Fig. 18-10). Hence, it is a condylar synovial joint.

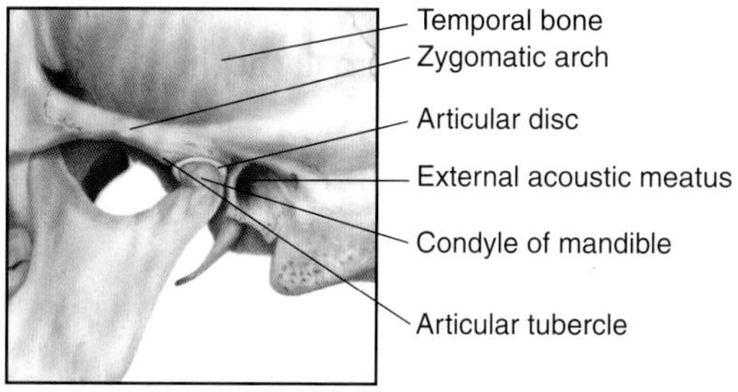

FIGURE 18-10 Bony structures of the temporomandibular joint.

Muscle Groups and Additional Structures

The principal muscles opening the mouth are the *external pterygoids* (Fig. 18-11). The muscles closing the mouth are the *masseter*, the *temporalis* and the *internal pterygoids*. All are innervated by cranial nerve V, the trigeminal nerve (see Chapter 20).

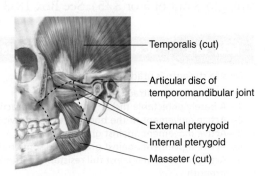

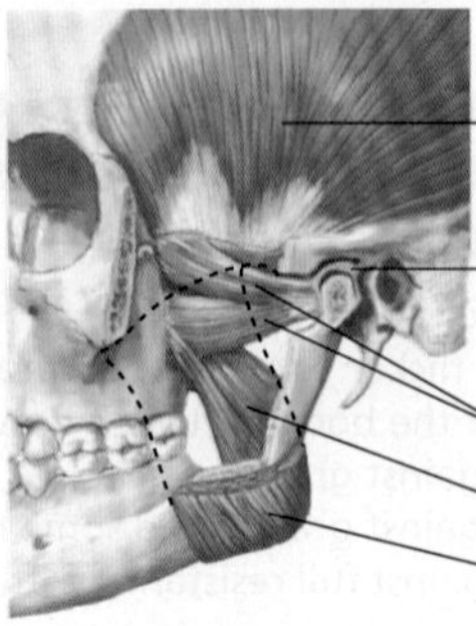

FIGURE 18-11 Muscles of the temporomandibular joint.

Physical Examination

Inspection and Palpation

Inspect the face for symmetry. Inspect the TMJ for swelling or redness. Swelling may appear as a rounded bulge approximately 0.5 cm anterior to the external auditory meatus.

CLINICAL TIP
Facial asymmetry associated with *TMJ syndrome.* Typical features are unilateral chronic pain with chewing, jaw clenching, or teeth grinding, often associated with stress (may also present as headache).

To locate and palpate the joint, place the tips of your index fingers just in front of the tragus of each ear and ask the patient to open their mouth (Fig. 18-12). The fingertips should drop into the joint spaces as the mouth opens. Check for smooth range of motion; note any swelling or tenderness. Snapping or clicking may be felt or heard in people without TMJ issues.

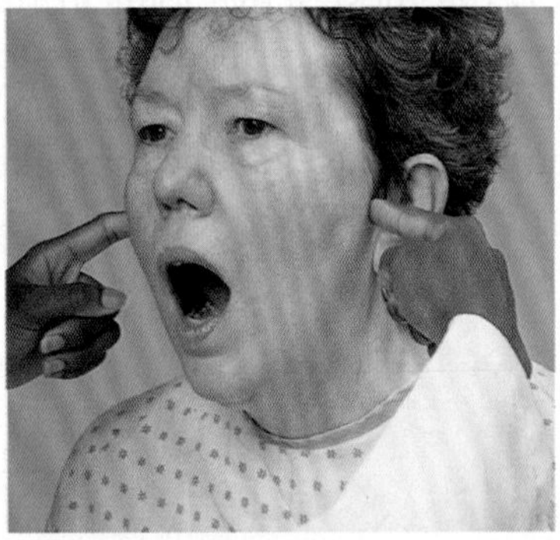

FIGURE 18-12 The nurse palpates the temporomandibular joint.

Dislocation of the TMJ may be seen in trauma. Palpable crepitus or clicking occurs with poor occlusion, meniscus injury, or synovial swelling from trauma.

Palpate the muscles of mastication for tenderness:

- The *masseters*, externally at the angle of the mandible

Pain and tenderness of the masseters on palpation occurs in *TMJ syndrome.*

- The *temporal muscles*, externally during clenching and relaxation of the jaw

Range of Motion and Maneuvers

The TMJ has glide and hinge motions in its upper and lower portions, respectively. Chewing consists primarily of gliding movements in the upper compartments.

Range of motion is threefold: ask the patient to demonstrate opening and closing, protrusion and retraction (by jutting the jaw forward), and lateral, or side-to-side, motion. Normally as the mouth is opened wide, three fingers can be inserted between incisors. During normal protrusion of the jaw, the bottom teeth can be placed in front of the upper teeth.

Muscle Strength

If the patient complains of difficulty chewing or jaw weakness, test muscle strength by asking them to perform the range-of-motion maneuvers, projection, lateral motion, and opening of mouth against your resistance.

THE SHOULDER

Overview

The glenohumeral joint of the shoulder is distinguished by wide ranging movement in all directions. This joint is largely uninhibited by bony structure. The shoulder derives its mobility from a complex interconnected structure of four joints, three large bones, and three principal muscle groups, often referred to as the **shoulder girdle**.

Bony Structures

The bony structures of the shoulder include the humerus, the clavicle, and the scapula (Fig. 18-13).

In Figure 18-13, identify the *manubrium*, the *sternoclavicular joint*, and the *clavicle*. Then identify the *tip of the acromion*, the *greater tubercle of the*

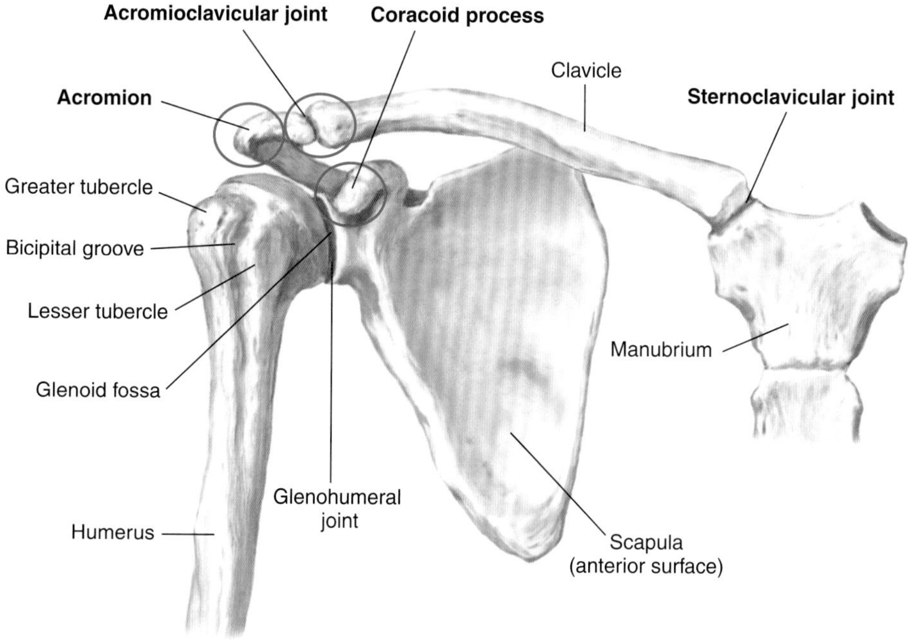

FIGURE 18-13 Bones of the shoulder.

humerus, and the *coracoid process*, which are important landmarks of shoulder anatomy.

Joints

Three joints articulate at the shoulder:

- The *glenohumeral joint*—In this joint, the head of the humerus articulates with the shallow glenoid fossa of the scapula. This joint is deeply situated and not normally palpable. It is a ball-and-socket joint, allowing the arm its wide arc of movement—**flexion** (a movement that decreases the angle between two body parts); **extension** (a movement that increases the angle between two body parts); **abduction** (movement away from the trunk); **adduction** (movement toward the trunk); **rotation** (the **movement of the limbs around their long axes**); and **circumduction** (movement of a limb in a circular manner).
- The *sternoclavicular joint*—The convex medial end of the clavicle articulates with the concave hollow in the upper sternum.
- The *acromioclavicular joint*—The lateral end of the clavicle articulates with the acromion process of the scapula.

Muscle Groups

Three groups of muscles attach at the shoulder: the scapulohumeral group, the axioscapular group (Fig. 18-14), and the axiohumeral group.

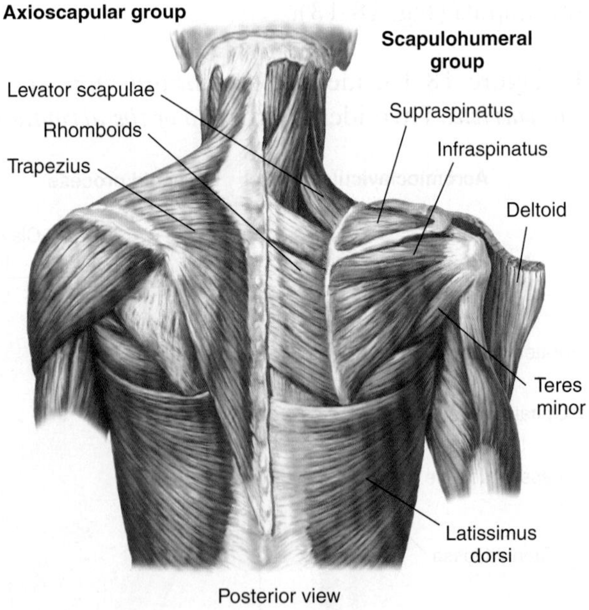

FIGURE 18-14 The scapulohumeral and axioscapular muscle groups of the shoulder, posterior view.

The Scapulohumeral Group

The scapulohumeral group extends from the scapula to the humerus and includes the muscles inserting directly on the humerus, known as *"SITS muscles"* of the *rotator cuff*:

- *S*upraspinatus
- *I*nfraspinatus
- *T*eres minor
- *S*ubscapularis (not illustrated)

The Axioscapular Group

The axioscapular group attaches the trunk to the scapula and includes the trapezius, rhomboids, serratus anterior, and levator scapulae. These muscles rotate the scapula and pull the shoulder posteriorly.

The Axiohumeral Group

The axiohumeral group attaches the trunk to the humerus and includes the pectoralis major and minor and the latissimus dorsi (Fig. 18-15). These muscles produce internal rotation of the shoulder.

The biceps and triceps, which connect the scapula to the bones of the forearm, are also involved in shoulder movement, especially forward flexion (biceps) and extension (triceps).

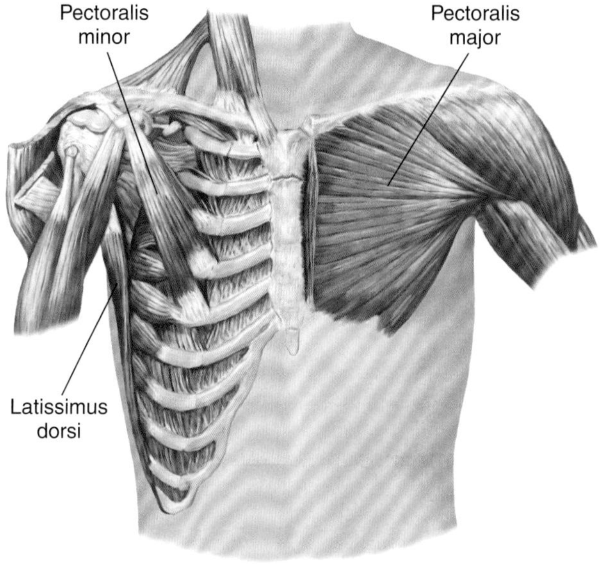

FIGURE 18-15 The axiohumeral muscle group of the shoulder, anterior view.

Additional Structures

Surrounding the glenohumeral joint is a fibrous *articular capsule* formed by the tendon insertions of the rotator cuff and other capsular muscles.

The long head of the biceps tendon runs in the bicipital groove of the humerus between the greater and lesser tubercles. To locate this tendon, rotate your arm externally and find the tendinous cord that runs just medial to the greater tubercle. The tendon will roll under your fingers.

The principal bursa of the shoulder is the *subacromial bursa*, positioned between the acromion and the head of the humerus and overlying the supraspinatus tendon (Fig. 18-16). Normally, the supraspinatus tendon and the subacromial bursa are not palpable.

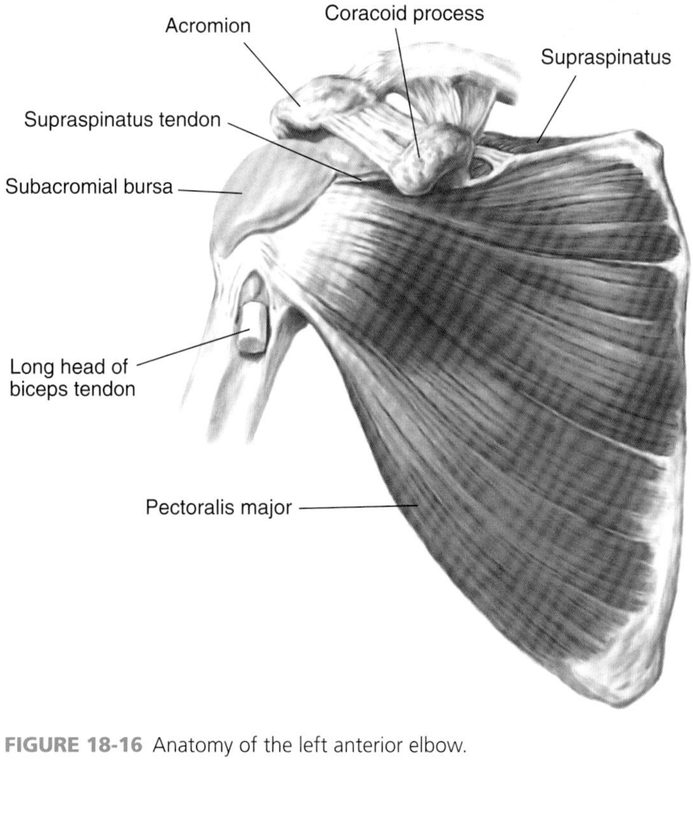

FIGURE 18-16 Anatomy of the left anterior elbow.

Physical Examination

Inspection

Observe the shoulder and shoulder girdle anteriorly, and inspect the scapulae and related muscles posteriorly.

Scoliosis may cause elevation of one shoulder. With *anterior dislocation of the shoulder*, the rounded lateral aspect of the shoulder appears flattened (McGee, 2018c).

Note any swelling, deformity, muscle atrophy or fasciculations, or abnormal positioning.

Atrophy of supraspinatus and infraspinatus over posterior scapula with increased prominence of scapular spine indicate a *rotator cuff tear.*

Inspect the entire upper extremity for color change, skin alteration, or unusual bony contours.

Palpation

Begin by palpating the bony landmarks of the shoulder; then palpate any area of pain (Table 18-5).

- Beginning medially, at the *sternoclavicular joint*, trace the clavicle laterally with your fingers.
- Now, from behind, follow the bony spine of the scapula laterally and upward until it becomes the acromion (Point A in Fig. 18-17), the summit of the shoulder. Its upper surface is rough and slightly convex. Identify the anterior tip of the acromion.

Review the bones of the shoulder in Figure 18-13.

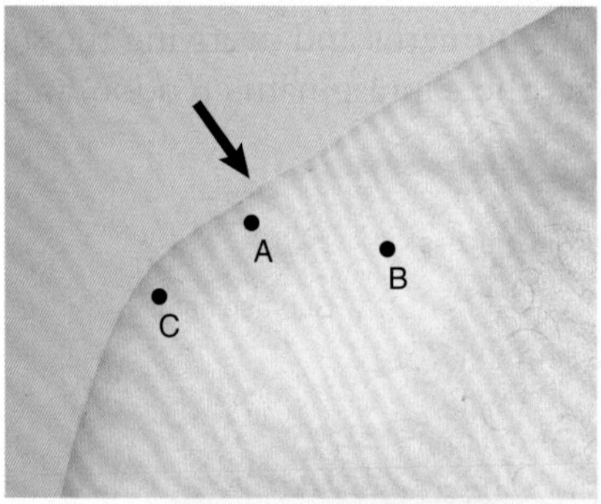

FIGURE 18-17 Surface anatomy landmarks of the right shoulder: the acromion (A), the coracoid process (B), and the greater tubercle (C).

- With your index finger on top of the acromion, just behind its tip, press medially with your thumb to find the slightly elevated ridge that marks the distal end of the clavicle at the *acromioclavicular joint* (the arrow in Fig. 18-17). Move your thumb medially and down a short step to the next bony prominence, the *coracoid process* (Point B in Fig. 18-17) of the scapula.
- Now, with your thumb on the coracoid process, allow your fingers to fall on and grasp the lateral aspect of the humerus to palpate the *greater tubercle* (Point C in Fig. 18-17), where the SITS muscles insert.

Range of motion is restricted with *bursitis, capsulitis, rotator cuff tears* or *sprains*, and *tendinitis*.

TABLE 18-5 Painful Shoulders

Rotator Cuff Tendinitis

Repeated shoulder motion, as in throwing or swimming, can cause edema and hemorrhage followed by inflammation, most commonly involving the supraspinatus tendon. Acute, recurrent, or chronic pain may result, often aggravated by activity. Patients report sharp catches of pain, grating, and weakness when lifting the arm overhead. When the supraspinatus tendon is involved, tenderness is maximal just below the tip of the acromion. In older adults, bone spurs on the undersurface of the acromion may contribute to symptoms. Patients are typically athletically active.

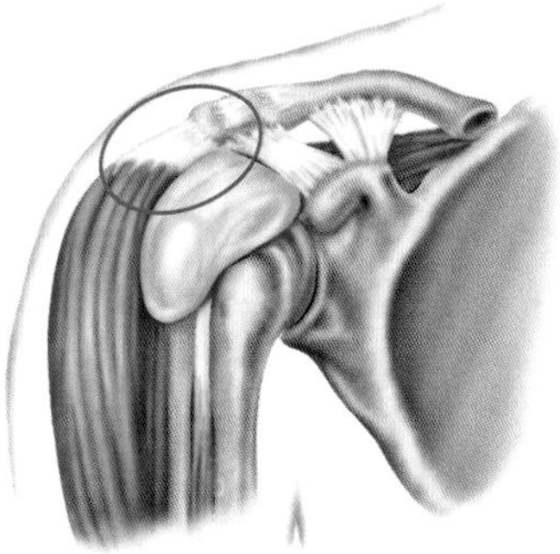

Rotator Cuff Tears

The rotator cuff muscles and tendons keep the head of the humerus in place against the concave glenoid fossa and strengthen arm movement—the subscapularis is used with internal rotation, the supraspinatus with elevation, and the infraspinatus and teres minor with external rotation. Injury from a fall or repeated impingement of muscle or tendon against a bone may weaken the rotator cuff, causing a partial or complete tear, usually after age 40. Weakness, atrophy of the supraspinatus and infraspinatus muscles, pain, crepitus and tenderness may ensue. In a complete tear of the supraspinatus tendon (illustrated), active abduction and forward flexion at the glenohumeral joint are severely impaired, producing a characteristic shrugging of the shoulder and a positive "drop arm" sign.

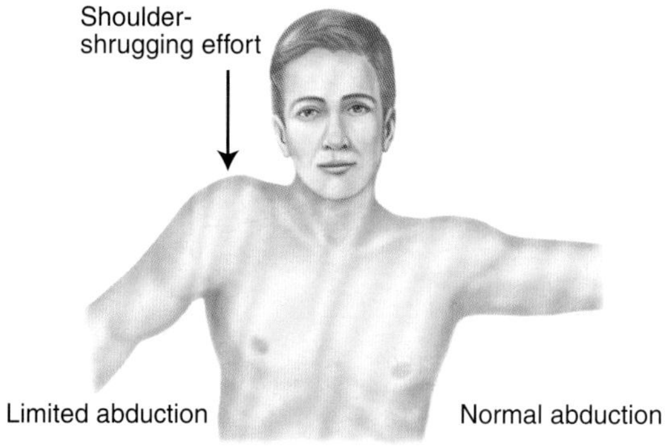

Anterior Dislocation of the Humerus

Shoulder instability from anterior dislocation of the humerus usually results from a fall or forceful throwing motion, then becomes recurrent. The shoulder seems to "slip out of the joint" when the arm is abducted and externally rotated, causing a *positive apprehension sign* for anterior instability when the examiner places the arm in this position. Any shoulder movement may cause pain, and patients hold the arm in a neutral position. The rounded lateral aspect of the shoulder appears flattened. Dislocations may also be inferior, posterior (relatively rare), and multidirectional.

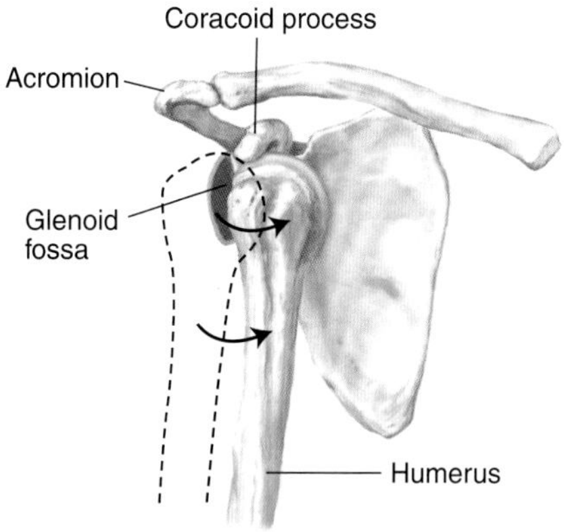

Range of Motion and Special Maneuvers

Range of Motion

The six motions of the shoulder girdle are flexion, extension, abduction, adduction, and internal and external rotation.

Standing in front of the patient, watch for smooth fluid movement as the patient performs the range of motions outlined Table 18-6. Table 18-6 includes clear, simple instructions that prompt the patient and the muscles responsible for each movement.

TABLE 18-6 Assessing Range of Motion of the Shoulders

Shoulder Movement	Patient Instructions	Principal Muscles Affecting Movement
Flexion 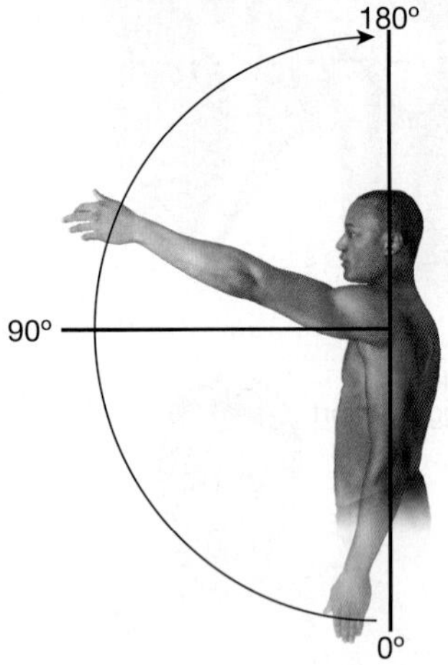	*"Raise your arms in front of you and overhead."*	Anterior deltoid, pectoralis major (clavicular head), coracobrachialis, biceps brachii (short head)
Hyperextension 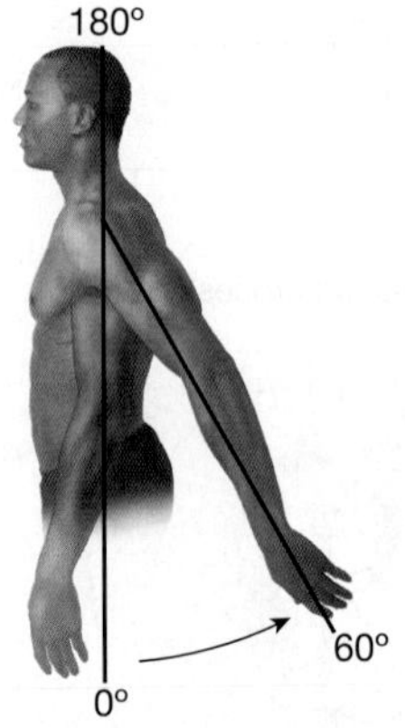	*"Raise your arms behind you."*	Latissimus dorsi, teres major, posterior deltoid, triceps brachii (long head)
Abduction 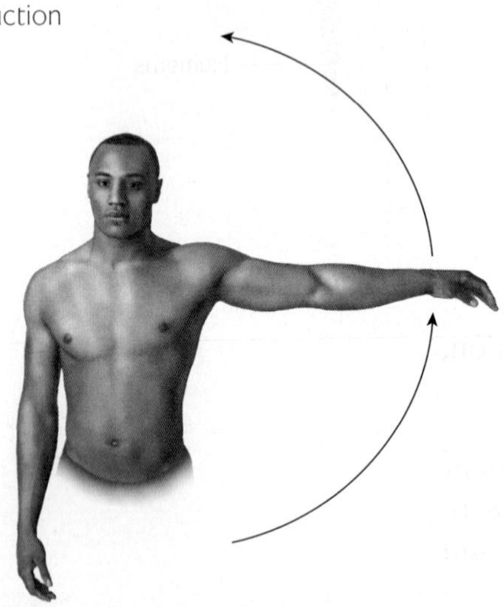	*"Raise your arms out to the side and overhead."* Note that to test *pure glenohumeral motion*, the patient should raise the arms to shoulder level at 90 degrees with palms facing down. To test *scapulothoracic motion*, the patient should turn the palms up and raise the arms an additional 60 degrees. The final 30 degrees test combined glenohumeral and scapulothoracic motion.	Supraspinatus, middle deltoid, serratus anterior (via upward rotation of the scapula)

Shoulder Movement	Patient Instructions	Principal Muscles Affecting Movement
Adduction 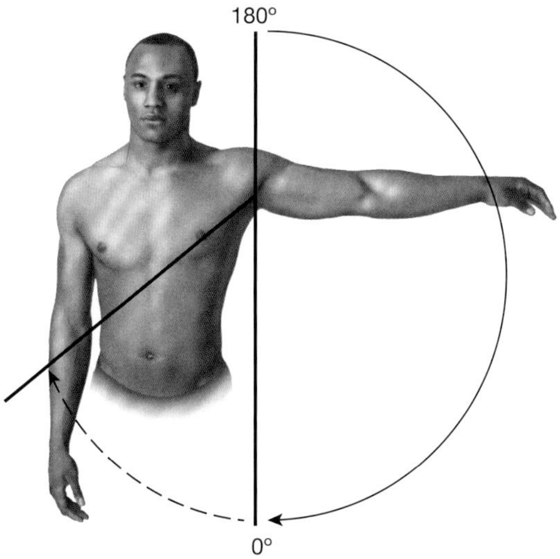	*"Lower your arms to your sides, then bring them across your body."*	Pectoralis major, coracobrachialis, latissimus dorsi, teres major, subscapularis
Internal rotation 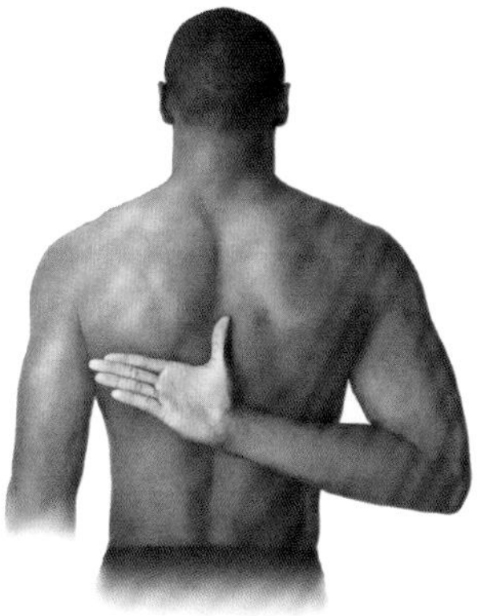	*"Place one hand behind your back and touch your shoulder blade."* Identify the highest midline spinous process the patient is able to reach.	Subscapularis, anterior deltoid, pectoralis major, teres major, latissimus dorsi
External rotation 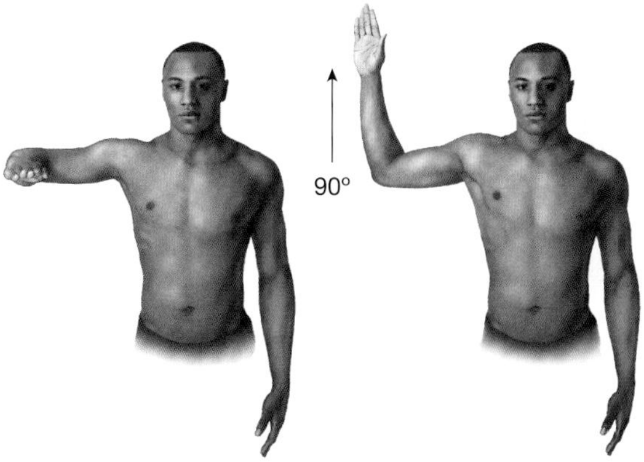	*"Raise your arm to shoulder level; bend your elbow and rotate your forearm toward the ceiling."* or *"Place one hand behind your neck or head as if you are brushing your hair."*	Infraspinatus, teres minor, posterior deltoid

Maneuvers to Assess Shoulder Function

When the patient complains of shoulder pain or weakness, carry out the special maneuvers described in Table 18-7. If any of these common maneuvers are positive, the patient should be referred to a specialist for further testing and diagnosis. The most common cause of shoulder pain involves the rotator cuff, usually the supraspinatus tendon.

In a patient aged 60 or older, a positive dropped-arm test is the individual finding most likely to identify a rotator cuff tear.

TABLE 18-7 Special Maneuvers for Examining the Shoulder

Structure	Technique	Illustration
Acromioclavicular joint	Palpate and compare both joints for swelling or tenderness. Adduct the patient's arm across the chest, sometimes called the *"crossover test."*	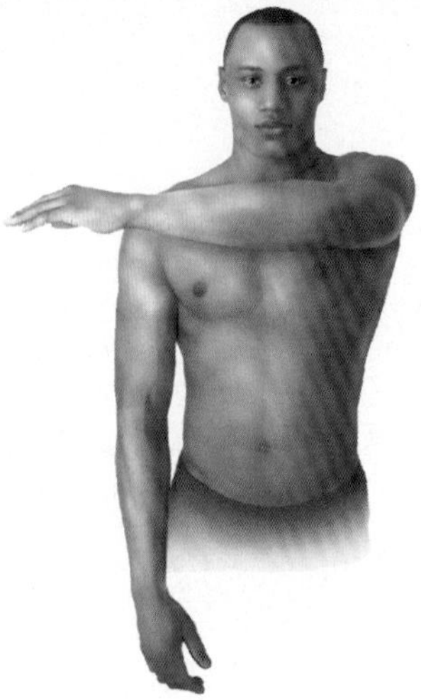
Overall shoulder rotation	Ask the patient to touch the opposite scapula using the two motions shown below (the Apley scratch test).	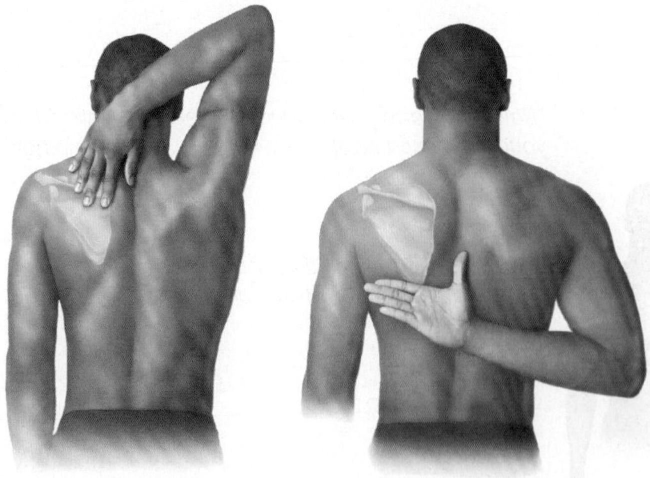

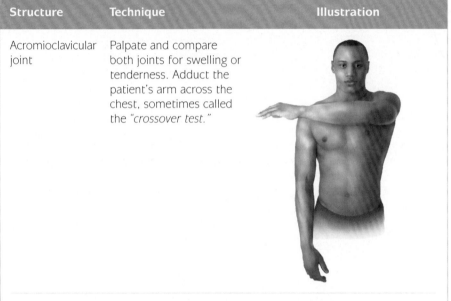

See Table 18-5, "Painful Shoulders." Pain with adduction is positive for a rotator cuff tear.

Pain during these motions suggests *rotator cuff disorder* or *adhesive capsulitis.*

Structure	Technique	Illustration	
Rotator cuff	Test for the *"drop-arm" sign*. Ask the patient to fully abduct the arm to shoulder level (or up to 90 degrees) and lower it slowly. (Note that abduction above shoulder level, from 90 degrees to 120 degrees, reflects action of the deltoid muscle.)	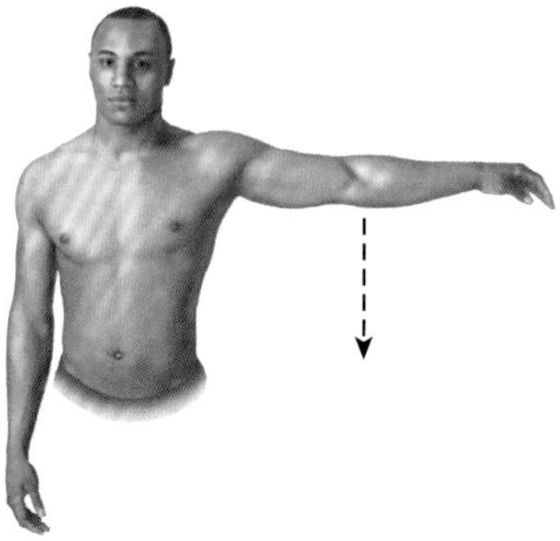	If the patient cannot hold the arm fully abducted at shoulder level, the test is *positive*, indicating a *rotator cuff tear* (McGee, 2018b).
Muscle strength tests	Test *supraspinatus strength* (sometimes called the "empty can test"). Elevate the arms to 90 degrees and internally rotate the arms with the thumbs pointing down, as if emptying a can. Ask the patient to resist as you place downward pressure on the arms.	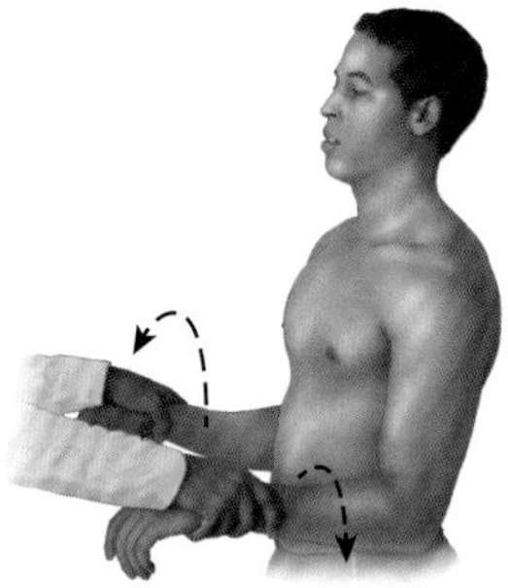	Weakness during this maneuver is a *positive test* for a supraspinatus *rotator cuff tear.*
	External rotation resistance test. Ask the patient to place arms at the side and flex the elbows to 90 degrees with the thumbs turned up. Provide resistance as the patient presses the forearms outward.	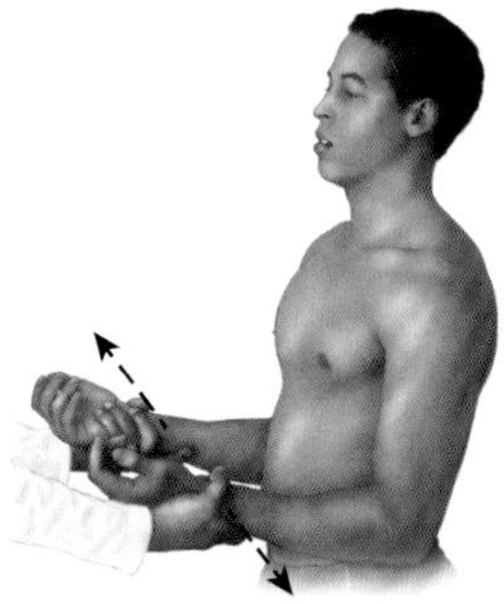	Pain or weakness during this maneuver is a positive test for an *infraspinatus disorder.* Limited external rotation points to *glenohumeral disease* or *adhesive capsulitis.*
Pain provocation test	Painful arc test. Fully adduct the patient's arm from 0 degrees to 180 degrees.	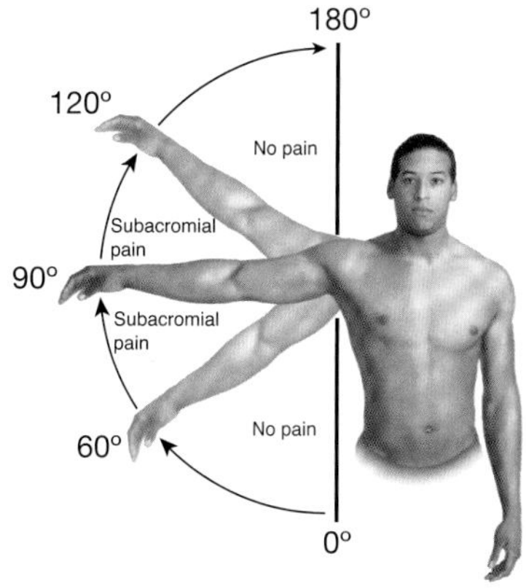	Shoulder pain from 60 degrees to 120 degrees is a *positive test* for a *subacromial impingement/rotator cuff tendinitis disorder.*

THE ELBOW

Overview, Bony Structures, and Joints

The elbow helps position the hand in space and stabilizes the lever action of the forearm. The elbow joint is formed by the humerus and the two bones of the forearm, the radius, and the ulna. Identify the medial and lateral epicondyles of the humerus and the olecranon process of the ulna.

These bones have three articulations: the *humeroulnar joint*, the *radiohumeral joint*, and the *radioulnar joint*. All three share a large common articular cavity and an extensive synovial lining.

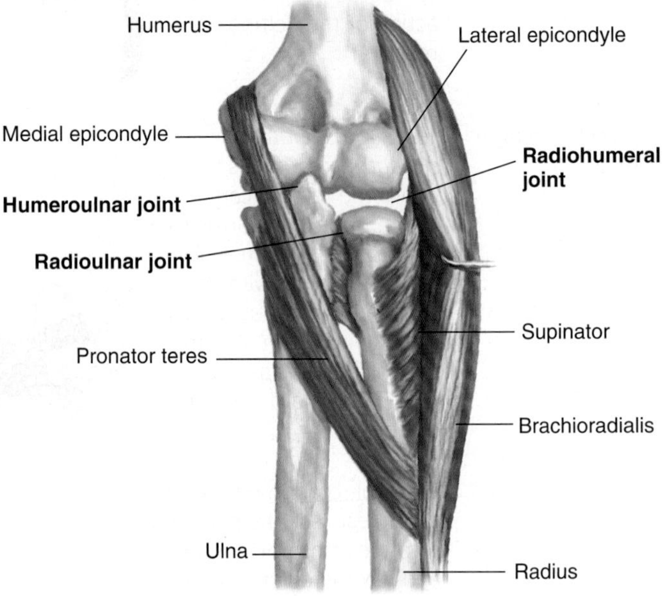

FIGURE 18-18 Anatomy of the left anterior elbow.

Muscle Groups and Additional Structures

Muscles traversing the elbow include the *biceps* and *brachioradialis* (flexion), the *triceps* (extension), the *pronator teres* (pronation), and the *supinator* (supination). Figure 18-18 illustrates these structures.

Note the location of the *olecranon bursa* between the olecranon process and the skin (Fig. 18-19). The bursa is not normally palpable but swells and becomes tender when inflamed. The *ulnar nerve* runs posteriorly in the ulnar groove between the medial epicondyle and the olecranon process. On the ventral forearm, the *median nerve* is just medial to the brachial artery.

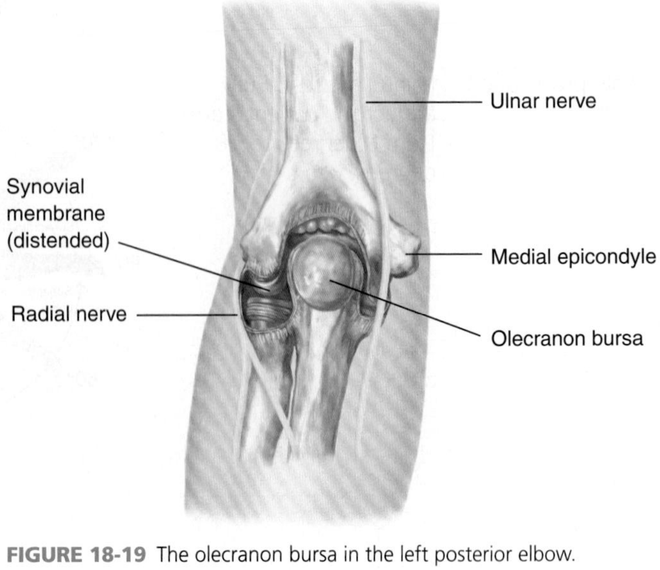

FIGURE 18-19 The olecranon bursa in the left posterior elbow.

Physical Examination

Inspection

Support the patient's forearm with your opposite hand so the elbow is flexed to about 70 degrees. Identify the medial and lateral epicondyles and the olecranon process of the ulna. Inspect the contours of the elbow, including the extensor surface of the ulna and the olecranon process. Note any nodules or swelling.

Swelling over the olecranon process occurs in olecranon bursitis, inflammation or synovial fluid in arthritis.

Palpation

Palpate the olecranon process and press over the epicondyles for tenderness (Fig. 18-20). Note any displacement of the olecranon.

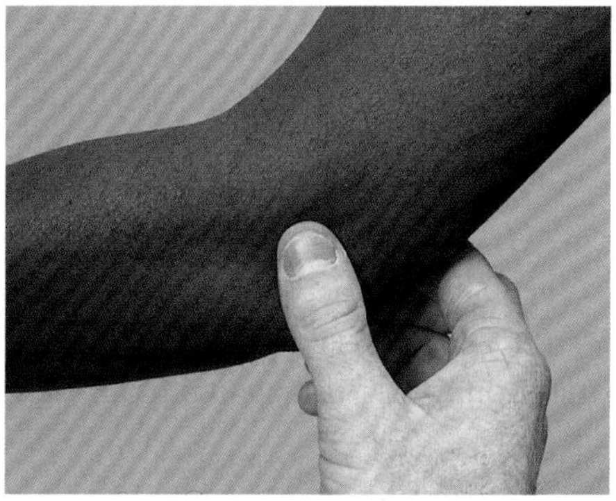

FIGURE 18-20 Palpating the epicondyles for swelling or tenderness.

Tenderness distal to the epicondyle occurs in *lateral epicondylitis* (tennis elbow) and less commonly in *medial epicondylitis* (pitcher's or golfer's elbow).

Palpate the grooves between the epicondyles and the olecranon, noting any tenderness, swelling, or thickening. The synovium is most accessible to examination between the olecranon and the epicondyles. (Normally neither synovium nor bursa is palpable.) The sensitive ulnar nerve can be felt posteriorly between the olecranon process and the medial epicondyle.

The olecranon is displaced posteriorly in *posterior dislocation of the elbow* and *supracondylar fracture* (Fig. 18-21).

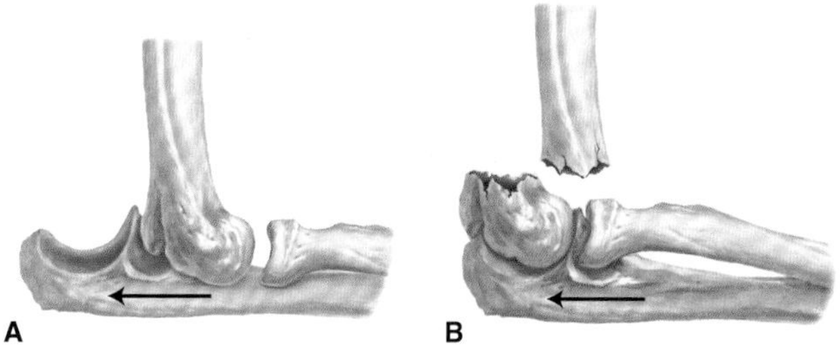

FIGURE 18-21 **A.** Posterior dislocation of the elbow. **B.** Supracondylar fracture of the elbow.

Range of Motion

Range of motion includes flexion and extension at the elbow and pronation and supination of the forearm (Fig. 18-22). Refer to Table 18-8 for clear, simple instructions that prompt the patient and the muscles responsible for each movement.

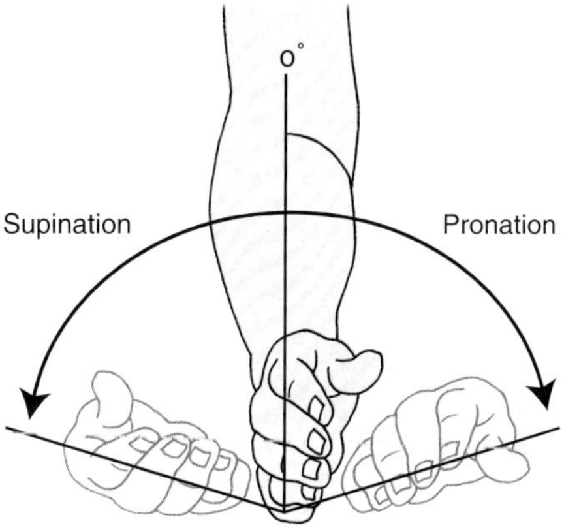

FIGURE 18-22 Supination and pronation of the forearm.

After injury, preservation of active range of motion (AROM) and full elbow extension makes fracture unlikely.

TABLE 18-8 Assessing Elbow Movement

Elbow Movement	Patient Instructions	Primary Muscles Affecting Movement
Flexion	*"Bend your elbow."*	Biceps brachii, brachialis, brachioradialis
Extension	*"Straighten your elbow."*	Triceps brachii, anconeus
Supination	*"Turn your palms up, as if carrying a bowl of soup."*	Biceps brachii, supinator
Pronation	*"Turn your palms down."*	Pronator teres, pronator quadratus

Muscle Strength Tests

Test flexion (C5, C6—biceps; Fig. 18-23) *and extension* (C6, C7, C8—triceps; Fig. 18-24) *at the elbow* by having the patient pull and push against your hand.

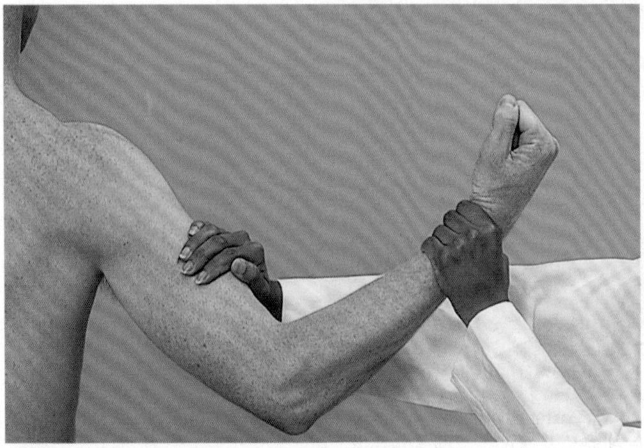

FIGURE 18-23 Testing muscle strength by having the patient flex the elbow.

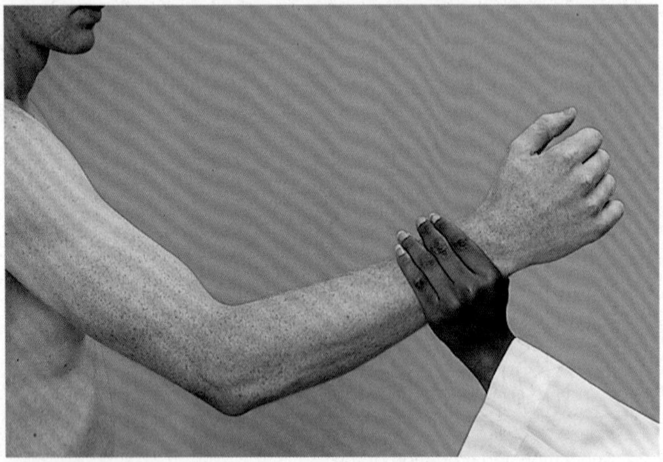

FIGURE 18-24 Testing muscle strength by having the patient extend the elbow.

THE WRIST AND HANDS

The wrist and hands form a complex unit of small, highly active joints used almost continuously during waking hours. There is little protection from overlying soft tissue, increasing vulnerability to trauma and disability.

Bony Structures

The wrist includes the distal radius and ulna and eight small carpal bones (Fig. 18-25). At the wrist, identify the bony tips of the radius and the ulna.

The carpal bones lie distal to the wrist joint within each hand. Identify the carpal bones, each of the five metacarpals, and the proximal, middle, and distal phalanges. Note that the thumb lacks a middle phalanx.

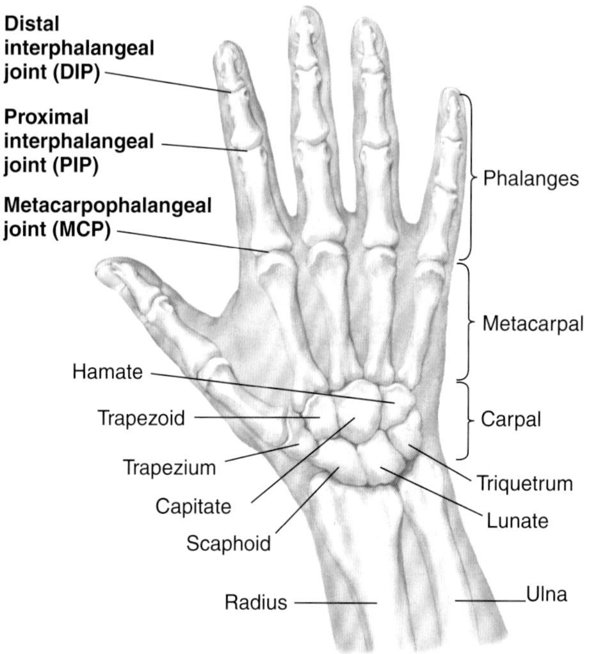

FIGURE 18-25 Bones of the wrist and hand.

Joints

The numerous joints of the wrist and hand lend unique dexterity to the hands:

- *Wrist joints*—The wrist joints include the *radiocarpal* or *wrist joint*, the *distal radioulnar joint*, and the *intercarpal joints* (Fig. 18-26). The joint capsule, articular disc, and synovial membrane of the wrist join the radius to the ulna and to the proximal carpal bones. On the dorsum of the wrist, locate the groove of the *radiocarpal joint*, which provides most of the flexion and extension at the wrist because the ulna does not articulate directly with the carpal bones.
- *Hand joints*—The joints of the hand include the *metacarpophalangeal (MCP) joints*, the *proximal interphalangeal (PIP) joints*, and the *distal interphalangeal (DIP) joints*. Flex the hand and find the groove marking the MCP joint of each finger (Fig. 18-27). It is distal to the knuckle and is best felt on either side of the extensor tendon.

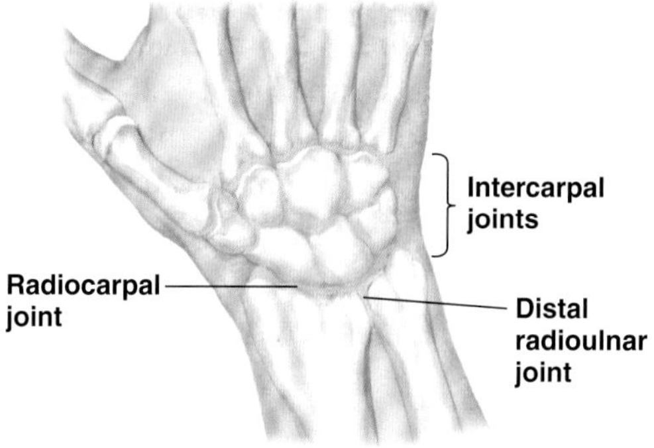

FIGURE 18-26 Joints of the wrist.

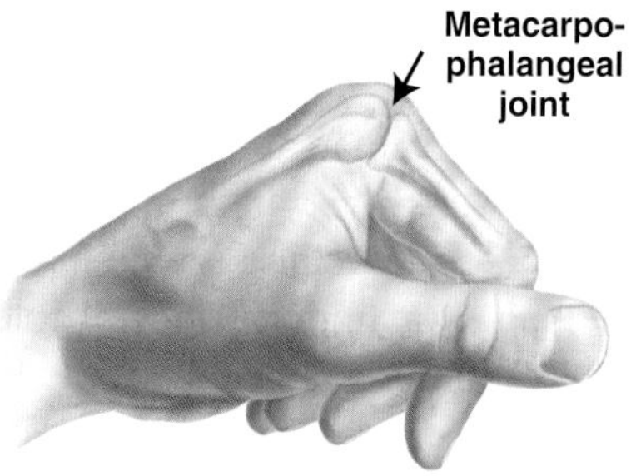

FIGURE 18-27 A metacarpophalangeal joint.

Muscle Groups

Wrist flexion arises from the two carpal muscles located on the radial and ulnar surfaces. Two radial and one ulnar muscle provide wrist extension. Supination and pronation result from muscle contraction in the forearm.

The thumb is powered by three muscles that form the thenar eminence and provide flexion, abduction, and opposition. The muscles of extension are at the base of the thumb along the radial margin. Movement in the digits depends on action of the flexor and extensor tendons of muscles in the forearm and wrist.

The intrinsic muscles of the hand attaching to the metacarpal bones are involved in flexion (*lumbricals*), abduction (*dorsal interossei*), and adduction (*palmar interossei*) of the fingers.

Additional Structures

Soft tissue structures, especially tendons and tendon sheaths, are especially important to movement of the wrist and hand. Six extensor tendons and two flexor tendons pass across the wrist and hand to insert on the fingers. Through much of their course, these tendons travel in tunnel-like sheaths, generally palpable only when swollen or inflamed.

Understanding the structures in the *carpal tunnel* is important. It is a channel beneath the palmar surface of the wrist and proximal hand. The channel contains the sheath and flexor tendons of the forearm muscles and the *median nerve*.

Holding the tendons and tendon sheath in place is a transverse ligament, the *flexor retinaculum*. The median nerve lies between the flexor retinaculum and the tendon sheath (Fig. 18-28). It provides sensation to the palm and the palmar surface of most of the thumb, the second and third digits, and half of the fourth digit. It also innervates the thumb muscles of flexion, abduction, and opposition.

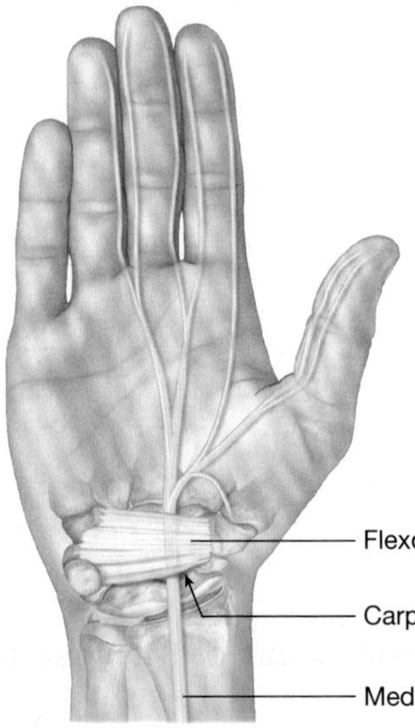

FIGURE 18-28 The carpal tunnel of the hand.

Physical Examination

Inspection

Observe the position of the hands in motion to see if movements are smooth and natural. At rest, the fingers should be slightly flexed and aligned almost in parallel.

Guarded movement suggests injury. Poor finger alignment is seen in flexor tendon damage.

Inspect the palmar and dorsal surfaces of the wrist and hand carefully for swelling over the joints. Diffuse swelling is seen in arthritis (Table 18-9) or infection; local swelling is seen in cystic ganglion. Note any deformities of the wrist, hand, or finger bones (Table 18-10), as well as any angulation from radial or ulnar deviation.

In *osteoarthritis,* Heberden nodes are seen at the DIP joints and Bouchard nodes at the PIP joints. In *rheumatoid arthritis,* symmetric deformity in the PIP, MCP, and wrist joints with ulnar deviation is present.

TABLE 18-9 Arthritis in the Hands

Acute Rheumatoid Arthritis

Tender, painful, stiff joints in *rheumatoid arthritis*, usually with *symmetric* involvement on both sides of the body. The proximal interphalangeal, metacarpophalangeal, and wrist joints are the most frequently affected. Note the fusiform or spindle-shaped swelling of the proximal interphalangeal joints in acute disease.

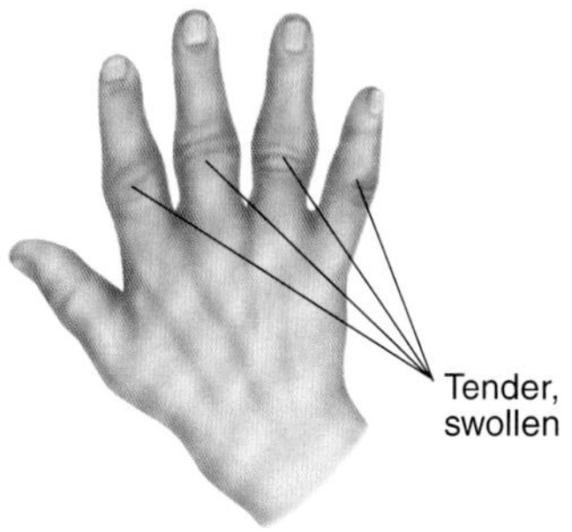

Chronic Rheumatoid Arthritis

In chronic disease, note the swelling and thickening of the metacarpophalangeal and proximal interphalangeal joints. Range of motion becomes limited, and fingers may deviate toward the ulnar side. The interosseous muscles atrophy. The fingers may show *"swan neck" deformities* (hyperextension of the proximal interphalangeal joints with fixed flexion of the distal interphalangeal joints). Less common is a *boutonnière deformity* (persistent flexion of the proximal interphalangeal joint with hyperextension of the distal interphalangeal joint). Rheumatoid nodules are seen in the acute or the chronic stage.

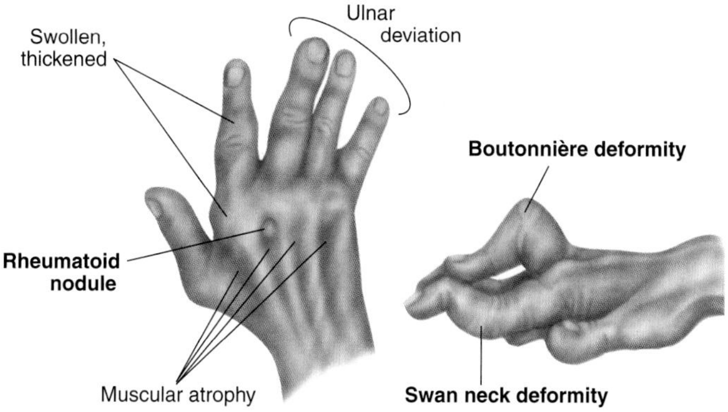

Osteoarthritis *(Degenerative Joint Disease)*

Heberden nodes on the dorsolateral aspects of the distal interphalangeal joints from bony overgrowth of osteoarthritis. Usually hard and painless, they affect middle-aged or older adults; often associated with arthritic changes in other joints. Flexion and deviation deformities may develop. *Bouchard nodes* on the proximal interphalangeal joints are less common. The metacarpophalangeal joints are spared.

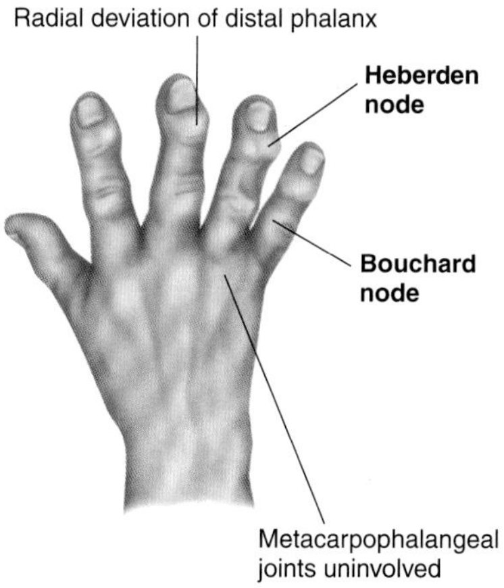

Chronic Tophaceous Gout (American College of Physicians, 2012)

The deformities of long-standing chronic tophaceous gout can mimic rheumatoid arthritis and osteoarthritis. Joint involvement is usually not as symmetric as in rheumatoid arthritis. Acute inflammation may be present. Knobby swellings around the joints ulcerate and discharge white chalk-like urates.

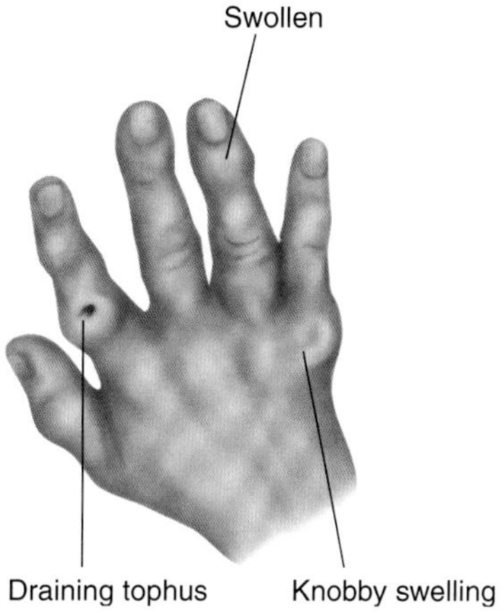

TABLE 18-10 Swellings and Deformities of the Hands

Dupuytren Contracture

The first sign of a *Dupuytren contracture* is a thickened plaque overlying the flexor tendon of the ring finger and possibly the little finger at the level of the distal palmar crease. Subsequently, the skin in this area puckers, and a thickened fibrotic cord develops between palm and finger. Flexion contracture of the fingers may gradually develop.

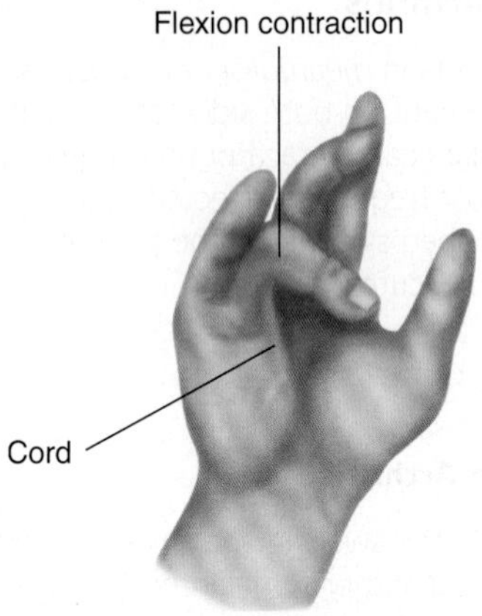

Trigger Finger

Caused by a painless nodule in a flexor tendon in the palm near the metacarpal head. The nodule is too big to enter easily into the tendon sheath during extension of the fingers from a flexed position. With extra effort or assistance, the finger extends and flexes with a palpable and audible snap as the nodule pops into the tendon sheath. Watch, listen, and palpate the nodule as the patient flexes and extends the fingers.

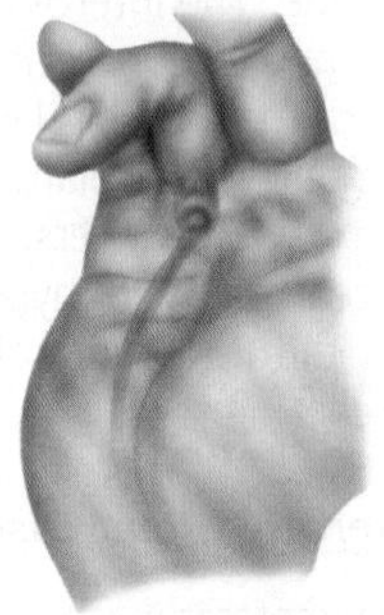

Thenar Atrophy

Thenar atrophy suggests a *median nerve disorder* such as *carpal tunnel syndrome*. Hypothenar atrophy suggests an *ulnar nerve disorder*.

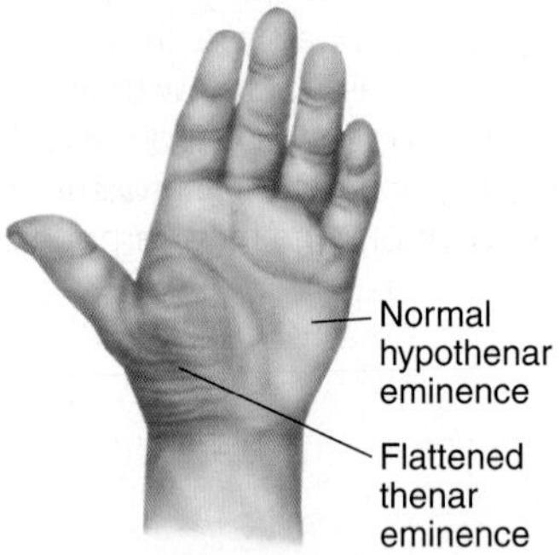

Ganglion

Ganglia are cystic, round, usually nontender swellings along tendon sheaths or joint capsules, frequently at the dorsum of the wrist. The cyst contains synovial fluid. Flexion of the wrist makes ganglia more prominent; extension tends to obscure them. Ganglia may also develop elsewhere on the hands, wrists, ankles, and feet. They can disappear spontaneously.

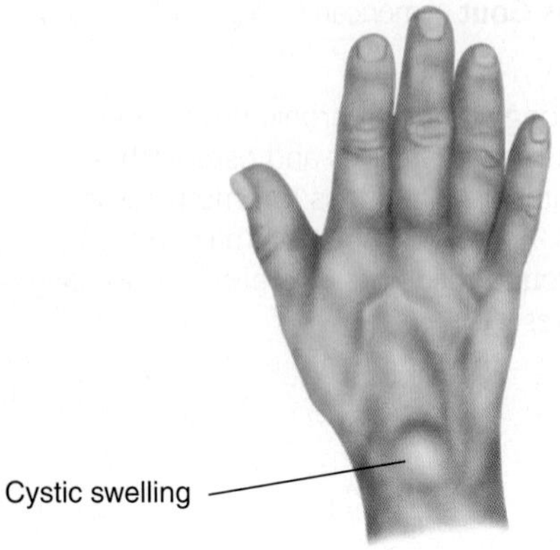

Observe the contours of the palm, namely, the thenar and hypothenar eminences.

Thenar atrophy may be due to median nerve compression from *carpal tunnel syndrome*; hypothenar atrophy is seen in *ulnar nerve compression.*

Note any thickening of the flexor tendons or flexion contractures in the fingers.

Flexion contractures in the ring, fifth, and third fingers, or *Dupuytren contractures*, arise from thickening of the palmar fascia.

Palpation

At the wrist, palpate the distal radius and ulna on the lateral and medial surfaces. Palpate the groove of each wrist joint with your thumbs on the dorsum of the wrist, your fingers beneath it (Fig. 18-29). Note any swelling, bogginess, or tenderness.

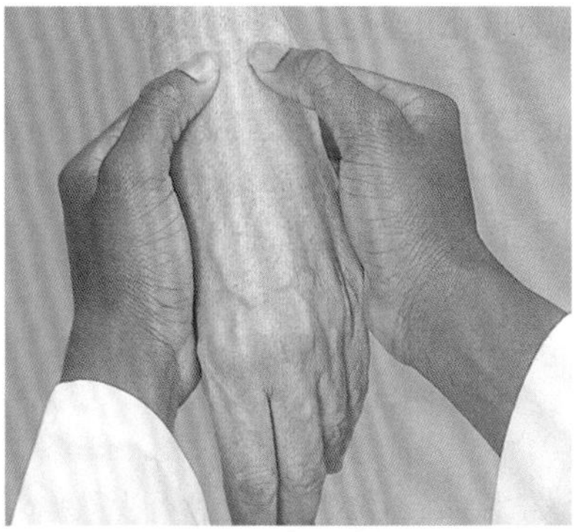

FIGURE 18-29 Palpating the wrist.

Any tenderness or bony step-offs are suspicious for fracture.

Swelling and/or tenderness suggest *rheumatoid arthritis* if bilateral and of several weeks' duration.

Palpate the radial styloid bone and the *anatomic snuffbox*, a hollowed depression just distal to the radial styloid process formed by the abductor and extensor muscles of the thumb (Fig. 18-30). The "snuffbox" becomes more visible with lateral extension of the thumb away from the hand.

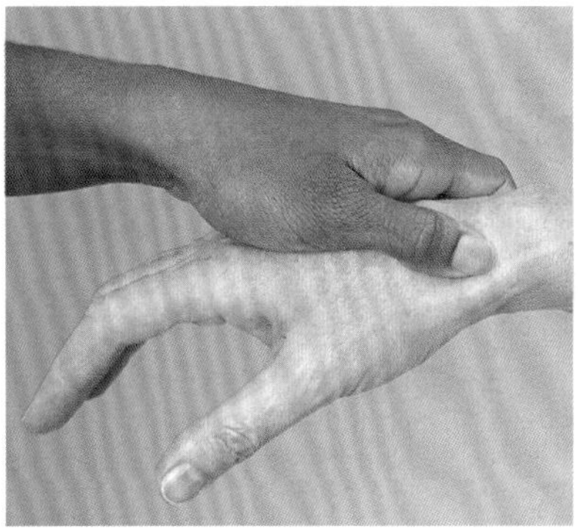

FIGURE 18-30 Palpating the anatomic snuffbox.

Tenderness over the "snuffbox" occurs in *scaphoid fracture,* the most common injury of the carpal bones.

Palpate the eight carpal bones lying distal to the wrist joint, and then each of the five metacarpals and the proximal, middle, and distal phalanges (Fig. 18-31).

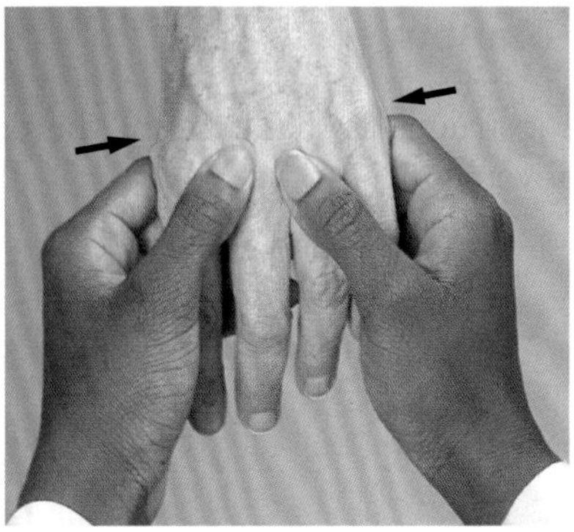

FIGURE 18-31 Palpating the MCP joints (*arrows*) of the hand.

Synovitis in the MCP joints is painful with this pressure, which will cause pain when shaking hands.

Palpate any other area where you suspect an abnormality.

The MCP joints are often boggy or tender in *rheumatoid arthritis* (but rarely involved in osteoarthritis).

Compress the MCP joints by squeezing the hand from each side between the thumb and fingers. Alternatively, use your thumb to palpate each MCP joint just distal to and on each side of the knuckle as your index finger feels the head of the metacarpal in the palm. Note any swelling, bogginess, or tenderness.

Now examine the fingers and thumb. Palpate the medial and lateral aspects of each PIP joint between your thumb and index finger, again checking for swelling, bogginess, bony enlargement, or tenderness.

Bouchard nodes (bony enlargements) are seen with *osteoarthritis* at the PIP joints.

Using the same techniques, examine the DIP joints (Fig. 18-32). Hard dorsolateral nodules on the DIP joints (Fig. 18-33), or *Heberden nodes*, are common in osteoarthritis.

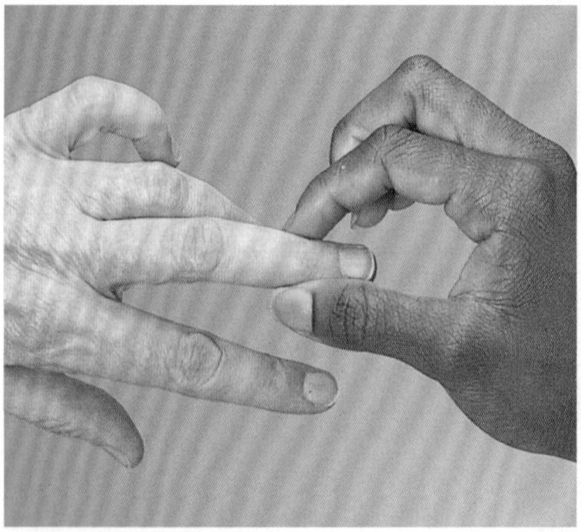

FIGURE 18-32 Palpating the DIP joints.

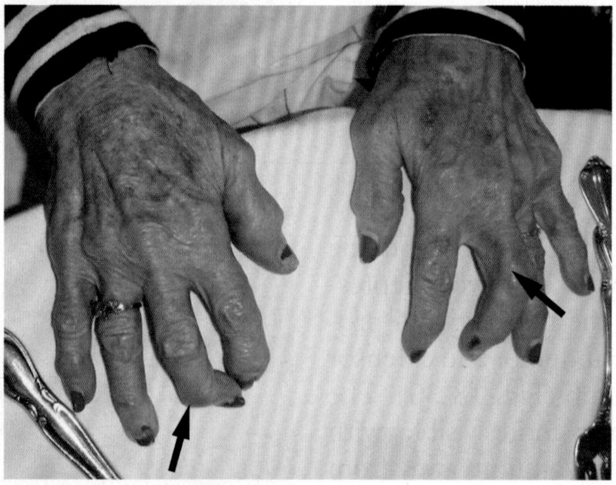

FIGURE 18-33 Heberden and Bouchard nodes seen in osteoarthritis. (Courtesy of Beth Hogan-Quigley, MSN, RN, CRNP, University of Pennsylvania School of Nursing, Philadelphia, PA.)

In any area of swelling or inflammation, palpate along the tendons inserting on the thumb and fingers.

Wrists: Range of Motion and Maneuvers

Refer to Table 18-11 for clear, simple instructions that prompt the patient and the muscles responsible for each movement.

Conditions that impair range of motion include *arthritis*, *tenosynovitis*, and *Dupuytren contracture*. See Table 18-10.

TABLE 18-11 Assessing Wrist Movement

Wrist Movement	Patient Instructions	Primary Muscles Affecting Movement	Illustration
Flexion	*"With your palms down, point your fingers toward the floor."*	Flexor carpi radialis, flexor carpi ulnaris	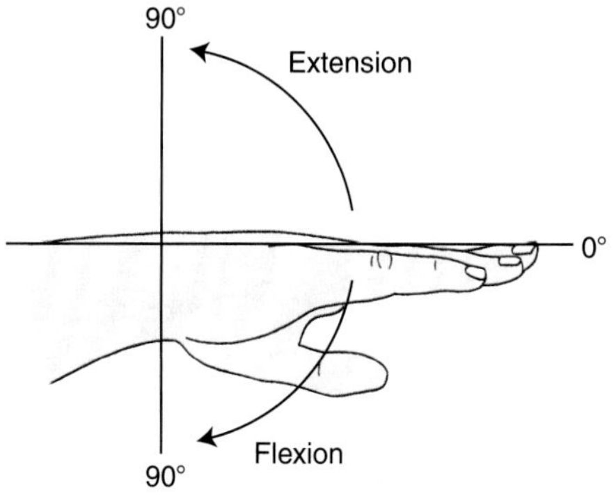
Extension	*"With your palms down, point your fingers toward the ceiling."*	Extensor carpi ulnaris, extensor carpi radialis longus, extensor carpi radialis brevis	
Adduction (radial deviation)	*"With your palms down, bring your fingers toward the midline."*	Flexor carpi ulnaris	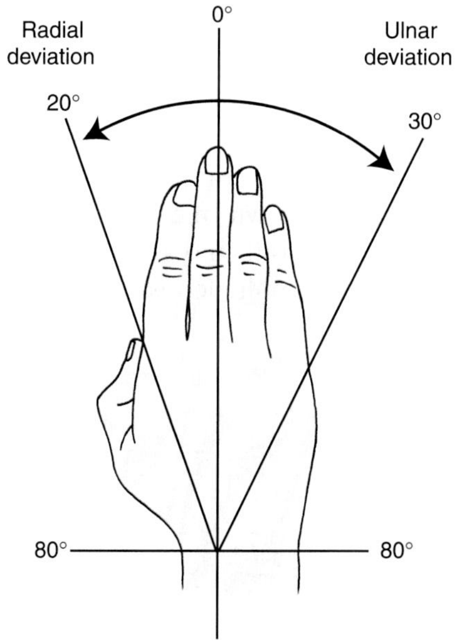
Abduction (ulnar deviation)	*"With your palms down, bring your fingers away from the midline."*	Flexor carpi radialis	

Muscle Strength Tests

Test extension at the wrist (C6, C7, C8, radial nerve—extensor carpi radialis longus and brevis). Ask the patient to make a fist; place your hand on top of the patient's fist; ask the patient to resist your effort to push down his fist (Fig. 18-34).

Weakness of extension is seen in peripheral nerve disease such as radial nerve damage and in central nervous system disease producing hemiplegia, as in *stroke* or *multiple sclerosis.*

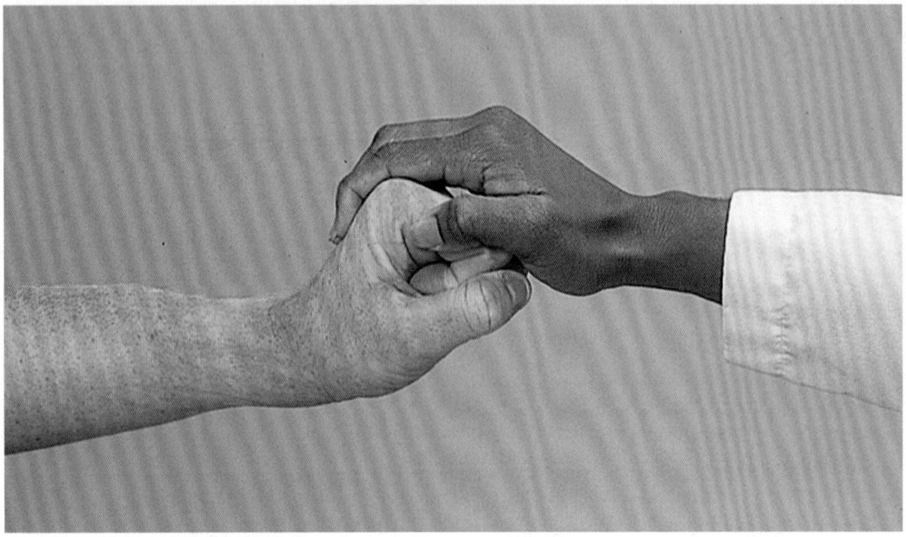

FIGURE 18-34 Testing extension at the wrist.

Test the grip (C7, C8, T1). Ask the patient to squeeze two of your fingers as hard as possible and not let them go (Fig. 18-35). (To avoid getting hurt by hard squeezes, place your own middle finger on top of your index finger.) You should normally have difficulty removing your fingers from the patient's grip. Testing both grips simultaneously with the arms extended or in the lap facilitates comparison.

A weak grip may be present in cervical radiculopathy, *carpal tunnel syndrome,* arthritis, and epicondylitis.

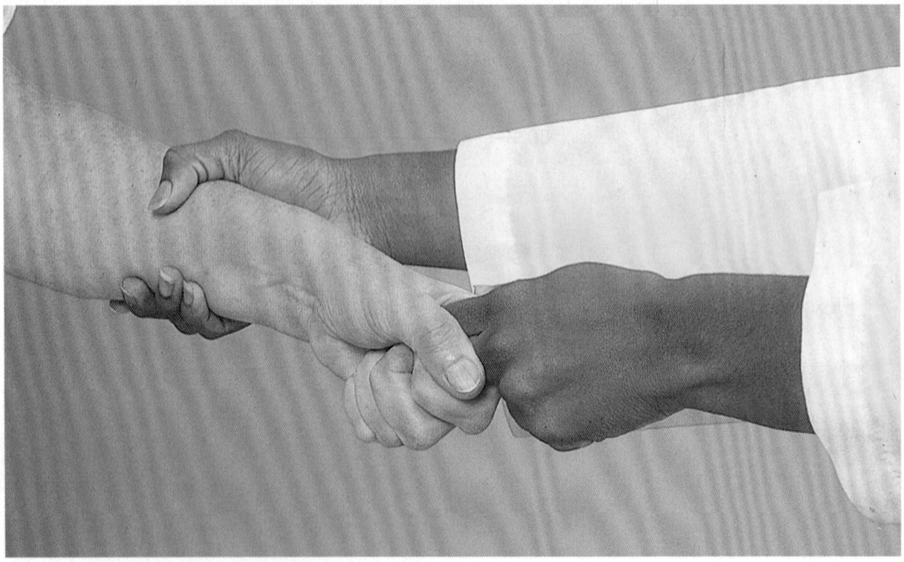

FIGURE 18-35 Testing hand grip strength.

Maneuvers to Test for Carpal Tunnel Syndrome

Several maneuvers useful for assessing common complaints relating to the wrist follow. For complaints of dropping objects, inability to twist lids off jars, aching at the wrist or even the forearm, and numbness of the first three digits, use the tests for assessing *carpal tunnel syndrome*. Note the distribution of the median, radial, and ulnar nerve innervations of the wrist and hand in Figure 18-36.

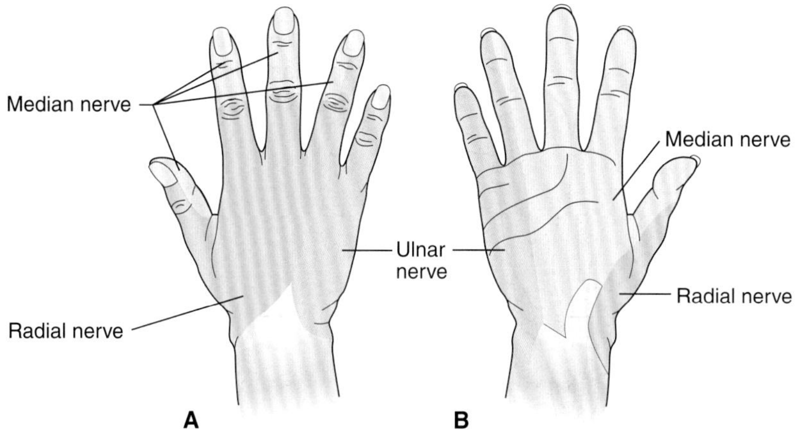

FIGURE 18-36 Dorsal view (**A**) and palmar view (**B**) of peripheral innervation of the hand.

CLINICAL TIP
Onset of *carpal tunnel syndrome* is often related to repetitive motion with wrists flexed (as in keyboard use, mail sorting), pregnancy, rheumatoid arthritis, diabetes, and hypothyroidism. Thenar atrophy may also be present. Decreased sensation in the median nerve distribution is common in *carpal tunnel syndrome*.

Test sensation of:

- the index finger pad—median nerve.
- the fifth finger pad—ulnar nerve.
- dorsal web space of the thumb and index finger—radial nerve.

Test *thumb abduction* by asking the patient to raise the thumb straight up as you apply downward resistance (Fig. 18-37) (McGee, 2018d; Sauvé et al., 2014).

Weak thumb abduction and decreased sensation indicate carpal tunnel disease.

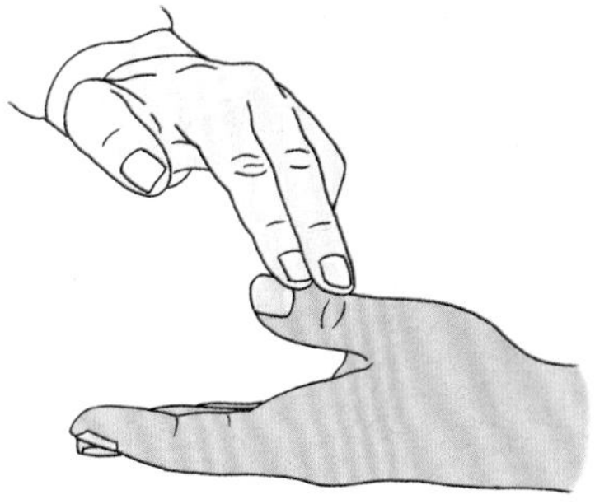

FIGURE 18-37 Testing thumb abduction.

Test for the *Tinel sign* for median nerve compression by tapping lightly over the course of the median nerve in the carpal tunnel as shown in Figure 18-38 (McGee, 2018d; Sauvé et al., 2014).

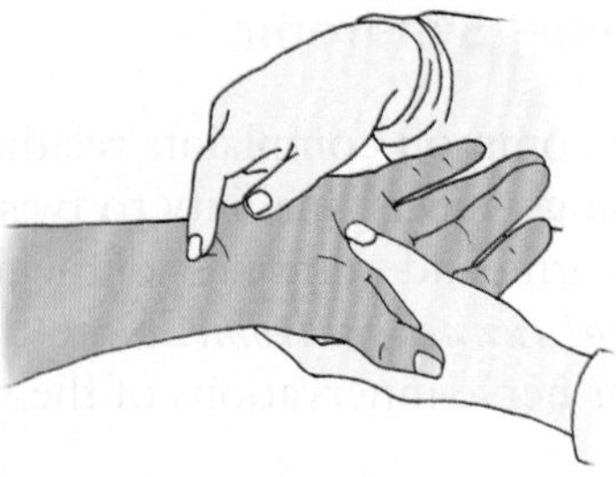

FIGURE 18-38 Testing for the Tinel sign.

Aching and numbness in the median nerve distribution is a *positive test.*

Test the *Phalen sign* for median nerve compression by asking the patient to hold the wrists in flexion for 60 seconds. Alternatively, ask the patient to press the backs of both hands together to form right angles (Fig. 18-39). These maneuvers compress the median nerve (McGee, 2018d; Sauvé et al., 2014).

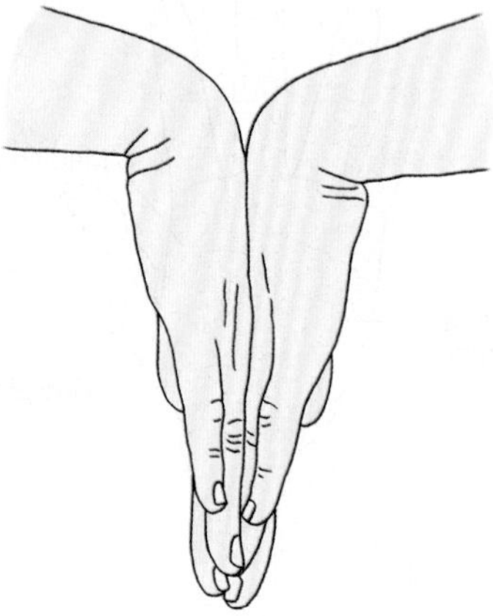

FIGURE 18-39 Compressing the median nerve to test for carpal tunnel syndrome.

Numbness and tingling in the median nerve distribution within 60 seconds is a *positive test result.*

Fingers and Thumbs: Range of Motion

Fingers

Assess *flexion*, *extension*, *abduction*, and *adduction* of the fingers:

- *Flexion and extension*—For *flexion* (Fig. 18-40A), to test the finger flexor muscles, ask the patient to "*Make a tight fist with each hand, thumb across the knuckles.*" For *extension,* to test the finger extensor muscles, ask the patient to "*Extend and spread the fingers.*" The fingers should open and close easily.
- *Abduction and adduction*—Ask the patient to spread the fingers apart (abduction from dorsal interossei, Fig. 18-40B) and back together (adduction from palmar interossei). Check for smooth, coordinated movement.

Impaired hand movement occurs in arthritis, trigger finger, and Dupuytren contracture.

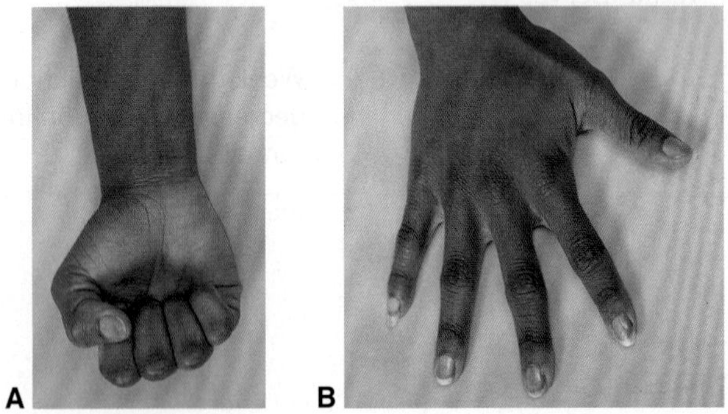

FIGURE 18-40 **A.** Flexion of the fingers. **B.** Abduction of the fingers.

Thumbs

At the *thumb*, assess *flexion*, *extension*, *abduction*, *adduction*, and *opposition*. Each of these movements is powered by a related muscle of the thumb. Ask the patient to move the thumb across the palm and touch the base of the fifth finger to test *flexion* (Fig. 18-41A), and then to move the thumb back across the palm and away from the fingers to test *extension* (Fig. 18-41B).

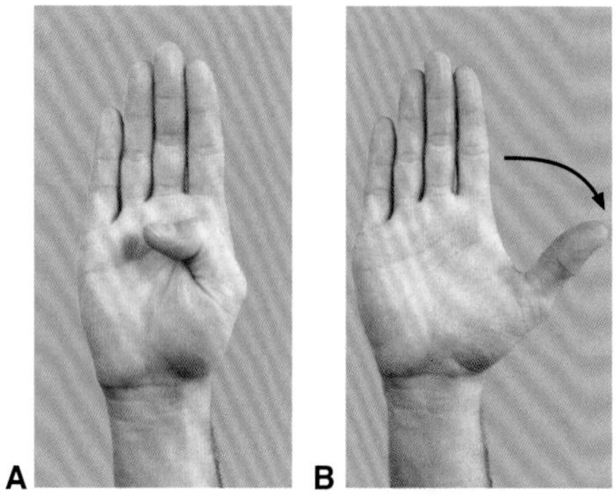

FIGURE 18-41 **A.** Flexion of the thumb. **B.** Extension of the thumb.

Next, ask the patient to place the fingers and thumb in the neutral position with the palm up; then have the patient move the thumb anteriorly away from the palm to assess *abduction* and back down for *adduction* (Fig. 18-42A). To test *opposition* or movements of the thumb across the palm, ask the patient to touch the thumb to the base of the small finger (Fig. 18-42B).

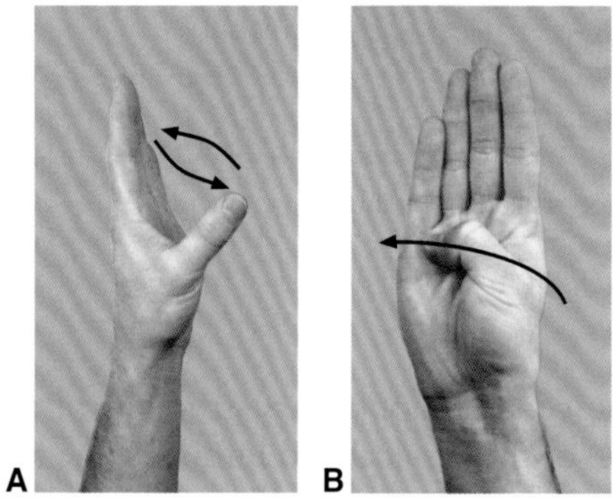

FIGURE 18-42 **A.** Abduction and adduction of the thumb. **B.** Opposition of the thumb.

Finger Muscle Strength Tests

Test finger abduction (C8, T1, ulnar nerve). Position the patient's hand with palm down and fingers spread. Instructing the patient not to let you move the fingers, try to force them together (Fig. 18-43).

Weak finger abduction occurs in ulnar nerve disorders.

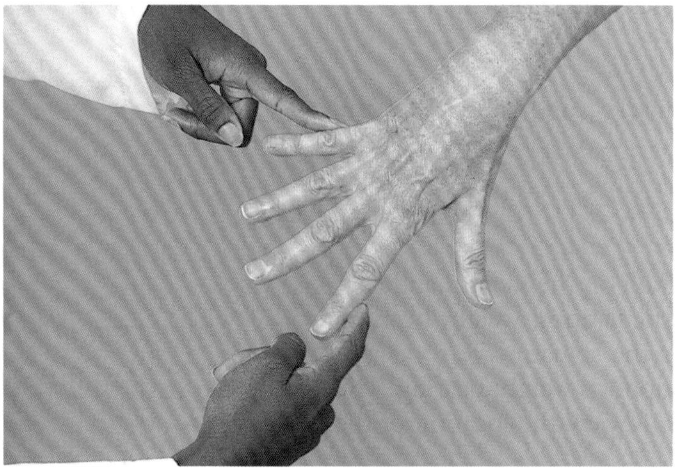
FIGURE 18-43 Testing strength with finger abduction.

Test opposition of the thumb (C8, T1, median nerve). The patient should try to touch the tip of the little finger with the thumb, against your resistance (Fig. 18-44).

Weak opposition of the thumb occurs in median nerve disorders such as *carpal tunnel syndrome*.

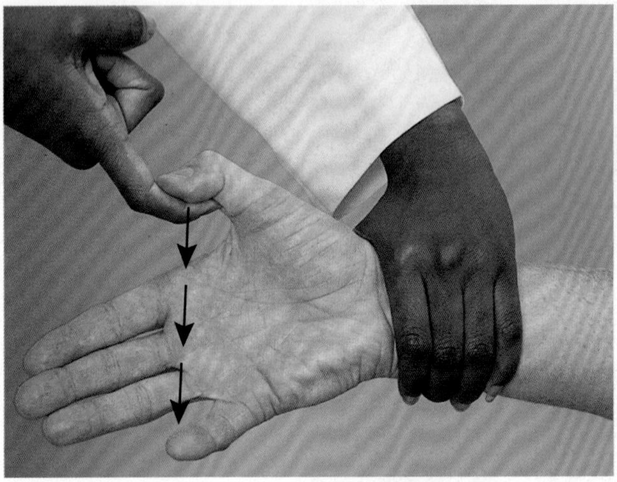

FIGURE 18-44 Testing strength of opposition of the thumb.

THE SPINE

The vertebral column, or spine, is the central supporting structure of the trunk and back. Note the *concave curves* of the cervical and lumbar spine and the *convex curves* of the thoracic and sacrococcygeal spine. These curves help distribute upper body weight to the pelvis and lower extremities and cushion the concussive impact of walking or running.

The complex mechanics of the back reflect the coordinated action of:

- the vertebrae and intervertebral discs.
- an interconnecting system of ligaments between anterior and posterior vertebrae, ligaments between the spinous processes, and ligaments between the lamina of two adjacent vertebrae.
- large superficial muscles, deeper intrinsic muscles, and muscles of the abdominal wall.

Bony Structures

The vertebral column contains 24 vertebrae stacked on the sacrum and coccyx. A typical vertebra contains sites for joint articulations, weight bearing, and muscle attachments, as well as foramina for the spinal nerve roots and peripheral nerves. Anteriorly, the *vertebral body* supports weight bearing. The posterior *vertebral arch* encloses the spinal cord. Review the location of the vertebral processes and foramina: Note:

- The *spinous process* projecting posteriorly in the midline and the two transverse processes. Muscles attach at these processes.

- The *articular processes*—two on each side of the vertebra, one facing up and one facing down, allow the vertebrae to articulate with each other, therefore often called *articular facets.*

- The *vertebral foramen*, which encloses the spinal cord, the *intervertebral foramen*, formed by the inferior and superior articulating process of adjacent vertebrae, creating a channel for the spinal nerve roots; and in the cervical vertebrae, the *transverse foramen* for the vertebral artery.

Figures 18-45 and 18-46 show examples of cervical and lumbar vertebrae.

The proximity of the spinal cord and spinal nerve roots to their bony vertebral casing and the intervertebral discs makes them especially vulnerable to disc herniation, impingement from degenerative changes in the vertebrae, and trauma.

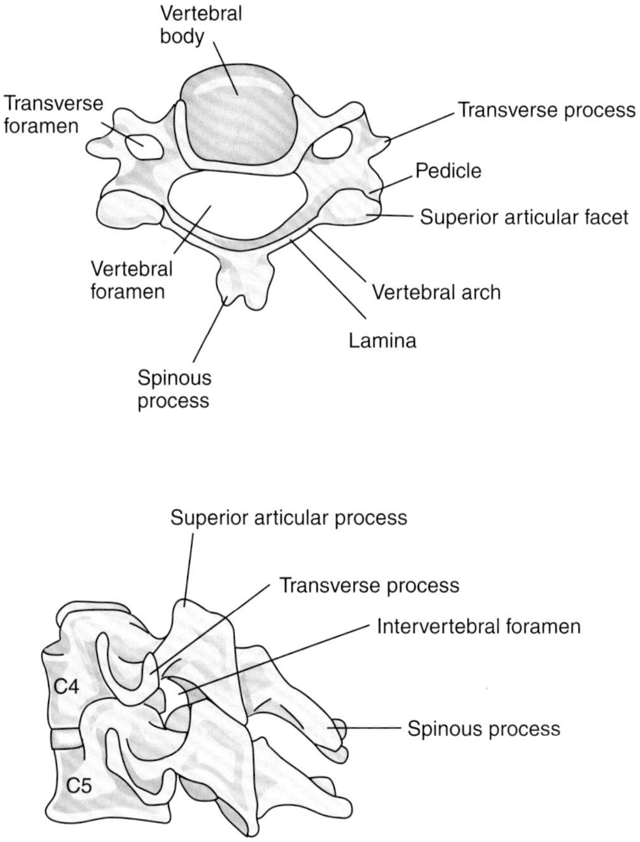

FIGURE 18-45 Coronal and lateral views of cervical vertebrae C4 and C5.

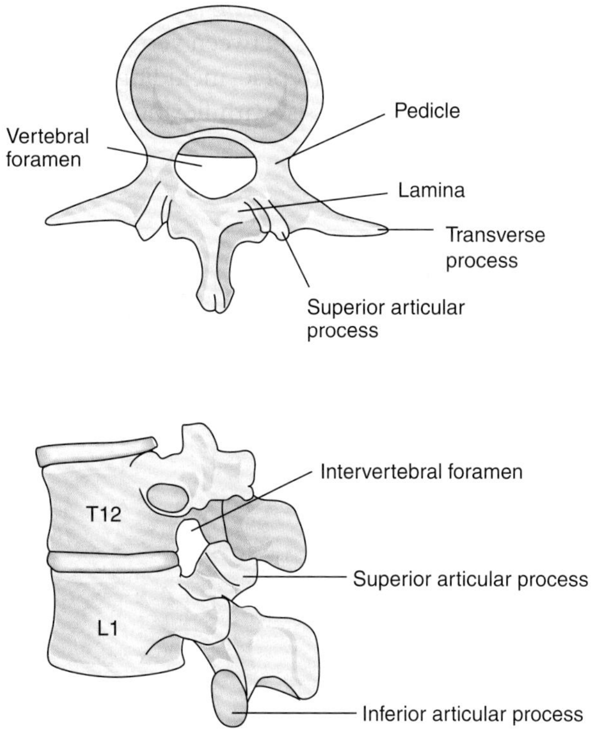

FIGURE 18-46 Coronal and lateral views of thoracic and lumbar vertebrae T12 and L1.

Joints

The spine has slightly movable cartilaginous joints between the vertebral bodies and between the articular facets. Between the vertebral bodies are the ***intervertebral discs,*** each consisting of a soft mucoid central core, the ***nucleus pulposus,*** rimmed by the tough fibrous tissue of the ***annulus fibrosis.*** The intervertebral discs cushion movement between vertebrae and allow the vertebral column to curve, flex, and bend (Fig. 18-47).

Note that the vertebral column angles sharply posterior at the ***lumbosacral junction*** and becomes immovable. The mechanical stress at this angulation contributes to the risk for disc herniation and subluxation, or slippage, of L5 on S1.

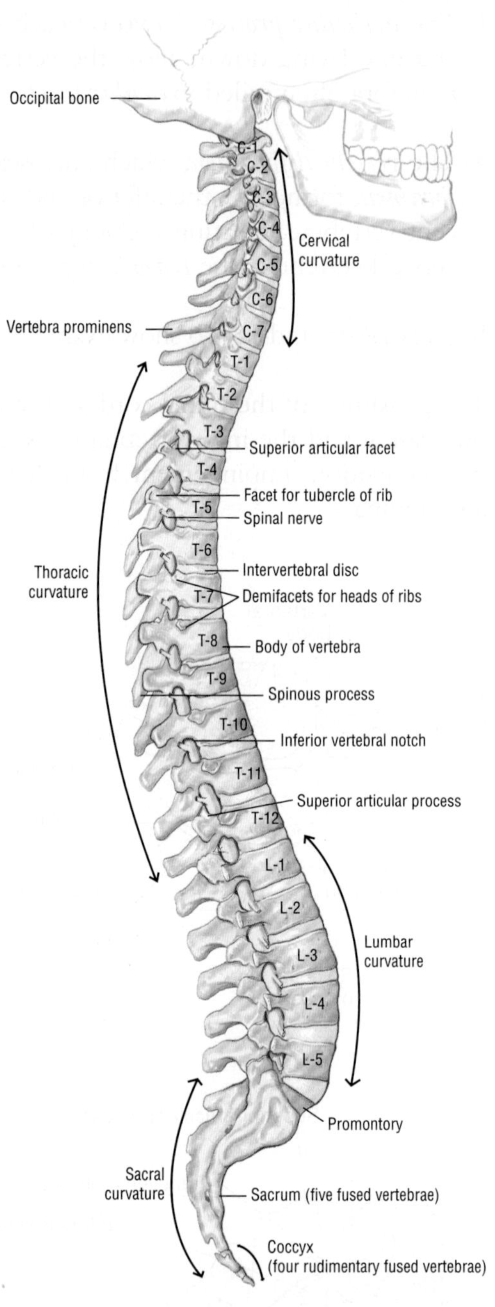

FIGURE 18-47 The cervical, thoracic, lumbar, and sacral curves of the spine.

Muscle Groups

The ***trapezius*** and ***latissimus dorsi*** form the large outer layer of muscles attaching to each side of the spine (Fig. 18-48). They overlie two deeper muscle layers—a layer attaching to the head, neck, and spinous processes (*splenius capitis, splenius cervicis,* and *sacrospinalis*) and a layer of smaller intrinsic muscles between vertebrae. Muscles attaching to the anterior surface of the vertebrae, including the *psoas* muscle and muscles of the abdominal wall, assist with flexion.

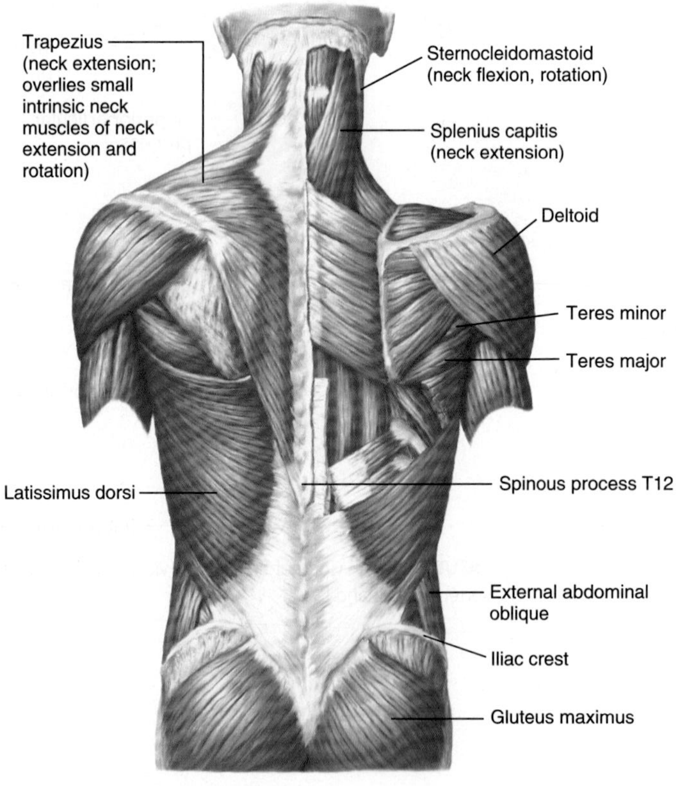

FIGURE 18-48 Muscles of the back.

Physical Examination

Inspection

Begin by observing the patient's posture, including the position of both the neck and trunk, when entering the room.

Assess the patient for erect position of the head; smooth, coordinated neck movement; and ease of gait.

Neck stiffness may signal arthritis, muscle strain, or other underlying pathology.

Drape or gown the patient to expose the entire back for complete inspection. If possible, the patient should be upright in the natural standing position, with feet together and arms hanging at the sides. The head should be midline in the same plane as the sacrum, and the shoulders and pelvis should be level.

Lateral deviation and rotation of the head suggest *torticollis* from contraction of the sternocleidomastoid muscle.

Viewing the patient from behind (Fig. 18-49), identify the following landmarks:

- Spinous processes of C7 and T1 are usually more prominent with forward neck flexion
- Paravertebral muscles on either side of the midline
- Iliac crests
- Posterior superior iliac spines, usually marked by skin dimples

A line drawn above the posterior iliac crests crosses the spinous process of L4.

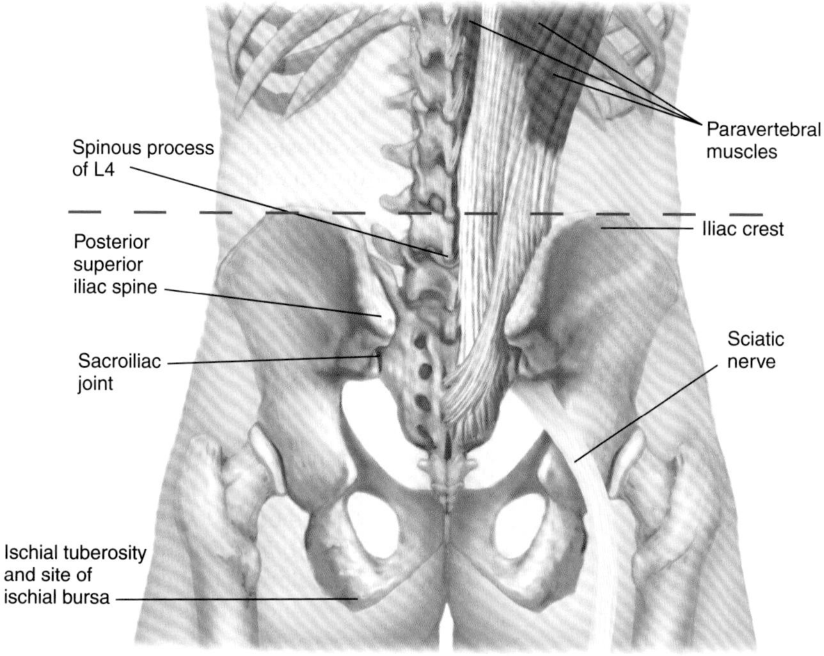

FIGURE 18-49 Anatomy of the lower back.

Inspect the patient from the side and from behind. Evaluate the spinal curvatures and the features described in Table 18-12.

TABLE 18-12 Inspection of the Spine

View of Patient	Focus of Inspection	Illustration
From the Side	Cervical, thoracic, and lumbar curves Kyphosis—increased thoracic curvature Lordosis—increased lumbar curvature	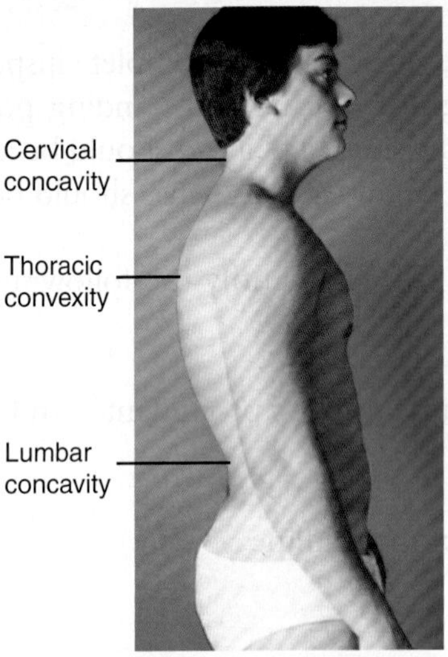
From Behind	Upright spinal column (an imaginary line should fall straight from C7 through the gluteal cleft) Alignment of the shoulders, the iliac crests, and the skin creases below the buttocks (gluteal folds) Scoliosis—lateral curvature of the spine **CLINICAL TIP** ***Unequal shoulder heights*** **are seen in scoliosis.** ***Unequal heights of the iliac crests,*** **or** ***pelvic tilt,*** **suggest scoliosis. Unequal leg lengths also cause pelvic tilt. The tilt will disappear when a block is placed under the short leg and foot.** If scoliosis is suspected, perform the Adam forward bend test and use a scoliometer to test for the degree of scoliosis. See further discussion in Chapter 23, "Assessing Children: Infancy through Adolescence." Note any skin markings, tags, or masses.	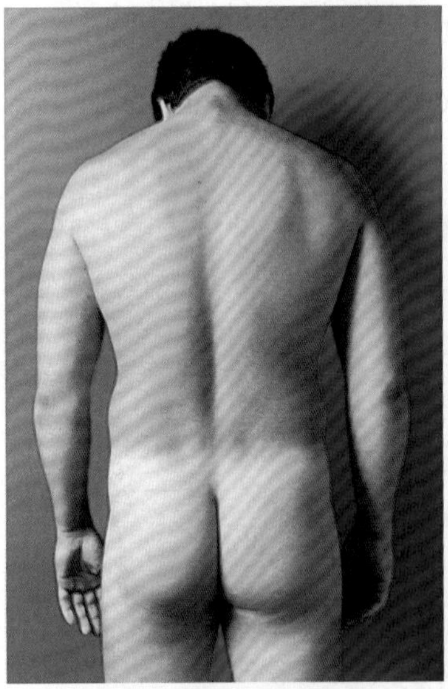

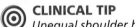

Increased *thoracic kyphosis* often occurs with aging. In children, a correctable structural deformity should be referred to an advanced practitioner.

In *scoliosis*, there is lateral and compensatory curvature of the spine to bring the head back to midline. Scoliosis often becomes evident during adolescence.

Birthmarks, port wine stains, hairy patches, and lipomas often overlie bony defects such as *spina bifida.* Café-au-lait spots (discolored patches of skin), skin tags, and fibrous tumors are seen in *neurofibromatosis*

Palpation

From a sitting or standing position, palpate the spinous processes of each vertebra with your thumb. Note any tenderness and/or whether any spinous process appears more forward or recessed from its neighbor.

Tenderness suggests fracture or dislocation if preceded by trauma; if no trauma, suspect infection or arthritis. Forward slippage of one of the lumbar vertebra may compress the spinal cord.

Palpate over the *sacroiliac joint*, often identified by the dimple overlying the posterior superior iliac spine.

Inspect and palpate the *paravertebral muscles* for tenderness and spasm. Muscles in spasm feel firm and knotted and may be visible.

Spasm occurs in degenerative and inflammatory processes of muscles, prolonged contraction from abnormal posture, or anxiety.

With the hip flexed and the patient lying on the opposite side, palpate the *sciatic nerve* (Fig. 18-50), the largest nerve in the body, consisting of nerve roots from L4, L5, S1, S2, and S3. The nerve lies midway between the greater trochanter and the ischial tuberosity as it leaves the pelvis through the sciatic notch.

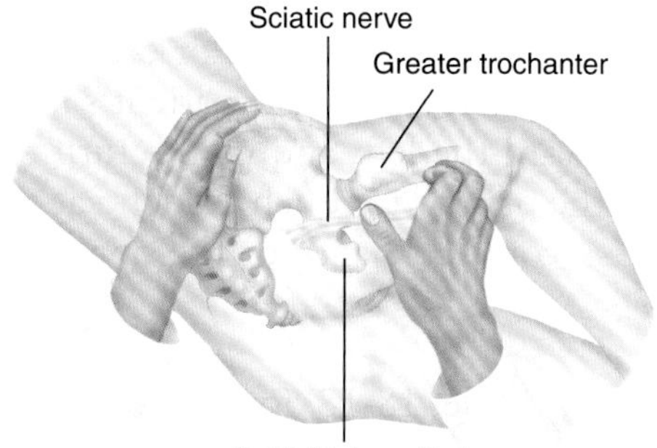

FIGURE 18-50 Palpating the sciatic nerve.

Sciatic nerve tenderness suggests a herniated disc or mass lesion impinging on the contributing nerve roots.

Herniated intervertebral discs, most common at L5-S1 or L4-L5, may produce tenderness of the spinous processes, the intervertebral joints, the paravertebral muscles, the sacrosciatic notch, and the sciatic nerve.

Palpate for tenderness in any other areas (Fig. 18-51) that are suggested by the patient's symptoms.

Rheumatoid arthritis may also cause tenderness of the intervertebral joints.

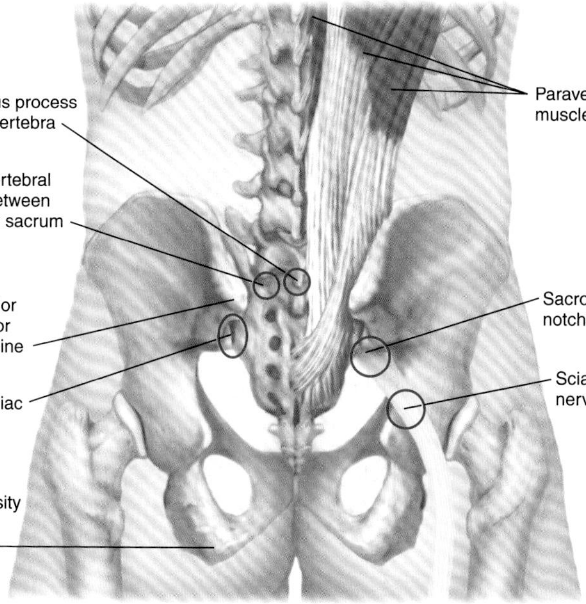

FIGURE 18-51 Other areas of the lower back to palpate for tenderness.

CLINICAL TIP
Remember that tenderness in the costovertebral angles may signify kidney infection rather than a musculoskeletal problem.

See Table 18-3, "Low Back Pain."

Range of Motion and Maneuvers

Range of Motion of the Neck

The neck is the most mobile portion of the spine, remarkable for its seven fragile vertebrae supporting the 10- to 15-lb head. *Flexion* and *extension* occur primarily between the skull and C1, the atlas; *rotation* at C1 to C2, the axis; and *lateral bending* at C2 to C7.

Limitations in range of motion can arise from stiffness from arthritis, pain from trauma, or muscle spasm such as *torticollis.*

Muscle Strength Test of the Neck

Muscle strength of the neck may be tested with range of motion by the examiner placing a hand to resist the motion of the patient. For example, to test rotation, place your right hand on the left side of the patient's face and ask the patient to rotate the head toward the left, and then return to midline; then, to test lateral flexion, ask the patient to touch the left ear to the shoulder against your resistance. Use your left hand for the opposite side.

Assess neck range of motion referring to Table 18-13 for clear, simple instructions that prompt the patient and the muscles responsible for each movement.

Neck, shoulder, or arm pain or numbness may indicate cervical cord or nerve root compression. See Table 18-4, "Pains in the Neck."

If the patient has tenderness, loss of sensation, muscle weakness or impaired movement, perform neurologic testing of the neck and upper extremities.

TABLE 18-13 Assessing Range of Motion of the Neck

Neck Movement	Patient Instructions	Primary Muscles Affecting Movement
Flexion	*"Bring your chin to your chest."*	Sternocleidomastoid, scalene, prevertebral muscles
Extension	*"Look up at the ceiling."*	Splenius capitis and cervicis, small intrinsic neck muscles
Rotation	*"Look over one shoulder, and then the other."*	Sternocleidomastoid, small intrinsic neck muscles
Lateral flexion	*"Bring your ear to your shoulder."*	Scalenes and small intrinsic neck muscles

Range of Motion: The Spinal Column

Next assess range of motion in the spinal column. Refer to Table 18-14 for clear, simple instructions that prompt the patient and the muscles responsible for each movement.

TABLE 18-14 Assessing Range of Motion of the Spinal Column

Back Movement	Patient Instructions	Primary Muscles Affecting Movement	Illustration
Flexion To measure flexion of the spine, mark the spine at the lumbosacral junction, then 10 cm above and 5 cm below the first mark. A 4-cm increase between the two upper marks is normal; the distance between the lower two marks should be unchanged.	*"Bend forward and try to touch your toes."* Note the smoothness and symmetry of movement, the range of motion, and the curve in the lumbar area. As flexion proceeds, the lumbar concavity should flatten out.	Psoas major, psoas minor, quadratus lumborum; abdominal muscles attaching to the anterior vertebrae, such as the internal and external obliques and rectus abdominis	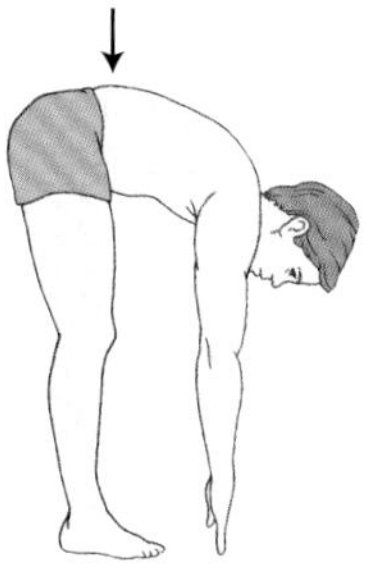 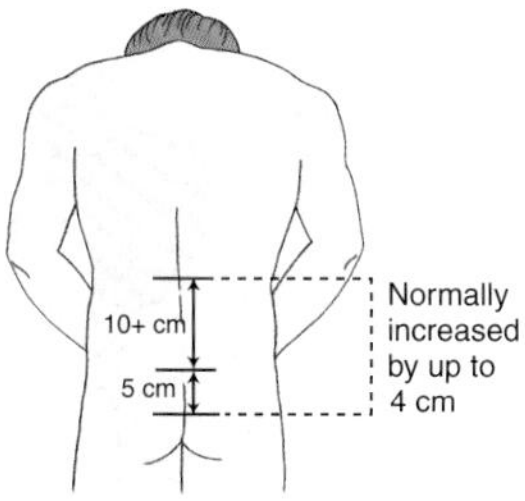
Extension	*"Bend back as far as possible."* Support the patient by placing your hand on the posterior superior iliac spine, with your fingers pointing toward the midline.	Deep intrinsic muscles of the back, such as the erector spinae and transversospinalis groups	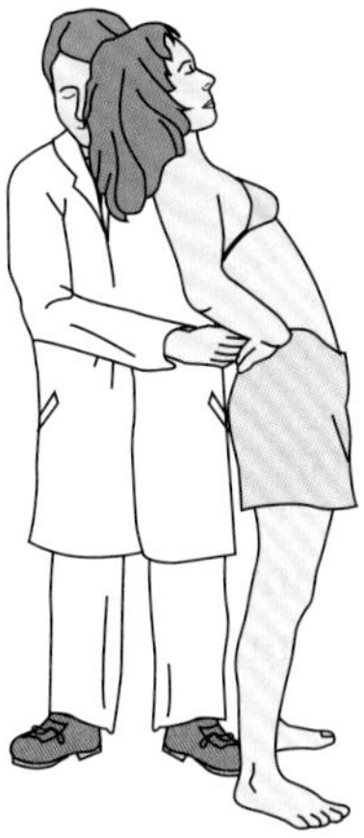

(continued)

Deformity of the thorax on forward bending is seen in *scoliosis.*

Persistence of lumbar lordosis with flexion suggests muscle spasm or *ankylosing spondylitis.*

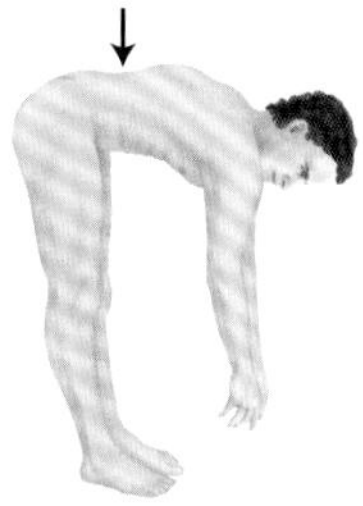

Provide support to patient if they are unsteady while bending backward.

TABLE **18-14** **Assessing Range of Motion of the Spinal Column** (*Continued*)

Back Movement	Patient Instructions	Primary Muscles Affecting Movement	Illustration
Rotation	*"Rotate from side to side."* Stabilize the patient's pelvis by placing one hand on the patient's hip and the other on the opposite shoulder. Then rotate the trunk by pulling the shoulder and then the hip posteriorly. Repeat these maneuvers for the opposite side.	Abdominal muscles, intrinsic muscles of the back	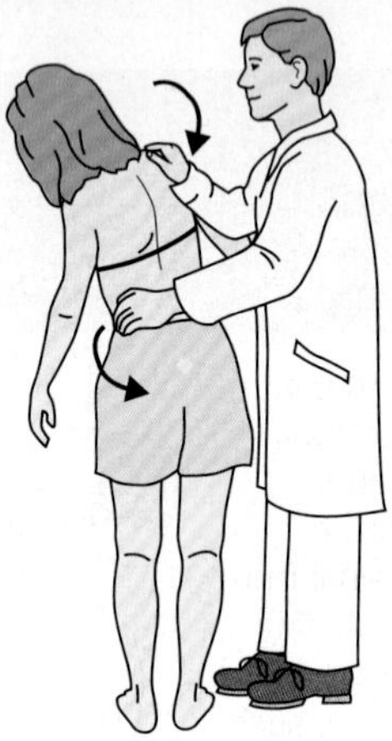
Lateral flexion	*"Bend to the side from the waist."* Stabilize the patient's pelvis by placing your hand on the patient's hip. Repeat for the opposite side.	Abdominal muscles, intrinsic muscles of the back	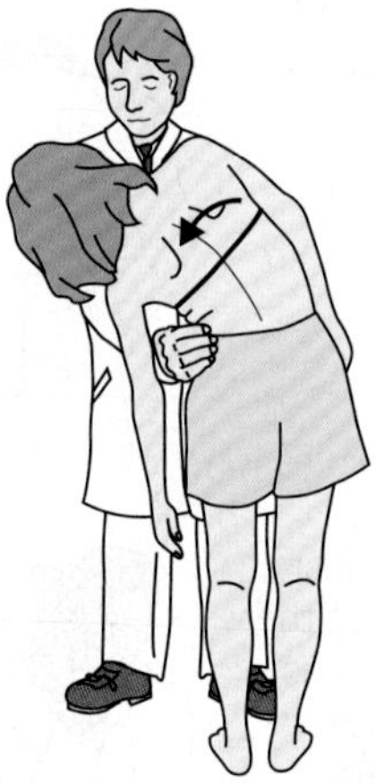

Decreased *spinal mobility* is seen in *osteoarthritis* and *ankylosing spondylitis.*

Muscle Strength Test: The Spinal Column

Assessment of muscle strength of the spinal column may also be performed during the range-of-motion assessment by having the patient flex, extend, and flex laterally against resistance.

Pain or tenderness with these maneuvers, particularly with radiation into the leg, warrants neurologic testing of the lower extremities and referral to an advanced practitioner or physician.

Pain may indicate cord or nerve root compression. Arthritis or infection in the hip, rectum, or pelvis may cause symptoms in the lumbar spine. See Table 18-3, "Low Back Pain." See also Chapter 20, "The Nervous System."

THE HIP

The hip joint is deeply embedded in the pelvis and is notable for its strength, stability, and wide range of motion. The stability of the hip joint, so essential for weight bearing, arises from the deep fit of the head of the femur into the *acetabulum*, its strong fibrous articular capsule, and the powerful muscles crossing the joint and inserting below the femoral head, providing leverage for movement of the femur.

Bony Structures and Joints

The hip joint lies below the middle third of the inguinal ligament but in a deeper plane. It is a ball-and-socket joint—note how the rounded head of the femur articulates with the cup-like cavity of the acetabulum. Because of its overlying muscles and depth, it is not readily palpable. Review the bones of the pelvis—the *acetabulum*, the *ilium*, and the *ischium*—and the connection inferiorly at the *symphysis pubis* and posteriorly with the sacroiliac bone (Fig. 18-52).

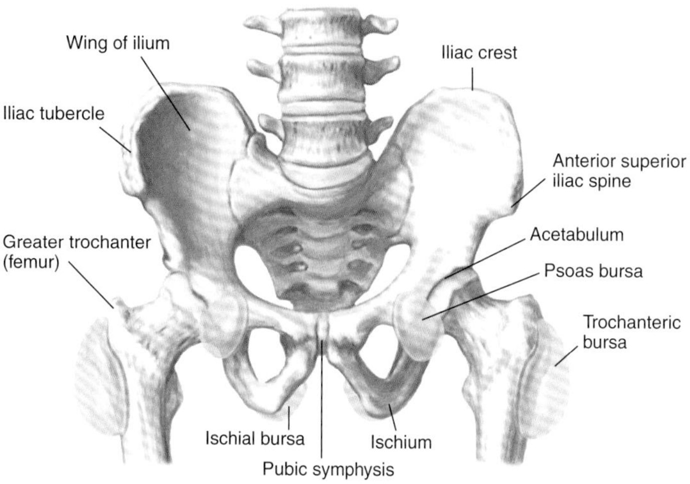

FIGURE 18-52 Anatomy of the pelvis, anterior view.

On the *anterior surface of the hip*, locate the following bony landmarks:

- The iliac crest at the level of L4
- The iliac tubercle
- The anterior superior iliac spine
- The greater trochanter
- The pubic symphysis

On the *posterior surface of the hip* (Fig. 18-53), locate the following:

- The posterior superior iliac spine
- The greater trochanter
- The ischial tuberosity
- The sacroiliac joint

Note that an imaginary line between the posterior superior iliac spines crosses the joint at S2.

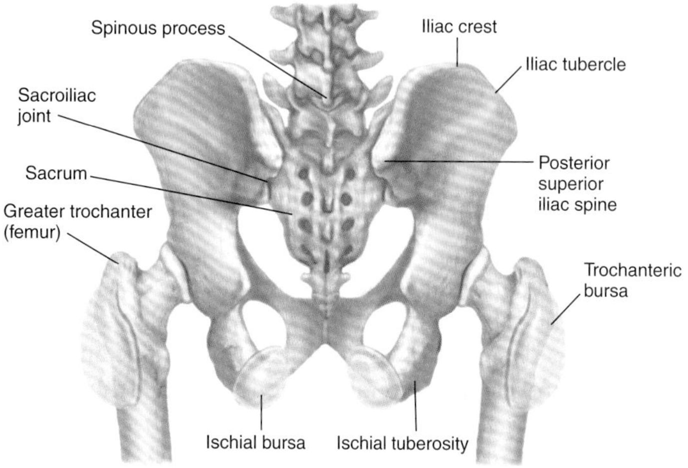

FIGURE 18-53 Anatomy of the pelvis, posterior view.

Muscle Groups

Four powerful muscle groups move the hip.

The *flexor group* lies anteriorly and flexes the thigh (Fig. 18-54). The primary hip flexor is the *iliopsoas*, extending from above the iliac crest to the lesser trochanter. The *extensor group* lies posteriorly and extends the thigh (Fig. 18-55). The *gluteus maximus* is the primary extensor of the hip. It forms a band crossing from its origin along the medial pelvis to its insertion below the trochanter.

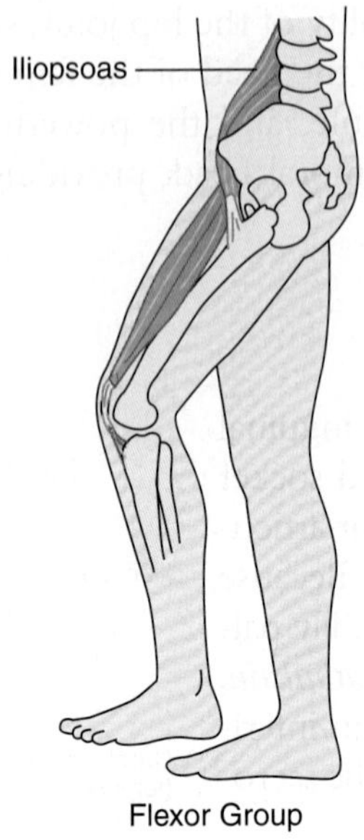

FIGURE 18-54 Flexor muscles of the hip.

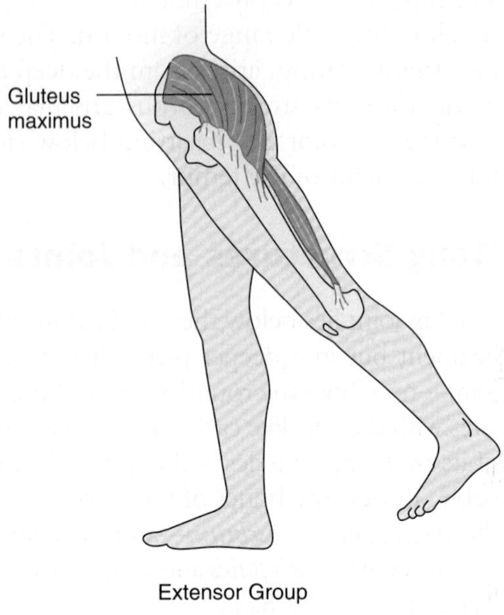

FIGURE 18-55 Extensor muscles of the hip.

The *adductor group* is medial and swings the thigh toward the body (Fig. 18-56). The muscles in this group arise from the rami of the pubis and ischium and insert on the posteromedial aspect of the femur. The *abductor group* is lateral, extending from the iliac crest to the head of the femur, and moves the thigh away from the body (Fig. 18-57). This group includes the *gluteus medius* and *minimus.* These muscles help stabilize the pelvis during the stance phase of gait.

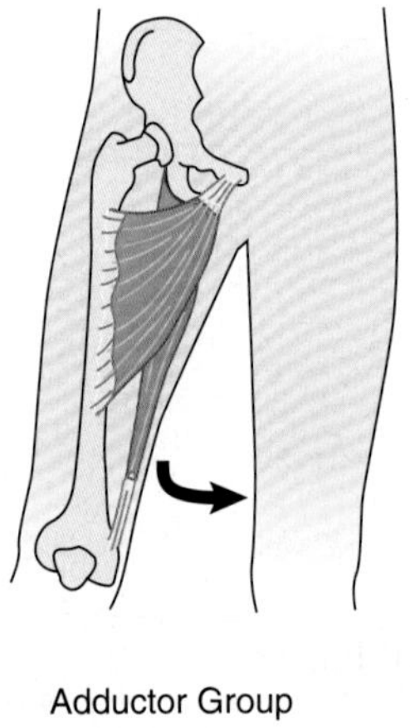

FIGURE 18-56 Adductor muscles of the hip.

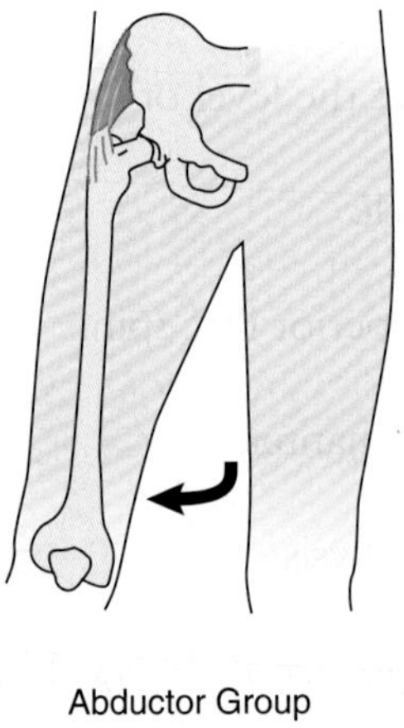

FIGURE 18-57 Abductor muscles of the hip.

Additional Structures

A strong, dense articular capsule, extending from the acetabulum to the femoral neck, encases and strengthens the hip joint, reinforced by three overlying ligaments and lined with synovial membrane. There are three principal bursae at the hip. Anterior to the joint is the *psoas* (also termed *iliopectineal* or *iliopsoas*) *bursa,* overlying the articular capsule and the psoas muscle. Find the bony prominence lateral to the hip joint—the *greater trochanter* of the femur. The large multilocular *trochanteric bursa* lies on its posterior surface. The *ischial* (or *ischiogluteal*) *bursa*—not always present—lies under the *ischial tuberosity,* on which a person sits. Note its proximity to the sciatic nerve, as shown in Figure 18-51.

Physical Examination

Inspection

Inspection of the hip begins with careful observation of the patient's gait on entering the room. Observe the two phases of gait, stance and swing:

- *Stance*—The gait phase that lasts from heel strike to push-off and accounts for 60% of a single gait cycle (Fig. 18-58).

Most problems appear during the weight-bearing stance phase.

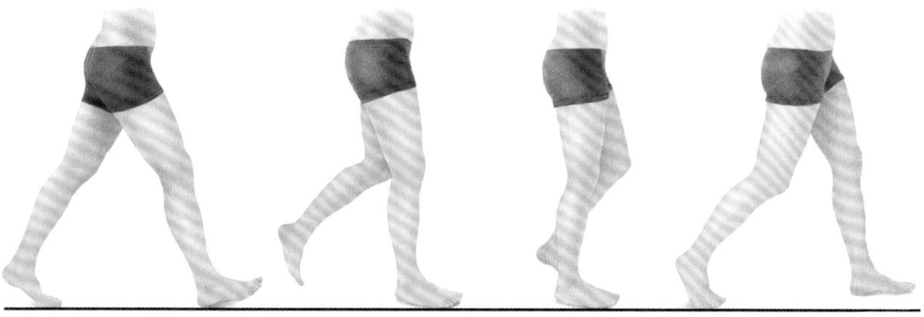

FIGURE 18-58 The stance phase of the gait.

- *Swing*—The gait phase in which the foot does not touch the ground and swings forward without bearing weight; accounts for 40% of the cycle.

Observe the gait for the width of the base (*distance between the feet*), the shift of the pelvis, and flexion of the knee. The width of the base should be 2 to 4 in from heel to heel (Fig. 18-59). Normal gait has a smooth, continuous rhythm. The knee should be flexed throughout the stance phase, except when the heel strikes the ground to counteract motion at the ankle. The ankle should dorsiflex so that the foot does not drag the ground during the swing phase.

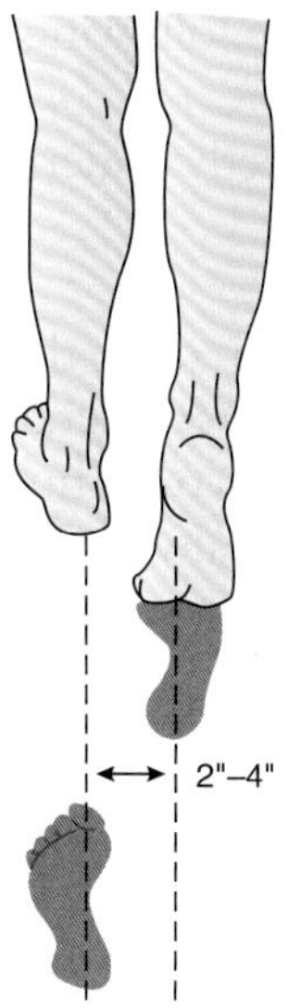

FIGURE 18-59 Observe the distance between the patient's feet when ambulating.

A wide base suggests cerebellar disease or foot problems. Pain during weight bearing or examiner strike on the heel occurs in *femoral neck stress fractures* (Neubauer et al., 2016).

Hip dislocation, arthritis, or abductor weakness can cause the pelvis to drop on the opposite side, producing a waddling gait.

CLINICAL TIP
Lack of knee flexion interrupts the smooth pattern of gait. The leg swings out to the side, as the patient walks (*circumduction*).

Inspect the lumbar portion of the spine for slight lordosis and with the patient supine, assess the length of the legs for symmetry. (To measure leg length, see the "Special Techniques: Measuring the Length of Legs" section.)

Lack of dorsiflexion may be due to footdrop. The patient will compensate by lifting the knee higher when walking.

Inspect the anterior and posterior surfaces of the hip for any areas of muscle atrophy or bruising.

Changes in leg length are seen in *scoliosis*. Leg shortening and external rotation suggest *hip fracture*.

Palpation

Bony Landmarks

Palpate the surface landmarks of the hip identified in Figures 18-52 and 18-53. On the *anterior aspect* of the hips, palpate the following key structures.

- Identify the *iliac crest* at the upper margin of the pelvis at the level of L4.
- Follow the downward anterior curve and locate the *iliac tubercle*, marking the widest point of the crest, and continue tracking downward to the *anterior superior iliac spine.*
- Place your thumbs on the anterior superior spines, and move your fingers downward from the iliac tubercles to the *greater trochanter* of the femur.
- Then move your thumbs medially and obliquely to the *pubic symphysis*, which lies at the same level as the greater trochanter.

On the *posterior aspect* of the hips, palpate the following bony landmarks:

- Palpate the *posterior superior iliac spine* directly underneath the visible dimples just above the buttocks.
- Placing your left thumb and index finger over the posterior superior iliac spine, next locate the *greater trochanter* laterally with your fingers at the level of the gluteal fold, and place your thumb medially on the *ischial tuberosity*. The *sacroiliac joint* is not always palpable. Note that an imaginary line along the posterior superior iliac spines crosses the joint at S2.

Note any tenderness or deformity during palpation.

Inguinal Structures

With the patient supine, ask the patient to place the heel of the leg being examined on the opposite knee. Then palpate along the *inguinal ligament*, which extends from the anterior superior iliac spine to the pubic tubercle (Fig. 18-60). The femoral nerve, artery, and vein bisect the overlying inguinal ligament; lymph nodes lie medially. The mnemonic "NAVEL" may help you remember the lateral-to-medial sequence of *n*erve, *a*rtery, *v*ein, *e*mpty space, and *l*ymph node.

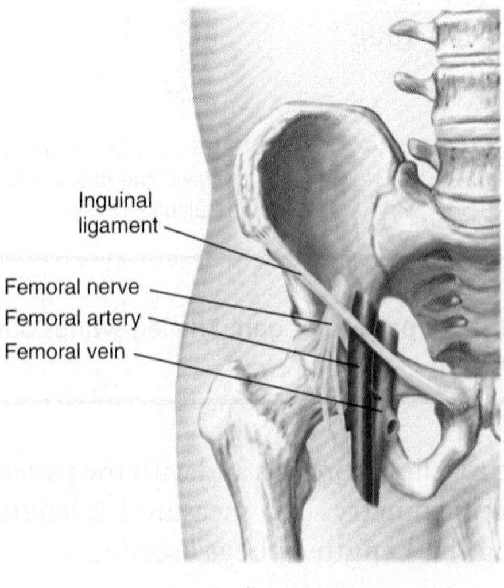

FIGURE 18-60 Inguinal anatomy.

Bulges along the ligament may suggest an *inguinal hernia* or, on occasion, an *aneurysm*. Enlarged lymph nodes suggest infection in the lower extremity or pelvis. Tenderness in the groin area may be from *synovitis* of the hip joint, *bursitis*.

Range of Motion and Muscle Strength Testing

Active Range of Motion

Now assess hip range of motion, referring to Table 18-15 for clear, simple instructions that prompt the patient and the muscles responsible for each movement.

TABLE 18-15 Assessing Range of Motion of the Hip

Hip Movement	Patient Instructions	Primary Muscles Affecting Movement
Flexion	*"Lie on your back. Bend your knee to your chest, and pull it against your abdomen."*	Iliopsoas
Hyperextension	*"Lie face down, and then bend your knee and lift it up."* *Or "Lying flat on your stomach, move your lower leg away from the midline and down over the side of the table."*	Gluteus maximus
Abduction	*"Lying flat on your back, move your lower leg away from the midline."*	Gluteus medius and minimus
Adduction	*"Lying flat, bend your knee and move your lower leg toward the midline."*	Adductor brevis, adductor longus, adductor magnus, pectineus, gracilis
External rotation	*"Lying flat on your back, bend your knee and hip 90 degrees and turn your ankle and foot across your opposite leg."*	Internal and external obturators, quadratus femoris, superior and inferior gemelli
Internal rotation	*"Lying flat on your back, bend your knee and hip 90 degrees and turn your lower ankle and foot away from your body."*	Gluteus medius and minimus

Active range of motion is the amount of motion at a given joint when the patient moves the part voluntarily without assistance from another body part, person, or device.

CLINICAL TIP

Before performing range of motion on patients who have had hip replacement surgery, ascertain whether they have hip motion limitations. To prevent hip dislocation, patients may have limited range of motion, which is different for an anterior versus a posterior surgical approach.

Passive Range of Motion

Passive range of motion (PROM) is the amount of motion at a given joint when the joint is moved by an external force or person. If it is necessary to assist the patient with hip range of motion, follow the instructions in the following sections for knee flexion, abduction, adduction, and external and internal rotation.

Flexion

With the patient supine, place your hand under the patient's lumbar spine. Ask the patient to bend each knee one at a time up to the chest and pull it firmly against the abdomen (Fig. 18-61). Note that the hip can flex further when the knee is flexed. When the back touches your hand, indicating normal flattening of the lumbar lordosis, further flexion arises from the hip joint itself.

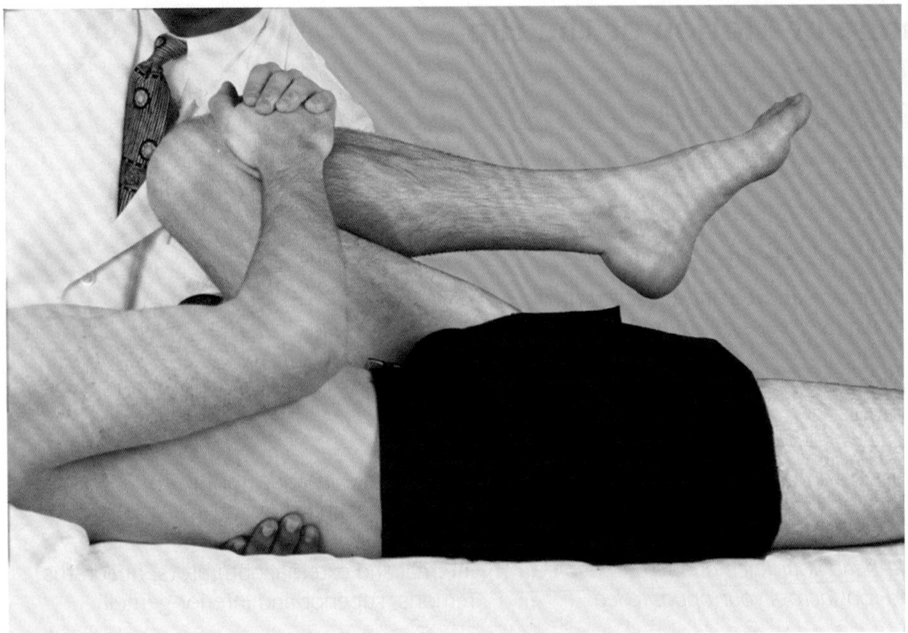

FIGURE 18-61 Testing hip flexion.

If the patient is unable to keep the opposite leg extended when one leg is flexed, it suggests a *flexion deformity of the opposite leg's hip*, as seen in Figure 18-62.

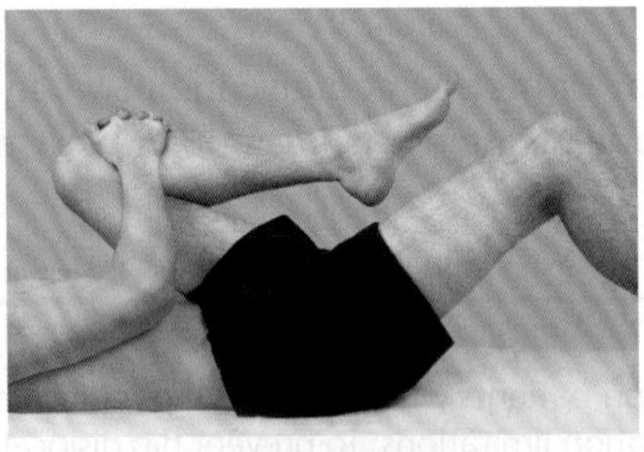

FIGURE 18-62 Positive flexion deformity of the opposite leg's hip.

As the thigh is held against the abdomen, observe the degree of flexion at the hip and knee. Normally, the anterior portion of the thigh can almost touch the chest wall. Note whether the opposite thigh remains fully extended, resting on the table.

Flexion deformity may be masked by an increase, rather than flattening, in lumbar lordosis and an anterior pelvic tilt.

Extension

With the patient lying face down, extend the thigh toward you in a posterior direction. Alternatively, carefully position the supine patient near the edge of the table and extend the leg posteriorly.

Abduction

Stabilize the pelvis by pressing down on the opposite anterior superior iliac spine with one hand. With the other hand, grasp the ankle and abduct the extended leg until you feel the iliac spine move (Fig. 18-63). This movement marks the limit of hip abduction.

Restricted abduction is common in hip *osteoarthritis.*

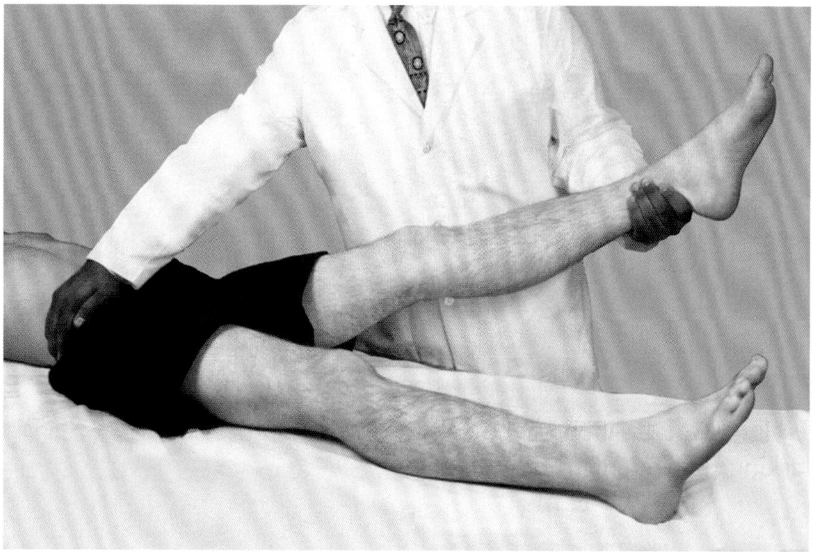

FIGURE 18-63 Testing hip abduction.

Alternatively, stand at the foot of the table, grasp both ankles, and spread them maximally, abducting both extended legs at the hips. This method provides easy comparison of two sides when movements are restricted, but it is impractical when range of motion is full.

Adduction

With the patient supine, stabilize the pelvis, hold one ankle, and move the leg medially across the body and over the opposite extremity (Fig. 18-64).

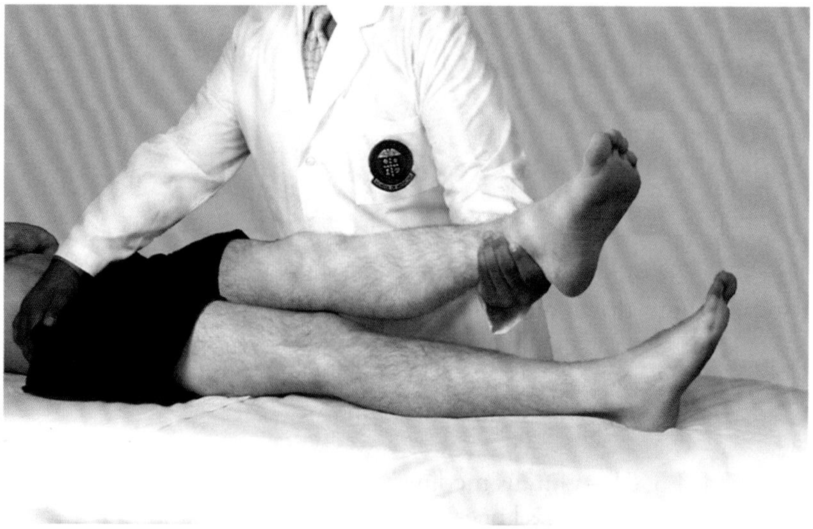

FIGURE 18-64 Testing hip adduction.

External and Internal Rotation

Flex the leg to 90 degrees at hip and knee, stabilize the thigh with one hand, grasp the ankle with the other, and swing the lower leg medially for external rotation at the hip (Fig. 18-65) and laterally for internal rotation. Although confusing at first, it is the motion of the head of the femur in the acetabulum that identifies these movements.

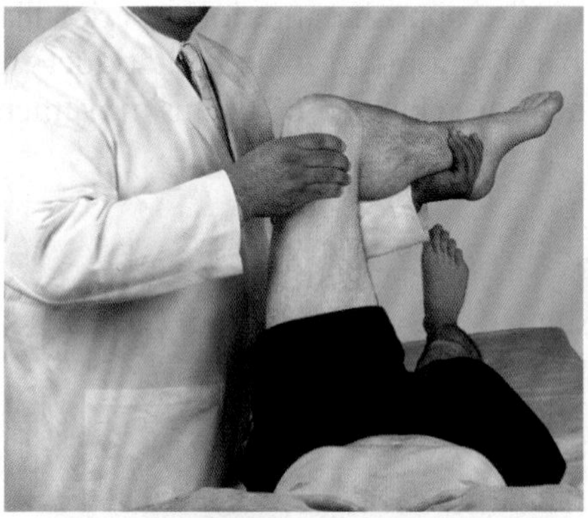

FIGURE 18-65 Testing the external rotation of the hip.

Restrictions of internal and external rotation are indicators of hip disease such as arthritis.

Muscle Strength Tests

Flexion

Test muscle strength during flexion at the hip (L2, L3, L4—iliopsoas) by placing your hand on the patient's thigh and asking the patient to raise the leg against your hand (Fig. 18-66).

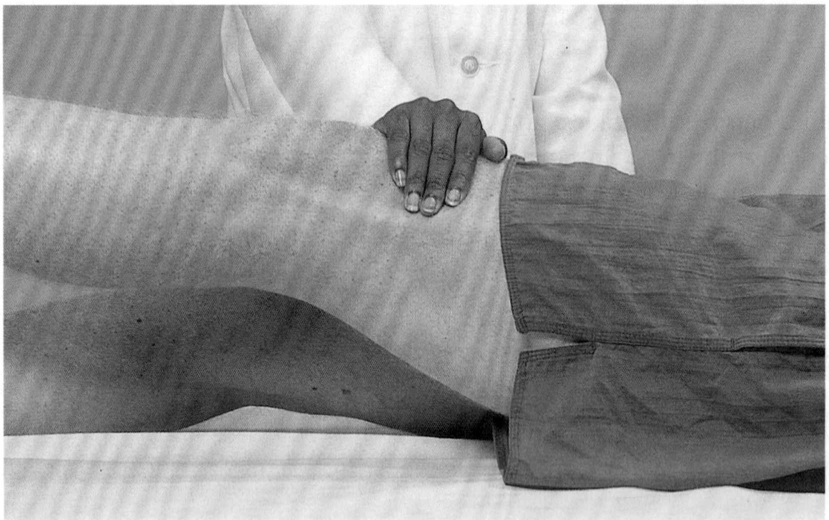

FIGURE 18-66 Testing muscle strength with hip flexion.

Extension

Test muscle strength during extension at the hips (S1—gluteus maximus) by having the supine patient push the posterior thigh down against your hand.

Abduction

Test muscle strength during abduction at the hips (L4, L5, S1—gluteus medius and minimus) by placing your hands on the outside of the patient's knees and asking the patient to press their knees outward against your hands.

Adduction

Test muscle strength during adduction at the hips (L2, L3, L4—adductors) by placing your hands firmly on the bed between the patient's knees. Ask the patient to bring both legs together.

Symmetric weakness of the proximal muscles suggests a *myopathy* or muscle disorder; symmetric weakness of distal muscles suggests a *polyneuropathy,* or disorder of peripheral nerves.

THE KNEE

The knee joint is the largest joint in the body. It is a hinge joint involving three bones: the femur, the tibia, and the patella (or knee cap), with three articular surfaces—two between the femur and the tibia and one between the femur and the patella. Note how the two rounded condyles of the femur rest on the relatively flat tibial plateau (Fig. 18-67). There is no inherent stability in the knee joint itself, making it dependent on ligaments to hold its articulating bones in place. This feature, in addition to the lever action of the femur on the tibia and lack of padding from fat or muscle, makes the knee highly vulnerable to injury.

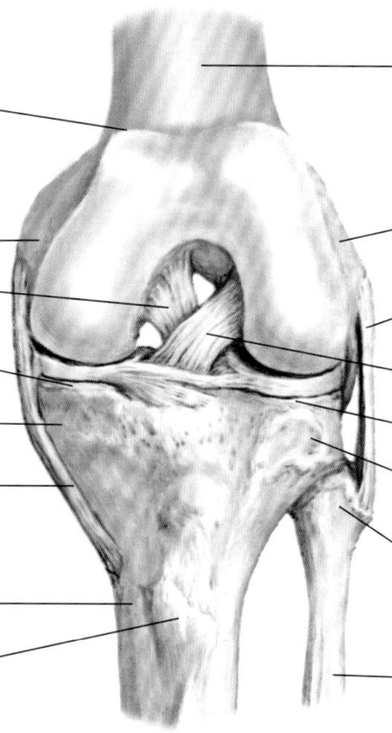

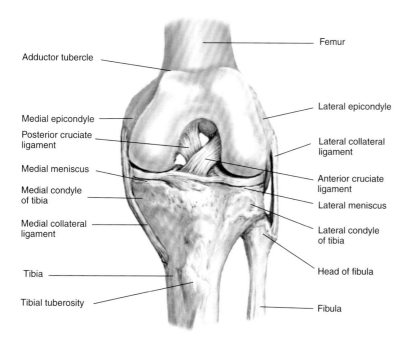

FIGURE 18-67 Anatomy of the knee, anterior view.

Bony Structures

Review the bony landmarks in and around the knee (see Fig. 18-67) before you examine the knee. On the *medial surface*, identify the *medial epicondyle* of the femur and the *medial condyle* of the tibia.

On the *anterior surface*, identify the patella, which rests on the anterior articulating surface of the femur midway between the epicondyles, embedded in the tendon of the quadriceps muscle. This tendon continues below the knee joint as the *patellar tendon*, which inserts distally on the *tibial tuberosity*.

On the *lateral surface*, find the *lateral epicondyle* of the femur and the *lateral condyle* of the tibia.

Joints

Two condylar *tibiofemoral joints* are formed by the convex curves of the medial and lateral condyles of the femur as they articulate with the concave condyles of the tibia. The third articular surface is the *patellofemoral joint.* The patella slides on the groove of the anterior aspect of the distal femur, called the *trochlear groove*, during flexion and extension of the knee.

Muscle Groups

Powerful muscles move and support the knee. The *quadriceps femoris* extends the leg, covering the anterior, medial, and lateral aspects of the thigh (Fig. 18-68A). The *hamstring muscles* lie on the posterior aspect of the thigh and flex the knee (Fig. 18-68B).

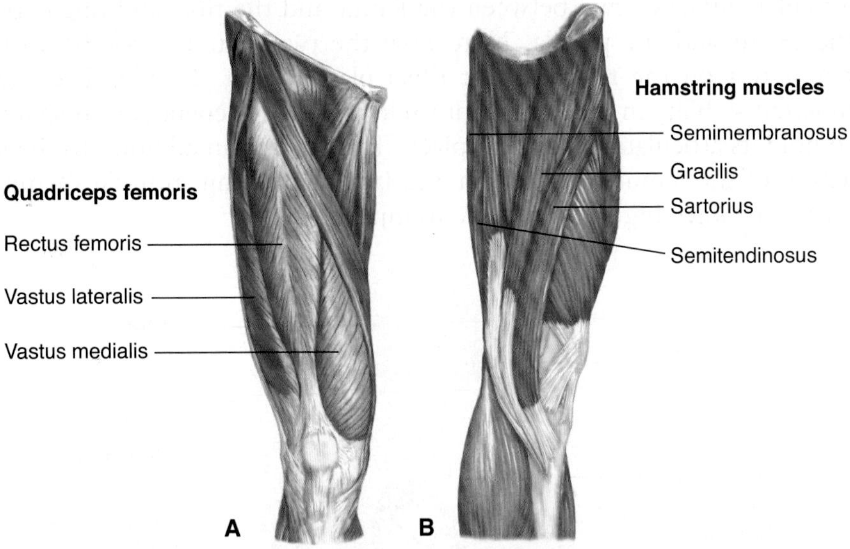

FIGURE 18-68 A. Quadriceps femoris of the anterior lower extremity. **B.** Hamstring muscles of the posterior lower extremity.

Additional Structures

The menisci and two important pairs of ligaments, the collaterals and the cruciates, are crucial to stability of the knee. Identify these structures in Figure 18-69.

- The *medial and lateral menisci* cushion the action of the femur on the tibia. These crescent-shaped fibrocartilaginous discs add a cup-like surface to the otherwise flat tibial plateau.
- The *medial collateral ligament (MCL)*, not easily palpable, is a broad, flat ligament connecting the medial femoral epicondyle to the medial condyle of the tibia. The medial portion of the MCL also attaches to the medial meniscus.
- The *lateral collateral ligament (LCL)* connects the lateral femoral epicondyle and the head of the fibula. The MCL and LCL provide medial and lateral stability to the knee joint.

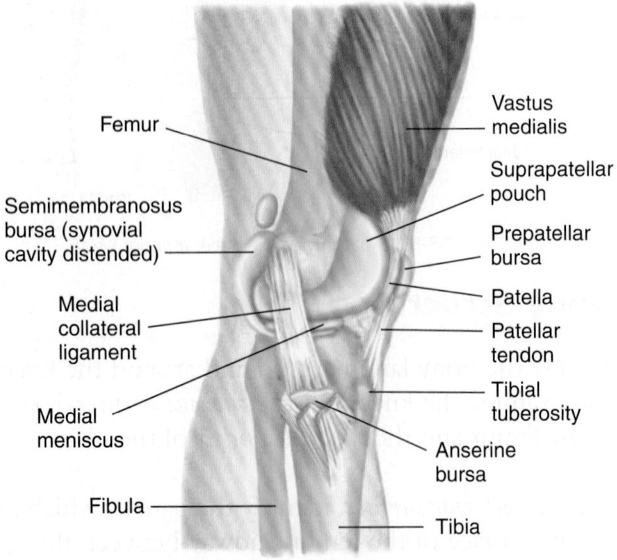

FIGURE 18-69 A medial view of the menisci and ligaments of the left knee.

- The *anterior cruciate ligament (ACL)* crosses obliquely from the *anterior* medial tibia to the lateral femoral condyle, preventing the tibia from sliding forward on the femur.

- The *posterior cruciate ligament (PCL)* crosses from the *posterior* tibia and lateral meniscus to the medial femoral condyle, preventing the tibia from slipping backward on the femur.

Because these ligaments lie within the knee joint, they are not palpable. They are nonetheless crucial to the anteroposterior stability of the knee.

Physical Examination

Inspection

Observe the gait for a smooth, rhythmic flow as the patient enters the room. The knee should be extended at heel strike and flexed at all other phases of swing and stance.

Stumbling or pushing the knee into extension with the hand during heel strike suggests *quadriceps weakness.*

Check the alignment and contours of the knees. Observe any atrophy of the quadriceps muscles.

Bowlegs (*genu varum*) and knock-knees (*genu valgum*) can be observed; flexion contracture (inability to extend fully) occurs with limb paralysis.

Look for loss of the normal hollows around the patella, a sign of swelling in the knee joint and suprapatellar pouch; note any other swelling in or around the knee.

Swelling over the patella suggests *prepatellar bursitis.* Swelling over the tibial tubercle suggests *infrapatellar* or, if more medial, *anserine bursitis.*

Palpation

Ask the patient to sit on the edge of the examining table with the knees in flexion. In this position, bony landmarks are more visible, and the muscles, tendons, and ligaments are more relaxed, making them easier to palpate.

Pay special attention to any areas of tenderness. Pain is a common complaint in knee problems, and localizing the structure causing pain is important for accurate evaluation.

Tibiofemoral Joint

Palpate the *tibiofemoral joint.* Facing the knee, place your thumbs in the soft tissue depressions on either side of the *patellar tendon* (Fig. 18-70). Identify the groove of the tibiofemoral joint. Note that the patella lies just above this joint line. As you press your thumbs downward, feel the edge of the tibial plateau. Follow it medially, then laterally, until you are stopped by the converging femur and tibia. By moving your thumbs upward toward the midline to the top of the patella, you can follow the articulating surface of the femur and identify the margins of the joint. Note any irregular bony ridges along the joint margins.

Osteoarthritis is likely when there are tender bony ridges along the joint margins, genu varum deformity, and stiffness lasting 30 minutes or less (McGee, 2018a). Crepitus may also be present.

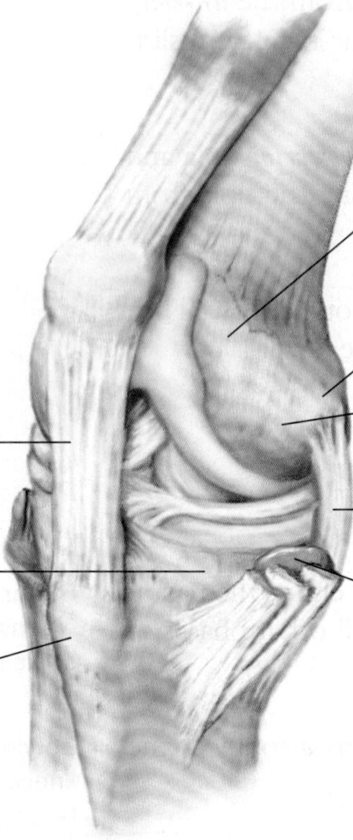

FIGURE 18-70 Structures in the medial compartment in the right knee.

Now locate the *patella* and trace the *patellar tendon* distally until you palpate the *tibial tuberosity*. Ask the patient to extend the leg to make sure the patellar tendon is intact.

Tenderness over the tendon or inability to extend the leg suggests a partial or complete tear of the patellar tendon.

With the patient supine and the knee extended, compress the patella against the underlying femur. Ask the patient to tighten the quadriceps as the patella moves distally in the trochlear groove. Check for a smooth sliding motion (the *patellofemoral grinding test*).

Pain and crepitus suggest roughening of the patellar undersurface that articulates with the femur. Similar pain may occur with climbing stairs or getting up from a chair.

Pain with compression and with patellar movement during quadriceps contraction suggests *chondromalacia,* or degenerative patella (the *patellofemoral syndrome*).

Suprapatellar Pouch, Prepatellar Bursa, and Anserine Bursa

Palpate for thickening or swelling in the *suprapatellar pouch* and along the margins of the patella (Fig. 18-71). Start 10 cm above the superior border of the patella, well above the pouch, and feel the soft tissues between your thumb and fingers. Move your hand distally in progressive steps, trying to identify the pouch. Continue your palpation along the sides of the patella. Note any tenderness or warmth greater than in the surrounding tissues.

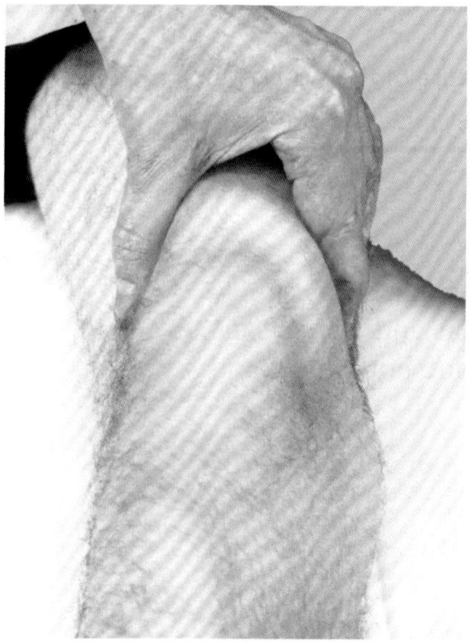

FIGURE 18-71 Palpating the suprapatellar pouch of the knee.

Swelling above and adjacent to the patella suggests synovial thickening or **effusion** (escape of fluid into a body cavity) in the knee joint (Fig. 18-72).

Thickening, bogginess, or warmth in these areas indicates synovitis or nontender effusions from osteoarthritis.

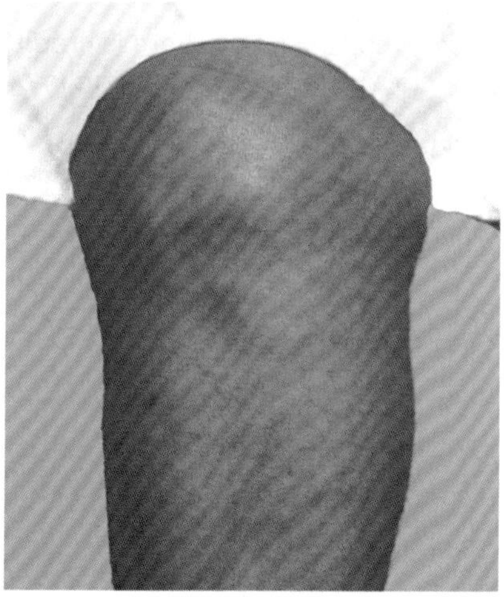

FIGURE 18-72 Effusion of the knee joint.

Gastrocnemius and Soleus Muscles, Achilles Tendon

Palpate the *gastrocnemius* and *soleus muscles* on the posterior surface of the lower leg. Their common tendon, the Achilles, is palpable from about the lower third of the calf to its insertion on the calcaneus.

A defect in the muscles with tenderness and swelling occur in a *ruptured Achilles tendon*; tenderness and thickening of the tendon above the calcaneus, sometimes with a protuberant posterolateral bony process of the calcaneus occur in *Achilles tendinitis*.

To test the integrity of the *Achilles tendon*, place the patient prone with the knee and ankle flexed at 90 degrees. Alternatively, ask the patient to kneel on a chair. Squeeze the calf and watch for plantar flexion at the ankle.

CLINICAL TIP
Absence of plantar flexion is a positive test indicating rupture of the Achilles tendon.

Range of Motion

Now assess knee range of motion. Refer to Table 18-16 for clear, simple instructions that prompt the patient through the motion and the specific muscles responsible for each movement. Be sure to examine both knees and compare findings.

TABLE 18-16 Assessing Range of Motion of the Knee

Knee Movement	Patient Instructions	Primary Muscles Affecting Movement
Flexion	*"Bend or flex your knee." Or "Squat down to the floor."*	Hamstring group: biceps femoris, semitendinosus, and semimembranosus
Extension	*"Straighten your leg." Or "After you squat down to the floor, stand up."*	Quadriceps: rectus femoris, vastus medialis, lateralis, and intermedius
Internal rotation	*"While sitting, swing your lower leg toward the midline."*	Sartorius, gracilis, semitendinosus, semimembranosus
External rotation	*"While sitting, swing your lower leg away from the midline."*	Biceps femoris

There is crepitus with flexion and extension in osteoarthritis (McGee, 2018a).

Muscle Strength Test

Test muscle strength during extension at the knee (L2, L3, L4—quadriceps). Support the knee in flexion and ask the patient to straighten the leg against your hand (Fig. 18-73). The quadriceps is the strongest muscle in the body, so expect a forceful response.

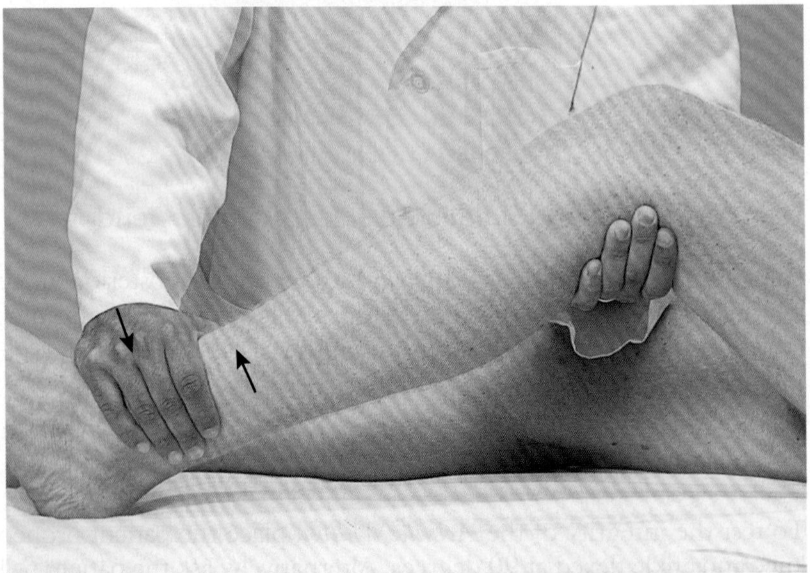

FIGURE 18-73 Testing muscle strength with knee extension.

Test flexion at the knee (L4, L5, S1, S2—hamstrings) as shown in Figure 18-74. Place the patient's leg so that the knee is flexed with the foot resting on the bed. Tell the patient to keep the foot down as you try to straighten the leg.

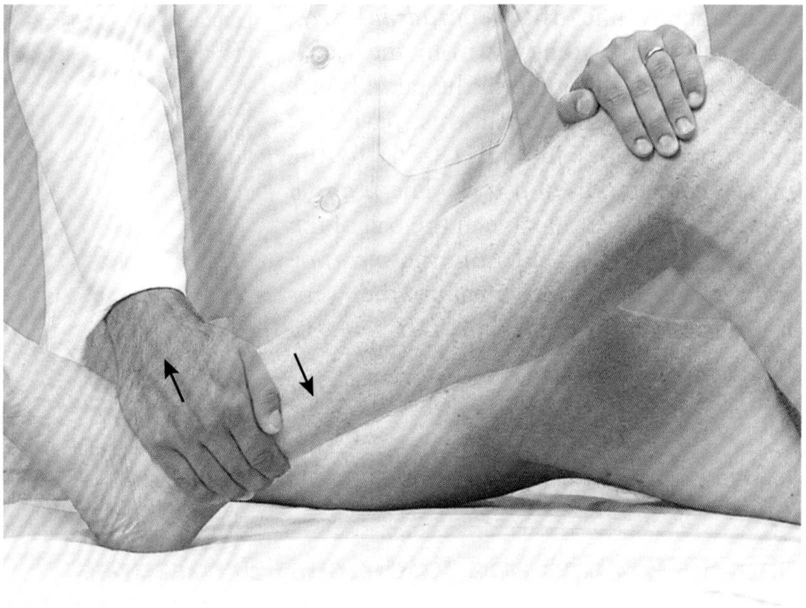

FIGURE 18-74 Testing muscle strength with knee flexion.

THE ANKLE AND FOOT

The total weight of the body is transmitted through the ankle to the foot. The ankle and foot must balance the body and absorb the impact of the heel strike and gait. Despite thick padding along the toes, sole, and heel and stabilizing ligaments at the ankles, the ankle and foot are frequent sites of sprain and bony injury.

Bony Structures and Joints

The ankle is a hinge joint formed by the *tibia*, the *fibula*, and the *talus*. The tibia and fibula act as a mortise, stabilizing the joint while bracing the talus like an inverted cup.

The principal joints of the ankle are the *tibiotalar joint*, between the tibia and the talus, and the *subtalar (talocalcaneal) joint*.

Note the principal landmarks of the ankle (Fig. 18-75): the *medial malleolus*, the bony prominence at the distal end of the tibia, and the *lateral malleolus* at the distal end of the fibula. Lodged under the talus and jutting posteriorly is the *calcaneus*, or heel.

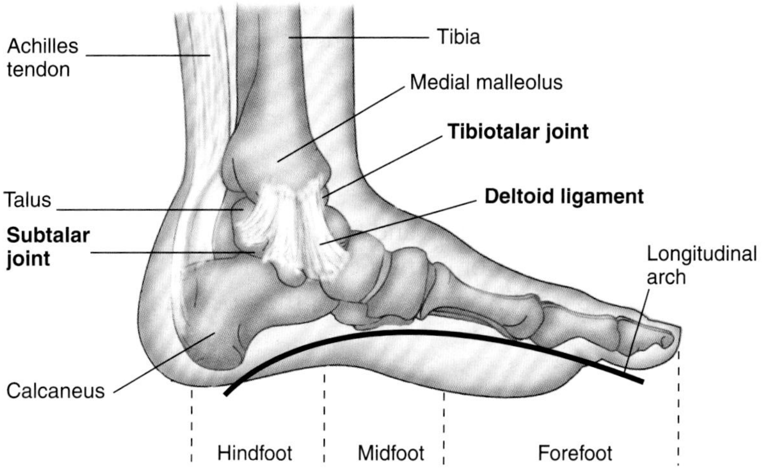

FIGURE 18-75 Anatomy of the ankle, medial view.

An imaginary line, the *longitudinal arch*, spans the foot, extending from the calcaneus of the hind foot along the tarsal bones of the midfoot (see cuneiforms, navicular, and cuboid bones in Fig. 18-76) to the forefoot metatarsals and toes. The *heads of the metatarsals* are palpable in the ball of the foot. In the forefoot, identify the *metatarsophalangeal joints,* proximal to the webs of the toes, and the *PIP and DIP joints* of the toes.

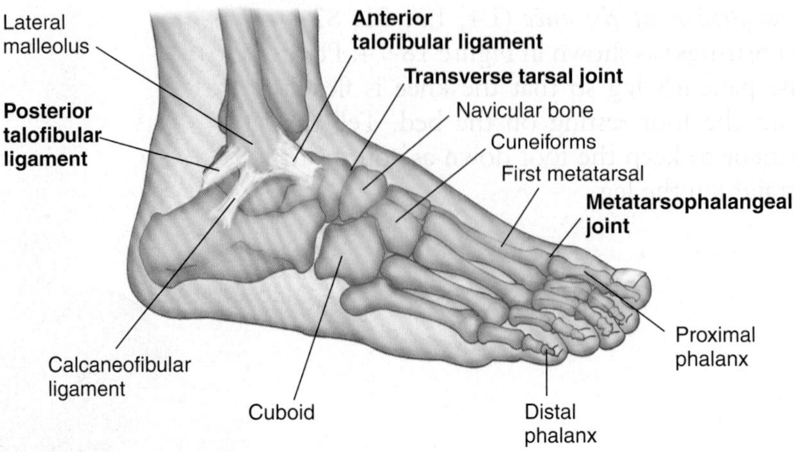

FIGURE 18-76 Anatomy of the ankle, lateral view.

Muscle Groups and Additional Structures

Movement at the tibiotalar ankle joint is limited to dorsiflexion and plantar flexion. *Plantar flexion (pointing the toe)* is powered by the gastrocnemius, the posterior tibial muscle, and the toe flexors. Their tendons run behind the malleoli. The *dorsiflexors* include the anterior tibial muscle and the toe extensors. They lie prominently on the anterior surface, or dorsum, of the ankle, anterior to the malleoli.

Ligaments extend from each malleolus onto the foot:

- Medially, the triangle-shaped *deltoid ligament* fans out from the inferior surface of the medial malleolus to the talus and proximal tarsal bones, protecting against stress from eversion (ankle bowing inward).
- Laterally, the three ligaments are less substantial, with higher risk for injury: the *anterior talofibular ligament*—most at risk in injury from inversion (ankle bows outward) injuries; the *calcaneofibular ligament*; and the *posterior talofibular ligament.* The strong Achilles tendon attaches the gastrocnemius and soleus muscles to the posterior calcaneus. The plantar fascia inserts on the medial tubercle of the calcaneus.

Physical Examination

Inspection

Observe all surfaces of the ankles and feet, noting any erythema, deformities, nodules, swelling, calluses, or corns. See Table 18-17, "Abnormalities of the Feet" and Table 18-18, "Abnormalities of the Toes and Soles."

TABLE 18-17 Abnormalities of the Feet

Acute Gouty Arthritis

The metatarsophalangeal joint of the great toe is the initial joint involved in 50% of episodes of *acute gouty arthritis*. It is characterized by a very painful and tender, hot, dusky red swelling that extends beyond the margin of the joint. It is easily mistaken for a cellulitis. Acute gout may also involve the dorsum of the foot.

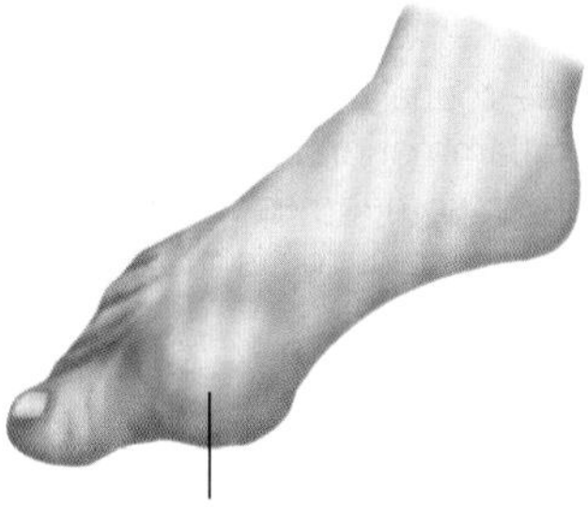

Flat Feet

Signs of *flat feet* may be apparent only when the patient stands, or they may become permanent. The longitudinal arch flattens so that the sole approaches or touches the floor. The normal concavity on the medial side of the foot becomes convex. Tenderness may be present from the medial malleolus down along the medial-plantar surface of the foot. Swelling may develop anterior to the malleoli. Inspect the shoes for excess wear on the inner sides of the soles and heels.

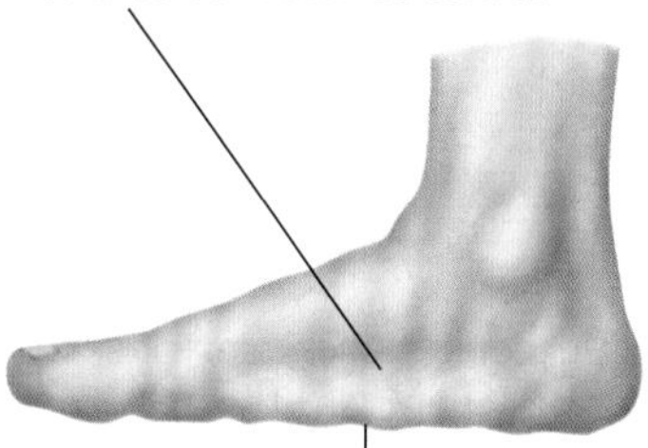

Hallux Valgus

In *hallux valgus*, there is lateral deviation of the great toe and enlargement of the head of the first metatarsal on its medial side, forming a bursa or bunion. This bursa may become inflamed. Biologic women are more likely to be affected than are biologic men.

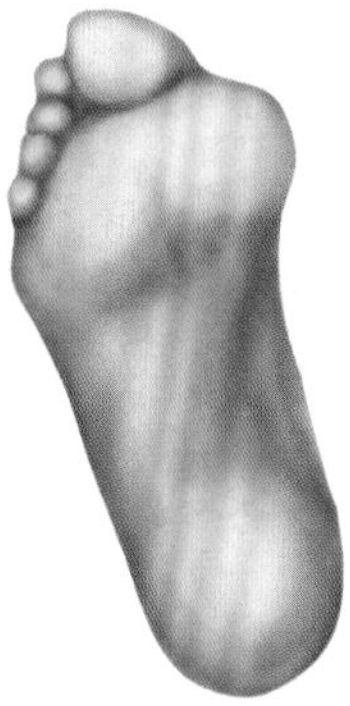

Morton Neuroma

Tenderness is seen over the plantar surface between the third and fourth metatarsal heads from perineural fibrosis of the common digital nerve due to irritation. (It is not a true neuroma.) Pain radiates to the toes when you press on the plantar interspace while squeezing the toes with your other hand. Symptoms include hyperesthesia, numbness, aching, and burning from the metatarsal heads into the third and fourth toes.

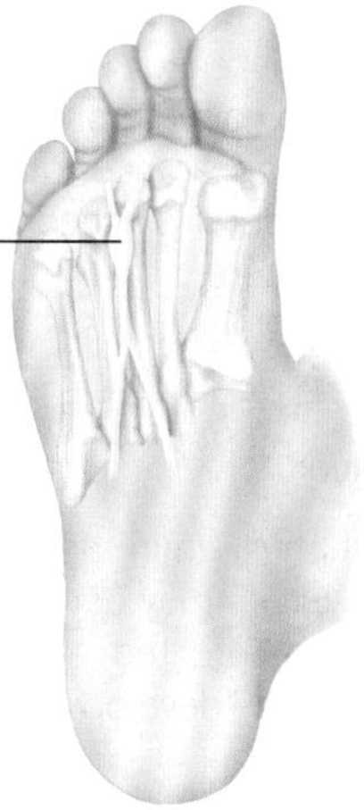

TABLE 18-18 Abnormalities of the Toes and Soles

Ingrown Toenail

The sharp edge of a toenail may dig into and injure the lateral nail fold, resulting in inflammation and infection. A tender, reddened, overhanging nail fold, sometimes with granulation tissue and purulent discharge, results. The great toe is most often affected.

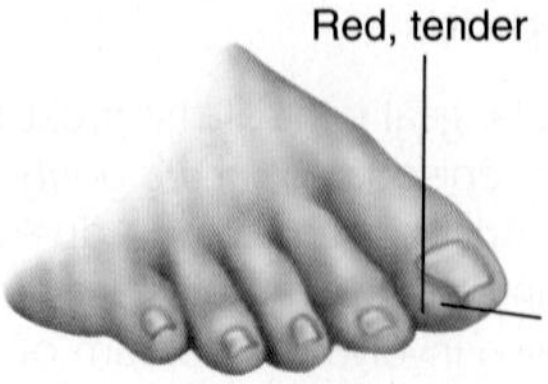

Hammer Toe

Most commonly involving the second toe, a hammer toe is characterized by hyperextension at the metatarsophalangeal joint with flexion at the proximal interphalangeal joint. A corn frequently develops at the pressure point over the proximal interphalangeal joint.

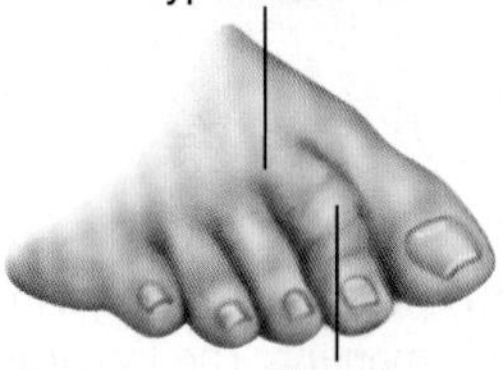

Corn

A corn is a painful conical thickening of skin that results from recurrent pressure on normally thin skin. The apex of the cone points inward and causes pain. Corns characteristically occur over bony prominences such as the fifth toe. When located in moist areas such as pressure points between the fourth and fifth toes, they are called soft corns.

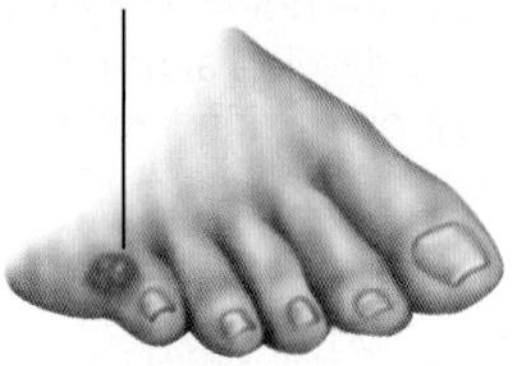

Callus

Like a corn, a callus is an area of greatly thickened skin that develops in a region of recurrent pressure. Unlike a corn, a callus involves skin that is normally thick, such as the sole, and is usually painless. If a callus is painful, suspect an underlying plantar wart.

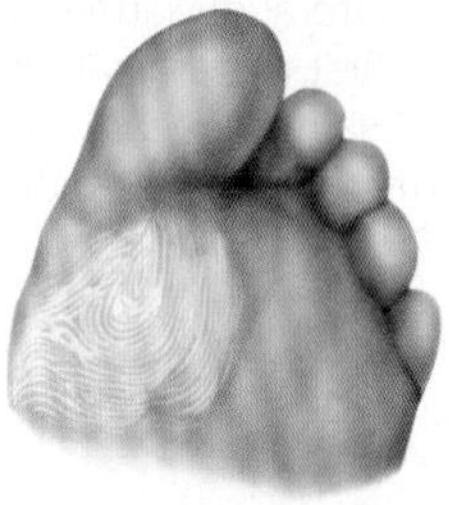

Plantar Wart

A plantar wart is a common wart caused by the *human papillomavirus* and located in the thickened skin of the sole. It may look like a callus or even be covered by one. Look for the characteristic small dark spots that give a stippled appearance to a wart. Normal skin lines stop at the wart's edge. It is tender if pinched from the side, whereas a callus is tender to direct pressure.

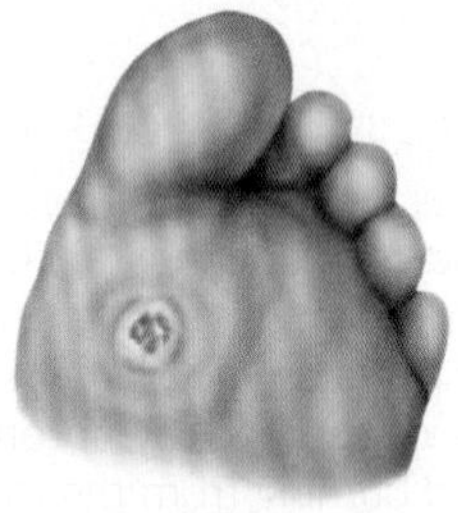

Neuropathic Ulcer

When pain sensation is diminished or absent, as in diabetic neuropathy, neuropathic ulcers may develop at pressure points on the feet. Although often deep, infected, and indolent, they are painless. Underlying osteomyelitis may develop.

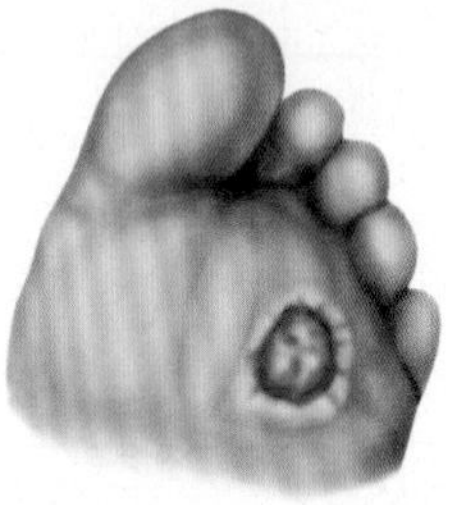

Palpation

With your thumbs, palpate the anterior aspect of each *ankle joint,* noting any bogginess, swelling, or tenderness (Fig. 18-77).

Localized tenderness is found in arthritis, ligamentous injury, or infection of the ankle.

Feel along the *Achilles tendon* for nodules and tenderness.

Nodules occur with rheumatoid arthritis; tenderness in Achilles is seen in tendinitis, bursitis, or partial tear from trauma.

Palpate the heel, especially the posterior and inferior calcaneus, and the plantar fascia for tenderness.

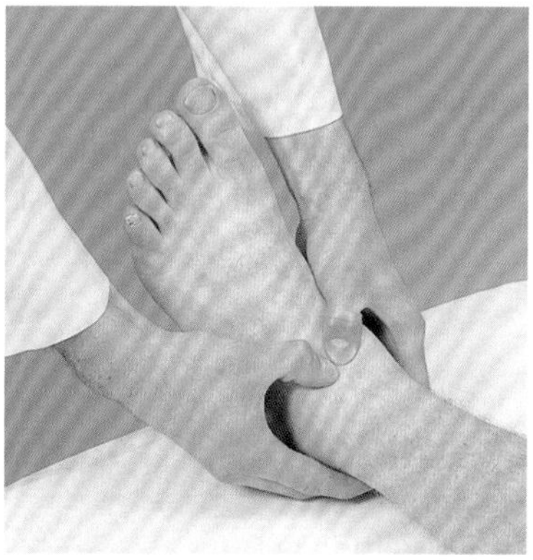

FIGURE 18-77 Palpating the anterior aspect of the ankle joint.

Bone spurs may be present on the calcaneus. Focal heel pain on palpation of the plantar fascia suggests *plantar fasciitis* (Young, 2012), seen in prolonged standing or heel-strike exercise, also in *rheumatoid arthritis, gout.*

Palpate for tenderness over the medial and lateral malleolus, especially in cases of trauma.

After trauma, inability to bear weight after four steps and tenderness over the posterior aspects of either malleolus, especially the medial malleolus, is suspicious for ankle fracture.

Palpate the *metatarsophalangeal joints* for tenderness (Fig. 18-78). Compress the forefoot between the thumb and fingers. Exert pressure just proximal to the heads of the first and fifth metatarsals.

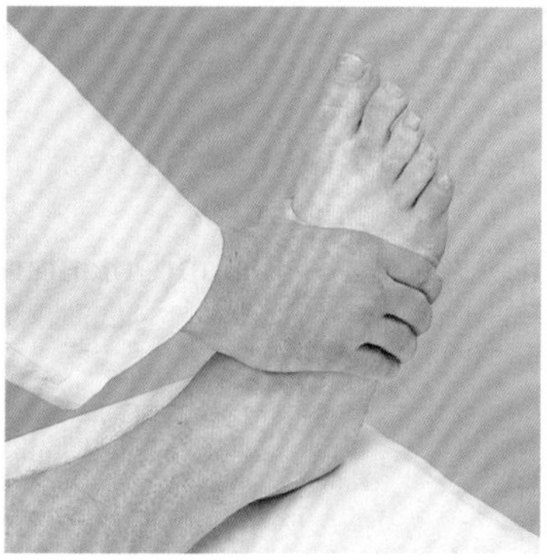

FIGURE 18-78 Palpating the metatarsophalangeal joints.

Tenderness on compression is an early sign of *rheumatoid arthritis.* Acute inflammation of the first metatarsophalangeal joint is seen in *gout.*

Palpate the heads of the five metatarsals and the grooves between them with your thumb and index finger (Fig. 18-79). Place your thumb on the dorsum of the foot and your index finger on the plantar surface.

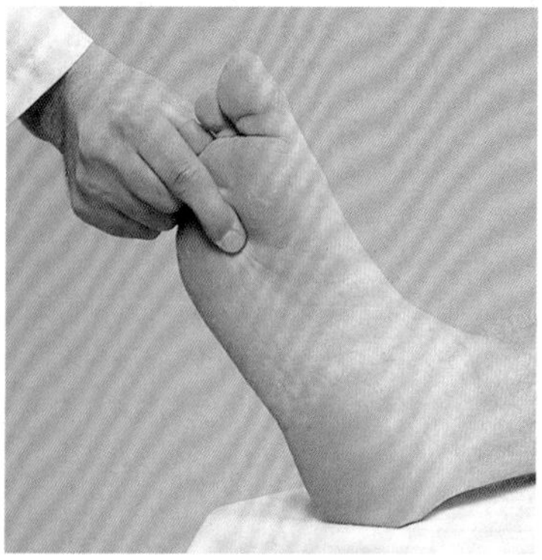

FIGURE 18-79 Palpating the metatarsal heads and grooves.

Pain and tenderness, called *metatarsalgia,* occurs with trauma, arthritis, and vascular compromise.

Range of Motion and Muscle Strength Tests

Active Range of Motion

Assess flexion and extension at the tibiotalar (ankle) joint. In the foot, assess inversion and eversion at the subtalar and transverse tarsal joints. Ask the patient to follow your directions according to Table 18-19 to assess ankle range of motion.

TABLE 18-19 Assessment of Ankle and Foot Range of Motion

Ankle and Foot Movement	Patient Instructions	Primary Muscles Affecting Movement
Ankle flexion (plantar flexion)	*"Point your foot toward the floor."*	Gastrocnemius, soleus, plantaris, tibialis posterior
Ankle extension (dorsiflexion)	*"Point your foot toward the ceiling."*	Tibialis anterior, extensor digitorum longus, and extensor hallucis longus
Inversion	*"Bend your heel inward."*	Tibialis posterior and anterior
Eversion	*"Bend your heel outward."*	Peroneus longus and brevis

Passive Range of Motion Maneuvers

If the patient cannot perform AROM, test for PROM as follows:

- *The ankle (tibiotalar) joint*—Dorsiflex (Fig. 18-80) and plantar flex the foot at the ankle.

Pain during movements of the ankle and the foot helps localize possible arthritis.

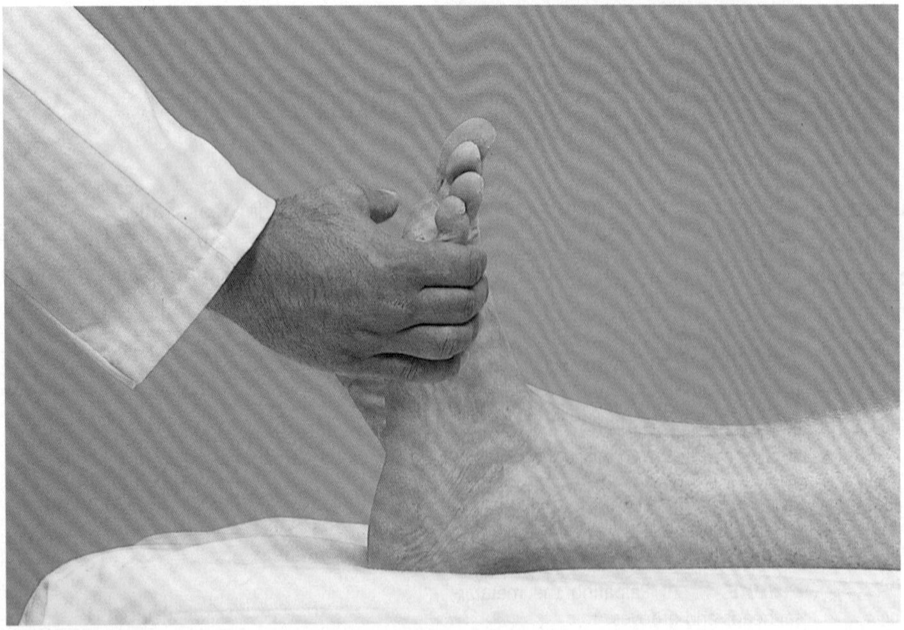

FIGURE 18-80 Testing dorsiflexion at the ankle.

- *The subtalar (talocalcaneal) joint*—Stabilize the ankle with one hand, grasp the heel with the other, and invert and evert the foot (Fig. 18-81).

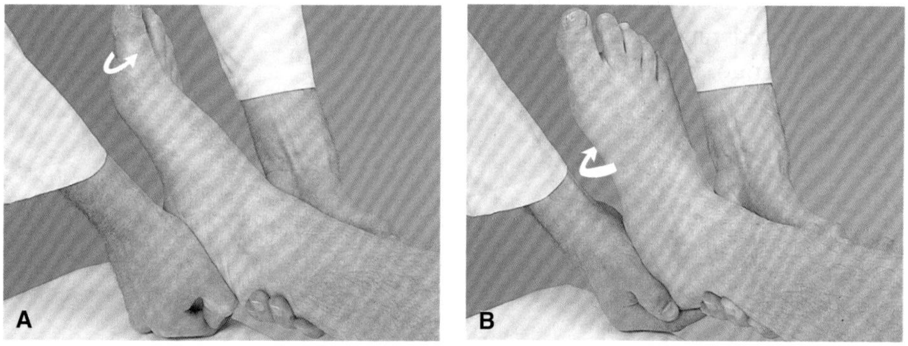

FIGURE 18-81 Testing the integrity of the subtalar (talocalcaneal) joint by inverting (**A**) and everting (**B**) the foot at the heel.

CLINICAL TIP
An arthritic joint is frequently painful when moved in any direction, whereas a ligamentous sprain produces maximal pain when the ligament is stretched. For example, in a common form of sprained ankle, inversion and plantar flexion of the foot cause pain, whereas eversion and plantar flexion are relatively pain-free.

- *The transverse tarsal joint*—Stabilize the heel and invert and evert the forefoot (Fig. 18-82).
- *The metatarsophalangeal joints*—Flex the toes in relation to the feet.

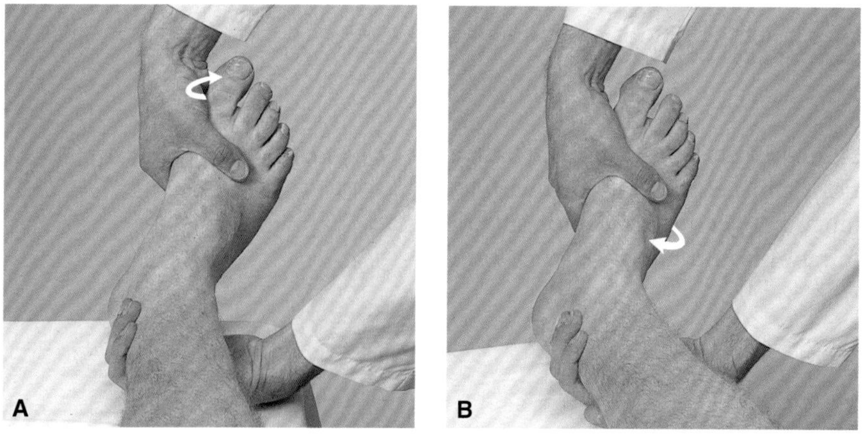

FIGURE 18-82 Testing the integrity of the transverse tarsal joint by inverting (**A**) and everting (**B**) the forefoot.

Muscle Strength Tests

Test muscle strength during dorsiflexion (mainly L4, L5, tibialis anterior) and *plantar flexion* (mainly S1, gastrocnemius, soleus) at the ankle by asking the patient to pull up and push down against your hand.

Describing Limited Motion of a Joint

Although measurement of motion is seldom necessary, limitations can be described in degrees. Pocket goniometers are available for this purpose. In Figure 18-83, the red lines indicate the limited range of the patient's movement, and the black lines show the normal range. Observations may be described in several ways (see Fig. 18-83).

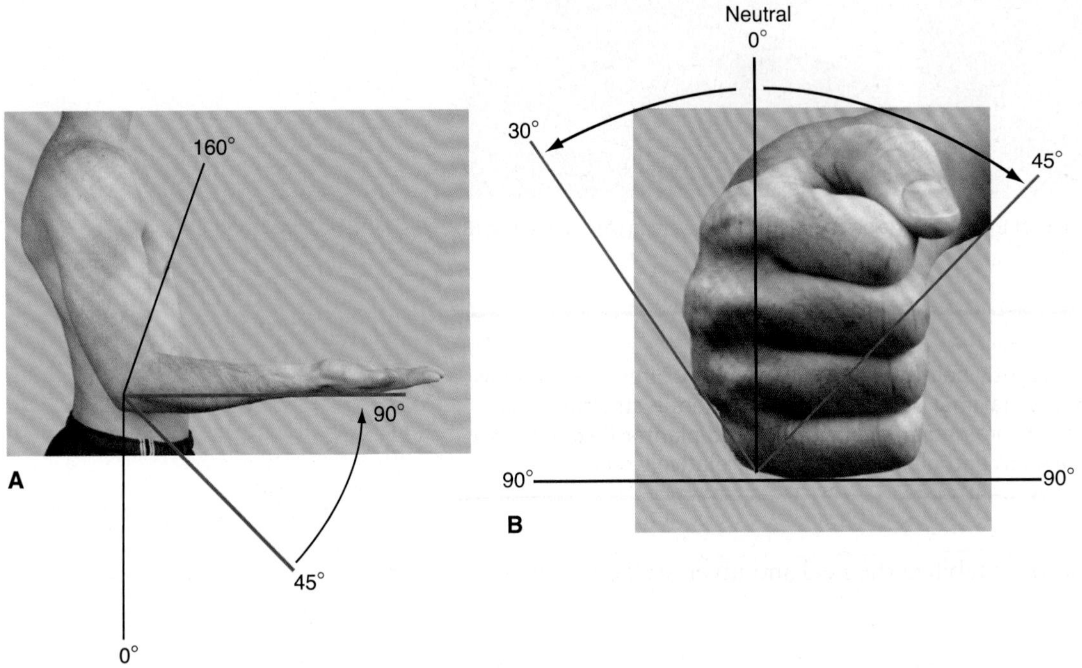

FIGURE 18-83 **A.** The elbow flexes from 45 to 90 degrees or elbow flexion is limited to 45 to 90 degrees. **B.** Supination at the elbow is limited to 30 degrees or pronation at the elbow is limited to 45 degrees.

SPECIAL TECHNIQUES: MEASURING THE LENGTH OF LEGS

If you suspect that the patient's legs are unequal in length, measure them. Have the patient relax in the supine position, symmetrically aligned with legs extended. With a tape, measure the distance between the anterior superior iliac spine and the medial malleolus. The tape should cross the knee on its medial side (Fig. 18-84).

Unequal leg length may explain a scoliosis.

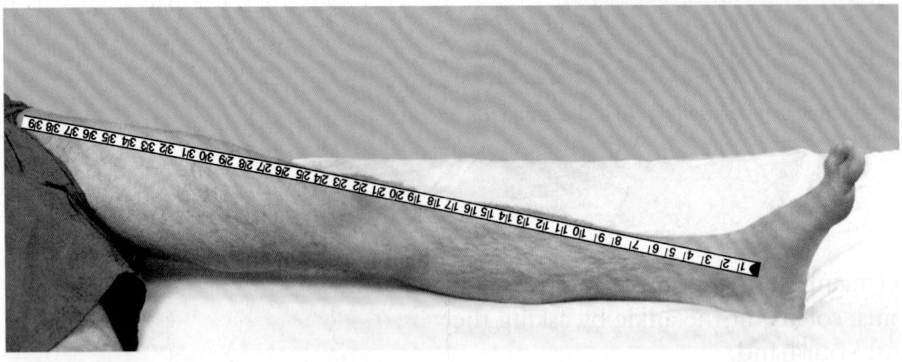

FIGURE 18-84 Measuring leg length from the anterior superior iliac spine to the medial malleolus.

RECORDING YOUR FINDINGS

The examples in Box 18-4 contain phrases appropriate for most write-ups. Note that use of the anatomic terms specific to the structure and function of individual joint problems makes your write-up of musculoskeletal findings more meaningful and informative. Additional terms to describe patterns of pain associated with musculoskeletal conditions are included throughout Table 18-20.

BOX 18-4 RECORDING THE EXAMINATION—THE MUSCULOSKELETAL SYSTEM

"FROM (Full range of motion) in all joints with muscle strength 5/5. No erythema, warmth, swelling, or deformity."

OR

"FROM in all joints except hands, with inability to fully close fists. Heberden nodes noted at the DIP joints of hand, Bouchard nodes at PIP joints bilaterally; hand muscle strength 4/5 bilaterally; hand pain 4/10 with flexion of fingers. Hip pain 2/10 bilaterally with flexion, extension, and rotation; hip muscle strength 5/5. FROM in the knees, with moderate crepitus; strength 5/5. Hallux valgus bilaterally at the first MTP joints."

Suggests *osteoarthritis*

HEALTH PROMOTION AND COUNSELING

Important topics for health promotion and counseling regarding the musculoskeletal system include:

- Nutrition, exercise, and weight
- Low back pain
- Fall prevention
- Osteoporosis screening and prevention

Maintaining the integrity of the musculoskeletal system brings many aspects of daily life into play—balanced nutrition, regular exercise, and appropriate body weight. Each joint has its own specific vulnerabilities to trauma and wear. Care with lifting, avoidance of falls, household safety measures, and exercise help to protect and preserve well-functioning muscles and joints and prevent or delay the onset of arthritis, chronic back pain, and osteoporosis, all important targets of Healthy People 2030 (U.S. Department of Health and Human Services. Office of Disease Prevention and Health Promotion, n.d.c).

Nutrition, Exercise, and Weight

Healthy habits directly benefit the skeleton and muscles. Good nutrition supplies calcium needed for bone mineralization and bone density. Exercise maintains and possibly increases bone mass in addition to improving outlook

TABLE 18-20 Patterns of Pain in and Around the Joints

Problem	Process	Common Locations	Pattern of Spread	Onset	Progression and Duration
Rheumatoid Arthritis (American College of Physicians, 2012; Anderson et al., 2012; Davis & Matteson, 2012)	Chronic inflammation of *synovial membranes* with secondary erosion of adjacent cartilage and bone, and damage to ligaments and tendons	Hands (proximal interphalangeal and metacarpophalangeal joints), feet (metatarsophalangeal joints), wrists, knees, elbows, ankles	Symmetrically additive: progresses to other joints while persisting in the initial ones	Usually insidious	Often chronic, with remissions and exacerbations
Osteoarthritis (Degenerative Joint Disease) (Gelber, 2014)	Degeneration and progressive loss of *cartilage* within the joints, damage to underlying bone, and formation of new bone at the margins of the cartilage	Knees, hips, hands (distal, sometimes proximal interphalangeal joints), cervical and lumbar spine, and wrists (first carpometacarpal joint); also joints previously injured or diseased	Additive; however, only one joint may be involved.	Usually insidious	Slowly progressive with temporary exacerbations after periods of overuse
Gouty Arthritis (Mead et al., 2014; Neogi, 2011; Sauvé et al., 2014) *Acute Gout*	An inflammatory reaction to microcrystals of sodium urate	Base of the big toe (the first metatarsophalangeal joint), the instep or dorsa of feet, the ankles, knees, and elbows	Early attacks usually confined to one joint	Sudden, often at night, often after injury, surgery, fasting, or excessive food or alcohol intake	Occasional isolated attacks lasting days up to 2 wk; they may get more frequent and severe, with persisting symptoms
Fibromyalgia Syndrome (Clauw, 2014)	Widespread musculoskeletal pain and tender points. May accompany other diseases. Mechanisms unclear	"All over," but especially in the neck, shoulders, hands, low back, and knees	Usually insidious	Variable	Chronic, with "ups and downs"

The vagueness of these characteristics is in itself a clue to the fibromyalgia syndrome

Associated Symptoms				
Swelling	**Redness, Warmth, and Tenderness**	**Stiffness**	**Limitation of Motion**	**Generalized Symptoms**
Frequent swelling of synovial tissue in joints or tendon sheaths; also subcutaneous nodules	Tender, often warm, but seldom red	Prominent, often for an hour or more in the mornings, also after inactivity	Often develops	Weakness, fatigue, weight loss, and low fever are common
Small effusions in the joints may be present, especially in the knees; also bony enlargement	Possibly tender, seldom warm, and rarely red	Frequent but brief (usually 5–10 min), in the morning and after inactivity	Often develops	Usually absent
Present within and around the involved joint	Exquisitely tender, hot, and red	Not evident	Motion is limited primarily by pain	Fever may be present
None	Multiple specific and symmetric tender "trigger points," often not recognized until the examination	Present, especially in the morning	Absent, though stiffness is greater at the extremes of movement	A disturbance of sleep, usually associated with morning fatigue; overlaps with depression

and management of stress (Fig. 18-85). Weight appropriate to height and body frame reduces excess mechanical wear on weight-bearing joints such as hips and knees. Of adults aged 18 years and older, 25.4% engaged in no leisure-time physical activity in 2018.

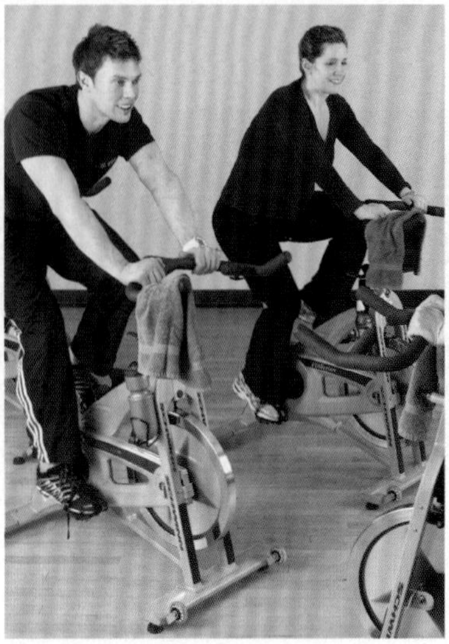

FIGURE 18-85 Stationary biking is a low-impact cardiovascular and muscle-strengthening activity.

The Healthy People 2030 objectives set goals for physical activity aimed at increasing the proportion of adults meeting guidelines for aerobic and muscle-strengthening physical activity (U.S. Department of Health and Human Services. Office of Disease Prevention and Health Promotion, n.d.a). These goals are based on the 2018 *Physical Activity Guidelines for Americans* 2nd edition (Office of Disease Prevention and Health Promotion, 2018), an evidence-based report that highlights the benefits of physical activity, including risk reduction for early death, cardiovascular disease, hypertension, type 2 diabetes, breast and colon cancer, obesity, osteoporosis, falls, and depression (Box 18-5). Physical activity also helps improve sleep quality and cognitive function in older adults.

BOX 18-5 PHYSICAL ACTIVITY GUIDELINES FOR AMERICANS

- Adults should participate in at least 2 hours and 30 minutes to 5 hours a week of moderate-intensity or 1 hour and 15 minutes to 2 hours and 30 minutes of vigorous-intensity aerobic physical activity a week or an equivalent combination of moderate- and vigorous-intensity aerobic activity. Preferably, aerobic activity should be spread throughout the week.
- Adults should also participate in muscle-strengthening activities of moderate or greater intensity and that involve all major muscle groups on 2 or more days a week, as these activities provide additional health benefits.

Source: Office of Disease Prevention and Health Promotion. (2018). *Physical activity guidelines for Americans* (2nd ed.). Retrieved April 15, 2021, from https://health.gov/our-work/physical-activity/current-guidelines

The report includes guidelines to help sedentary people gradually build up their activity level, starting with 10 minutes of exercise a day. Guided exercise regimens help reduce sports and exercise injuries, which are a significant source of musculoskeletal disorders.

Low Back Pain Prevention

Low back pain may feel dull like a constant ache or sudden and sharp. Most patients with acute low back pain are better within 6 weeks with medication and therapy. Back pain can result from (NIH. National Institute of Arthritis, 2019; NIH. National Institute of Neurological Disorders and Stroke, 2020):

See Table 18-3, "Low Back Pain," for common causes of low back pain.

- An accident
- A fall
- Lifting something heavy
- Changes that happen in the spine with aging
- A spinal disorder or medical condition

Nurses should educate healthy patients on strategies (NIH. National Institute of Arthritis, 2019) to prevent back pain. These include:

- Diet—The patient should be counseled to maintain a healthy weight as excess weight puts strain on the back. The diet should contain calcium and vitamin D to maintain bone strength. Osteoporosis in the spine can lead to back pain.
- Exercise—Flexion, extension, stretching, and aerobic exercise are recommended. Exercises such as tai chi and yoga or any weight-bearing exercise that challenges one's balance are helpful.
- Maintaining good posture and avoiding heavy lifting—Education on lifting strategies, posture, and the biomechanics of injury is prudent for people doing repetitive lifting such as nurses, heavy-machinery operators, and construction workers, for example.

Preventing Falls

Among older people in the United States, *falls* exact a heavy toll in morbidity and mortality. They are the leading cause of nonfatal injuries and account for a dramatic rise in death rates after 65 years of age. One out of three older people fall each year and one out of five falls causes a serious injury such as a broken bone or a head injury. More than 95% of hip fractures are caused by falling, usually by falling sideways. Each year, over 300,000 older adults are hospitalized for hip fractures. For those living independently before a hip fracture, 15% to 25% will still be in long-term care institutions a year after their fracture. Falls are the most common cause of traumatic brain injuries (TBIs) (Centers for Disease Control and Prevention [CDC], 2020).

Fall risk factors are both cognitive and physiologic, including unstable gait, imbalanced posture, reduced strength, previous fall, impaired mobility, medications, incontinence, hypertension, cognitive loss as in dementia, altered mental status, deficits in vision and proprioception, and osteoporosis. Poor lighting, stairs, chairs at awkward heights, slippery or irregular surfaces, and ill-fitting shoes are environmental dangers that can often be corrected. Nurses should work with patients and families to help modify such risks whenever possible. Home health assessments have proven useful in reducing environmental hazards, as have exercise programs to improve patient balance and strength. There are a number of fall risk assessment tools, such as the Hendrich II, that are helpful for identifying individuals at risk for falling.

See Chapter 24, "Assessing Older Adults."

Osteoporosis

Screening

Osteoporosis is a common U.S. health problem: 5.1% of men and 24.5% of women over age 65 have osteoporosis at the femoral neck or lumbar spine (U.S. Department of Health and Human Services. Office of Disease Prevention and Health Promotion, n.d.b).

Osteoporosis is a disease marked by reduced bone strength leading to an increased risk of fractures (broken bones). The osteoporosis objectives in Healthy People 2030 track bone mineral density as a measure of the major risk factor for fractures, and hip fractures, the major and most serious of osteoporosis-related fractures (U.S. Department of Health and Human Services. Office of Disease Prevention and Health Promotion, n.d.b). *Bone strength* reflects both *bone density* and *bone quality*. *Bone density* is determined by the interaction of bone mass (highest in the second decade), new bone formation, and bone resorption or loss. *Bone quality* refers to architecture, turnover, damage accumulation from microfractures, and mineralization. Osteoporosis typically arises from bone loss during aging, but reduced bone mass from suboptimal bone growth in childhood and adolescence can also cause osteoporosis.

Measuring Bone Density

Bone strength depends on bone quality, bone density, and overall bone size. Because there is no direct measurement of bone strength, bone mineral density, which accounts for approximately 70% of bone strength, is used as a proxy measure. The World Health Organization uses bone density to define osteopenia and osteoporosis:

- *Osteopenia*—Bone density T score between –2.5 and –1.0 (1.0–2.5 standard deviations below the young adult mean)

A T score is a standard deviation, a mathematical term that calculates how much a measurement varies from the mean.

- *Osteoporosis*—T score less than –2.5 (bone density 2.5 or more standard deviations below the young adult mean)

Bone densitometry scoring also includes Z scores representing comparisons with age-matched controls. These measurements are useful for determining whether bone loss is caused by an underlying disease or condition.

Bone density is measured at the hip, femoral neck, Ward triangle at the femoral neck, greater trochanter, and total hip, which includes all the measurements. A 10% drop in bone density, equivalent to 1.0 standard deviation, is associated with a 20% increase in risk for fracture.

CLINICAL TIP

Bone density peaks by age 30. Bone loss from age-related declines in estrogen and testosterone is initially rapid, then slows and becomes continuous.

Screening Recommendations

The U.S. Preventive Services Task Force (USPSTF, 2018) gives a grade B recommendation supporting osteoporosis screening for women aged 65 and older and for younger women whose 10-year fracture risk equals or exceeds that of an average-risk 65-year-old woman. The USPSTF finds that evidence about risks and benefits for men is insufficient for recommending routine screening. However, the American College of Physicians recommends that clinicians periodically assess older men for osteoporosis risk and measure bone density for those at increased risk who are candidates for drug therapy (Qaseem et al., 2008). Box 18-6 outlines risk factors for osteoporosis.

BOX 18-6 RISK FACTORS FOR OSTEOPOROSIS

- Postmenopausal status in women
- Age ≥50 years
- Low body mass index
- Low dietary calcium intake
- Vitamin D deficiency
- Prior fragility fracture
- Osteoporosis in a first-degree relative, especially with a prior fragility fracture
- Sedentary lifestyle or extended bed rest
- Tobacco and excessive alcohol use
- Inflammatory disorders of the musculoskeletal, pulmonary, or gastrointestinal systems, including celiac sprue, chronic renal disease, organ transplantation, diabetes, HIV hypogonadism, multiple myeloma, anorexia nervosa, and rheumatologic and autoimmune diseases
- Medications such as oral and high-dose inhaled corticosteroids, anticoagulants (long-term use), aromatase inhibitors for breast cancer, methotrexate, selected antiseizure medications, immunosuppressive agents, proton-pump inhibitors (long-term use), and antigonadal therapy for prostate cancer

The USPSTF recommends using a fracture risk assessment tool such as the World Health Organization's Fracture Risk Assessment Tool (FRAX) calculator. The FRAX calculator generates a 10-year osteoporotic fracture risk based on age; gender; weight; height; parental fracture history; use of glucocorticoids; presence of rheumatoid arthritis (RA) or conditions associated with secondary osteoporosis; tobacco and heavy alcohol use; and when available, femoral neck bone mineral density (BMD). The FRAX calculator also provides a 10-year hip fracture risk.

A previous low-impact fracture from standing height or less is the greatest risk factor for subsequent fracture.

FRAX has been validated for African American, Hispanic, and Asian women in the United States and has calculators that are continent and country-specific.

The website for the FRAX calculator for assessing fracture risk for the United States is http://www.shef.ac.uk/FRAX/tool.jsp?country=9

Prevention and Treatment

The therapeutic uses of available agents and options for preventing and treating osteoporosis are briefly summarized as follows.

Adequate calcium intake at all ages is necessary to prevent osteoporosis (National Institutes of Health [NIH], 2019). By the time teenagers finish growing, 90% of adult bone mass is established. For the older adult, increased calcium intake reduces age-related hyperparathyroidism and increases mineralization of newly formed bone. The nurse should assess calcium intake with the history.

There are two main forms of calcium supplements, calcium carbonate and calcium citrate. Supplements contain variable amounts of elemental calcium. Patients can read these amounts on the supplement facts panel of the containers. Calcium carbonate is less expensive and should be consumed with food. Calcium citrate is absorbed more easily in individuals with reduced levels of stomach acid and can be taken with or without food. Calcium absorption depends on the total amount consumed at one time—absorption diminishes at higher doses. Counsel patients to take doses of 500 mg at two separate times each day. Vitamin D supplements are available in two forms, D_2 (ergocalciferol) and D_3 (cholecalciferol); D_3 increases serum 25(OH)D levels more effectively than D_2 (NIH, 2019, 2021; NIH. Osteoporosis and Related Bone Diseases National Resource Center, 2018). Recommended daily intakes of calcium and vitamin D are listed in Table 18-21.

CLINICAL TIP
Patients on proton-pump inhibitor medicine have reduced stomach acid levels and should take calcium citrate supplements.

TABLE 18-21 Recommended Calcium and Vitamin D Intakes

Age Group	Calcium (mg/day)	Vitamin D (IU/day)
Infants 0–6 months	200	400
Infants 6–12 months	260	400
1–3 years old	700	600
4–8 years old	1,000	600
9–13 years old	1,300	600
14–18 years old	1,300	600
19–30 years old	1,000	600
31–50 years old	1,000	600
51–70-year-old males	1,000	600
51–70-year-old females	1,200	600
>70 years old	1,200	800
14–18 years old, pregnant/lactating	1,300	600
19–50 years old, pregnant/lactating	1,000	600

mg, milligrams; IU, International units.
Source: NIH. Osteoporosis and Related Bone Diseases National Resource Center. (2018, October). Calcium and Vitamin D: Important at every age. https://www.bones.nih.gov/health-info/bone/bone-health/nutrition/calcium-and-vitamin-d-important-every-age#d

Up to two thirds of patients with hip fractures are deficient in vitamin D, essential for calcium absorption and muscle strength. Vitamin D is synthesized in the skin through exposure to sunlight. Many people obtain enough vitamin D naturally by receiving 15 minutes of sunlight each day. Studies show that vitamin D production decreases in older adults, people who are housebound, and for most people during the winter. They may need vitamin D supplements to achieve the recommended daily intake. Food sources of vitamin D include egg yolks, saltwater fish, and liver (NIH, 2021).

Antiresorptive agents inhibit osteoclast activity and slow bone remodeling, allowing better mineralization of bone matrix and stabilization of the trabecular microarchitecture. These agents include bisphosphonates, selective estrogen receptor modulators (SERMs), calcitonin, and postmenopausal estrogen, now in question because of associated risks of breast cancer and vascular problems.

Bisphosphonates have been linked to osteonecrosis of the jaw and atypical femur fractures. SERMs increase the risk for thromboembolic events. Postmenopausal estrogen replacement is linked to increased risk of breast cancer and venous thromboembolism.

Anabolic agents such as parathyroid hormone stimulate bone formation by acting primarily on osteoblasts but require subcutaneous administration and monitoring for hypercalcemia. They are reserved for moderate to severe cases of osteoporosis (T scores less than −3.5 or less than −2.5 with a fragility fracture) or those who have failed or not tolerated other therapies (Thompson et al., 2020).

Regular exercise that includes weight bearing and resistance training can increase bone density and muscle strength but has not yet been shown to reduce fracture risk (USPSTF, 2018). Multidisciplinary programs to improve strength, balance, and home and medication safety can help prevent falls.

Alcohol prevents absorption of calcium. Women should limit alcohol to one drink per day and men to two drinks per day. Limit caffeine in the diet. Caffeine causes increased calcium excretion.

Bibliography

CITATIONS

American College of Physicians. (2012). Approach to the patient with rheumatic disease, in rheumatology. In V. Collier (Ed.), *Medical knowledge self-assessment program (MKSAP) 16*. American College of Physicians.

Anderson, J., Caplan, L., Yazdany, J., Robbins, M. L., Neogi, T., Michaud, K., Saag, K. G., O'Dell, J. R., & Kazi, S. (2012). Rheumatoid arthritis disease activity measures: American College of Rheumatology recommendations for use in clinical practice. *Arthritis Care & Research (Hoboken)*, *64*(5), 640–647.

Assassi, S., Weisman, M. H., Lee, M., Savage, L., Diekman, L., Graham, T. A., Rahbar, M. H., Schall, J. I., Gensler, L. S., Deodhar, A. A., Clegg, D. O., Colbert, R. A., & Reveille, J. D. (2014). New population-based reference values for spinal mobility measures based on the 2009–2010 National Health and Nutrition Examination Survey. *Arthritis & Rheumatology*, *66*(9), 2628–2637.

Bono, C. M., Ghiselli, G., Gilbert, T. J., Kreiner, D. S., Reitman, C., Summers, J. T., Baisden, J. L., Easa, J., Fernand, R., Lamer, T., Matz, P. G., Mazanec, D. J., Resnick, D. K., Shaffer, W. O., Sharma, A. K., Timmons, R. B., & Toton, J. F.; North American Spine Society. (2011). North American Spine Society. An evidence-based clinical guideline for the diagnosis and treatment of cervical radiculopathy from degenerative disorders. *The Spine Journal*, *11*, 64–72.

Centers for Disease Control and Prevention (CDC). (2020, March 3). Older adult fall prevention. https://www.cdc.gov/homeandrecreationalsafety/falls/index.html

Chou, R. (2014). In the clinic. Low back pain. *Annals of Internal Medicine*, *160*, ITC6-1.

Chou, R., & Shekelle, P. (2010). Will this patient develop persistent disabling low back pain? *JAMA*, *303*, 1295–1302.

Clauw, D. J. (2014). Fibromyalgia: A clinical review. *JAMA*, *311*, 1547–1555.

Davis, J. M. 3rd, & Matteson, E. L.; American College of Rheumatology; European League Against Rheumatism. (2012). My treatment approach to rheumatoid arthritis. *Mayo Clinic Proceedings*, *87*, 659–673.

Gelber, A. C. (2014). In the clinic. Osteoarthritis. *Annals of Internal Medicine*, *161*, ITC1-1.

Golub, A. L., & Laya, M. B. (2015). Osteoporosis: Screening, prevention, and management. *The Medical Clinics of North America*, *99*, 587–606.

McGee, S. (2018a). Examination of the musculoskeletal system: The knee. In *Evidence-based physical diagnosis* (4th ed., pp. 503–504). Elsevier Saunders.

McGee, S. (2018b). Examination of the musculoskeletal system: The shoulder. In *Evidence-based physical diagnosis* (4th ed., p. 493). Elsevier Saunders.

McGee, S. (2018c). Examination of the musculoskeletal system: The shoulder. In *Evidence-based physical diagnosis* (4th ed., p. 483). Elsevier Saunders.

McGee, S. (2018d). Peripheral nerve injury: Diagnosis of carpal tunnel syndrome. In *Evidenced-based physical diagnosis* (4th ed., pp. 603–604). Elsevier Saunders.

Mead, T., Arabindoo, K., & Smith, B. (2014). Managing gout: There's more we can do. *Journal of Family Practice*, *63*, 707–713.

National Institutes of Health (NIH). (2019). Osteoporosis and related bone diseases National Resource Center. Osteoporosis overview. Retrieved October, 2019, from https://www.bones.nih.gov/health-info/bone/osteoporosis/overview

National Institutes of Health (NIH). (2021). Office of Dietary Supplements. Vitamin D. https://ods.od.nih.gov/factsheets/VitaminD-HealthProfessional/

Neogi, T. (2011). Gout. *The New England Journal of Medicine*, *364*, 443–452.

Neubauer, T., Brand, J., Lidder, S., & Krawany, M. (2016). Stress fractures of the femoral neck in runners: A review. *Research in Sports Medicine*, *24*(3), 283–297.

NIH. National Institute of Arthritis. (2019, July). Musculoskeletal and skin diseases. Back pain: Can I prevent back pain? https://www.niams.nih.gov/health-topics/back-pain#tab-prevention

NIH. National Institute of Neurological Disorders and Stroke. (2020, April 27). Low back pain fact sheet. https://www.ninds.nih.gov/disorders/patient-caregiver-education/fact-sheets/low-back-pain-fact-sheet

NIH. Osteoporosis and Related Bone Diseases National Resource Center. (2018, October). Calcium and Vitamin D: Important at every age. https://www.bones.nih.gov/health-info/bone/bone-health/nutrition/calcium-and-vitamin-d-important-every-age#d

Office of Disease Prevention and Health Promotion. (2018). *Physical activity guidelines for Americans* (2nd ed.). Retrieved April 15, 2021, from https://health.gov/our-work/physical-activity/current-guidelines

Onks, C. A., & Billy, G. (2013). Evaluation and treatment of cervical radiculopathy. *Primary Care*, *40*, 837–848.

Qaseem, A., Snow, V., Shekelle, P., Hopkins, R., Jr, Forciea, M. A., & Owens, D. K. (2008). Screening for osteoporosis in men: A clinical practice guideline from the American College of Physicians. *Annals of Internal Medicine*, *148*(9), 680–684. https://doi.org/10.7326/0003-4819-148-9-200805060-00008

Raychaudhuri, S. P., & Deodhar, A. (2014). The classification and diagnostic criteria of ankylosing spondylitis. *Journal of Autoimmunity*, *48*, 128–133.

Ropper, A. H., & Zafonte, R. D. (2015). Sciatica. *The New England Journal of Medicine*, *372*, 1240–1248.

Rozenberg, S., Foltz, V., & Fautrel, B. (2012). Treatment strategy for chronic low back pain. *Joint Bone Spine*, *79*, 555–559.

Sauvé, P. S., Rhee, P. C., Shin, A. Y., & Lindau, T. (2014). Examination of the wrist: Radial-sided wrist pain. *The Journal of Hand Surgery*, *39*(10), 2089–2092.

Thompson, J. C., Wanderman, N., Anderson, P. A., & Freedman, B. A. (2020). Abaloparatide and the spine: A narrative review. *Clinical Interventions in Aging*, *15*, 1023–1033.

U.S. Department of Health and Human Services. Office of Disease Prevention and Health Promotion. (n.d.a). Healthy People 2030: Physical activity. Retrieved April 15, 2021 from https://health.gov/healthypeople/objectives-and-data/browse-objectives/physical-activity

U.S. Department of Health and Human Services. Office of Disease Prevention and Health Promotion. (n.d.b). Healthy People 2030: Osteoporosis. Retrieved April 15, 2021, from https://health.gov/healthypeople/objectives-and-data/browse-objectives/osteoporosis

U.S. Department of Health and Human Services. Office of Disease Prevention and Health Promotion. (n.d.c). Healthy People 2030. Retrieved April 15, 2021, from https://health.gov/healthypeople

U.S. Preventive Services Task Force (USPSTF). (2018, June 26). Final recommendation statement: Osteoporosis to prevent fractures: Screening. https://www.uspreventiveservicestaskforce.org/uspstf/document/RecommendationStatementFinal/osteoporosis-screening

Young, C. (2012). In the clinic. Plantar fasciitis. *Annals of Internal Medicine*, *156*, ITC1-1.

19 MENTAL STATUS AND MENTAL HEALTH ASSESSMENT

KEY TERMS

affect	insight	orientation
bradykinesia	judgment	thought content
dementia	level of consciousness	thought processes
hyperkinesia	mental status	

Learning Objectives

The student will:

1. Obtain a mental status history for a patient.
2. Describe the major components assessed in the mental status examination.
3. Document the findings of the mental status assessment.
4. Identify the screening, health promotion, and counseling tools for mental health concerns.

Mental status and mental health assessments are complex and should be woven into every aspect of care. For the purpose of this chapter, the **mental status** is the overall observation and screening of a patient's behavior and cognitive function. The mental health assessment incorporates an assessment of presenting symptoms and behaviors utilizing screening tools in an effort to promote well-being. As nurses, we are uniquely positioned to screen, detect, and investigate clues of mental status and behavioral health changes, including harmful behaviors. Nurses are on the frontlines and poised to encourage health-promoting behaviors. Empathic listening and close observation offer a perspective to the patient's outlook, concerns, and habits. Nevertheless, health care providers, including nurses, may miss subtle clues and dysfunctional behaviors in patients. Recognizing mental health changes in behaviors or coping mechanisms throughout the entire assessment and not specific to one system is especially important given the significant prevalence and morbidity, the high likelihood of treatment, the shortage of mental health care providers, and the increasing importance of primary care clinicians as the first to encounter the patient's distress (Olfson, 2016). Mental health disorders affect almost 50 million adults in the United States, and only about 35 million of those obtain treatment (Substance Abuse and Mental Health Services Administration, 2019). Of those individuals, adherence to treatment guidelines in primary care offices is less than 50% and is disproportionately lower for ethnic minorities (Poghosyan et al., 2019) and members of the LGBTQIA community (Substance Abuse and Mental Health Services Administration, 2019). Social determinants of health paired with lack of mental health resources indicate appropriate care is urgent. Health practitioner awareness of subtle signs and symptoms and knowledge of availability and access to resources are necessary to support the community served (Doornbos et al., 2020).

This chapter introduces:

- Common symptoms and behaviors suggestive of changes in mental status and mental health
- Concepts that guide history taking and the general assessment of mental status
- Components of the mental status examination that should be conducted when behavioral problems are potential indications of mental health changes
- Priorities for mental health promotion and counseling

It is important for nurses to assess for both mental and physical changes. Mental health disorders are commonly masked by other clinical conditions, calling for sensitive and careful inquiry. Questions addressing specific areas are available and utilized to guide the mental status examination as needed. Early recognition of a disorder is paramount. The astute assessment and documentation of findings are crucial to formulate the best plan for each individual patient.

Many of the terms pertinent to the mental health history and the mental status examination are familiar to you from social conversation. It is important to learn their precise meanings in the context of formal evaluation of mental status, as detailed in Table 19-1.

TABLE 19-1 Mental Status Examination Terminology

Level of Consciousness	Alertness or State of Awareness of the Environment
Attention	The ability to focus or concentrate over time on one task or activity; an inattentive or distractible person with impaired consciousness has difficulty giving a history or responding to questions.

Level of Consciousness	Alertness or State of Awareness of the Environment
Memory	The process of registering or recording information, tested by asking for immediate repetition of material followed by storage or retention of information. Recent or short-term memory covers minutes, hours, or days; remote or long-term memory refers to intervals of years.
Orientation	Awareness of personal identity, place, time and situation; requires both memory and attention.
Perceptions	Sensory awareness of objects in the environment and their interrelationships (external stimuli); also refers to internal stimuli such as dreams or hallucinations.
Thought processes	The logic, coherence, and relevance of the patient's thought as it leads to select goals or how people think.
Thought content	What the patient thinks about, including level of insight and judgment.
Insight	Awareness that symptoms or disturbed behaviors are normal or abnormal; for example, distinguishing between daydreams and hallucinations that seem real.
Judgment	Process of comparing and evaluating alternatives when deciding on a course of action; reflects values that may or may not be based on reality and social conventions or norms.
Affect	An observable, usually episodic, feeling or tone expressed through voice, facial expression, and demeanor.
Mood	A more sustained emotion that may color a person's view of the world (mood is to affect as climate is to weather).
Language	A complex symbolic system for expressing, receiving, and comprehending words; as with consciousness, attention, and memory, language is essential for assessing other mental functions.
Higher cognitive functions	Assessed by vocabulary, amount of information, abstract thinking, calculations, and construction of objects that have two or three dimensions.

THE HEALTH HISTORY

Common or concerning symptoms related to mental status and mental health identified during the health history are listed in Box 19-1.

BOX 19-1 COMMON OR CONCERNING SYMPTOMS

- Changes in attention, mood, or speech
- Changes in orientation or insight
- Changes in memory
- Medical symptoms without an explanation

Your assessment of mental status begins when you first meet the patient (Fig. 19-1). As you gather the health history, you will quickly observe the patient's level of alertness and orientation, mood, attention, speech, and memory. As the history unfolds, you will learn about the patient's insight and judgment as well as any recurring or unusual thoughts or perceptions. You may gain a glimpse or understanding of how this impacts the person or how they are dealing with what is occurring. These components will alert you to conditions that may require more detailed follow-up, including a formal mental status examination and possible referral.

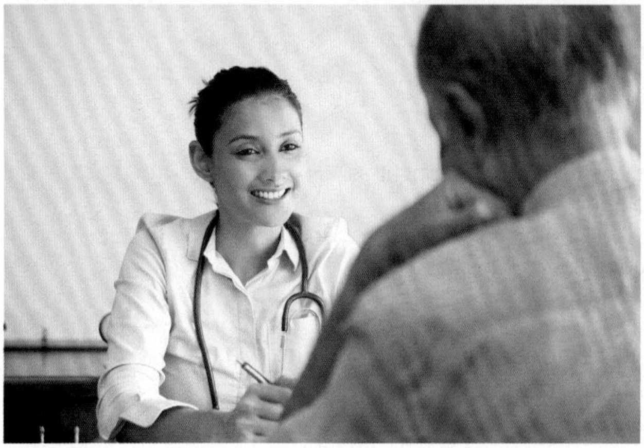

FIGURE 19-1 Your assessment of mental status begins when you first meet the patient. (AshTproduction/Shutterstock.)

If a family member or friend accompanies the patient to the visit, consultation with them may prove informative, especially if the patient and examiner do not speak the same language and cultural implications can facilitate better understanding. A medical interpreter is most beneficial for understanding the exact words from the patient rather than a layperson's interpretations. Make sure the patient has adequate time to talk and be heard and family members do not take over the interview (Armitage, 2015).

Attention, Mood, and Speech; Insight and Orientation

Assess the patient's level of consciousness, general appearance, mood, and ability to pay attention, remember, understand, and speak. Place the patient's vocabulary and general knowledge and information in the context of the cultural and educational background. The patient's account of illness and life circumstances often tell you about insight and judgment. Asking questions such as, "How did the COVID-19 pandemic impact you?" If you suspect a problem in orientation and memory, you can ask, "When was your last clinic appointment?" "And the date today?" Try to integrate your evaluation of mental status into the history, and it will seem less like an interrogation. The flow comes more easily with practice and interactions with a variety of patients (Martinez-Martinez et al., 2019).

See Chapter 20, "The Nervous System," Table 20-8, "Disorders of Speech."

Memory Changes

There are many reasons for changes in memory. A detailed health history can assist in targeting the origin of change and the plan for it. Often if the memory is wavering, family members or close friends may be instrumental in recalling events or situations. Inclusion of the person and use of therapeutic communication techniques and compassion assist in the discussion of memory changes.

Open-ended questions, such as "Have you (or anyone else) noticed any changes in your memory?" "Do feel as though you are misplacing items?" and "Are you feeling forgetful?" start the conversation.

If the person or someone in their inner circle confirms memory loss, then ask about onset and duration. "When did you notice the forgetfulness initially? Did this occur suddenly or over a period of time?"

Additional information should be collected about any changes in socialization, personality, wandering or getting lost in familiar areas, and activities of daily living like eating, dressing, toileting, ambulating, buying groceries, cooking, and/or paying bills. This information is necessary to assess the situation to keep the person safe and provide necessary support to maintain a quality life.

Neurocognitive disorders other than delirium are divided into two categories: major cognitive disorders, including **dementia** (a chronic disorder of mental processes characterized by memory loss, personality changes, and impaired reasoning), and less severe levels of cognitive impairment, now termed mild neurocognitive disorders, which may apply to younger individuals with impairment from traumatic brain injury or HIV infection, for example. These varying levels and reconfigurations have impacted clinicians on many levels from education of patients to reimbursement for care.

The term *dementia* is to be documented in parenthesis due to widespread clinical usage.

A wide range of factors warrant assessment of mental status; brain injuries, psychiatric symptoms, reports from family members of vague or changed behavior, subtle behavioral changes, difficulty taking medications as prescribed, problems attending to household chores or paying bills, and loss of interest in their usual activities are some examples. Other patients may have changes related to the hospitalization or medications and behave differently or have a change in orientation after surgery or during an acute illness. Each change should be identified and assessed as expeditiously as possible. The nurse is the patient's advocate, and the person who can alleviate unexpected problems identified during prompt assessment that can impact the patient and family on many levels such as relationships or finances.

Screening for neurocognitive disorders such as delirium and dementia can be found in Chapter 24.

See Table 24-1, "Delirium and Dementia."

Medical Symptoms without an Explanation

For beginning nurses, the challenge is to sort out the array of symptoms encountered. Symptoms may be psychological, relating to mood change or an emotional state, or physical, relating to a body sensation such as pain, fatigue, or palpitations. Physical symptoms are also known as somatic. Common somatic complaints include pain from headache, backache, or musculoskeletal conditions; gastrointestinal symptoms; sexual or reproductive symptoms; and neurologic symptoms such as dizziness or loss of balance (Martinez-Martinez et al., 2019).

Approximately 5% of somatic symptoms are acute, triggering immediate evaluation (Kroenke, 2014). Another 70% to 75% are minor or self-limited and resolve in 6 weeks. Nevertheless, approximately 25% of patients have persisting and recurrent symptoms that elude assessment through the history and physical examination and fail to improve. Overall, 30% of symptoms are medically unexplained. Some of them involve single complaints that appear to persist longer than others such as back pain, headache, or musculoskeletal pain. Others occur in clusters presenting as functional syndromes, such as irritable bowel syndrome, fibromyalgia, chronic fatigue, temporomandibular joint disorder, or multiple chemical sensitivity.

Two thirds of patients with depression, for example, present with physical complaints, and half report multiple unexplained physical or somatic symptoms (Kroenke, 2014). Often both occur together and have overlapping symptoms (Kroenke, 2009).

A physical symptom can be explained physically or medically or can be unexplained; a somatoform symptom lacks an adequate medical or physical explanation (Kroenke, 2014).

Understanding Symptoms

Physical and psychological symptoms may be intertwined and present as both medical and mental health issues (Kroenke, 2009). Evidence shows that symptom etiology is often multifactorial, lacking a single cause and with several related symptoms or symptom clusters rather than single complaints. Astute assessment, verbal cues, and attention to subtle, nonverbal communication, in addition to input from family or friends are important for a comprehensive history.

Failure to recognize a mix of physical symptoms and functional syndromes with common mental health disorders such as anxiety, depression, unexplained or somatoform physical symptoms, and substance use disorder may contribute to loss of the patient's quality of life and impaired treatment outcomes. Often these patients may need to use the health care system frequently and have significant disability. Treating the signs and symptoms of mental health disorders with complete attention and compassion is key (Tranter & Robertson, 2019).

PHYSICAL EXAMINATION

Important Areas of the Mental Status Examination

The assessment of mental status is challenging and complex as it assesses both the patient's behavior and cognitive function. Changes in mental status warrant careful evaluation for underlying pathologic and pharmacologic causes. The patient's personality, psychodynamics, family and life experiences, and cultural background all factor into the mental status assessment. The nervous system, mental status, and brain structure and function are intimately intertwined. The assessment of mental status is an integral component of the assessment of the nervous system, and the first segment of the nervous system documentation. With practice, you will learn to describe the patient's mood, speech, behavior, and cognition and relate these findings to your examination of the cranial nerves, motor and sensory systems, and reflexes.

Novice nurses may feel reluctant to perform mental status examinations, wondering if the examinations will upset patients or invade their privacy. Such concerns are understandable. An insensitive examination may alarm a patient, and even a skillful examination may bring to conscious awareness a deficit that the patient is trying to ignore. Discuss concerns with your instructor or other experienced nurses. Remember that patients appreciate an understanding listener.

The components of the mental status examination (Table 19-2) can help organize your observations, but they are not intended as a step-by-step

TABLE 19-2 Components of the Mental Status Examination

Components	Observations
Appearance and behavior	• Level of consciousness • Dress, grooming, personal hygiene • Posture and motor behavior • Facial expression
Speech and language	• Quantity, rate, and volume of speech • Articulation of words • Fluency
Mood and affect	• Mood is the emotional makeup or feeling and how it varies with life events. • Affect is how the emotions are expressed.
Thought process and content	• Logic, relevance, organization, and coherence of a patient's thought • Abnormalities in thought content or perception • Insight and judgment
Cognitive function	• Orientation to person, place, time, and situation • Attention/concentration: digit span, serial 7's, spelling backward • Remote and recent memory • New learning ability • Higher cognitive function: information and vocabulary, calculations, abstract thinking and constructional ability

guide. When a full examination is indicated, be flexible in approach but thorough. In some situations, however, sequence is important. If, during the initial interview, the patient's consciousness, attention, comprehension of words or ability to speak seems impaired, assess this observation promptly. If a patient cannot give a reliable history, testing many other mental functions will be difficult and warrants an evaluation for acute causes.

Appearance and Behavior

Utilize all the relevant observations made throughout the course of the history and examination.

Level of Consciousness

Is the patient awake and alert? Does the patient seem to understand the questions and respond appropriately and reasonably quickly, or is there a tendency to lose track of the topic and fall silent or even asleep?

If the patient does not respond to your questions, escalate the stimulus with the following steps:

- Speak to the patient by name and in a loud voice.
- Touch the patient gently, as if awakening someone sleeping.
- If there is no response to these stimuli, promptly assess the patient for stupor or coma as this is a severe reduction in level of consciousness.

A patient's **level of consciousness** is based on the response and as outlined in Table 19-3.

TABLE 19-3 Categorizing Level of Consciousness

Level of Consciousness	Patient Response
Alert	Patient is awake, eyes open and looks when spoken to in a normal tone of voice. Responds appropriately and fully.
Lethargy	Patients appear drowsy, look at you, respond to question, and then fall asleep.
Obtunded	Patients open their eyes and look at you, but slowly respond and are somewhat confused.
Stupor	Patients arouse from sleep only after painful stimuli. Verbal responses are slow or absent. Go back to unresponsive state after stimulus stops. Minimal awareness of self or environment.
Coma	Patients are unconscious and do not respond to painful stimuli or voice and do not open their eyes.

Dress, Grooming, and Personal Hygiene

Note if the person appears to be their stated age or if they look older or younger than the actual age. Compare one side of the body with the other as you assess the patient and think about these additional components:

One-sided neglect may result from a lesion in the opposite parietal cortex, usually the nondominant side.

- How is the patient dressed?
- Is the clothing clean and appropriate for patient's age and the weather?
- Scars?
- Note the grooming of the patient's hair, nails, teeth, skin, and, if present, facial hair. How does the grooming and hygiene compare with peers of comparable age, lifestyle, culture, and socioeconomic group?

Grooming and personal hygiene may deteriorate in depression, schizophrenia, and dementia. Excessive fastidiousness may be seen in obsessive–compulsive disorder.

Posture and Motor Behavior

Assess if the patient prefers to sit, lie quietly, or walk around. Observe the patient's posture and ability to relax. Note the pace, range, and type of movement. Are movements voluntary, spontaneous, and fluid? Are any limbs immobile, flaccid, or fixed in position? Are posture and motor activity affected by topics under discussion, type of activity, pain, or who is in the room?

CLINICAL TIP
Look for the tense posture and restlessness of anxiety; the fidgeting; crying, pacing, and hand wringing of agitated depression; the hopeless, slumped posture, and slowed movements of depression; the agitated and expansive movements of a manic episode.

Observe the patient's gait:

- Slowed psychomotor: **bradykinesia** (slow movement, shuffle or drags feet when walking, limited or no facial expression)

A person with a neurocognitive disorder or depression may exhibit *bradykinesia.*

- Agitated psychomotor: **hyperkinesia** (excess abnormal movements)

A person under the influence of a stimulant drug or having a manic episode may exhibit *hyperkinesia.*

- Shuffle, ataxic, or stiff

A person who is shuffling, ataxic, or stiff may have a neurologic disease.

Facial Expression

Observe the face, both at rest and when communicating with others. Watch for variations in expression with topics under discussion. Are they appropriate for the topics being discussed? Is the face relatively immobile throughout?

CLINICAL TIP
Note expressions of anxiety, depression, apathy, anger, elation; facial immobility as seen in Parkinson disease. Look for the anger, hostility, suspiciousness, or evasiveness of paranoia; the elation and euphoria of mania; the flat affect and remoteness of schizophrenia; the apathy (dulled affect with detachment and indifference) of dementia; and anxiety or depression.

Speech and Language

Throughout the interview, note the characteristics of the patient's speech, including the following.

Quantity

Is the patient talkative or silent? Is this a change? Is this related to cultural background? Are comments spontaneous or limited to direct questions?

Rate

Is speech fast or slow?

Note the slow speech of depression and the accelerated, louder speech of mania.

Loudness

Is speech loud or soft?

Articulation of Words

Are the words clear and distinct? Does the speech have a nasal quality? Dysarthria refers to defective articulation. Aphasia is a disorder of language. Dysphonia results from impaired volume, quality, or pitch of the voice. See Chapter 20, "The Nervous System," Table 20-8, "Disorders of Speech."

Fluency

Fluency reflects the flow and melody of speech and the content and use of words. Watch for abnormalities of spontaneous speech such as:

- Hesitancies and gaps in the flow and rhythm of words
- Disturbed inflections, such as a monotone
- Circumlocutions, in which phrases or sentences are substituted for a word the person cannot think of, such as "what you write with" for "pen"
- Paraphasias, in which words are malformed ("I write with a den"), wrong ("I write with a bar"), or invented ("I write with a dar")

These abnormalities suggest aphasia from cerebrovascular infarction. Aphasia may be receptive (impaired comprehension with fluent speech) or expressive (with preserved comprehension and slow nonfluent speech). If the patient's speech lacks meaning or fluency, proceed with further testing as outlined in Table 19-4.

TABLE 19-4 Testing for Aphasia

Word comprehension	Ask the patient to follow a one-stage command, such as "Point to your nose." Try a two-stage command: "Point to your mouth then your knee."
Repetition	Ask the patient to repeat a phrase of one-syllable words (the most difficult repetition task): "No ifs, ands, or buts."
Naming	Ask the patient to name the parts of a watch.
Reading comprehension	Ask the patient to read a paragraph aloud.
Writing	Ask the patient to write a sentence.

The prompts in Table 19-4 help identify the type of aphasia. Check for deficits in vision, hearing, intelligence, and education; these may affect responses. Two common kinds of aphasia—receptive (Wernicke) and expressive (Broca)—are compared in Table 20-8, "Disorders of Speech."

A person who can write a correct sentence does not have aphasia.

Mood and Affect

Mood

Ask the person to describe their mood, including usual mood level and how it has varied with life events. "How did you feel about that?" for example, or more generally, "How is your overall mood?" The reports of relatives and friends may be of great value.

Moods include sadness and deep melancholy; contentment, joy, euphoria, and elation; anger and rage; anxiety and worry; and detachment and indifference.

Has the mood been intense and unchanging or labile? How long has it lasted? Is it appropriate to the patient's circumstances or situation? If depressed, have there been episodes of an elevated mood, suggesting a bipolar disorder?

If you suspect depression, assess its severity and any risk of suicide. The following series of questions is useful, proceeding as far as the patient's positive answers warrant:

- Do you feel discouraged (or depressed, blue) or not yourself?
- How low do you feel?

- What do you see for yourself in the future?
- Do you ever feel that life is not worth living or that you want to be dead?
- Have you ever thought of killing yourself?
- How did (do) you think you would do it? Do you have a plan?
- What do you think would happen after you were dead?

Directly asking about suicidal thoughts does not implant the idea in the patient's mind, and it may be the only way to get the information. Although you may feel uneasy about direct questions, many patients discuss their thoughts and feelings freely, sometimes with considerable relief. By open discussion, you demonstrate your interest and concern for a possibly life-threatening problem. It is your responsibility to ask directly about suicidal thoughts. This may be the only way to uncover suicidal ideation and plans that indicate immediate intervention and treatment.

Affect

Affect is a collation of a number of components of the mental status examination and should be assessed in the context of what is currently occurring and past visits. Using your observations of facial expressions, voice, and body movements, assess the patient's **affect,** or external expression of the inner emotional state.

- Does it vary appropriately with topics being discussed, or is it labile, blunted, or flat?
- Does it seem inappropriate or extreme at certain points? If so, how?
- Note the patient's openness, approachability, and reactions to others and to the surroundings.
- Does the patient seem to hear or see things that you do not? Does the patient seem to be talking with someone who is not present?

Thought Process and Content

Thought Process

Assess the logic, relevance, organization, and coherence of the patient's **thought processes** throughout the interview. Does speech progress logically toward a goal? Listen for patterns of speech that suggest disorders of thought processes, as outlined in Table 19-5.

TABLE 19-5 Variations in Thought Process

Name	Explanation	Occurrence
Circumstantiality	Speech with unnecessary detail, indirection, and delay in reaching the point. Some topics may have a meaningful connection. People without mental disorders may have circumstantial speech.	Obsessions
Blocking	Sudden interruption of speech in midsentence or before the idea is completed, attributed to "losing the thought." Blocking occurs in people with normal mental health statuses.	Schizophrenia, manic episodes, or other psychotic disorders
Flight of ideas	An almost continuous flow of accelerated speech with abrupt changes from one topic to the next. Changes are based on understandable associations, plays on words, or distracting stimuli, but ideas are not well connected.	Most frequently noted in manic episodes
Confabulation	Fabrication of facts or events in response to questions to fill in the gaps from impaired memory.	Dementia, schizophrenia, psychotic disorders, or aphasia
Incoherence	Speech that is incomprehensible and illogic with lack of meaningful connections, abrupt changes in topic, or disordered grammar or word use. Flight of ideas, when severe, may produce incoherence.	Severe psychotic disturbances (usually schizophrenia)
Derailment (loosening of associations)	"Tangential" speech with shifting topics that are loosely connected or unrelated. The patient is unaware of the lack of association.	Schizophrenia
Neologisms	Invented or distorted words, words with new and highly idiosyncratic meanings.	Korsakoff syndrome from alcoholism
Perseveration	Persistent repetition of words or ideas.	Schizophrenia or other psychotic disorders
Echolalia	Repetition of the words and phrases of others.	Manic episodes or schizophrenia
Clanging	Speech with choice of words based on sound rather than meaning, as in rhyming and punning. For example, "Look at my eyes and nose, wise eyes and rosy nose. Two to one, the ayes have it!"	Schizophrenia or manic episodes

Thought Content

Thought content is what the person is thinking and is assessed during the interaction. To assess thought content, follow appropriate leads as they occur rather than asking scripted lists of specific questions. For example, "You mentioned that a neighbor was responsible for your entire illness. Can you tell me more about that?" Or in another specific situation, "What do you think about at times like these?"

For more focused inquiries, be tactful and accepting. Patients may experience changes in thought content that may indicate certain medical disorders. By framing questions in such a way that guides the patient (Table 19-6), the nurse can find out additional information adding clarity to a possible mental disorder diagnosis while working with the health care team.

TABLE 19-6 Assessment of Thought Content

Delusions	Do you think people are talking about you? Do you feel like you are not a good person? Are people taking things from you? What are your super powers?
Obsessions	Do you have thoughts or pictures in your head that will not go away?
Phobias	Are you extremely afraid of anything that other people do not fear as much?
Suicidal	Do you ever feel that life is not worth living? Have you ever thought about killing yourself?

Perceptions

Inquire about false perceptions in a manner similar to that used for thought content. For example, "When you heard the voice speaking to you, what did it say? How did it make you feel?" Or, "After you have been drinking a lot, do you ever see things that are not really there?" Or, "Sometimes after major surgery like this, people hear peculiar or frightening things. Has anything like this ever happened to you?" In these ways, find out about abnormal perceptions (Table 19-7).

TABLE 19-7 Abnormalities of Perception

Name	Explanation	Occurrence
Illusions	Misinterpretations of real external stimuli, such as mistaking rustling leaves for the sound of voices	Grief reactions, delirium, acute and posttraumatic stress disorders, schizophrenia
Hallucinations	Perception-like experiences that seem real, but unlike illusions, lack actual external stimulation. The person may or may not recognize the experiences as false. Hallucinations may be auditory, visual, olfactory, gustatory, tactile, or somatic. False perceptions associated with dreaming, falling asleep, and awakening are not classified as hallucinations.	Delirium, dementia (less commonly), posttraumatic stress disorder, schizophrenia, alcoholism

Source: American Psychiatric Association. (2013). *Diagnostic and statistical manual of mental disorders* (5th ed.). American Psychiatric Press.

Insight and Judgment

Insight

Insight is the ability to understand a situation and is often intuitive. Some of the first interview questions to the patient often yield important information about insight: "What brings you to the hospital?" "What seems to be the trouble?" "What do you think is wrong?" Note whether the patient is aware that a particular mood, thought, or perception is abnormal or potentially part of an illness.

Patients with psychotic disorders often lack insight into their illnesses. Denial of impairment may accompany some neurologic disorders.

Judgment

Judgment is the ability to make an appropriate decision after careful thought. These attributes are usually best assessed during the interview. Assess judgment by noting the patient's responses to family situations, jobs, use of money, and interpersonal conflicts. "How do you plan to get the help you will need after leaving the hospital?" "What are your plans if you lose your job?" "If your partner starts to abuse you again, what will you do?" "Who will attend to your financial affairs while you are in long-term care?"

CLINICAL TIP
Judgment may be poor in delirium, dementia, intellectual disabilities, and psychotic states. Anxiety, mood disorders, intelligence, education, income, and cultural values also influence judgment.

Note whether decisions and actions are based on reality or impulse, wish fulfillment, or disordered thought content. What insights and values seem to underlie the patient's decisions and behaviors? Allowing for cultural variations, how do these compare with mature adult standards? Because judgment reflects maturity, it may be variable and unpredictable during adolescence.

Poor judgment may occur when memory or attention is impaired, as in delirium.

Cognitive Functions

Orientation

The patient's **orientation** can usually be determined in the context of the interview. For example, you can naturally ask for clarification about specific dates and times, the patient's address and telephone number, the names of family members, or the route taken or why they are in the hospital. At times, direct questions are necessary to determine if the person is oriented to all four of the following components:

- Person—the patient's own name and the names of relatives and professional personnel

"Can you tell me your name?"

- Place—the patient's residence, city, and state

"What is your address?"

- Time—the time of day, day of the week, month, season, date and year, duration of hospitalization

"Can you tell me what time it is now? What day it is?"

- Situation—what just happened/is happening (frequently used after an accident or anesthesia)

"Can you tell me what just happened?"

When choosing the questions, be sure you know the correct answer or be able to validate it. Otherwise, the person may answer appropriately, but it may or may not be correct.

Attention/Concentration

The following tests of attention are commonly used.

Digit Span

Explain that you would like to test the patient's ability to concentrate, perhaps adding that this can be difficult if the patient is in pain or ill. Recite a series of numbers, starting with two at a time and speaking each number clearly at a rate of about one per second. Ask the patient to repeat the numbers back to you. If this repetition is accurate, try a series of three numbers, then four, as long as the patient responds correctly. Jot down the numbers as you say them to ensure your own accuracy. If the patient makes a mistake, try once more with another series of the same length. Stop after a second failure in a single series.

Causes of poor performance include delirium, dementia, intellectual disability, and performance anxiety.

When choosing digits, you may use street numbers, zip codes, telephone numbers, and other numerical sequences that are familiar to you, but avoid consecutive numbers, easily recognized dates, and sequences that are possibly familiar to the patient.

Now, starting again with a series of two, ask the patient to repeat the numbers to you backward. Normally, a person should be able to repeat correctly at least five numbers forward and four backward.

Serial 7s

Instruct the patient, "Starting from 100, subtract 7, and keep subtracting 7." Note the effort required and the speed and accuracy of the responses. After five correct answers, the patient has a positive serial 7 response. Writing down the answers helps you keep up with the arithmetic. Normally, a person can complete serial 7s in 1½ minutes, with fewer than four errors. If the patient cannot do serial 7s, try 3s or counting backward.

Poor performance may result from delirium, late-stage dementia, intellectual disability, loss of calculating ability, anxiety, or depression. Also consider educational level.

Spelling Backward

This can substitute for serial 7s. Say a five-letter word, spell it, for example, "W-O-R-L-D," and ask the patient to spell it backward.

Memory

Remote Memory

Inquire about birthdays, anniversaries, social security number, names of schools attended, jobs held, or past historical events such as wars relevant to the patient's past.

Remote memory may be impaired in the late stage of dementia.

Recent Memory

Recent memory assessment can involve the events of the day. Ask questions with answers you can check against other sources to see if the patient is confabulating or making up facts to compensate for memory difficulty. These might include the day's weather, today's appointment time, and medications or laboratory tests taken during the day. Asking what the patient had for breakfast may be a waste of time unless you can check the accuracy of the answer.

CLINICAL TIP

Recent memory is impaired in dementia and delirium. Amnestic disorders impair memory or new learning ability significantly and reduce a person's social or occupational functioning, but they do not have the global features of delirium or dementia. Anxiety, depression, and intellectual disability may also impair recent memory.

New Learning Ability

Give the patient three or four words such as "table, flower, purple, and hamburger." Ask the patient to repeat them so that you know that the information has been heard and registered. This step, like digit span, tests retention of information and immediate recall. Then proceed to other parts of the examination. After about 3 to 5 minutes, ask the patient to repeat the words. Note the accuracy of the response, awareness of whether it is correct, and any tendency to confabulate. Normally, a person should be able to remember the words.

Higher Cognitive Functions

Information and Vocabulary

If clinically observed in the context of cultural and educational background, information and vocabulary provide a rough estimate of the patient's baseline abilities. Begin assessing the patient's knowledge and vocabulary during the interview. Ask about work, hobbies, reading, favorite television programs, or current events. Start with simple questions, then to more difficult questions. Note the person's grasp of information, the complexity of the ideas, and choice of vocabulary.

CLINICAL TIP
Information and vocabulary are relatively unaffected by psychiatric disorders except in the most severe cases. Testing may help distinguish adults with lifelong intellectual impairment (whose information and vocabulary are limited) from those with mild or moderate dementia (whose information and vocabulary are fairly well preserved).

More directly, ask about specific facts such as:

- The name of the president, vice president, or governor
- The names of the last four or five presidents
- The names of five large cities in the country

Calculation Ability

Test the patient's ability to do arithmetic calculations, starting at the rote level with simple addition ("What is 4 + 3? 8 + 7?") and multiplication ("What is 5 × 6? 9 × 7?"). Proceed to more difficult tasks by using two-digit numbers ("15 + 12? 25 × 6?") or longer, written examples.

Poor performance suggests dementia or aphasia but must be measured against knowledge and education. Alternatively, pose practical and functionally important questions, such as "If something costs 78 cents and you give the clerk a dollar bill, how much money should you get back?"

Abstract Thinking

Test the capacity to think abstractly in two ways, with proverbs and similarities. Abstract thinking is an understanding of words at a higher cognitive level and more than the literal interpretation of a word.

Concrete responses are often given by people with an intellectual disability, delirium, or dementia but may also be a function of limited education, culture, or exposure. Patients are thinking of the literal meaning of the word. Patients with schizophrenia may respond concretely or with personal, bizarre interpretations.

Proverbs

Ask the patient what the following proverbs mean:

- People who live in glass houses should not throw stones.
- Don't count your chickens before they're hatched.
- A rolling stone gathers no moss.
- The squeaky wheel gets the grease.

Note the relevance of the answers and their degree of concreteness or abstractness. For example, "Don't throw stones at glass or it will break" is concrete, whereas "Someone who repeatedly does something (e.g., is late) should not criticize someone else when they are late" is abstract. Average patients should give abstract or semiabstract responses.

These types of questions should take into consideration age, educational level, native language, and culture as proverbs are not widely used today and patients with healthy cognitive functioning may not be familiar with the phrases.

Similarities

Ask the patient to tell you how the following are alike:

- An orange and an apple
- A cat and a mouse
- A church and a theater
- A piano and a violin
- Wood and coal

Note the accuracy and relevance of the answers and their degree of concreteness or abstractness. For example, "A cat and a mouse are both animals" is abstract. "They both have tails" is concrete. "A cat chases a mouse" is not relevant.

Constructional Ability

The task here is to copy figures of increasing complexity onto a piece of blank unlined paper (Fig. 19-2). Show each figure one at a time and ask the patient to copy it as well as possible.

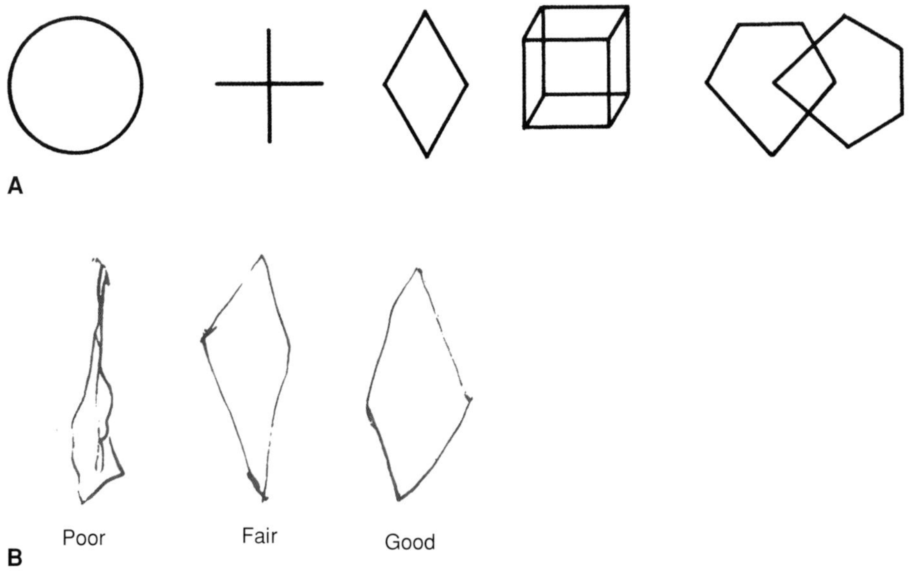

FIGURE 19-2 A. Figures the patient should copy to demonstrate constructional ability. **B.** Three patient diamond drawings.

In another approach, ask the patient to draw a clock face complete with numbers and hands as rated in Figure 19-3 (Louis et al., 2015).

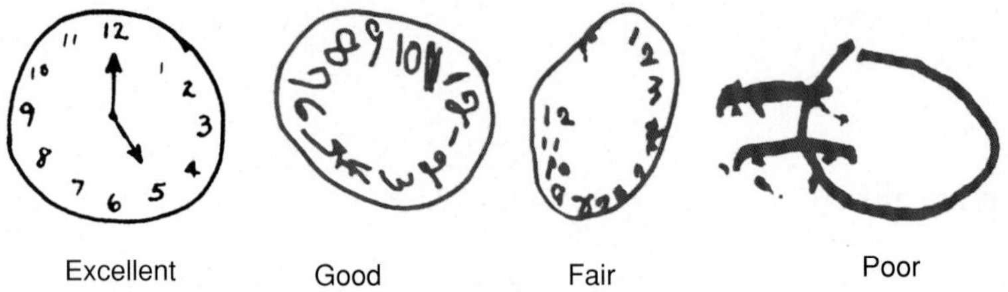

FIGURE 19-3 Clock face drawings to assess constructional ability.

If vision and motor ability are intact, poor constructional ability suggests dementia or parietal lobe damage. Cognitive disability may also impair performance.

RECORDING YOUR FINDINGS

Box 19-2 includes examples of documentation of mental status assessment findings.

BOX 19-2 RECORDING BEHAVIOR AND MENTAL STATUS

"Mental status: Alert and oriented to person, place, time, and situation, well groomed, cheerful. Speech fluent, words clear. Thought processes coherent, insight intact. Serial 7s accurate; recent and remote memory intact. Calculations intact."

Alert and oriented to person, place, time, and situation can be abbreviated: A&O × 4

OR

"Mental status: O × 2 (person and place). Appears sad, fatigued; clothes wrinkled. Speech slow, words mumbled. Thought processes coherent but insight into current life problems is limited. Digit span, serial 7s, and calculations accurate but responses delayed. Clock drawing appropriate."

Suggests depression

HEALTH PROMOTION AND COUNSELING

The Mini-Mental State Examination

The Mini-Mental State Examination (MMSE) is a brief questionnaire that is widely used to screen adult patients for cognitive dysfunction or dementia. Patients are asked a series of questions to test orientation, registration, attention, calculation, recall, language, and the ability to follow simple instructions. The MMSE follows mental ability/decline over time and can be used in patients who are fluent in English and have a minimum of an eighth-grade education. The maximum score is 30 points and as cognition declines, so does the score. A person who scores 0 to 17 points would have severe cognitive impairment (Folstein et al., 1975).

Although several versions are available on the internet, copyright permission for use and reproduction is required. More detailed information regarding the MMSE can be found through a variety of sources online and are available in many languages.

Health promotion screenings during a mental status assessment may include:

- Screening for anxiety
- Screening for posttraumatic stress disorder (PTSD)
- Screening for depression
- Screening for risk of suicide
- Screening for substance use disorders, including alcohol and prescription drugs

All screening tools need to be age appropriate.

Mental health disorders can cause significant suffering. A serious mental illness is a behavioral, mental, or emotional disorder that severely impacts life. Attention to additional needs of diverse communities is crucial as they may be adversely affected by language barriers and access to care. Mental health issues are common causes of hospitalization in the United States, and mental illness is associated with increased risks for chronic medical conditions, decreased life expectancy, disability, substance use, and suicide (National Institute of Mental Health, 2020) (Box 19-3).

BOX 19-3 PATIENT INDICATORS FOR MENTAL HEALTH SCREENING

- Medically unexplained physical symptoms—more than half have a depression or anxiety disorder
- Multiple physical or somatic symptoms or "high symptom count"
- High severity of the presenting somatic symptom(s)
- Chronic pain
- Symptoms for more than 6 weeks
- Rating as a "difficult encounter"
- Recent stress
- Low self-rating of health
- High use of health care services
- Substance abuse

Chronic pain may be a spectrum disorder in patients with anxiety, depression, and/or somatic symptoms.

Anxiety

Anxiety disorders affect 40 million people each year in the United States, but only 37% receive treatment (Center of Excellence for Integrated Health Solutions, 2020). An anxiety disorder interrupts daily life, and the American Psychological Association (APA) includes symptoms of feelings of being tense or on edge, uncontrolled worrying, difficulty concentrating, sleep disruption, and physical changes such as nausea or increased blood pressure (Center of Excellence for Integrated Health Solutions, 2020). There are several types of anxiety disorders as described by the *Diagnostic and Statistical Manual of Mental Disorders, 5th Edition* (*DSM-5*) including: general

BOX 19-4 **GENERALIZED ANXIETY DISORDER (GAD-7) SCREENING QUESTIONS**

Questions to ask if the patient reports anxiety symptoms over the last 2 weeks include:

- Have you been feeling nervous, anxious, or on edge?
- Have you been unable to stop or control worrying?
- Have you found yourself worrying too much about various things?
- Have you experienced difficulty relaxing?
- Have you felt restless to the point of being unable to sit still?
- Have you felt annoyed or irritable?
- Have you felt fearful that something bad may occur?

For additional information, including how to score the tool: https://patient.info/doctor/generalised-anxiety-disorder-assessment-gad-7
Adapted from Spitzer, R. L., Kroenke, K., Williams, J. B. W., & Lowe, B. (2006). A brief measure for assessing generalized anxiety disorder. *Archives of Internal Medicine, 166*, 1092–1097. Copyright held by Pfizer Inc

anxiety disorder (Box 19-4), panic disorder, phobias, mutism (unable to speak from physical, functional, or psychological cause), social anxiety, and separation anxiety disorder. The causes are multifaceted and may include environmental factors, genetic factors, medical factors, and chemical factors, including withdrawal. Anxiety disorders may not occur in isolation. Holistic treatments are available including relaxation techniques, stress management, support systems, exercises, counseling, and medications (Center of Excellence for Integrated Health Solutions, 2020).

Posttraumatic Stress Disorder

PTSD was previously classified as an anxiety disorder in the *DSM-IV*, but it is now listed as a trauma and stress-related disorder in the *DSM-5* (American Psychiatric Association, 2013). PTSD results from the exposure to a traumatic event, threatening the patient with death, serious injury, and/or combat or sexual violence (Center for Substance Abuse Treatment [US] | Substance Abuse and Mental Health Services Administration [US], 2020). One in 11 individuals will experience PTSD at some time in their lives (American Psychiatric Association, 2020). Symptoms include flashbacks, nightmares, isolation, disruptive behavior, fear, and anger. Triggers, such as a touch or noise, may remind patients of the causal event (American Psychiatric Association, 2020).

The Primary Care-PTSD (PC-PTSD-5) screening tool is used in primary care and medical facilities, including the Veterans Affairs network, to identify people exposed to traumatic events that may need assistance. The tool has five items and asks if the person who has had an upsetting, frightening, or terrible experience has experienced the following in the last month:

1. Had nightmares about the event(s) or thought about the event(s) when you did not want to?
2. Tried hard not to think about the event(s) or went out of your way to avoid situations that reminded you of the event(s)?
3. Been constantly on guard, watchful, or easily startled?
4. Felt numb or detached from people, activities, or your surroundings?

5. Felt guilty or unable to stop blaming yourself or others for the event(s) or any problems the event(s) may have caused?

If the answer is "yes" to three of these questions, this tool is sensitive to probable PTSD and additional follow-up is necessary (Prins et al., 2015).

Depression

There are more than 264 million people living with depression throughout the world (GBD Disease and Injury Incidence and Prevalence Collaborators, 2018). The World Health Organization has identified depression as a leading contributing factor to disabilities worldwide (World Health Organization, 2020). More than 17 million adult Americans have major depression, and of those, almost 50% also have a coexisting anxiety disorder (National Institute on Drug Abuse, 2020). Depression is nearly twice as common in women as in men (National Institute on Drug Abuse, 2020). Depression frequently accompanies chronic medical illness. High-risk patients may have subtle early signs of depression, including low self-esteem, loss of pleasure in daily activities (*anhedonia*), sleep disorders, and difficulty concentrating or making decisions. Look carefully for symptoms of depression in vulnerable patients, especially those who are young, female, single, divorced or separated, seriously or chronically ill, bereaved, or who have other psychiatric disorders, including substance abuse. A personal or family history of depression also places patients at risk. The U.S. Preventive Services Task Force (USPSTF) recommends screening all adults over 18 years regardless of risk factors (Siu et al., 2020). The Patient Health Questionnaire (PHQ) (Spitzer et al., 1999) is commonly used for screening in adults (Box 19-5).

BOX 19-5 THE PATIENT HEALTH QUESTIONNAIRE (PHQ) QUESTIONS

- Have you felt little interest or pleasure in doing things?
- Have you been feeling down, depressed, or hopeless?
- Have you had trouble falling or staying asleep or sleeping too much?
- Have you been feeling tired or having little energy?
- Have you experienced poor appetite or overeating?
- Have you been feeling bad about yourself or that you are a failure or have let yourself or your family down somehow?
- Have you had trouble concentrating on things, such as reading the newspaper or watching television?
- Have you been moving or speaking so slowly that other people have noticed? Or are you so fidgety or restless that you have been moving around more than usual?
- Have you had thoughts that you would be better off dead or thoughts of hurting yourself in some way?

For additional information, including how to score the tool: https://www.mdcalc.com/phq-9-patient-health-questionnaire-9#creator-insights.
Adapted from Spitzer, R. L., Kroenke, K., & Williams, J. B. W.; for the Patient Health Questionnaire Primary Care Study Group. (1999). Validation and utility of a self-report version of PRIME-MD: The PHQ primary care study. *JAMA*, *282*(18), 1737–1744. Copyright held by Pfizer Inc.

The nurse may opt to use the Geriatric Depression Scale for older adults (see Chapter 24) and the Edinburgh Postnatal Depression Scale (EDS) for pregnant and postnatal women at https://www.mombaby.org/wp-content/uploads/2016/03/Edinburgh.pdf (Cox et al., 1987; Wisner et al., 2002).

Suicide

Preventing suicide is a global public health initiative established by the World Health Organization (World Health Organization, 2014). Suicide deaths in the United States alone account for over 800,000 deaths each year (Hedegaard et al., 2018). Annually, the prevalence is 10.8 per 100,000 and is the second leading cause of death among 10- to 34-year-olds (Nock et al., 2008).

Men have suicide success rates nearly four times higher than women, though women are three times more likely to attempt suicide. Men are most likely to use firearms to commit suicide, while women are most likely to use poison. Overall, suicides in non-Hispanic White individuals account for about 90% of all suicides, though Native American/Alaska Native women ages 15 to 24 years old have the highest suicide rates of any racial/ethnic group. An estimated 25 attempts are made for each death by suicide, with ratios of 100:1 to 200:1 among young adults (Bethel, 2013; Bolster et al., 2015). Each year, more than two million young people attempt suicide and of these almost 90% are unbeknownst to parents (Bethel, 2013). Nurses may be the first in contact with a person contemplating suicide. Pursue any clinical suspicion of suicide by asking patients directly about suicidal ideations or plans and refer at-risk patients immediately for psychiatric care (Substance Abuse and Mental Health Services Administration, 2020). The Suicide Safe app assists health care providers with incorporating strategies for prevention using the Suicide Assessment Five-Step Evaluation and Triage (SAFE-T) (Bolster et al., 2015). The number for the national suicide prevention hotline is 1-800-272-8255(TALK) and is available 24 hours a day every day of the week.

Substance Use Disorders, Including Alcohol and Prescription Drugs

The interactions and comorbidity of alcohol and substance use disorders and suicide are extensive and profound. Alcohol, tobacco, and illicit drugs account for more illness, deaths, and disabilities than any other preventable condition. The National Survey on Drug Use and Health reported that 139.8 million people over the age of 12 in the United States drank in the past month, 67.1 million people reported binge drinking, and 16.6 million were heavy drinkers (Substance Abuse and Mental Health Services Administration, 2019).

Over 53.2 million Americans reported use of a drug, not prescribed or not for medicinal purposes during the year prior to the survey, and this has continued to increase each year. This translates into approximately 19.4% or almost one in five people who have used a drug without medical input in the past year (Substance Abuse and Mental Health Services Administration, 2019). The breakdown of drug use includes approximately 43.5 million marijuana users. The second leading use was prescription drugs with 16.9 million people using them for nonmedicinal purposes with 1.7 million Americans battling opioid use disorder (OUD)

(Scholl et al., 2018). Approximately 3.7 million of these individuals received any form of substance use treatment with only 2.4 million receiving treatment at a specialty facility for a drug or alcohol problem in the past year (Substance Abuse and Mental Health Services Administration, 2019). Rates of drug-induced deaths continue to increase and are highest among White Americans and Native American/Alaska Natives. The Centers for Disease Control and Prevention reports that prescription drugs are now the leading cause of drug-induced deaths (Centers for Disease Control and Prevention, 2020). Every patient should be asked about alcohol use, substance use, and misuse of prescription drugs with the universal screening questions outlined in Box 19-6.

BOX 19-6 UNIVERSAL SCREENING FOR SUBSTANCE USE DISORDERS

Alcohol: National Institute on Alcohol Abuse and Alcoholism (NIAAA)		
	None	**One or more**
Men: How many times in the past year have you had five or more drinks in a day?		
Women: How many times in the past year have you had four or more drinks in a day?		
Drugs: National Institute on Drug Abuse (NIDA)		
	None	**One or more**
How many times in the past year have you used a recreational drug or a prescription drug for a nonmedical reason?		

Depending on the results of the brief screen, the full screening tools are the Alcohol Use Disorder Identification Test (AUDIT) and the Drug Abuse Screening Test (DAST).

See Chapter 4, "The Health History," "Alcohol and Illicit Drugs," and Chapter 16, "The Gastrointestinal and Renal Systems," "Screening for Alcohol Misuse."

BIBLIOGRAPHY

American Psychiatric Association. (2013). *Diagnostic and statistical manual of mental disorders* (5th ed.). American Psychiatric Press.

American Psychiatric Association. (2020). *What is posttraumatic stress disorder?* Retrieved May 14, 2020, from https://www.psychiatry.org/patients-families/ptsd/what-is-ptsd

Armitage, A. (2015). *Advanced practice nursing guide to the neurological exam*. Springer Publishing Company.

Bethel, J. (2013). Assessment of suicidal intent in emergency care. *Nursing Stand*, *28*(4), 52–58.

Bolster, C., Holliday, C., Oneal, G., & Shaw, M. (2015). Suicide assessment and nurses: What does the evidence show? *Online Journal of Issues in Nursing [Electronic Resource]*, *20*(1), 2.

Center of Excellence for Integrated Health Solutions. (2020). *Screening*. Retrieved June 3, 2020, from https://www.integration.samhsa.gov/clinical-practice/screening

Center for Substance Abuse Treatment (US) | Substance Abuse and Mental Health Services Administration (US). (2020). Treatment Improvement Protocol (TIP) Series, No. 57. 2014. *Trauma-informed care in behavioral health services*. Retrieved May 14, 2020, from https://www.ncbi.nlm.nih.gov/books/NBK207191/box/part1_ch3.box16

Centers for Disease Control and Prevention. (2020). *Wide-ranging online data for epidemiologic research (WONDER)*. CDC, National Center for Health Statistics. Retrieved May 5, 2020, from http://wonder.cdc.gov

Cox, J. L., Holden, J. M., & Sagovsky, R. (1987). Detection of postnatal depression: Development of the 10-item Edinburgh Postnatal Depression Scale. *British Journal of Psychiatry*, *150*,

782–786. https://www.mombaby.org/wp-content/uploads/2016/03/Edinburgh.pdf

Doornbos, M. M., Zandee, G. L., Timmermans, B., Moes, J., Heitsch, E., Quist, M., Heetderks, E., Houskamp, C., & VanWolde, A. (2020). Factors impacting attrition of vulnerable women from a longitudinal mental health intervention study. *Public Health Nursing, 37*(1), 73–80. https://doi.org/10.1111/phn.12687

Folstein, M. F., Folstein, S. E., & McHugh, P. R. (1975). "Mini-mental state". A practical method for grading the cognitive state of patients for the clinician. *Journal of Psychiatric Research, 12*(3), 189–198.

GBD Disease and Injury Incidence and Prevalence Collaborators. (2018). Disease and injury global, regional and national incidence, prevalence, and years lived with disability to 354 diseases and injuries for 195 countries and territories, 1990–2017: A systematic analysis for the global burden of disease study. 2018. *The Lancet: Global Health Metrics, 392*(10159), 1789–1858.

Hedegaard, H., Curtin, S., & Warner, M. (2018). *Suicide rates in the United States continue to increase.* National Center for Health Statistics.

Kroenke, K. (2009). Unburdening the difficult clinical encounter. *Archives of Internal Medicine, 169*(4), 333–334.

Kroenke, K. (2014). A practical and evidence-based approach to common symptoms: A narrative review. *Annals of Internal Medicine, 161*, 579–586.

Louis, E. D., Mayer, S. A., & Rowland, L. P. (2015). *Merritt's neurology* (13th ed.). Wolters Kluwer.

Martinez-Martinez, C., Sanchez-Martinez, V., Sales-Orts, R., Dinca, A., Richart-Martinez, M., & Ramos-Pichardo, J. D. (2019). Effectiveness of direct contact intervention with people with mental illness to reduce stigma in nursing students. *International Journal of Mental Health Nursing, 28*(3), 735–743. https://doi.org/10.1111/inm.12578

National Institute of Mental Health. (2020). *Transforming the understanding and treatment of mental illnesses.*

National Institute on Drug Abuse. (2020). *National survey on drug use and health.* Retrieved May 13, 2020, from https://www.drugabuse.gov/related-topics/trends-statistics/national-survey-drug-use-health-nsduh

Nock, M. K., Borges, G., Bromet, E. J., Cha, C. B., Kessler, R. C., & Lee, S. (2008). Suicide and suicidal behavior. *Epidemiologic Reviews, 30*, 133–154.

Olfson, M. (2016). Building the mental health workforce capacity needed to treat adults with serious mental illnesses. *Health Affairs, 35*(6), 983–990. Retrieved May 13, 2020, from https://doi.org/10.137/hlthaff.2015.1619

Poghosyan, L., Norful, A. N., Ghaffari, A., George, M., Chhabra, S., & Olfson, M. (2019). Mental health delivery in primary care: The perspectives of primary care providers. *Archives of Psychiatric Nursing, 33*(5), 63–67. Retrieved May 13, 2020, from https://doi.org/10.1016/j.apnu.2019.08.001

Prins, A., Bovin, M. J., Kimerling, R., Kaloupek, D. G., Marx, B. P., Pless Kaiser, A., & Schnurr, P. P. (2015). *Primary care PTSD screen for DSM-5 (PC-PTSD-5) [Measurement instrument].* Retrieved June 3, 2020, from https://www.ptsd.va.gov/professional/assessment/screens/pc-ptsd.asp

Scholl, L., Seth, P., Kariisa, M., Wilson, N., & Baldwin, G. (2018). Drug and opioid-involved overdose deaths—United States, 2013–2017. *MMWR Morbidity and Mortality Weekly Report, 67*(5152), 1419–1427. https://doi.org/10.15585/mmwr.mm675152e1

Siu, A., & U.S. Preventive Services Task Force. (2020). *Screening for depression in adults: U.S. Preventive Services Task Force recommendation statement.* Retrieved May 13, 2020, from https://www.uspreventiveservicestaskforce.org/home/getfilebytoken/BnHj53HwgSBNXMvnyavxfS

Spitzer, R. L., Kroenke, K., & Williams, J. B. W.; for the Patient Health Questionnaire Primary Care Study Group. (1999). Validation and utility of a self-report version of PRIME-MD: The PHQ primary care study. *JAMA, 282*(18), 1737–1744.

Spitzer, R. L., Kroenke, K., Williams, J. B. W., & Lowe, B. (2006). A brief measure for assessing generalized anxiety disorder. *Archives of Internal Medicine, 166*, 1092–1097.

Substance Abuse and Mental Health Services Administration. (2019). *Key substance use and mental health indicators in the United States: Results from the 2018 National Survey on Drug Use and Health (HHS Publication No. PEP19-5068, NSDUH Series H-54).* Center for Behavioral Health Statistics and Quality, Substance Abuse and Mental Health Services Administration. Retrieved June 3, 2020, from https://www.samhsa.gov/data

Substance Abuse and Mental Health Services Administration. (2020). *Suicide assessment five-step evaluation and triage (SAFE-T).* Retrieved May 8, 2020, from https://www.integration.samhsa.gov/images/res/SAFE_T.pdf

Tranter, S., & Robertson, M. (2019). Improving the physical health of people with a mental illness: Holistic nursing assessments. *Mental Health Practice, 22*(4), 34–41.

Wisner, K. L., Parry, B. L., & Piontek, C. M. (2002). Postpartum depression. *New England Journal of Medicine, 347*(3), 194–199.

World Health Organization. (2014). *Preventing suicide: A global imperative.* World Health Organization. Retrieved May 13, 2020, from http://www.who.int/mental_health/suicide-prevention/world_report_2014/en

World Health Organization. (2020). *Depression.* Retrieved May 14, 2020, from https://www.who.int/news-room/fact-sheets/detail/depression

20

THE NERVOUS SYSTEM

KEY TERMS

aphasia
ataxia
bradykinesia
clonus
coma
deep tendon reflex
dermatome
diplopia
dysarthria
dysesthesias
fasciculations
Glasgow Coma Scale
hemianopsia
hemiplegia
kinesthesia
muscle stretch reflex
myelinated
nystagmus
paresthesia
peripheral neuropathy
proprioception
stereognosis
stroke
syncope
tonic–clonic
vasovagal syncope
vertigo

Learning Objectives

The student will:

1. Describe the structure and function of the nervous system.
2. Identify the cranial nerves and the motor and sensory functions.
3. Obtain a history of the nervous system.
4. Perform a screening neurologic examination.
5. Describe the use of the Glasgow Coma Scale in an unresponsive patient.
6. Document the findings of the nervous system examination.
7. Discuss risk reduction and health promotion strategies to prevent strokes.

Evaluation of the cranial nerves (CNs), motor system, sensory system, and reflexes is the focus of this chapter. The complex anatomy and physiology of the nervous system make examination and assessment challenging but attainable with practice and dedication. Taking a detailed history provides essential clues to tailor your physical examination, nursing interventions, and patient education.

ANATOMY AND PHYSIOLOGY

The Central Nervous System

The Brain

The brain has four regions: the cerebrum, the diencephalon, the brainstem, and the cerebellum (Fig. 20-1). Each cerebral hemisphere is subdivided into frontal, parietal, temporal, and occipital lobes (Fig. 20-2).

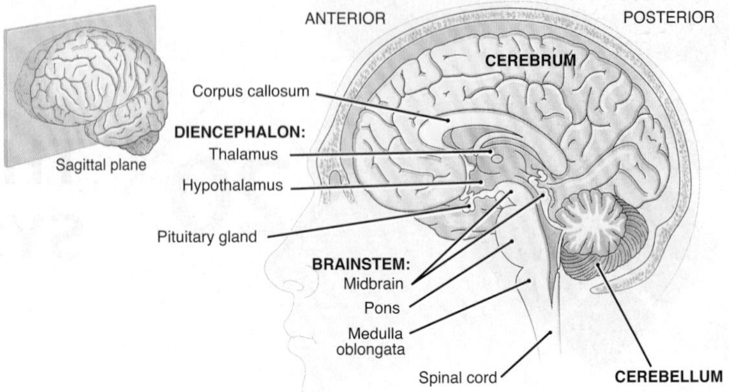

FIGURE 20-1 Four regions of the brain.

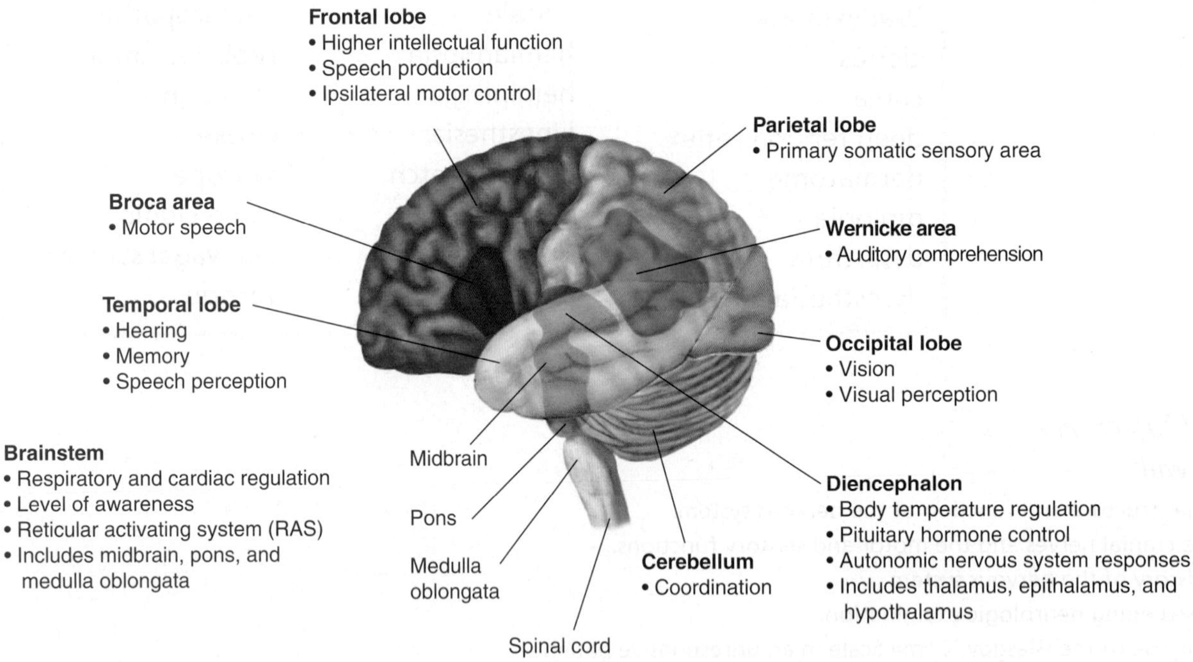

FIGURE 20-2 Left lateral view of the brain.

The central nervous system (CNS) of the brain is a vast network of interconnecting nerve cells, or *neurons*, consisting of cell bodies and their *axons*—single long fibers that conduct impulses to other parts of the nervous system.

Brain tissue may be gray or white. *Gray matter* consists of aggregations of neuronal cell bodies. It rims the surfaces of the cerebral hemispheres, forming the cerebral cortex. *White matter* consists of neuronal axons that are coated with myelin. The myelin sheaths, which create the white color, allow nerve impulses to travel more rapidly.

Deep in the brain lie additional clusters of gray matter (Fig. 20-3). These include the *basal ganglia*, which affect movement, and the thalamus and the hypothalamus, structures in the diencephalon. The *thalamus* processes sensory impulses and relays them to the cerebral cortex. The *hypothalamus* maintains homeostasis and regulates temperature, heart rate, and blood pressure. The hypothalamus affects the endocrine system and governs emotional behaviors such as anger and sexual drive. Hormones secreted in the hypothalamus act directly on the pituitary gland.

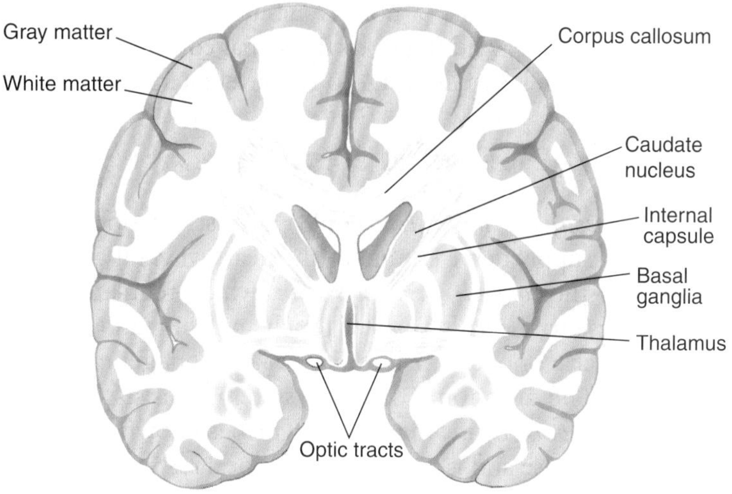

FIGURE 20-3 Coronal section of the brain.

The *internal capsule* is a white-matter structure where **myelinated** fibers converge from all parts of the cerebral cortex and descend into the brainstem. The *brainstem*, which connects the upper part of the brain with the spinal cord, has three sections: the midbrain, the pons, and the medulla.

Consciousness depends on the interaction between intact cerebral hemispheres and an important structure in the diencephalon and upper brainstem, the *reticular activating (arousal) system*.

The *cerebellum*, which lies at the base of the brain, coordinates all movements and helps maintain the body upright in space.

The Spinal Cord

Below the medulla, the CNS extends itself as the elongated *spinal cord*, encased within the bony vertebral column and terminating at the first or second lumbar vertebra. The cord provides a series of segmental relays with the periphery, serving as a conduit for information flow to and from the brain. The motor and sensory nerve pathways relay neural signals that enter and exit the cord through posterior and anterior nerve roots through the spinal and peripheral nerves.

The spinal cord is divided into five segments (Fig. 20-4): cervical, from C1 to C8; thoracic, from T1 to T12; lumbar, from L1 to L5; sacral, from S1 to S5; and coccygeal. The cervical spinal cord contains nerve tracts to and from both the upper and lower extremities. Note that the spinal cord is not as long as the vertebral canal. The lumbar and sacral roots travel the longest intraspinal

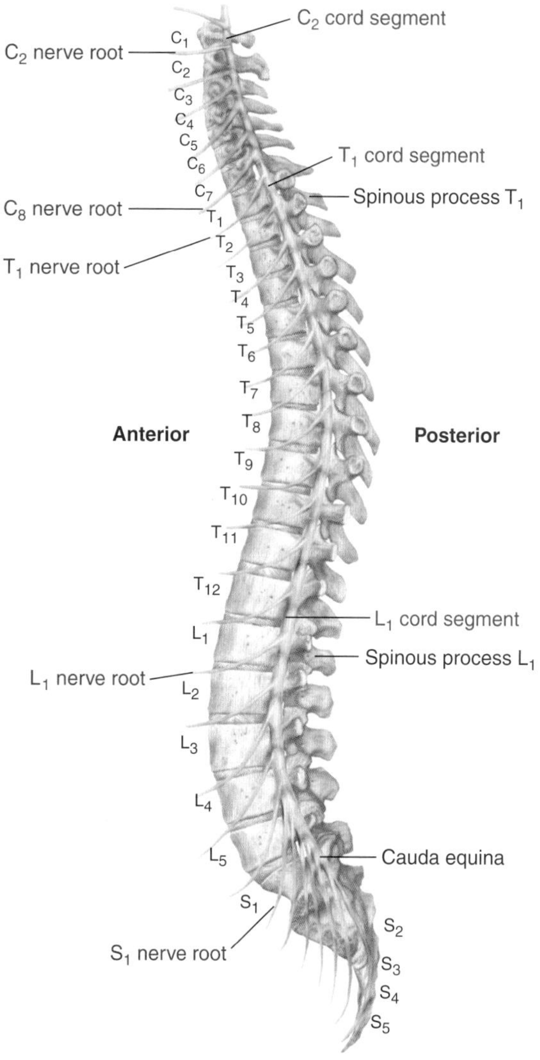

FIGURE 20-4 The spinal cord, lateral view.

distance and fan out like a horse's tail at L1 to L2, giving rise to the term *cauda equina*. To avoid injury to the spinal cord, most lumbar punctures are performed at the L3 to L4 or L4 to L5 vertebral interspaces (Bilal et al., 2020).

Peripheral Nervous System

The *peripheral nervous system* (PNS) consists of both CNs and peripheral nerves that supply nerve stimuli to the heart, visceral organs, skin, and limbs. It controls the *somatic nervous system*, which regulates muscle movements and response to the sensations of touch and pain, and the *autonomic nervous system*, which connects to internal organs and generates autonomic reflex responses. The autonomic nervous system consists of complementary systems, the *sympathetic nervous system*, which is known for mobilizing the fight-or-flight response and is responsible for local responses such as sweating with increased temperatures, and the *parasympathetic nervous system*, which keeps the body calm and relaxed, handling routine activities such food digestion.

The Cranial Nerves

Twelve pairs of special nerves called the *CNs* emerge from within the cranial vault through skull foramina and canals to structures in the head and neck. They are numbered sequentially with Roman numerals. CNs I and II are fiber tracts emerging from the brain. CNs III through XII arise from the diencephalon and the brainstem, as illustrated in Figure 20-5. Some CNs are limited to general motor or sensory functions, while others are specialized and have both motor and sensory functions. CNs relevant to physical examination are summarized in Table 20-1.

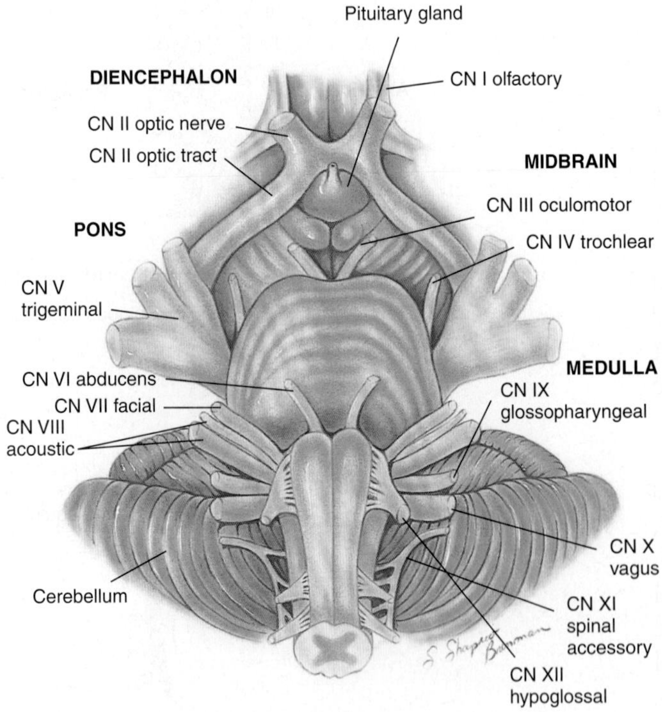

FIGURE 20-5 Cranial nerves visible from the inferior surface of the brain.

TABLE 20-1 Cranial Nerves

Number	Name	Function	Type of Impulse
I	Olfactory	Sense of smell	Sensory
II	Optic	Vision	Sensory
III	Oculomotor 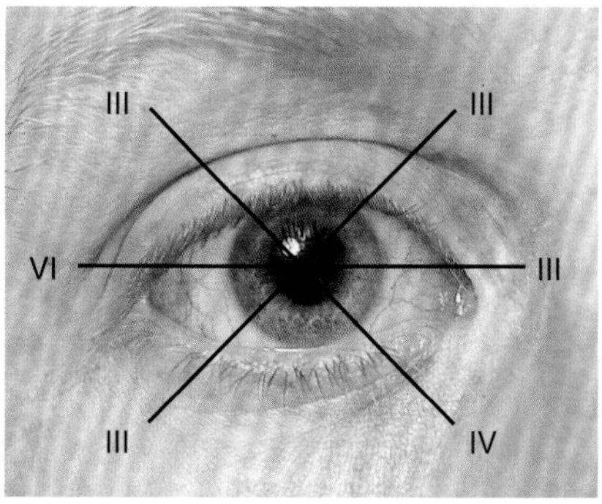 Right eyes (CN III, IV, VI).	Pupillary constriction, opening the eye (lid elevation), and most extraocular (outside the eye) movements	Motor
IV	Trochlear	Downward, internal rotation of the eye	Motor
V	Trigeminal 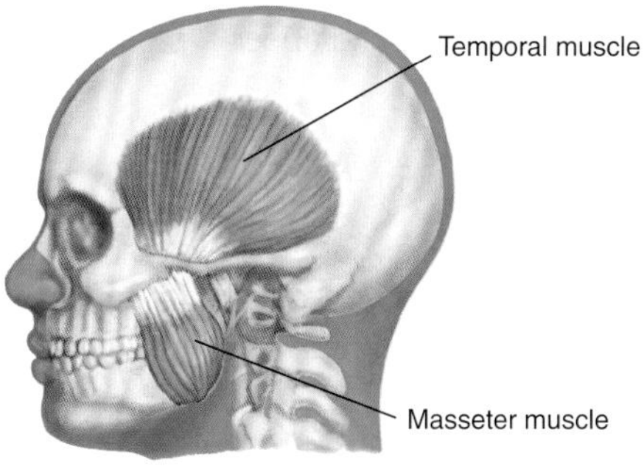 CN V, motor. 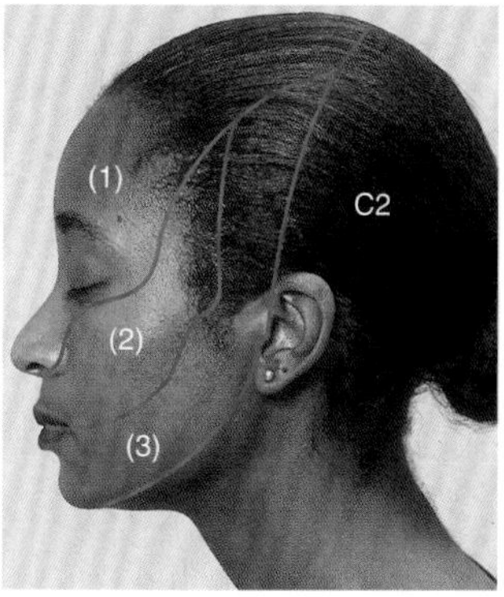 CN V, sensory.	*Motor*—temporal and masseter muscles (jaw clenching), lateral pterygoids (lateral jaw movement) *Sensory*—facial; the nerve has three divisions: (1) ophthalmic, (2) maxillary, and (3) mandibular	Both (motor, sensory)

(continued)

TABLE 20-1 **Cranial Nerves** *(Continued)*

Number	Name	Function	Type of Impulse
VI	Abducens	Lateral deviation of the eye	Motor
VII	Facial	*Motor*—facial movements, including those of facial expression, closing the eye, and closing the mouth *Sensory*—taste for salty, sweet, sour, and bitter substances on the anterior two thirds of the tongue	Both (motor, sensory)
VIII	Acoustic	Hearing (cochlear division) and balance (vestibular division)	Sensory
IX	Glossopharyngeal	*Motor*—pharynx *Sensory*—posterior portions of the ear-drum and ear canal, the pharynx, and the posterior tongue, including taste (salty, sweet, sour, bitter)	Both (motor, sensory)
X	Vagus	*Motor*—palate, pharynx, and larynx *Sensory*—pharynx and larynx	Both (motor, sensory)
XI	Spinal accessory 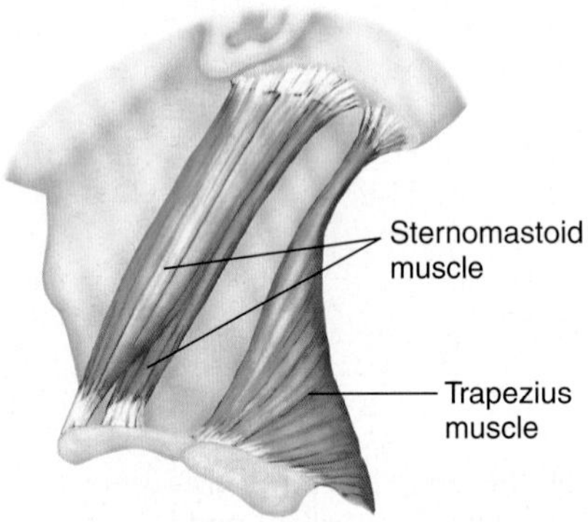	*Motor*—the sternomastoid and upper portion of the trapezius	Motor
XII	Hypoglossal	*Motor*—tongue	Motor

The Peripheral Nerves

The PNS includes spinal and peripheral nerves that carry impulses to and from the spinal cord. Thirty-one pairs of nerves attach to the spinal cord: eight cervical, twelve thoracic, five lumbar, five sacral, and one coccygeal. Each nerve has an anterior (ventral) root containing motor fibers and a posterior (dorsal) root containing sensory fibers. The anterior and posterior roots merge to form a short *spinal nerve*, less than 5 mm long. Spinal nerve fibers mix with similar fibers from other levels in plexuses outside the cord from which *peripheral nerves emerge*. Most peripheral nerves contain both *sensory* (afferent) and *motor* (efferent) fibers.

Like the brain, the spinal cord contains both gray matter and white matter. The gray matter consists of an aggregation of nerve cell nuclei and dendrites that are surrounded by white tracts of nerve fibers connecting the brain to the PNS. Note the butterfly appearance of the gray-matter nuclei with anterior and posterior horns (Fig. 20-6).

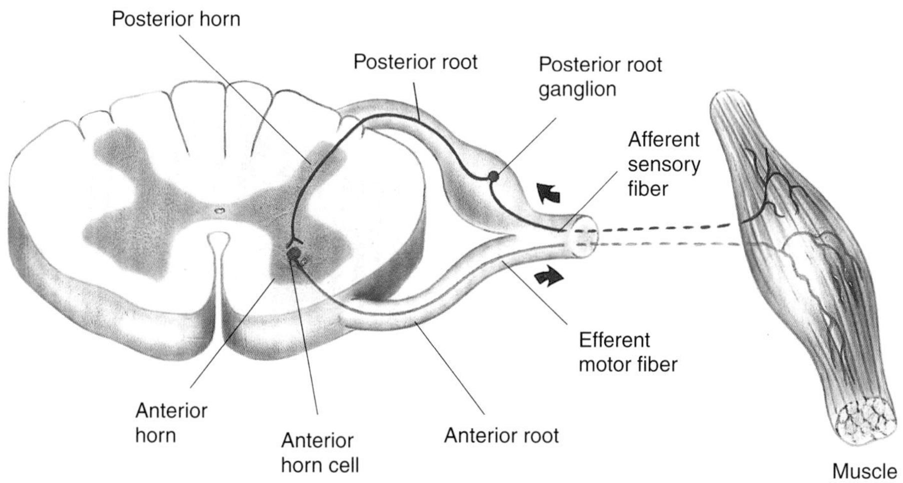

FIGURE 20-6 Cross-section of the spinal cord.

Motor Pathways

Motor pathways are complex avenues extending from *upper motor* neurons through long white-matter tracts, to synapses with lower motor neurons, and into the periphery (outward regions) through peripheral nerve structures. *Upper motor neurons* or nerve cell bodies lie in the motor strip of the cerebral cortex and in several brainstem nuclei; their axons synapse with motor nuclei in the brainstem (for CNs) and in the spinal cord (for peripheral nerves). *Lower motor neurons* have cell bodies in the spinal cord, called anterior horn cells; their axons transmit impulses through the anterior roots and spinal nerves into peripheral nerves, terminating at the neuromuscular junction.

Three kinds of motor pathways (Box 20-1) impinge on the anterior horn cells: the corticospinal tract, the basal ganglia system, and the cerebellar system. Additional pathways originating in the brainstem control flexor and extensor tone in limb movement and posture, most notably in coma.

BOX 20-1 THE PRINCIPAL MOTOR PATHWAYS

- The *corticospinal (pyramidal) tract*—The corticospinal tracts control voluntary movement and integrate skilled, complicated, or delicate movements by stimulating selected muscular actions and inhibiting others. They also carry impulses that inhibit *muscle tone*, the slight tension maintained by normal muscle even when it is relaxed. The corticospinal tracts originate in the motor cortex of the brain. Motor fibers travel down into the lower medulla, where they form an anatomic structure resembling a pyramid. There, most of these fibers cross to the opposite or *contralateral* side of the medulla, continue downward, and synapse with anterior horn cells or with intermediate neurons. Tracts synapsing in the brainstem with motor nuclei of the cranial nerves are termed *corticobulbar*.
- The *basal ganglia system*—This complex system includes motor pathways between the cerebral cortex, basal ganglia, brainstem, and spinal cord. It helps maintain muscle tone and control body movements, especially automatic movements such as walking.
- The *cerebellar system*—The cerebellum receives both sensory and motor input and coordinates motor activity, maintains equilibrium, and helps control posture.

These higher motor pathways affect movement only through the lower motor neuron systems, sometimes called the "final common pathway." Any movement, whether initiated voluntarily in the cortex (Fig. 20-7), "automatically" in the basal ganglia, or reflexively in the sensory receptors, must ultimately be translated into action via the anterior horn cells. A lesion in any of these areas will affect movement or reflex activity.

When the corticospinal tract is damaged or destroyed, its functions are reduced or lost below the level of injury. When upper motor neuron systems are damaged above the crossover of its tracts in the medulla, motor impairment develops on the opposite (or contralateral) side. In damage below the crossover, motor impairment occurs on the same (or ipsilateral) side of the body. The affected limb becomes weak or paralyzed; and skilled, complicated, or delicate movements are performed especially poorly when compared with large movements.

When there is an upper motor neuron lesion, muscle tone is increased, and deep tendon reflexes (DTRs) are exaggerated. Damage to the lower motor neuron systems causes ipsilateral weakness and paralysis, but in this case, muscle tone and reflexes are decreased or absent.

Disease of the basal ganglia system or cerebellar system does not cause paralysis but can be disabling. Damage to the basal ganglia system

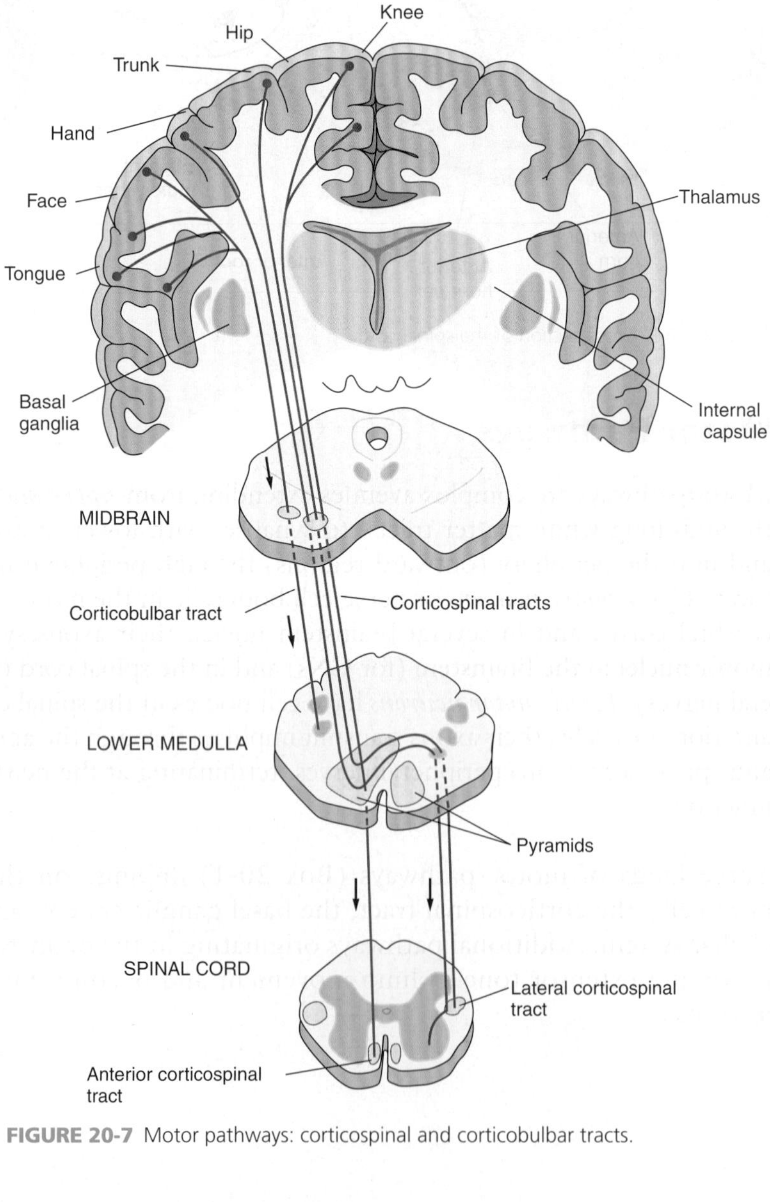

FIGURE 20-7 Motor pathways: corticospinal and corticobulbar tracts.

produces changes in muscle tone (most often an increase), disturbances in posture and gait, a slowness or lack of spontaneous and automatic movements termed **bradykinesia**, and various involuntary movements. Cerebellar damage impairs coordination, gait, and equilibrium and decreases muscle tone.

Sensory Pathways

Sensory impulses participate not only in reflex activity, as previously described, but also give rise to conscious sensation, calibrate body position in space, and help regulate internal autonomic functions like blood pressure, heart rate, and respiration.

A complex system of sensory receptors relays impulses from skin, mucous membranes, muscles, tendons, and viscera that travel through peripheral projections into the posterior root ganglia, where a second projection of the ganglia directs impulses centrally into the spinal cord. Sensory impulses then travel to the sensory cortex of the brain via one of two pathways: the *spinothalamic tract*, consisting of smaller sensory neurons with unmyelinated or thinly myelinated axons, and the *posterior columns*, which have larger neurons with heavily myelinated axons (Fig. 20-8).

Myelin is a mixture of proteins and phospholipids which form a sheath around nerve fibers and increases the conduction of nerve impulses.

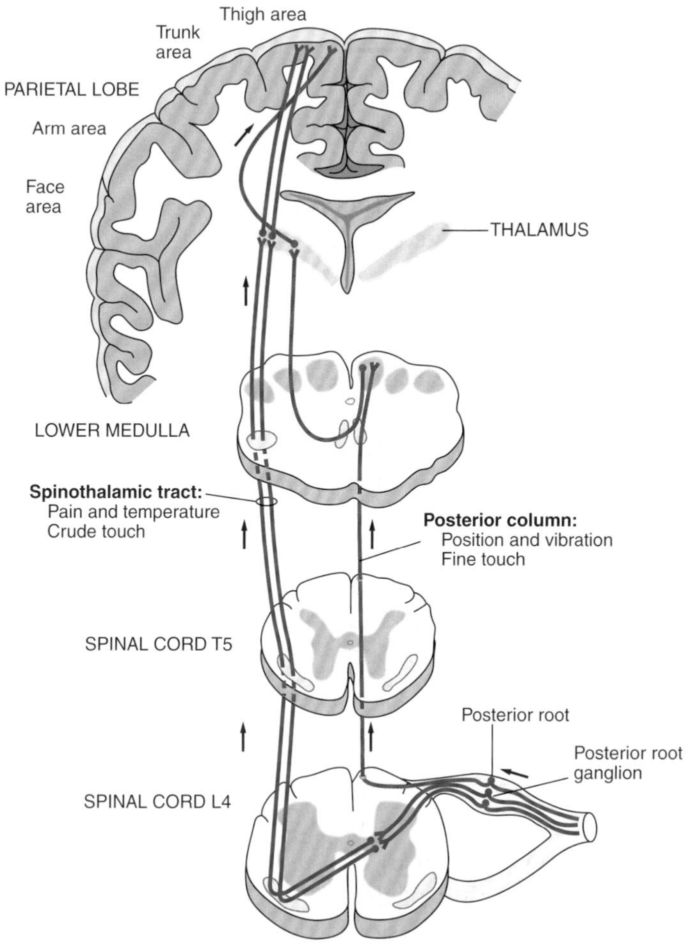

FIGURE 20-8 Sensory pathways: spinothalamic tract and posterior columns.

The peripheral component of the small fiber *spinothalamic tract* arises in free nerve endings in the skin that register *pain*, *temperature*, and *crude touch*. Within one or two spinal segments from their entry into the cord, these fibers pass into the posterior horn and synapse with secondary sensory neurons. The secondary neurons then cross to the opposite side and pass upward into the thalamus.

In the *posterior column* system, the peripheral large fiber projections of the dorsal root ganglia transmit the sensations of *vibration*, *proprioception*, *kinesthesia*, *pressure*, and *fine touch* from skin and joint position receptors to the dorsal root ganglia, where they travel through central projections in the posterior columns to second-order sensory neurons in the medulla. **Proprioception** is a sense of position of parts of the body and the strength necessary to move. **Kinesthesia** means the sense of movement. Fibers projecting from secondary neurons cross to the opposite side at the medullary level and continue on to the thalamus.

CLINICAL TIP

Patients with diabetes with small fiber neuropathy report sharp, burning, or shooting foot pain, whereas those with large fiber neuropathy experience numbness and tingling or even no sensation at all (Braffett et al., 2020; Pop-Busui et al., 2017).

At the *thalamic level*, the general quality of sensation is perceived (e.g., pain, cold, pleasant, unpleasant), but fine distinctions are not made. For full perception, a third group of sensory neurons sends impulses from the thalamus to the *sensory cortex* of the brain. Here stimuli are localized and higher-order discriminations are made.

Lesions at different points in the sensory pathways produce different kinds of sensory loss. Patterns of sensory loss, together with their associated motor findings, help identify where the lesions might be that are causing the loss. A lesion in the sensory cortex may not impair the perception of pain, touch, and position, for example, but does impair finer discrimination. A patient with this lesion cannot appreciate the size, shape, or texture of an object by feeling it and therefore cannot identify the object. Loss of position and vibration sense with preservation of other sensations points to disease of the posterior columns, whereas loss of all sensations from the waist down, together with paralysis and hyperactive reflexes in the legs, indicates transection of the spinal cord. Crude and light touch are often preserved despite partial damage to the cord, because impulses originating on one side of the body travel up both sides of the cord.

A *dermatome* is the band of skin innervated (receiving nerve impulse) by the sensory root of a single spinal nerve. Knowledge and testing of dermatomes help identify which specific spinal cord segment has the lesion. The dermatome "maps" are outlined in the "Dermatomes" section.

Spinal Reflexes: The Muscle Stretch and Deep Tendon Reflexes

The **muscle stretch reflex** is a monosynaptic reflex, a simple reflex that relays information from a sensory neuron to a motor neuron across a single synapse. The monosynaptic reflex regulates muscle length via nerve stimulation at the muscle spindles. The alpha motor neurons cause the contraction to resist stretching, and the gamma motor neurons control tension and sensitivity. The effect of the stretch reflex is muscle contraction in response to increased length/stretch of the muscle. Muscle stretch reflexes are common in skeletal muscle and important for both balance and posture.

The patella reflex is the most common muscle stretch reflex or monosynaptic reflex.

The **deep tendon reflex** (DTR), or Golgi tendon reflex, is polysynaptic and relays information from a sensory neuron to a motor neuron across two or more synapses inducing muscle relaxation/lengthening in response to increased tension in the muscle. The reflex controls muscle tension through relaxation so that the muscle force or contraction does not become so strong that the tendon is torn. This protection from tissue damage is instrumental, as is the precision and control of motor activity that the DTRs provide.

The muscle stretch reflex and the DTR can be elicited by a brisk tap to the area of a partially stretched muscle/tendon. For the reflex to fire, all components of the reflex arc must be intact: sensory nerve fibers, spinal cord synapse, motor nerve fibers, neuromuscular junction, and muscle fibers. Tapping activates special sensory fibers in the partially stretched muscle/tendon, triggering a sensory impulse that travels to the spinal cord via a peripheral nerve. The stimulated sensory fiber synapses directly with the anterior horn cell innervating the same muscle. When the impulse crosses the neuromuscular junction, the muscle suddenly contracts, completing the reflex arc.

Because each DTR involves specific spinal segments together with their sensory and motor fibers, an abnormal reflex can help locate a pathologic lesion. Learn the segmental levels of the DTRs (Table 20-2). They can be remembered by their numerical sequence in ascending order from ankle to triceps: S1 to L2, 3, 4 to C5, 6, 7.

Often, all reflexes are referred to as DTRs.

TABLE 20-2 Deep Tendon Reflexes and Muscle Stretch Reflexes

Reflex	Spinal Segment
Ankle reflex (Achilles)	Sacral 1 primarily
Knee reflex (patellar)	Lumbar 2, 3, 4
Supinator (brachioradialis) reflex	Cervical 5, 6
Biceps reflex	Cervical 5, 6
Triceps reflex	Cervical 6, 7

Reflexes may be initiated by stimulating skin as well as muscle. Stroking the skin of the abdomen, for example, produces a localized muscular twitch. Superficial (cutaneous) reflexes and their corresponding spinal segments are listed in Table 20-3.

TABLE 20-3 Cutaneous Stimulation Reflexes

Reflex	Spinal Segment
Abdominal reflexes, upper	Thoracic 8, 9, 10
Abdominal reflexes, lower	Thoracic 10, 11, 12
Cremasteric reflex	Lumbar 1, 2
Plantar responses	Lumbar 5, sacral 1
Anal reflex	Sacral 2, 3, 4

THE HEALTH HISTORY

Two of the most common symptoms in neurologic disorders are *headache* and *dizziness.* Review the health history pertinent to headaches. Additional common and concerning symptoms related to the neurologic history are listed in Box 20-2.

See Table 10-1, "Primary Headaches," and Table 10-2, "Secondary Headaches and Cranial Neuralgias."

BOX 20-2 COMMON OR CONCERNING SYMPTOMS

- Headache
- Head injury
- Dizziness or vertigo
- Weakness (generalized, proximal, or distal weakness)
- Numbness, abnormal or loss of sensations
- **Syncope** (fainting) and near syncope (blacking out)
- Seizures
- Tremors or involuntary movements

Headache

Headaches have many causes ranging from benign to life-threatening; they always warrant thorough assessment. Neurologic causes such as subarachnoid hemorrhage, meningitis, or mass lesions, are especially ominous. Pay close attention to the headache history and your examination findings.

CLINICAL TIP

Primary headaches include migraine, tension-type, trigeminal autonomic *cephalalgias,* and *other headaches*; *secondary headaches* arise from underlying structural, systemic, and infectious causes or substance withdraw and may be life-threatening (González-Quintanilla & Pascual, 2019; Headache Classification Committee of the International Headache Society [IHS], 2018).

Ask about the severity of the headache and its onset, location, duration, and any associated symptoms such as double vision, visual changes, weakness, or loss of sensation (Veenstra et al., 2016). Does the headache get worse with coughing, sneezing, or sudden head movements, which can alter intracranial pressure? Is there fever, stiff neck, or an ear, sinus, or throat infection that may signal meningitis (Iguchi et al., 2020; D'Souza, 2015)?

Subarachnoid hemorrhage is classically described by patients as "the worst headache of my life" with instantaneous onset (D'Souza, 2015; Sahraian et al., 2019). Severe headache and stiff neck accompany *meningitis* (Iguchi et al., 2020; Richie & Josephson, 2015).

Dull headache increased by coughing and sneezing, especially when reoccurring in the same location, occurs in mass lesions such as *brain* tumors or *abscess* (Chirchiglia et al., 2019).

An atypical (not usual) presentation of the patient's usual migraine may be suspicious for stroke, especially in biologic women using hormonal contraceptives (Ferreira et al., 2017).

CLINICAL TIP

Migraine headache is often preceded by an aura or prodrome and is highly likely if three of the five "POUND" features are present: *p*ulsatile or throbbing; *o*ne-day duration, or lasts 4 to 72 hours if untreated; *u*nilateral; *n*ausea or vomiting; *d*isabling or intensity causing interruption of daily activity (Lee et al., 2018).

Always look for unusual headache warning signs, such as sudden onset "like a thunderclap," onset after age 50, and associated symptoms such as fever and stiff neck. Examine for papilledema and focal neurologic signs.

Dizziness or Vertigo

Dizziness and *lightheadedness* are common but vague complaints that can have many meanings. You will need to elicit the patient's experience through a specific history and neurologic examination (Kim et al., 2012).

Does the patient feel faint or about to fall or pass out (*presyncope*)? Are they unsteady and off balance (*disequilibrium* or *ataxia*)? Or is there true **vertigo**, a spinning sensation within the patient or of the surroundings? If there is true vertigo, establish the time course of symptoms, which helps distinguish among different types of peripheral vestibular disorders.

Feeling lightheaded, weak in the legs, or about to faint points to *presyncope* from vasovagal stimulation, orthostatic hypotension, arrhythmia, or side effects from blood pressure and other medications.

Vertigo often reflects vestibular disease, usually from peripheral causes in the inner ear such as *benign positional vertigo*, *labyrinthitis*, or *Ménière disease* (Hankey, 2017).

See Table 12-1, "Dizziness and Vertigo."

Formulating subjective questions is important to differentiate whether the patient is experiencing dizziness or vertigo. Begin with an open-ended prompt like, "Tell me about the dizziness." When eliciting additional information regarding a sign or symptom, use the "OLD CART" mnemonic to focus on specific questions so that the sequence of events will become clearer:

- *Onset:* When did this feeling of "dizziness" begin?
- *Location:* Does it seem to occur on one side of the head or the other?
- *Duration:* How often does the dizziness occur?
  How long does it last?
  Does it go away?
  Does it come and go?
- *Characteristic symptoms:* What does it feel like?
  Is the room spinning?
  Are you spinning?
  Is the room rotating?
  Are you lightheaded?
  Do you feel faint?
- *Associated manifestations:* Does anything else occur when you feel dizzy?
  Do you have double vision (diplopia)? If there are localizing symptoms or signs like double vision (*diplopia*), difficulty forming words (*dysarthria*), or problems with gait or balance (*ataxia*), investigate the central causes of vertigo.
  Do you feel nauseous?
  Do you experience difficulty forming words (**dysarthria**)?
  Are there times when you have difficulty with balance or walking (**ataxia**)?
  Have you taken any new medications? Prescribed? Over-the-counter?
- *Relieving factors:* Does anything make the dizziness go away? Decrease?
  What makes it feel better?
- *Treatment:* Have you taken any medications to relieve the dizziness?
  Have you used any therapies to help treat it, like aromatherapy, a chiropractor, or acupuncture? Any others?
  Have you talked to your health care provider previously about the dizziness?

Diplopia, dysarthria, ataxia in vertebrobasilar *transient ischemic attack* (TIA) or *stroke* (Dolmans et al., 2019; Hankey, 2017; Hurford et al., 2019).

Weakness

Weakness is another common symptom with many causes that bears careful investigation. It is important to clarify what the patient means by "weakness": fatigue, apathy, drowsiness, or actual loss of strength. True motor weakness can arise from the CNS, a peripheral nerve, the neuromuscular junction, or a muscle. Time course and location are especially relevant. Is the onset sudden, gradual, or chronic over a long period of time?

CLINICAL TIP

Abrupt onset of motor and sensory deficits occurs in *TIA* and *stroke* (Simonenko et al., 2020; Yu & Kapral, 2019). Progressive onset of lower extremity weakness suggests *Guillain–Barré syndrome (GBS)*. GBS has also been seen 5 to 10 days after a diagnosis of *COVID-19* (Lim et al., 2020; Toscano et al., 2020). Chronic, more gradual onset of lower extremity weakness occurs in primary and metastatic spinal cord tumors.

Explore the weakness further using "OLD CART:"

- *Onset:* When did the weakness begin?
  Did it start slowly or suddenly?
- *Location:* What areas of the body are involved?
  Does the weakness affect one or both sides?
  What movements are affected?

Focal or asymmetric weakness has both central (ischemic, vascular, or mass lesions) and peripheral causes ranging from neuromuscular junction disorders to myopathies.

For weakness without lightheadedness, try to distinguish between proximal and distal weakness.

- *Proximal*—in the shoulder and/or hip girdle, for example
- *Distal*—in the hands and/or feet
- *Symmetric*—in the same areas on both sides of the body
- *Asymmetric*—types of weakness include focal, in a portion of the face or extremity; monoparesis, in one extremity; paraparesis, in both lower extremities; and hemiparesis, in one side of the body

Proximal limb weakness, when symmetric with intact sensation, occurs in myopathies from alcohol, drugs like glucocorticoids, and inflammatory muscle disorders like *polymyositis* and *dermatomyositis*. In the neuromuscular junction disorder *myasthenia gravis*, there is proximal typically asymmetric weakness that gets worse with effort (fatigability), often with associated *bulbar symptoms* such as diplopia, ptosis, dysarthria, and dysphagia (Jordan & Freimer, 2018; Mantegazza et al., 2018).

- *Duration:* Has it progressed? How so?
  How long does it last?
  Does it go away?
  Does it come and go?
- *Characteristic symptoms*
  - If assessing for proximal weakness:
    Are you able to reach something on a high shelf?
    Do you have difficulty getting out of a chair?
    How does it feel when you brush your hair?
    Are you able to walk up steps? How many?
    Does the weakness increase with repeated effort?
    Does it improve with rest?
  - If assessing for distal weakness in the arms:
    Have you noticed any changes in hand movements?
    Do you have any difficulty opening jars or cans?
    Has it become more cumbersome to use scissors, screwdrivers, or pliers?
  - If assessing for distal weakness in the legs:
    Have you noticed yourself tripping?
- *Associated manifestations:* Are there any sensations you experience when the weakness occurs?
  Have you noticed that there are some activities that you are not able to participate in any longer? Or need assistance completing?
  Do you experience any other symptoms when the weakness occurs, like nausea or vomiting? Headaches? Double vision? Difficulty swallowing? Slurred speech? Rash?
  Have you recently changed medications?
- *Relieving factors:* Does anything relieve the weakness?
  What improves it? Rest? Caffeine? Exercise?
  Have you noticed you are sleeping or resting more?

- *Treatment:* Have you taken any medications to relieve the weakness? Have you talked to your health care provider previously about the weakness?

Change in or Loss of Sensation

In a patient who reports numbness, ask the patient to be more precise. Is there tingling like "pins and needles"? These altered sensations are called **paresthesias**. These commonly occur when an arm or leg "goes to sleep" following compression of a nerve and may be described as tingling, prickling, or feelings of warmth, coldness, or pressure. **Dysesthesias** are distorted sensations in response to a stimulus and may last longer than the stimulus itself. For example, a person may perceive a light touch or pinprick as a burning or tingling sensation that is irritating or unpleasant. *Pain* may arise from neurologic causes but is usually reported with symptoms of other body systems, such as the head and neck or the musculoskeletal system.

See Table 18-3, "Lower Back Pain," and Table 18-4, "Pains in the Neck."

CLINICAL TIP

Sensory changes can arise at several levels: local nerve compression or "entrapment," seen in hand numbness in distributions specific to the median, ulnar, or radial nerve; nerve root compression with dermatomal sensory loss from vertebral bone spurs or herniated discs; or central lesions from *stroke* or *multiple sclerosis*.

Burning pain occurs in painful *sensory neuropathies* from conditions like diabetes (Feldman et al., 2019; Stino & Smith, 2017).

Ask the patient if they have noticed any change in sensation. If so, use "OLD CART" to ask further questions:

- *Onset:* When did this begin?
- *Location:* What part(s) of the body experience this change or loss in sensation?
- *Duration:* How long does it last? Is it continuous or does it come and go?
- *Characteristic symptoms:* Describe what it feels like (e.g., pins and needles, goes to sleep, tingling, prickling, pressure, warmth, cold, burning, irritating).
- *Associated manifestations:* Have you noticed any other changes (e.g., vision changes, difficulty eating)?
- *Relieving factors:* Does anything make it feel better?
- *Treatment:* What treatments or medications have you tried? What were the results?

Near Syncope and Syncope

Patient reports of fainting or "passing out" are common and warrant a meticulous history to guide management and possible hospital admission (İdil & Kılıc, 2019). Begin by finding out whether the patient has experienced syncope or near syncope. In syncope, the patient has actually lost consciousness and postural tone from transient global hypoperfusion of the brain. While in near syncope, the patient feels lightheaded or weak but fails to lose consciousness. True syncope is a more serious symptom (İdil & Kılıc, 2019).

Causes include seizures, "neurocardiogenic" conditions such as **vasovagal syncope**, *postural orthostatic tachycardia syndrome (POTS)*, *carotid sinus syncope*, *orthostatic hypotension*, and cardiac disease causing arrhythmias, especially ventricular tachycardia and bradyarrhythmias (Shen et al., 2017). Stroke and subarachnoid hemorrhage are unlikely causes of syncope unless both hemispheres are affected.

Get as complete and unbiased a description of the event as possible:

- What brought on the episode?
- Were there any warning symptoms?
- Was the patient standing, sitting, or lying down when the episode began?
- How long did it last?
- Could voices be heard while passing out and waking up?
- How rapidly did the patient recover?
- In retrospect, were onset and offset slow or fast?

Also ask if anyone observed the episode. If so, ask:

- What did the patient look like before losing consciousness, during the episode, and afterward?
- Was there any seizure-like movement of the arms or legs?
- Any incontinence of the bladder or bowel?
- Any drowsiness or impaired memory after the episode ended?

In *vasovagal syncope*, the most common type of syncope, look for the prodrome of nausea, diaphoresis, and pallor triggered by a fearful or unpleasant event, then vagally mediated hypotension, often with slow onset and offset. In syncope from arrhythmias, onset and offset are often sudden, reflecting loss and recovery of cerebral perfusion.

Seizures

A *seizure* is a paroxysmal disorder caused by sudden excessive electrical discharge in the cerebral cortex or its underlying structures. Seizures can be of several types (Table 20-4). Depending on the type, there may or may not be loss of consciousness. With some types of seizures, there may be abnormal feelings, thought processes, and sensations, including smells as well as abnormal movements. Asking "Have you ever had any seizures or 'spells'?" and "Any fits or convulsions?" can open the discussion.

TABLE 20-4 Seizure Disorders

The International League Against Epilepsy (ILAE) reclassified seizures in 2017. Some seizures have been reclassified from generalized to focal seizures. Additional generalized seizure types have been included with the use of "unknown" to classify seizures when unable to determine the onset. These changes better reflect current scientific understanding. Terminology changes have been refined for a better understanding such as use of the word "awareness" for consciousness. The complexities of the reclassification scheme are best explored by turning to the report of the ILAE Commission on Classification and Terminology, cited below, and to more detailed references. This table presents only basic concepts from this report.

Focal Seizures

Focal seizures are conceptualized as originating within networks limited to one hemisphere. They may be discretely localized or more widely distributed. Focal seizures may originate in subcortical structures. For each seizure type, ictal onset is consistent from one seizure to another, with preferential propagation patterns that can involve the contralateral hemisphere. In some cases, however, there is more than one network, and more than one seizure type, but each individual seizure type has a consistent site of onset.

Problem	Clinical Manifestations	Postictal State
Focal seizures without loss of consciousness	Involuntary movements of a body part that start unilaterally in the hand, foot, or face and spread to other body parts May alter emotions, visibility, or other senses (taste, smell, feel, sound) A "funny feeling" tingling, flashing lights, or dizziness or lightheadedness	Normal consciousness
Focal seizures with subjective sensory or psychic phenomena	The seizure may or may not start with the autonomic or psychic symptoms outlined above. Consciousness is impaired, and the person appears confused. Automatisms include automatic motor behaviors such as chewing, smacking the lips, walking about, and unbuttoning clothes; also more complicated and skilled behaviors such as driving a car Partial seizures that become generalized resemble tonic–clonic seizures (see next page). Unfortunately, the patient may not recall the focal onset, and observers may overlook it	Normal consciousness
Focal seizures with impaired awareness	Consciousness is impaired, and the person appears confused and stares into space. Automatisms include automatic motor behaviors such as chewing, smacking the lips, walking about, and unbuttoning clothes as well as more complicated and skilled behaviors such as driving a car	The patient may remember initial autonomic or psychic symptoms (which are then termed an *aura*) but is amnesic for the rest of the seizure. Temporary confusion and headache may occur

Generalized Seizures

Generalized seizures seem to involve all brain areas, and the location and lateralization are not consistent from one seizure to another. Generalized seizures can be asymmetric. They may begin with body movements, impaired consciousness, or both. When tonic–clonic seizures begin after age 30, suspect either a partial seizure that has become generalized or a general seizure caused by a toxic or metabolic disorder. Toxic and metabolic causes include withdrawal from alcohol or other sedative drugs, uremia, hypoglycemia, hyperglycemia, hyponatremia, and bacterial meningitis.

Problem	Clinical Manifestations	Postictal (Postseizure) State
Generalized seizures	The person loses consciousness suddenly, sometimes with a cry, and the body stiffens into tonic extensor rigidity. Breathing stops, and the person becomes cyanotic. A clonic phase of rhythmic muscular contraction follows. Breathing resumes and is often noisy, with excessive salivation. Injury, tongue biting, and urinary incontinence may occur A sudden brief lapse of consciousness, with momentary blinking, staring, or movements of the lips and hands but no falling. Two subtypes are recognized. *Typical absences* last less than 10 s and stop abruptly. *Atypical absences* may last more than 10 s	Unresponsive, confusion, frightened, very tired, and sore
Tonic–clonic (previously known as grand mal seizures)	Sudden brief, rapid jerks involving the trunk or limbs Associated with a variety of disorders	Confusion, drowsiness, fatigue, headache, muscular aching, and sometimes the temporary persistence of bilateral neurologic deficits such as hyperactive reflexes and Babinski responses. The person has amnesia for the seizure and recalls no aura
Absence	Sudden loss of consciousness, staring into space. Subtle body movement (e.g., eye blinks, lip smacking)	No aura recalled. Previously known as petit mal seizures. In absences, a prompt return to normal; in atypical absences, some postictal confusion
Myoclonic	Varies in intensity and frequency; can be sudden, brief, and involuntary; can be localized or all over the body	Variable
Atonic (drop attack)	The movements may have personally symbolic significance and often do not follow a neuroanatomic pattern. Injury is uncommon	Either a prompt return to normal or a brief period of confusion
Tonic	Stiffening of the muscles usually in the arms, legs, and back. May cause falling to the ground	
Clonic	Jerking, rhythmic muscle movements, usually in the face, neck, and arms	

Data from Fisher, R. S., Helen Cross, J., D'Souza, C., French, J. A., Haut, S. R., Higurashi, N., Hirsch, E., Jansen, F. E., Lagae, L., Moshe, S. L., Peltola, J., Perez, E. R., Scheffer, I. E., Schulze-Bonhage, A., Somerville, E., Sperling, M., Yacubian, E. M., & Zuberi, S. M. (2017). Instruction manual for the ILAE 2017 operational classification of seizure types. *Epilepsia*, *58*(4), 531–542.

Common causes of *acute symptomatic seizures* include: epilepsy; head trauma; alcohol, cocaine, and other drugs; withdrawal from alcohol, benzodiazepines, and barbiturates; metabolic insults from low or high glucose or low calcium or sodium; acute stroke; and meningitis or encephalitis.

Tonic–clonic motor activity, bladder or bowel incontinence, and *postictal state* suggest a generalized *seizure*. **Tonic–clonic** seizures are disturbances in both sides of the brain. There are two stages; the *tonic* stage is when the muscles stiffen, consciousness is lost, and the person may fall down. The *clonic* stage consists of rapid muscle contractions and convulsions. Unlike syncope, injury such as tongue biting or bruising of limbs may occur (Alguire, 2016; Kuhlmann et al., 2018).

Ictus is a sudden seizure, attack, or stroke; *postictal* is the state of consciousness after the seizure, attack, or stroke.

If the patient reports a history of seizures, ask:

- *Onset:* At what age did the seizures begin?
  When was the last seizure?
  Has there been a change in frequency?
- *Location:* Do you lose consciousness when you have a seizure?
  Does it affect your entire body?
- *Duration:* How often do the seizures occur?
  How long do the seizures last?
- *Characteristic symptoms:* What are the precipitating circumstances or warnings prior to a seizure?
  What are the behaviors and feelings that occur during the seizure?
  What occurs after the seizure? How do you feel?
- *Associated manifestations:* What is causing the seizures?
  Is there a history of a head injury or other condition that may be related to the seizures?
- *Relieving factors:* What can be done to relieve the actual seizure?
  What is instrumental in relieving the symptoms associated with the actual seizure or postictal period?
- *Treatment:* What medications are currently being administered?
  What has been used previously?
  Who is monitoring your medications and condition?

Tremors

Tremors and other *involuntary movements* occur with or without additional neurologic manifestations. Ask about any trembling, shakiness, or body movements that the patient seems unable to control (Table 20-5).

Low-frequency unilateral resting tremor, rigidity, and bradykinesia are seen in *Parkinson disease* (Bäckström et al., 2018; Blauwendraat et al., 2019). *Essential tremors* are high-frequency, bilateral, upper extremity tremors that occur with both limb movement and sustained posture and subside when the limb is relaxed; head, voice, and leg tremor may also be present (Kwon et al., 2018).

Distinct from these symptoms is *restless legs syndrome*, also known as Willis-Ekbom disease, described as an unpleasant sensation or pain in the legs, an urge to move, especially late in the afternoon or at night. The symptoms get worse with rest and improve with movement of the symptomatic limb(s) (Trenkwalder et al., 2016).

Reversible causes of restless legs syndrome include pregnancy, renal disease, and iron deficiency (Trenkwalder et al., 2016).

TABLE 20-5 Tremors and Involuntary Movements

Tremors are rhythmic oscillatory movements, which may be roughly subdivided into three groups: resting (or static) tremors, postural tremors, and intention tremors.

Resting (Static) Tremors

These tremors are most prominent at rest and may decrease or disappear with voluntary movement. Illustrated is the common, relatively slow, fine, pill-rolling tremor of Parkinsonism, about five per second.

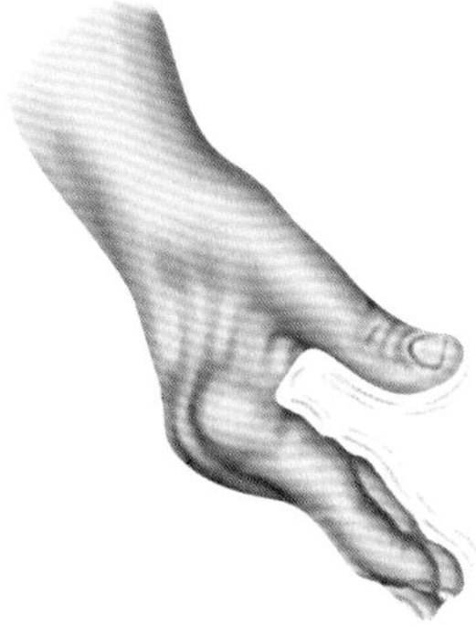

Postural (Action) Tremors

These tremors appear when the affected part is actively maintaining a posture. Examples include the fine rapid tremor of hyperthyroidism, the tremors of anxiety and fatigue, and benign essential (and sometimes familial) tremor. Tremor may worsen somewhat with intention.

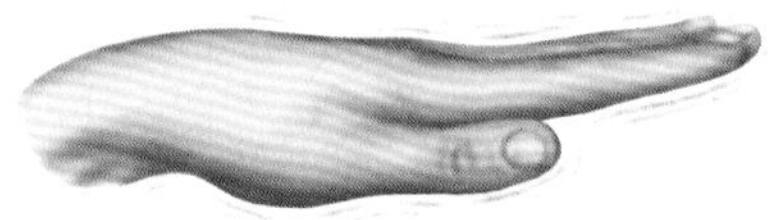

Intention Tremors

Intention tremors, absent at rest, appear with activity and often get worse as the target is neared. Causes include disorders of cerebellar pathways, as in multiple sclerosis.

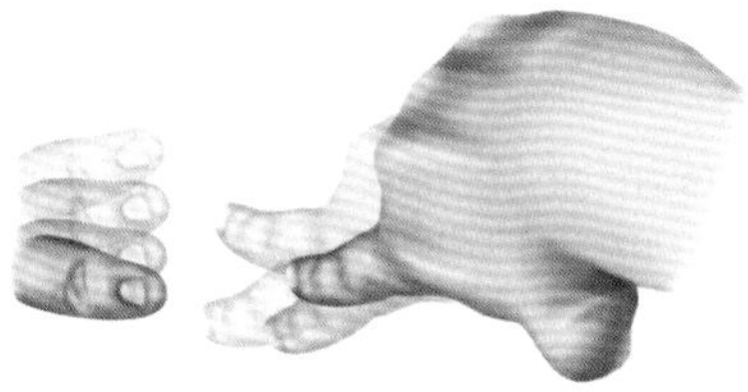

Oral-Facial Dyskinesias

Oral–facial dyskinesias are rhythmic, repetitive, bizarre movements that chiefly involve the face, mouth, jaw, and tongue—grimacing, pursing of the lips, protrusions of the tongue, opening and closing of the mouth, and deviations of the jaw. The limbs and trunk are involved less often. These movements may be a late complication of psychotropic drugs such as phenothiazines, termed *tardive* (late) dyskinesias. They also occur in long-standing psychoses, in some older adults, and in some edentulous individuals (without teeth).

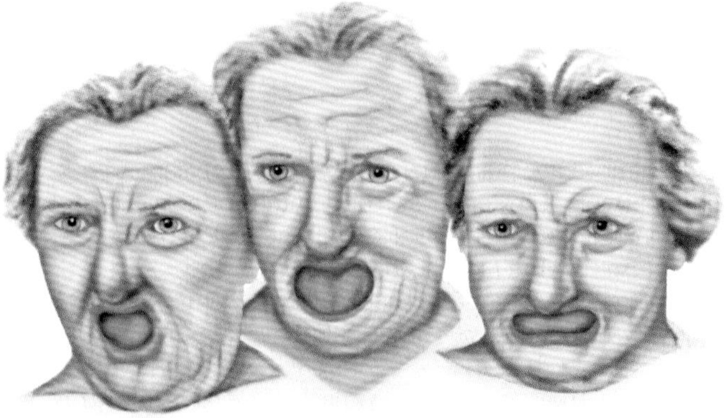

(*continued*)

TABLE 20-5 Tremors and Involuntary Movements *(Continued)*

Tics

Tics are brief, repetitive, stereotyped, coordinated movements occurring at irregular intervals. Examples include repetitive winking, grimacing, and shoulder shrugging. Causes include Tourette syndrome and drugs such as phenothiazines and amphetamines.

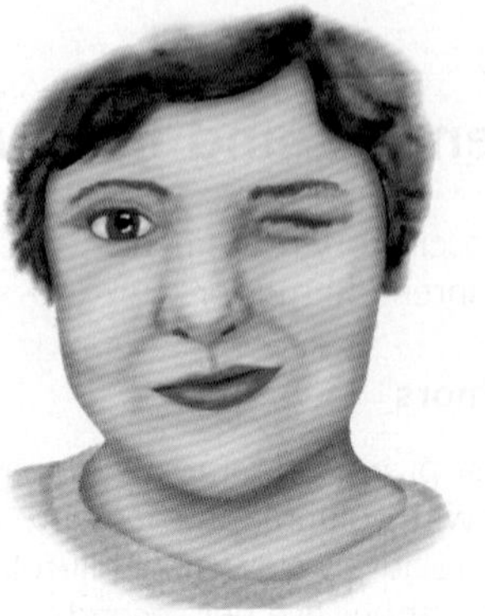

Dystonia

Dystonic movements are similar to athetoid movements, but often involve larger portions of the body, including the trunk. Grotesque, twisted postures may result. Causes include drugs such as phenothiazines, primary torsion dystonia, and as illustrated, spasmodic torticollis.

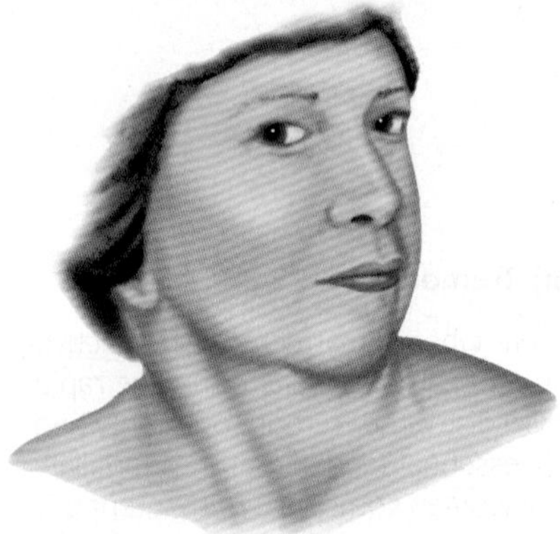

Athetosis

Athetoid movements are slower and more twisting and writhing than choreiform movements, and have larger amplitude. They most commonly involve the face and the distal extremities. Athetosis is often associated with spasticity. Causes include cerebral palsy.

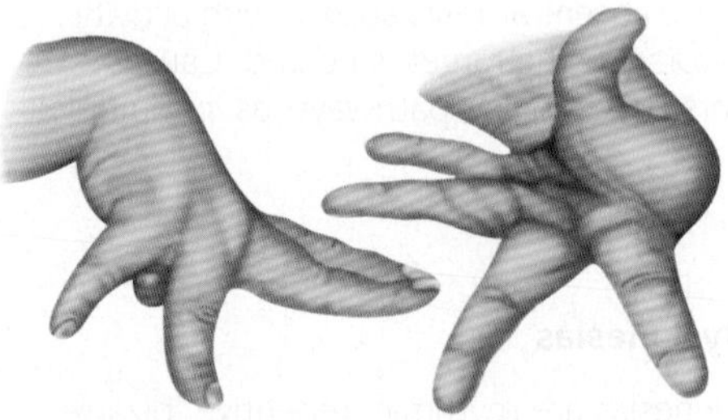

Chorea

Choreiform movements are brief, rapid, jerky, irregular, and unpredictable. They occur at rest or interrupt normal coordinated movements. Unlike tics, they seldom repeat themselves. The face, head, lower arms, and hands are often involved. Causes include Sydenham chorea (with rheumatic fever) and Huntington disease.

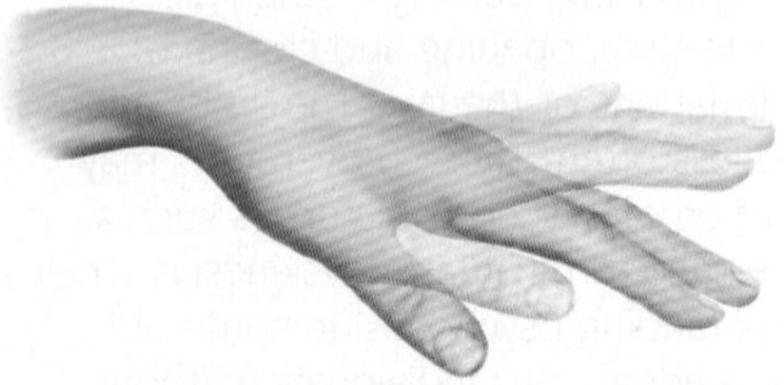

Source: Bentley, P., & Lovell, B. (2019). Endocrinology. *Memorizing Medicine: A Revision Guide*, 313–374. https://doi.org/10.1201/9780429446405-7; and Solomon, T., & Manji, H. (2020). Neurologic diseases. In E. Ryan, D. Hill, T. Solomon, T. Endy, & N. Aronson (Eds.), *Neurologic diseases* (10th ed., pp. 86–98). Elsevier.

PHYSICAL EXAMINATION

Assessment of the nervous system calls for many complex skills of examination and clinical reasoning. You have already learned the principles and techniques for assessing mental status, a critical component of the nervous system examination. As you saw in Chapter 19, "Mental Status and Mental Health Assessment," often the patient's mental status offers clues about delirium, memory disorders, and other neurologic conditions. As you study this chapter, let three important questions guide the approach to this challenging clinical area:

- Is mental status intact?
- Are right-sided and left-sided examination findings symmetric?
- If the findings are asymmetric or otherwise abnormal, does the lesion lie in the *CNS*, consisting of the brain and spinal cord, or in the *PNS*, consisting of the 12 pairs of CNs and the spinal and peripheral nerves?

Patient symptoms or signs point to the affected area of the nervous system.

Equipment needs vary according to the parts of the neurologic examination:

- CN examination
  - Penlight
  - Snellen chart
  - Newspaper or hand-held newsprint
  - Ophthalmoscope
  - Cotton swab
  - Tongue depressor
  - Gloves
  - Scent stimuli for olfactory assessment (e.g., vanilla, cinnamon, coffee, lemon juice, soap)
  - Tuning fork
- Sensory examination
  - Objects to feel (e.g., coin, paper clip)
  - Tuning fork

- Hot and cold water in test tubes or glass
- Cotton swab

- Muscle stretch response/DTRs
  - Reflex hammer
  - Tongue blade

Important areas of examination to perform include:

- Mental status, as in Chapter 19
- CNs I through XII
- Motor system: coordination, gait, and stance; also, muscle strength, bulk, and tone, as in Chapter 18, "The Musculoskeletal System"
- Sensory system: pain and temperature, position and vibration, light touch, and discrimination
- Deep tendon, abdominal, and plantar reflexes

This section presents the techniques you need for a practical and reasonably comprehensive examination of the nervous system. It is important to master the techniques for a thorough examination. Be active in your learning and ask your instructors to review your skills.

The amount of detail in an appropriate neurologic examination varies widely. In healthy patients, the examination will be relatively brief. If abnormal findings are detected, the examination will become more comprehensive. Be aware that neurologists may use many other techniques in specific situations. Whether you conduct a comprehensive or screening examination, organize your approach into five categories: (1) mental status, speech, and language; (2) CNs; (3) the motor system; (4) the sensory system; and (5) reflexes. If your findings are abnormal, begin to group them into patterns of central or peripheral disorders.

For efficiency, integrate the neurologic assessment with other parts of the examination. Survey the patient's mental status and speech during the interview, even though further testing may be necessary during the neurologic examination. Assess the CNs as you examine the head and neck and any neurologic abnormalities in the arms and legs as you evaluate the peripheral vascular and musculoskeletal systems. Chapter 22 provides an outline of an integrated approach. Think about and describe your findings, however, in terms of the nervous system as a unit. A screening neurologic examination is outlined in Box 20-3.

BOX 20-3 A SCREENING NEUROLOGIC EXAMINATION

A screening neurologic examination should be performed in all patients, even those without neurologic complaints, to detect any significant neurologic disease. The exact sequence of such screening may vary; however, it should cover the major components of the full examination: mental status, cranial nerves, motor system (strength, gait, and coordination), sensation, and reflexes. An example of a screening examination is as follows:

Mental Status

- Level of alertness
- Appropriateness of responses
- Orientation to date and place

Cranial Nerves

- Vision—visual fields, funduscopic examination
- Pupillary light reflex
- Eye movements
- Hearing
- Facial strength—smile, eye closure

Sensory System

- Light touch
- Pain/Temperature
- Proprioception

Motor System

- Muscle strength—shoulder abduction, elbow extension, wrist extension, finger abduction, hip flexion, knee flexion, ankle dorsiflexion
- Muscle bulk and tone
- Gait—casual, heel walk, toe walk, tandem walk
- Coordination—fine finger movements, finger-to-nose, heel to shin

Reflexes

- Muscle stretch response/deep tendon reflexes
- Plantar responses

Note: If there is reason to suspect neurologic disease based on the patient's history or the results of any components of the screening examination, a more complete neurologic examination is necessary.
Source: Jameson, J., Fauci, A., Kasper, D., Hauser, S., Longo, D., Loscalzo, J., & Harrison, T. (2015). *Harrison's principles of internal medicine*. The McGraw-Hill Education.

The Cranial Nerves

The examination of the CNs can be summarized as in the following sections.

Cranial Nerve I—Olfactory

Test the *sense of smell* by presenting the patient with familiar and nonirritating odors. First, make sure that each nasal passage is patent by compressing one side of the nose and asking the patient to sniff through the other. Then ask the patient to close both eyes. Occlude one nostril and test smell in the other side with substances such as cloves, coffee, soap, or vanilla. Avoid noxious odors like ammonia that might stimulate CN V. Ask the patient to

Loss of smell may occur in sinus conditions, head trauma, smoking, aging, COVID-19, *Parkinson disease*, or with cocaine use.

identify the odor. Test smell on the other side with a different odor. Normally a patient perceives odors on each side and identifies them correctly.

Cranial Nerve II—Optic

Test *visual acuity* (see Chapter 11). Inspect the *optic fundi* with your ophthalmoscope, paying special attention to the optic discs.

Inspect each disc carefully for bulging and blurred margins (*papilledema*); pallor (*optic atrophy*); and cup enlargement (*glaucoma*).

Test the visual fields by confrontation (see Chapter 11). Test each eye separately and both eyes together. Occasionally in stroke patients, for example, patients will complain of partial loss of vision, and testing of both eyes reveals a *visual field defect*, an abnormality in peripheral vision, such as *homonymous hemianopsia*. Testing one eye would not confirm the finding.

See Table 11-2, Visual Field Defects.

CLINICAL TIP

Check for prechiasmal, or anterior defects found in *glaucoma, retinal emboli, optic neuritis* (visual acuity poor), bitemporal **hemianopsia** (vision loss over half the field of vision). From defects at the optic chiasm, usually from *pituitary tumor* or homonymous hemianopsias or quadrantanopsia in postchiasmal lesions, usually in the *parietal lobe*, with associated findings of stroke (Fuller et al., 2017; Kuang et al., 2015).

Cranial Nerves II and III—Optic and Oculomotor

Inspect the size and shape of the pupils and compare one side with the other. *Anisocoria*, or a difference of no more than 1 mm in the diameter of one pupil compared to the other, is seen in up to 20% of healthy individuals. Test the *pupillary reactions to light*. Anisocoria not due to a medical condition is called physiologic anisocoria (Jenkins et al., 2019).

See Table 11-6, "Pupillary Abnormalities."

CLINICAL TIP

If the large pupil reacts poorly to light or anisocoria worsens in light, the large pupil has abnormal pupillary constriction, seen in *CN III palsy.* If ptosis (drooping eyelid) and *ophthalmoplegia* (eyes not aligned) are also present, consider *intracranial aneurysm* if the patient is awake and *transtentorial herniation* (a life-threatening situation when the medial temporal lobe is squeezed by a unilateral mass across and under the tentorium that supports the temporal lobe) if the patient is comatose.

Also check the *near reaction* or accommodation (p. 276), which tests pupillary constriction (pupillary constrictor muscle), convergence (medial rectus muscle), and accommodation of the lens (ciliary muscle).

If both pupils react to light and anisocoria worsens in darkness, the small pupil has abnormal pupillary dilation seen in *Horner syndrome* and *simple anisocoria* (Kanagalingam & Miller, 2015).

Cranial Nerves III, IV, and VI—Oculomotor, Trochlear, and Abducens

Test the *extraocular movements* in the six cardinal directions of gaze and look for loss of conjugate movements in any of the six directions, which causes **diplopia** (double vision). Ask the patient which direction makes the diplopia worse and inspect the eye closely for asymmetric deviation of movement. Determine if the diplopia is *monocular* or *binocular* by asking the patient to cover one eye, or perform the cover–uncover test (see Table 11-7, "Dysconjugate Gaze").

Monocular diplopia occurs in local problems with glasses or contact lenses; cataracts; astigmatism; and ptosis. Binocular diplopia occurs in *CN III, IV, VI neuropathy* and eye muscle disease from *myasthenia gravis, trauma, thyroid ophthalmopathy*, and *internuclear ophthalmoplegia* (Khanna & Holmes, 2017).

Check convergence of the eyes. Identify any **nystagmus**, an involuntary jerking movement of the eyes with quick and slow components (Table 20-6). Note the direction of gaze in which it appears, the plane of the nystagmus (horizontal, vertical, rotary, or mixed), and the direction of the quick and slow components (see Chapter 11). *Nystagmus is named for the direction of the quick component.* Ask the patient to fix their vision on a distant object and observe if the nystagmus increases or decreases.

Nystagmus occurs in *cerebellar disease*, especially with gait ataxia and dysarthria (increases with retinal fixation) and *vestibular disorders* (decreases with retinal fixation).

TABLE 20-6 Nystagmus

Nystagmus is a rhythmic oscillation of the eyes, analogous to a tremor in other parts of the body. Its causes are multiple, including impairment of vision in early life, disorders of the labyrinth and the cerebellar system, and drug toxicity. Nystagmus occurs normally when a person watches a rapidly moving object (e.g., a passing train). Study the characteristics of nystagmus described in this table to correctly identify the type of nystagmus.

Direction of Gaze in Which Nystagmus Appears

Nystagmus Present (Right Lateral Gaze)

Although nystagmus may be present in all directions of gaze, it may appear or become accentuated only on deviation of the eyes (e.g., to the side or upward). On extreme lateral gaze, the normal person may show a few beats resembling nystagmus. Avoid making assessments in such extreme positions, and *observe for nystagmus only within the field of full binocular vision.*

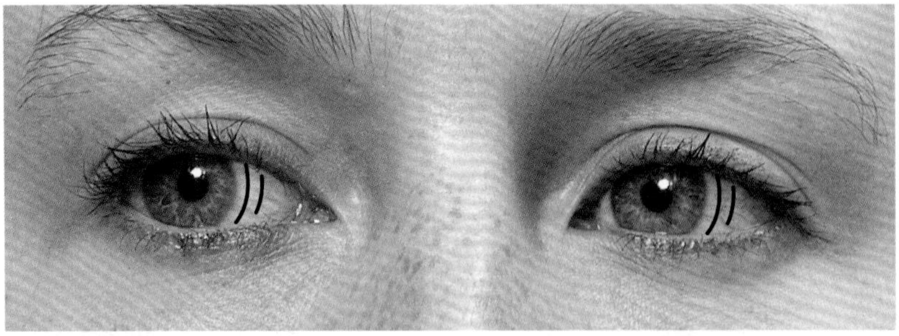

Nystagmus Not Present (Left Lateral Gaze)

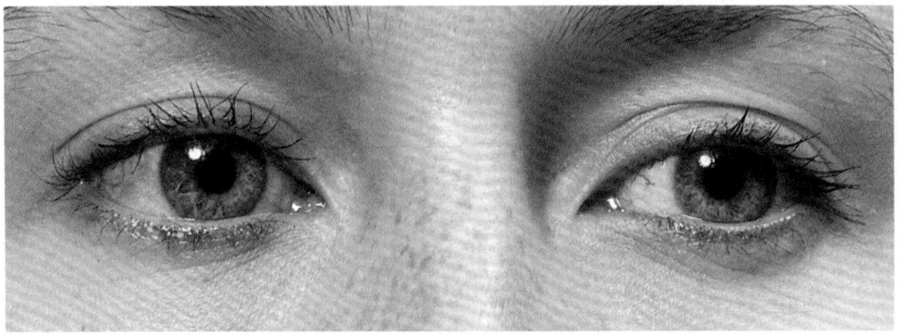

(continued)

TABLE 20-6 Nystagmus (*Continued*)

Direction of the Quick and Slow Components

Left-Beating Nystagmus—a Quick Jerk to the Left in Each Eye, Then a Slow Drift to the Right

Nystagmus usually has both slow and fast movements but *is defined by its fast phase.* For example, if the eyes jerk quickly to the patient's left and drift back slowly to the right, the patient is said to have *left-beating nystagmus.* Occasionally, nystagmus consists only of coarse oscillations without quick and slow components. It is then said to be *pendular.*

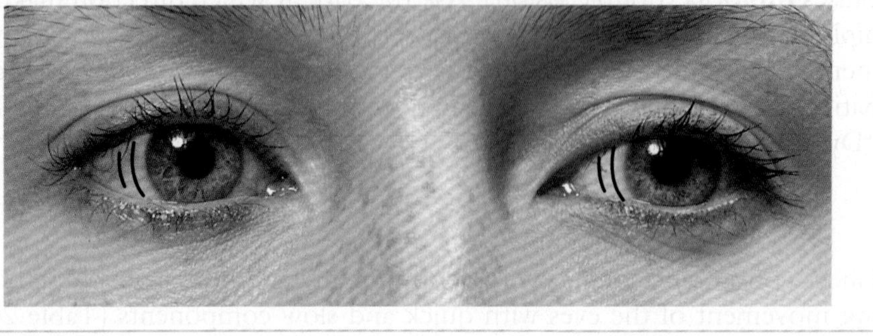

Look for *ptosis* (drooping of the upper eyelids). A slight difference in the width of the palpebral fissures may be a normal variation in approximately one third of all people.

Ptosis occurs in *third nerve palsy* (CN III), *Horner syndrome* (ptosis, meiosis, anhidrosis), or *myasthenia gravis.*

Cranial Nerve V—Trigeminal

Motor

While palpating the temporal (Fig. 20-9) and masseter (Fig. 20-10) muscles, ask the patient to clench the teeth. Note the strength of the muscle contraction and whether the strength is equal bilaterally or stronger or weaker unilaterally. Ask the patient to move the jaw side to side.

Difficulty clenching the jaw or moving it to the opposite side occurs in masseter and lateral pterygoid muscle weakness, respectively. Jaw deviation during opening points to weakness on the deviating side.

Look for unilateral weakness in CN V lesions in the pons and bilateral weakness in cerebral hemispheric disease because of bilateral cortical innervation.

CNS patterns from stroke include facial and body sensory loss on the same side (ipsilateral) but from the opposite side (contralateral) in a cortical or thalamic lesion; ipsilateral face but contralateral body sensory loss occurs in brainstem lesions.

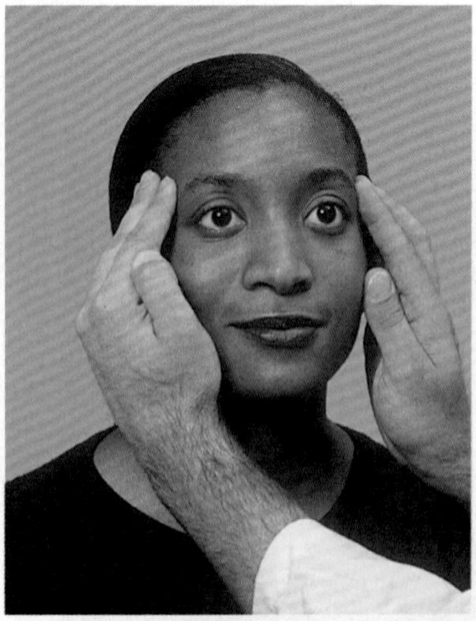

FIGURE 20-9 Palpating the temporal muscles.

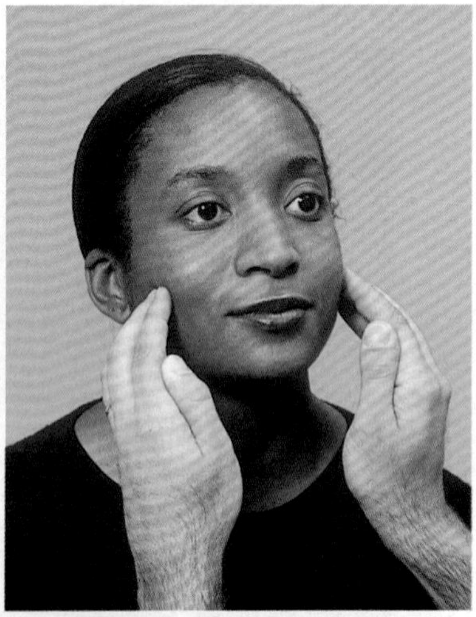

FIGURE 20-10 Palpating the masseter muscles.

Sensory

Sensation is tested on the forehead, cheeks, and chin on each side for *pain sensation*, as shown in the circled areas in Figure 20-11. The patient's eyes should be closed during the actual test; but prior to the examination, demonstrate what sharp and dull each feels like. Use an appropriate sharp object, such as a sharp wood splinter by breaking or twisting a tongue depressor for the sharp sensation and the use end of a cotton swab as a dull stimulus. Ask the patient to report whether it is "sharp" or "dull" and to compare sides.

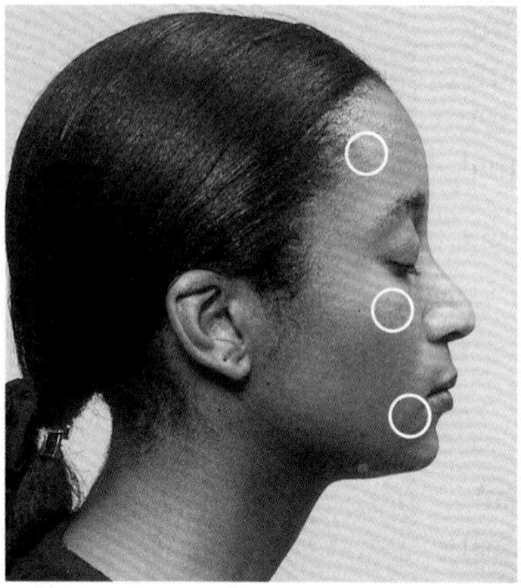

FIGURE 20-11 Sensory assessment.

Isolated facial sensory loss occurs in peripheral nerve disorders including lesions of the *trigeminal neuralgia.*

If you detect sensory loss, confirm it by testing *temperature sensation*. Two test tubes, filled with hot and ice-cold water, are the traditional stimuli. A tuning fork may also be used. It usually feels cool. If you are near running water, the fork is easily made cold or warm. Dry it before use. Touch the skin and ask the patient to identify "hot" or "cold."

Then test for *light touch,* using a fine wisp of cotton. Ask the patient to respond whenever you touch the skin.

Corneal Reflex

Test the *corneal reflex*. Ask the patient to look up and away from you and approach from the opposite side, out of the patient's line of vision. Avoiding the eyelashes, lightly touch the cornea (not just the conjunctiva) with a fine wisp of cotton. If the patient is apprehensive, touching the conjunctiva first may be helpful.

Inspect for blinking of the eyes, the normal reaction to this stimulus. The sensory limb of this reflex is carried in CN V and the motor response in CN VII. Use of contact lenses frequently diminishes or abolishes this reflex and therefore is not used as frequently.

Blinking is absent in both eyes in CN V lesions and on the side of weakness in lesions of CN VII. Absent blinking and sensorineural hearing loss occur in *acoustic neuroma.*

Concept Mastery Alert

The Trigeminal Nerve

The trigeminal nerve has two functions—motor and sensory—with one branch innervating the eye and triggering a blink.

Cranial Nerve VII—Facial

Inspect the face, both at rest and during conversation with the patient. Note any asymmetry (e.g., of the nasolabial folds), and observe any tics or other abnormal movements.

Ask the patient to:

1. raise both eyebrows.
2. frown.
3. close both eyes tightly so that you cannot open them. Test muscular strength by trying to open them (Fig. 20-12).
4. show both the upper and lower teeth.
5. smile.
6. puff out both cheeks.

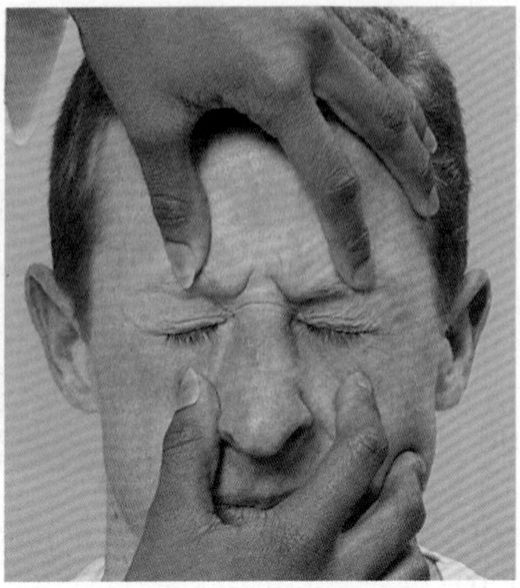

FIGURE 20-12 Testing muscular strength in the face.

Flattening of the nasolabial fold and drooping of the lower eyelid suggest facial weakness.

A peripheral injury to CN VII, as seen in *Bell palsy*, affects both the upper and lower face; a central lesion affects mainly the lower face. Loss of taste, *hyperacusis* (increased sensitivity to noise), and increased or decreased tearing also occur in Bell palsy (Rao et al., 2020).

In unilateral facial paralysis, the mouth droops on the paralyzed side when the patient smiles or grimaces.

Types of facial paralysis are outlined in Table 20-7.

TABLE 20-7 Types of Facial Paralysis

Facial weakness or paralysis may result either (1) from a peripheral lesion of CN VII, the facial nerve, anywhere from its origin in the pons to its periphery in the face, or (2) from a central lesion involving the upper motor neuron system between the cortex and the pons. A peripheral lesion of CN VII, exemplified here by a Bell palsy, is compared with a central lesion, exemplified by a left hemispheric cerebrovascular accident. These can be distinguished by their different effects on the upper part of the face.

The lower part of the face is normally controlled by upper motor neurons located on only one side of the cortex—the opposite side. *Left-sided damage to these pathways, as in a stroke, paralyzes the right lower face.* The upper face, however, is controlled by pathways from both sides of the cortex. Even though the upper motor neurons on the left are destroyed, others on the right remain, and the right upper face continues to function fairly well.

CN VII—Peripheral Lesion	CN VII—Central Lesion
Peripheral nerve damage to CN VII paralyzes the entire right side of the face, including the forehead.	

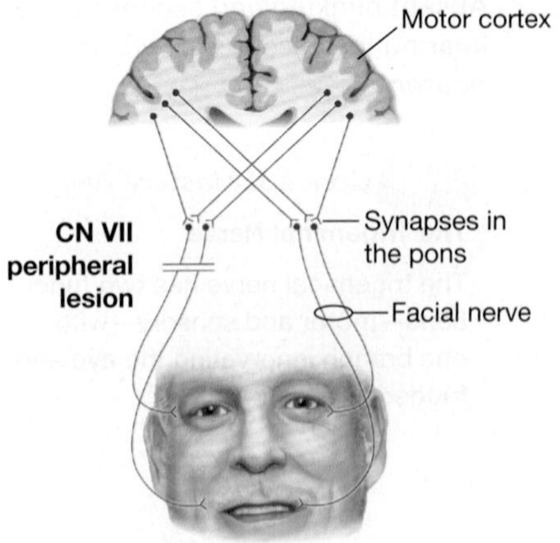

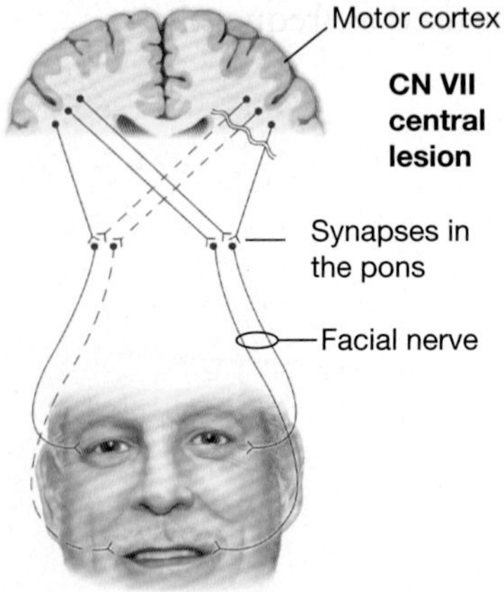

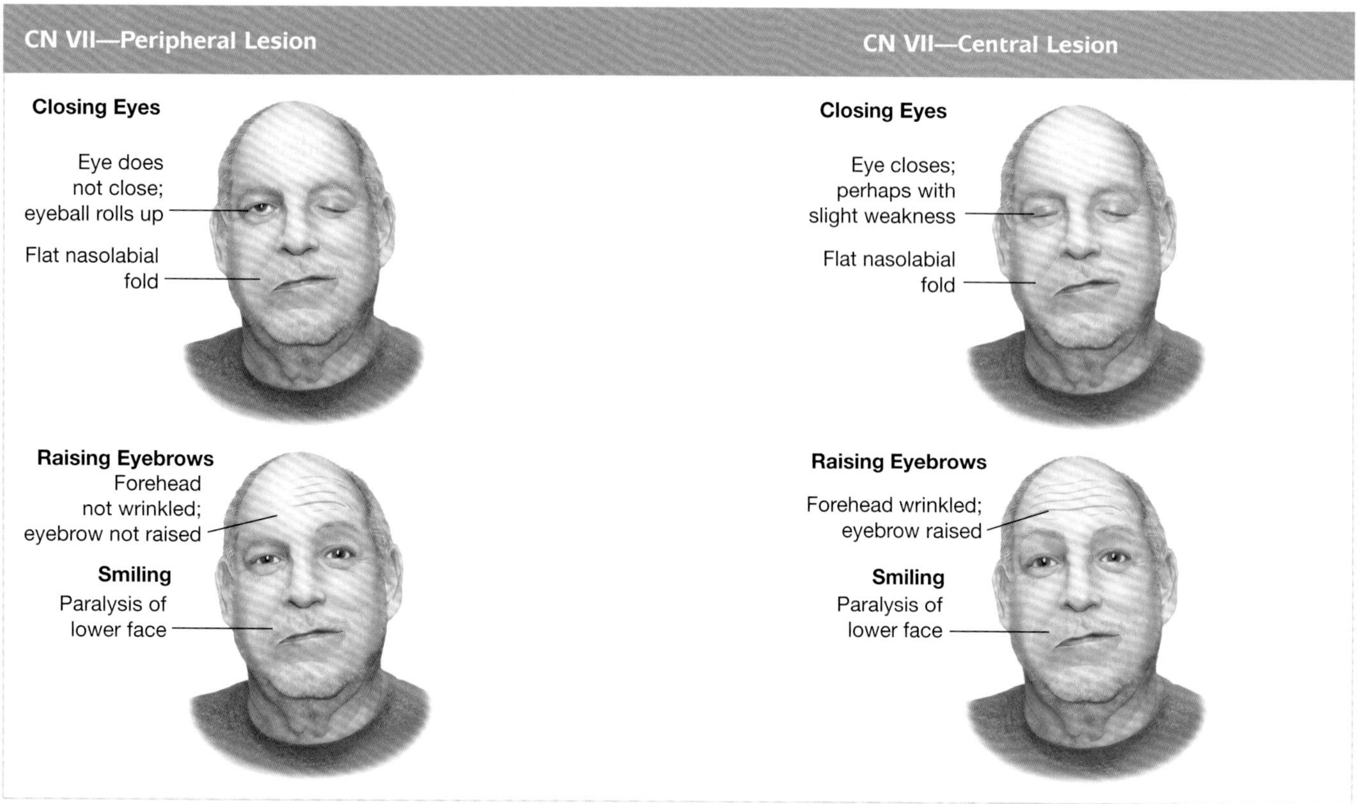

Cranial Nerve VIII—Acoustic

Assess hearing with the whispered voice test. Ask the patient to repeat numbers whispered into one ear while pressing on the tragus. Another technique is to stand behind the patient and rub your fingers next to the contralateral ear.

The finger rub has a 91% sensitivity rate, and the whisper test is 79% sensitive; specificity was higher for the whisper test (Strawbridge & Wallhagen, 2017).

If hearing loss is present, determine if the loss is *conductive*, from impaired "air through ear" transmission, or *sensorineural*, from damage to the cochlear branch of CN VIII. Test for *air and bone conduction* using the Rinne test and *lateralization* using the Weber test.

See the techniques for the Weber and Rinne tests in Chapter 12 and Table 12-4, "Patterns of Hearing Loss."

CLINICAL TIP

Excess cerumen, otosclerosis, and *otitis media* occur in conductive hearing loss and *presbycusis* from aging, most commonly in sensorineural hearing loss.

Specific tests of the vestibular function of CN VIII are rarely included in the typical neurologic examination.

Vertigo occurs with hearing loss and nystagmus in *Ménière disease*—see Table 12-1, "Dizziness and Vertigo," and Table 20-6, "Nystagmus."

Cranial Nerves IX and X—Glossopharyngeal and Vagus

Listen to the patient's *voice.* Is it hoarse, or does it have a nasal quality?

Hoarseness occurs in vocal cord paralysis, a nasal voice in paralysis of the palate.

Is there difficulty in swallowing?

Difficulty swallowing suggests pharyngeal or palatal weakness.

Ask the patient to say "ah" or to yawn as you watch the *movements of the soft palate and the pharynx.* The soft palate normally rises symmetrically, the uvula remains in the midline, and each side of the posterior pharynx moves medially, like a curtain. The slightly curved uvula seen occasionally as a normal variation should not be mistaken for a uvula deviated by a lesion of CN IX or X.

The palate fails to rise with a bilateral lesion of CN X. In unilateral paralysis, one side of the palate fails to rise and, together with the uvula, is pulled toward the normal side.

Warn the patient when testing the *gag reflex,* which consists of elevation of the tongue and soft palate and constriction of the pharyngeal muscles. Stimulate the back of the throat lightly on each side in turn and note the gag reflex. It may be symmetrically diminished or absent in some normal people. If a patient is healthy and swallowing is intact, checking a gag reflex is not necessary.

Unilateral absence of this reflex suggests a lesion of CN IX and perhaps CN X.

Cranial Nerve XI—Spinal Accessory

Look for atrophy or *fasciculations* in the trapezius muscles, and compare one side with the other when standing behind the patient. **Fasciculations** are fine flickering irregular movements in small groups of muscle fibers. Ask the patient to shrug both shoulders upward against your hands. Note the strength and contraction of the trapezii. See Figure 20-13.

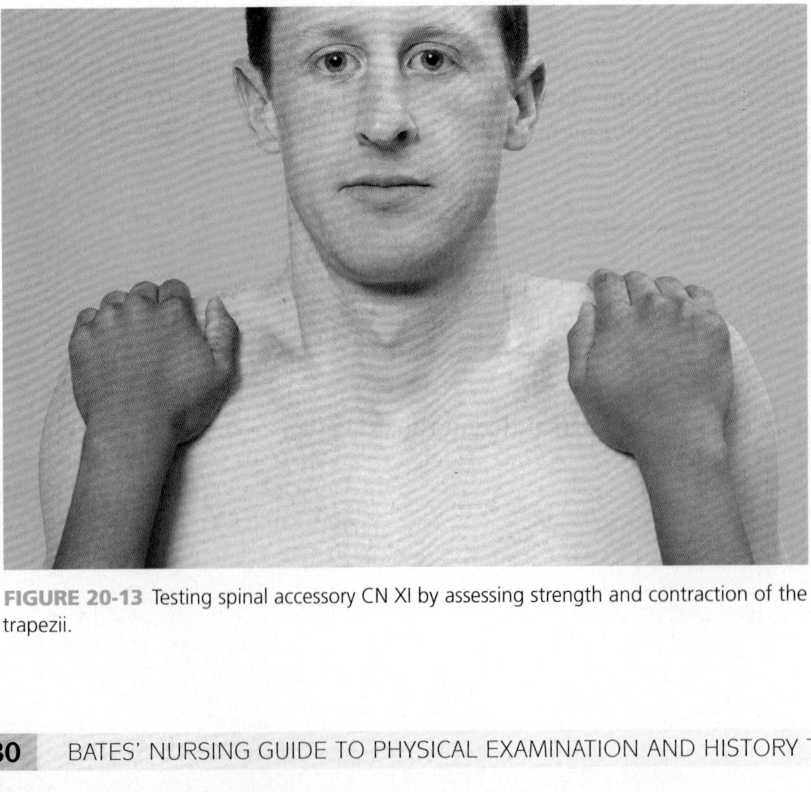

FIGURE 20-13 Testing spinal accessory CN XI by assessing strength and contraction of the trapezii.

CLINICAL TIP

Trapezius weakness with atrophy and fasciculations indicates a peripheral nerve disorder. In trapezius muscle paralysis, the shoulder droops, and the scapula is displaced downward and laterally.

Ask the patient to turn the head to each side against your hand (Fig. 20-14). Observe the contraction of the opposite sternocleidomastoid and note the force of the movement against your hand.

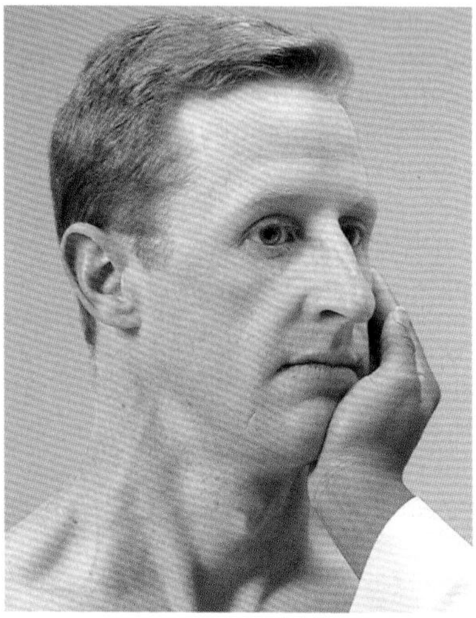

FIGURE 20-14 Assessing spinal accessory CN XI by testing the patient's ability to turn the head.

A supine patient with bilateral weakness of the sternocleidomastoid has difficulty raising their head off the pillow.

Cranial Nerve XII—Hypoglossal

Listen to the articulation of the patient's words. This depends on CNs V, VII, IX, and X as well as XII. Inspect the patient's tongue as it lies on the floor of the mouth. Look for any atrophy or *fasciculations.* Some coarser restless movements are often seen in a normal tongue. Then, with the patient's tongue protruded, look for asymmetry, atrophy, or deviation from the midline. Ask the patient to move the tongue from side to side and note the symmetry of the movement. In ambiguous cases, ask the patient to push the tongue against the inside of each cheek in turn as you palpate externally for strength. For poor articulation, or *dysarthria,* see Table 20-8, "Disorders of Speech." Tongue atrophy and fasciculations occur in *amyotrophic lateral sclerosis* and a history of *polio.*

In a unilateral cortical lesion, the protruded tongue deviates away from the side of the cortical lesion. In CN XII lesions, the tongue deviates to the weak side.

TABLE 20-8 Disorders of Speech

Disorders of speech fall into three groups: those affecting (1) phonation of the voice, (2) the articulation of words, and (3) the production and comprehension of language.

Aphonia—Refers to a loss of voice that accompanies disease affecting the larynx or its nerve supply. *Dysphonia* refers to less severe impairment in the volume, quality, or pitch of the voice. For example, a person may be hoarse or only able to speak in a whisper. Causes include laryngitis, laryngeal tumors, and a unilateral vocal cord paralysis (cranial nerve X).

Dysarthria—Refers to a defect in the muscular control of the speech apparatus (lips, tongue, palate, or pharynx). Words may be nasal, slurred, or indistinct, but the central symbolic aspect of language remains intact. Causes include motor lesions of the central or peripheral nervous system, parkinsonism, and cerebellar disease.

Aphasia—Refers to a disorder in producing or understanding language. It is often caused by lesions in the dominant cerebral hemisphere, usually the left.

Compared below are two common types of aphasia: (1) Wernicke, a fluent (receptive) aphasia, and (2) Broca, a nonfluent (or expressive) aphasia. There are other less common kinds of aphasia, which are distinguished by differing responses on the specific tests listed. Neurologic consultation is usually indicated.

(continued)

TABLE 20-8 Disorders of Speech (*Continued*)

	Wernicke Aphasia (Receptive)	Broca Aphasia (Expressive)
Qualities of Spontaneous Speech	Fluent; often rapid, voluble, and effortless. Inflection and articulation are good, but sentences lack meaning and words are malformed (paraphasias) or invented (neologisms). Speech may be totally incomprehensible.	Nonfluent; slow, with few words and laborious effort. Inflection and articulation are impaired but words are meaningful with nouns, transitive verbs, and important adjectives. Small grammatical words are often dropped.
Word Comprehension	Impaired	Fair to good
Repetition	Impaired	Impaired
Naming	Impaired	Impaired, though the patient recognizes objects
Reading Comprehension	Impaired	Fair to good
Writing	Impaired	Impaired
Location of Lesion	Posterior superior temporal lobe	Posterior inferior frontal lobe

Although it is important to recognize aphasia early in the encounter with a patient, its full diagnostic meaning does not become clear until integrated with the neurologic examination.

The Motor System

As you assess the motor system, focus on body position, involuntary movements, characteristics of the muscles (bulk, tone, and strength), and coordination. You can use this sequence for assessing overall motor function, or check each component in the arms, legs, and trunk. If you detect an abnormality, identify the muscle(s) involved and if it originates centrally or peripherally. Know which nerves innervate the major muscle groups.

Body Position

Observe the patient's body position during movement and at rest.

CLINICAL TIP
Abnormal positions alert you to conditions such as paresis or hemiparesis from stroke.

Involuntary Movements

Watch for involuntary movements such as tremors, tics, chorea, or fasciculations. Note their location, quality, rate, rhythm, and amplitude, and their relation to posture, activity, fatigue, emotion, and other factors.

See Table 20-5, "Tremors and Involuntary Movements."

Muscle Bulk, Tone, and Strength

Muscle bulk, tone, and strength are detailed in Chapter 18, "The Musculoskeletal System." Table 20-9 outlines disorders of muscle tone.

TABLE 20-9 Disorders of Muscle Tone

	Spasticity	Rigidity	Flaccidity	Paratonia (Generalized Increased Motor Tone)
Location of Lesion	Upper motor neuron of the corticospinal tract at any point from the cortex to the spinal cord	Basal ganglia system	Lower motor neuron system at any point from the anterior horn cell to the peripheral nerves	Both hemispheres, usually in the frontal lobes
Description	A form of muscular hypertonicity with increased resistance to stretch	Condition of hardness, stiffness, or inflexibility	Loss of muscle tone (*hypotonia*), causing the limb to be loose or floppy. The affected limbs may be hyperextensible or even flail-like. Flaccid muscles are also weak	Sudden changes in tone with passive range of motion. Sudden loss of tone that increases the ease of motion is called *mitgehen* (moving with). Sudden increase in tone making motion more difficult is called *gegenhalten* (holding against)
Common Cause	Stroke, especially late or chronic stage	Parkinsonism	Guillain–Barré syndrome; also initial phase of spinal cord injury (spinal shock) or stroke	Dementia

Coordination

Coordination of muscle movement requires four areas of the nervous system to function in an integrated way:

- The motor system—for muscle strength
- The cerebellar system (also part of the motor system)—for rhythmic movement and steady posture
- The vestibular system—for balance and for coordinating eye, head, and body movements
- The sensory system—for position sense

In cerebellar disease, look for nystagmus, dysarthria, hypotonia, and ataxia.

To assess coordination, observe the patient performing:

- Rapid alternating movements
- Point-to-point movements

- Gait and other related body movements
- Standing in specified ways

Rapid Alternating Movements

Arms

Show the patient how to strike one hand on the thigh, raise the hand, turn it over, and then strike the back of the hand down on the same place (Fig. 20-15). Urge the patient to repeat these alternating movements as rapidly as possible.

Observe the speed, rhythm, and smoothness of the movements. Repeat with the other hand. The nondominant hand often does not perform as well.

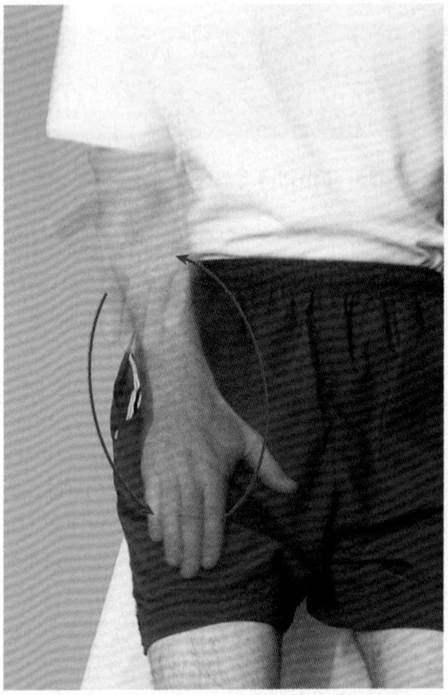

FIGURE 20-15 Rapid alternating movements of the arm.

CLINICAL TIP

In cerebellar disease, instead of alternating quickly, these movements are slow, irregular, and clumsy, an abnormality called *dysdiadochokinesis.* Upper motor neuron weakness and basal ganglia disease may also impair rapid alternating movements but not in the same manner.

Show the patient how to tap the distal joint of the thumb with the tip of the index finger, again as rapidly as possible (Fig. 20-16). Again, observe the speed, rhythm, and smoothness of the movements. The nondominant side often does not perform as well.

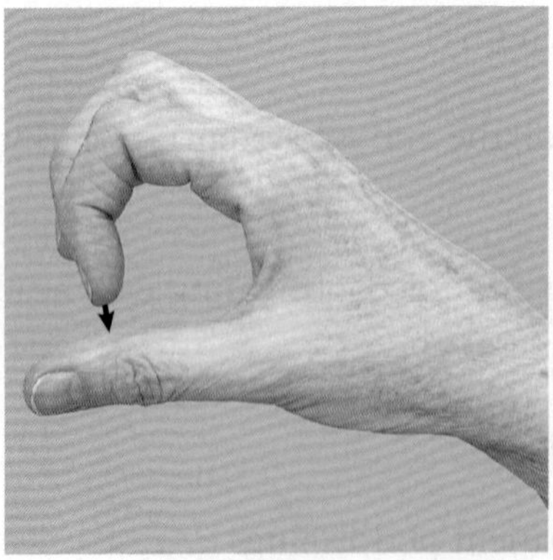

FIGURE 20-16 Rapid alternating movements of the finger.

Legs

Ask the patient to tap your hand or the floor as quickly as possible with the ball of each foot in turn. Note any slowness or awkwardness. Normally the feet do not perform as well as the hands.

Point-to-Point Movements

Arms: Finger-to-Nose Test

Ask the patient to touch your index finger and then their nose alternately several times (Fig. 20-17). Move your finger position so that the patient has to alter directions. Observe the accuracy and smoothness of movements and watch for any tremor. Normally, the patient's movements are smooth and accurate.

In cerebellar disease, movements are clumsy, unsteady, and inappropriately variable in their speed, force, and direction. In *dysmetria*, the patient's finger may initially overshoot the mark but then reach it fairly well. An *intention tremor* may appear toward the end of the movement. See Table 20-5, "Tremors and Involuntary Movements."

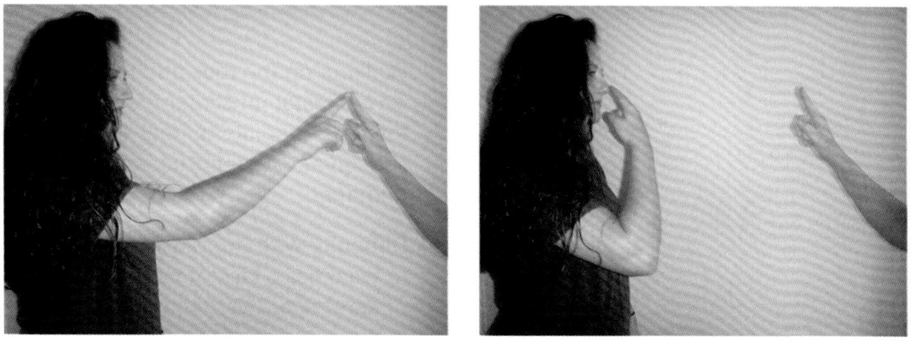

FIGURE 20-17 Finger-to-nose test. (Courtesy of Beth Hogan-Quigley, DNP, MSN, RN, CRNP.)

Now hold your finger in one place so that the patient can touch it with one arm and finger outstretched. Ask the patient to raise their arm overhead and lower it again to touch your finger. After several repeats, ask the patient to close both eyes and try several more times. Repeat on the other side. Normally a person can touch the examiner's finger successfully with eyes open or closed. These maneuvers test position sense and the functions of both the labyrinth of the inner ear and the cerebellum.

In cerebellar disease, incoordination modestly worsens with the eyes closed, indicating loss of position sense. Consistent deviation to one side which worsens with the eyes closed, referred to as *past pointing*, suggests cerebellar or vestibular disease.

Legs: Heel-to-Shin Test

Ask the patient to place one heel on the opposite knee, and then run it down the shin to the big toe (Fig. 20-18). Observe the smoothness and accuracy of the movements. Repetition with the patient's eyes closed tests for position sense. Repeat on the other side.

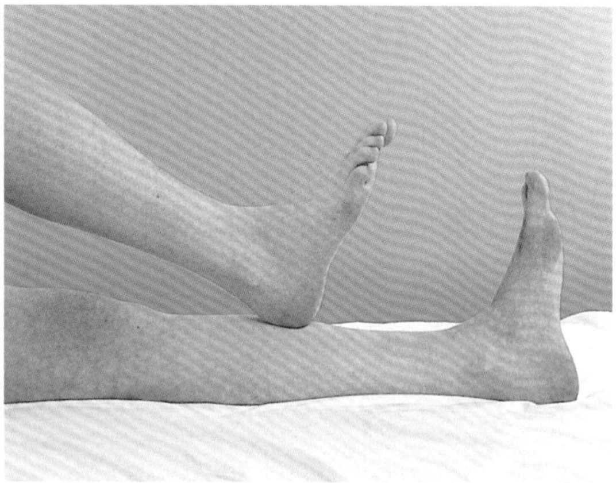

FIGURE 20-18 Heel-to-shin test.

In cerebellar disease, the heel may overshoot the knee and then oscillate from side to side down the shin. If position sense is absent, the heel lifts too high and the patient tries to look. With eyes closed, performance is poor.

Gait

Ask the patient to:

- *Walk across the room* or down the hall, then turn, and come back. Observe posture, balance, swinging of the arms, and movements of the legs. Normally balance is easy, the arms swing at the sides, and turns are accomplished smoothly.

Abnormalities of gait increase risk of falls.

CLINICAL TIP
A gait that lacks coordination with reeling and instability is called *ataxic.* Ataxia may be due to cerebellar disease, loss of position sense, or intoxication.

- *Walk heel-to-toe* in a straight line, a pattern called *tandem walking* (Fig. 20-19).

Tandem walking may reveal an ataxia not previously obvious.

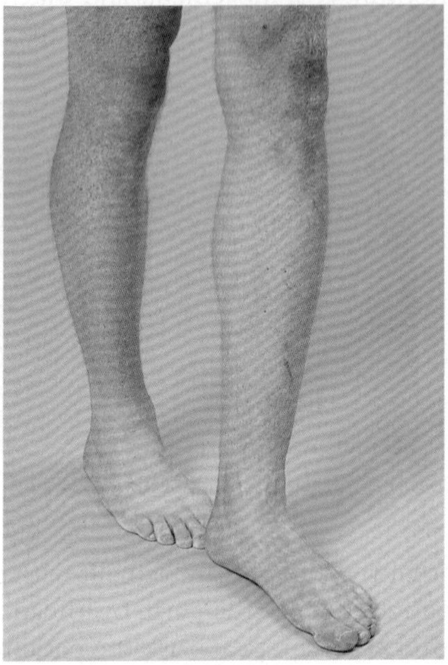

FIGURE 20-19 Assessing gait as the patient walks heel to toe.

- *Walk on the toes* then *on the heels*—sensitive tests, respectively, for plantar flexion and dorsiflexion of the ankles, as well as for balance.

Walking on the toes and heels may reveal distal muscular weakness in the legs. Inability to heel-walk is a sensitive test for corticospinal tract damage.

- *Hop in place* on each foot in turn (if the patient is not too ill). Hopping involves the proximal muscles of the legs as well as the distal ones and requires both good position sense and normal cerebellar function.

Difficulty with hopping may be due to weakness, lack of position sense, or cerebellar dysfunction.

- *Do a shallow knee bend*—first on one leg, then on the other (Fig. 20-20). Support the patient's elbow if you think the patient is in danger of falling.

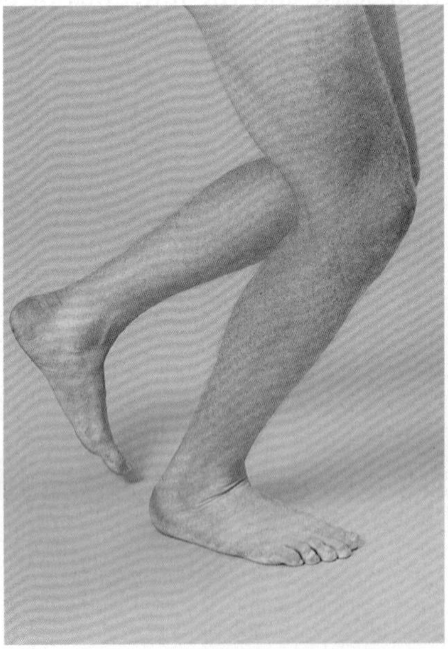

FIGURE 20-20 A shallow knee bend test.

CLINICAL TIP
Difficulty with the shallow knee bend suggests proximal weakness (extensors of the hip), weakness of the quadriceps (the extensor of the knee), or both.

- *Rising from a sitting position* without arm support and *stepping up* on a sturdy stool are more suitable tests than hopping or knee bends if the patient is unsteady, neurologically impaired, or frail.

Proximal muscle weakness involving the pelvic girdle and legs causes difficulty with both rising from sitting and stepping up.

Abnormalities of gait and posture are summarized in Table 20-10.

TABLE 20-10 Abnormalities of Gait and Posture

Spastic Hemiparesis

Seen in corticospinal tract lesion in stroke, causing poor control of flexor muscles during swing phase. Affected arm is flexed, immobile, and held close to the side with elbow, wrists, and interphalangeal joints flexed. Affected leg extensors spastic; ankle plantar flexed and inverted. Patients may drag toe, circle leg stiffly outward and forward (*circumduction*), or lean trunk to contralateral side to clear affected leg during walking.

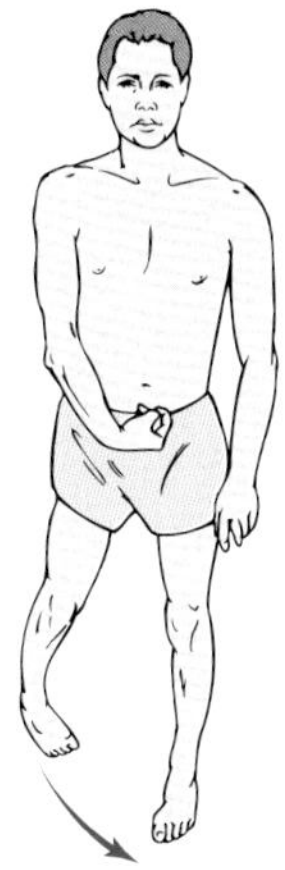

Scissors Gait

Seen in spinal cord disease causing bilateral lower extremity spasticity, including adductor spasm, and abnormal proprioception. Gait is stiff. Patients advance each leg slowly, and the thighs tend to cross forward on each other at each step. Steps are short. Patients appear as if walking through water.

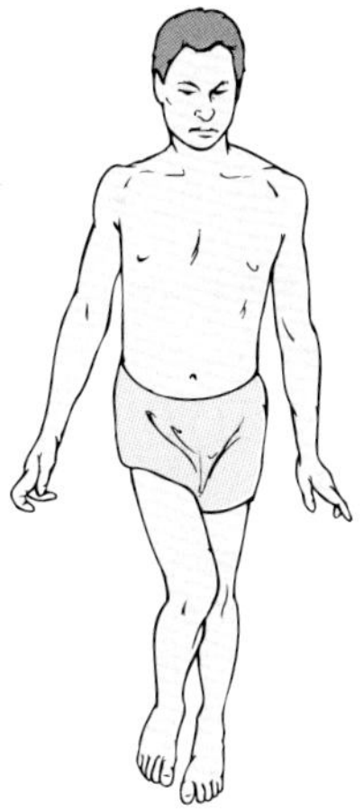

Steppage Gait

Seen in foot drop, usually secondary to peripheral motor unit disease. Patients either drag the feet or lift them high with knees flexed and bring them down with a slap onto the floor, thus appearing to be walking up stairs. They cannot walk on their heels. The steppage gait may involve one or both legs. Tibialis anterior and toe extensors are weak.

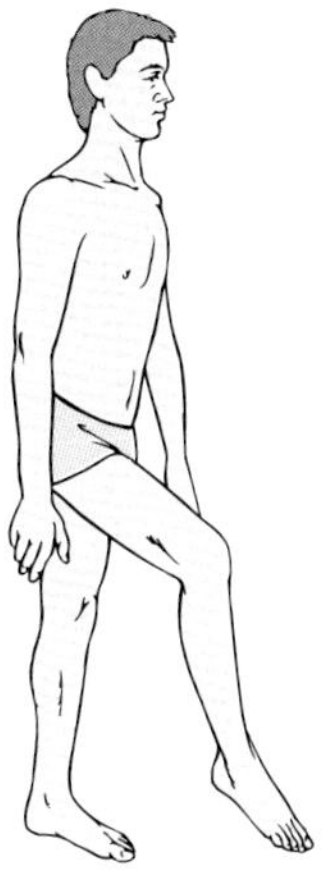

(*continued*)

TABLE 20-10 Abnormalities of Gait and Posture (*Continued*)

Parkinsonian Gait

Seen in the basal ganglia defects of Parkinson disease. Posture is stooped, with flexion of head, arms, hips, and knees. Patients are slow getting started. Steps are short and shuffling, with involuntary hastening (*festination*). Arm swings are decreased, and patients turn around stiffly—"all in one piece." Postural control is poor (*anteropulsion* or *retropulsion*).

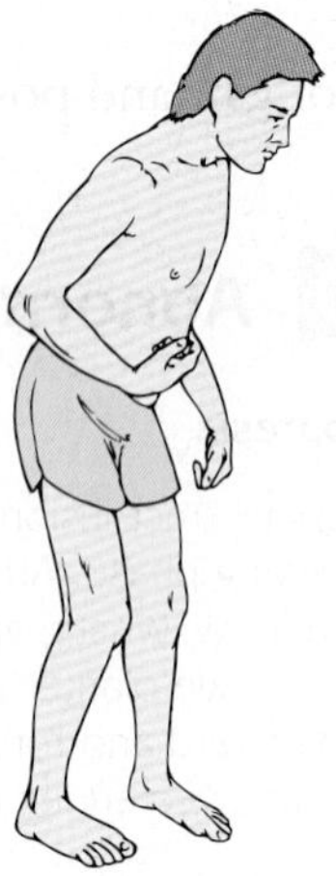

Cerebellar Ataxia

Seen in disease of the cerebellum or associated tracts. Gait is staggering, unsteady, and wide-based with exaggerated difficulty on turns. Patients cannot stand steadily with feet together, whether eyes are open or closed. Other cerebellar signs are present such as dysmetria, nystagmus, and intention tremor.

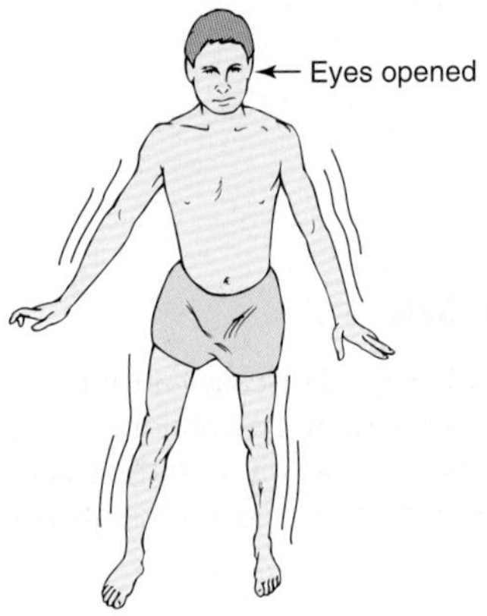

Sensory Ataxia

Seen in loss of position sense in the legs (with polyneuropathy or posterior column damage). Gait is unsteady and wide-based. Patients throw their feet forward and outward and bring them down, first on the heels and then on the toes, with a double tapping sound. They watch the ground for guidance when walking. With eyes closed, they cannot stand steadily with feet together (positive Romberg sign), and the staggering gait worsens.

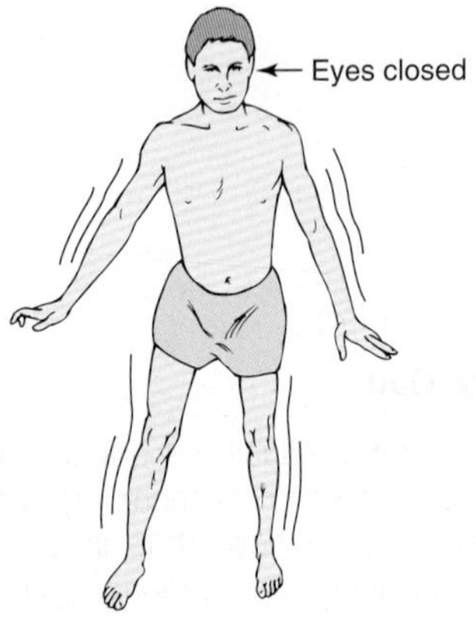

Stance

The following tests can often be performed concurrently. They differ only in the patient's arm position and in what is assessed. In each case, stand close enough to the patient to prevent a fall.

The Romberg Test

The Romberg test is mainly a test of position sense. The patient should first stand with feet together and eyes open and then close both eyes for 30 to 60 seconds without support. The nurse should stand next to the patient without touching them in case of loss of balance, with arms in front and back of the patient. Note the patient's ability to maintain an upright posture. Normally only minimal swaying occurs.

CLINICAL TIP
In ataxia from dorsal column disease and loss of position sense, vision compensates for the sensory loss. The patient stands easily with eyes open but loses balance when they are closed, a *positive Romberg sign.* In *cerebellar ataxia*, the patient has difficulty standing with feet together whether the eyes are open or closed.

Test for Pronator Drift

The patient should stand for 20 to 30 seconds with both arms out straight forward, palms up, and eyes closed. A person who cannot stand may be tested for a pronator drift in the sitting position. In either case, a person with normal functioning can hold this arm position well.

CLINICAL TIP
Pronator drift is the pronation of one forearm. It is both sensitive and specific for a corticospinal tract lesion originating in the contralateral hemisphere. Downward drift of the arm with flexion of fingers and elbow may also occur (Weaver, 2020; Wills, 2016).

Now, instructing the patient to keep the arms up and eyes shut, as shown in Figure 20-21, *tap the arms briskly downward*. The arms normally return smoothly to the horizontal position. This response requires muscular strength, coordination, and a good sense of position.

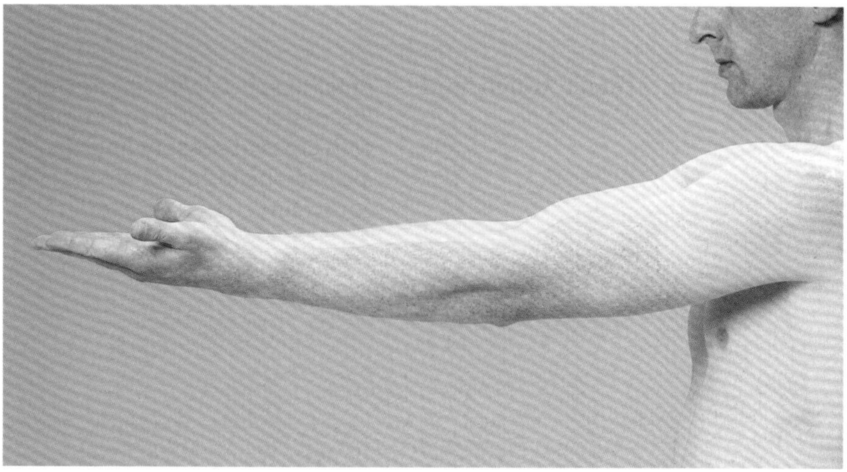

FIGURE 20-21 Negative pronator drift.

In *loss of position sense*, the arms drift sideward or upward (Fig. 20-22), sometimes with writhing movements of the hands; the patient may not recognize the displacement and when asked, corrects it poorly. In *cerebellar incoordination*, the arm returns to its original position but overshoots and bounces.

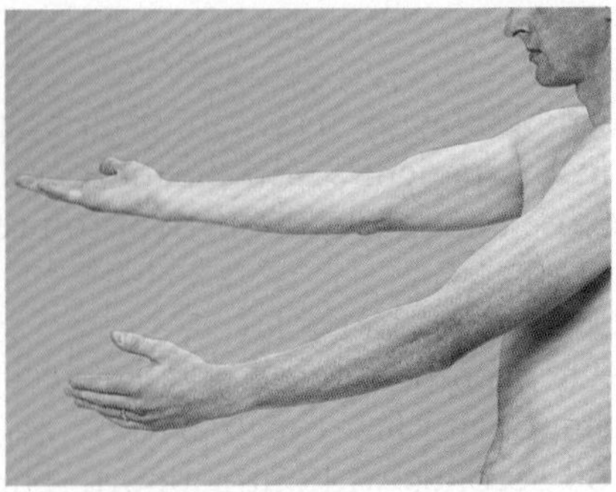

FIGURE 20-22 Positive pronator drift.

The Sensory System

To evaluate the sensory system, you will test several kinds of sensation:

- Pain and temperature (spinothalamic tracts)
- Position and vibration (posterior columns)
- Light touch (both spinothalamic and posterior)
- Discriminative sensations, which depend on some of the previously mentioned sensations but also involve the cortex

When abnormal findings are detected, correlate them with motor and reflex activity. See Table 20-11 for CNS and PNS disorders.

Assess the patient carefully as the following questions are considered:

- Is the underlying lesion central or peripheral?
- Is the sensory loss bilateral or unilateral?
- Does it have a pattern suggesting a dermatomal distribution, a polyneuropathy, or a spinal cord syndrome?
- Is there a loss of pain and temperature sensation? Intact touch and vibration?

Refer to specialty textbooks for discussion of *spinal cord syndromes* with crossed sensory findings, both ipsilateral and contralateral to the cord injury.

TABLE 20-11 Disorders of the Central and Peripheral Nervous Systems

Central Nervous System Disorders

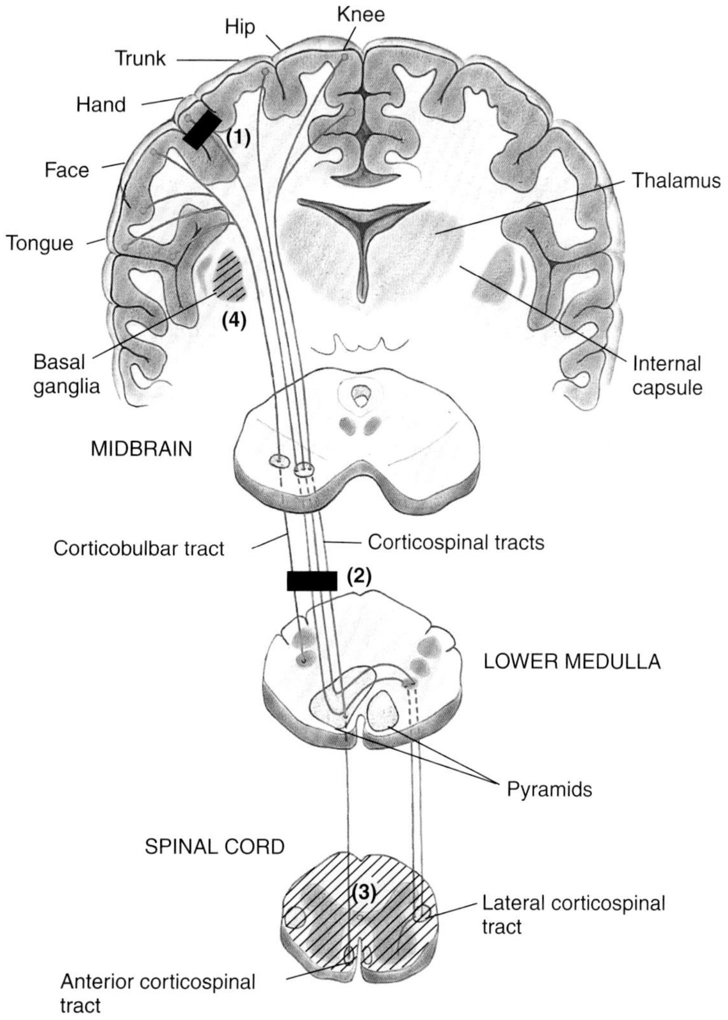

Location of Lesion	Typical Findings: Motor	Typical Findings: Sensory	Typical Findings: Deep Tendon Reflexes	Examples of Cause
Cerebral cortex (1)	Chronic contralateral corticospinal-type weakness and spasticity. Flexion is stronger than extension in the arm, plantar flexion is stronger than dorsiflexion in the foot, and the leg is externally rotated at the hip.	Contralateral sensory loss in the limbs and trunk on the same side as the motor deficits	Increased	Cortical stroke

(continued)

TABLE 20-11 Disorders of the Central and Peripheral Nervous Systems *(Continued)*

	Typical Findings			
Location of Lesion	**Motor**	**Sensory**	**Deep Tendon Reflexes**	**Examples of Cause**
Brainstem (2)	Weakness and spasticity as above, plus cranial nerve deficits such as diplopia (from weakness of the extraocular muscles) and dysarthria	Variable; no typical sensory findings	Increased	Brainstem stroke, acoustic neuroma
Spinal cord (3)	Weakness and spasticity as above, but often affecting both sides (when cord damage is bilateral), causing paraplegia or quadriplegia depending on the level of injury	Dermatomal sensory deficit on the trunk bilaterally at the level of the lesion, and sensory loss from tract damage below the level of the lesion	Increased	Trauma, causing cord compression
Subcortical gray matter: basal ganglia (4)	Slowness of movement (bradykinesia), rigidity, and tremor	Sensation not affected	Normal or decreased	Parkinsonism
Cerebellar (not illustrated)	Hypotonia, ataxia, and other abnormal movements, including nystagmus, dysdiadochokinesis, and dysmetria	Sensation not affected	Normal or decreased	Cerebellar stroke, brain tumor

Peripheral Nervous System Disorders

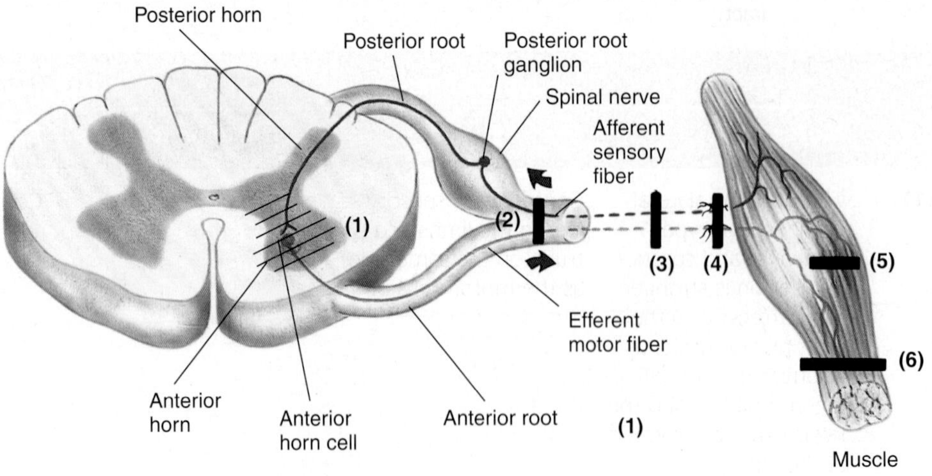

Location of Lesion	Typical Findings: Motor	Typical Findings: Sensory	Typical Findings: Deep Tendon Reflexes/ Muscle Stretch Reflex	Examples of Cause
Anterior horn cell (1)	Weakness and atrophy in a segmental or focal pattern; fasciculations	Weakness and atrophy in a segmental or focal pattern; fasciculations	Decreased	Polio, amyotrophic lateral sclerosis
Spinal roots and nerves (2)	Weakness and atrophy in a root-innervated pattern; sometimes with fasciculations	Weakness and atrophy in a root-innervated pattern; sometimes with fasciculations	Decreased	Herniated cervical or lumbar disc
Peripheral nerve—mononeuropathy (3)	Weakness and atrophy in a peripheral nerve distribution; sometimes with fasciculations	Weakness and atrophy in a peripheral nerve distribution; sometimes with fasciculations	Decreased	Trauma
Peripheral nerve—polyneuropathy (4)	Weakness and atrophy more distal than proximal; sometimes with fasciculations	Weakness and atrophy more distal than proximal; sometimes with fasciculations	Decreased	Peripheral polyneuropathy of alcoholism, diabetes
Neuromuscular junction (5)	Fatigability more than weakness	Fatigability more than weakness	Normal	Myasthenia gravis
Muscle (6)	Weakness usually more proximal than distal; fasciculations rare	Weakness usually more proximal than distal; fasciculations rare	Normal or decreased	Muscular dystrophy

Patterns of Testing

Because sensory testing quickly fatigues many patients and can produce unreliable results, conduct the examination as efficiently as possible. Focus on areas that have numbness or pain, motor or reflex abnormalities suggesting a lesion of the spinal cord or PNS, and trophic changes such as absent or excessive sweating, atrophic skin, or cutaneous ulceration. You will often need to retest at another time to confirm abnormalities.

CLINICAL TIP

Meticulous sensory mapping helps establish the level of a spinal cord lesion and to determine whether a more peripheral lesion is in a nerve root, a major peripheral nerve, or one of its branches.

The patterns of testing listed in Box 20-4 help you identify sensory deficits accurately and efficiently.

BOX 20-4 TIPS FOR DETECTING SENSORY DEFICITS

- *Compare symmetric areas* on the two sides of the body, including the arms, legs, and trunk.

CLINICAL TIP
Hemisensory loss pattern suggests a lesion in the contralateral cerebral hemisphere; a *sensory level* (when one or more sensory modalities are reduced below a dermatome on one or both sides) suggests a *spinal cord lesion.*

- For pain, temperature, and touch sensation, *compare the distal to the proximal areas* of the extremities. Scatter the stimuli to sample most of the dermatomes and major peripheral nerves. One suggested pattern is to include:
  - Both shoulders (C4)
  - The inner and outer aspects of the forearms (C6 and T1)
  - The thumbs and little fingers (C6 and C8)
  - Fronts of both thighs (L2)
  - The medial and lateral aspects of both calves (L4 and L5)
  - The little toes (S1)
  - The medial aspect of each buttock (S3)
- For vibration and position sensation, test the fingers and toes first. If these are normal, it is safe to assume that more proximal areas will also be normal.
- *Vary the pace of your testing so* the patient does not merely respond to the repetitive rhythm.
- When you detect an area of sensory loss or hypersensitivity, *map out its boundaries* in detail. Stimulate first at a point of reduced sensation, then in progressive steps until the patient reports a change to normal sensation.

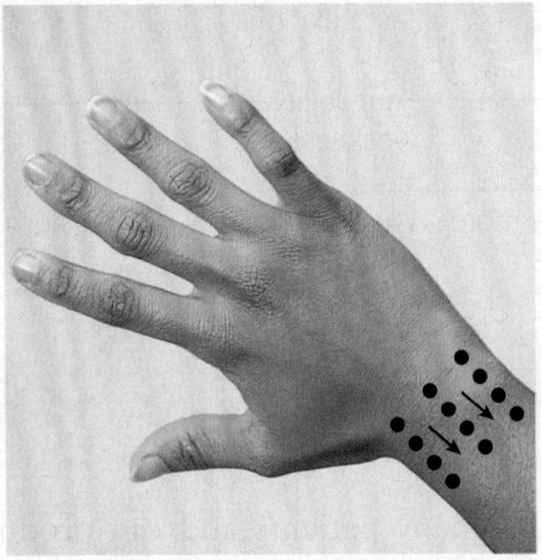

Symmetric distal sensory loss suggests a diabetic *polyneuropathy.* This finding may be missed unless the distal and proximal areas are compared.

In the figure in Box 20-4, all sensation in the hand is lost. Repetitive testing in a proximal direction reveals a gradual return to normal sensation at the wrist. This pattern does not fit either a peripheral nerve damage or dermatomal loss. If bilateral, it suggests the "glove" of the "stocking-glove" sensory loss of a *polyneuropathy,* often seen in *alcoholism and diabetes.*

Before each of the tests in the following sections, show the patient what you plan to do and explain how you would like the patient to respond. The patient's eyes should be closed during actual testing.

Pain

Use a broken tongue blade, cotton swab, or other suitable tool. Occasionally, substitute the blunt end for the point.

Ask the patient, "Is this sharp or is this dull?" When making comparisons, ask "Does this feel the same as this?" by touching the patient. Apply the lightest pressure needed for the stimulus to feel sharp, and do not draw blood.

Analgesia refers to absence of pain sensation, *hypoalgesia* to decreased sensitivity to pain, and *hyperalgesia* to increased sensitivity.

Temperature

Testing is often omitted if pain sensation is normal. If there are sensory deficits, use two test tubes, filled with hot and cold water, or a tuning fork heated or cooled by running water. Have the patient close their eyes and touch the skin. Ask the patient to identify "hot" or "cold."

Light Touch

With a fine wisp of cotton, touch the skin lightly, avoiding pressure. Ask the patient to close their eyes and respond whenever a touch is felt and to compare one area with another. Avoid testing calloused skin, which is normally relatively insensitive.

Anesthesia is absence of touch sensation, *hypesthesia* is decreased sensitivity, and *hyperesthesia* is increased sensitivity.

Vibration

Use a relatively low-pitched tuning fork of 128 Hz. Ask the patient to close their eyes and respond whenever the vibration is felt. Tap it on the heel of your hand, place it firmly over a distal interphalangeal joint of the patient's finger, and test over the interphalangeal joint of the big toe (Fig. 20-23). Ask what the patient feels. If you are uncertain whether it is pressure or vibration, ask the patient to tell you when the vibration stops, and then touch the fork to stop it. If vibration sense is impaired, proceed to more proximal bony prominences (e.g., wrist, elbow, medial malleolus, patella, anterior superior iliac spine, spinous processes, and clavicles).

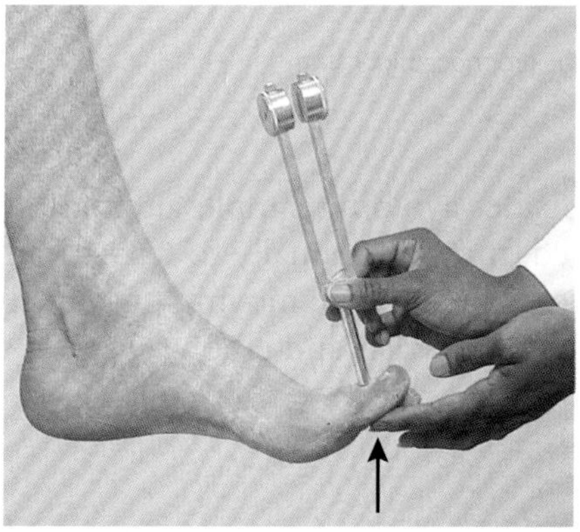

FIGURE 20-23 Testing vibration sense over the big toe.

CLINICAL TIP

Vibration sense is often the first sensation to be lost in a peripheral neuropathy. Common causes include *diabetes* or *alcoholism.* Vibration sense is also lost in posterior column disease, as in *tertiary syphilis* or *vitamin B_{12} deficiency* (Alanazy et al., 2018). Testing vibration sense in the trunk may be useful in estimating the level of a cord lesion.

Proprioception (Joint Position Sense)

Grasp the patient's big toe, holding it by its sides between the thumb and index finger, and then pull it away from the other toes (Fig. 20-24). This prevents extraneous tactile stimuli from affecting testing. Demonstrate "up" and "down" as you move the patient's toe clearly upward and downward. Then, with the patient's eyes closed, ask for a response of "up" or "down" when moving the large toe in a small arc.

Loss of position sense, like loss of vibration sense, occurs in *tabes dorsalis, multiple sclerosis*, or *B_{12} deficiency* from posterior column disease, and in diabetic neuropathy.

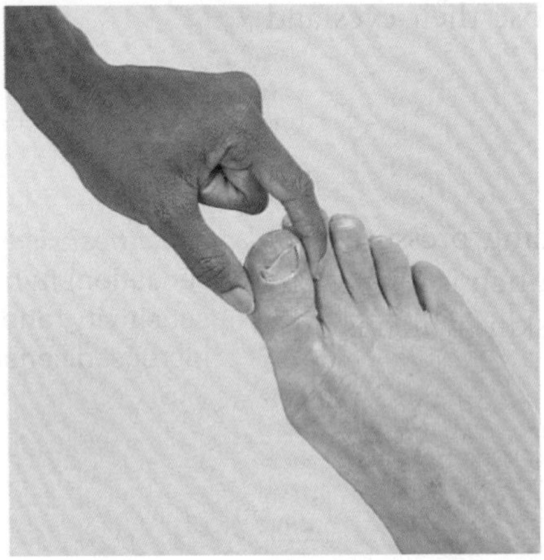

FIGURE 20-24 Testing proprioception with the big toe.

Repeat the test several times on each side, avoiding simple alternation of the stimuli. If position sense is impaired, move proximally to test the ankle joint. In a similar fashion, test position in the fingers, moving proximally if indicated to the metacarpophalangeal joints, wrist, and elbow.

Discriminative Sensations

Several additional techniques test the ability of the sensory cortex to correlate, analyze, and interpret sensations. Because discriminative sensations depend on touch and position sense, they are useful only when these sensations are either intact or only slightly impaired.

If touch and position sense are normal, decreased or absent discriminative sensation indicates a lesion in the sensory cortex. Stereognosis, number identification, and two-point discrimination are also impaired in posterior column disease.

Screen a patient with stereognosis and proceed to other methods if indicated. The patient's eyes should be closed during all these tests.

- **Stereognosis** refers to the ability to identify an object by feeling it. Place a familiar object such as a coin, paper clip, key, pencil, or cotton ball, in the patient's hand, and ask the patient to tell you what it is. Normally a patient will manipulate it skillfully and identify it correctly within 5 seconds. Asking the patient to distinguish "heads" from "tails" on a coin is a sensitive test of stereognosis.

Astereognosis refers to the inability to recognize objects placed in the hand.

- *Number identification (graphesthesia)*—If arthritis or other conditions prevent the patient from manipulating an object well enough to identify it, test the ability to identify numbers. With the blunt end of a pen or pencil, draw a large number in the patient's palm (Fig. 20-25). A person can generally identify most numbers.

The inability to recognize numbers, or *graphesthesia,* indicates a lesion in the sensory cortex.

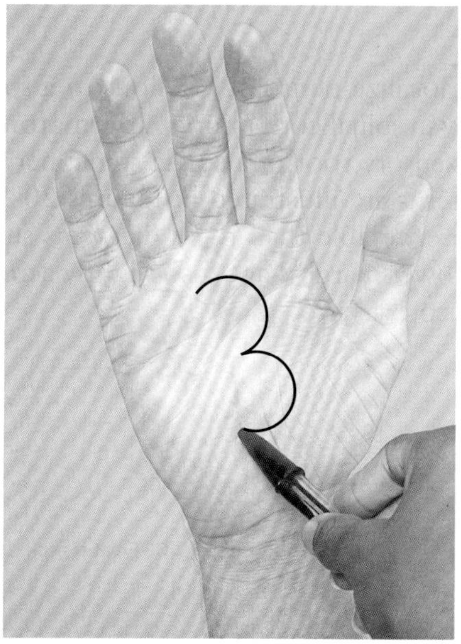

FIGURE 20-25 Testing graphesthesia.

- *Two-point discrimination*—Using the two ends of an opened paper clip, touch a finger pad in two places simultaneously (Fig. 20-26). Alternate the double stimulus irregularly with a one-point touch. Be careful to not cause pain.

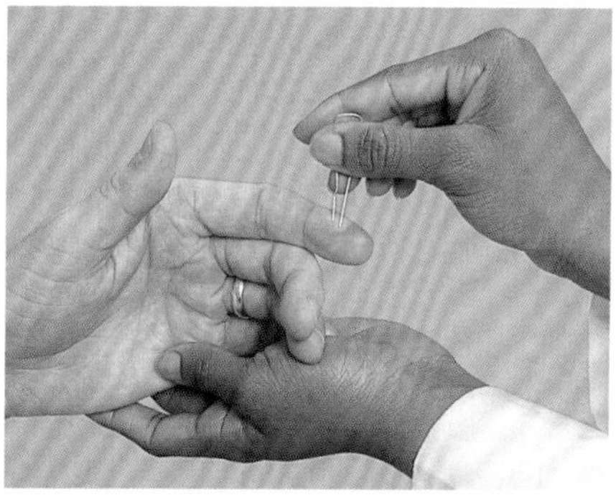

FIGURE 20-26 Testing two-point discrimination.

- Find the minimal distance at which the patient can discriminate one from two points (normally <5 mm on the finger pads). This test may be used on other parts of the body, but normal distances vary widely from one body region to another.

Lesions of the sensory cortex increase the distance between two recognizable points.

- *Point localization*—Briefly touch a point on the patient's skin. Then ask the patient to open both eyes and point to the place touched. Generally, a person can do so accurately. This test, together with the test for extinction, is especially useful on the trunk and the legs.

Lesions of the sensory cortex impair the ability to localize points accurately.

- *Extinction*—Simultaneously stimulate corresponding areas on both sides of the body. Ask where the patient feels your touch. Normally both stimuli are felt.

With lesions of the sensory cortex, only one stimulus may be recognized. The stimulus on the side opposite the damaged cortex is extinguished.

Dermatomes

Knowledge of dermatomes helps you localize neurologic lesions to a specific level of the spinal cord, particularly in spinal cord injury. A **dermatome** is the band of skin innervated by the sensory root of a single spinal nerve. Dermatome and peripheral nerve patterns are illustrated in Figures 20-27 and 20-28. Dermatome levels are more variable than these diagrams suggest. They overlap at their upper and lower margins and also slightly across the midline (Kishner et al., 2020; Stecco et al., 2019).

In spinal cord injury, the sensory level may be several segments *lower* than the spinal lesion for reasons that are not well understood. Percussing for the level of vertebral pain may be helpful (Stecco et al., 2019).

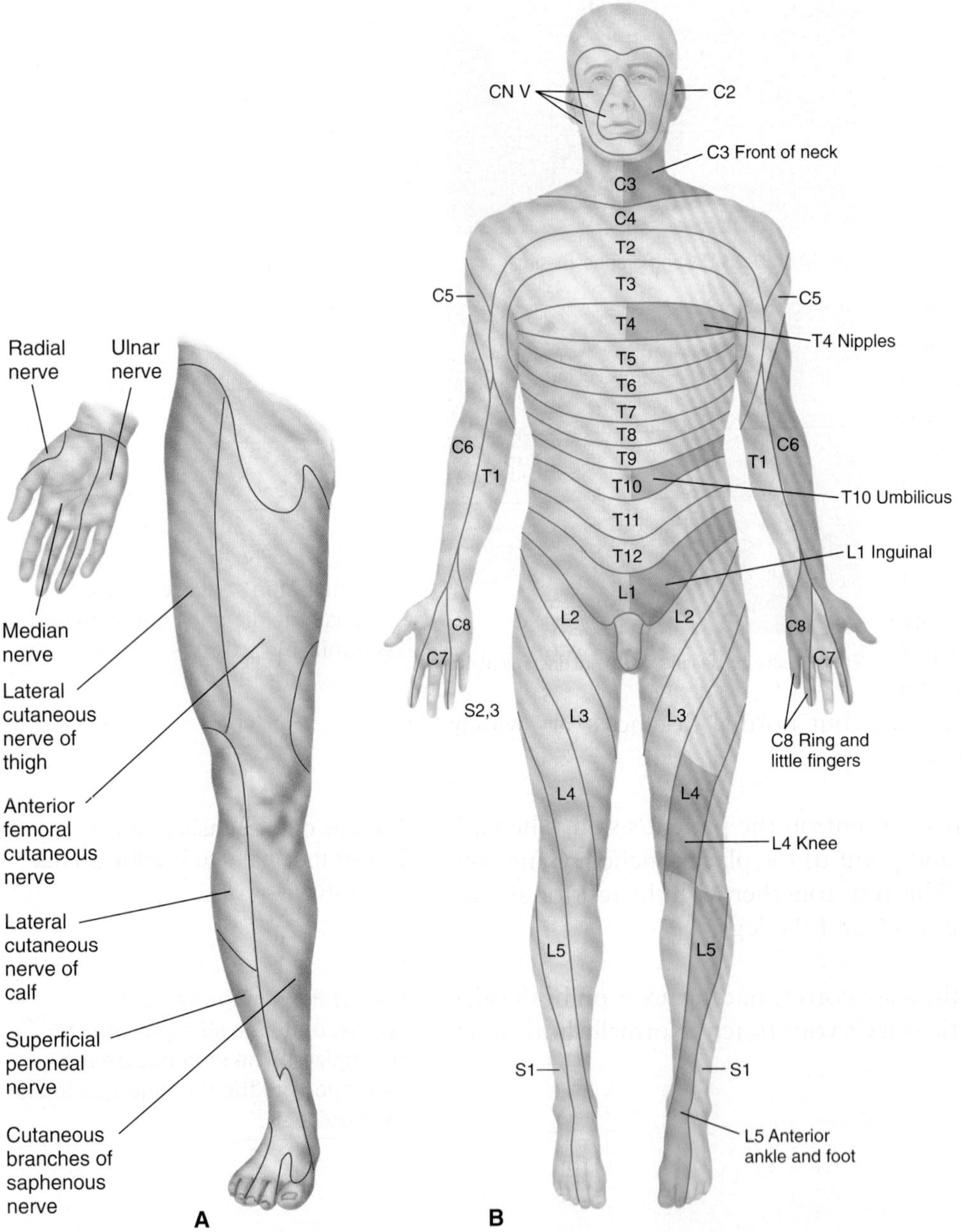

FIGURE 20-27 Anterior view of (**A**) areas innervated by peripheral nerves and (**B**) dermatomes innervated by posterior roots.

Do not try to memorize all the dermatomes. Instead, focus on learning selected dermatomes such as those specifically named in Figures 20-27 and 20-28. The distribution of a few key peripheral nerves is shown Figures 20-27A and 20-28A.

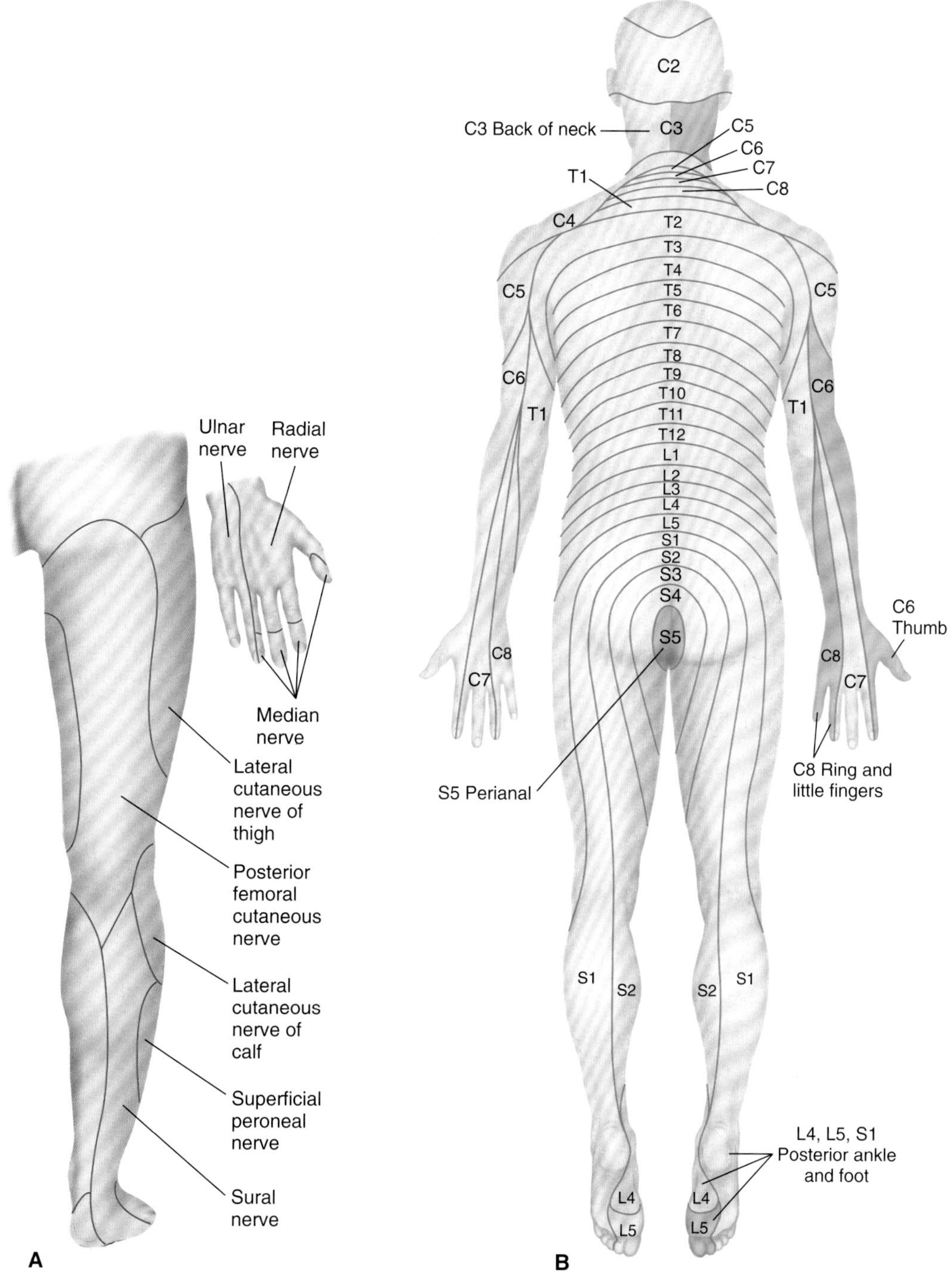

FIGURE 20-28 Posterior view of (**A**) areas innervated by peripheral nerves and (**B**) dermatomes innervated by posterior roots.

Muscle Stretch Reflexes (Deep Tendon Reflexes)

Eliciting *muscle stretch reflexes* requires special handling of the reflex hammer. Select a properly weighted reflex hammer and learn the different uses of the pointed end and the flat end. For example, the pointed end is useful for striking small areas, such as your finger as it overlies the biceps tendon. Test the reflexes as follows:

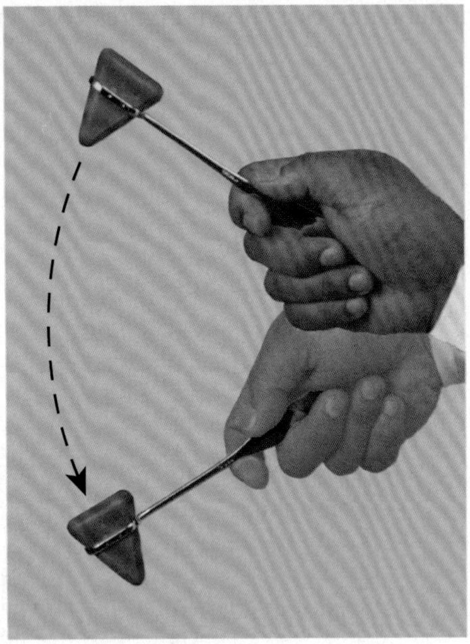

FIGURE 20-29 Use of the reflex hammer.

- Encourage the patient to relax, then position the limbs properly and symmetrically.
- Hold the reflex hammer loosely between your thumb and index finger so that it swings freely in an arc within the limits set by your palm and other fingers (Fig. 20-29).
- With your wrist relaxed, strike the tendon briskly using a rapid wrist movement. Your strike should be quick and direct, not glancing.
- Note the speed, force, and amplitude of the reflex response and grade the response using the scale in Table 20-12. Always compare the response of one side with the other. Reflexes are usually graded on a 0 to 4 scale (Reschechtko & Pruszynski, 2020).

Hyperactive reflexes (hyperreflexia) occur with CNS lesions along the descending corticospinal tract. Look for associated upper motor neuron findings of weakness, spasticity, or a Babinski sign.

TABLE 20-12 Scale for Grading Reflexes

4+	Very brisk, hyperactive, with *clonus* (rhythmic oscillations between flexion and extension)
3+	Brisker than average; possibly but not necessarily indicative of disease
2+	Average; normal
1+	Somewhat diminished; low normal
0	No response

Reflex response depends partly on the force of your stimulus. Use only enough force to provoke a definite response. Differences between sides are usually easier to assess than symmetric changes. Symmetrically increased, diminished, or even absent reflexes can be normal.

Reinforcement

If the patient's reflexes are symmetrically diminished or absent, use *reinforcement*, a technique involving isometric contraction of other muscles for up to 10 seconds that may increase reflex activity (Fig. 20-30). In testing arm reflexes, for example, ask the patient to clench their teeth or to squeeze one thigh with the opposite hand. If leg reflexes are diminished or absent, reinforce them by asking the patient to lock fingers and pull one hand against the other. Tell the patient to pull just before you strike the tendon. Students often find it difficult to elicit the muscle tendon reflexes. Continue to find the location and use a loose grip on the reflex hammer. Although one side (tip or flat) of the hammer may be recommended, trying the other side is an option in addition to reinforcement and distraction techniques.

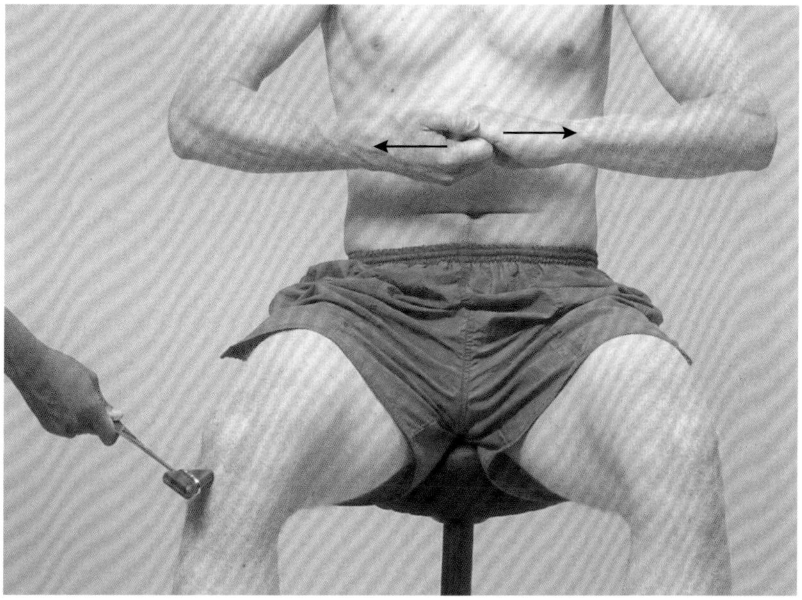

FIGURE 20-30 Using reinforcement to increase reflex activity.

The Biceps Reflex (C5, C6)

The patient's elbow should be partially flexed and the forearm pronated with palm down. Place your thumb or finger firmly on the biceps tendon. Aim the strike with the reflex hammer directly through your digit toward the biceps tendon (Fig. 20-31).

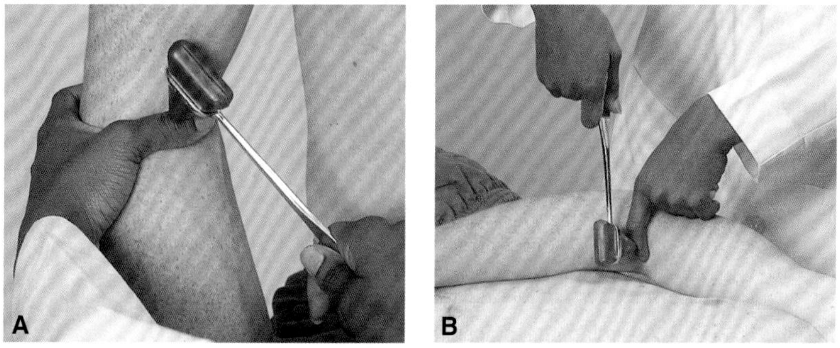

FIGURE 20-31 Assessing the biceps reflex with the patient sitting (**A**) and lying down (**B**).

Observe flexion at the elbow, and watch for and feel the contraction of the biceps muscle.

The Triceps Reflex (C6, C7)

The patient may be sitting or supine for testing the triceps reflex (Fig. 20-32). Flex the patient's arm at the elbow, with palm toward the body, and pull it slightly across the chest. Strike the triceps tendon with a direct blow directly behind and just above the elbow. Watch for contraction of the triceps muscle and extension at the elbow.

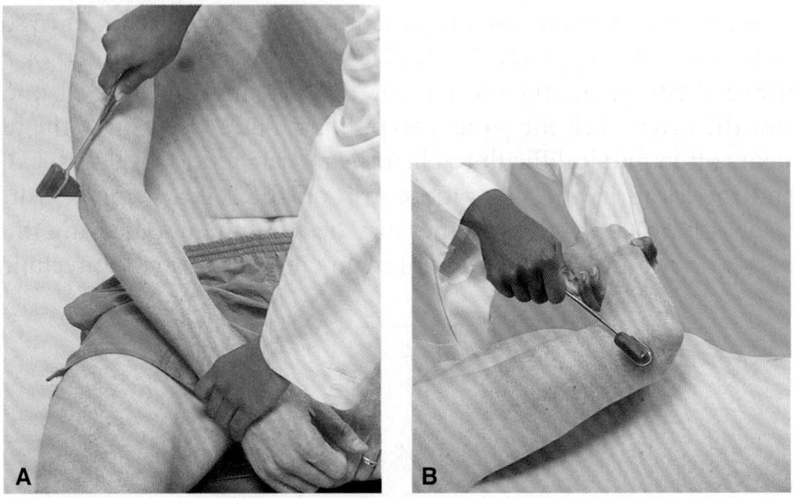

FIGURE 20-32 Assessing the triceps reflex with the patient sitting (**A**) and lying down (**B**).

If you have difficulty getting the patient to relax, try supporting the upper arm (Fig. 20-33). Ask the patient to let the arm go limp, as if it were "hung up to dry." Then strike the triceps tendon.

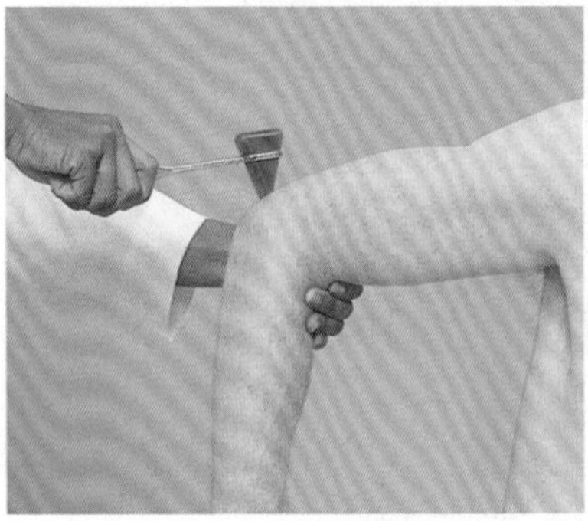

FIGURE 20-33 Assessing the triceps reflex while supporting the upper arm.

The Brachioradialis Reflex (C5, C6)

The patient's hand should rest on the abdomen or the lap with the forearm partly pronated for the brachioradialis reflex test (Fig. 20-34). Strike the radius with the point or flat edge of the reflex hammer, about 1 to 2 in above the wrist. Watch for flexion and supination of the forearm.

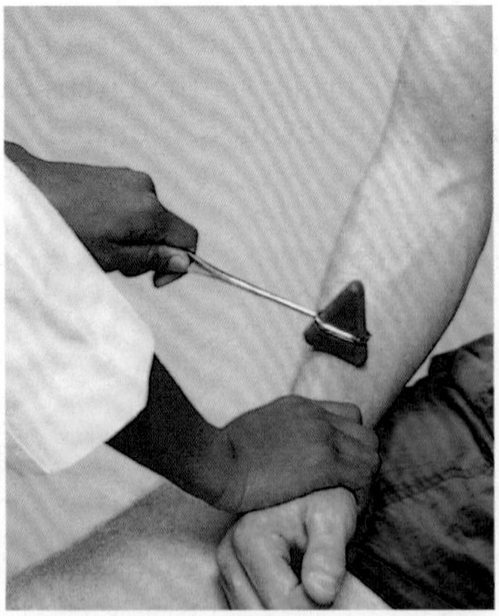

FIGURE 20-34 Assessing the brachioradialis reflex.

The Quadriceps (Patellar) Reflex (L2, L3, L4)

The patient may be either sitting or lying down for the patellar reflex test as long as the knee is flexed. Briskly tap the patellar tendon just below the patella (Fig. 20-35). Note contraction of the quadriceps with extension at the knee. Place your hand on the patient's anterior thigh to feel this reflex.

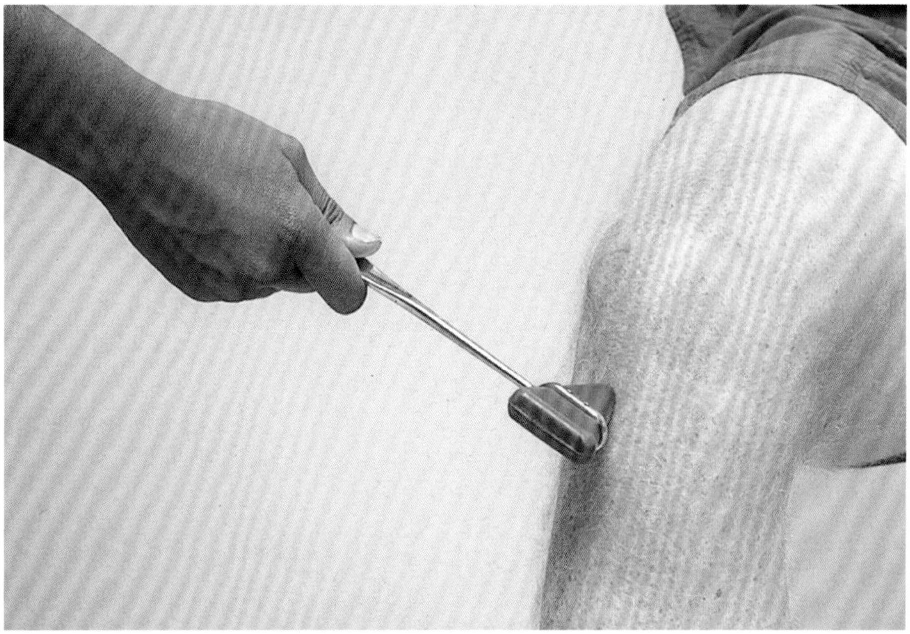

FIGURE 20-35 Assessing the patellar reflex with the patient in a sitting position.

There are two options for examining the supine patient. Supporting both knees at once (Fig. 20-36A) allows you to assess small differences between quadriceps reflexes by repeatedly testing one reflex and then the other. If supporting both legs is uncomfortable for you or the patient, you can place your supporting arm under the patient's leg (Fig. 20-36B). Some patients find it easier to relax with this method.

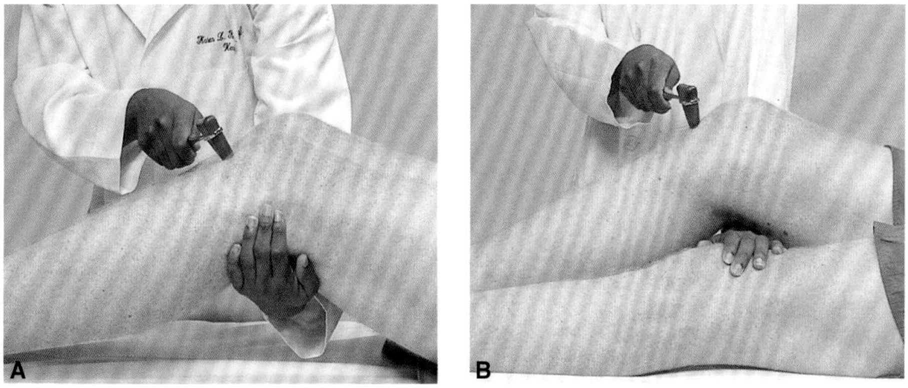

FIGURE 20-36 Assessing the patellar reflex of a supine patient while supporting both knees at once (**A**) or one knee at a time (**B**).

The Achilles (Ankle) Reflex (Primarily S1)

If the patient is sitting, partially dorsiflex the foot at the ankle (Fig. 20-37). Persuade the patient to relax. Strike the Achilles tendon and watch and feel for plantar flexion at the ankle. Also note the speed of relaxation after muscular contraction.

The slowed relaxation phase of reflexes in *hypothyroidism* is often best detected during the ankle reflex.

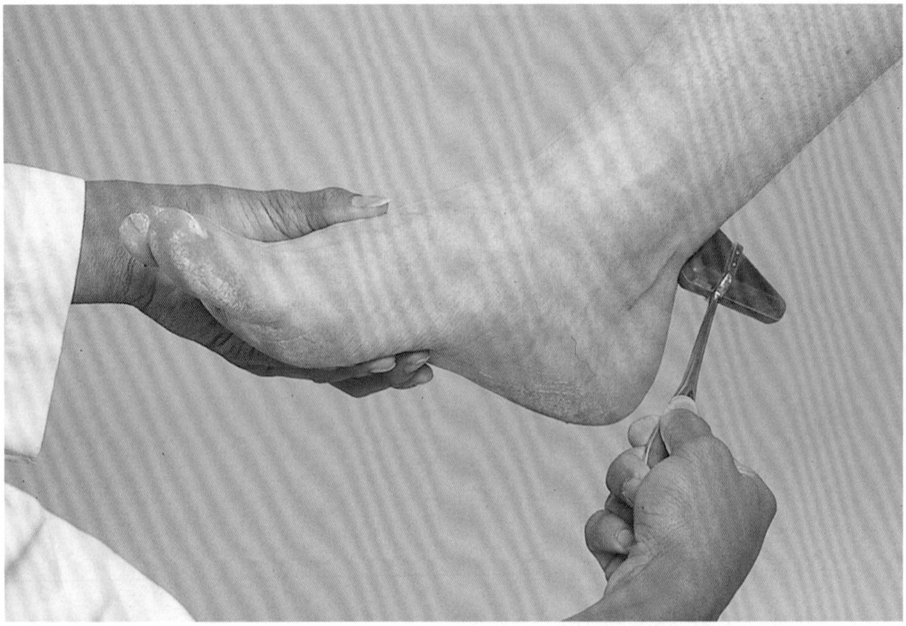

FIGURE 20-37 Testing the Achilles reflex in a sitting patient.

When the patient is lying down, flex one leg at both hip and knee and rotate it externally so that the lower leg rests across the opposite shin (Fig. 20-38). Then dorsiflex the foot at the ankle and strike the Achilles tendon.

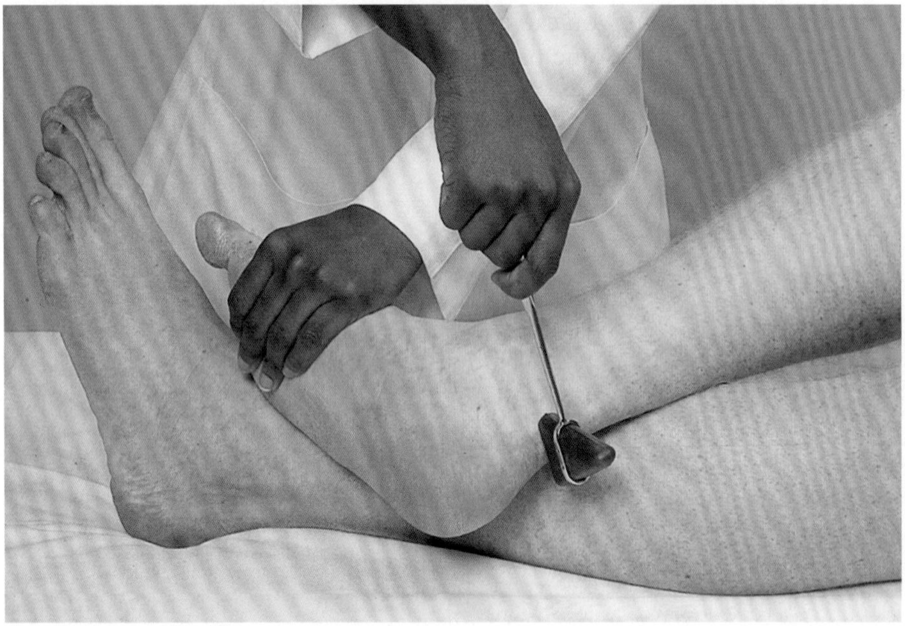

FIGURE 20-38 Testing the Achilles reflex in a patient who is lying down.

These reflex assessments are summarized in Table 20-13.

TABLE 20-13 Deep Tendon Reflex Assessment

Muscle Stretch Reflex	Spinal Cord Location	Assessment	Expectation
Biceps	C5, C6	Elbow is slightly flexed and pronated.	Elbow flexion
		Place your thumb over the tendon, and strike with the tip of the hammer.	Bicep muscle contraction
Triceps	C6, C7	Support the patient's flexed, relaxed arm and strike the tendon (located above elbow joint) with the tip of the hammer.	Contraction of triceps muscle Extension of elbow
Brachioradialis	C5, C6	With arm resting on lap or abdomen and partially pronated, use either end of the hammer to strike the radius ~2 in above the wrist.	Flexion and supination of forearm
Patellar	L2, L3, L4	Flexed knee.	Quadriceps contraction
		Use either side of the hammer to strike the tendon below the patella.	Knee extension
Achilles	S1 mainly	Firmly support the patient's relaxed foot in the dorsiflexion position.	Plantar flexion
		Strike the Achilles tendon.	

Clonus

If the reflexes seem hyperactive, test for ankle **clonus** (rhythmic oscillations). Support the knee in a partly flexed position. With your other hand, dorsiflex and plantar flex the foot a few times while encouraging the patient to relax, and then sharply dorsiflex the foot and maintain it in dorsiflexion (Fig. 20-39). Look and feel for rhythmic oscillations between dorsiflexion and plantar flexion. Normally the ankle does not react to this stimulus. There may be a few clonic beats if the patient is tense or has exercised.

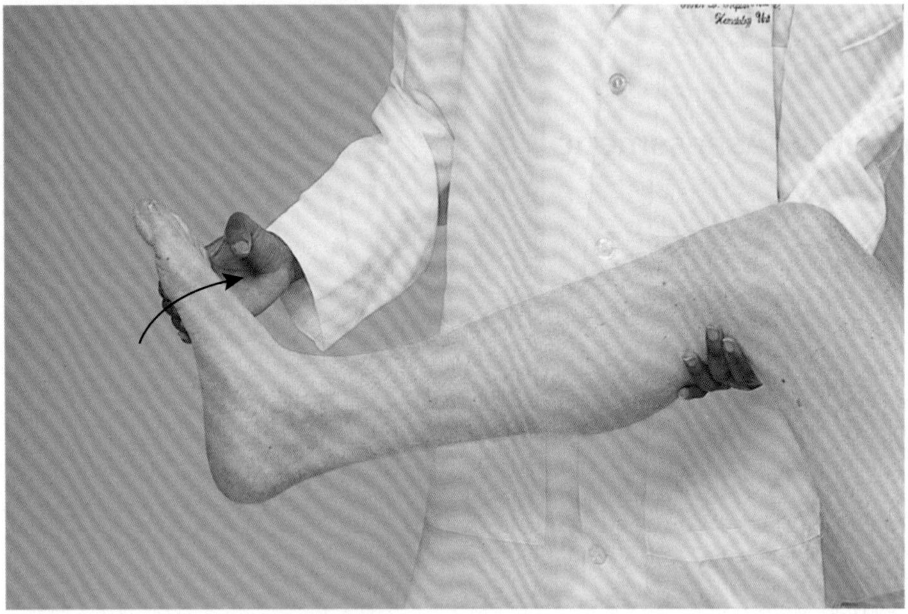

FIGURE 20-39 Assessing for ankle clonus.

CLINICAL TIP

Sustained clonus indicates CNS disease. The ankle plantar flexes and dorsiflexes repetitively and rhythmically. Clonus must be present for a reflex to be graded 4.

Clonus may also be elicited at other joints. A sharp downward displacement of the patella, for example, may elicit patellar clonus in the extended knee (Mirza et al., 2020).

Cutaneous or Superficial Stimulation Reflexes

The Abdominal Reflexes

With the patient lying on their back, test the abdominal reflexes by lightly but briskly stroking each side of the abdomen, above (T8, T9, T10) and below (T10, T11, T12) the umbilicus, in the directions illustrated in Figure 20-40. Use a key, the wooden end of a cotton-tipped applicator, or a tongue blade twisted and split longitudinally. Note the contraction of the abdominal muscles and deviation of the umbilicus toward the stimulus. Obesity may mask an abdominal reflex. In this situation, use your finger to retract the patient's umbilicus away from the side to be stimulated. Feel with your retracting finger for the muscular contraction.

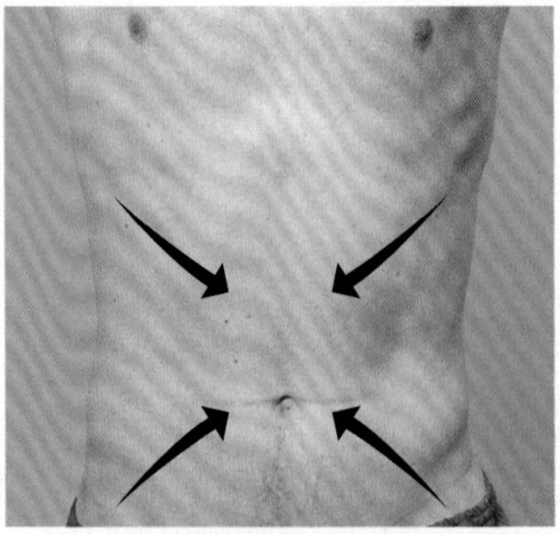

FIGURE 20-40 Direction of strokes for assessing abdominal reflexes.

Abdominal reflexes may be absent in both central and peripheral nerve disorders.

The Plantar Response (L5, S1)

With a key, the wooden end of an applicator stick, or the end of a tongue blade, stroke from the heel moving up toward the small toe to the ball of the foot, curving medially across the ball. Use the lightest stimulus that will provoke a response but increase firmness if necessary. Closely observe movement of the big toe; normally, plantar flexion with the toes curving down and inward is seen (Fig. 20-41A). Dorsiflexion of the big toe and fanning of the other toes are a *"present" Babinski response* (Fig. 20-41B), arising from a CNS lesion affecting the corticospinal tract. The Babinski response can be transiently found in unconscious states from drug or alcohol intoxication and during the postictal period following a seizure.

A Babinski response is either present or not present though often documented as "positive" or "negative."

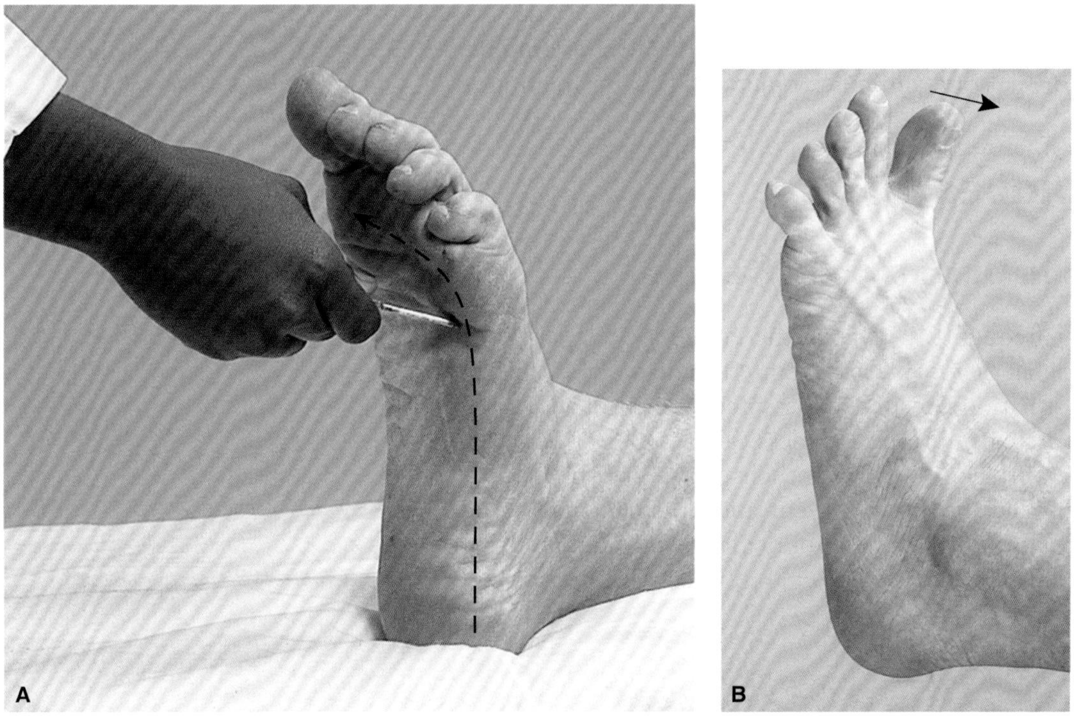

FIGURE 20-41 **A.** An absent/negative Babinski response. **B.** A present/positive Babinski response.

Some patients withdraw from this stimulus by flexing the hip and the knee. Hold the ankle, if necessary, to complete your observation. It is sometimes difficult to distinguish withdrawal from a Babinski response (Qu et al., 2020).

A marked Babinski response is occasionally accompanied by reflex flexion at hip and knee.

Further Examination

As you proceed to the *general physical examination*, include the following assessments. Check for unusual odors.

Consider alcohol, liver failure, or uremia.

- Look for abnormalities of the skin, including color, moisture, evidence of bleeding disorders, needle marks, and other lesions.

Note any jaundice, cyanosis, or the cherry-red color of carbon monoxide poisoning.

- Inspect the scalp and skull for signs of trauma.

Check for bruises, lacerations, or swelling.

- Examine the fundi carefully.

Examine closely for *hypertensive retinopathy* and *papilledema*, an important sign of elevated intracranial pressure.

- Test the corneal reflexes to make sure they are intact. Remember that contact lenses may abolish these reflexes.

Corneal reflex loss occurs in coma and lesions affecting CN V or CN VII.

- Inspect the ears and nose, and examine the mouth and throat.

Blood or cerebrospinal fluid in the nose or the ears suggests a skull fracture; otitis media suggests a possible brain abscess.

- Be sure to evaluate the heart, lungs, and abdomen.

Tongue injury suggests a seizure.

As you complete the neurologic examination, check for facial asymmetry and asymmetries in motor, sensory, and reflex function. Test for meningeal signs if indicated.

Meningeal signs are suspicious for *meningitis or subarachnoid hemorrhage* (Fellner et al., 2020).

SPECIAL TECHNIQUES

Assessment of the Unconscious Patient

The unconscious patient frequently arrives in the emergency department. A history with as much detail as possible is warranted to help determine the cause and extent of the situation. Accurate assessment is critical (Cooksley et al., 2018). **Coma** is a state of unresponsiveness (Table 20-14). The person cannot be aroused and they do not open their eyes even when stimulated. This is a potentially life-threatening event and possible causes are a stroke, brain tumor, intoxication from alcohol or drugs, a traumatic brain injury, or an underlying infection (Cooksley et al., 2018).

TABLE 20-14 Metabolic and Structural Coma

Although there are many causes of coma, most can be classified as either *structural* or *metabolic*. Findings vary widely in individual patients; the features listed are general guidelines rather than strict diagnostic criteria. Remember that psychiatric disorders may mimic coma.

	Toxic-Metabolic	Structural
Pathophysiology	Arousal centers poisoned or critical substrates depleted	Lesion destroys or compresses brainstem arousal areas, either directly or secondary to more distant expanding mass lesions
Clinical Features		
Respiratory patternt	If regular, may be normal or hyperventilation; if irregular, usually Cheyne–Stokes	Irregular, especially Cheyne–Stokes or ataxic breathing; also with selected stereotypical patterns like "apneustic" respiration (peak inspiratory arrest) or central hyperventilation

	Toxic-Metabolic	Structural
Pupillary size and reaction	Equal, reactive to light; if *pinpoint* from opiates or cholinergics, you may need a magnifying glass to see the reaction May be unreactive if *fixed and dilated* from anticholinergics or hypothermia	Unequal or unreactive to light (fixed) *Midposition, fixed*—suggests midbrain compression *Dilated, fixed*—suggests *compression* of CN III from herniation
Level of consciousness	Changes *after* pupils change	Changes *before* pupils change
Possible Causes	Uremia, hyperglycemia, alcohol, drugs, liver failure, hypothyroidism, hypoglycemia, anoxia, ischemia, meningitis, encephalitis, hyperthermia, hypothermia	Epidural, subdural, or intracerebral hemorrhage; cerebral infarct or embolus; tumor, abscess; brainstem infarct, tumor, or hemorrhage; cerebellar infarct, hemorrhage, tumor, or abscess

Prior to taking a history, performing a physical examination, and running laboratory tests, the "ABCDE" steps should be performed: *a*irway, *b*reathing, *c*irculation, *d*isability, and *e*valuation.

Airway, Breathing, and Circulation

First assess and stabilize the ABCs: airway, breathing, and circulation.

Assess the airway by quickly checking the patient's color and pattern of breathing. Inspect the posterior pharynx and listen over the trachea for stridor to make sure the airway is clear. If respirations are slowed or shallow or if the airway is obstructed by secretions, consider intubating the patient as soon as possible while stabilizing the cervical spine.

Assess breathing by observing the rate, rhythm, and pattern of respirations. Because neural structures that govern breathing in the cortex and brainstem overlap those that govern consciousness, abnormalities of respiration often occur in coma.

See Table 20-14, "Metabolic and Structural Coma," and Table 13-5, "Abnormalities in Rate and Rhythm of Breathing."

Assess circulation by checking the remaining vital signs: pulse, blood pressure, and *rectal* temperature. If hypotension or hemorrhage is present, establish intravenous access and begin intravenous fluids. Further emergency management and laboratory studies are beyond the scope of this text.

Level of Consciousness (Disability)

Level of consciousness primarily reflects the patient's capacity for arousal or wakefulness. Testing these targets is at the level of activity that the patient can be aroused to perform in response to escalating stimuli from the examiner.

The Glasgow Coma Scale

The **Glasgow Coma Scale** (GCS) is a standardized tool for objective assessment. GCS is a tool with a numeric value assigned to three different components: eye opening, motor response, and verbal response (Table 20-15). Each area receives a score and all the scores are then added together to determine the level of brain function and assess levels of consciousness (Table 20-16) and coma.

TABLE 20-15 Glasgow Coma Scale

Activity	Response	Scoring	Patient's Score
	Spontaneously: Eyes open, not necessarily aware	4	
Opens eyes	To speech: Nonspecific response, not necessarily to command	3	
	To pain: Pain from sternum/limb/supraorbital pressure	2	
	None: No response, even to supraorbital pressure	1	
	Obeys: Follows simple commands	6	
	Localizes pain: Arm attempts to remove supraorbital/ chest pressure	5	
Motor response	Withdrawal: Arm withdraws to pain, shoulder abducts	4	
	Flexor response: Withdrawal response or assumes hemiplegic posture	3	
	Extension: Shoulder adducted and shoulder and forearm internally rotated	2	
	None: No verbalization of any type	1	
	Oriented: Converses and is oriented	5	
	Confused: Converses but confused, disoriented	4	
Verbal response	Inappropriate: Intelligible, no sustained sentences	3	
	Incomprehensible: Moans/Groans, no speech	2	
	None: No verbalization of any type	1	
			Total (3–15) ________

Interpretation: Patients with scores of 3 to 8 are usually considered to be in a coma.
A score of 15 is a fully alert and functioning person.
A score of 3 is the lowest possible score and denotes "no response" in any of the three areas assessed (Teasdale & Jennett, 1974).

TABLE 20-16 Levels of Consciousness: Arousal Techniques and Patient Responses

Level	Technique	Abnormal Responses
Alertness	Speak to the patient in a normal tone of voice. An alert patient opens the eyes, looks at you, and responds fully and appropriately to stimuli (arousal intact).	None
Lethargy	Speak to the patient in a loud voice. For example, call the patient's name or ask, "How are you?"	A lethargic patient appears drowsy but opens the eyes and looks at you, responds to questions, and then falls asleep.
Obtunded	Shake the patient gently as if awakening a sleeper.	An obtunded patient opens the eyes and looks at you but responds slowly and is somewhat confused. Alertness and interest in the environment are decreased.
Stupor	Apply a painful stimulus. For example, pinch a tendon, rub the sternum, or roll a pencil across a nail bed. (No stronger stimuli necessary.)	A patient in a stupor arouses from sleep only after painful stimuli. Verbal responses are slow or even absent. The patient lapses into an unresponsive state when the stimulus ceases. There is minimal awareness of self or the environment.
Coma	Apply repeated painful stimuli.	A comatose patient remains unarousable with eyes closed. There is no evident response to inner needs or external stimuli.

Evaluation of the Unconscious Patient

Perform the neurologic evaluation. Identify any focal or asymmetric findings to determine possible causes of impaired consciousness. Interview the relatives, friends, or witnesses to establish the speed of onset and duration of unconsciousness. The warning symptoms, precipitating factors, previous episodes, and the prior appearance and behavior of the patient are helpful. Any history of past medical and psychiatric illnesses is also useful.

Pupils

Observe the size and equality of the pupils (Table 20-17) and test their reaction to light. The presence or absence of the light reaction is one of the most important signs distinguishing structural from metabolic causes of coma. The light reaction often remains intact in metabolic coma.

Structural lesions from stroke, bleeding, abscess, or tumor mass may lead to asymmetric pupils and loss of light reaction due to pressure on the CNs.

TABLE 20-17 Pupils in Comatose Patients

Pupillary size, equality, and light reactions help in assessing the cause of coma and in determining the region of the brain that is impaired. Remember that unrelated pupillary abnormalities, including miotic drops for glaucoma or mydriatic drops for a better view of the ocular fundi, may have preceded the coma.

Small or Pinpoint Pupils

Bilaterally small pupils (1–2.5 mm) suggest (1) damage to the sympathetic pathways in the hypothalamus or (2) metabolic encephalopathy (a diffuse failure of cerebral function that has many causes, including drugs). Light reactions are usually normal.

Pinpoint pupils (<1 mm) suggest (1) a hemorrhage in the pons or (2) the effects of morphine, heroin, or other narcotics. The light reactions may be seen with a magnifying glass.

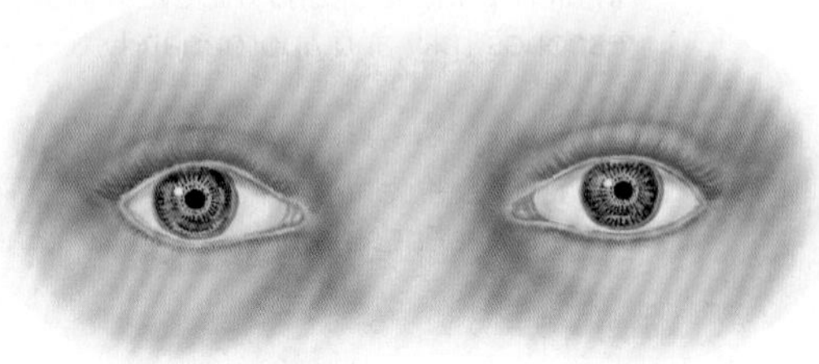

Midposition Fixed Pupils

Pupils that are in the *midposition or slightly dilated* (4–6 mm) and are *fixed to light* suggest structural damage in the midbrain.

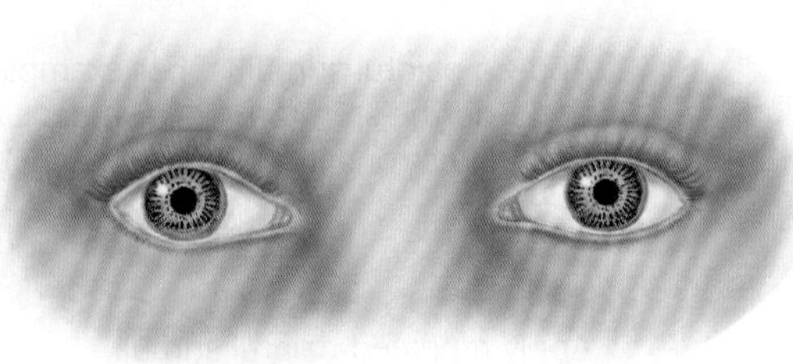

Large Pupils

Bilaterally fixed and dilated pupils may be due to severe anoxia and its sympathomimetic effects, as seen after cardiac arrest. They may also result from atropine-like agents, phenothiazines, or tricyclic antidepressants.

Bilaterally large reactive pupils may be due to cocaine, amphetamine, LSD, or other sympathetic nervous system agonists.

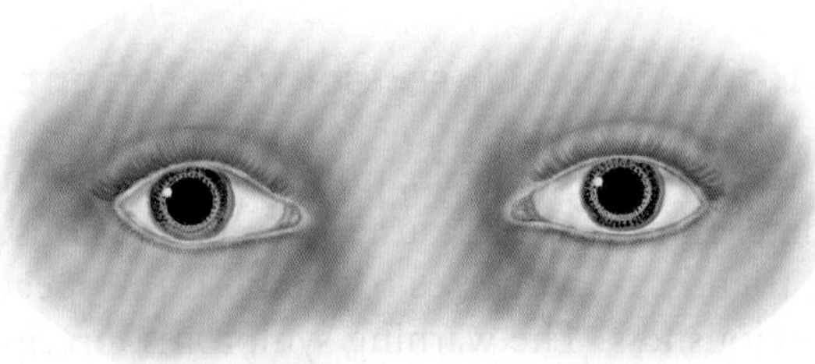

One Large Pupil

A pupil that is *fixed and dilated* warns of herniation of the temporal lobe, causing compression of the oculomotor nerve and midbrain. A single large pupil is commonly seen in diabetic patients with infarction of CN III. Diabetic CN III palsy often spares pupillary function.

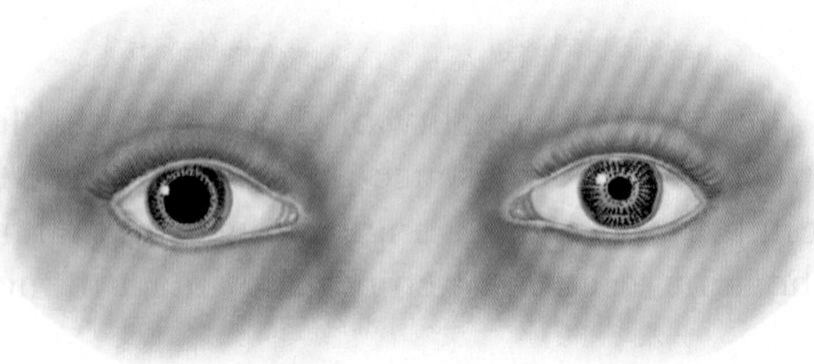

Ocular Movement

Observe the position of the eyes and eyelids at rest. Check for horizontal deviation of the eyes to one side (*gaze preference*). When the oculomotor pathways are intact, the eyes look straight ahead.

CLINICAL TIP
In structural hemispheric lesions, the eyes "look at the lesion" in the affected hemisphere. In irritative lesions from epilepsy or early cerebral hemorrhage, the eyes "look away" from the affected hemisphere.

This reflex helps to assess brainstem function in a comatose patient. Holding open the upper eyelids so that you can see the eyes (Fig. 20-42), turn the head quickly, first to one side and then to the other. Make sure the patient has no neck injury before performing this test.

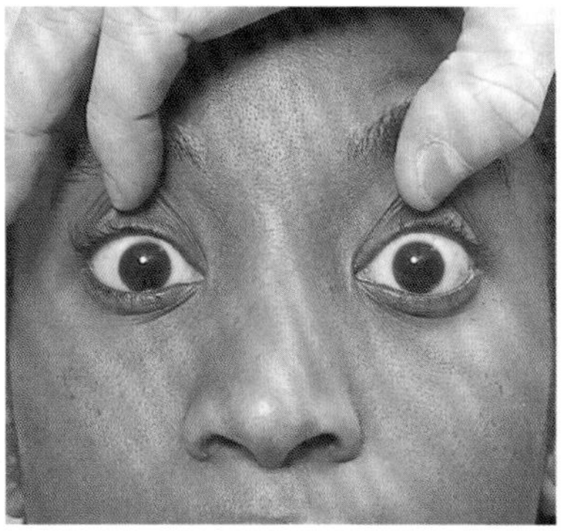

FIGURE 20-42 Holding open the eyelids to assess brainstem function.

In a comatose patient with an intact brainstem, as the head is turned, the eyes move toward the opposite side (the doll's eye movements). In Figure 20-43, for example, the patient's head has been turned to the right; her eyes have moved to the left. Her eyes still seem to gaze at the camera. The doll's eye movements are intact.

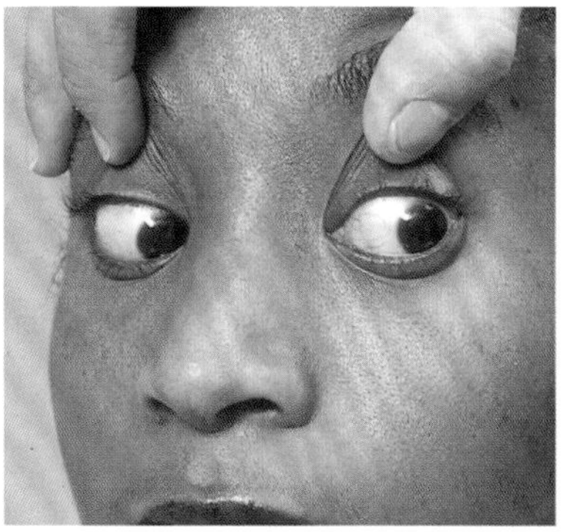

FIGURE 20-43 The doll's eyes movements are intact.

In a comatose patient with absence of doll's eye movements, the ability to move both eyes to one side is lost, suggesting a lesion of the midbrain or pons (Fig. 20-44).

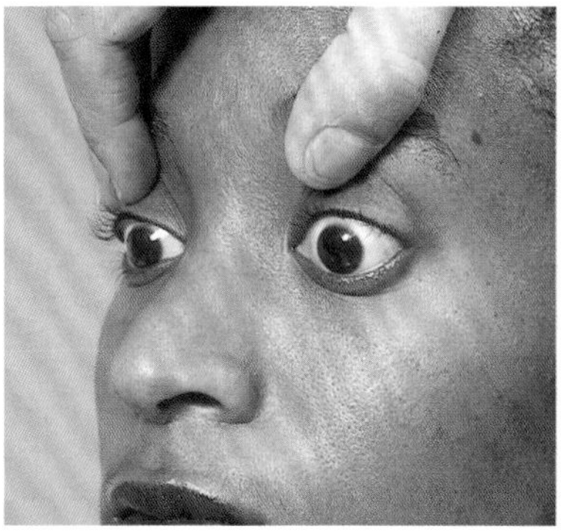

FIGURE 20-44 The doll's eyes movements are absent.

Posture and Muscle Tone

Observe the patient's posture (Table 20-18). If there is no spontaneous movement, you may need to apply a painful stimulus. Classify the resulting pattern of movement as:

- *Normal-avoidant*—the patient pushes the stimulus away or withdraws.
- *Stereotypic*—the stimulus evokes abnormal postural responses of the trunk and extremities.
- *Flaccid paralysis or no response*

TABLE 20-18 Abnormal Postures in Comatose Patients

Decorticate Rigidity (Abnormal Flexor Response)

In *decorticate rigidity*, the upper arms are flexed tight to the sides with elbows, wrists, and fingers flexed. The legs are extended and internally rotated. The feet are plantar flexed. This posture implies a destructive lesion of the corticospinal tracts within or near the cerebral hemispheres. When unilateral, this is the posture of chronic spastic hemiplegia.

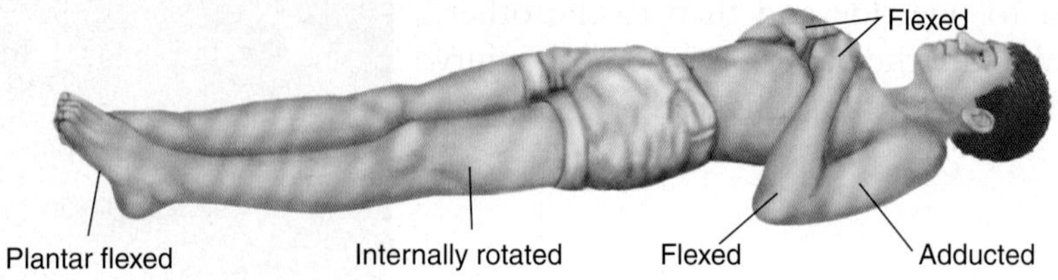

Hemiplegia (Early)

Sudden unilateral brain damage involving the corticospinal tract may produce *hemiplegia* (one-sided paralysis), which early in its course is flaccid. Spasticity will develop later. The paralyzed arm and leg are slack. They fall loosely and without tone when raised and dropped to the bed. Spontaneous movements or responses to noxious stimuli are limited to the opposite side. The leg may lie externally rotated. One side of the lower face may be paralyzed, and that cheek puffs out on expiration. Both eyes may be turned away from the paralyzed side.

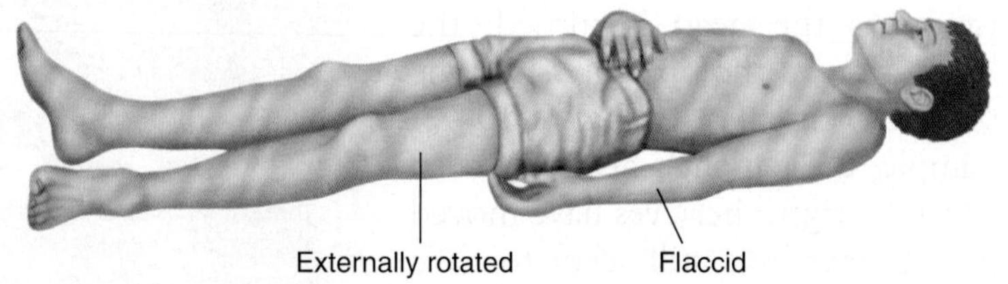

Decerebrate Rigidity (Abnormal Extensor Response)

In *decerebrate rigidity*, the jaws are clenched and the neck is extended. The arms are adducted and stiffly extended at the elbows with forearms pronated and wrists and fingers flexed. The legs are stiffly *extended at the knees* with the feet plantar flexed. This posture may occur spontaneously or only in response to external stimuli such as light, noise, or pain. It is caused by a lesion in the diencephalon, midbrain, or pons, though it may also arise from severe metabolic disorders such as hypoxia or hypoglycemia.

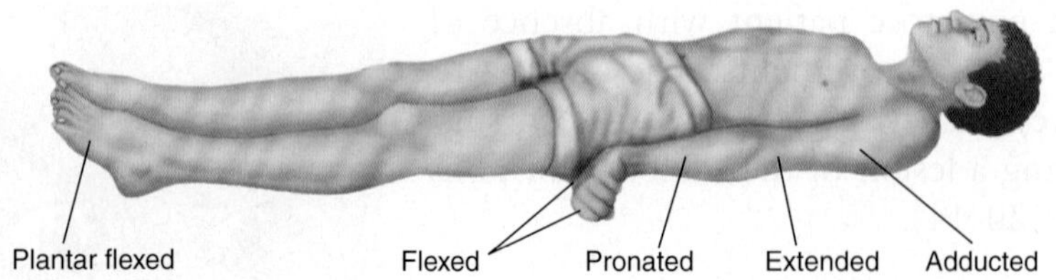

Test muscle tone by grasping each forearm near the wrist and raising it to a vertical position. Note the position of the hand, which is usually only slightly flexed at the wrist (Fig. 20-45).

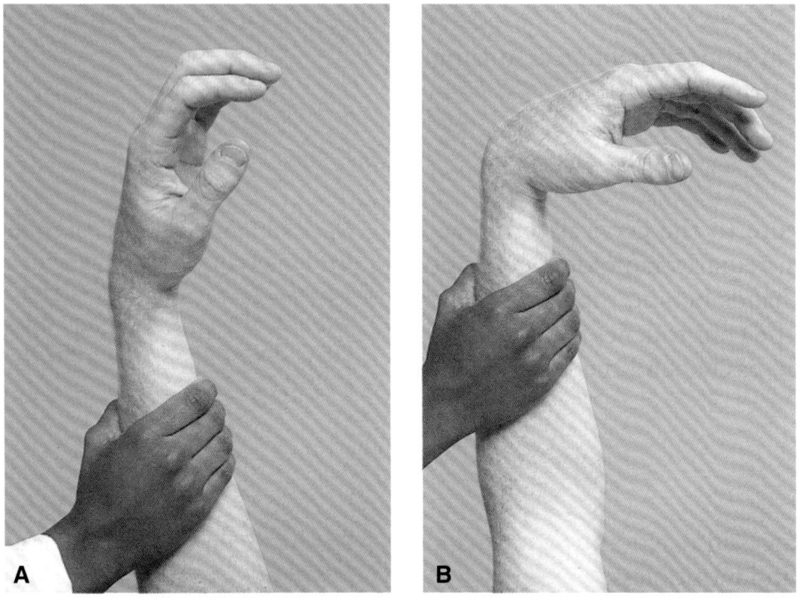

FIGURE 20-45 **A.** Muscle tone with slight flexion of the wrist. **B.** Lack of muscle tone in a flaccid wrist.

CLINICAL TIP

The **hemiplegia** (paralysis of one side of the body) of sudden cerebral accidents is usually flaccid at first. The limp hand drops to form a right angle with the wrist.

Then lower the arm to about 12 or 18 in off the bed and drop it. Watch how it falls. A normal arm drops somewhat slowly.

A flaccid arm drops rapidly like a rock.

Support the patient's flexed knees. Then extend one leg at a time at the knee and let it fall (Fig. 20-46). Compare the speed with which each leg falls.

In *acute hemiplegia*, the flaccid leg falls more rapidly.

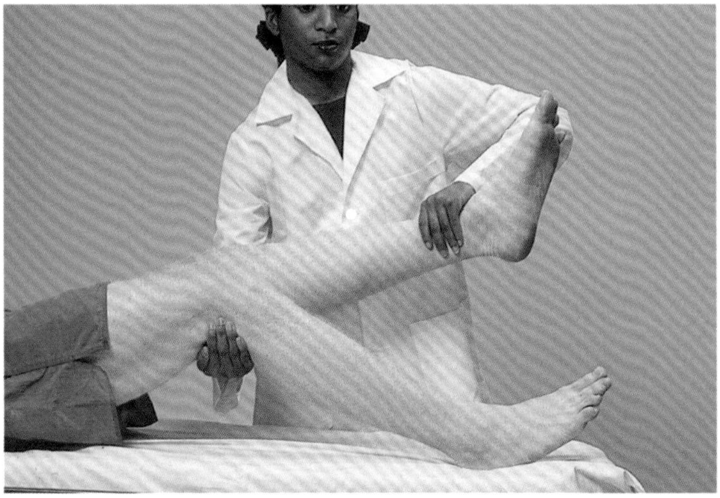

FIGURE 20-46 Assessing muscle tone of the leg.

Flex both legs so that the heels rest on the bed and then release them. The normal leg returns slowly to its original extended position.

In acute hemiplegia, the flaccid leg falls rapidly into extension with external rotation at the hip.

Meningeal Signs

Test for these important signs whenever you suspect meningeal inflammation from meningitis or subarachnoid hemorrhage.

Neck Mobility/Nuchal Rigidity

First make sure there is no injury or fracture to the cervical vertebrae or cervical cord. In trauma settings, this often requires radiologic evaluation. Then, with the patient supine, place your hands behind the patient's head and flex the neck forward if possible until the chin touches the chest. Normally the neck is supple, and the patient can easily bend the head and neck forward.

Neck stiffness and resistance to flexion occurs in patients with *acute bacterial meningitis* and *subarachnoid hemorrhage* (Singer, 2020; Solomon & Manji, 2020).

Brudzinski Sign

As you flex the neck, watch the hips and knees in reaction to your maneuver. Normally they should remain relaxed and motionless.

Flexion of the hips and knees is a *positive Brudzinski sign* and suggests meningeal inflammation (Singer, 2020; Solomon & Manji, 2020).

Kernig Sign

Flex the patient's leg at both the hip and the knee, and then straighten the knee (Fig. 20-47). Discomfort behind the knee during full extension occurs in many healthy people, but this maneuver should not produce pain.

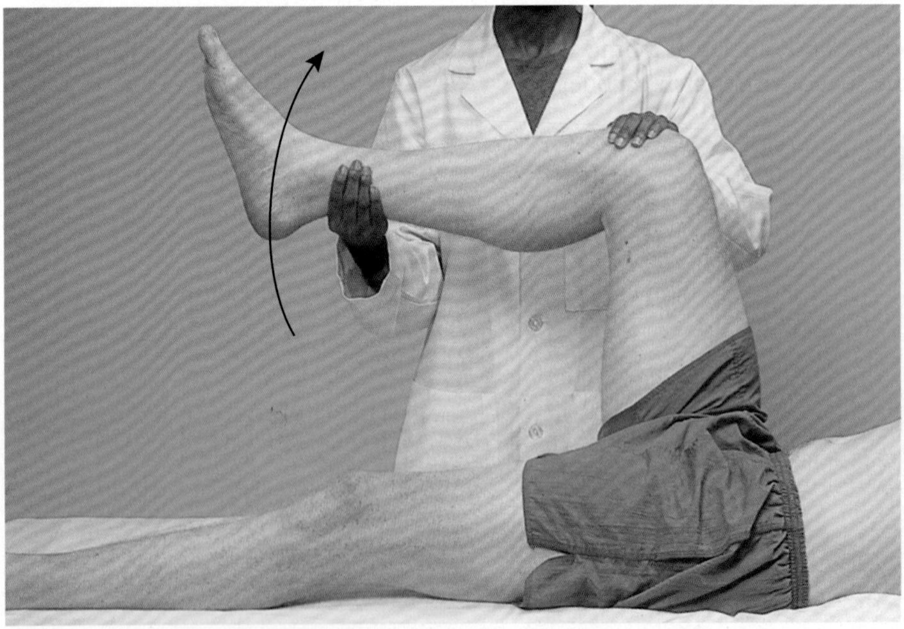

FIGURE 20-47 Assessing for the Kernig sign.

CLINICAL TIP

Pain and increased resistance to extending the knee are *positive Kernig signs.* When bilateral, it suggests meningeal irritation (Singer, 2020; Solomon & Manji, 2020).

Compression of a lumbosacral nerve root may also cause resistance together with pain in the low back and the posterior thigh. Only one leg is usually involved.

During the examination of a comatose patient, remember two cardinal don'ts:

- *Don't* dilate the pupils, the single most important clue to the underlying cause of coma (structural versus metabolic).
- *Don't* flex the neck if there is any question of trauma to the head or neck. Immobilize the cervical spine and get an x-ray first to rule out fractures of the cervical vertebrae that could compress and damage the spinal cord.

Reducing the Risk of Diabetic Peripheral Neuropathy

Diabetes causes several types of **peripheral neuropathy** (damage to the peripheral nerves) (Bentley & Lovell, 2019). Maintaining optimal glycemic control can prevent or delay the onset of neuropathy, particularly from type 1 diabetes.

Distal symmetric sensorimotor polyneuropathy—This is the most common type of diabetic neuropathy. It is slowly progressive, often asymptomatic, and a risk factor for ulcerations, arthropathy, and amputation. Symptomatic patients report burning electrical pain in the lower extremities, usually at night.

Autonomic dysfunction, *mononeuropathies*, and *polyradiculopathies*, including *diabetic amyotrophy*, initially cause unilateral thigh pain and proximal lower extremity weakness.

Patients with diabetes should have their feet examined regularly for neuropathy, including testing pinprick sensation, ankle reflexes, vibration perception (with a 128-Hz tuning fork), and plantar light touch sensation (with a Semmes–Weinstein monofilament), as well as checking for skin breakdown, poor circulation, and musculoskeletal abnormalities (American Diabetes Association, 2015).

The lower extremity amputation prevention (LEAP)/Semmes-Weinstein test detects the loss of protective sensation using a 5.07 monofilament nylon wire with 10 g of force on designated sites on the plantar surface of the feet (Fig. 20-48 and Box 20-5). The test is positive for peripheral neuropathy if the patient cannot feel the monofilament.

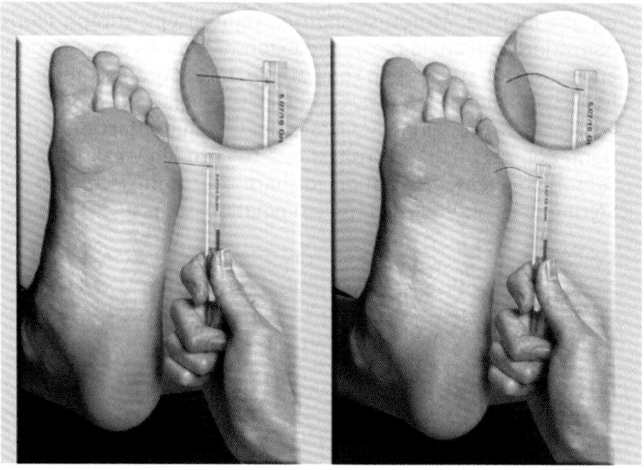

FIGURE 20-48 Assessing for peripheral neuropathy using the LEAP test.

BOX 20-5 STEPS FOR THE MONOFILAMENT (LEAP) EXAMINATION

1. Explain the rationale for the examination.
2. Patient's shoes and socks are removed.
3. Demonstrate what the monofilament feels like on the patient's hand or arm.
4. Ask the patient to respond "yes" each time they feel the pressure of the monofilament.
5. Have the patient close their eyes and hold the monofilament perpendicular to the patient's foot.
6. Press the monofilament until it bends in a "C" shape on the designated areas (the patient should sense the monofilament by the time it bows). See Figure 20-48.
7. Hold the monofilament in place for 1 to 2 seconds. Press so that it buckles one of two times and say "time one" or "time two." The patient identifies which time the foot was touched.
8. Randomize the site sequence.
9. Test both feet on the plantar surface of the distal hallux and third toe, and the first, third, and fifth metatarsal heads. Avoid ulcers, calluses, or corns.

RECORDING YOUR FINDINGS

Note that initially you may use sentences to describe your findings; later you will use phrases. Box 20-6 contains phrases appropriate for most write-ups. Note the five components of the examination and write-up of the nervous system.

BOX 20-6 RECORDING THE NEUROLOGIC EXAMINATION—EXAMPLES

"*Mental Status:* Alert, relaxed, and cooperative. Thought process coherent. O×4 (person, place, time, and situation). Detailed cognitive testing deferred. *Cranial Nerves:* I—not tested; II through XII intact. *Motor:* Good muscle bulk and tone. Strength 5/5 throughout. Cerebellar—Rapid alternating movements (RAMs), finger-to-nose, heel-to-shin intact bilaterally. Gait rhythmic, with smooth alternating arm swing and stable base. Romberg—maintains balance with eyes closed. No pronator drift. *Sensory:* Sharp/dull, light touch, position, and vibration intact bilaterally. *Reflexes* (biceps, triceps, brachioradialis, knee, and ankle): 2+ and symmetric with bilateral plantar responses."

OR

Mental Status: Patient alert and tries to answer questions but has difficulty finding words. *Cranial Nerves:* I—not tested; II—visual acuity intact, visual fields full; III, IV, VI—extraocular movements intact; V motor—temporal and masseter strength intact; VII motor—prominent right facial droop and flattening of right nasolabial fold, left facial movements intact, sensory—taste not tested; VIII—hearing intact bilaterally to whispered voice; IX, X—gag intact; XI—strength of sternomastoid and trapezius muscles 5/5; XII—tongue midline. *Motor:* strength in right biceps, triceps, iliopsoas, gluteals, quadriceps, hamstring, and ankle flexor and extensor muscles 3/5 with good bulk but increased tone and spasticity; strength in comparable muscle groups on the left 5/5 with good bulk and tone. Gait—unable to test. Cerebellar—unable to test on right due to right arm and leg weakness; RAMs, Finger → Nose, Heel → Shin intact on left, unable to perform on the right. Romberg—unable to test due to right leg weakness. Right pronator drift present. *Sensory:* decreased sensation to sharp over right face, arm, and leg; intact on the left. Stereognosis and two-point discrimination not tested. *Reflexes* per table:

	Biceps	Triceps	Brach	Knee	Ankle	Plantar
Right	4+	4+	4+	4+	4+	↑
Left	2+	2+	2+	2+	1+	↓

Suggests left hemispheric cerebrovascular accident in distribution of the left middle cerebral artery with right-sided hemiparesis.

HEALTH PROMOTION AND COUNSELING

Preventing stroke and transient ischemic attacks (TIAs) is a focus of health promotion and counseling during the neurologic assessment.

Strokes are the fourth leading cause of death in the United States and are a leading cause of long-term disability (ninds.nih.gov, 2020). A **stroke** is a sudden neurologic deficit caused by lack of blood circulation to the brain due to either cerebrovascular ischemia (80%) or hemorrhage (ninds.nih.gov, 2020).

- *Hemorrhagic stroke* is bleeding into the brain.
- *Ischemic stroke* is when the blood flow is blocked. Strokes may be silent (asymptomatic) or apparent (symptomatic).

Blockages in ischemic strokes can be caused by a:

- *Thrombus*—A blood clot in the blood vessel in the brain or neck.
- *Embolus*—A blood clot moving from another area of the body (e.g., heart) to the brain.
- *Stenosis*—Narrowing of an artery leading to or in the brain (Aplin & Morphett, 2020; ninds.nih.gov, 2020).

CLINICAL TIP

The American Heart Association/American Stroke Association (AHA/ASA) cites the well-validated *"ABCD2" scoring system* for predicting ischemic stroke within 2, 7, and 90 days after TIA: *a*ge 60 years or over; initial *b*lood pressure 140/90 mm Hg or higher; *c*linical features of focal weakness or impaired speech without focal weakness; *d*uration 10 to 59 minutes or 60 minutes or more; and *d*iabetes (Aplin & Morphett, 2020).

Types of strokes are outlined in Table 20-19.

TABLE 20-19 Types of Stroke

Assessment of stroke requires careful history taking and a detailed physical examination and should focus on three fundamental questions: *What brain area and related vascular territory explain the patient's findings? Is the stroke ischemic or hemorrhagic? If ischemic, is the mechanism thrombus or embolus?* Stroke is a medical emergency, and timing is of the essence. Answers to these questions are critical to patient outcomes and use of antithrombotic therapies in acute ischemic stroke.

In *acute ischemic stroke*, ischemic brain injury begins with a central core of very low perfusion and often irreversible cell death. This core is surrounded by an *ischemic penumbra* of metabolically disturbed cells that are still potentially viable, depending on restoration of blood flow and duration of ischemia. Because most irreversible damage occurs in the first 3–6 h after onset of symptoms, therapies targeted to the 3-h window achieve the best outcomes, with recovery in up to 50% of patients in some studies (www.stroke.org, 2020).

(continued)

TABLE 20-19 Types of Stroke *(Continued)*

Clinical Features and Vascular Territories of Stroke		
Clinical Finding	**Vascular Territory**	**Additional Comments**
Contralateral leg weakness	*Anterior circulation*—anterior cerebral artery (ACA)	Includes stem of circle of Willis connecting internal carotid artery to ACA, and the segment distal to ACA and its anterior choroidal branch
	Anterior circulation—middle cerebral artery (MCA)	Largest vascular bed for stroke
Contralateral face, arm and leg weakness, sensory loss, vision field cut, aphasia	Left MCA	
Apraxia	Right MCA	
Contralateral motor or sensory deficit without cortical signs	*Subcortical circulation*—lenticulostriate deep penetrating branches of MCA	Small vessel subcortical *lacunar infarcts* in internal capsule, thalamus, or brainstem. Four common syndromes: pure motor hemiparesis; pure sensory hemianesthesia; ataxic hemiparesis; clumsy hand-dysarthria syndrome
Contralateral field cut	*Posterior circulation*—posterior cerebral artery (PCA)	Includes paired vertebral and basilar artery, paired posterior cerebral arteries. Bilateral PCA infarction causes cortical blindness but preserves pupillary light reaction
Dysphagia, dysarthria, tongue/palate deviation and/or ataxia with crossed sensory/motor deficits (= ipsilateral face with contralateral body)	*Posterior circulation*—brainstem, vertebral, or basilar artery branches	
Oculomotor deficits and/or ataxia with crossed sensory/motor deficits	*Posterior circulation*—basilar artery	Complete basilar artery occlusion—"locked-in syndrome" with intact consciousness but with inability to speak and quadriplegia

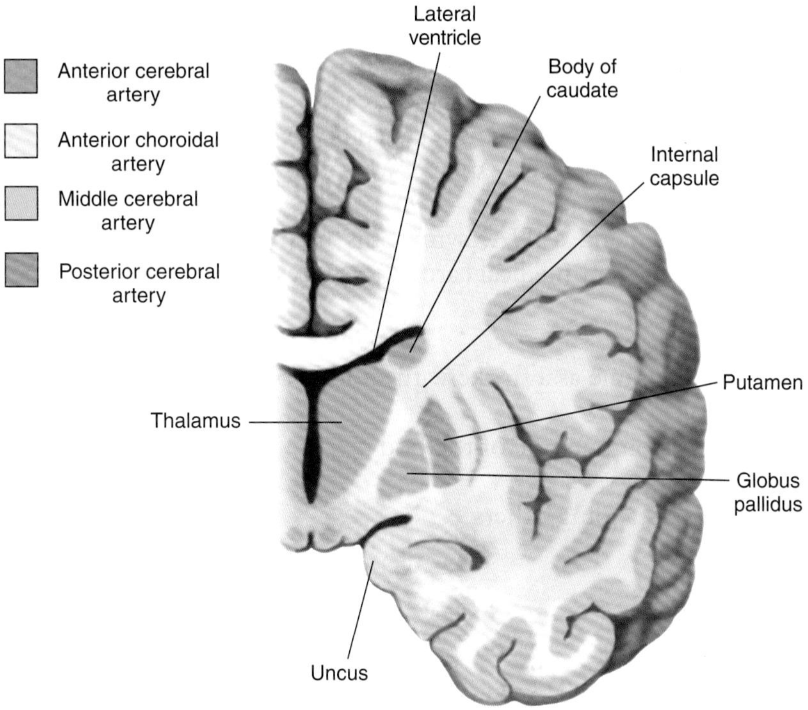

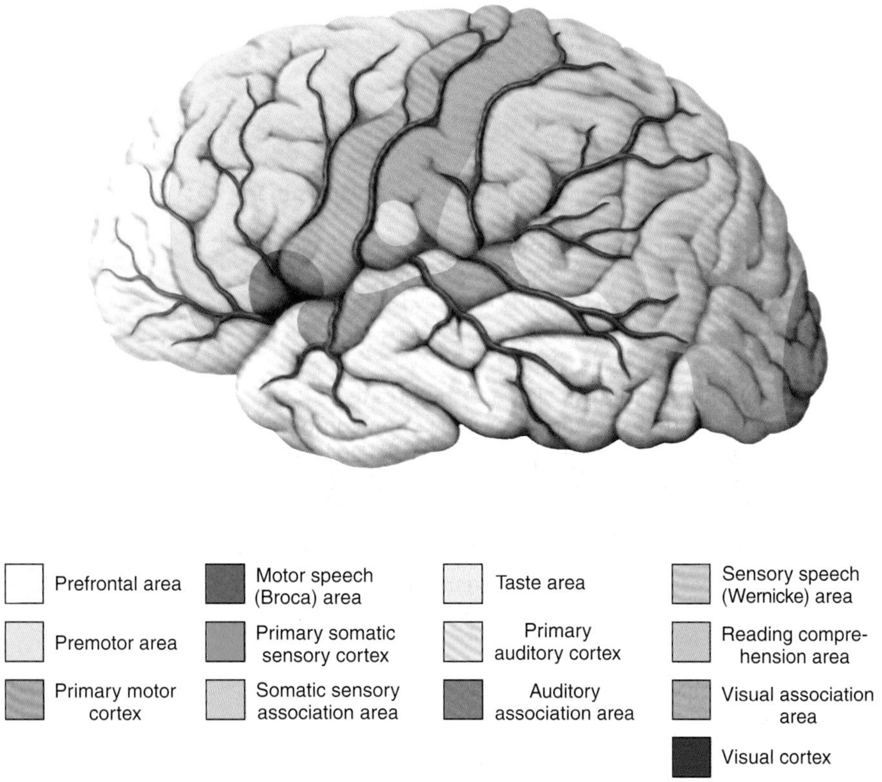

One can differentiate cortical from subcortical involvement. *Subcortical or lacunar syndromes* do not affect higher cognitive function, language, or visual fields.

Data from American College of Physicians. (2012). *Stroke, in neurology. Medical knowledge self-assessment program (MKSAP) 14*. American College of Physicians.

TIAs are a major risk factor for stroke and are sometimes called "mini strokes." The symptoms may last a few minutes or hours before disappearing. These TIAs may be a warning prior to a stroke; TIAs occurs in approximately 12% of all strokes. The 90 days following a TIA present the greatest chance of having a stroke (Aplin & Morphett, 2020), and the risk of a completed stroke following a TIA can be up to 15% in the first week (Aplin & Morphett, 2020).

If a patient thinks they are experiencing a TIA, symptoms may resolve quickly, but it is not safe to assume urgent medical care is not necessary. In fact, they should call 911 right away.

The warning signs for a TIA are the same as a stroke with sudden onset of:

- weakness, numbness, or paralysis on one side of the body.
- slurred speech or difficulty understanding others.
- blindness in one or both eyes.
- dizziness.
- severe headache with no apparent cause.

Key facts for stroke prevention are outlined in Box 20-7.

BOX 20-7 KEY FACTS FOR PREVENTION AND PATIENT EDUCATION

- Stroke affects nearly 800,000 Americans each year, including more than 600,000 suffering a first stroke, and accounts for about one in every 20 deaths.
- The total annual costs associated with stroke are estimated to be about $46 billion.
- Stroke prevalence is twice as high among Black Americans compared to White Americans, and Black Americans have the highest mortality rate due to stroke.

CLINICAL TIP

Cardiovascular causes of death, including stroke, are the greatest contributors to the 5-year disparity in life expectancy for Black men compared to White men and the 4-year racial disparity for women (Hall et al., 2012; Virani et al., 2020). However, the racial gap in life expectancy has recently been declining.

- Death rates due to strokes have decreased among all racial/ethnic groups with the exception of the Hispanic community, which has experienced an increase.
- Of all people admitted to the hospital for strokes, 34% were younger than 65 years.
- Only 51% of the U.S. population is aware of the five stroke warning signs and would call 911 if they thought someone was having a stroke.
- Stroke outcomes improve significantly when thrombolytic therapy is given within 3 to 4.5 hours of symptom onset; however, only a minority of those suffering a stroke reaches an emergency room within this time window.

Source: Virani, S. S., Alonso, A., Benjamin, E. J., Bittencourt, M. S., Callaway, C. W., Carson, A. P., Chamberlain, A. M., Chang, A. R., Cheng, S., Delling, F. N., Djousse, L., Elkind, M., Ferguson, J. F., Fornage, M., Khan, S. S., Kissela, B. M., Knutson, K. L., Kwan, T. W., Lackland, D. T., … Tsao, C. W.; American Heart Association Council on Epidemiology and Prevention Statistics Committee and Stroke Statistics Subcommittee. (2020). Heart disease and stroke statistics—2020 update: A report from the American Heart Association. *Circulation*, *141*(9), e139–e596. https://doi.org/10.1161/CIR.0000000000000757

Symptoms and signs of stroke depend on the vascular territory affected in the brain. The most common cause of ischemic symptoms is occlusion of the *middle cerebral artery*, which causes *visual field cuts* and *contralateral hemiparesis and sensory deficits*. Occlusion of the *left middle cerebral artery* often produces **aphasia (loss of ability to understand or express speech)**; and occlusion of the right middle cerebral artery, *neglect* or *inattention* to the opposite side of the body.

See Table 20-8, "Disorders of Speech," for a discussion of *aphasia*. See also Table 20-19, "Types of Strokes."

Stroke Warning Signs

The AHA and the ASA urge patients to seek immediate care for any of the warning signs. It is important to teach these stroke warning signs and symptoms to your patients; they are listed in Box 20-8.

BOX 20-8 AHA/ASA STROKE WARNING SIGNS AND SYMPTOMS

Use the acronym "FAST" to remember warning signs and symptoms of stroke.

- F: Face drooping—Does one side of the face droop or is it numb? Ask the person to smile. Is the person's smile uneven?
- A: Arm weakness—Is one arm weak or numb? Ask the person to raise both arms. Does one arm drift downward?
- S: Speech difficulty—Is speech slurred? Is the person unable to speak or hard to understand? Ask the person to repeat a simple sentence, like "The sky is blue." Is the sentence repeated correctly?
- T: Time to call 911—If someone shows any of these symptoms, even if the symptoms go away, call 911 and get the person to the hospital immediately. Check the time so you'll know when the first symptoms appeared.

Beyond FAST: Other important symptoms include:

- Sudden numbness or weakness of the leg, arm, or face
- Sudden confusion or trouble understanding
- Sudden trouble seeing in one or both eyes
- Sudden trouble walking, dizziness, loss of balance, or coordination
- Sudden severe headache with no known cause

Source: Centers for Disease Control and Prevention (CDC). (2008). Awareness of stroke warning symptoms–13 States and the District of Columbia, 2005. *MMWR. Morbidity and Mortality Weekly Report*, *57*(18), 481–485; and www.stroke.org. (2020). Stroke symptoms. Retrieved 11 October, 2020, from https://www.stroke.org/en/about-stroke/stroke-symptoms

Stroke Risk Factors—Primary Prevention

Recognizing that stroke and coronary heart disease share common cardiovascular risk factors and threats to health, Healthy People 2030 and the AHA presented a revised concept of cardiovascular health that encompasses seven health behaviors and health factors, and a revised set of combined impact goals for the coming decade: *By 2030, one of the Healthy People 2030 goals is to improve the cardiovascular health of all Americans while reducing deaths from cardiovascular disease and stroke* (HealthyPeople.gov, 2020).

For primary prevention, target documented modifiable risk factors, detailed in Table 20-20. Learn the indications for using aspirin in healthy and individuals with diabetes (HealthyPeople.gov, 2020; www.stroke.org, 2020).

TABLE 20-20 Stroke Risk Factors—Primary Prevention for Ischemic Stroke

Hypertension	Hypertension is the leading determinant of risk for both ischemic and hemorrhagic strokes. Pharmacologic reduction of blood pressure of blood pressure significantly reduces stroke risk, particularly among Black people and older adults (Kernan et al., 2014).
Smoking	Smoking is associated with doubling the risk of ischemic stroke and a two- to fourfold increased risk of subarachnoid hemorrhage. Smoking cessation rapidly reduces the risk of stroke but never to the level of never smokers.
Dyslipidemia	Statin treatment reduces the risk of all strokes.
Diabetes	Stroke risk is doubled with diabetes; 20% of patients with diabetes will die of stroke. Blood pressure control and statin therapy reduce stroke risk in patients with diabetes.
Weight	Obesity doubles the risk of ischemic stroke by 64%.
Diet and nutrition	Dietary factors affect stroke risk primarily by elevating blood pressure. Decreasing salt and saturated fat intake and diets emphasizing fruits, vegetables, nuts, and low-fat dairy products may reduce stroke risk.
Physical inactivity	Moderate exercise, like brisk walking for 150 min a week or 30 min on most days, improves cardiovascular health.
Alcohol use	Alcohol use has a direct dose-dependent effect on the risk of hemorrhagic stroke. Heavy alcohol use increases the risk for all types of stroke due to effects on hypertension, hypercoagulable states, cardiac arrhythmias, and reduced cerebral blood flow.
Disease-Specific Risk Factors	
Atrial fibrillation	Valvular (rheumatic) and nonvalvular atrial fibrillation increases risk of stroke between two- to sevenfold and 17-fold, respectively, compared to the general population. Antiplatelet agents and anticoagulants can reduce the risk for ischemic stroke. When considering antithrombotic therapy, experts recommend individual risk stratification into high-, moderate-, and low-risk groups to balance risk of stroke against risk of bleeding. "$CHADS_2$" is a commonly used scoring system based on *c*ongestive heart failure, *h*ypertension, *a*ge 75 y or older, *d*iabetes, and prior stroke/TIA. The CHA_2DS_2-VASc, which adds an age category of 65–74 y, female sex, and vascular disease to the scoring system, improves risk stratification for individuals estimated as low or moderate risk with $CHADS_2$ (Kernan et al., 2014).
Carotid artery disease	The estimated prevalence of clinically important carotid artery stenosis in the U.S. population over age 65 is 1%. Medical therapy, including statins, antiplatelet agents, treatment of diabetes and hypertension, and smoking cessation, has reduced the risk of stroke in individuals with asymptomatic carotid artery stenosis to less than 2% annually. Experts recommend carotid endarterectomy for selected asymptomatic patients with carotid artery stenosis >60%—provided that the surgeon and center have very low perioperative risks for stroke and mortality (www.stroke.org, 2020).
Obstructive sleep apnea	Sleep apnea is an independent risk factor for stroke, particularly in men. Stroke risk increases with increasing sleep apnea severity as measured by the number of respiratory events (cessation or air flow reduction) per hour. Sleep apnea is usually treated with continuous positive airway pressure (CPAP), though its effectiveness for reducing stroke risk is unknown.

Source: Denny, M., Ramadan, A., Savitz, S., & Grotta, J. (2019). Ischemic stroke etiology and secondary prevention. *Acute Stroke Care*, 119–152. https://doi.org/10.1017/9781108759823.008; Kernan, W. N., Ovbiagele, B., Black, H. R., Bravata, D. M., Chimowitz, M. I., Ezekowitz, M. D., Fang, M. C., Fisher, M., Furie, K. L., Heck, D. V., Johnston, S. C., Kasner, S. E., Kittner, S. J., Mitchell, P. H., Rich, M. W., Richardson, D., Schwamm, L. H., & Wilson, J. A.; American Heart Association Stroke Council, Council on Cardiovascular and Stroke Nursing, Council on Clinical Cardiology, & Council on Peripheral Vascular Disease. (2014). Guidelines for the prevention of stroke in patients with stroke and transient ischemic attack: A guideline for healthcare professionals from the American Heart Association/American Stroke Association. *Stroke*, *45*(7), 2160–2236. https://doi.org/10.1161/STR.0000000000000024; and www.stroke.org. (2020). Stroke symptoms. Retrieved 11 October, 2020, from https://www.stroke.org/en/about-stroke/stroke-symptoms

Optimal blood pressure control is essential for preventing *hemorrhagic stroke*. Additional risk factors for the most common cause of hemorrhagic stroke—ruptured aneurysms in the circle of Willis—include smoking, alcohol use, oral contraceptives, and family history in a first-degree relative.

TIA and Stroke—Secondary Prevention

For the patient who has already suffered a TIA or stroke, focus on identifying the underlying cause including noncardiac emboli, cardiac emboli, and carotid artery stenosis; reducing cardiovascular risk factors, including inactivity, hyperlipidemia, poorly controlled diabetes or hypertension, smoking, and heavy alcohol consumption; and identifying the most appropriate interventions for secondary prevention, including antiplatelet agents, anticoagulants, and carotid revascularization (www.stroke.org, 2020). Strokes in young adults often have a different set of causes—patent foramen ovale and less commonly, carotid or vertebral/basilar artery dissection, hypercoagulable states, or cocaine and illicit drug use (Aplin & Morphett, 2020).

BIBLIOGRAPHY

CITATIONS

Alanazy, M. H., Alfurayh, N. A., Almweisheer, S. N., Aljafen, B. N., & Muayqil, T. (2018). The conventional tuning fork as a quantitative tool for vibration threshold. *Muscle & Nerve*, *57*(1), 49–53. https://doi.org/10.1002/mus.25680

Alguire, P. C., & American College of Physicians. (2016). Epilepsy syndromes and their diagnosis. In *MKSAP 15 Medical knowledge self-assessment program: Nephrology* (pp. 74). American College of Physicians.

American Diabetes Association (2015). 9. Microvascular complications and foot care. *Diabetes Care*, *38*(Suppl 1), S58–S66. https://doi.org/10.2337/dc15-S012

Aplin, P., & Morphett, M. (2020). Stroke and transient ischaemic attacks. In *Textbook of adult emergency medicine* (5th ed., pp. 356–364). Elsevier.

Bäckström, D., Granåsen, G., Domellöf, M. E., Linder, J., Jakobson Mo, S., Riklund, K., Zetterberg, H., Blennow, K., & Forsgren, L. (2018). Early predictors of mortality in Parkinsonism and Parkinson disease: A population-based study. *Neurology*, *91*(22), e2045–e2056. https://doi.org/10.1212/WNL.0000000000006576

Bentley, P., & Lovell, B. (2019). Endocrinology. *Memorizing Medicine: A Revision Guide*, 313–374. https://doi.org/10.1201/9780429446405-7

Bilal, B., Urfalıoğlu, A., Öksüz, G., Arslan, M., Boran, Ö. F., & Doğaner, A. (2020). Ultrasonographic measurement of the ligamentum flavum at different angles in the lateral tilt position. *Journal of Clinical Monitoring and Computing*, *34*(4), 821–825. https://doi.org/10.1007/s10877-019-00353-5

Blauwendraat, C., Heilbron, K., Vallerga, C. L., Bandres-Ciga, S., von Coelln, R., Pihlstrøm, L., Simón-Sánchez, J., Schulte, C., Sharma, M., Krohn, L., Siitonen, A., Iwaki, H., Leonard, H., Noyce, A. J., Tan, M., Gibbs, J. R., Hernandez, D. G., Scholz, S. W., Jankovic, J., Shulman, L. M., ... Singleton, A. B.; International Parkinson's Disease Genomics Consortium (IPDGC). (2019).Parkinson's disease age at onset genome-wide association study: Defining heritability, genetic loci, and α-synuclein mechanisms. *Movement Disorders*, *34*(6), 866–875. https://doi.org/10.1002/mds.27659

Braffett, B. H., Gubitosi-Klug, R. A., Albers, J. W., Feldman, E. L., Martin, C. L., White, N. H., Orchard, T. J., Lopes-Virella, M., Lachin, J. M., & Pop-Busui, R.; DCCT/EDIC Research Group. (2020). Risk factors for diabetic peripheral neuropathy and cardiovascular autonomic neuropathy in the diabetes control and complications trial/epidemiology of diabetes interventions and Complications (DCCT/EDIC) Study. *Diabetes*, *69*(5), 1000–1010. https://doi.org/10.2337/db19-1046

Centers for Disease Control and Prevention (CDC). (2008). Awareness of stroke warning symptoms–13 States and the District of Columbia, 2005. *MMWR. Morbidity and Mortality Weekly Report*, *57*(18), 481–485.

Chirchiglia, D., Chirchiglia, P., & Marotta, R. (2019). Migraine aura-like headache in occipital lobe brain tumors. *Romanian Journal of Neurology*, *18*(4), 174–176. https://doi.org/10.37897/rjn.2019.4.3

Cooksley, T., Rose, S., & Holland, M. (2018). A systematic approach to the unconscious patient. *Clinical Medicine (London, England)*, *18*(1), 88–92. https://doi.org/10.7861/clinmedicine.18-1-88

Denny, M., Ramadan, A., Savitz, S., & Grotta, J. (2019). Ischemic stroke etiology and secondary prevention. *Acute Stroke Care*, 119–152. https://doi.org/10.1017/9781108759823.008

Dolmans, L. S., Hoes, A. W., Bartelink, M., Koenen, N., Kappelle, L. J., & Rutten, F. H. (2019). Patient delay in TIA: A systematic review. *Journal of Neurology, 266*(5), 1051–1058. https://doi.org/10.1007/s00415-018-8977-6

D'Souza, S. (2015). Aneurysmal subarachnoid hemorrhage. *Journal of Neurosurgical Anesthesiology, 27*(3), 222–240. https://doi.org/10.1097/ANA.0000000000000130

Feldman, E. L., Callaghan, B. C., Pop-Busui, R., Zochodne, D. W., Wright, D. E., Bennett, D. L., Bril, V., Russell, J. W., & Viswanathan, V. (2019). Diabetic neuropathy. *Nature Reviews. Disease Primers, 5*(1), 41. https://doi.org/10.1038/s41572-019-0092-1

Fellner, A., Goldstein, L., Lotan, I., Keret, O., & Steiner, I. (2020). Meningitis without meningeal irritation signs: What are the alerting clinical markers? *Journal of the Neurological Sciences, 410*, 116663. https://doi.org/10.1016/j.jns.2019.116663

Ferreira, K. S., Guilherme, G., Faria, V. R., Borges, L. M., & Uchiyama, A. A. (2017). Women living together have a higher frequency of menstrual migraine. *Headache, 57*(1), 135–142. https://doi.org/10.1111/head.12969

Fisher, R. S., Cross, J. H., D'Souza, C., French, J. A., Haut, S. R., Higurashi, N., Hirsch, E., Jansen, F. E., Lagae, L., Moshé, S. L., Peltola, J., Roulet Perez, E., Scheffer, I. E., Schulze-Bonhage, A., Somerville, E., Sperling, M., Yacubian, E. M., & Zuberi, S. M. (2017). Instruction manual for the ILAE 2017 operational classification of seizure types, *Epilepsia, 58*(4), 531–542. https://doi.org/10.1111/epi.13671

Fuller, M. L., Briceño, C. A., Nelson, C. C., & Bradley, E. A. (2017). Tangent screen perimetry in the evaluation of visual field defects associated with ptosis and dermatochalasis. *PloS one, 12*(3), e0174607. https://doi.org/10.1371/journal.pone.0174607

González-Quintanilla, V., & Pascual, J. (2019). Other primary headaches: An update. *Neurologic Clinics, 37*(4), 871–891. https://doi.org/10.1016/j.ncl.2019.07.010

Hall, M. J., Levant, S., & DeFrances, C. J. (2012). Hospitalization for stroke in U.S. hospitals, 1989–2009. *NCHS Data Brief*, (95), 1–8.

Hankey, G. (2017). Stroke. *The Lancet, 389*(10069), 641–654. https://doi.org/10.1016/s0140-6736(16)30962-x

Headache Classification Committee of the International Headache Society (IHS). (2018). The International Classification of Headache Disorders, 3rd edition. *Cephalalgia, 38*(1), 1–211. https://doi.org/10.1177/0333102417738202

HealthyPeople.gov. (2020). *Healthy People 2030: Heart disease and stroke.* Retrieved 5 June, 2021, from https://health.gov/healthypeople/objectives-and-data/browse-objectives/heart-disease-and-stroke

Hurford, R., Li, L., Lovett, N., Kubiak, M., Kuker, W., & Rothwell, P. M.; Oxford Vascular Study. (2019). Prognostic value of "tissue-based" definitions of TIA and minor stroke: Population-based study. *Neurology, 92*(21), e2455–e2461. https://doi.org/10.1212/WNL.0000000000007531

İdil, H., & Kılıc, T. Y. (2019). Diagnostic yield of neuroimaging in syncope patients without high-risk symptoms indicating neurological syncope. *The American Journal of Emergency Medicine, 37*(2), 228–230. https://doi.org/10.1016/j.ajem.2018.05.033

Iguchi, M., Noguchi, Y., Yamamoto, S., Tanaka, Y., & Tsujimoto, H. (2020). Diagnostic test accuracy of jolt accentuation for headache in acute meningitis in the emergency setting. *The Cochrane Database of Systematic Reviews, 6*(6), CD012824. https://doi.org/10.1002/14651858.CD012824.pub2

Jameson, J., Fauci, A., Kasper, D., Hauser, S., Longo, D., Loscalzo, J., & Harrison, T. (2015). *Harrison's principles of internal medicine.* The McGraw-Hill Education.

Jenkins, E., Webb, D. W., & Regan, M. O. (2019). An eye-opening case aniscoria. *Archives of Disease in Childhood, 104*, A354.

Jordan, A., & Freimer, M. (2018). Recent advances in understanding and managing myasthenia gravis. *F1000Research, 7*, F1000 Faculty Rev-1727. https://doi.org/10.12688/f1000research.15973.1

Kanagalingam, S., & Miller, N. R. (2015). Horner syndrome: Clinical perspectives. *Eye and Brain, 7*, 35–46. https://doi.org/10.2147/EB.S63633

Kernan, W. N., Ovbiagele, B., Black, H. R., Bravata, D. M., Chimowitz, M. I., Ezekowitz, M. D., Fang, M. C., Fisher, M., Furie, K. L., Heck, D. V., Johnston, S. C., Kasner, S. E., Kittner, S. J., Mitchell, P. H., Rich, M. W., Richardson, D., Schwamm, L. H., & Wilson, J. A.; American Heart Association Stroke Council, Council on Cardiovascular and Stroke Nursing, Council on Clinical Cardiology, & Council on Peripheral Vascular Disease. (2014). Guidelines for the prevention of stroke in patients with stroke and transient ischemic attack: A guideline for healthcare professionals from the American Heart Association/American Stroke Association. *Stroke, 45*(7), 2160–2236. https://doi.org/10.1161/STR.0000000000000024

Khanna, C. L., & Holmes, J. M. (2017). Strabismus and binocular diplopia due to advanced glaucomatous visual field loss. *Journal of AAPOS, 21*(4), 263–267. https://doi.org/10.1016/j.jaapos.2017.06.009

Kim, A. S., Sidney, S., Klingman, J. G., & Johnston, S. C. (2012). Practice variation in neuroimaging to evaluate dizziness in the ED. *The American Journal of Emergency Medicine, 30*(5), 665–672. https://doi.org/10.1016/j.ajem.2011.02.038

Kishner, S., McMyne, R., & Comeaux, J. (2020). Dermatomes anatomy. https://emedicine.medscape.com/article/1878388-overview

Kuang, T. M., Zhang, C., Zangwill, L. M., Weinreb, R. N., & Medeiros, F. A. (2015). Estimating lead time gained by optical coherence tomography in detecting glaucoma before development of visual field defects. *Ophthalmology, 122*(10), 2002–2009. https://doi.org/10.1016/j.ophtha.2015.06.015

Kuhlmann, L., Lehnertz, K., Richardson, M. P., Schelter, B., & Zaveri, H. P. (2018). Seizure prediction – ready for a new era. *Nature Reviews. Neurology, 14*(10), 618–630. https://doi.org/10.1038/s41582-018-0055-2

Kwon, K. Y., Ryu, H. S., Lee, H. M., Kim, M. J., Shin, H. W., Park, H. K., You, S., Sung, Y. H., Chung, S. J., & Koh, S. B. (2018). Hand tremor questionnaire: A useful screening tool for differentiating patients with hand tremor between Parkinson's disease and essential tremor. *Journal of Clinical*

Neurology (Seoul, Korea), *14*(3), 381–386. https://doi.org/10.3988/jcn.2018.14.3.381

Lee, V., Ang, L. L., Soon, D., Ong, J., & Loh, V. (2018). The adult patient with headache. *Singapore Medical Journal*, *59*(8), 399–406. https://doi.org/10.11622/smedj.2018094

Lim, A., Singhal, S., Lavallee, P., Amarenco, P., Rothwell, P., Albers, G., Sharma, M., Brown, R. Jr, Ranta, A., Maddula, M., Kleinig, T., Dawson, J., Elkind, M. S. V., Guarino, M., Coutts, S. B., Clissold, B., Ma, H., & Phan, T. (2020). An International report on the adaptations of rapid transient ischaemic attack pathways during the COVID-19 pandemic. *Journal of Stroke and Cerebrovascular Diseases*, *29*(11), 105228. https://doi.org/10.1016/j.jstrokecerebrovasdis.2020.105228

Mantegazza, R., Bernasconi, P., & Cavalcante, P. (2018). Myasthenia gravis. *Current Opinion in Neurology*, *31*(5), 517–525. https://doi.org/10.1097/wco.0000000000000596

Mirza, A. B., Akhbari, M., Lavrador, J. P., & Maratos, E. C. (2020). Atypical cauda equina syndrome with lower limb clonus: A literature review and case report. *World Neurosurgery*, *134*, 507–509. https://doi.org/10.1016/j.wneu.2019.10.198

ninds.nih.gov. (2020). Brain basics: Preventing stroke. Retrieved 11 October, 2020, from https://www.ninds.nih.gov/Disorders/Patient-Caregiver-Education/Preventing-Stroke

Pop-Busui, R., Boulton, A. J., Feldman, E. L., Bril, V., Freeman, R., Malik, R. A., Sosenko, J. M., & Ziegler, D. (2017). Diabetic neuropathy: A position statement by the American Diabetes Association. *Diabetes Care*, *40*(1), 136–154. https://doi.org/10.2337/dc16-2042

Qu, J. F., Chen, Y. K., Luo, G. P., Qiu, D. H., Liu, Y. L., Zhong, H. H., & Wu, Z. Q. (2020). Does the Babinski sign predict functional outcome in acute ischemic stroke? *Brain and Behavior*, *10*(4), e01575. https://doi.org/10.1002/brb3.1575

Rao, D., Fiester, P., Rahmathulla, G., Makary, R., & Tavanaiepour, D. (2020). A case of a facial nerve venous malformation presenting with crocodile tear syndrome. *Surgical Neurology International*, *11*, 3. https://doi.org/10.25259/SNI_570_2019

Reschechtko, S., & Pruszynski, J. A. (2020). Stretch reflexes. *Current Biology: CB*, *30*(18), R1025–R1030. https://doi.org/10.1016/j.cub.2020.07.092

Richie, M. B., & Josephson, S. A. (2015). A practical approach to meningitis and encephalitis. *Seminars Neurology*, *35*(6), 611–620. https://doi.org/10.1055/s-0035-1564686.

Sahraian, S., Beheshtian, E., Haj-Mirzaian, A., Alvin, M. D., & Yousem, D. M. (2019). "Worst Headache of Life" in a Migraineur: Marginal value of emergency department CT scanning. *Journal of the American College of Radiology: JACR*, *16*(5), 683–690. https://doi.org/10.1016/j.jacr.2018.11.014

Shen, W. K., Sheldon, R. S., Benditt, D. G., Cohen, M. I., Forman, D. E., Goldberger, Z. D., Grubb, B. P., Hamdan, M. H., Krahn, A. D., Link, M. S., Olshansky, B., Raj, S. R., Sandhu, R. K., Sorajja, D., Sun, B. C., & Yancy, C. W. (2017). 2017 ACC/AHA/HRS guideline for the evaluation and management of patients with syncope: Executive summary: A report of the American College of Cardiology/American Heart Association Task Force on Clinical Practice Guidelines and the Heart Rhythm Society. *Journal of the American College of Cardiology*, *70*(5), 620–663. https://doi.org/10.1016/j.jacc.2017.03.002

Simonenko, V., Shirokov, E., & Ovchinnikov, Y. (2020). Acute coronary syndrome and transient ischemic attacks: Clinical and therapeutic parallels. *Clinical Medicine (Russian Journal)*, *98*(4), 245–250. https://doi.org/10.30629/0023-2149-2020-98-4-245-250

Singer, A. (2019). Meningitis. In *Textbook of adult emergency medicine* (5th ed., pp. 395–400). Elsevier.

Solomon, T., & Manji, H. (2020). Neurologic diseases. In E. Ryan, D. Hill, T. Solomon, T. Endy, & N. Aronson (Eds.), *Neurologic diseases* (10th ed., pp. 86–98). Elsevier.

Stecco, C., Pirri, C., Fede, C., Fan, C., Giordani, F., Stecco, L., Foti, C., & De Caro, R. (2019). Dermatome and fasciatome. *Clinical anatomy (New York, N.Y.)*, *32*(7), 896–902. https://doi.org/10.1002/ca.23408

Stino, A. M., & Smith, A. G. (2017). Peripheral neuropathy in prediabetes and the metabolic syndrome. *Journal of Diabetes Investigation*, *8*(5), 646–655. https://doi.org/10.1111/jdi.12650

Strawbridge, W. J., & Wallhagen, M. I. (2017). Simple tests compare well with a hand-held audiometer for hearing loss screening in primary care. *Journal of the American Geriatrics Society*, *65*(10), 2282–2284. https://doi.org/10.1111/jgs.15044

Teasdale, G., & Jennett, B. (1974). Assessment of coma and impaired consciousness. A practical scale. *Lancet (London, England)*, *2*(7872), 81–84. https://doi.org/10.1016/s0140-6736(74)91639-0

Toscano, G., Palmerini, F., Ravaglia, S., Ruiz, L., Invernizzi, P., Cuzzoni, M. G., Franciotta, D., Baldanti, F., Daturi, R., Postorino, P., Cavallini, A., & Micieli, G. (2020). Guillain-Barré syndrome associated with SARS-CoV-2. *The New England Journal of Medicine*, *382*(26), 2574–2576. https://doi.org/10.1056/NEJMc2009191

Trenkwalder, C., Allen, R., Högl, B., Paulus, W., & Winkelmann, J. (2016). Restless legs syndrome associated with major diseases: A systematic review and new concept. *Neurology*, *86*(14), 1336–1343. https://doi.org/10.1212/WNL.0000000000002542

Veenstra, P., Kollen, B. J., de Jong, G., Baarveld, F., & van den Berg, J. P. (2016). Nurses improve migraine management in primary care. *Cephalalgia*, *36*(8), 772–778. https://doi.org/10.1177/0333102415612767

Virani, S. S., Alonso, A., Benjamin, E. J., Bittencourt, M. S., Callaway, C. W., Carson, A. P., Chamberlain, A. M., Chang, A. R., Cheng, S., Delling, F. N., Djousse, L., Elkind, M., Ferguson, J. F., Fornage, M., Khan, S. S., Kissela, B. M., Knutson, K. L., Kwan, T. W., Lackland, D. T., ... Tsao, C. W.; American Heart Association Council on Epidemiology and Prevention Statistics Committee and Stroke Statistics Subcommittee. (2020). Heart disease and stroke statistics—2020 update: A report from the American Heart Association. *Circulation*, *141*(9), e139–e596. https://doi.org/10.1161/CIR.0000000000000757

Weaver, D. (2020). Rotator drift: A sign of upper motor neuron leg weakness. *Clinical Neurology and Neurosurgery*,

197, 106084. https://doi.org/10.1016/j.clineuro.2020.106084

Wills, A. (2016). How to perform a basic neurological examination. *Medicine*, *44*(8), 464–468. https://doi.org/10.1016/j.mpmed.2016.05.009

www.stroke.org. (2020). Stroke symptoms. Retrieved 11 October, 2020, from https://www.stroke.org/en/about-stroke/stroke-symptoms

Yu, A., & Kapral, M. (2019). More people are surviving after acute stroke. *BMJ*, l2150. https://doi.org/10.1136/bmj.l2150

21 REPRODUCTIVE SYSTEMS

KEY TERMS

amenorrhea
cryptorchidism
cystocele
dysmenorrhea
dyspareunia
enterocele
hernia
menarche
menopause
menstruation
rectocele

Learning Objectives

The student will:

1. Describe the anatomy and physiology of the female and male reproductive systems.
2. Obtain history of the reproductive system.
3. Discuss developmental, psychosocial, cultural, and environmental factors that affect the reproductive systems.
4. Explain appropriate techniques for examining external reproductive structures.
5. Differentiate between normal and abnormal findings in the reproductive system.
6. Document subjective and objective findings related to the reproductive system using the appropriate terminology.

The reproductive system is intimately intertwined with a person's self-concept. Cultural and religious beliefs and attitudes also influence a person's reproductive knowledge and health care. Lesbian, gay, bisexual, transgender, queer/questioning, intersexual, and/or asexual (LGBTQIA) patients have fewer visits and interactions with providers, underscoring the importance of sensitive care for all patients by all nurses. Although internal pelvic and rectal examinations are not within the role of the generalist nurse, it is important for the nurse to explain the anatomy and physiology of the reproductive systems to patients; interview a patient for a thorough system history; and recognize normal and abnormal external genitalia. This knowledge will allow the nurse to educate patients about their reproductive systems in order to promote optimal health and function; assist with family planning; prevent the spread of sexually transmitted infections (STIs); and promote early recognition of problems for referral to an advanced practice nurse or physician. It is not uncommon for a hospital or clinic patient who has developed a relationship with the nurse to feel more comfortable discussing intimate concerns with the nurse rather than family or the physician. For example, an adolescent may be uncomfortable discussing reproductive function with their parents. This chapter will provide the generalist nurse with the ability to carry out this role. The chapter is organized into the female reproductive system and the male reproductive system for ease of reading.

FEMALE REPRODUCTIVE SYSTEM

ANATOMY AND PHYSIOLOGY

The anatomy of the external female genitalia (Fig. 21-1), or *vulva*, includes the *mons pubis*, a hair-covered fat pad overlying the symphysis pubis; the *labia majora*, rounded folds of adipose tissue; the *labia minora*, thinner pinkish-red folds that extend anteriorly to form the *prepuce*; and the *clitoris*. The *vestibule* is the boat-shaped channel, or fossa, between the labia minora. In its posterior portion lies the vaginal opening, the *introitus*, which in a woman who has never had intercourse may be hidden by the *hymen*. The *perineum* is the tissue between the introitus and the anus.

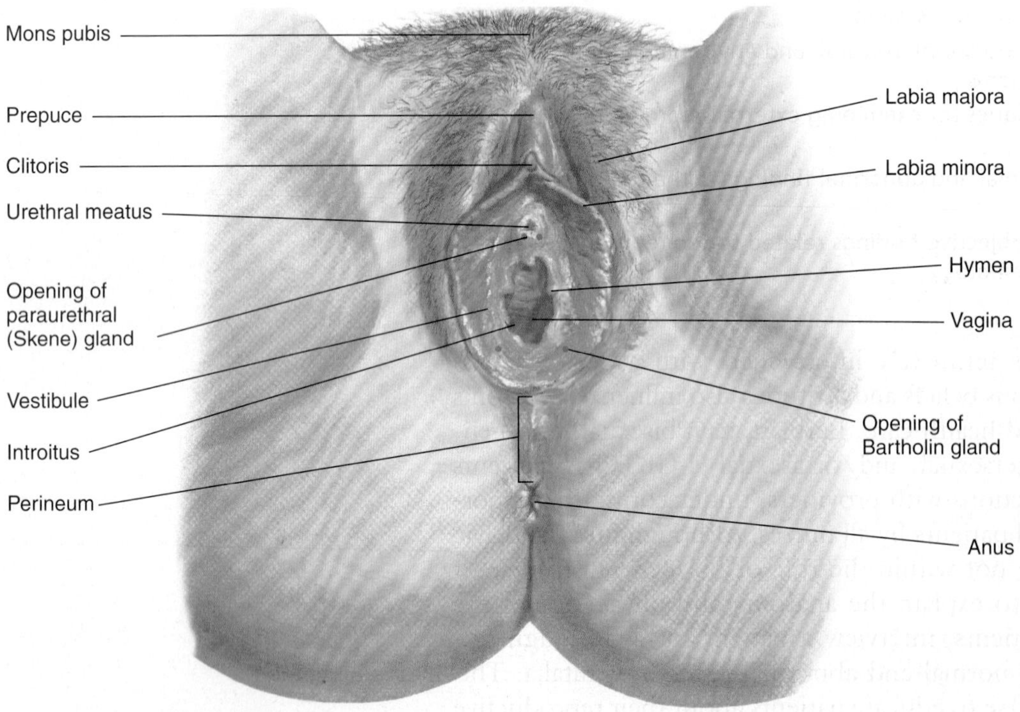

FIGURE 21-1 The external female genitalia.

The *urethral meatus* opens into the vestibule between the clitoris and the vagina. Just posterior to the meatus on either side are the openings of the *paraurethral (Skene) glands.*

The openings of the *Bartholin glands* are located posteriorly on both sides of the vaginal opening but are not usually visible (Fig. 21-2). Bartholin glands themselves are situated more deeply. Both the Skene glands and the Bartholin glands provide lubrication during sexual intercourse.

The *vagina* is a musculomembranous tube extending upward and posteriorly between the urethra and the rectum. The vaginal mucosa lies in transverse folds, or rugae.

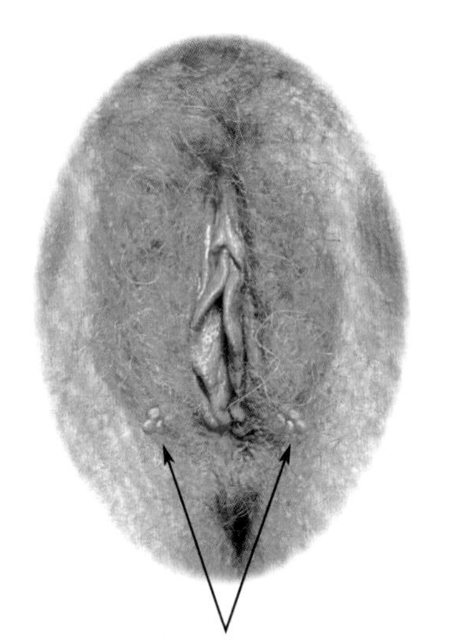

FIGURE 21-2 The locations of the Bartholin glands.

The vagina lies almost at a right angle to the *uterus*, a thick-walled fibromuscular structure shaped like an inverted pear (Fig. 21-3). Its convex upper surface is the uterine *fundus.* The body of the uterus, or *corpus*, and the cylindrical *cervix* inferiorly are joined at the *isthmus.* The uterine walls contain three layers: the *perimetrium*, with its serosal coating from the perineum; the *myometrium* of distensible smooth muscle; and the *endometrium*, the adherent inner coating. The distal cervix protrudes into the vagina, dividing the upper vagina into three recesses, the *anterior*, *posterior*, and *lateral fornices.*

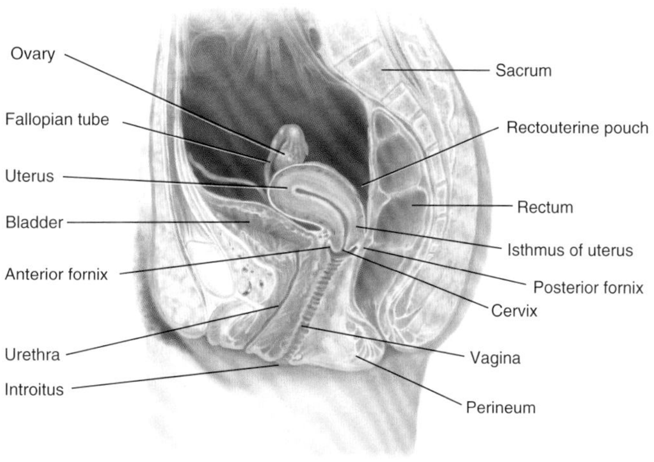

FIGURE 21-3 The internal female genitalia.

The vaginal surface of the cervix, the *ectocervix* (Fig. 21-4), is seen easily with the help of a speculum. At its center is a round, oval, or slitlike depression, the *external os* of the cervix, which marks the opening into the endocervical canal. The ectocervix is covered by the plushy, red *columnar epithelium* that surrounds the os and lines the endocervical canal, and by a shiny pink *squamous epithelium* continuous with the vaginal lining. The *squamocolumnar junction* forms the boundary between these two types of epithelium. The squamocolumnar junction migrates toward the os, creating the *transformation zone.* This is the area at risk for later dysplasia and cancer, which is sampled by the Papanicolaou (Pap) smear.

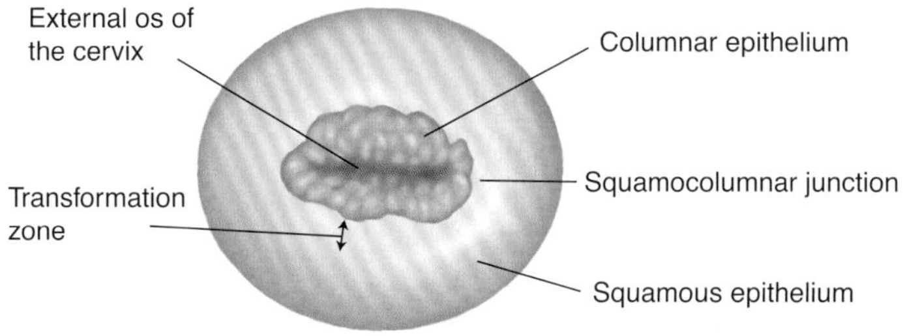

FIGURE 21-4 The cervical epithelia and transformation zone.

A *fallopian tube* with a fan-like tip, the fimbria, extends from the ovary to each side of the uterus and conducts the oocyte from the periovarian peritoneal cavity to the uterine cavity. The two ovaries are almond-shaped glands that vary considerably in size but average approximately 3.5 by 2 by 1.5 cm from adulthood through menopause. The ovaries are palpable on pelvic examination in roughly half of women during the reproductive years. Normally, fallopian tubes are not palpable. The term *adnexa*, a plural Latin word meaning appendages, refers to the ovaries, tubes, and supporting tissues.

The ovaries have two primary functions: the production of oocytes and the secretion of hormones, including estrogen, progesterone, and testosterone. Increased hormonal secretion during puberty stimulates the growth of the uterus and its endometrial lining, enlargement of the vagina, and thickening of the vaginal epithelium and the development of secondary sex characteristics, including the breasts and pubic hair.

The pelvic organs are supported by a sling of tissues composed of muscle, ligaments, and endopelvic fascia, called the *pelvic floor*, which helps support the pelvic organs. The urethra, vagina, and rectum all pass through the pelvic floor. Pelvic floor muscles also aid in sexual function, urinary and fecal continence, and stabilization of connecting joints.

Weakness of the pelvic floor muscles may cause pain, urinary incontinence, fecal incontinence, and prolapse of the pelvic organs that can produce a **cystocele** (protrusion of the bladder into the vagina); **rectocele** (protrusion of the posterior vaginal wall into the rectum); or **enterocele** (protrusion of the small bowel into the vagina). Risk factors are advancing age, prior pelvic surgery or trauma, number of pregnancies and childbirth, medical conditions (e.g., diabetes, multiple sclerosis, Parkinson disease), medications (e.g., anticholinergics, alpha adrenergic blockers), and chronically increased intra-abdominal pressure from chronic obstructive pulmonary disease (COPD), chronic constipation, or obesity (Johnson et al., 2015).

Assessment of sexual maturity in girls, as classified by Tanner, depends not on internal examination, but on the growth of pubic hair and the development of breasts. Tanner stages, or sexual maturity ratings as they relate to pubic hair and breasts, are shown in Chapter 23, "Assessing Children: Infancy through Adolescence."

In most women, pubic hair spreads downward in a triangular pattern, pointing toward the vagina. In 10% of women, it may form an inverted triangle, pointing toward the umbilicus. This growth is usually not completed until the middle 20s or later.

Just before menarche, there is a physiologic increase in vaginal secretions—a normal change that sometimes causes concern in a girl or her mother. As menses become more regular, these increased secretions (*leukorrhea*) coincide with ovulation. They also accompany sexual arousal. These normal kinds of discharges must be differentiated from those of infectious processes.

Lymph from the vulva and lower vagina drains into the inguinal nodes. Lymph from the internal genitalia, including the upper vagina, flows into the pelvic and abdominal lymph nodes, which are not palpable.

THE HEALTH HISTORY

There are three parts to a female reproductive history: menstrual history, obstetric history, and sexual history. It is usually more comfortable for the patient if the nurse begins with the menstrual and obstetric history and saves the sexual history questions for last. However, if the patient comes to you with a sexual problem, it is appropriate to follow their lead with questions relating to the issue.

There are five phases of a female reproductive health: prepuberty (premenstruation); puberty (menarche); childbearing (menstruation); perimenopausal; and menopausal. The nurse must incorporate the needs of each phase into the assessment process as appropriate for the individual.

When a woman reports a problem in the reproductive system, the "OLD CART" mnemonic may be used to elicit a full history of the problem. If no problem is reported, obtain a baseline reproductive history starting with the menstrual history.

Box 21-1 lists common concerns that may arise during health history of the female reproductive system.

BOX 21-1 COMMON CONCERNS

- Menarche, menstruation, menopause, postmenopausal bleeding
- Dysmenorrhea (painful menses)
- Pregnancy
- Contraception
- Vulvovaginal symptoms
- Sexual preference and sexual response
- STIs

Menstrual History

Describe menstrual patterns using the terms in Box 21-2.

Questions about *menarche*, *menstruation*, and *menopause* often provide the nurse an opportunity to explore the patient's concerns and attitudes about the body. When talking with an adolescent, for example, opening questions might include: "How did you first learn about monthly periods? How did you feel when they started?" Many worry when their periods are not regular or come late. "Has anything like that bothered you?" You can explain that girls in the United States usually begin **menstruation** (monthly bleeding) between the ages of 9 and 16 years, and often it takes 1 year or more before menstrual cycles settle into a regular pattern. Age at **menarche** (when menstruation begins) is variable, depending on genetic endowment, socioeconomic status, and nutrition.

BOX 21-2 THE MENSTRUAL HISTORY—HELPFUL DEFINITIONS

1. Menses—monthly flow of bloody fluid from the uterus
   - *Menarche*—Onset of menses
   - *Menopause*—Absence of menses for 12 consecutive months, usually occurring between 48 and 55 years
   - *Perimenopause*—Period of years marking the transition to menopause
   - *Postmenopausal bleeding*—Bleeding occurring 6 months or more after cessation of menses
   - *Amenorrhea*—Absence of menses
   - *Dysmenorrhea*—Pain with menses, often with bearing down, aching, or cramping sensation in the lower abdomen or pelvis
   - *Premenstrual syndrome (PMS)*—A cluster of emotional, behavioral, and physical symptoms occurring 5 days before menses for three consecutive cycles
   - *Abnormal uterine bleeding*—Bleeding between menses or infrequent, excessive, prolonged, or postmenopausal bleeding
2. Frequency—Measured from the first day of one menses to the first day of the next menses. The interval between periods ranges roughly from 24 to 32 days
3. Duration—Number of days the flow lasts, usually 3 to 7 days

For the menstrual history, ask the patient:

- How old were you when your menstrual periods began (age at *menarche*)?
- When did your last period start? If possible, the one before that?

The dates of previous periods can signal possible pregnancy or menstrual irregularities.

- How often do you have periods?
- How long do they last?
- What color is the flow?

Unlike the normal dark red menstrual discharge, excessive flow tends to be bright red and may include "clots" (not true fibrin clots).

- How heavy is the flow?

Flow can be assessed roughly by the number of pads or tampons used daily. Because people vary in their practices for sanitary measures, however, ask the patient whether they usually soak a pad or tampon, spots it lightly, etc. Further, do they use more than one at a time? Do they have any bleeding between periods? Any bleeding after intercourse?

Up to 50% of women report **dysmenorrhea**, or pain with menses. Ask the patient:

- Do you have any discomfort or pain before or during your periods?

- If so, what is it like? How long does it last, and does it interfere with your daily usual activities?
- Are there other associated symptoms?

Dysmenorrhea may be *primary*, without an organic cause, or *secondary*, with an organic cause.

Primary dysmenorrhea results from increased prostaglandin production during the luteal phase of the menstrual cycle when estrogen and progesterone levels decline. Uterine prostaglandin causes the uterus to contract.

CLINICAL TIP
Causes of *secondary dysmenorrhea* include endometriosis, adenomyosis, pelvic inflammatory disease, and endometrial polyps.

PMS includes emotional and behavioral symptoms such as depression, angry outbursts, irritability, anxiety, confusion, crying spells, changes in sexual desire, sleep disturbance, poor concentration, and/or social withdrawal (American College of Obstetricians & Gynecologists, 2015, May). Ask about signs such as bloating and weight gain, swelling of the hands and feet, and generalized aches and pains. Criteria for diagnosis are symptoms and signs in the 5 days prior to menses for at least three consecutive cycles, cessation of symptoms and signs within 4 days after the onset of menses, and interference with daily activities.

Amenorrhea refers to the absence of periods. Failure of periods to initiate is called *primary amenorrhea*, and the cessation of periods after they have been established is termed *secondary amenorrhea*. Pregnancy, lactation, and menopause are physiologic causes of secondary amenorrhea.

CLINICAL TIP
Other causes of *secondary amenorrhea* include low body weight from any cause, including malnutrition, anorexia nervosa, stress, chronic illness, or hypothalamic-pituitary-ovarian dysfunction.

Ask about any abnormal bleeding. The term *abnormal uterine bleeding* encompasses several patterns:

Causes vary by age group and include pregnancy, cervical or vaginal infection, cancer, cervical or endometrial polyps or hyperplasia, fibroids, bleeding disorders, hormonal contraception, or replacement therapy. *Postcoital bleeding* suggests cervical polyps or cancer, or in an older woman, atrophic vaginitis.

- *Polymenorrhea*, or intervals of fewer than 21 days between menses
- *Oligomenorrhea*, or infrequent bleeding
- *Menorrhagia*, or excessive flow
- *Metrorrhagia*, or intermenstrual bleeding
- Postcoital bleeding

Menopause usually occurs between 48 and 55 years of age. It is defined retrospectively as cessation of menses for 12 months, progressing through several stages of erratic cyclical bleeding. These stages of variable cycle length, often with vasomotor symptoms like hot flashes, flushing, and sweating, represent *perimenopause*. The ovaries stop producing estradiol and progesterone, and estrogen levels drop significantly, though some testosterone synthesis persists (North American Menopause Society, 2021). If the patient is *perimenopausal,* ask about such vasomotor symptoms as hot flashes, flushing, and sweating. Sleep disturbances are also common. After menopause, there may be vaginal dryness and **dyspareunia** (painful intercourse); hair loss; and mild hirsutism as the androgen-to-estrogen ratio increases. Urinary symptoms may also occur in the absence of infection because of atrophy of the urethra and urinary trigone.

CLINICAL TIP
Women may ask about many alternative compounds and botanicals for relief of menopause-related symptoms. Many are poorly studied and not proven to be beneficial. Estrogen replacement relieves symptoms but poses other health risks (North American Menopause Society, 2017).

Ask a middle-aged or older woman:

- Have you stopped menstruating? When?
- Did you have any symptoms at that time?
- Have you had any bleeding since?
- How do (did) you feel about not having your period anymore?
- Has it affected your life in any way?
- Have you had any bleeding or spotting since menopause?

CLINICAL TIP
Postmenopausal bleeding may occur in endometrial cancer, hormone replacement therapy, uterine and cervical polyps.

Obstetric History

Pregnancy

Questions relating to pregnancy include:

- Have you ever been pregnant? How many times?
- What years did you give birth (or miscarry)?
- How many living children do you have?

- Did you have any difficulties during pregnancy?
- Have you ever had a miscarriage? An abortion?

CLINICAL TIP
The term *abortion* is used by health care providers to mean either a spontaneous or an induced termination of a pregnancy before the fetus is viable. *Miscarriage* is a lay term for the spontaneous loss of a pregnancy. Be sure to clarify whether an abortion is spontaneous or therapeutic (i.e., induced).

- When did this occur?
- What were the circumstances around the miscarriage or abortion?
- How did you cope with these losses?

Obstetricians commonly record the pregnancy history using the "gravida-para" system (Box 21-3).

BOX 21-3 THE GRAVIDA-PARA NOTATION

- G = gravida, or total number of pregnancies
- P = para, or outcomes of pregnancies; after "P," you will often see the notations "F" (full-term), "P" (premature), "A" (abortion), and "L" (living child).

A woman who has had two living children and one miscarriage would be documented as "G3 P2 F2 A1."

If amenorrhea suggests a *current pregnancy*, inquire about the date of last intercourse and *common early symptoms*: tenderness, tingling, or increased size of the breasts; urinary frequency; nausea and vomiting; easy fatigability; and sensations that the baby is moving, usually present at about 20 weeks. Be considerate of the patient's feelings about discussing these topics and explore them when the patient has specific concerns.

CLINICAL TIP
Amenorrhea followed by heavy bleeding suggests a *threatened abortion* or *dysfunctional uterine bleeding* related to lack of ovulation.

Contraception

Inquire about methods of contraception used by the patient and partner. Is the patient satisfied with the method chosen? Are there any questions about the options available?

Vulvovaginal Symptoms

The most common vulvovaginal symptoms are *vaginal discharge* (Table 21-1) and local *itching*. Use the "OLD CART" approach to obtain a thorough history. If the patient reports a discharge, inquire about its amount, color, consistency, and odor. Ask about any local *sores* or *lumps* in the vulvar area

TABLE 21-1 Vaginal Discharge

Discharge from a vaginal infection must be distinguished from a physiologic discharge. A physiologic discharge is clear or white and may contain white clumps of epithelial cells; it is not malodorous. It is also important to distinguish vaginal from cervical discharges. The examiner will use a large cotton swab to wipe off the cervix. If no cervical discharge is present in the os, a vaginal origin is suspected and consider the causes below. Note that the diagnosis of cervicitis or vaginitis hinges on careful collection and analysis of the appropriate laboratory specimens.

	Trichomonal Vaginitis	Candidal Vaginitis	Bacterial Vaginosis
Illustration	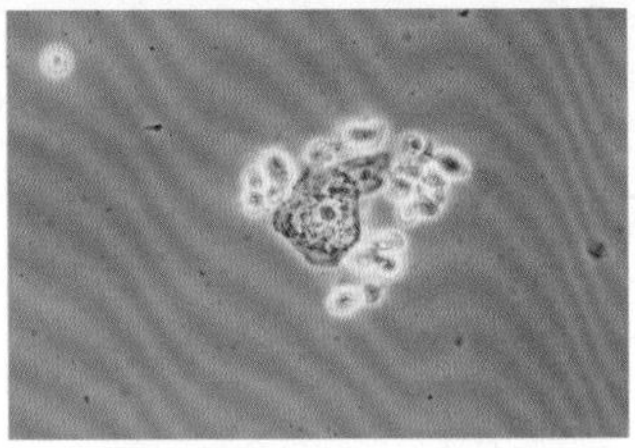	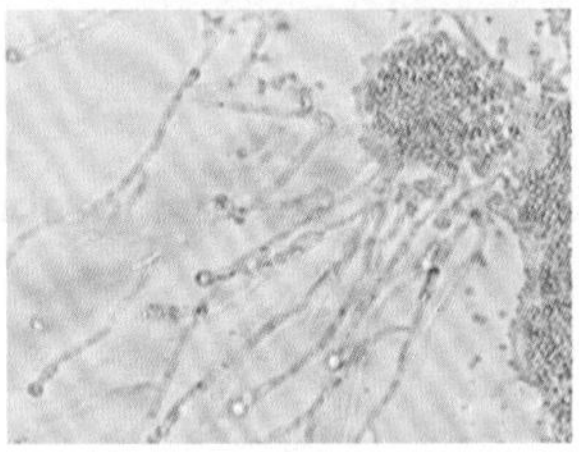	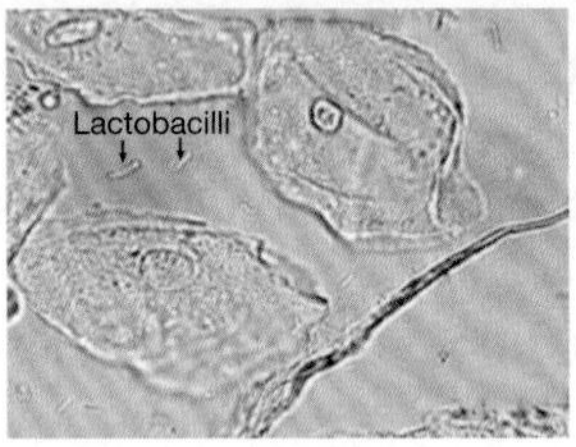
Cause	*Trichomonas vaginalis*, a protozoan; often but not always acquired sexually	*Candida albicans*, a yeast (normal overgrowth of vaginal flora); many factors predispose, including antibiotic therapy	Bacterial overgrowth probably from anaerobic bacteria; often transmitted sexually
Discharge	Yellowish green or gray, possibly frothy; often profuse and pooled in the vaginal fornix; may be malodorous	White and curdy; may be thin but typically thick; not as profuse as in trichomonal infection; not malodorous	Gray or white, thin, homogeneous, malodorous; coats the vaginal walls; usually not profuse, may be minimal
Other Symptoms	Pruritus (though not usually as severe as with *Candida* infection); pain on urination (from skin inflammation or possibly urethritis); dyspareunia	Pruritus; vaginal soreness; pain on urination (from skin inflammation); dyspareunia	Unpleasant fishy or musty genital odor reported to occur after intercourse
Vulva and Vaginal Mucosa	Vestibule and labia minora erythematous. The vaginal mucosa may be diffusely reddened. Vaginal mucosa may be diffusively reddened, with small red granular spots or petechiae in the posterior fornix. In mild cases, the mucosa looks normal.	The vulva and even the surrounding skin are often inflamed and sometimes swollen to a variable extent. The vaginal mucosa is often reddened with white, often tenacious patches of discharge. The mucosa may bleed when these patches are scraped off. In mild cases, the mucosa looks normal.	The vulva and vaginal mucosa usually appear normal.
Laboratory Evaluation	Scan saline wet mount for trichomonads	Scan potassium hydroxide (KOH) preparation for the branching hyphae of *Candida*.	Scan saline wet mount for *clue cells* (epithelial cells with stippled borders); sniff for fishy odor after applying KOH ("whiff test"); test the vaginal secretions for pH >4.5.

(Table 21-2). Are they painful or not? Because patients vary in their understanding of anatomic terms, be prepared to try alternative phrasing such as "Any itching (or other symptoms) near your vagina? Between your legs? Where you urinate?"

TABLE 21-2 Lesions of the Vulva

Epidermoid Cyst

A small, firm, round cystic nodule in the labia suggests an epidermoid cyst. These are yellowish in color. Look for the dark punctum marking the blocked opening of the gland.

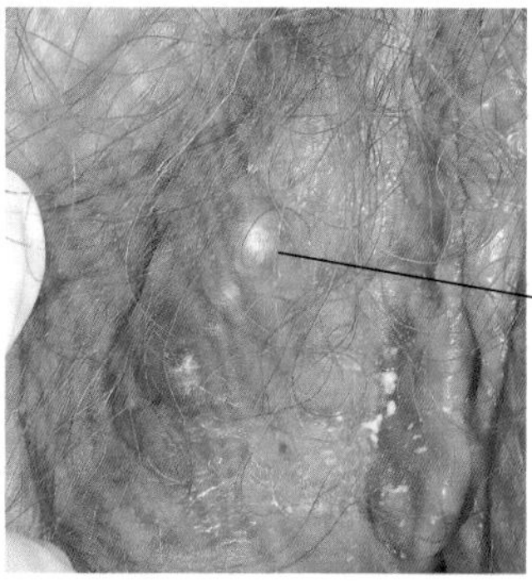

Venereal Wart (Condyloma Acuminatum)

Warty lesions on the labia and within the vestibule are often condyloma acuminata from infection with *human papillomavirus*.

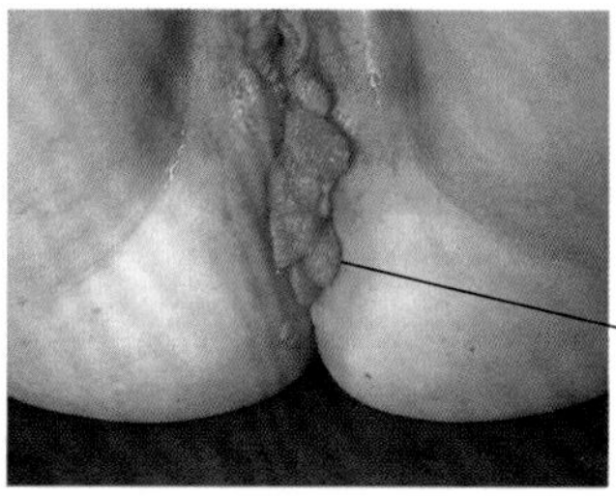

Syphilitic Chancre

This firm painless ulcer from primary syphilis forms ~21 days after exposure to *Treponema pallidum*. It may remain hidden and undetected in the vagina, and heals regardless of treatment in 3–6 wk.

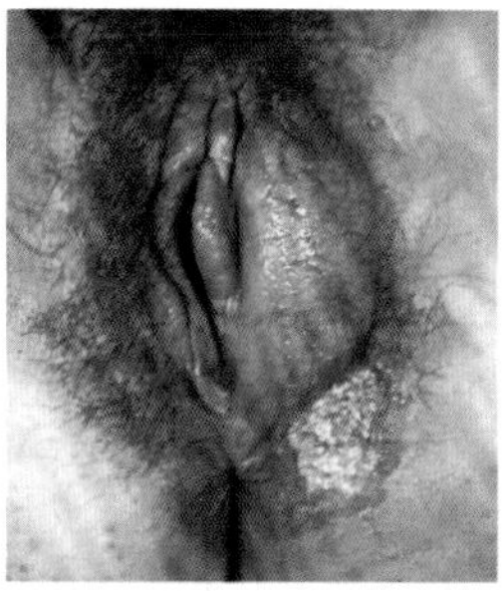

Uterine Prolapse

Uterine prolapse occurs when the uterus protrudes into the vagina.

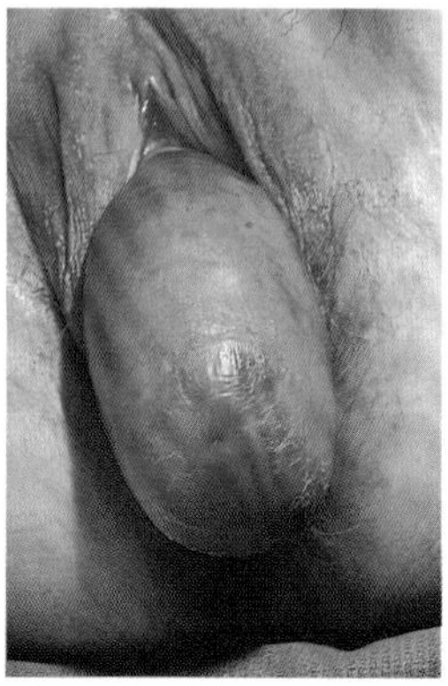

(continued)

TABLE 21-2 Lesions of the Vulva (*Continued*)

Genital Herpes

Shallow, small, painful ulcers on red bases point to infection from genital herpes simplex virus 1 or 2. Ulcers may take 2–4 wk to heal. Recurrent outbreaks of localized vesicles, which may progress to ulcers, are common.

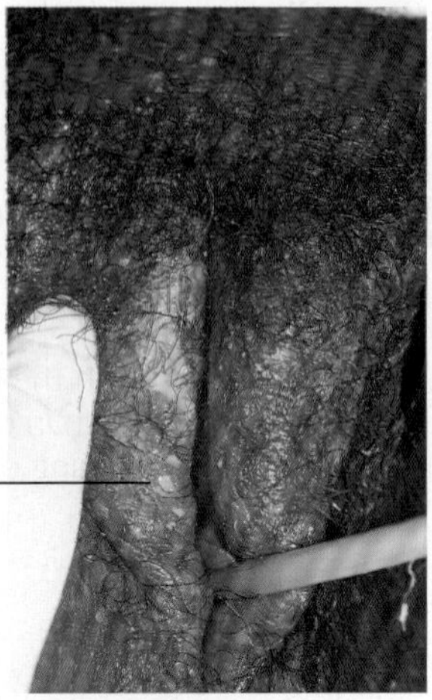

Bartholin Gland Infection

Causes of a Bartholin gland infection include trauma, gonococci anaerobes like bacteroides and peptostreptococci, and *Chlamydia trachomatis*. Acutely, the gland appears as a tense, hot, very tender abscess. Look for pus emerging from the duct or erythema around the duct opening. Chronically, a nontender cyst felt may be large or small.

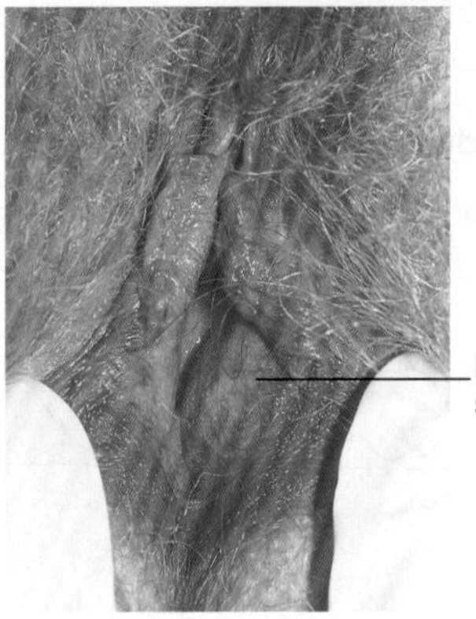

Sexual Health

Sexual health plays an important role in overall well-being. Patients will immediately sense your receptiveness to their concerns in this sensitive and vital area. Maintaining a neutral, nonjudgmental tone helps your patients feel safe and trust you with their concerns. Many patients have strong beliefs about sexual behavior related to their upbringing, faith, ethnicity, educational level, and past experiences. Reassure them that sex in a mature consensual relationship is healthy, and that you explore sexual health with all your patients. Be aware of your own body language, facial expressions, and tone of voice so that you create an open environment for discussion. In younger patients and adolescents, consider asking the parents to leave the room so patients feel free to answer questions without fear of parental disapproval or repercussions, especially when discussing possible sexual abuse.

Review tips for taking the sexual history in Box 21-4. Using neutral and nonjudgmental questions, ask about your patient's relationship status. If they are living (or have lived) with a partner, ask what their relationship is to that person, then follow up using the patient's language. (Loss of a partner can sometimes be determined by asking about whom they have lived with in the past.)

For example, you can begin with a general statement such as, "To provide good care, I need to review your sexual health and see if you are at risk for any STIs. I know this is a sensitive area. Any information you share is confidential."

BOX 21-4 TIPS FOR TAKING THE SEXUAL HISTORY

- Explain why you are taking the sexual history.
- Note that you realize this information is highly personal, and encourage the patient to be open and direct.
- Relate that you gather this history from all your patients.
- Affirm that your conversation is confidential.

Sexual Orientation and Gender Identity

Direct questions about sexual orientation may be difficult to answer. Patients with same-sex partners or who have been in same-sex relationships may be more anxious or fearful during clinical encounters because of past experiences. A reassuring manner will help them express concerns about their sexual health and activity.

As you talk with patients, begin with neutral questions about *sexual orientation* and *gender identity*:

- Are you currently dating? Sexually active? In a relationship? How would you identify your sexual orientation?

The range of responses includes heterosexual or straight, lesbian, gay, women who have sex with women (WSW), men who have sex with men (MSM), bisexual and queer/questioning, among others.

- How would you describe your gender identity?

Responses may include male, female, transgender, intersex, nonbinary, female-to-male, male-to-female, unsure or questioning, or "prefer not to answer."

- Do you have sex with men, women, or both?
- Do you use birth control? What method?
- Do you use protection against STIs? What method?
- Has anyone ever tried to touch or have sex with you without your consent?
- How is sex for you?
- Are you having any problems with sex?
- Are you satisfied with your sex life as it is now?

- Has there been any significant change in your sex life in the last few years?
- Are you satisfied with your ability to perform sexually?
- How satisfied do you think your partner is?
- Do you feel that your partner is satisfied with the frequency of sexual activity?
- Are you comfortable with your partner's sexual practices?

Sexual Response

If the patient has concerns about sexual activity; ask them to tell you about them. Direct questions help you assess each phase of the sexual response: desire, arousal, and orgasm:

Sexual dysfunction is classified by the phase of sexual response. A patient may lack desire, may fail to become aroused and attain adequate vaginal lubrication, or despite adequate arousal, may be unable to reach orgasm. Causes may include lack of estrogen, medical illness, trauma or abuse, surgery, pelvic anatomy, or psychiatric conditions.

"Do you have an interest in sex?" inquires about the desire phase.

For the arousal phase, ask:

- Do you get sexually aroused?
- Do you lubricate easily (get wet or slippery)?
- Do you stay too dry?

If patient reports dryness, ask about the use of lubricant.

For the orgasmic phase, ask:

- Are you able to reach climax (reach an orgasm or "come")?
- Is it important for you to reach climax?

Ask also about *dyspareunia* (pain or discomfort during intercourse). If present, try to localize the symptom. Is it near the outside, occurring at the start of intercourse, or is it farther in when the partner is pushing deeper? *Vaginismus* refers to an involuntary spasm of the muscles surrounding the vaginal orifice that makes penetration during intercourse painful or impossible.

CLINICAL TIP

Superficial pain suggests local inflammation, atrophic vaginitis, or inadequate lubrication; deeper pain may be from pelvic disorders or pressure on a normal ovary. The cause of *vaginismus* may be physical or psychological.

In addition to ascertaining the nature of a sexual problem, ask about its:

- Onset
- Severity
- Persistence or sporadic nature
- Setting where it occurs in
- Factors that make it better or worse
- What the patient thinks is the cause
- What the patient has tried to do about it and what the goals are

The factors surrounding sexual dysfunction is an important but complicated topic, involving the patient's general health; medications and drugs, including use of alcohol; the patient's and the partner's knowledge of sexual practices and techniques; the patient's attitudes, values, and fears; the relationship and communication between partners; and the setting in which sexual activity takes place.

A sexual problem may be related to situational or psychosocial factors.

Sexually Transmitted Infections

Local symptoms or findings on physical examination may raise the possibility of *STIs*. After establishing the usual attributes of any symptoms, elicit the sexual history. Inquire about sexual contacts and establish the number of sexual partners in the past 3 to 6 months. Ask if the patient has concerns about human immunodeficiency virus (HIV) infection, has been tested for HIV previously, desires HIV testing, or has current or past partners at risk. Also ask about oral and anal sex and if indicated, about symptoms involving the mouth, throat, anus, and rectum. Review the past history of STIs. "Have you ever had herpes? Any other problems such as gonorrhea? Syphilis? Chlamydia Pelvic infections?" What does the patient and partner use to prevent STIs? Continue with the more general questions suggested previously.

PHYSICAL EXAMINATION

Box 21-5 lists important areas for examination of the female reproductive system.

BOX 21-5 EXTERNAL EXAMINATION

- Mons pubis
- Labia majora and minora
- Urethral meatus, clitoris
- Vaginal introitus
- Perineum

The generalist nurse may prepare a female patient for or assist with an internal pelvic examination. In addition, the nurse may inspect the external genitalia during a procedure, such as urinary catheterization; during postpartum or postabortion care; while following up on a patient complaint; or while giving a complete bed bath. Therefore, the nurse must know the normal appearance of the external genitalia.

Approach to the Pelvic Examination

Many women feel anxious or uncomfortable before and during pelvic examinations. Some women have had painful, embarrassing, or even demeaning experiences during previous examinations, and others may be facing a pelvic examination for the first time. Some are fearful about what the clinician may find and how findings may affect their lives. Asking the patient's permission to perform the examination shows courtesy and respect.

Patients having their first pelvic examination may not know what to expect. Show them the equipment and let them handle the speculum. Use three-dimensional models to explain each step of the exam in advance. During the examination explain each step again. This can help them learn about their body and be more comfortable. Careful and gentle technique is especially important in minimizing any pain or discomfort during the first pelvic examination.

Patients' responses to the pelvic examination may reveal clues about their feelings about the examination and their sexuality. If the patient pulls away, adducts their thighs, or reacts negatively to the examination, you can gently comment, "I notice you are having some trouble relaxing. Is it just being here, or are you troubled by the examination? Is anything worrying you?" Behaviors that seem to present an obstacle may lead to a better understanding of your patient's concerns. Adverse reactions may signal prior or current abuse and should be explored.

Indications for a pelvic examination during adolescence include menstrual abnormalities such as amenorrhea, excessive bleeding, or dysmenorrhea; unexplained abdominal pain; vaginal discharge; the prescription of contraceptives; bacteriologic and cytologic studies in a sexually active patient; and the patient's own request for assessment.

See Chapter 23, "Assessing Children: Infancy through Adolescence."

Helping the patient relax is essential for an adequate examination. Adopting the tips in Table 21-3 will help ensure the patient's comfort. Raising the head of the examination table and supplying a mirror for the patient to observe the examination helps them understand the process.

Note that all examiners should be accompanied by an appropriate chaperone.

Rape Victims

Regardless of age, *rape* merits special evaluation, usually requiring medical consultation and documentation. Often there is a special rape kit provided in many emergency departments that must be used to ensure a chain of custody for evidence. Specimens must be labeled carefully with name, date, and time. Additional information may be needed for further legal investigation.

TABLE 21-3 Tips for the Successful Pelvic Examination

The Patient	The Nurse
• Avoids intercourse, douching, or use of vaginal suppositories or creams for 24–48 hours before examination • Empties bladder before examination • Lies supine, with head and shoulders elevated, arms at sides or folded across chest to enhance eye contact and reduce tightening of abdominal muscles	• Obtains permission; acts as chaperone • Explains each step of the examination in advance • Drapes patient from midabdomen to knees; folds drape between knees to provide eye contact with patient • Warms speculum with tap water • Monitors comfort of the examination by watching the patient's face

Equipment

Be sure the examiner has a good light, gloves, a vaginal speculum of appropriate size, water-soluble lubricant, and equipment for taking samples for Papanicolaou smears, bacteriologic cultures and DNA probes, or other diagnostic tests.

Specula are either metal (Fig. 21-5) or plastic and come in two basic shapes, named Pedersen and Graves. Both are available in small, medium, and large sizes. The medium Pedersen speculum is usually most comfortable for sexually active women.

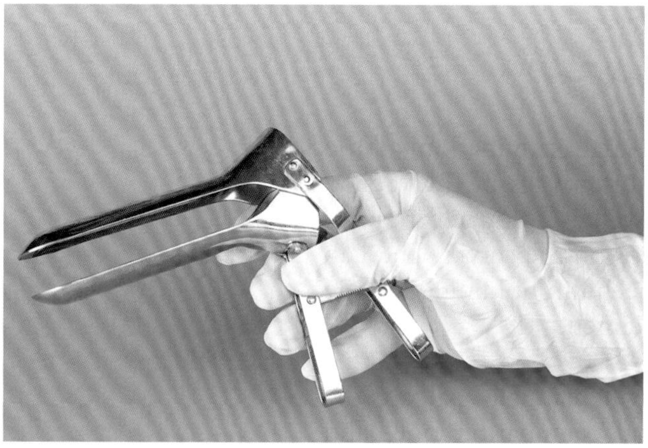

FIGURE 21-5 A metal speculum. (Olivka888/Shutterstock.)

Positioning the Patient

Drape the patient appropriately and then assist into the lithotomy position by placing one heel and then the other into the stirrups. The patient may be more comfortable with shoes or socks on than with bare feet. Ask the person to slide all the way down the examining table until the buttocks extend slightly beyond the edge. The thighs should be flexed, abducted, and externally rotated at the hips. Make sure a pillow supports the patient's head.

External Examination

Assess the Sexual Maturity of an Adolescent Patient

You can assess pubic hair during either the abdominal or the pelvic examination. Note its character and distribution, and rate it according to the Tanner stages.

Delayed puberty is often familial or related to chronic illness. It may also reflect disorders of the hypothalamus, anterior pituitary gland, or ovaries.

Examine the External Genitalia

Advise the patient that you will be touching the genital area. Inspect the mons pubis, labia, and perineum. Separate the labia and inspect the:

Excoriations or itchy, small, red maculopapules suggest *pediculosis pubis* (lice or "crabs"). Look for nits or lice at the bases of the pubic hairs.

- Labia minora
- Clitoris

An enlarged clitoris is seen in masculinizing conditions.

- Urethral meatus
- Vaginal opening, or introitus

Note any inflammation, ulceration, discharge, swelling, lacerations, bruising, or nodules.

Herpes simplex, Behçet disease, syphilitic chancre, epidermoid cyst may be observed. See Table 21-2.

Lacerations and/or bruising may indicate sexual abuse.

Internal Examination

The internal pelvic examination consists of a visual examination of the vagina and cervix with a speculum that separates the walls of the vagina. The examiner can assess vaginal muscle tone as well as color, ulcerations, inflammation, discharge, or masses in the vagina or on the cervix. The Pap smear sample is obtained at this time also. The speculum holding open the vagina prevents contamination of the cervical specimen.

After the speculum is removed, the examiner will manually palpate the organs of the reproductive system. In the bimanual examination, one hand is placed on the lower abdomen and two fingers of the other hand are inserted into the vagina. The cervix and uterus can be palpated for position, size, mobility, shape, regularity, masses, and tenderness. In slender, relaxed women, the ovaries may be palpated for size, position, regularity, and tenderness. Normally the fallopian tubes cannot be felt unless infection or a tubal pregnancy exists. A rectal examination may also be performed at this time.

RECORDING YOUR FINDINGS

Examples of documentation taken during a pelvic examination of the female genitalia are included in Box 21-6.

BOX 21-6 RECORDING THE PELVIC EXAMINATION—FEMALE GENITALIA

"No inguinal adenopathy. External genitalia without erythema, lesions, or masses."
OR
"Bilateral shotty inguinal adenopathy. External genitalia without erythema or lesions. Thin, white vaginal homogeneous discharge with mild fishy odor present."

HEALTH PROMOTION AND COUNSELING

Important Topics for health promotion and counseling related to the female reproductive system include:

- Reproductive system education
- Changes with menopause
- Cervical cancer screening: Pap smear and human papillomavirus (HPV) infection
- Early prenatal care
- Options for family planning
- STIs including HIV

Reproductive System Education

An accurate understanding of the normal appearance and function of the reproductive system will enable patients to take control of their reproductive health through family planning and disease prevention; to recognize pregnancy, problems, and maturational changes; and to seek appropriate care in a timely fashion. The use of three-dimensional models and charts is helpful to convey the structure and function of the system.

Changes with Menopause

Inform the patient of the psychological and physiologic changes of menopause—mood shifts and changes in self-concept; vasomotor changes ("hot flashes"); accelerated bone loss; increases in total and low-density lipoprotein (LDL) cholesterol; and vulvovaginal atrophy leading to symptoms of vaginal drying, dysuria, and at times, dyspareunia. Refer the patient to a midwife or gynecologist for treatment options for symptoms causing discomfort.

Cervical Cancer Screening: The Pap Smear and HPV Infection

Incidence and mortality rates for cervical cancer have dropped by more than 50% since the mid-1970s largely due to screening with the *Pap smear*, which can identify cervical changes before they become cancerous. In 2020, an estimated 13,800 women will be diagnosed with invasive cervical cancer. Most cases of cervical cancer occur in women who have not had appropriate screening (American Cancer Society, 2021b; American Society of Clinical Oncology, 2021, January).

The goal of cytologic screening is to sample the transformation zone of the cervix, the area where physiologic transformation from columnar endocervical epithelium to squamous (ectocervical) epithelium takes place and where dysplasia and cancer arise. HPV infection with high-risk oncogenic subtypes is found in virtually all cervical cancers (NIH, National Cancer Institute, 2021a). Of HPV infections, 90% are asymptomatic and resolve within 2 years. The most important risk factor for cervical cancer is *persistent infection with high-risk HPV subtypes*, especially HPV 16 or HPV 18. These two subtypes cause roughly 70% of cervical cancers worldwide. Even the 10% of people with persistent infection rarely progress to cervical cancer if they undergo regular screening, since the average estimated time for a high-grade HPV lesion to progress to cervical cancer is 10 years, allowing a long interval for detection and treatment (NIH, National Cancer Institute, 2021b). Genital infection with low-risk subtypes, such as HPV 6 and HPV 11, is associated with genital warts.

Two notable risk factors for cervical cancer include *failure to undergo screening*, which accounts for roughly half of women diagnosed with cervical cancer, and *multiple sexual partners*. Other risk factors include cigarette smoke exposure, immunosuppression from any cause, long-term use of oral contraceptives, high parity, sexual activity before 17 years, diethylstilbestrol (DES) exposure in utero, and prior cervical cancer (NIH, National Cancer Institute, 2021a).

Cervical Cancer Screening Guidelines

Guidelines for cervical cancer screening are outlined in Table 21-4.

The HPV Vaccine

The Advisory Committee on Immunization Practices (ACIP) of the Centers for Disease Control and Prevention (CDC) and the American Academy of Pediatrics recommend a routine two-dose vaccination series with the second dose given 6 to 12 months after the first with either the quadrivalent or bivalent vaccine for *girls and boys at ages 11 or 12* before their first sexual encounter. The series can begin as early as age 9. However, some adults ages 27 through 45 may decide to get the HPV vaccine based on discussion with their clinicians. A three-dose schedule is recommended for people who get the first dose on or after their 15th birthday and for people with

TABLE 21-4 Current Cervical Cancer Screening Guidelines for Average-Risk Women[a] from the U.S. Preventive Services Task Force and Centers for Disease Control and Prevention

Variable	Recommendation
Age at which to begin screening	21 y
Screening method and interval	Age 21–65 y: cytology every 3 y OR Age 21–29 y: cytology every 3 y Age 30–65 y: cytology every 3 y alone, every 5 y with high-risk human papillomavirus (hrHPV) testing alone, or every 5 y with hrHPV testing alone, or every 5 y with cotesting
Age at which to end screening	>65 y, assuming 3 consecutive negative results on cytology or 2 consecutive negative results on cytology plus HPV testing within 10 y before cessation of screening, with the most recent test performed within 5 y
Screening after hysterectomy	Not recommended with removal of the cervix

[a]Definition of Average Risk: No history of high-grade, precancerous cervical lesion (cervical intraepithelial neoplasia grade 2 or a more severe lesion) or cervical cancer; not immunocompromised (including being HIV-infected); and no in utero exposure to diethylstilbestrol.

Source: Sawaya, G. F., Kulasingam, S., Denberg, T., Qaseem, A., & Clinical Guidelines Committee of American College of Physicians. (2015). Cervical cancer screening in average-risk women: Best practice advice from the Clinical Guidelines Committee of the American College of Physicians. *Annals of Internal Medicine*, *162*(12), 851–859; Centers for Disease Control and Prevention (CDC). (2021a). 2015 sexually transmitted diseases treatment guidelines. HPV associated cancers and precancers. Screening recommendations: Cervical cancer. https://www.cdc.gov/std/treatment/default.htm; and U.S. Preventive Services Task Force (USPSTF). (2018b). Final recommendation statement: Cervical cancer: Screening. Retrieved March 6, 2021, from https://www.uspreventiveservicestaskforce.org/uspstf/recommendation/cervical-cancer-screening

certain immunocompromising conditions. In a three-dose series, the second dose should be given 1 to 2 months after the first dose, and the third dose should be given 6 months after the first dose (CDC, 2020b).

The quadrivalent vaccine prevents infection from HPV subtypes 16 and 18, as well as 6 and 11, which cause 90% of genital warts. The bivalent vaccine prevents infection from subtypes 16 and 18. The nine-valent HPV vaccine protects against more than 99% of HPV disease related to genotypes 6, 11, 16, and 18 and up to 96.7% for HPV disease related to genotypes 31, 33, 45, 52, and 58. Vaccination with the quadrivalent or nine-valent HPV vaccine is also recommended for the prevention of cervical, vulvar, and vaginal cancers and precancers in females, as well as anal cancers and precancers and genital warts in both females and males (NIH, National Cancer Institute, n.d.a).

Vaccination is recommended for females ages 13 through 26 and for males ages 13 through 21 who have not had prior vaccination or completed the three-dose series. Males ages 22 through 26 may also be vaccinated. If females or males reach age 27 before completing the series, the second and/or third vaccine doses can be administered after age 26 to complete the series. Prevaccination assessments to establish the need for a Pap smear or high-risk HPV DNA testing are not recommended.

The HPV vaccine is recommended for gay and bisexual men (or any man who has sex with men) and people with compromised immune systems, including HIV infection, through age 26 if they have not been fully vaccinated when younger.

Starting HPV vaccination early is important. According to the *National Youth Risk Survey, 2017*, 40% of high school students surveyed had had sexual intercourse (CDC, 2021b). Vaccinated females should still get cervical cancer screening since the vaccines do not prevent all HPV subtypes. Consistent use of condoms does not eliminate risk of cervical HPV infection (CDC, 2013, March 5).

Early Prenatal Care

The 2018 infant mortality rate was 5.7 deaths per 1,000 live births and the preterm (before 37 weeks of gestation) rate was 10% of live births (CDC, 2020c). Early prenatal care and preparation for pregnancy, such as stopping alcohol use and smoking, weight loss in obese women, and taking folic acid and calcium supplements, lower the perimortality rate. Women who express a desire to become pregnant or who are at risk for pregnancy should have a gynecologic examination to identify possible problems before pregnancy and be counseled on how to best prepare for pregnancy. If the history indicates the woman may be pregnant, she should be encouraged to obtain prenatal care as soon as possible.

Options for Family Planning

It is important to counsel patients, particularly adolescents, about the timing of ovulation in the menstrual cycle and how to plan or prevent pregnancy. The CDC notes that "Teen pregnancy has declined to the lowest rates in seven decades, yet still rank highest among the developed countries" (CDC, 2019, March 1). Significant health disparities remain: in non-Hispanic Black, Hispanic, and Native American/Alaska Native teens, birth rates were two times higher than the rate for non-Hispanic White teens. Nurses should be familiar with the numerous options for contraception and their effectiveness in order to explain contraception methods to patients. Take the time to understand the patient or family's concerns and preferences and respect these preferences whenever possible. Continued use of a preferred method is superior to a more effective method that is abandoned. For teenagers, a confidential setting eases discussion of topics that may seem private and difficult to explore (Santa Maria et al., 2017).

Sexually Transmitted Infections

Chlamydia trachomatis is the most commonly reported STI in the United States. In 2018, a total of 1,758,668 cases were reported to the CDC. Often symptoms are subtle, and the infection remains undiagnosed. If untreated, women may develop pelvic inflammatory disease (PID), a polymicrobial infection with an 8% to 40% risk of tubal infertility depending on the number of episodes. Rates of reported chlamydia are highest among adolescent and young adults. In 2018, almost two thirds of all reported chlamydia cases were among people aged 15 to 24 years (CDC, 2021c). As with other STIs, risk factors are age younger than 24 and sexually active; prior infection with *Chlamydia* or other STIs; new or multiple partners; inconsistent condom use; and occupational sex work.

Concept Mastery Alert

Pelvic Inflammatory Disease

PID is most commonly caused by STIs, such as chlamydia. Vaginal infections are not a common cause because they are usually confined to the tissues of the vagina and are prevented from moving into the uterus by the cervix.

HIV infections continue to be a public health problem. In 2018, 37,968 new cases were diagnosed in the United States. In the United States, HIV is mainly spread by having sex or sharing syringes and other injection equipment with someone who is infected with HIV. Substance use can contribute to these risks indirectly because alcohol and other drugs can lower inhibitions and make people less likely to use condoms.

To improve detection and treatment, the CDC (CDC, 2015) and the USPSTF (USPSTF, 2019) strongly recommend screening for STIs as summarized in Box 21-7.

BOX 21-7 CDC STI AND HIV SCREENING RECOMMENDATIONS 2015

- *Chlamydia* and *gonorrhea screening* annually for *all sexually active women younger than age 25 and older women with risk factors* such as new or multiple sex partners, or a sex partner infected with an STI. Retest 3 months after treatment.
- *Chlamydia, syphilis, hepatitis B,* and *HIV screening* for *all pregnant women,* and *gonorrhea screening* for *at-risk pregnant women* starting early in pregnancy with repeat testing as needed to protect the health of mothers and their infants.
- *Chlamydia, gonorrhea,* and *syphilis screening* at least once a year for *all sexually active gay, bisexual, and other MSM.* MSM who have multiple or anonymous partners should be screened more frequently for STIs (i.e., at 3- to 6-month intervals).
- *HIV testing* at least once for *all adults and adolescents from ages 13 to 64. Pregnant women* should be tested at the first prenatal visit and retested if at high risk. All people who seek evaluation or treatment for STDs should be tested for HIV.
- *HIV testing* at least once a year for *anyone having unsafe sex or using injection drug equipment.* Sexually active gay and bisexual men may benefit from testing every 3 to 6 months.

Nurses should assess risk factors for STIs and HIV infection by taking a careful sexual history and counseling patients about spread of disease and how to reduce high-risk practices. Key to effective clinician counseling are respect, compassion, a nonjudgmental attitude, and use of open-ended and understandable questions like "Tell me about any new sex partners" and "Have you ever had anal sex, meaning 'penis in rectum/anus sex?'" The USPSTF review of evidence notes that successful counseling includes: "prevalence, transmission, and details on how to reduce the risk for transmission; help in identifying personal risk for STIs; training in common behavior change processes, such as problem solving, decision making, and goal-setting; training in communication surrounding condom use and safe sex; and hands-on practice with condoms" (USPSTF, 2020). The CDC recommends interactive client-centered counseling, tailored to the person's specific risk factors and situation. Training in prevention counseling improves effectiveness. Information is available from the CDC at https://effectiveinterventions.cdc.gov/en/home.aspx.

See Chapter 4, "The Health History," discussion on eliciting the sexual history.

MALE REPRODUCTIVE SYSTEM

ANATOMY AND PHYSIOLOGY

Review the anatomy of the male genitalia illustrated in Figure 21-6.

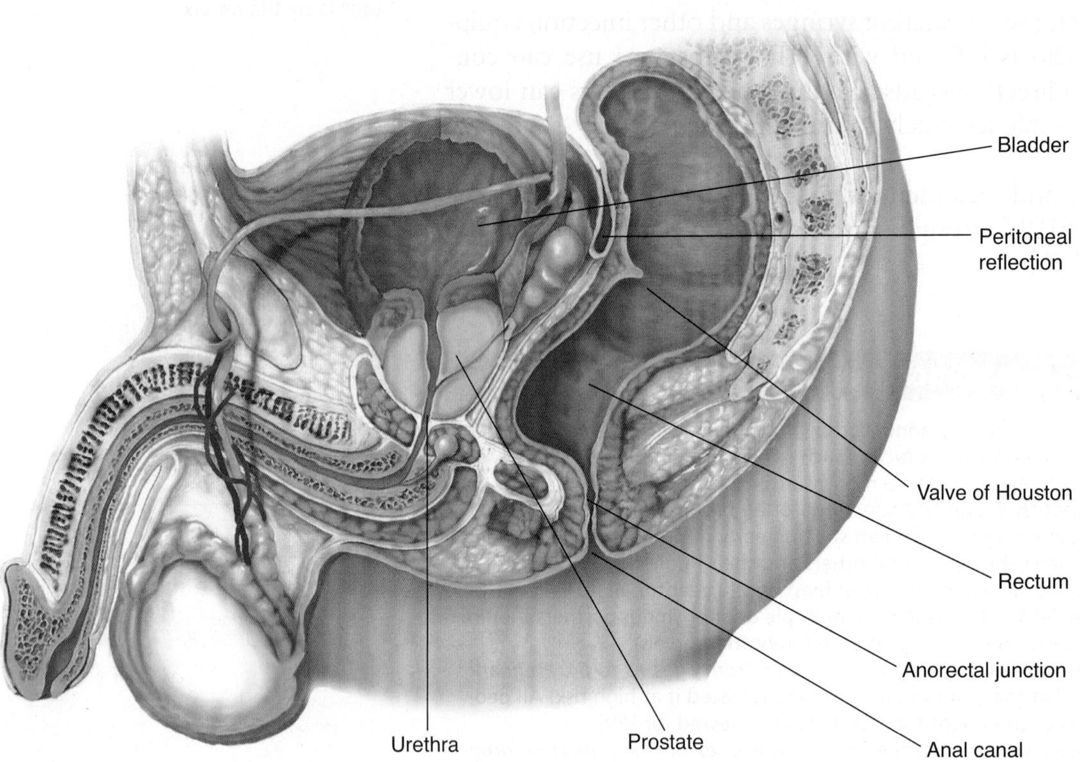

FIGURE 21-6 The male genitalia.

The *shaft of the penis* is formed by three columns of vascular erectile tissue: the *corpus spongiosum*, containing the urethra, and two *corpora cavernosa*. The corpus spongiosum extends from the bulb of the penis to the cone-shaped *glans* with its expanded base, or *corona*. In uncircumcised men, the glans is covered by a loose, hood-like fold of skin called the *prepuce* or *foreskin*, where *smegma*, or secretions of the glans, may collect. The urethra is located in the ventral midline of the shaft of the penis; urethral abnormalities may sometimes be felt there. The urethra opens into the vertical, slitlike *urethral meatus*, located somewhat ventrally at the tip of the glans.

The *testes* are paired ovoid glands consisting primarily of seminiferous tubules and interstitial tissue, covered by a fibrous outer coating, the *tunica albuginea*. The testes are normally 1.5 to 2 cm in length for prepubertal boys and 4 to 5 cm postpuberty. The left testis usually lies lower than the right. The testes produce spermatozoa and testosterone. Testosterone stimulates the pubertal growth of the male genitalia, prostate, and seminal vesicles. It also stimulates the development of masculine secondary sex characteristics, including facial hair, body hair, musculoskeletal growth, and enlargement of the larynx with its associated lower-pitched voice.

Surrounding or appended to the testes are several structures. The *scrotum* is a loose, wrinkled pouch divided into two compartments, each containing a testis or testicle. Covering the testis, except posteriorly, is the serous membrane of the *tunica vaginalis*. On the posterolateral surface of each testis is the softer, comma-shaped *epididymis*, consisting of tightly coiled tubules emanating from the testis that become the *vas deferens*. The epididymis provides a reservoir for storage, maturation, and transport of sperm from the testis to the *vas deferens*.

During ejaculation, the *vas deferens*, a cord-like structure, transports sperm from the tail of the epididymis along a somewhat circular route to the urethra. The *vas* ascends from the scrotal sac into the pelvic cavity through the inguinal canal, then loops anteriorly over the ureter to the prostate behind the bladder. There it merges with the *seminal vesicle* to form the *ejaculatory duct*, which traverses the prostate and empties into the urethra. Secretions from the *vas deferens*, the seminal vesicles, and the prostate all contribute to the seminal fluid. Within the scrotum, each vas is closely associated with blood vessels, nerves, and muscle fibers. These structures make up the *spermatic cord*.

Male sexual function depends on normal levels of testosterone, arterial blood flow from the internal iliac artery to the internal pudendal artery and its penile artery and branches, and intact neural innervation from alpha-adrenergic and cholinergic pathways. Erection from venous engorgement of the corpora cavernosa results from two types of stimuli. Visual, auditory, or erotic cues trigger sympathetic outflow from higher brain centers to the T11 through L2 levels of the spinal cord. Tactile stimulation initiates sensory impulses from the genitalia to the S2 to S4 reflex arcs and the parasympathetic pathways through the pudendal nerve. Both sets of stimuli appear to increase levels of nitric oxide and cyclic guanosine monophosphate (GMP), resulting in local vasodilation.

Lymphatics

Lymph drainage from the *penis* passes primarily to the deep inguinal and external inguinal nodes. Lymph vessels from the *scrotum* drain into the superficial inguinal lymph nodes. When an inflammatory or possibly malignant lesion is found on these surfaces, assess the inguinal nodes for enlargement or tenderness. Lymphatic drainage from the *testes* parallels their venous drainage: the left testicular vein empties into the left renal vein, and the right testicular vein empties into the inferior vena cava. The connecting abdominal lymph nodes are clinically undetectable. See Chapter 15 for further discussion of the inguinal nodes.

Anatomy of the Groin

A **hernia** is a condition in which part of an organ is displaced and protrudes through the wall of the cavity containing it, (e.g., part of the intestine through the abdominal musculature). Because hernias are relatively common, it is important to understand the anatomy of the groin (Fig. 21-7). The basic landmarks are the anterior superior iliac spine, the pubic tubercle, and the inguinal ligament that runs between them.

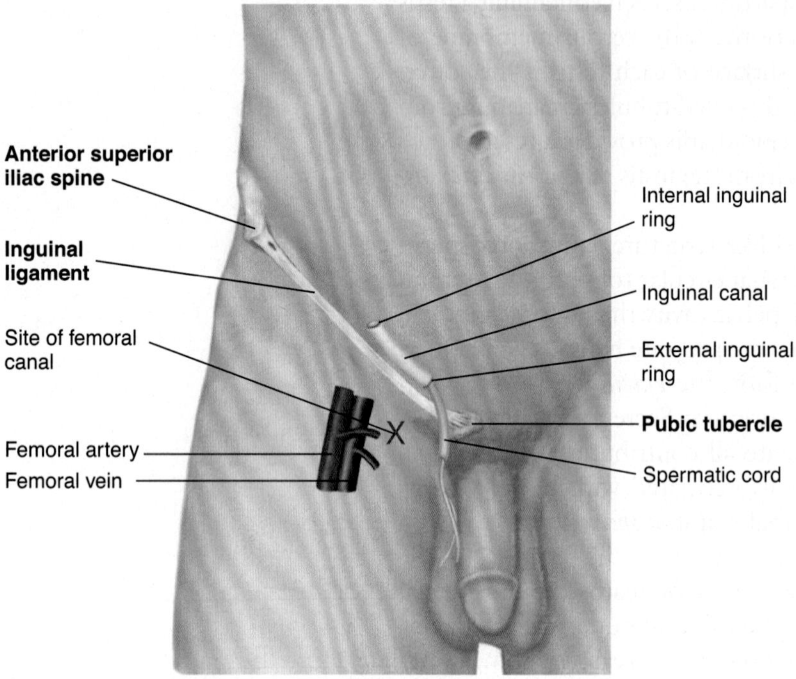

FIGURE 21-7 Anatomic landmarks of the right groin.

The *inguinal canal*, which lies medial to and approximately parallel to the inguinal ligament, forms a tunnel for the vas deferens as it passes through the abdominal muscles. The exterior opening of the tunnel—the *external inguinal ring*—is a triangular, slitlike structure palpable just above and lateral to the pubic tubercle. The internal opening of the canal—or *internal inguinal ring*—is approximately 1 cm above the midpoint of the inguinal ligament. Neither canal nor internal ring is palpable through the abdominal wall. When loops of bowel force their way through weak areas of the inguinal canal, they produce *inguinal hernias*, as illustrated in Table 21-5, "Course, Presentation, and Differentiation of Hernias in the Groin."

Indirect inguinal hernias develop at the internal inguinal ring, where the spermatic cord exits the abdomen. *Direct inguinal hernias* arise more medially due to weakness in the floor of the inguinal canal and are associated with straining and heavy lifting.

Another potential route for a herniating mass is the *femoral canal*. This lies below the inguinal ligament. Although this canal is not visible, you can estimate its location by placing your right index finger, pointing toward the patient's head, on the right femoral artery. Your middle finger will then overlie the femoral vein; your ring finger will overlie the femoral canal. Femoral hernias protrude at this location.

Femoral hernias are more likely to present as emergencies with bowel incarceration or strangulation.

TABLE 21-5 Course, Presentation, and Differentiation of Hernias in the Groin

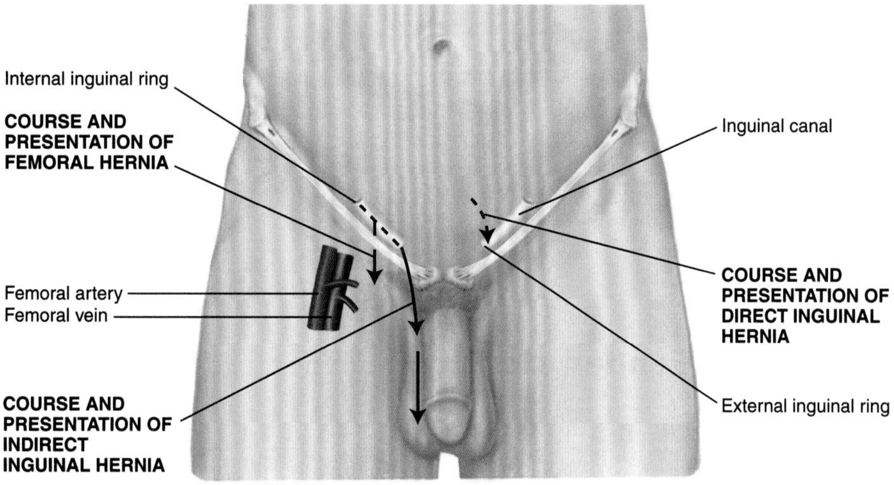

	Inguinal Hernias: Indirect	Inguinal Hernias: Direct	Femoral Hernias
Illustration	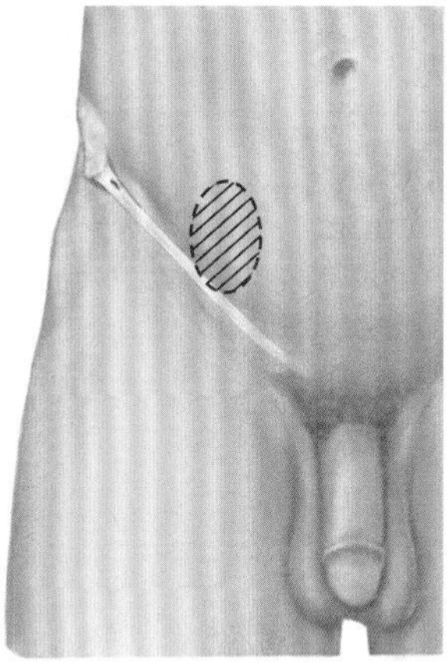	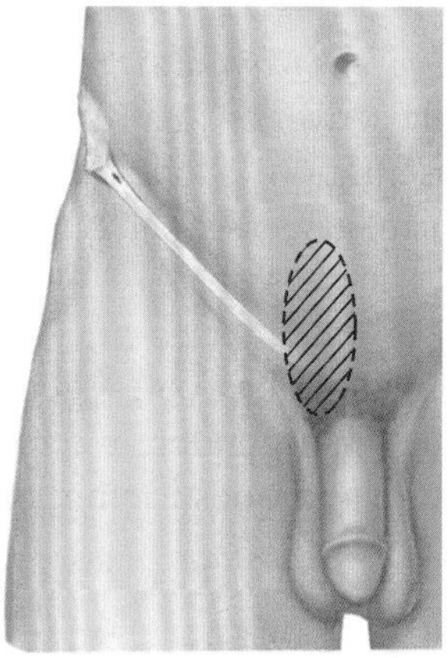	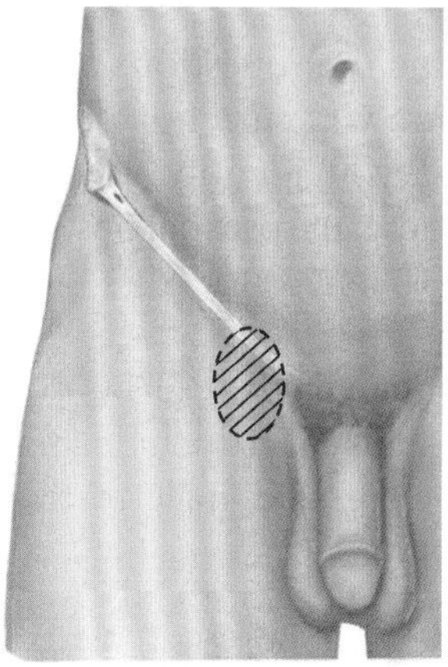
Frequency, Age, and Sex	Most common, all ages, both sexes Often in children; may occur in adults	Less common Usually in men older than 40; rare in women	Least common More common in women than in men
Point of Origin	Above inguinal ligament, near its midpoint (the internal inguinal ring)	Above inguinal ligament, close to the pubic tubercle (near the external inguinal ring)	Below the inguinal ligament; appears more lateral than an inguinal hernia Can be hard to differentiate from lymph nodes
Course (Examining finger in inguinal canal during coughing or straining)	Often into the scrotum The hernia comes down the inguinal canal and touches the fingertip.	Rarely into the scrotum The hernia bulges anteriorly and pushes the side of the finger forward.	Never into the scrotum The inguinal canal is empty.

THE HEALTH HISTORY

Common or concerning symptoms related to the health history of the male reproductive system are listed in Box 21-8.

BOX 21-8 COMMON OR CONCERNING SYMPTOMS

- Sexual orientation and gender identity
- Penile discharge or lesions
- Scrotal pain, swelling, or lesions
- Problems with urination

Sexual Orientation and Gender Identity

Review the tips for taking the sexual history in Box 21-4.

Discussing sexual orientation and gender identity touches a vital and multifaceted core of your patients' lives. Reflect on any biases you may have so they do not interfere with professional responses to your patients' disclosures and concerns. A neutral supportive approach is essential for exploring your patients' health and well-being.

- Pose neutral questions about *sexual orientation* and *gender identity* such as: "Are you currently dating, sexually active, or in a relationship?" "How would you identify your sexual orientation?" The range of responses includes heterosexual or straight, lesbian, gay, bisexual, queer/questioning, and others.

- Continue with "How would you describe your gender identity?" Responses may include male, female, transgender, intersex, nonbinary, female-to-male, male-to-female, unsure and questioning, and "prefer not to answer."

Sexual Response

Explore the patient's sexual response:

- How is sex for you?

- How is your current relationship?

- How is your ability to perform sexually? Are you satisfied with your relationship and your sexual activity? Has your partner ever hurt you or forced you to have sex?

- Are you comfortable with your partner's sexual practices?

If the patient expresses relational or sexual concerns, explore both their psychological and physiologic dimensions:

- What does this relationship mean to you?
- Have you experienced any changes in desire or frequency of sexual activity?
- What is your view of the cause, what responses have you tried, and what are your goals?

Direct questions help assess each phase of the sexual response.

To assess *libido*, or desire, ask, "Have you maintained interest in sex?"

Low libido may arise from depression, endocrine dysfunction, or side effects of medications.

For the *arousal phase*, ask, "Can you achieve and maintain an erection?"

CLINICAL TIP
Erectile dysfunction may be from psychogenic causes, especially if early-morning erection is preserved. It can also result from decreased testosterone, decreased blood flow in the hypogastric arterial system, or impaired neural innervation (Gareri et al., 2014).

Explore the timing, severity, setting, and any other factors that may contribute to the issue:

- Have any changes in the relationship with your partner or in your life circumstances coincided with onset of a problem?
- Are there circumstances when erection is normal, for example, on awakening in the early morning or during the night? With other partners? With masturbation?

Ask questions that relate to the phase of *orgasm* and *ejaculation* of semen.

If ejaculation is premature, or early and out of control, ask:

- About how long does intercourse last?
- Do you climax too soon?
- Do you feel you have control over climaxing?
- Do you think your partner would like intercourse to last longer?

CLINICAL TIP
Premature ejaculation is common, especially in young men. Less common is reduced or absent ejaculation affecting middle-aged or older men. Possible causes are medications, surgery, neurologic deficits, or lack of androgen. Lack of orgasm with ejaculation is usually psychogenic.

For reduced or absent ejaculation, ask, "Do you find that you cannot reach orgasm even though you can have an erection?"

Try to determine whether the problem involves the pleasurable sensation of orgasm, the ejaculation of seminal fluid, or both. Review the frequency and setting of the symptoms, medications, surgery, and possible neurologic causes.

Penile Discharge or Lesions

To assess the possibility of genital infection from STIs, ask, "Have you had any discharge, leaking, or dripping from your penis or staining on your underwear?"

If the patient reports discharge, ask:

- When did it start?
- Is it continuous or intermittent?
- How much discharge is there? A teaspoon? A tablespoon?
- What color is the discharge?

Penile discharge may accompany gonococcal (usually yellow) and nongonococcal urethritis (may be clear or white).

- Is the discharge thick or thin?
- Have you had any sores or growths on the penis or scrotum? Or pain or swelling in the scrotum?
- Have you had a fever, chills, rash, or any other symptoms?
- Have you ever had these symptoms before? If yes, how were they treated?

To assess further for STIs, ask, "Have you ever been diagnosed with an STI? Chlamydia? Herpes? Gonorrhea? Syphilis? HIV?"

Because STIs may involve other parts of the body, additional questions are often indicated. An introductory explanation may be useful. "STIs can involve any body opening where you have sex. It's important for you to tell me which openings you use. It's important for you to tell me if you have oral or anal sex." Ask about symptoms such as sore throat, diarrhea, rectal bleeding, anal itching, or anal pain.

Infections from oral–penile transmission include gonorrhea, chlamydia, syphilis, and herpes. Symptomatic or asymptomatic proctitis (*inflammation of the rectum and anus*) may follow anal intercourse.

Because many infected individuals do not have symptoms or risk factors, ask all patients, "Do you have any concerns about HIV infection?" Discuss the need for *universal testing for HIV* (USPSTF, 2019). Table 21-6 outlines STIs for the male genitalia.

TABLE 21-6 Sexually Transmitted Infections of Male Genitalia

Genital Warts (Condylomata Acuminata)

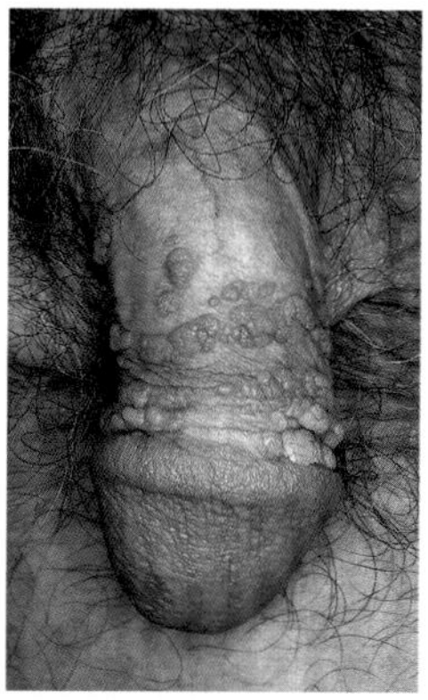

- *Appearance:* Single or multiple papules or plaques of variable shapes; may be round, acuminate (or pointed), or thin and slender. May be raised, flat, or cauliflower-like (verrucous)
- *Causative organism: Human papillomavirus (HPV),* usually from subtypes 6, 11; carcinogenic subtypes rare, approximately 5–10% of all anogenital warts
- *Incubation:* weeks to months; infected contact may have no visible warts
- Can arise on penis, scrotum, groin, thighs, anus; usually asymptomatic, occasionally cause itching and pain
- May disappear without treatment

Genital Herpes Simplex

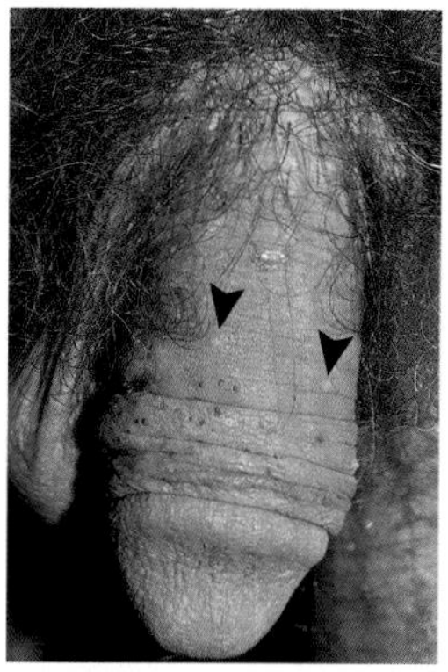

- *Appearance:* Small scattered or grouped vesicles, 1–3 mm in size, on glans or shaft of penis. Appear as erosions if vesicular membrane breaks
- *Causative organism:* Usually *herpes simplex virus 2* (90%), a double-stranded DNA virus
- *Incubation:* 2–7 days after exposure
- Primary episode may be asymptomatic; recurrence usually less painful, of shorter duration
- Associated with fever, malaise, headache, arthralgias; local pain and edema, lymphadenopathy
- Need to distinguish from genital herpes zoster (usually in older patients with dermatomal distribution) and candidiasis

Primary Syphilis

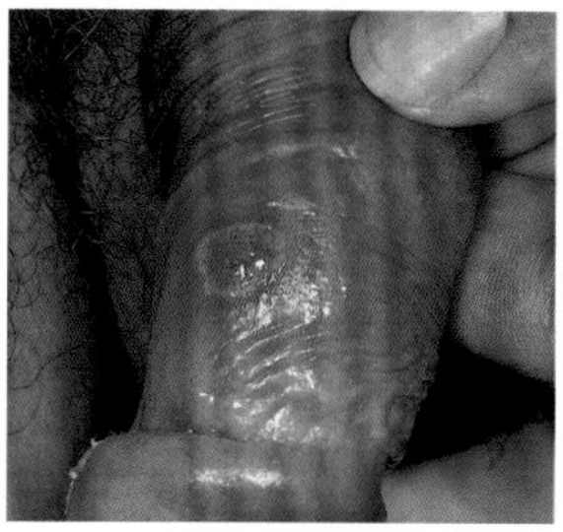

- *Appearance:* Small red papule that becomes a *chancre*, or *painless* erosion up to 2 cm in diameter. Base of chancre is clean, red, smooth, and glistening; borders are raised and indurated. Chancre heals within 3–8 wk
- *Causative organism: Treponema pallidum*, a spirochete
- *Incubation:* 9–90 days after exposure
- May develop inguinal lymphadenopathy within 7 days; lymph nodes are rubbery, nontender, mobile
- 20–30% of patients develop secondary syphilis while chancre still present (suggests coinfection with HIV)
- Distinguish from genital herpes simplex; chancroid; granuloma inguinale from *Klebsiella granulomatis* (rare in the United States; four variants, so difficult to identify)

Chancroid

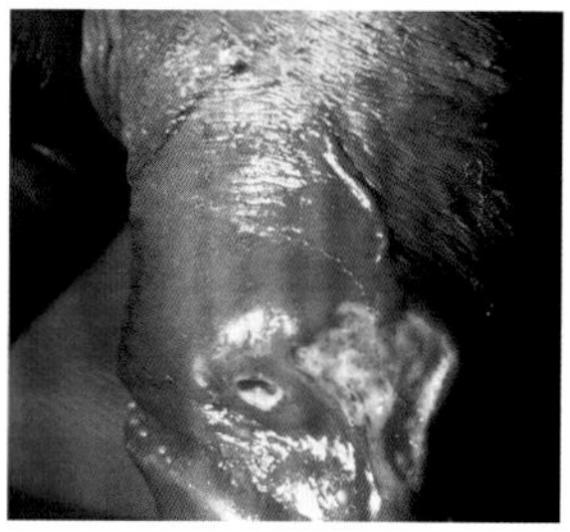

- *Appearance:* Red papule or pustule initially, then forms a *painful* deep ulcer with ragged nonindurated margins; contains necrotic exudate, has a friable base
- *Causative organism: Haemophilus ducreyi*, an anaerobic bacillus
- *Incubation:* 3–7 days after exposure
- Painful inguinal adenopathy; suppurative buboes in 25% of patients
- Need to distinguish from primary syphilis; genital herpes simplex; lymphogranuloma venereum, granuloma inguinale from *Klebsiella granulomatis* (both rare in the United States)

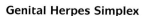

Scrotal Pain or Swelling

If the patient complains of pain or swelling in his scrotum, follow the "OLD CART" mnemonic to gather thorough information. A sudden onset of scrotal pain may indicate torsion of the testicle, which is an emergency. A painless lump may be cancer. Ask patients if they perform self-testicular examination and how often.

Inguinal Pain or Swelling

Inguinal pain or swelling may indicate an inguinal hernia. These hernias may be unilateral or bilateral. Ask the patient to point to the area of the pain and/or swelling and to describe it. "When did it begin? Is the pain continuous or intermittent? Achy or sharp? Does it occur with lifting heavy objects, standing, bending, or bearing down?"

Hernia pain and swelling are more likely to occur when internal abdominal pressure increases (e.g., when lifting).

Problems with Urination

The prostate gland wraps around the urethra. If the gland enlarges due to benign prostatic hyperplasia (BPH) or cancer, the patient may experience urinary symptoms. Men older than 70 are at the greatest risk. Therefore, the nurse should review the pattern of urination (see Chapter 16, "The Gastrointestinal and Renal Systems"). Ask the patient:

- Do you have any difficulty starting or holding back the urine stream?
- Is the flow weak?
- How often do you urinate during the day? At night?
- Is there any pain or burning as urine is passed?
- Is there any blood in the urine or in your semen? Any pain with ejaculation?
- Do you have any discomfort or heaviness in the prostate area at the base of the penis?

These symptoms suggest possible prostatitis.

PHYSICAL EXAMINATION

The generalist nurse does not perform prostate examinations or examine the genitalia by palpation of the male patient. However, the nurse may inspect the genitalia during a bed bath, a procedure such as urinary catheterization, or postoperative follow-up care of the genitourinary system. The nurse should be able to recognize abnormal conditions found on inspection that require referral or treatment. For younger patients, review the Tanner sexual maturity ratings in Chapter 23, "Assessing Children: Infancy through Adolescence."

Gloves should be worn. Occasionally male patients have erections during the examination or a procedure where the penis is touched. If this happens, explain that this is a normal response, and finish your examination with a calm demeanor.

The Penis

Inspect the penis, including:

- The *skin*. Inspect the skin on the ventral and dorsal surfaces and the base of the penis for excoriations or inflammation, lifting the penis when necessary.

- The *prepuce* (foreskin) (Fig. 21-8). If present, retract the prepuce or ask the patient to retract it. This step is essential for the detection of many chancres and carcinomas. Smegma, a cheesy, whitish material, may accumulate normally under the foreskin.

- The *glans*. Look for any ulcers, scars, nodules, or signs of inflammation.

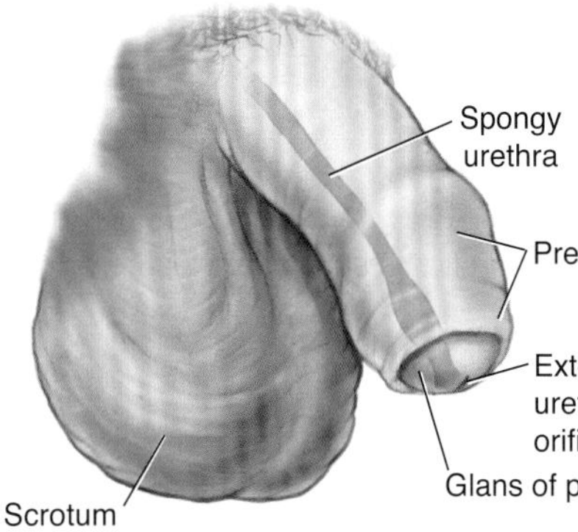

FIGURE 21-8 Anatomy of the male genitalia.

Phimosis is a tight prepuce that cannot be retracted over the glans. *Paraphimosis* is a tight prepuce that, once retracted, cannot be returned. Edema ensues.

Balanitis is inflammation of the glans. *Balanoposthitis* is inflammation of the glans and prepuce.

Check the skin around the base of the penis for excoriations or inflammation. Look for nits or lice at the bases of the pubic hairs.

Pubic or genital excoriations suggest the possibility of lice (crabs) or sometimes scabies.

Note the location of the urethral meatus.

Hypospadias is a congenital, ventral displacement of the meatus on the penis. See Table 21-7.

Inspect the penis for discharge. Normally there is none.

CLINICAL TIP

Profuse yellow discharge may indicate *gonococcal urethritis*; scanty white or clear discharge may indicate *nongonococcal urethritis*. Definitive diagnosis requires a Gram stain and culture.

If you retracted the foreskin, replace it before proceeding to examination of the scrotum. Table 21-7 outlines abnormalities of the penis and scrotum.

TABLE 21-7 Abnormalities of the Penis and Scrotum

Hypospadias

Congenital displacement of the urethral meatus to the inferior surface of the penis. A groove extends from the actual urethral meatus to its normal location on the tip of the glans.

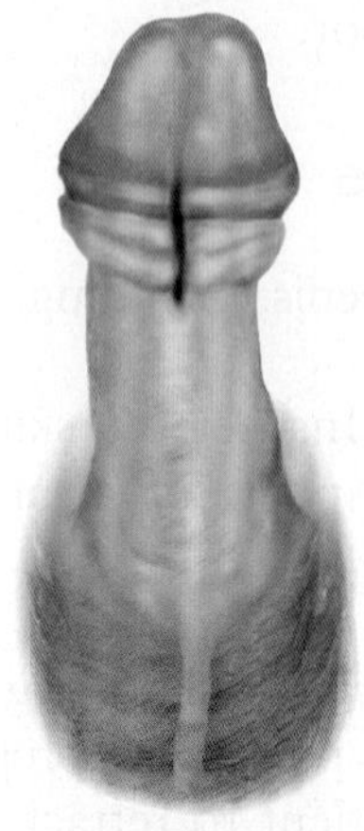

Scrotal Edema

Pitting edema may make the scrotal skin taut; seen in congestive heart failure or nephrotic syndrome.

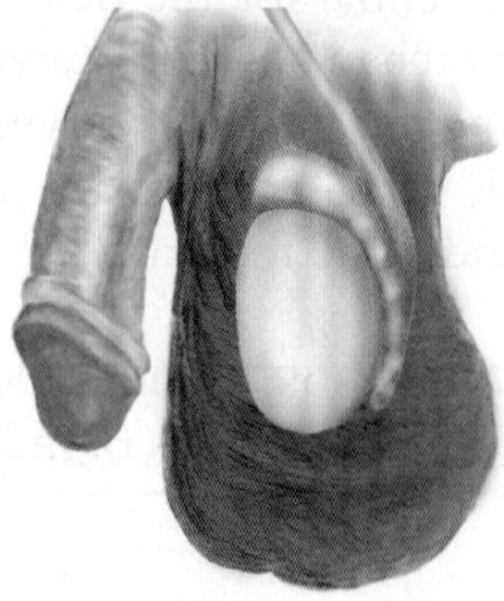

Epispadias

The urethral meatus is located on the top of the glans (dorsal side). This condition is a congenital defect and occurs rarely.

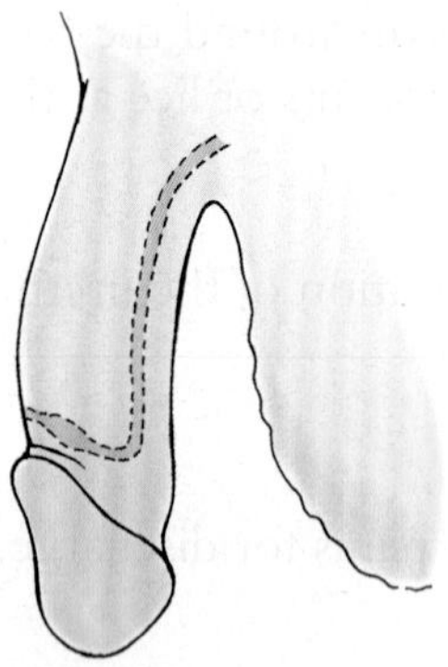

Hydrocele

A nontender, fluid-filled mass within the tunica vaginalis. It transilluminates, and the examining fingers can palpate above the mass within the scrotum.

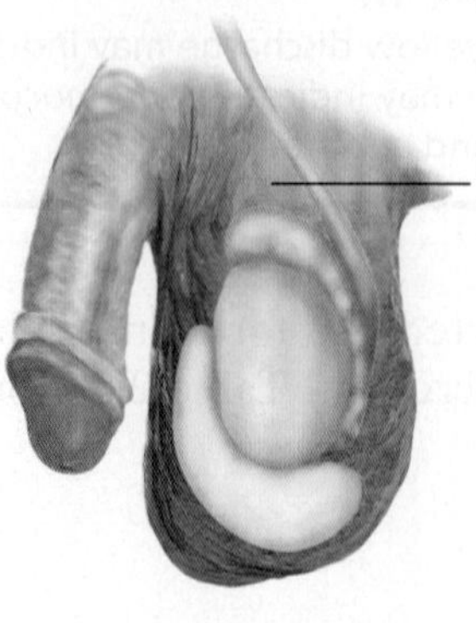

Carcinoma of the Penis

An indurated nodule or ulcer that is usually nontender. Limited almost completely to men who are not circumcised, it may be masked by the prepuce. Any persistent penile sore is suspicious.

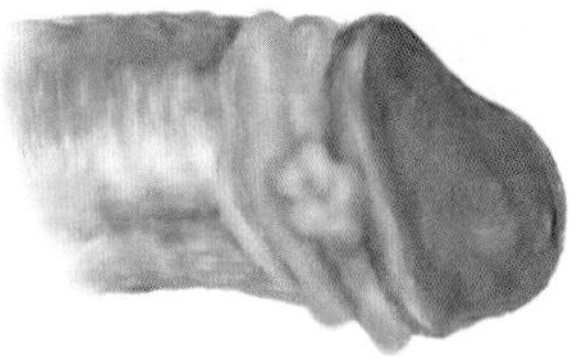

Scrotal Hernia

Usually an *indirect inguinal hernia* that comes through the external inguinal ring so the examining fingers cannot get above it within the scrotum.

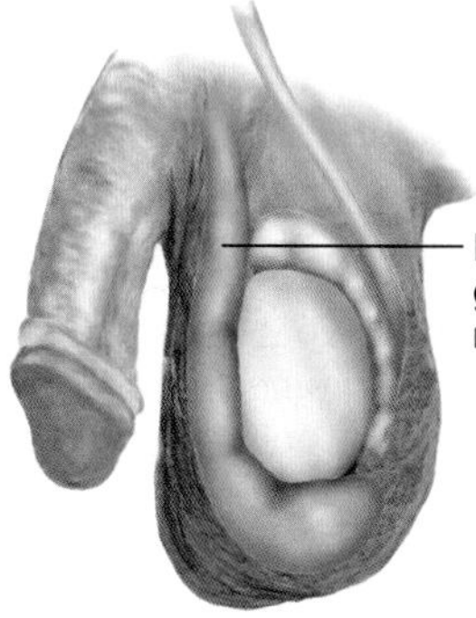

The Scrotum and Its Contents

Inspect the scrotum (see Table 21-7), including:

- The *skin*. Lift up the scrotum so that you can inspect its posterior surface. Note any lesions or scars. Inspect the pubic hair distribution.

Rashes, epidermoid cysts, and rarely skin cancer may be seen on the scrotum.

- The *scrotal contours*. Inspect for swelling, lumps, or veins bulging masses, or asymmetry of the left and right hemi-scrotum.
- The *inguinal areas*. Note any erythema, excoriation, or visible adenopathy.

Erythema and mild excoriation point to fungal infection, not uncommon in this moist area.

CLINICAL TIP
A poorly developed scrotum on one or both sides suggests **cryptorchidism** (an undescended testicle). Common scrotal swellings include indirect *inguinal hernias*, *hydroceles*, and *scrotal edema*.

There may be dome-shaped white or yellow papules or nodules formed by occluded follicles filled with keratin debris of desquamated follicular epithelium. Such *epidermoid cysts* are common, frequently multiple, and benign (Fig. 21-9).

Table 21-8 outlines abnormalities of the testis, and Table 21-9 outlines abnormalities of the epididymis and spermatic cord. These structures are housed in the scrotum.

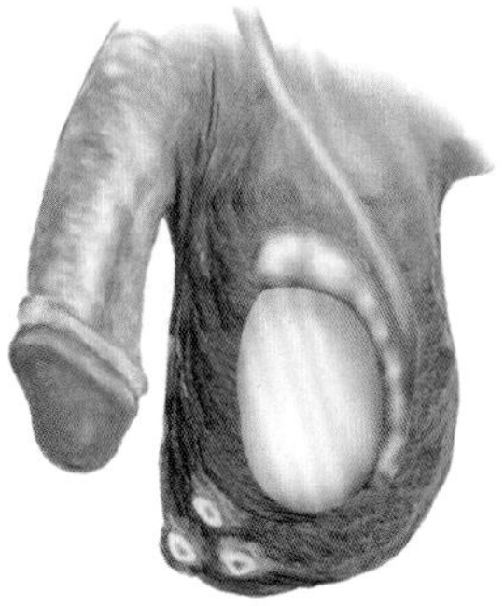

FIGURE 21-9 Epidermoid cysts.

TABLE 21-8 Abnormalities of the Testis

Cryptorchidism

The testis is atrophied and lies outside the scrotum in the inguinal canal, abdomen, or near the pubic tubercle; it may also be congenitally absent. In this illustration, there is no palpable left testis or epididymis in the unfilled scrotum. Cryptorchidism, even with surgical correction, markedly raises the risk for testicular cancer.

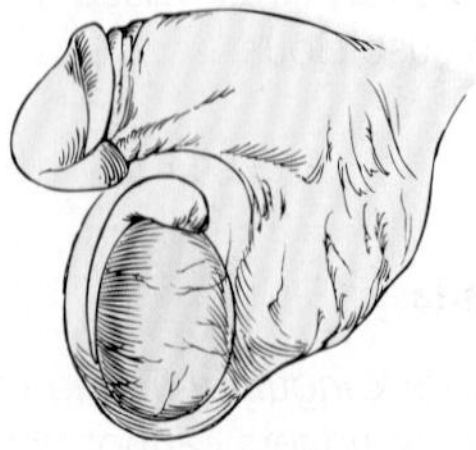

Small Testis

In adults, testicular length is usually ≤3.5 cm. Small, firm testes usually ≤2 cm suggest *Klinefelter syndrome*. Small, soft testes suggesting atrophy are seen in cirrhosis, myotonic dystrophy, use of estrogens, and hypopituitarism; may also follow orchitis.

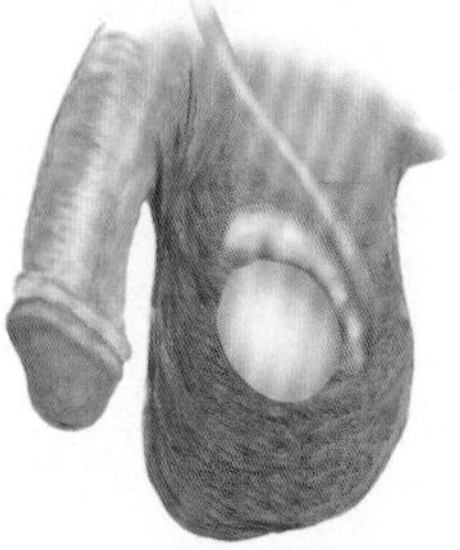

Acute Orchitis

The testis is acutely inflamed, painful, tender, and swollen. It may be difficult to distinguish from the epididymis. The scrotum may be reddened. Seen in mumps and other viral infections; usually unilateral.

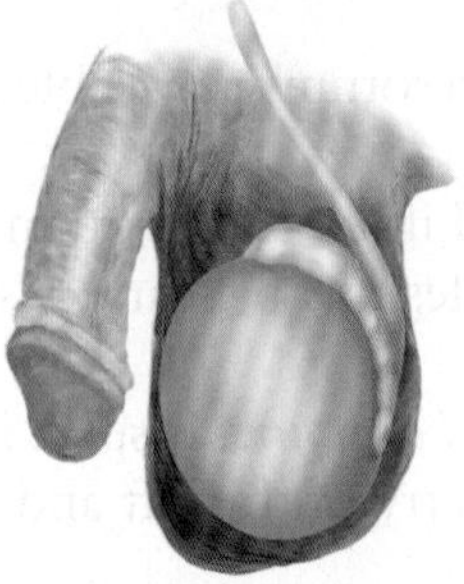

Tumor of the Testis

Usually appears as a painless nodule. Any nodule within the testis warrants investigation for malignancy.

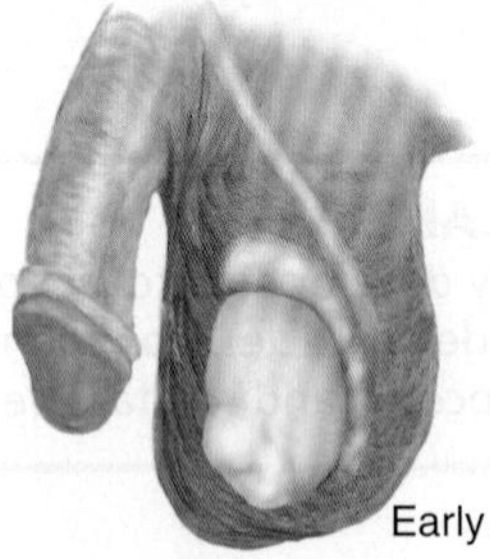

Early

As a testicular neoplasm grows and spreads, it may seem to replace the entire organ. The testicle characteristically feels heavier than normal.

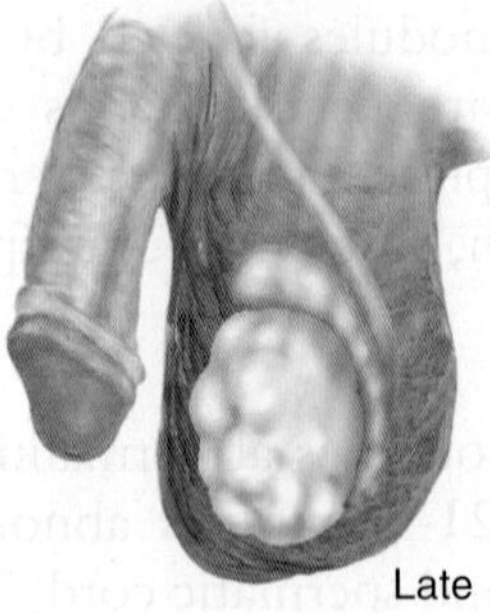

Late

TABLE 21-9 Abnormalities of the Epididymis and Spermatic Cord

Spermatocele and Cyst of the Epididymis

A painless, movable cystic mass just above the testis suggests a spermatocele or an epididymal cyst. Both transilluminate. The former contains sperm, and the latter does not, but they are clinically indistinguishable.

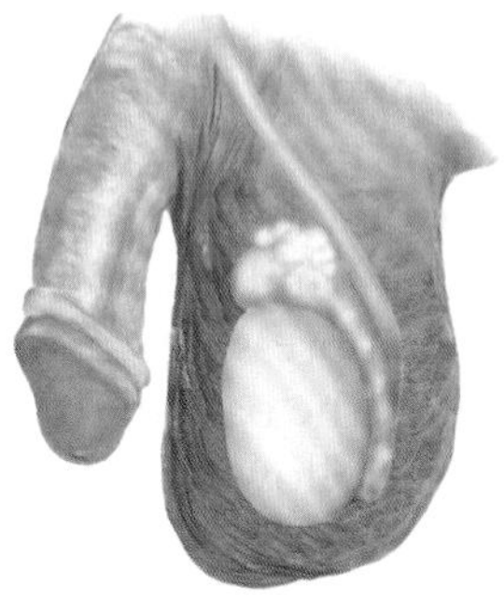

Varicocele of the Spermatic Cord

Varicocele refers to varicose veins of the spermatic cord, usually found on the left. It feels like a soft "bag of worms" in the spermatic cord above the testis, and if prominent, appears to distort the contours of the scrotal skin. A varicocele collapses in the supine position, so examination should be both supine and standing. If the varicocele does not collapse when the patient is supine, suspect a left spermatic vein obstruction within the abdomen.

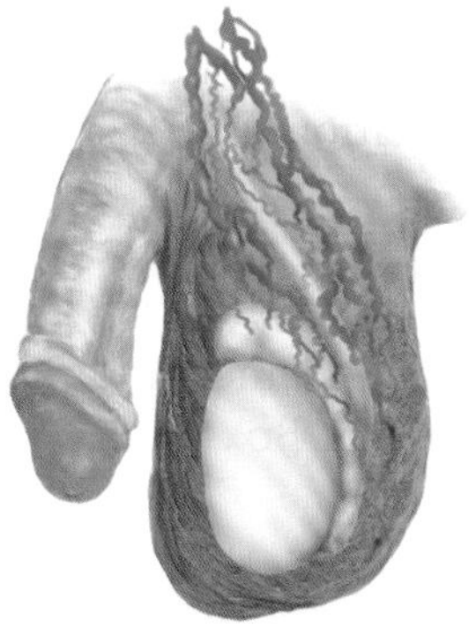

Acute Epididymitis

An acutely inflamed epididymis is indurated, swollen and notably tender, making it difficult to distinguish from the testis. The scrotum may be reddened and the vas deferens inflamed. Causes include infection from *Neisseria gonorrhoeae* and *Chlamydia trachomatis* in younger adults, *Escherichia coli* and *Pseudomonas* in older adults, trauma, and autoimmune disease. Barring urinary symptoms, urinalysis is often negative.

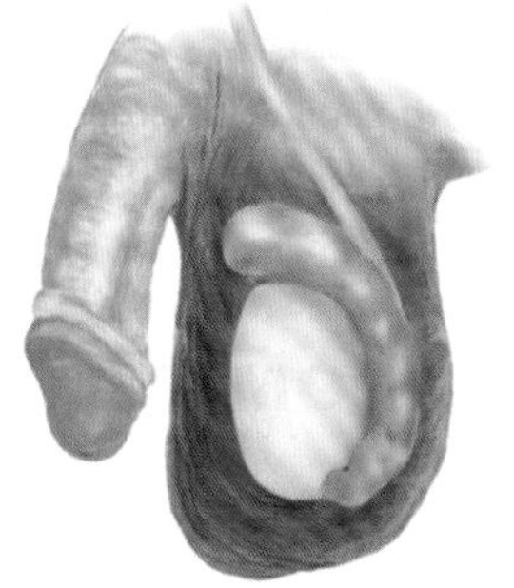

Torsion of the Spermatic Cord

Torsion, or twisting, of the testicle on its spermatic cord produces an acutely painful, tender, and swollen organ that is often retracted upward in the scrotum. If the presentation is delayed, the scrotum becomes red and edematous. There is no associated urinary infection. Torsion is most common in neonates and adolescents, but can occur at any age. It is a surgical emergency because of obstructed circulation.

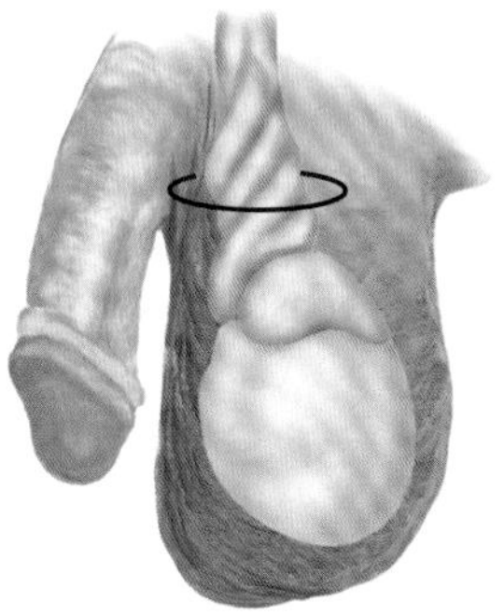

Hernias

If the patient has complained of a bulge or pain in his lower abdomen, especially with lifting or straining, he should be examined for hernias (see Table 21-5). Standing is the preferred position, because the upright position causes gravity to accentuate the bulge. Inspect the inguinal and femoral areas for bulging and asymmetry. As you observe, ask the patient to strain and bear down (the Valsalva maneuver) to increase intra-abdominal pressure, making it easier to observe a hernia. If a bulge is present, the patient should be referred to a physician or advanced practitioner for follow-up.

A bulge that appears with straining suggests a *hernia*.

Absence of a bulge during inspection does not guarantee absence of a hernia, especially in an obese patient. If suspicious history findings have been reported, the patient should be referred to an advanced practitioner for further examination.

RECORDING YOUR FINDINGS

An example of documentation of the assessment findings of the male genitalia is included in Box 21-9.

BOX 21-9 RECORDING THE PHYSICAL EXAMINATION—MALE GENITALIA AND HERNIAS

"Circumcised. No penile discharge or lesions. No scrotal swelling or discoloration. Testes descended bilaterally. No apparent inguinal or femoral hernias."

HEALTH PROMOTION AND COUNSELING

Topics for health promotion and counseling regarding the male reproductive system include:

- Prevention of STIs
- Testicular self-examination (TSE)
- Screening for prostate cancer

Prevention of Sexually Transmitted Infections

Review the information previously discussed in the section on STIs in the "Health Promotion and Counseling" portion of the "Female Reproductive System" section. Much of what applies to women applies to men as well.

As you counsel patients, encourage them to seek prompt attention for any genital lesions or penile discharge. Address preventive behaviors such as using condoms and dental dams, limiting the number of sexual partners, and establishing regular health care for treatment of STIs and HIV. *Correct use of male condoms* is highly effective in preventing the transmission of HIV, HPV, and other STIs (CDC, 2016). Key instructions should include:

- Using a new condom with each sex act
- Applying the condom before any sexual contact occurs
- Adding only water-based lubricants
- Immediate withdrawal if the condom breaks during sexual activity, and holding the condom during withdrawal to keep it from slipping off

The HPV vaccine can prevent HPV-related diseases in males (genital warts, anal cancer, and penile cancer) and can possibly reduce HPV transmission to female sex partners and lower the risk of oropharyngeal cancers. See Table 21-4 for age and dose recommendations.

CLINICAL TIP
Penile cancer usually forms on or under the foreskin. HPV causes about one third of penile cancer cases. When found early, penile cancer is usually curable (NIH, National Cancer Institute, n.d.b).

Testicular Cancer

It is estimated that 9,470 new cases of testicular cancer will be diagnosed in American men, and 440 will die of this disease in 2021 (American Cancer Society, 2021c). Testicular cancer is the most common cancer of young men between the ages of 15 and 34. White Americans have a four to five times higher risk than Black Americans or Asian Americans (American Cancer Society, 2018).

When detected early, testicular carcinoma has an excellent prognosis. Although the USPSTF and the American Cancer Society have not recommended routine TSE for screening, the nurse may wish to teach the patient how to perform a TSE to enhance health awareness and self-care, especially for men at high risk (Box 21-10). Risk factors include cryptorchidism, which confers a high risk for testicular carcinoma in the undescended testicle; a history of carcinoma in the contralateral testicle; HIV infection, DES exposure in utero; carcinoma in situ of the testicle; a hydrocele in childhood; and a positive family history. Teach men, especially young men, how to perform TSEs (PDQ® Screening & Prevention Editorial Board, 2021) and to seek physician evaluation for the following findings: any painless lump, swelling, or enlargement in either testicle; pain or discomfort in a testicle or the scrotum; a feeling of heaviness or a

BOX 21-10 PATIENT INSTRUCTIONS FOR THE TESTICULAR SELF-EXAMINATION

This examination is best performed after a warm bath or shower. This way the scrotal skin is warm and relaxed. It is best to do the test while standing.

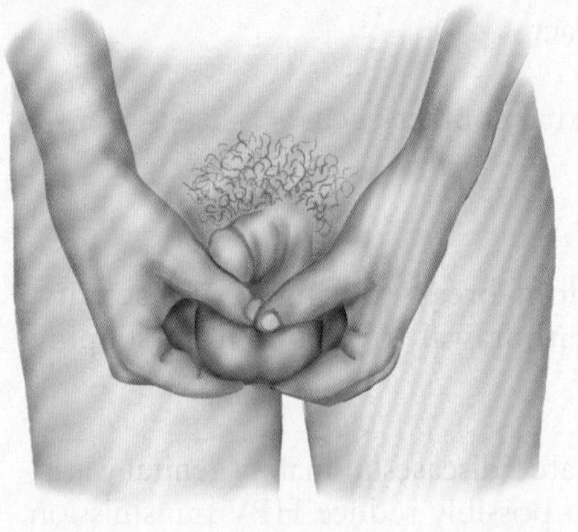

- Standing in front of a mirror, check for any swelling on the skin of the scrotum.
- With the penis out of the way, gently feel your scrotal sac to locate a testicle. Examine each testicle separately.
- Use one hand to stabilize the testicle. Using the fingers and thumb of your other hand, firmly but gently feel or roll the testicle between your fingers. Feel the entire surface. Find the epididymis. This is a soft, tube-like structure at the back of the testicle that collects and carries sperm; it is not an abnormal lump. Check the other testicle and epididymis the same way.
- If you find a hard lump, an absent or enlarged testicle, a painful swollen scrotum, or any other differences that do not seem normal, don't wait. See your health care provider right away.

As noted by the American Cancer Society, "It's normal for one testicle to be slightly larger than the other, and for one to hang lower than the other. You should also know that each normal testicle has a small, coiled tube (epididymis) that can feel like a small bump on the upper or middle outer side of the testicle. Normal testicles also have blood vessels, supporting tissues, and tubes that carry sperm. Some men may confuse these with abnormal lumps at first. If you have any concerns, ask your doctor."

Sources: American Cancer Society. (2018). Testicular self-exam. https://www.cancer.org/cancer/testicular-cancer/detection-diagnosis-staging/detection.html; U.S. National Library of Medicine, National Institutes of Health. (2021) MedlinePlus—Testicular self-exam. http://www.nlm.nih.gov/medlineplus/ency/article/003909.htm

sudden fluid collection in the scrotum; or a dull ache in the lower abdomen or the groin.

Prostate Cancer

Prostate cancer is the second leading cancer diagnosed in U.S. men after skin cancer. It is the second leading cause of cancer death in American men behind lung cancer. About one in nine men will be diagnosed with prostate cancer during his lifetime (American Cancer Society, 2018). Age, ethnicity, inherited mutations of the BRCA1 or BRCA2 genes, and family history are the primary risk factors:

- *Age*. Prostate cancer occurs mainly in older men. About 6 in 10 cases are diagnosed in men aged 65 or older, and it is rare before age 40. The average age at the time of diagnosis is about 66 (American Cancer Society, 2018).

- *Ethnicity*. For undetermined reasons, prostate cancer occurs more often in African American men and African Caribbean men than in men of other races. African American men are more than twice as likely to die of prostate cancer as are White men (American Cancer Society, 2020).
- *Family history*. Having a father or brother with prostate cancer doubles a man's risk. Inheritance of certain gene variations, such as BRCA1 and BRCA2, increase a man's risk of prostate cancer (American Cancer Society, 2020, June 9).

Prostate screening may be done with a prostate-specific antigen (PSA) blood test or a digital rectal examination (DRE) by an advanced practice health care provider. Both the PSA and DRE may yield false negatives or positives, potentially exposing the man to unnecessary further testing, surgery, or missed cancer diagnoses. The USPSTF, the American Cancer Society, and the American Urological Association offer guidelines for screening. All recommend the decision to be screened should be an individual one based on risk factors and the man's preference (American Cancer Society, 2021a; American Urological Association, 2018; Haseen & Kahn, 2020; USPSTF, 2018a).

For the American Urological Associations Guidelines go visit https://www.auanet.org/education/guidelines/prostate-cancer-detection.cfm

Men *with symptoms* of prostate disorders—incomplete emptying of the bladder, urinary frequency or urgency, weak or intermittent stream or straining to initiate flow, hematuria, nocturia, or bony pains in the pelvis—should be referred to a urologist. Men may be reluctant to report such symptoms but should be encouraged to seek evaluation and treatment early.

LGBTQIA Health Care

People who are LGBTQIA are members of every community. They are diverse, come from all walks of life, and include people of all races and ethnicities, ages, and socioeconomic statuses, and come from all parts of the country.

During clinical encounters, LGBTQIA patients often experience significant anxiety related to fears of being accepted. They may be uncomfortable disclosing their sexual behaviors and possibly still defining their sexual identity. When they experience bias or discrimination, they are unlikely to reveal their sexual identity or concerns. Transgender males who have vaginas, cervixes, and/or uteruses require routine gynecologic care and screenings. Transgender females who have penises and testicles should have testicular and prostate cancer screenings (Haseen & Kahn, 2020).

A useful resource for LGBTQIA care is Substance Abuse & Mental Health Services Administration (SAMHSA)'s "Top Health Issues for LGBT Populations" at: https://store.samhsa.gov/product/top-health-issues-lgbt-populations/sma12-4684 (SAMHSA, 2012).

BIBLIOGRAPHY

CITATIONS

American Cancer Society. (2018, May 17). Risk factors for testicular cancer. Retrieved May 2, 2021. https://www.cancer.org/cancer/testicular-cancer/causes-risks-prevention/risk-factors.html

American Cancer Society. (2020, June 9). Prostate cancer risk factors. https://www.cancer.org/cancer/prostate-cancer/causes-risks-prevention/risk-factors.html

American Cancer Society. (2021a). American Cancer Society recommendations for prostate cancer early detection. https://www.cancer.org/cancer/prostate-cancer/detection-diagnosis-staging/acs-recommendations.html

American Cancer Society. (2021b). Key statistics for cervical cancer. https://www.cancer.org/cancer/cervical-cancer/about/key-statistics

American Cancer Society. (2021c). Key statistics for testicular cancer. https://www.cancer.org/cancer/testicular-cancer/about/key-statistics.html

American College of Obstetricians and Gynecologists. (2015, May). Premenstrual syndrome. Retrieved May 2, 2021, from https://www.acog.org/patient-resources/faqs/gynecologic-problems/premenstrual-syndrome

American Society of Clinical Oncology. (2021, January). Cancer.net. Cervical cancer: Statistics. https://www.cancer.net/cancer-types/cervical-cancer/statistics#:~:text=This%20year%2C%20an%20estimated%2013%2C170%20women%20in%20the,can%20find%20cervical%20changes%20before%20they%20turn%20cancerous

American Urological Association. (2018). Prostate cancer: Early detection guidelines. Retrieved May 2, 2021, from https://www.auanet.org/guidelines/prostate-cancer-early-detection-guideline

Centers for Disease Control and Prevention (CDC). (2013, March 5). Condom effectiveness: Fact sheet for Public Health Personnel. Genital ulcer diseases and HPV infections. Retrieved May 1, 2021, from https://www.cdc.gov/condomeffectiveness/latex.htm

Centers for Disease Control and Prevention (CDC). (2015, June 4). 2015 Sexually Transmitted Diseases Treatment Guidelines. Screening Recommendations and Considerations. Retrieved May 3, 2021. https://www.cdc.gov/std/tg2015/screening-recommendations.htm

Centers for Disease Control and Prevention (CDC). (2016, August 12). Condom effectiveness. Retrieved May 2, 2021, from https://www.cdc.gov/condomeffectiveness/

Centers for Disease Control and Prevention (CDC). (2019, March 1). Reproductive health: Teen pregnancy. About teen pregnancy. Page last updated March 1, 2019. Retrieved May 1, 2021 from http://www.cdc.gov/teenpregnancy/about/index.htm

Centers for Disease Control and Prevention (CDC). (2020a). *HIV surveillance report, 2018 (Updated)*, vol. 31. Retrieved April 30, 2021, from https://www.cdc.gov/hiv/library/reports/hiv-surveillance.html

Centers for Disease Control and Prevention (CDC). (2020b). Vaccines and preventable diseases. Human papilloma virus (HPV) vaccination: What everyone should know. https://www.cdc.gov/vaccines/vpd/hpv/public/index.html

Centers for Disease Control and Prevention (CDC). (2020c). Reproductive health. Infant mortality. https://www.cdc.gov/reproductivehealth/maternalinfanthealth/infantmortality.htm

Centers for Disease Control and Prevention (CDC). (2021a). 2015 sexually transmitted diseases treatment guidelines. HPV associated cancers and precancers. Screening recommendations: Cervical cancer. https://www.cdc.gov/std/treatment/default.htm

Centers for Disease Control and Prevention (CDC). (2021b). Adolescent and school health: Sexual risk behaviors can lead to HIV, STDs, & Teen Pregnancy. https://www.cdc.gov/healthyyouth/sexualbehaviors/index.htm

Centers for Disease Control and Prevention (CDC). (2021c). Sexually transmitted disease surveillance 2019. https://www.cdc.gov/std/statistics/2019/default.htm

Gareri, P., Castagna, A., & Francomano, D. (2014). Erectile dysfunction in the elderly: An old widespread issue with novel treatment perspectives. *International Journal of Endocrinology, 2014*, 878670.

Haseen, B., Kahn, A., Belton, A., & Roth, B. C. (2020). Health Care for Transgender Men: What is missing in OB/GYN Care? *Journal of Lower Genital Tract Disease, 24*(2), 232–233. 10.1097/LGT.0000000000000507.

Johnson, C. T., Hallock, J. L., Bienstock, J. L., eds. (2015). Chapter 26: Anatomy of the female pelvis. *Johns Hopkins manual of gynecology and obstetrics* (5th ed.). Wolters Kluwer–Lippincott Williams and Wilkins; 338.

NIH. National Cancer Institute. (2021a). Cervical cancer treatment (PDQ®)–Health professional version: Risk factors. https://www.cancer.gov/types/cervical/hp/cervical-treatment-pdq#_392_toc

NIH. National Cancer Institute. (2021b). HPV and cancer: How does HPV cause cancer? https://www.cancer.gov/about-cancer/causes-prevention/risk/infectious-agents/hpv-and-cancer

NIH. National Cancer Institute. (n.d.a). HPV and cancer. Retrieved May 1, 2021, from https://www.cancer.gov/about-cancer/causes-prevention/risk/infectious-agents/hpv-and-cancer

NIH. National Cancer Institute. (n.d.b). Penile cancer-patient version. Retrieved March 7, 2021, from https://www.cancer.gov/types/penile

North American Menopause Society. (2017). The 2017 hormone therapy position statement of the North American Menopause Society. *Menopause, 24*(7), 728–753.

North American Menopause Society. (2021). Changes in hormone levels. https://www.menopause.org/for-women/sexual-health-menopause-online/changes-at-midlife/changes-in-hormone-levels

PDQ® Screening and Prevention Editorial Board. (2020, August 12). *PDQ testicular cancer screening*. National Cancer Institute. https://www.cancer.gov/types/testicular/hp/testicular-screening-pdq

Santa Maria, D., Guilamo-Ramos, V., Jemmott, L. S., Derouin, A., & Villarruel, A. (2017). Nurses on the front lines: Improving adolescent sexual and reproductive health across health care settings. *American Journal of Nursing*, *117*(1), 42–51.

Substance Abuse and Mental Health Services Administration (SAMHSA). (2012). Top health issues for LGBT populations. Information & Resource Kit. Retrieved March 7, 2021, from https://store.samhsa.gov/product/top-healthissues-lgbt-populations/sma12-4684

U.S. Preventative Services Task Force (USPSTF). (2018a). Prostate cancer screening: Final recommendation statement 2018. https://uspreventiveservicestaskforce.org/uspstf/recommendation/prostate-cancer-screening

U.S. Preventive Services Task Force (USPSTF). (2018b). Final recommendation statement: Cervical cancer: Screening. Retrieved March 6, 2021, from https://www.uspreventiveservicestaskforce.org/uspstf/recommendation/cervical-cancer-screening

U.S. Preventative Services Task Force (USPSTF). (2019). Human immunodeficiency virus (HIV) infection: Screening. Retrieved April 30, 2021, from https://www.uspreventiveservicestaskforce.org/uspstf/recommendation/human-immunodeficiency-virus-hiv-infection-screening?ds=1&s=HIV

U.S. Preventive Services Task Force (USPSTF). (2020). Sexually transmitted infections: Behavioral counseling. https://uspreventiveservicestaskforce.org/uspstf/recommendation/sexually-transmitted-infections-behavioral-counseling

22 PUTTING THE PHYSICAL EXAMINATION ALL TOGETHER

Learning Objectives

The student will:

1. Identify the components of the physical examination.
2. Identify the best approach for the physical examination based on individual patient needs.
3. Create an appropriate environment to ensure an accurate physical examination.
4. Demonstrate a head-to-toe physical examination.

The integration of history taking and physical examination makes up the health assessment. This combination of information from each body system provides the nurse with the knowledge of the individual to develop a plan of care and specific nursing interventions. The previous system chapters are structured for nurses to first ask questions to elicit the subjective information and then use the techniques of inspection, palpation, percussion, and auscultation to identify objective information. Learning each system in depth is important. Equally important is the integration of all systems into a complete physical examination, as well as the ability to critically evaluate the individual patient and decide which system or systems to focus on during the patient visit.

Assessments are performed with every patient contact. In general, a complete assessment is performed on new patients or new admissions to a health care facility (Fig. 22-1). The patient may be a healthy individual arriving at the clinic for a school physical or an ill patient admitted to the hospital.

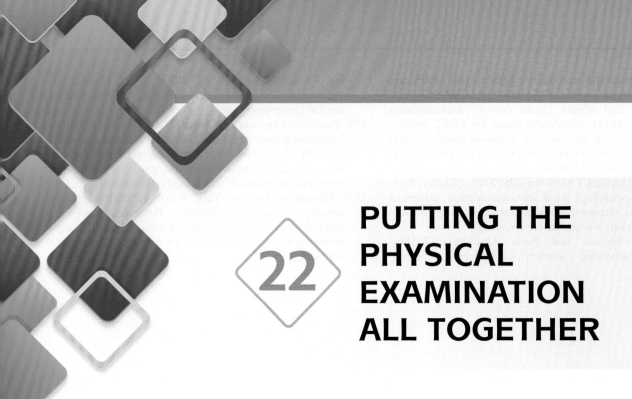

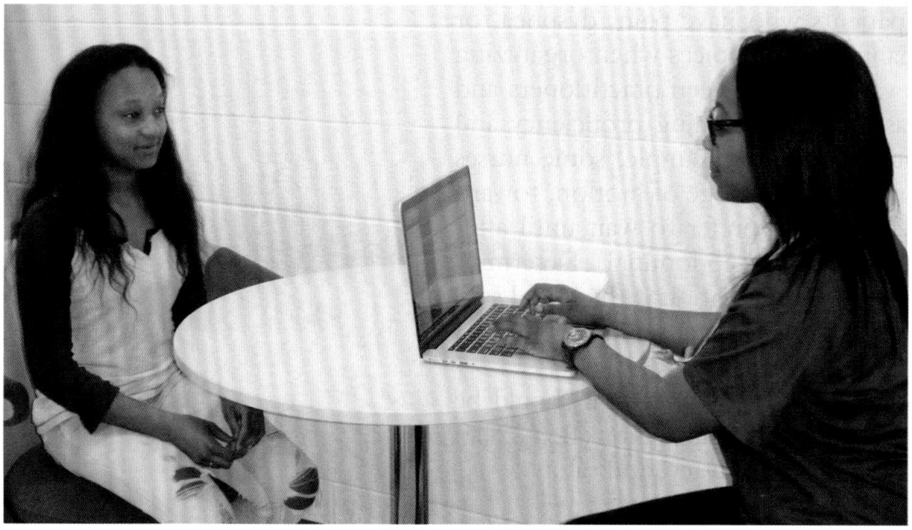

FIGURE 22-1 A complete assessment is performed on all new patients.

A focused assessment targets specific body systems. The decision to limit the number of systems assessed can be based on history findings, timing, severity of illness, or pain. The nurse caring for a patient who arrives with a chief complaint of a painful arm will focus on the following systems: musculoskeletal, cardiovascular, peripheral vascular, and neurologic. Based on the information obtained in the health history, systems may be excluded from the examination. If the pain was caused by an injury to the arm that did not impact the heart and there is no cardiac history, the cardiac examination may be eliminated, but musculoskeletal, neurologic, and peripheral vascular systems would still be important to evaluate. If however, the painful arm is not related to an injury and could be chest pain radiating to the arm, a cardiac assessment becomes a priority.

Initially, the complete examination may seem cumbersome and time-consuming. The student may wonder how to condense all the information and skills into an orchestrated, consistent examination or how to prioritize or choose specific systems for a focused exam. Students want to exude confidence and demonstrate comprehension of the examination; this will come with time and additional practice. During laboratory sessions, it is important to use the time with your partner and the guidance of your instructor to ensure proper technique and positioning for the examination. After laboratory sessions, it is imperative to take additional time for repeat practice. Repetition is necessary to refine skills and coordinate appropriate techniques into a thorough examination.

In general, a complete assessment is performed in a head-to-toe (cephalic to caudal) sequence comparing side to side (bilaterally) for symmetry. Prior to performing the head-to-toe examination, review the systems and plot the best flow for the examination. Some systems overlap and can be interwoven during the examination. Combining overlapping systems, limits the number of times patients need to change position from sitting to lying to standing, which can be difficult for patients who have pain, dyspnea, or limited range of motion. There are many correct choices when organizing the examination, and you will notice variations between practitioners and instructors. Continued practice will assist you in gaining proficiency and finding the best flow for you and the patient. For example, some nurses cover the musculoskeletal examination, including range of motion, toward the beginning of the examination, while others prefer to wait until after assessing the core components (cardiac, respiratory, abdominal). Determining the most efficient format for the physical examination is the initial step while remaining flexible based on individual patient needs and mobility.

It is time to prepare for the actual examination. The equipment should be available and in working order prior to the start of the examination (Box 22-1). The environment should be assessed for comfort, privacy, and safety.

BOX 22-1 EQUIPMENT

- Hand sanitizer
- Examination gloves
- Alcohol wipes
- Paper and pen, computer
- Draw sheet or drape
- Stadiometer
- Scale
- Examination light/gooseneck lamp
- Thermometer
- Watch with a second hand
- Sphygmomanometer
- Stethoscope
- Pulse oximeter
- Doppler
- Ophthalmoscope
- Otoscope/speculums
- Nasal speculum
- Stimulus to test sense of smell (e.g., mint, coffee, or alcohol swab if other scents not available)
- Snellen chart or visual acuity card to test distant vision
- Near vision card
- Opaque card
- Penlight
- Tongue depressors
- 2 × 2 gauze pads
- Cup of water
- Ruler and flexible tape measure, preferably marked in centimeters
- Goniometer
- Scoliometer
- Reflex hammer
- Tuning forks, 128 Hz and 512 Hz
- Q-tips, paper clips, or other disposable objects
- Cotton
- Mini-mental status examination tool
- Your note cards developed throughout the semester with highlights for individual systems

During the examination, remember to consider the patient's privacy. Close the door or curtain and use a sheet to cover parts of the body not being examined at that time. While examining the patient, explain procedures and findings throughout the entire examination. Letting the patient know what you are doing and your findings, such as taking a blood pressure, creates teaching and learning moments and develops a rapport with your patient.

Many students find it beneficial to make note cards, which can be used as cues for each system. Do not write too much or you might be distracted. As a new practitioner, a full head-to-toe examination of the patient should take less than 1 hour from start to finish. The following discussion provides a basic guide for conducting a physical examination while minimizing the number of position changes for the patient. Another sequence may work better for you, and this is acceptable as long as the examination proceeds in a logical flow, includes all the necessary components, and limits patient position changes. However, if an assessment is missed, it may be added later at another convenient time in the examination. The more you practice and repeat the techniques, the less likely this is to occur. Now assess your demeanor, and take a breath before entering the room.

As students become more proficient and comfortable with physical examination techniques and flow, the note cards can be rewritten with less detail.

A SAMPLE OF THE SEQUENCING FOR A HEAD-TO-TOE ASSESSMENT

Upon entering the room, the nurse should: wash their hands, introduce themselves and their purpose, and identify the patient including how they prefer to be addressed. Once the preliminaries have been completed, it is time to begin the history-taking component while the patient is dressed and sitting in a chair. During this conversation, the general survey and observation of the patient can be done simultaneously and throughout the examination.

Patient Seated

General Survey and Observation

- Assess the environment for:
  - Safety
  - Privacy
  - Noise and its impact on hearing
  - Lighting and its impact on sight
- Assess the individual for:
  - Age—stated age versus apparent age
  - Emotional state—compare verbal description and nonverbal
  - Developmental stage—compare with behavior

- Cultural background
- Health requirements and learning needs

Mental Status

Mental status is assessed throughout the history and examination beginning with the general survey; this includes assessment obtained when speaking to the patient. Assess the further aspects outlined in Table 22-1. If changes are noted, then a mini mental status examination should be performed.

TABLE 22-1 Mental Status Assessment

Appearance and behavior	• Level of consciousness • Dress, grooming, personal hygiene • Posture and motor behavior • Facial expression
Speech and language	• Quantity, rate, and volume of speech • Articulation of words • Fluency
Mood and affect	• Mood is the emotional makeup or feeling and how it varies with life events. • Affect is how emotions are expressed.
Thought process and content	• Logic, relevance, organization, and coherence of a patient's thought • Abnormalities in thought content or perception • Insight and judgment
Cognitive function	• Orientation to person, place, time, and situation • Attention/concentration: digit span, serial 7s, spelling backward • Remote and recent memory • New learning ability • Higher cognitive function: information and vocabulary, calculations, abstract thinking, constructional ability

Vital Signs

At the end of the history interview, ask the patient to change into a gown. This can be done before or after vital signs are taken as long as the arm can be exposed for the blood pressure. Vital signs to assess include:

- Temperature (Fig. 22-2)
- Pulse
- Respirations

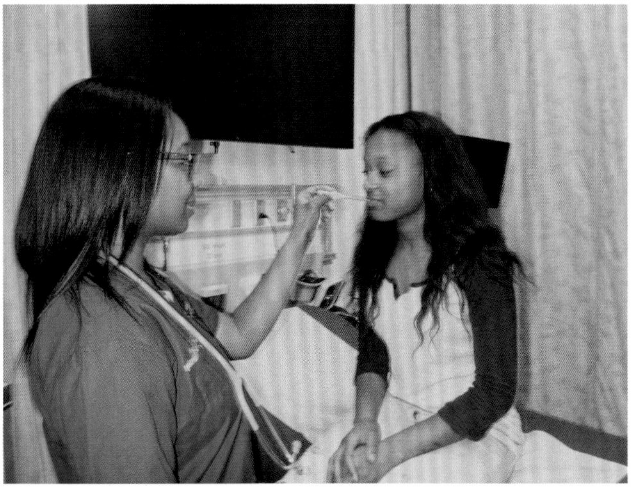

FIGURE 22-2 Taking the patient's temperature.

- Blood pressure—check each arm, position at heart level
- Pain

Body Measurements

Gowns should be on and shoes removed for height and weight to maintain consistency.

- Height
- Weight
- Body mass index and ideal body weight

Integument

Assess the skin throughout the examination as you examine each part of the body (Fig. 22-3):

- Inspect the hands and arms for color, lesions, scars, rashes, or any changes in the skin.
- Palpate for moisture, temperature, and texture.
- Palpate for skin turgor.

Hair

- Inspect the hair for color and distribution.
- Palpate hair for texture.

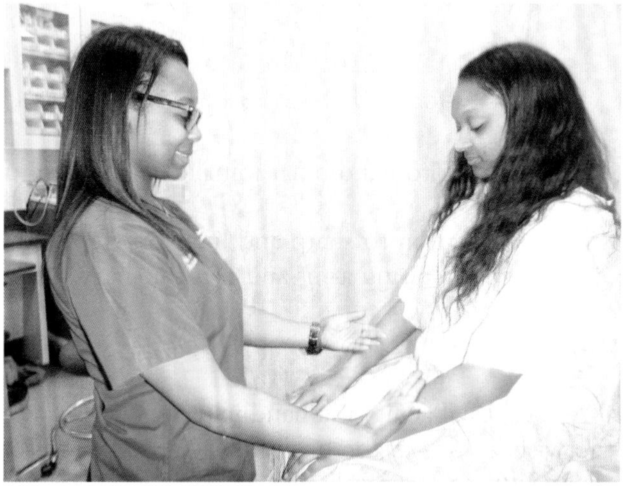

FIGURE 22-3 Assessing the skin.

Nails

- Inspect the nails for size, shape, angle, and color.
- Palpate nails for texture and capillary refill, and note any changes.

Head

- Inspect the skull for size and shape.
- Inspect the scalp for lesions and bumps.
- Palpate the scalp for tenderness, raised areas, or depressions.

Face

- Inspect facial features, movements, and expressions for symmetry.

Cranial nerve (CN) VII is the facial nerve: check symmetry of the face—raise eyebrows, frown, close eyes, smile, puff out cheeks.

- Palpate masseter and temporal muscle strength (Fig. 22-4).

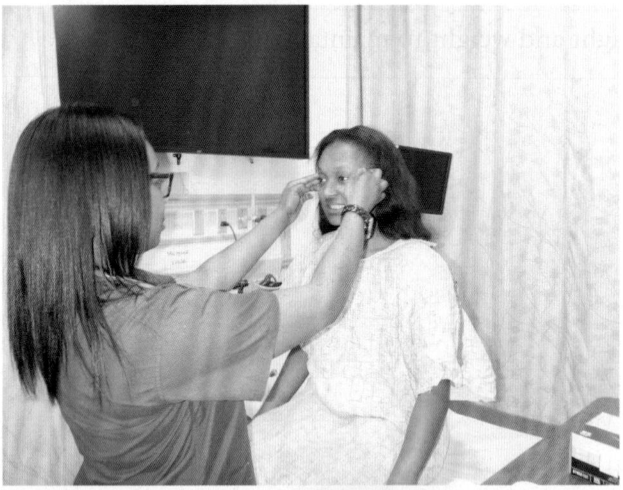

FIGURE 22-4 Palpating temporal muscle strength.

- Assess temporomandibular joint for pain, crepitus, and swelling.
- Assess sensation to sharp and light on face—forehead, cheeks, and chin (continue assessing arms and feet for sharp and light touch).

CN V is the trigeminal nerve.

Eyes

- Assess visual acuity if a handheld eye chart is available (Fig. 22-5). Otherwise do this in the beginning before the patient is seated or hold this part until the patient is standing for other parts of the assessment toward the end of the examination.

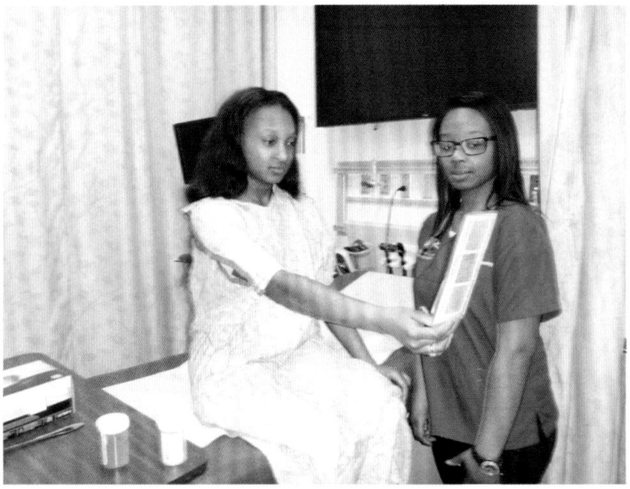

FIGURE 22-5 Assessing visual acuity.

- Inspect:
  - Eyelids for position, edema, color, lesions, and closure
  - Eyelashes for quantity, distribution
  - Eyebrows for quantity, distribution
  - Lacrimal apparatus for swelling, drainage, dryness, and crusting
  - Conjunctiva for color, nodules, or lesions
  - Sclera for color, vascular pattern, nodules, or lesions
  - Cornea and lens for opacities
  - Iris for color, crescentic shadow
  - Pupils for size, shape, symmetry, and direct and consensual light reaction

CN II is the optic nerve; CN III is the oculomotor nerve; CN IV is the trochlear nerve; and CN VI is the abducens nerve.

- Test visual fields by confrontation.
- Eye muscle examinations
  - Test six cardinal directions of gaze
  - Convergence
  - Near reaction (accommodation)
  - Cover–uncover test

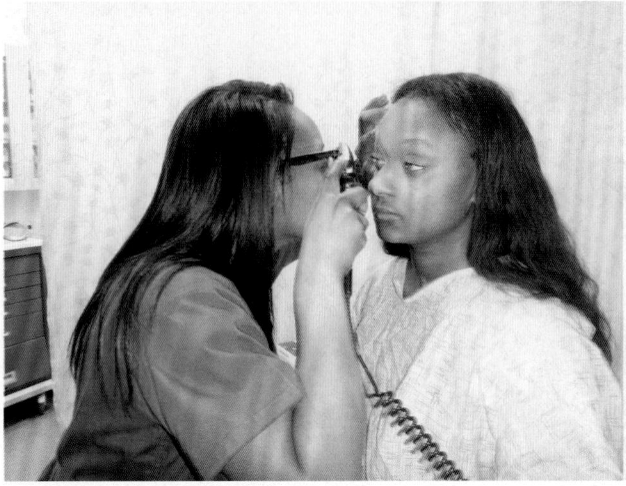

FIGURE 22-6 Ophthalmoscope examination.

- Ophthalmoscope examination (Fig. 22-6)—inspect:
  - Optic disc for color, size, shape
  - Retina for color, abnormalities
  - Arteries and veins for changes

Ears

- Inspect the pinna, lobe, and tragus for:
  - Position
  - Shape
  - Ulcers
  - Lesions
  - Discharge
- Palpate the pinna and tragus for:
  - Tenderness
  - Lumps
- Palpate the mastoid firmly for tenderness.

- Otoscopic examination—inspect:
  - Ear canal for color, swelling, lesions, discharge, and foreign bodies
  - Tympanic membrane for color and contour
  - Cone of light
- Hearing acuity
  - Whisper test
  - Weber (512 Hz on top of head; Fig. 22-7)
  - Rinne (512 Hz on mastoid bone and compare to air conduction)

CN VIII is the acoustic nerve.

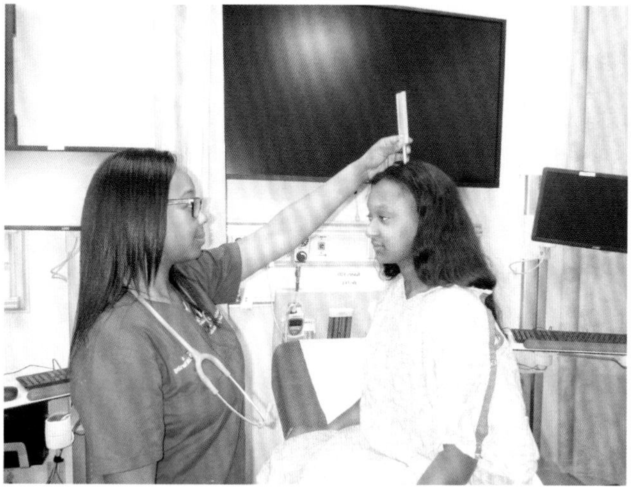

FIGURE 22-7 The Weber test.

Nose and Sinuses

- Inspect for:
  - Symmetry
  - Alignment
  - Deformity
- Palpate for tenderness and patency.
- Palpate the frontal and maxillary sinuses.

- Inspect the mucous membrane, septum, and turbinates for:
  - Inflammation
  - Polyps
  - Ulcers
  - Deviation
- Sense of smell—have patient identify two different scents with eyes closed (Fig. 22-8).

CN I is the olfactory nerve.

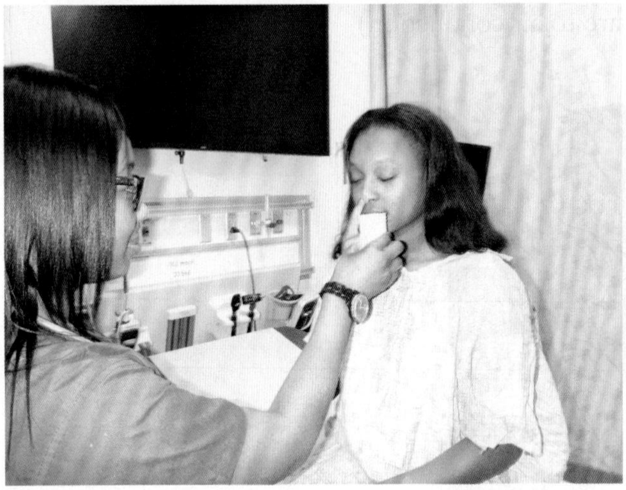

FIGURE 22-8 Testing the sense of smell.

Mouth and Pharynx

- Inspect the lips, oral mucosa, gums, roof of mouth, and floor of mouth for:
  - Color
  - Lesions
  - Moisture
- Inspect dentition for condition, number, and placement.
- Inspect the tongue for:
  - Size
  - Shape

- Color
- Moisture
- Lesions
- Texture

- Listen for articulation of words.

CN XII is the hypoglossal nerve.

- Tongue movement—assess at rest, when raised, when protruding, and side-to-side movements.
- Taste

CN VII is the facial nerve; CN IX is the glossopharyngeal nerve.

- Pharynx—inspect rise of palate and uvula (Fig. 22-9).

CN IX is the glossopharyngeal nerve; CN X is the vagus nerve.

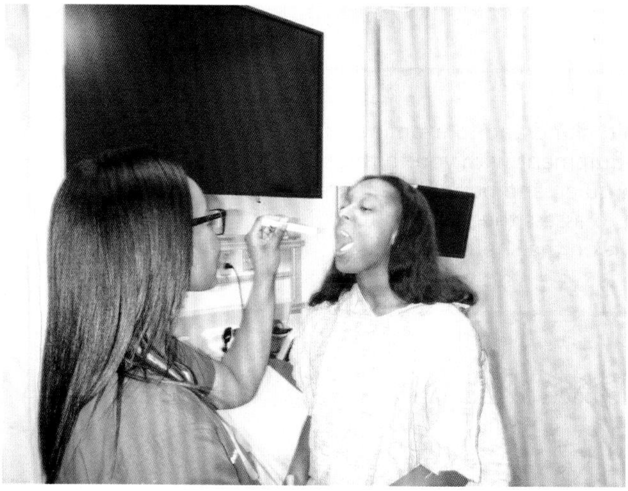

FIGURE 22-9 Inspecting the palate and uvula.

Neck

- Inspect the neck anteriorly for symmetry, masses, enlarged lymph nodes, or deviation.
- Inspect trachea position.
- Palpate the head and neck lymph nodes.
- Test sternocleidomastoid and lower trapezius muscle strength (Fig. 22-10).

CN XI is the spinal accessory nerve.

- Test head and neck range of motion (flexion, extension, rotation, and lateral flexion)

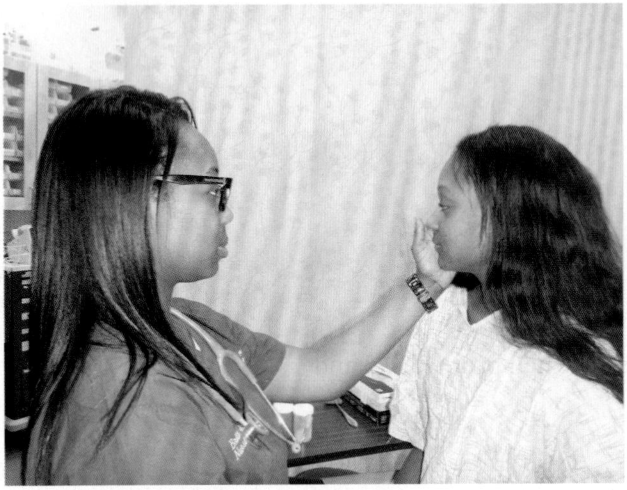

FIGURE 22-10 Testing neck strength.

- Inspect the thyroid.
- Palpate the thyroid (may be from the front or back of the patient).

CLINICAL TIP
Move behind the sitting patient to feel the thyroid gland and to examine the back, posterior thorax, and lungs. Take necessary equipment with you to the posterior to limit trips around the patient (stethoscope, ruler, and pen). Have the patient open the back of the gown to expose the back to assess the skin and to percuss and auscultate the lung fields, leaving the gown on the shoulders and covering the front of the patient.

The nurse will next move on to assessing from the back of the patient.

Posterior Thorax

- Inspect:
    - Shape
    - Deformities
    - Retractions
    - Symmetry
    - Skin integrity
- Palpate for:
    - Tenderness

- Tactile fremitus
- Respiratory expansion (Fig. 22-11)

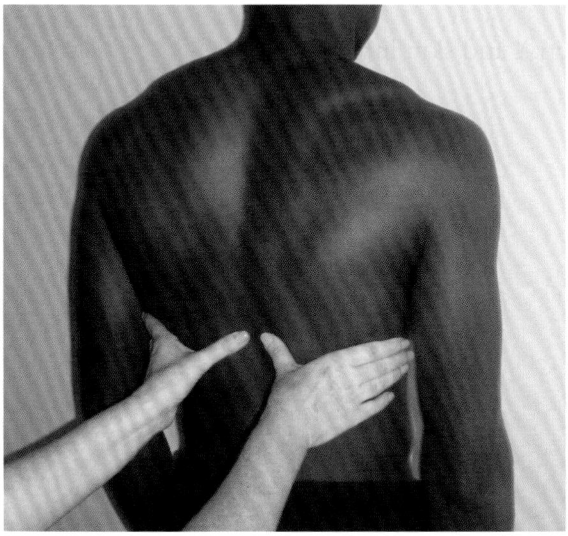

FIGURE 22-11 Assessing respiratory expansion.

- Percuss lung sounds in all fields and diaphragmatic excursion on both sides.
- Auscultate lung sounds and identify adventitious sounds and their locations (Fig. 22-12).
- Assess the cervical spine (with inspection, palpation).
- Assess for pain at the costovertebral angles (CVA tenderness).

Assess for CVA tenderness when the patient is standing or sitting.

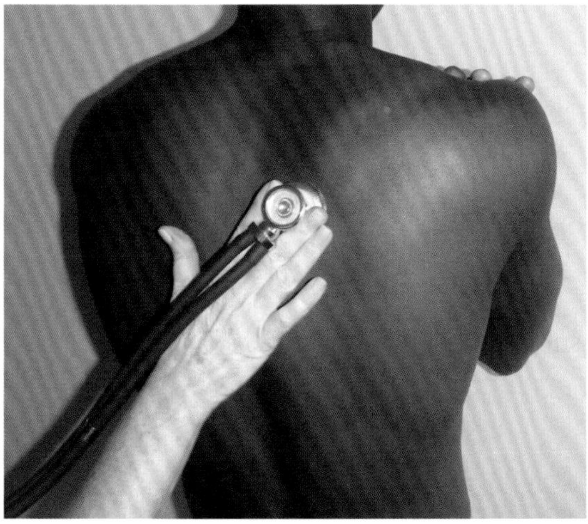

FIGURE 22-12 Auscultating lung sounds.

As the nurse returns to the front of the patient, some portions of the anterior thorax, cardiac, and breast examinations can be performed sitting or lying down.

Anterior Thorax

Assessment of the anterior thorax can be performed with the patient sitting or lying down based on the patient's condition or situation.

- Inspect for shape, deformities, retractions, symmetry, and skin integrity.
- Palpate for:
    - Tenderness
    - Tactile fremitus
    - Respiratory expansion
- Percuss sounds.
- Auscultate lung sounds.

Cardiac

The patient should be sitting for the cardiac assessment. Auscultate with the bell at the apical impulse while the patient is leaning forward to listen for aortic stenosis/murmur.

Breasts

The patient should be sitting for the inspection of the breasts. Inspect the patient with:

- The arms at the sides
- The arms raised over the head
- The hands pressed into the hips
- The patient leaning forward

Axillary Nodes

Palpate the axillary nodes (central, lateral, pectoral, subscapular).

Patient Lying Down

Cardiovascular

To assess the cardiovascular system, the head of bed or table should be elevated at a 30-degree angle. The use of tangential lighting assists with the visibility of pulsations (Fig. 22-13).

Typically, the examiner stands on the left side of the exam table next to the patient's right side.

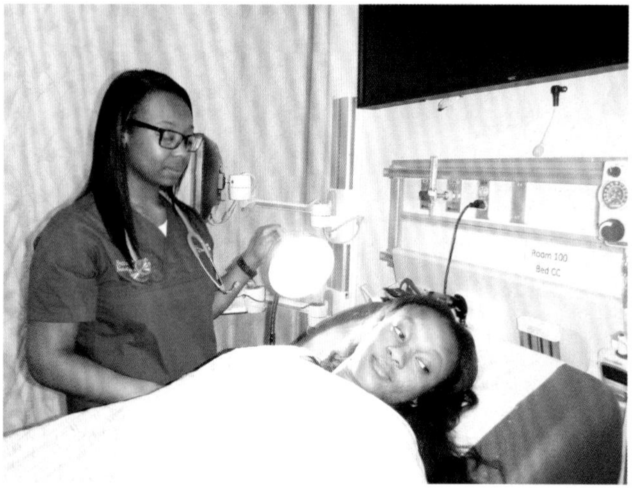

FIGURE 22-13 Table and lighting placement for assessing the cardiovascular system.

- Inspect the carotid arteries for pulsations.
- Palpate the carotid arteries.
- Auscultate the carotid artery for bruits with the bell while patient holds their breath (Fig. 22-14). Auscultate the other carotid artery with the breath held.

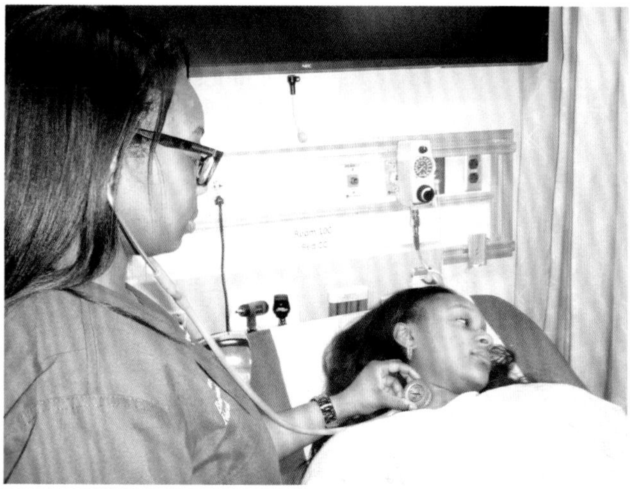

FIGURE 22-14 Auscultating the carotid artery.

- Inspect the external jugular vein.
- Inspect the precordium.
- Auscultate the heart (Fig. 22-15) with the diaphragm at the:
    - right sternal border (RSB) second intercostal space (ICS)
    - left sternal border (LSB) second ICS

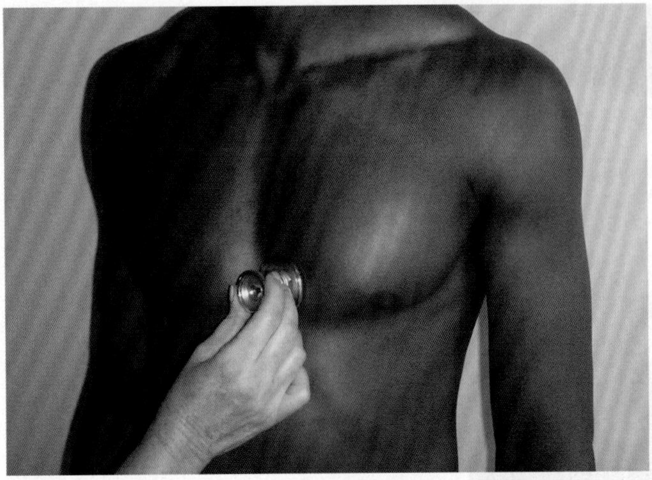

FIGURE 22-15 Auscultating the heart at the left sternal border, fourth intercostal space.

- LSB third ICS
- LSB fourth ICS
- LSB fifth ICS
- left midclavicular line (MCL) fifth ICS

- Auscultate the heart with the bell at the:
  - RSB second ICS
  - LSB second ICS
  - LSB third ICS
  - LSB fourth ICS
  - LSB fifth ICS
  - MCL fifth ICS

If patient is being followed for cardiac issues, assess the heart sounds in both the supine and left lateral positions.

- Auscultate with the bell at the apical impulse while in the left lateral decubitus position (listening for mitral murmur, S_3, S_4).

Breast Examination

- Before examining the breast, place the arm that is on the side of the breast being examined above the head and drape the opposite breast.
- Palpate the breast using the vertical pattern technique.

Abdomen

- Inspect for:
  - Contour
  - Pulsations
  - Bulges
  - Skin integrity
- Auscultate for bowel sounds and aortic pulsation (Fig. 22-16).

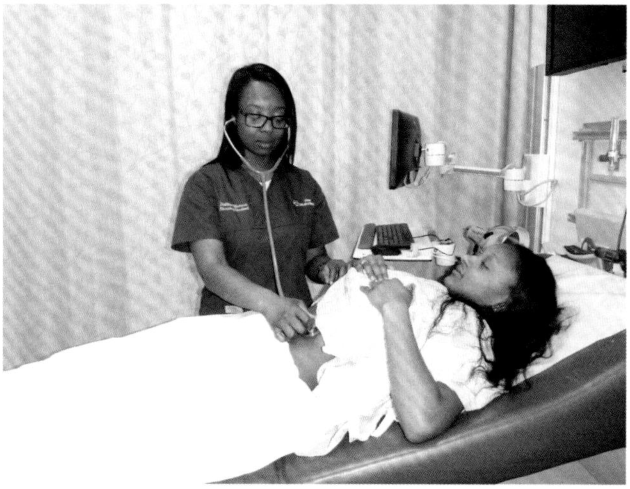

FIGURE 22-16 Auscultating the abdomen.

- Percuss abdominal sounds and liver, kidneys, and spleen.
- Abdominal reflex—lightly stroke inward in all quadrants.
- Lightly palpate all four quadrants noting masses, tenderness, and the patient's expression.
- Deeply palpate all four quadrants noting masses, tenderness, and the patient's expression.
- Palpate for the liver, kidneys, and spleen.

Peripheral Vascular

- Inspect the arms and legs for:
  - Symmetry
  - Color

  - Edema
  - Hair distribution
  - Nail bed color
- Palpate pulses
  - Radial
  - Brachial; at this time, also palpate the epitrochlear lymph nodes.
  - Femoral; at this time, also palpate the remaining lymph nodes (the inguinal vertical then horizontal groups)
  - Popliteal
  - Posterior tibial (Fig. 22-17)

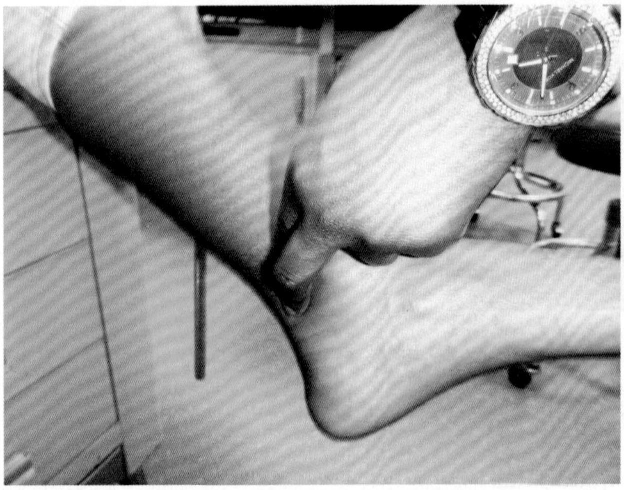

FIGURE 22-17 Palpating the posterior tibial pulse.

  - Dorsalis pedis
- Palpate for pitting edema in feet and legs.
- Palpate and assess capillary refill.

Musculoskeletal (Lower Body)

- Inspect for deformity, swelling, nodules, redness, and muscle bulk of the:
  - Hips

  - Knees
  - Ankles, feet, and toes
- Palpate for tenderness, crepitus, swelling, and increased warmth of the:
  - Hips
  - Knees
  - Ankles, feet, and toes
- Palpate strength and range of motion
  - Hips (flexion, extension, abduction, adduction, internal and external rotation)
  - Knees (flexion and extension)
  - Ankles (dorsiflexion, plantar flexion, inversion, eversion)
  - Toes (flexion, extension, abduction, adduction)

Patient Seated

Musculoskeletal—Upper Body

- Inspect for deformity, swelling, nodules, redness, and muscle bulk of the:
  - Shoulders
  - Elbows
  - Wrists, hands, and fingers
- Palpate for tenderness, crepitus, swelling, and increased warmth of the:
  - Shoulders
  - Elbows
  - Wrists, hands, and fingers
- Palpate strength and range of motion
  - Shoulders (flexion, extension, abduction, adduction, internal and external rotation)
  - Forearm (pronation, supination)

- Elbow (flexion, extension)
- Wrists (extension [dorsiflexion], flexion [palmar flexion], radial and ulnar deviation)
- Fingers (grip and flexion, extension, abduction, adduction; Fig. 22-18)
- Thumb (flexion, extension, opposition, abduction, adduction)

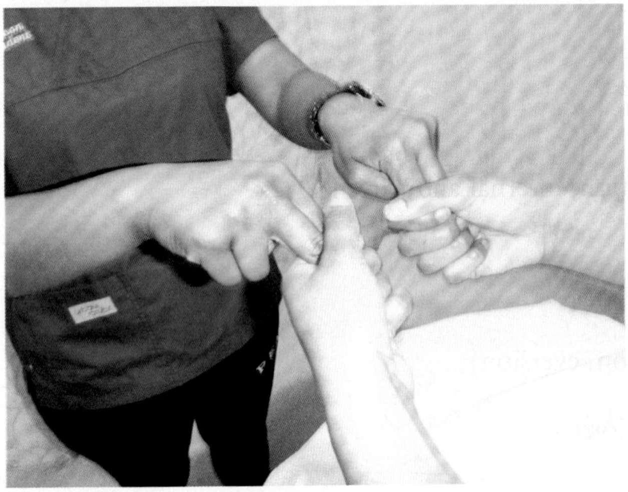

FIGURE 22-18 Assessing the patient's grip.

Neurologic—Motor

- Inspect body position, noting tremors.
- Deep tendon reflexes
  - Biceps
  - Triceps
  - Brachioradialis
  - Patellar
  - Achilles

Neurologic—Sensory

If sensory assessments were not incorporated previously, then complete them now.

- Pain and light touch—if the patient is unable to feel pain and light touch, then assess for vibration and temperature

- Position sense
- Vibration
- Stereognosis

Neurologic—Coordination

If coordination assessments were not incorporated previously, then complete them now.

- Rapid alternating movements
- Finger to nose (Fig. 22-19)

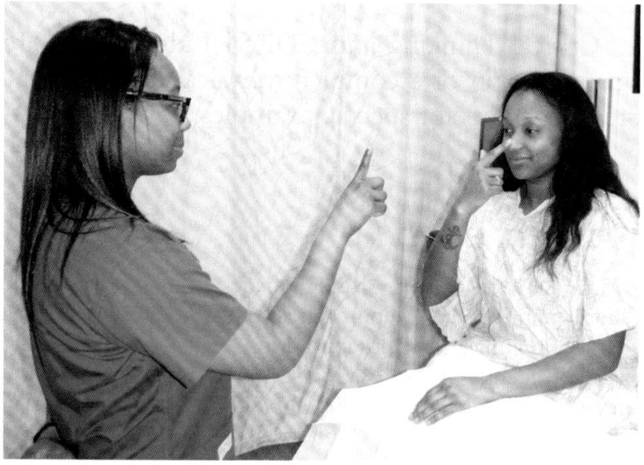

FIGURE 22-19 Finger-to-nose coordination assessment.

Patient Standing

Musculoskeletal—Spine

- Inspect for deformity, symmetry, and skin integrity.
- Palpate spinous processes.
- Assess range of motion (flexion, extension, lateral bends, rotation).

Neurologic

Perform the Romberg test (Fig. 22-20), pronator drift, gait, balance, and other appropriate neurologic screenings.

Visual Acuity

It is recommended that visual acuity be assessed at the beginning or at the end of the examination to alleviate the patient getting up another time.

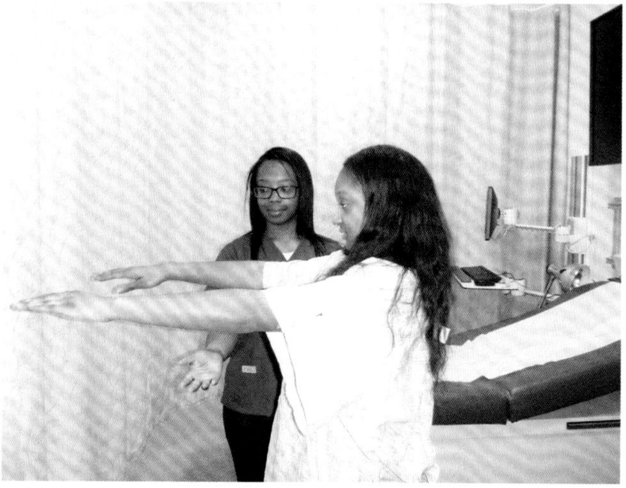

FIGURE 22-20 The Romberg test.

If a handheld Snellen chart is not available, then performing the visual acuity examination of the eye now is appropriate.

CN II is the optic nerve.

RECORDING YOUR FINDINGS

Continue to practice and refine your physical examination skills. The integration of the subjective and objective data guides the nurse in preparing the best nursing plan of care for the patient.

Refer to Chapter 2, "Critical Thinking and Clinical Judgment in Health Assessment," for documentation of a complete physical examination and each of the body systems chapters for specific examples.

ADDITIONAL READINGS

Geist, M. J., Sanders, R., Harris, K., Arce-Trigatti, A., & Hitchcock-Cass, C. (2019). Clinical immersion: An approach for fostering cross-disciplinary communication and innovation in nursing and engineering students. *Nurse Educator*, *44*(2), 69–73. https://doi.org/10.1097/NNE.0000000000000547

Kohtz, C., Brown, S. C., Williams, R., & O'Connor, P. A. (2017). Physical assessment techniques in nursing education: A replicated study. *Journal of Nursing Education*, *56*(5), 287–291. https://doi.org/10.3928/01484834-20170421-06

Osborne, S., Douglas, C., Reid, C., Jones, L., Gardner, G., & RBWH Patient Assessment Research Council. (2015). The primacy of vital signs–acute care nurses' and midwives' use of physical assessment skills: A cross sectional study. *International Journal of Nursing Studies*, *52*(5), 951–962.

Peitzman, S. J., & Cuddy, M. A. (2015). Performance in physical examination on the USMLE step 2 clinical skills examination. *Academic Medicine*, *90*(2), 209–213.

Storey, S., Wagnes, L., LaMothe, J., Pittman, J., Cohee, A., & Newhouse, R. (2019). Building evidence-based nursing practice capacity in a large statewide health system: A multimodal approach. *The Journal of Nursing Administration*, *49*(4), 208–214. https://doi.org/10.1097/nna.0000000000000739

Tawalbeh, L. I. (2017). Effect of simulation on the confidence of university nursing students in applying cardiopulmonary assessment skills: A randomized controlled trial. *The Journal of Nursing Research?: JNR*, *25*(4), 289–295. https://doi.org/10.1097/jnr.0000000000000170

Verghese, A., Charlton, B., Kassirer, J. P., Ramsey, M., & Ioannidis, J. P. A. (2015). Inadequacies of physical examination as a cause of medical errors and adverse events: A collection of vignettes. *The American Journal of Medicine*, *128*(12), 1322–1324.e3.

UNIT 3

Special Lifespan

23 ASSESSING CHILDREN: INFANCY THROUGH ADOLESCENCE

KEY TERMS

amblyopia	hypospadias	talipes equinovarus
Babinski response	metatarsus adductus	Tanner sexual maturity rating (SMR)
bronchiolitis	paradoxical breathing	thelarche
circumcision	pectus excavatum	thrills
diastasis recti	plagiocephaly	tibial torsion
edentulous	retractions	tripod position
hydrocele	scoliosis	
hydrocephalus	spina bifida occulta	

Learning Objectives

The student will:

1. Identify education topics for anticipatory guidance, health promotion, and risk reduction.
2. Perform a developmental assessment on infants, children, and adolescents.
3. Obtain a history of an infant, child, and adolescent.
4. Use age-appropriate techniques to perform a physical examination on infants, children, and adolescents.
5. Analyze findings against age-appropriate norms and standards.
6. Correctly document infant, child, and adolescent assessment findings.

This chapter begins with general principles of development and key components of health promotion. It then has sections on infants, young and school-aged children, and adolescents, with relevant discussions of history taking, development, physical examination, health promotion and counseling, and for each (Fig. 23-1).

Often, students are intimidated when approaching a tiny baby or a screaming child, especially under the critical eyes of anxious parents.

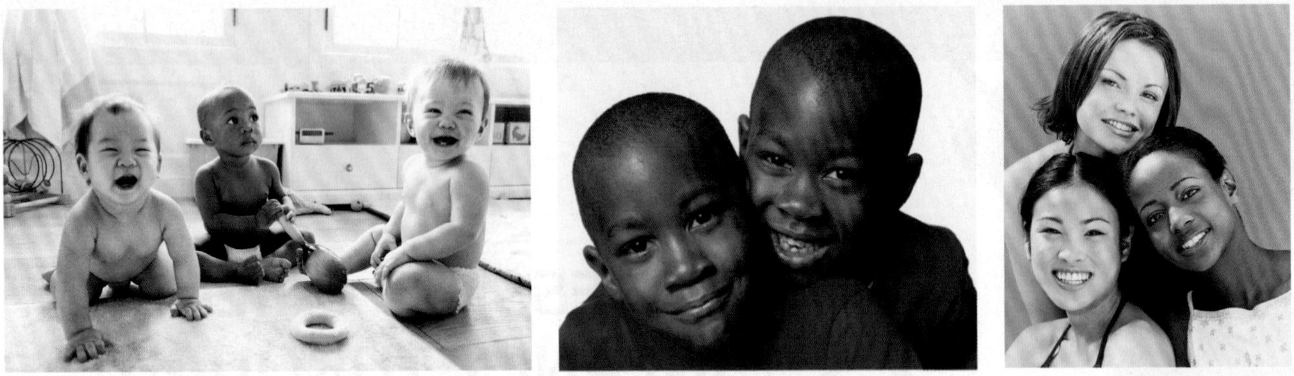

FIGURE 23-1 Health assessment varies for children of different ages. (Left: Rawpixel.com/Shutterstock)

When examining infants and children, the sequence should vary according to the child's age and comfort level. *Perform nondisturbing maneuvers early and potentially distressing maneuvers near the end of the examination.* For example, palpate the head and neck and auscultate the heart and lungs early (Fig. 23-2), and examine the ears and mouth and palpate the abdomen near the end. If the child reports pain in one area, examine that part last.

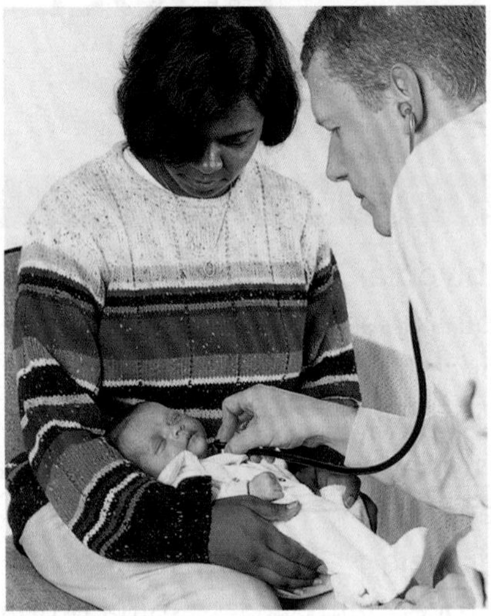

FIGURE 23-2 Auscultate the heart and lungs early, leaving more distressing maneuvers for the end of the examination.

The format of the pediatric medical record is the same as that of the adult record. Although the sequence of the physical examination may vary, convert your clinical findings into the traditional documentation format.

GENERAL PRINCIPLES OF CHILD DEVELOPMENT

Childhood is a period of remarkable physical, cognitive, and social growth—by far the greatest in a person's lifetime (Fig. 23-3). Within a few short years, a child's size increases 20-fold, they acquire sophisticated language and reasoning, they develop complex social interactions, and they progress toward mature adulthood.

Understanding the normal physical, cognitive, and social development of children facilitates effective interviews and physical examinations and helps nurses distinguish normal and abnormal findings.

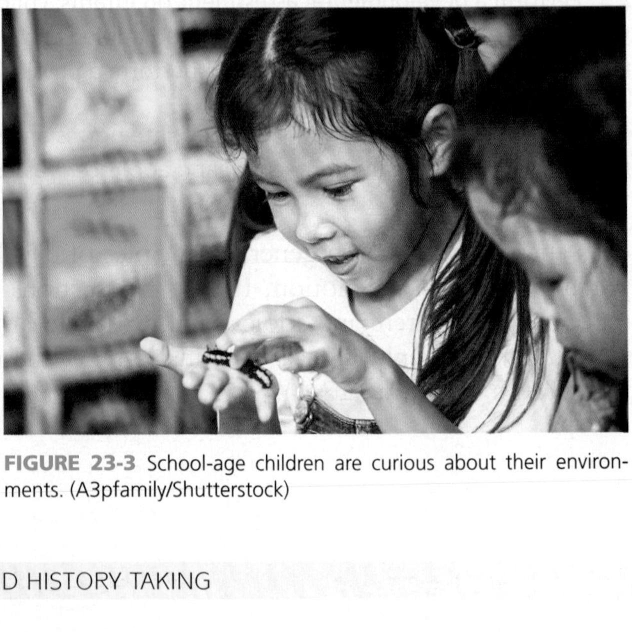

FIGURE 23-3 School-age children are curious about their environments. (A3pfamily/Shutterstock)

Four principles are true of child development:

1. Child development proceeds along a predictable pathway.
2. The range of normal development is wide.
3. Various physical, social, and environmental factors, as well as diseases, can affect child development and health.
4. The child's developmental level affects how you conduct the history and physical examination.

Child development proceeds along a predictable pathway governed by the maturing brain. You can measure age-specific milestones and characterize development as normal or abnormal according to the child's achievement of them (Fig. 23-4). Because the child's health visit and physical examination takes place at one point in time, determine where the child fits along a developmental trajectory. Milestones are achieved in an order that can be anticipated. Loss of milestones is always concerning.

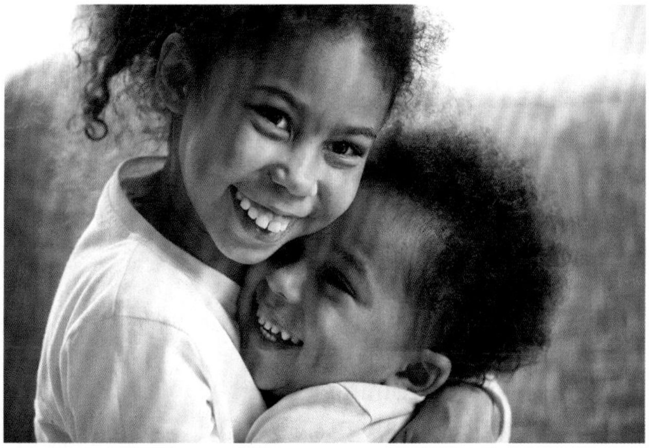

FIGURE 23-4 Developmental milestones are achieved in a predictable order. (fizkes/Shutterstock)

The range of normal development is wide. Children mature at different rates. Each child's physical, cognitive, and social development should fall within a broad developmental range.

Various physical, social, and environmental factors, as well as diseases, can affect child development and health. For example, chronic illnesses, child abuse, and poverty can all cause detectable physical abnormalities and alter the rate and course of development. Additionally, children with physical or cognitive disabilities may not follow the expected age-specific developmental trajectory (Fig. 23-5). Tailor the physical examination to the child's developmental level.

The child's developmental level affects how you conduct the history and physical examination. For example, interviewing a 5-year-old is fundamentally different than interviewing an adolescent. Before performing a physical examination, attempt to ascertain the child's approximate developmental level and adapt your physical examination to that level. An understanding of normal child development helps you make those decisions.

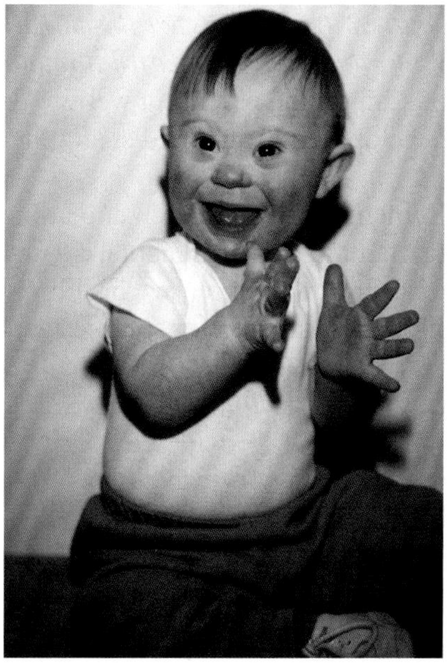

FIGURE 23-5 Child development is affected by many factors, including genetic conditions like Down syndrome.

HEALTH PROMOTION AND COUNSELING: KEY COMPONENTS

Benjamin Franklin noted that "an ounce of prevention is worth a pound of cure." This adage is particularly true for children and adolescents because prevention and health promotion at a young age can result in improved health outcomes for decades. Pediatric clinicians dedicate substantial time to health supervision visits and health promotion activities.

The American Academy of Pediatrics (AAP) has developed guidelines for health promotion for children (AAP, 2020; Hagan et al., 2017). Current concepts of health promotion for children include the detection and prevention of disease as well as active promotion of the well-being of children and their families, spanning physical, cognitive, emotional, and social health.

Children facing injury, surgery, hospitalization or invasive medical procedures may be frightened by the experience resulting in pediatric medical traumatic stress, "a set of psychological and physiological responses of children and their families to medical experiences". Nurses should consider the role of medical traumatic stress as well as the potential impact of prior trauma, when caring for pediatric patients and their families. More information can be found at www.HealthCareToolbox.org

Every interaction with a child and family is an opportunity for health promotion. From the interview to the physical examination, think about your interactions as opportunities for two things: the traditional detection of medical problems and the promotion of health. Capitalize on your examination to offer age-appropriate guidance about the child's development. Provide suggestions about reading, conversing, playing music, and optimizing opportunities for gross and fine motor development. Advise parents about upcoming developmental stages and strategies to encourage their child's development (Fig. 23-6). *Parents are the major agents of health promotion for children, and your advice is implemented through them.* The AAP created HealthyChildren.org, an online parenting website to provide information about healthy living, developmental ages and stages, health issues, and more.

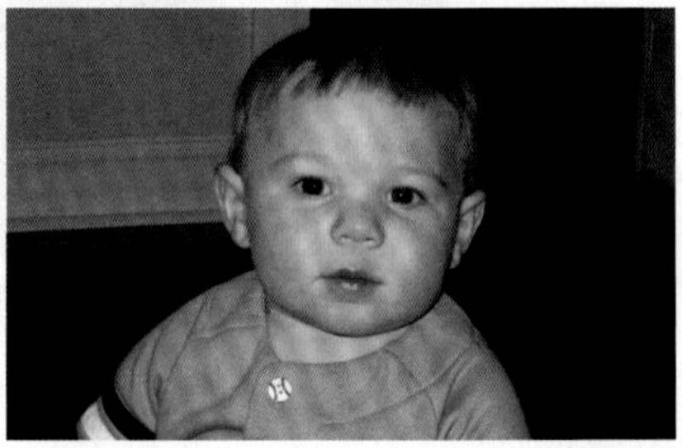

FIGURE 23-6 The older infant enjoys watching people.

Remember that children and adolescents who have chronic illnesses or high-risk family or environmental circumstances will probably require more frequent visits and more intensive health promotion. Key health promotion issues and strategies, tailored for specific age groups, are found throughout this chapter.

Integrate explanations of your physical findings with health promotion. For example, provide advice about expected maturational changes or how health behaviors can affect physical findings (e.g., exercise may reduce blood pressure and prevent obesity). Be sure to explain the relationship between healthy lifestyles and physical health.

Childhood immunizations are a mainstay of health promotion and have been praised as the most significant medical achievement of public health worldwide. The childhood immunization schedule changes yearly, and updates are published widely and disseminated on websites of the

Centers for Disease Control and Prevention (CDC) and the AAP (AAP, 2021; CDC, 2021). To view the most current immunization schedule, visit www.cdc.gov/vaccines.

Screening procedures are performed at specific ages. For all children, these include growth parameters and developmental screening at all ages—blood pressure after age 3, body mass index (BMI) screening after age 2, vision and hearing screening at key ages, and behavioral and mental health screening. Increasingly, standardized screening instruments are being used to assist clinicians in identifying abnormalities. In addition, screening procedures particularly recommended for all children at certain ages or for specific high-risk patients include tests for lead poisoning, tuberculosis exposure, anemia, dyslipidemia, urinary tract infections, and sexually transmitted infections. There is variation worldwide in recommendations for screening tests; the AAP recommendations are provided at www.aap.org.

Anticipatory guidance is a major component of the pediatric visit (AAP, 2020). Key areas for health promotion cover a broad range of topics, from purely "medical" to developmental, social, and emotional health (Box 23-1). All these factors affect children's health.

FIGURE 23-7 Infants usually learn to walk at about 1 year.

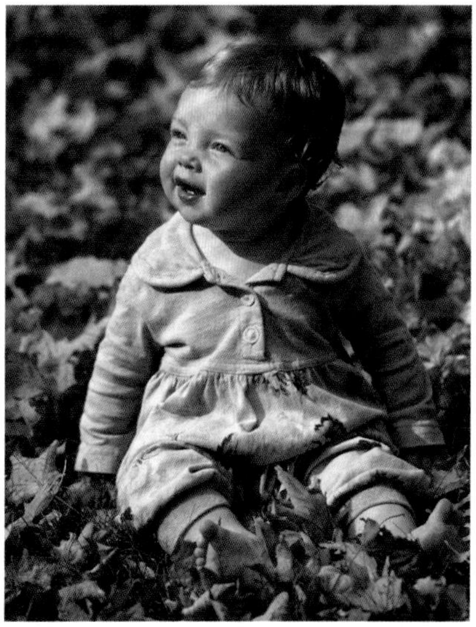

FIGURE 23-8 Exposing infants to new experiences promotes cognitive development.

BOX 23-1 KEY COMPONENTS OF PEDIATRIC HEALTH PROMOTION

1. Age-appropriate developmental achievement of the child
   - Physical (maturation, growth, puberty)
   - Motor (gross and fine motor skills) (Fig. 23-7)
   - Cognitive (achievement of milestones, language, school performance) (Fig. 23-8)
   - Emotional (self-regulation, mood, temperament, self-efficacy, self-esteem, independence)
   - Social (social competence, self-responsibility, integration with family and community, peer interactions)
2. Health supervision visits
   - Periodic assessment of medical and oral health
   - Children with special health care needs often require more frequent health supervision visits
3. Integration of physical examination findings with healthy lifestyle recommendations
4. Immunizations
5. Screening procedures
6. Anticipatory guidance (AAP, 2020)
   - Healthy habits
   - Nutrition and healthy eating
   - Safety and prevention of injury or illness
   - Sexual development and sexuality
   - Self-responsibility, efficacy, and healthy self-esteem
   - Family relationships (interactions, strengths, supports)
   - Positive parenting strategies
   - Emotional and mental health
   - Oral health
   - Recognition of illness
   - Sleep
   - Prevention of risky behaviors (e.g., tobacco, alcohol and drug use, unprotected sex)
   - School and vocation
   - Peer relationships
   - Community interactions
7. Partnership among health care provider, child/adolescent, and family

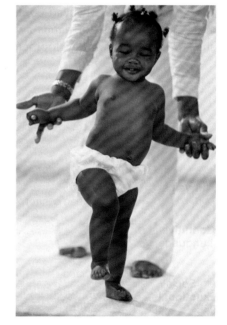

ASSESSING THE INFANT

Development

Physical Development (Johnson & Blasco, 1997)

Physical growth during infancy is faster than at any other age. By 1 year, the infant's birth weight should have tripled and height increased by 50% from birth.

Newborns have surprising abilities, such as fixing upon and following human faces. Neurologic development progresses centrally to peripherally. Thus, newborns learn head control before trunk control and use of arms and legs before use of hands and fingers. Figure 23-9 noting milestones shows the significant developmental progression in infancy.

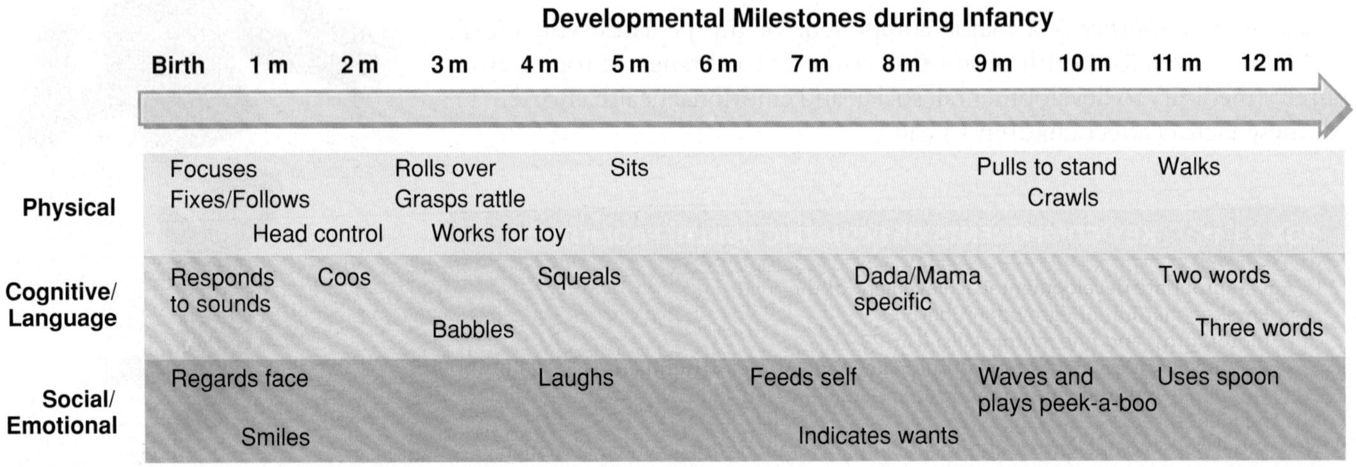

FIGURE 23-9 Developmental milestones during infancy.

Activity, exploration, and environmental manipulation contribute to learning. By 3 months, normal infants lift the head and clasp the hands. By 6 months, they roll over, reach for objects, turn to voices, and possibly sit with support. With increasing peripheral coordination, infants reach for objects, transfer them from hand to hand, crawl, stand by holding on, and play with objects by banging and grabbing. A 1-year-old child may be standing and putting objects in their mouth (Colson & Dworkin, 1997).

Cognitive and Language Development

Exploration fosters increased understanding of self and environment. Infants learn cause and effect (e.g., shaking a rattle produces sound), object permanence, and use of tools. By 9 months, they may recognize the examiner as a stranger deserving wary cooperation, seek comfort from parents during examinations, and actively manipulate reachable objects (e.g., equipment). Language development proceeds from cooing at 2 months, to babbling at 6 months, to saying one to three words by 1 year (Copelan, 1995).

Social and Emotional Development

Understanding of self and family also matures. Social tasks include bonding, attachment to caregivers, and trust that caregivers will meet their needs. Temperaments vary. Some infants are predictable, adaptable, and respond positively to new stimuli; others are less so and respond intensely or negatively. Because environment affects social development, observe the infant's interactions with caregivers.

The Health History

The health history is an important tool for assessing health, growth, and development. After a full history is obtained, subsequent visits should ask about the child's health, growth, development, and health patterns as well as other changes (e.g., family life) since the previous visit.

Birth History

At the initial appointment, ask the parent about the pregnancy and birth:

- Were there any problems during the pregnancy?
- Did the mother use alcohol during pregnancy? If yes, when, how often, and how much?
- Did the mother use any medications, drugs, or supplements during pregnancy? If yes, what, how much, and when?
- How close was the infant's birth to the due date?
- Were there any problems during labor or birth?
- Was the child born vaginally or by cesarean section (C-section)?

Past History

At the first visit of the infant to the health care practice or clinic, ask where the infant was seen before, when, and for what reasons. Also ask:

- Does the child have any allergies?
- Are they on any medications, including vitamins or fluoride drops?
- Have they had any illnesses? Ask the parent to describe the illness, treatment, and outcome.

Family History

The family history may reveal hereditary disease patterns. Inquire about the age and health status of siblings, parents, grandparents, aunts, and uncles. A genogram is helpful to trace patterns emerging within a family.

Also inquire about *family structure*. Who lives in the house with the infant? What is their relationship to the infant?

Health Maintenance

- *Immunizations*—What immunizations has the infant had? Did they have any reaction to the "shots"?
- *Safety measures*—Inquire about the baby's position during sleep, blankets or toys in crib, use of car seats, and presence of smoke and carbon monoxide detectors in the house.
- *Risk factors*—The infant's environment may be affected by the parent's behaviors; therefore, inquire about:
    - *Tobacco*—Do you smoke or vape? In the house? In the presence of the infant? Does anyone else in your house smoke?
    - *Alcohol*—Do you or your partner drink alcoholic beverages? How much alcohol do you drink per sitting and per week?
    - *Substance abuse*—Do you or your partner use marijuana, cocaine, heroin, or other recreational drugs?
    - *Environmental hazards*—Inquire about lead paint, asbestos insulation or tiles, or other household hazards.

Conduct a review of systems, asking the parent about each system in turn.

When the review is complete, ask the parent if they have any concerns about their infant. Then move on to the infant's developmental status according to the infant's age. For example, ask the parent of a 6-month-old if they can sit alone. Inquire at what age the infant achieved each milestone.

Health Patterns

Complete the history by asking about the infant's health patterns:

- *Nutrition*—What does the infant drink? How many ounces at one time? Or how long does the infant nurse at each breast? How many times a day? Does the infant eat cereal or other foods? Does the infant have any problems during or after feedings?

- *Elimination*—Describe your infant's typical urination pattern and bowel pattern, including amount, consistency, and number.

- *Sleep*—Tell me about your infant's sleep pattern (including time of day the infant sleeps and hours of sleep). Do you, another family member, or a pet ever sleep with the child?

- *Activity/Play*—What amuses your infant? How do you play with your infant?

Approaching the Infant

Use developmentally appropriate methods such as *distraction* and *play* to examine the infant. Because infants pay attention to one thing at a time, it is relatively easy to distract the infant's attention from the examination as it is being performed. Distract the infant with a moving object, a flashing light, a game of peek-a-boo, or any sort of noise. Tips for examining infants are summarized in Box 23-2.

If you cannot distract the infant or engage the awake infant with an object, your face, or a sound, consider a possible *visual* or *hearing deficit.*

BOX 23-2 TIPS FOR EXAMINING INFANTS

- Approach the infant gradually using a toy or object for distraction.
- Perform as much of the examination as possible with the infant in the parent's lap.
- Speak softly to the infant or mimic the infant's sounds to attract attention.
- If the infant is cranky, make sure they are well fed before proceeding.
- Ask the parent about the infant's strengths to elicit useful developmental and parenting information.
- Do not expect to do a head-to-toe examination in a specific order. Work with what the infant gives you and save the mouth and ear examination for last.

General Guidelines

Start with the infant sitting or lying in the parent's lap. If the infant is tired, hungry, or ill, ask the parent to hold the baby against the parent's chest. Make sure appropriate toys, a blanket, or other familiar objects are nearby (Fig. 23-10). A hungry infant may need to be fed before initiating the examination.

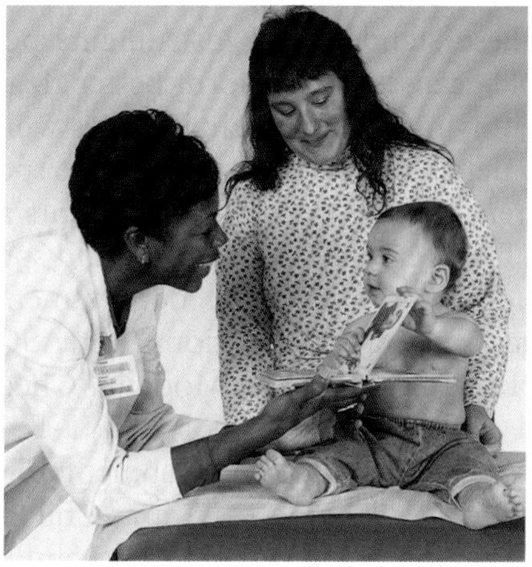

FIGURE 23-10 A toy or book can be used to distract the infant during the examination.

Close observation of an awake infant sitting on the parent's lap can reveal potential abnormalities such as *hypotonia* or *hypertonia,* conditions with abnormal skin color, jaundice or cyanosis, jitteriness, or respiratory problems.

Observe parent–infant interactions. Watch the parent's affect when talking about the infant. Note the parent's manner of holding, moving, dressing, and comforting the infant. Assess and comment on positive interactions, such as the pride in the parent's face in Figure 23-10.

Observation of the infant's communication with the parent can reveal abnormalities such as *developmental delay, language delay, hearing deficits,* or *inadequate parental attachment.* Likewise, such observations may identify maladaptive nurturing patterns that may stem from *maternal depression* or *inadequate social support.*

Infants usually do not object to having their clothing removed. To keep yourself and your surroundings dry, it is wise to leave the diaper in place throughout the examination; remove it only to examine the skin underneath, genitals, rectum, lower spine, and hips.

Testing for Developmental Milestones

Because you will want to measure the infant's best performance, checking milestones is best at the end of the interview, just before the examination. This "fun and games" interlude also enhances cooperation during the examination. Experienced nurses can weave the developmental examination into the other parts of the examination. Figure 23-9 shows some key physical or motor, cognitive or language, and social–emotional milestones during the first year. As an example, the infant in Figure 23-10 can sit unsupported, uses a thumb-finger grasp, and is indicating wants—an 8-month level.

Many disorders cause delays in more than one milestone. For most children with developmental delay, the causes are unknown. Some known causes include *abnormality in embryonic development* (e.g., prenatal insult, chromosomal problem), *hereditary and genetic disorders* (e.g., inborn errors, genetic abnormalities), *environmental and social problems* (e.g., insufficient stimulation), *pregnancy or perinatal problems* (e.g., placental insufficiency, prematurity), and *childhood diseases* (e.g., infection, trauma, chronic illness).

The AAP recommends health care providers use a standardized developmental screening instrument for infants as young as several months of age (Hagan et al., 2017). Several developmental screening instruments have been tested widely and validated in many nations (Perrin & Sheldrick, 2013). In general, these instruments assess *five critical domains of infant/child development: gross motor, fine motor, cognitive (or problem-solving), communication, and personal/social domains of development.* Pediatric health providers are recommended to use these standardized instruments periodically during preventive health visits because they perform better than a clinician's physical examination in identifying developmental delays which can often be subtle and challenging to determine because of the wide spectrum of normal development in children. These screening instruments are practical to use in clinical settings and have reasonable sensitivity and specificity for identifying developmental delays. Some useful developmental screening instruments include the Ages and Stages Questionnaire (ASQ), the Early Language Milestone Scale (ELM Scale-2), the Modified Checklist for Autism in Toddlers, Revised with Follow-Up (M-CHAT-R/F) (Dunlap & Filipek, 2020), the Parents' Evaluation of Developmental Status (PEDS), Denver II, and the Survey of Well-Being of Young Children (SWYC). Combined with your findings on interview and physical examination, results from these screening tests can help determine an appropriate management strategy.

If a cooperative infant fails items on a standardized developmental screening instrument, developmental delay is possible, necessitating more precise testing and evaluation.

Autism spectrum disorder (ASD) is a neurodevelopmental disorder that affects communication and behavior. People with ASD have difficulty with social communication and interaction, restricted interests, and repetitive behaviors. It is the fastest growing developmental disorder in the United States. Routine developmental screening is key to early identification. In 2016, the AAP recommended expanding routine screening to include ASD-specific screening (Christensen & Zubler, 2020; NIH. National Institute of Mental Health, 2018).

Parental reports of unusual behaviors have been found to be significant predictors of later ASD diagnoses. Symptoms generally appear in the first 2 years of life; therefore, it is important to begin screening children early. The M-CHAT-R/F can be used as a screening tool and is available at no cost at https://mchatscreen.com. It may also be taken online for free at https://www.autismspeaks.org/screen-your-child.

Use screening instruments as an adjunct to a comprehensive developmental examination. Suspected delays from the general examination or developmental screening instruments warrant further evaluation by a developmental pediatrician, child neurologist, and/or child psychiatrist or psychologist. For babies born prematurely, adjust expected developmental milestones for the gestational age up to approximately 24 months.

Physical Examination of the Infant

General Survey and Vital Signs

Measure the infant's body size (length, weight, and head circumference) and vital signs (blood pressure, starting age 3; pulse; respiratory rate; and temperature). Compare vital signs or body proportions with age-specific norms, because they change dramatically as children grow.

Pain Assessment

A child's pain may be due to disease, accident, surgery, or medical procedures. It may be acute or chronic. Unrelieved pain may lead to psychological stress and trauma. Pain may interrupt school, social, and family activities. Younger children may cry or hold still and try not to move. They may have poor appetite or be irritable or cranky. They may not be able to sleep well, or they may want to sleep a lot. When obtaining the history of an infant or young child, ask the parent how they know when their child is in pain. What word(s) does the child use for pain? A few common words to indicate pain are "hurt," "owie," and "boo-boo" (Freund & Bolick, 2019; Quinn et al., 2018).

Nurses must assess children's pain at regular intervals and whenever they observe changes in a child's behavior. There are many pain assessment tools for children; the nurse must select the best tool for the child's age, developmental level, cognitive level, and their level of consciousness.

The Neonatal Infant Pain Scale (NIPS) can be used in children younger than 1 year of age. The FLACC (face, legs, activity, cry, consolability) Pain Scale can be used for children 1 to 3 years of age.

Somatic Growth

Measurement of growth is one of the most important indicators of infant health. Deviations may provide an early indication of an underlying problem. Compare growth parameters with respect to:

- Normal values for age and sex
- Prior readings on the same child to assess trends

CLINICAL TIP
Variations beyond two standard deviations for age, or above the 95th percentile or below the 5th percentile, are indications for more detailed evaluation. These deviations may be the first and only indicators of disease.

Measure growth parameters carefully, using consistent technique and, optimally, the same scales to measure weight and a standardized infant length board to measure length.

A common cause of an apparent deviation in somatic growth is *measurement error,* attributed partly to the challenge of measuring a squirming infant or child. Confirm abnormalities with repeat measurement.

The most important tools for assessing somatic growth are the growth charts published by the National Center for Health Statistics and the World Health Organization (WHO) (CDC. National Center for Health Statistics, 2010, 2016). All charts include length, weight, and head circumference for age for children up to 36 months as well as height and weight for children 2 to 18 years of age. Charts plotting BMI are also available. These growth charts have percentile lines indicating the percentage of normally developed children above and below the child's measurement by chronologic age. Special growth charts are available for use in infants born prematurely to adjust for the earlier birth.

Although many healthy infants cross percentiles on growth charts, a sudden or significant change in growth may indicate systemic disease or inappropriate feeding.

Abnormalities that can cause deviation from normal growth patterns include *Down syndrome* or *prematurity.* Growth charts are also available for children with specific conditions such as *Down syndrome* or *Turner syndrome.*

The AAP, National Institutes of Health (NIH), and CDC now recommend that clinicians use the 2009 WHO international growth charts for children 0 to 2 years of age. CDC growth charts should be used in the United States to assess growth in children 2 to 19 years of age.

Length

For children younger than 2 years, two people are needed to measure body length. Place the child supine on a length board, as shown in Figure 23-11. Direct measurement of the infant using a tape measure or drawing on the paper on an examination table is inaccurate. Velocity growth curves are helpful for older children, especially those who are suspected of having endocrine disorders.

Reduced growth velocity, shown by a drop in height percentile on a growth curve, may signify a chronic condition. Comparison with normal standards is essential, because growth velocity normally is less during the second year than during the first year.

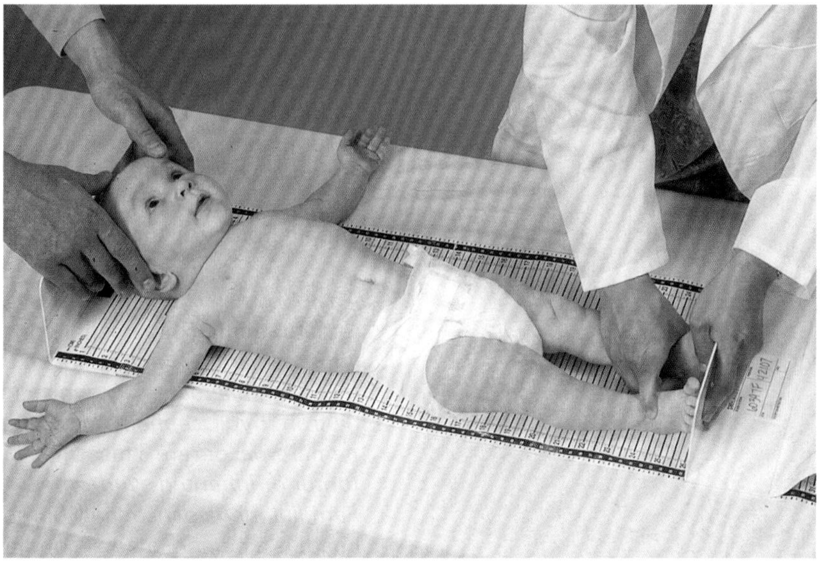

FIGURE 23-11 Two people are needed to accurately measure the infant's length.

Chronic conditions causing reduced length or height include *neurologic, renal, cardiac, gastrointestinal*, and *endocrine disorders* as well as *cystic fibrosis.*

Weight

Weigh infants directly with an infant scale (Fig. 23-12); this is more accurate than an indirect method based on weighing the parent and child together and subtracting the weight of the parent from the total weight. Infants should be clothed only in a dry diaper or weighed naked. The nurse should stand close to the scale, ready to prevent a fall by a squirming infant.

Failure to thrive is inadequate weight gain for age. Common scenarios are:

- Growth below fifth percentile for age
- Growth drop greater than two quartiles in 6 months
- Weight for height below fifth percentile

Causes include environmental or psychosocial factors and a variety of gastrointestinal, neurologic, cardiac, endocrine, renal, and other diseases.

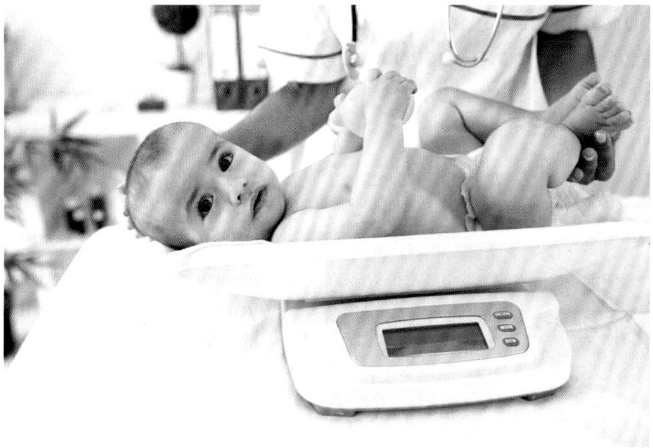

FIGURE 23-12 The nurse weighs an infant on an electronic infant scale. (didesign021/Shutterstock)

If the infant's weight is unexpectedly and significantly different than anticipated, redo the measurement to ensure accuracy.

Head Circumference

Head circumference should always be measured during the first 2 years of life, but measurement can be useful at any age to assess growth of the head. The head circumference in infants reflects the rate of growth of the cranium and the brain. Measuring the circumference of the head with a nonelastic tape measure just above the ears, as seen in Figure 23-13, produces the most accurate results.

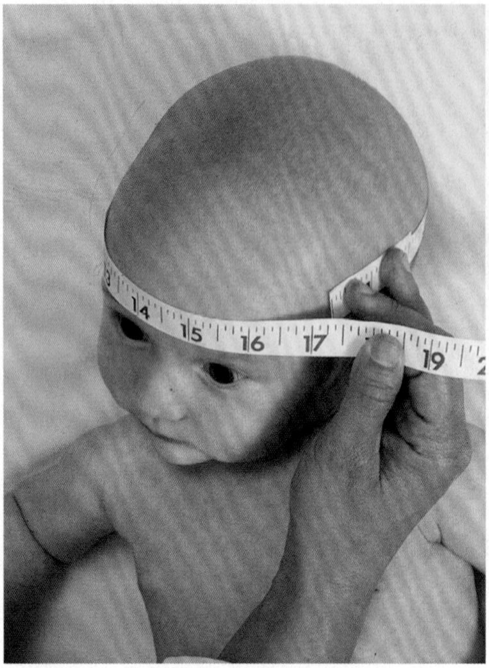

FIGURE 23-13 Measuring an infant's head circumference.

A small head size may be from premature closure of the sutures or microcephaly. Microcephaly may be familial or the result of various chromosomal abnormalities, congenital infections (e.g., Zika virus), maternal metabolic disorders, and neurologic insults.

An abnormally large head size (greater than 97th percentile or two standard deviations above the mean) is *macrocephaly,* which may be from *hydrocephalus, subdural hematoma,* or rare causes like *brain tumor or inherited syndromes. Familial megaloencephaly* (large head) is a benign familial condition with normal brain growth.

Vital Signs

Blood Pressure

Although obtaining accurate blood pressure readings in infants can be challenging, this measurement is nevertheless important for some high-risk infants and should be performed routinely after age 3. You will need your skills in distraction or play, as shown in Figure 23-14.

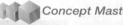

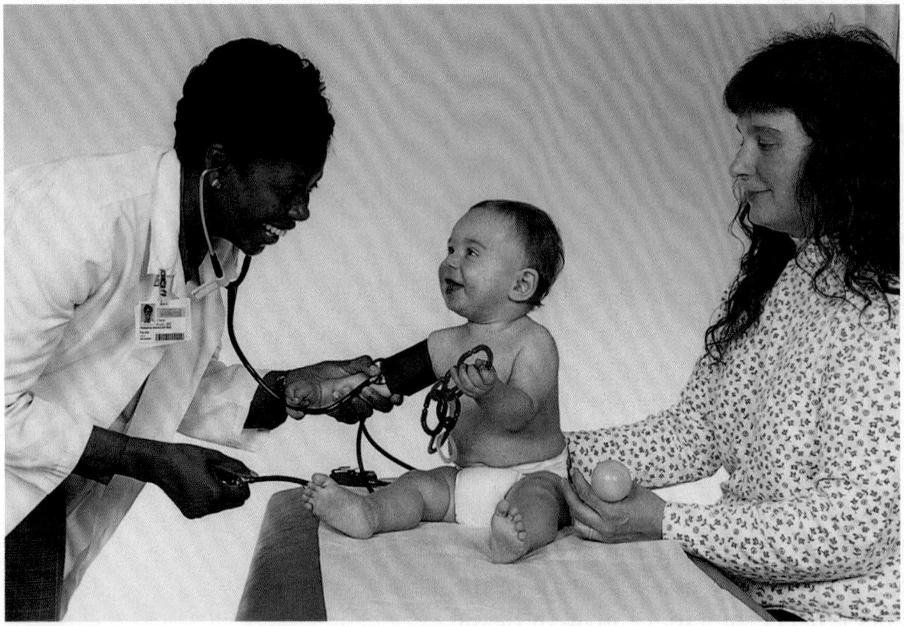

FIGURE 23-14 Using a toy to distract the infant during blood pressure measurement.

Concept Mastery Alert

Ensuring Blood Pressure Accuracy

In any patient, but especially a young child or infant, it is always important to further assess any abnormal finding, such as blood pressure to ensure that the finding is accurate. Before proceeding with checking the blood pressure in the other arm, the nurse should confirm that the blood pressure cuff was the correct size for the child. The nurse must ensure that the cuff covers two-thirds of the upper arm before completing a further assessment.

Electronic blood pressure machines are commonly used today for infants. Be sure to choose the correct size cuff, apply it correctly, and control the child's movement in order to obtain a correct measurement (Fig. 23-15).

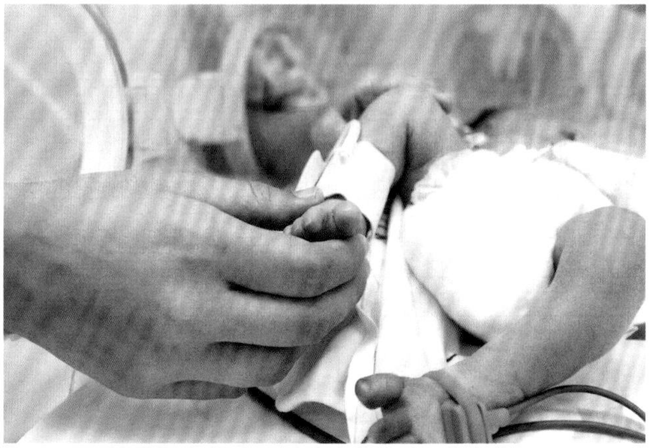

FIGURE 23-15 Using an electronic blood pressure machine for a neonate in an incubator. (July Semianovich/Shutterstock)

The systolic blood pressure gradually increases throughout childhood. For example, normal systolic pressure in male infants is about 70 mm Hg at birth, 85 mm Hg at 1 month, and 90 mm Hg at 6 months (NIH. National Heart, Lung, & Blood Institute, 2005). The prevalence of elevated blood pressure and hypertension in children and adolescents has increased over the past decade. This trend is most likely related to increases in primary hypertension associated with increasing obesity rates in children (Matossian, 2018).

Causes of *sustained hypertension* in infants include renal artery disease (stenosis, thrombosis), congenital renal malformations, and coarctation of the aorta.

Pulse

The heart rate of infants is more sensitive to the effects of illness, exercise, and emotion than that of adults. Average infant heart rates are listed in Table 23-1, and abnormalities in pulse and blood pressure are outlined in Table 23-2.

TABLE 23-1 Heart Rates from Birth to 1 Year

Age	Average Heart Rate	Range per min
Birth–2 mo	140	90–165
0–6 mo	130	80–175
6–12 mo	115	75–170

Source: Fleming, S., Thompson, M., Stevens, R., Heneghan, C., Plüddemann, A., Maconochie, I., Tarassenko, L., & Mant, D. (2011). Normal ranges of heart rate and respiratory rate in children from birth to 18 years of age: A systematic review of observational studies. *Lancet, 377*(9770), 1011–1018.

TABLE 23-2 Abnormalities in Heart Rhythm and Blood Pressure

Supraventricular Tachycardia

Paroxysmal supraventricular tachycardia (SVT) is the most common dysrhythmia in children. Some infants with SVT look well or may be somewhat pale with tachypnea but have a heart rate of 240 beats per minute or greater. Others are ill and in cardiovascular collapse.

SVT in infants is usually sustained, requiring medical therapy for conversion to a normal rate and rhythm. In older children, it is more likely to be truly paroxysmal, with episodes of varying duration and frequency.

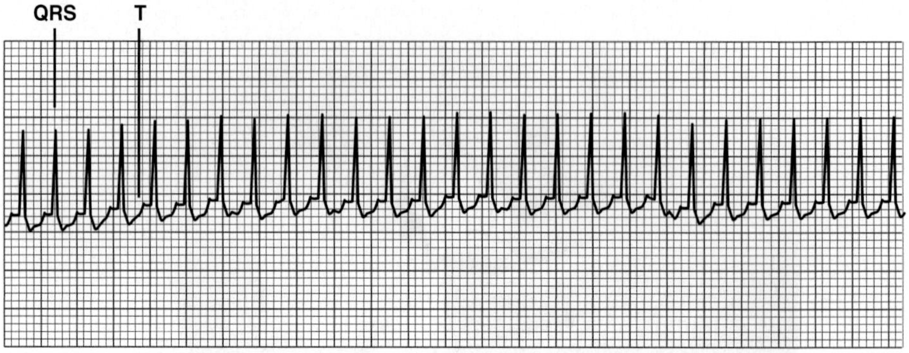

Hypertension in Childhood—A Typical Example

Hypertension can start in childhood (Ingelfinger, 2014). While elevated blood pressure in young children is more likely to have a renal, cardiac, or endocrine cause, adolescents with hypertension are most likely to have primary or essential hypertension.

This child developed hypertension and it continued into adulthood. Children tend to remain in the same percentile for blood pressure as they grow. When hypertension continues into adulthood, it supports the concept that adult essential hypertension often begins during childhood. The consequences of untreated hypertension can be severe and include cardiac, renal, and visual sequelae.

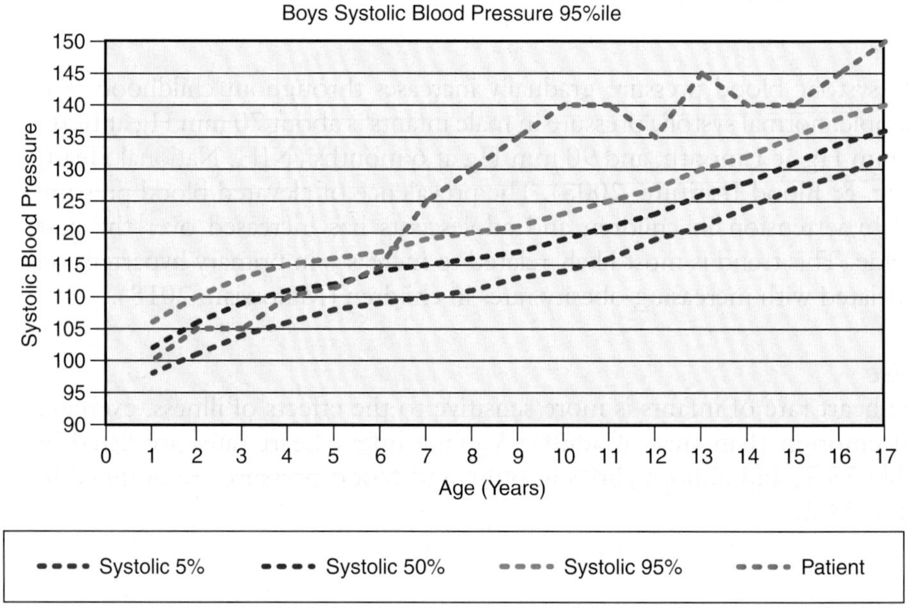

A pulse rate that is too rapid to count (usually greater than 180/min) may indicate *paroxysmal supraventricular tachycardia (PSVT).*

You may have trouble obtaining an accurate pulse rate in a squirming infant. The best strategy is to auscultate the heart or to palpate the femoral arteries in the inguinal area or the brachial arteries in the antecubital fossa. Take the infant's pulse while sleeping if possible or take it first before performing any uncomfortable assessments or procedures.

Bradycardia may be from drug ingestion, hypoxia, intracranial or neurologic conditions, or rarely cardiac dysrhythmia, such as heart block.

Respiratory Rate

The respiratory rate in infants has a greater range and is more responsive to illness, exercise, and emotion *than that of adults or older children*. The rate of respirations per minute ranges between 30 and 60 in the newborn.

Extremely rapid and shallow respiratory rates are seen in newborns with *cyanotic cardiac disease* and right-to-left shunting as well as metabolic acidosis.

The respiratory rate may vary considerably from moment to moment in the infant with alternating periods of rapid and slow breathing (called "periodic breathing"). The sleeping respiratory rate is most reliable. Respiratory rates during active sleep compared with quiet sleep may be up to 10 breaths per minute faster. The respiratory pattern should be observed for at least 60 seconds. In infancy and early childhood, diaphragmatic breathing is predominant; thoracic excursion is minimal.

Fever can raise respiratory rates in infants by up to 10 respirations per minute for each degree centigrade of fever.

Commonly accepted cutoffs for defining *tachypnea* are:

- Birth to 2 months, greater than 60/min
- 2 to 12 months, greater than 50/min

Tachypnea and increased respiratory effort in an infant are signs of lower respiratory disease such as *bronchiolitis* or *pneumonia.*

Temperature

Because fever is so common in infants and children, obtain an accurate body temperature when you suspect infection. The techniques for obtaining rectal, oral, temporal artery, and tympanic membrane temperatures in adults are described in the Chapter 7 section, "Beginning the Physical Examination." Oral temperatures are not recommended for infants.

Fever (greater than 38.0°C or 100.4°F) in infants younger than 2 to 3 months may be a sign of *serious infection* or *disease*. These infants should be evaluated promptly.

When necessary to obtain a rectal temperature on an infant, the technique differs slightly from the adult procedure. Place the infant prone, separate the buttocks with the thumb and forefinger on one hand, and with the other hand gently insert a well-lubricated digital rectal thermometer to a depth of 1.3 to 2.5 cm (0.5 to 1 in). Keep the thermometer in place until the thermometer signals completion.

Body temperature in infants and children is not as constant as in adults. The average rectal temperature is higher in infancy and early childhood, usually above 99.0°F (37.2°C) until after age 3. Body temperature may fluctuate as much as 3°F during a single day, approaching 101°F (38.3°C) in normal children, particularly in late afternoon and after vigorous activity.

Anxiety may elevate the body temperature of children. *Excessive bundling* of infants may elevate skin temperature but not core temperature.

Temperature instability in a newborn may result from sepsis, metabolic abnormality, or other serious conditions. Older infants rarely manifest temperature instability.

The Skin

Inspection

Carefully examine the infant's general color for cyanosis, paleness, ruddiness, or jaundice. To detect jaundice, apply pressure to blanch the skin of the normal pink or brown color (Fig. 23-16). A yellowish color indicates jaundice.

Central cyanosis in a baby or child of any age should raise suspicion of *congenital heart disease.* The best area to look for central cyanosis is the tongue and oral mucosa, not the nail beds, lips, or the extremities.

Jaundice that persists beyond 2 to 3 weeks should raise suspicions of *biliary obstruction* or *liver disease.*

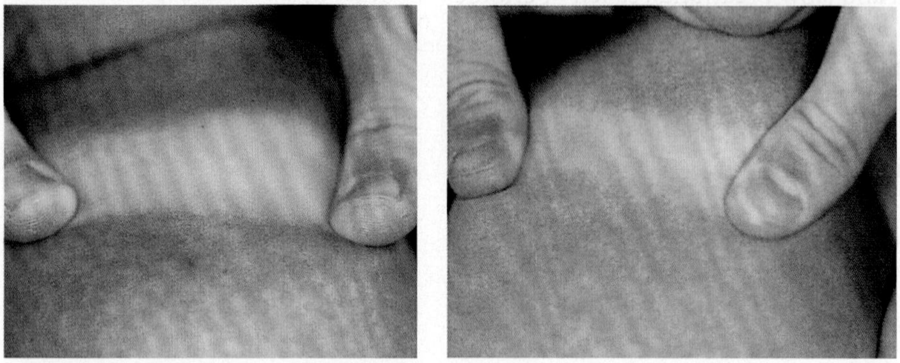

FIGURE 23-16 Pressing the red color from the skin allows better recognition of the yellow of jaundice. The infant on the *left* has no appreciable jaundice while the infant on the *right* has a bilirubin level of 13 mg/dL (222 mmol/L). (From Fletcher, M. [1998]. *Physical Diagnosis in Neonatology.* Lippincott-Raven.)

Next, examine the infant for normal and abnormal skin markings, such as birthmarks. Document their appearance and compare to the infant's last visit. Benign birthmarks are illustrated in Table 23-3. See also Table 23-4, "Common Skin Rashes and Skin Findings in Newborns and Infants" for examples of abnormal skin markings.

A dark or bluish pigmentation over the buttocks and lower lumbar regions is common in newborns of African, Asian, and Mediterranean descent (see Table 23-3). This is congenital dermal melanocytosis, formerly called Mongolian spots, due to pigmented cells in the deep layers of the skin; they become less noticeable with age and usually disappear during childhood. Document these pigmented areas to avoid later concern about bruising or abuse.

A common *vascular marking* is the "salmon patch" (also known as *nevus simplex,* telangiectatic nevus, or capillary hemangioma). These flat, irregular, light pink patches (see Table 23-3) are most often seen on the nape of the neck ("stork bite"), upper eyelids, forehead, or upper lip ("angel kisses"). They are not true nevi but instead result from distended capillaries. They almost all disappear by 1 year of age.

Palpation

Palpate the infant's skin to assess the degree of hydration, or *turgor.* Gently pinch a fold of loosely adherent skin on the abdominal wall between your thumb and forefinger to determine its consistency. The skin in well-hydrated infants returns to its normal position immediately upon release. Delay in return is a phenomenon called "tenting" and usually occurs in children with significant *dehydration.* See Chapter 9 "The Integumentary System."

Dehydration is a common problem in infants. Usual causes are insufficient intake or excess loss of fluids from diarrhea.

TABLE 23-3 Benign Birthmarks

Finding	Illustration
Eyelid Patch This birthmark fades, usually within the first year of life.	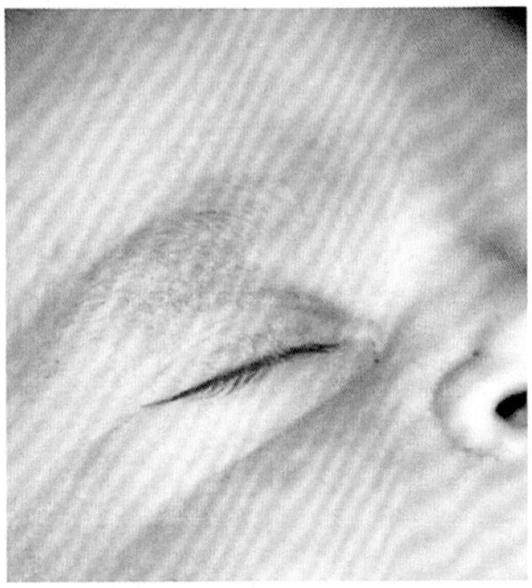
Salmon Patch Also called the "stork bite," this splotchy pink mark fades with age.	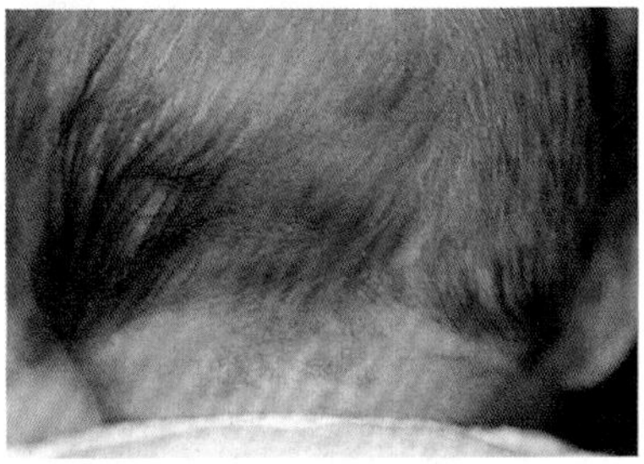
Café-Au-Lait Spots These light brown pigmented lesions usually have borders and are uniform. They are noted in more than 10% of Black infants. *If more than five café-au-lait spots exist, consider the diagnosis of neurofibromatosis.*	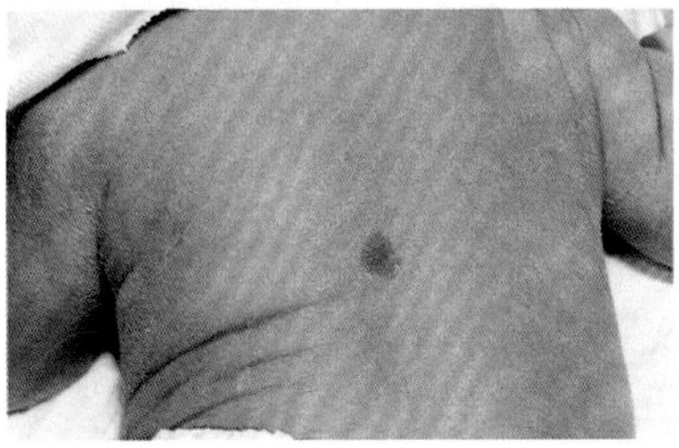
Congenital Dermal Melanocytosis (Mongolian Spots) These are more common among dark-skinned babies. It is important to note them so that they are not mistaken for bruises or abuse.	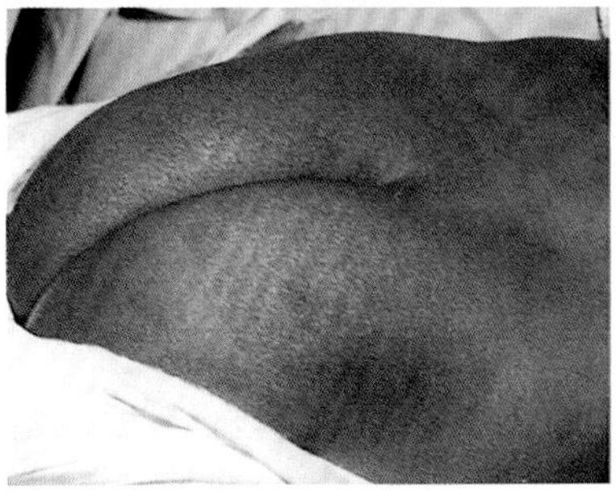

Pigmented light brown lesions (less than 1–2 cm at birth) are *café-au-lait spots.* Isolated lesions have no significance, but multiple lesions with sharp borders suggest *neurofibromatosis.*

Midline hair tufts over the lumbosacral spine region suggest a *spinal cord defect.*

TABLE 23-4 Common Skin Rashes and Skin Findings in Newborns and Infants

Face

Erythema Toxicum

These common yellow or white pustules are surrounded by a red base.

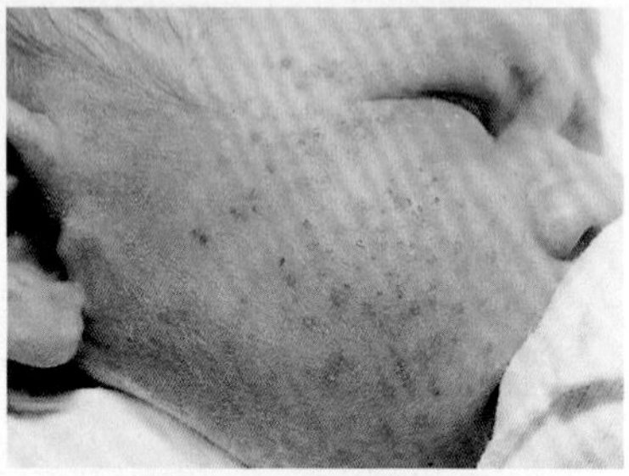

Neonatal Acne

Red pustules and papules are most prominent over the cheeks and nose of some normal newborns.

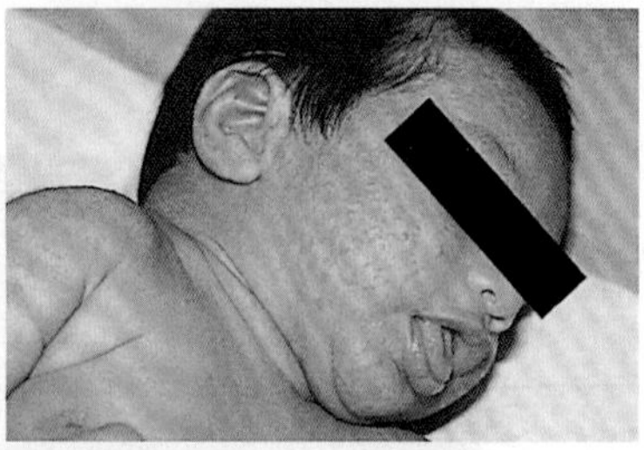

Seborrhea

The salmon red, scaly eruption often involves the face, neck, axilla, diaper area, and behind the ears.

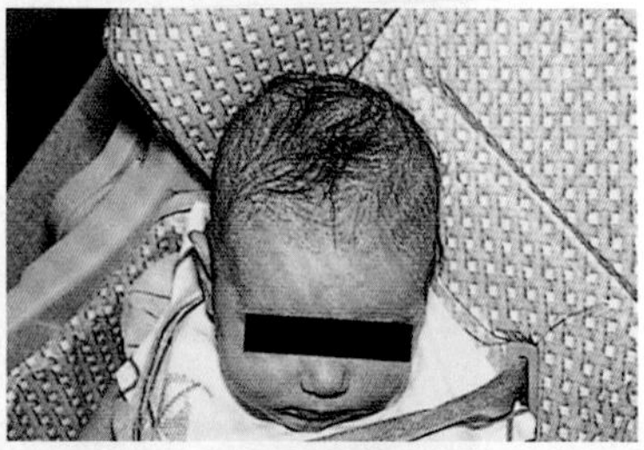

Body and Extremities

Atopic Dermatitis (Eczema)

Erythema, scaling, dry skin, and intense itching characterize this condition.

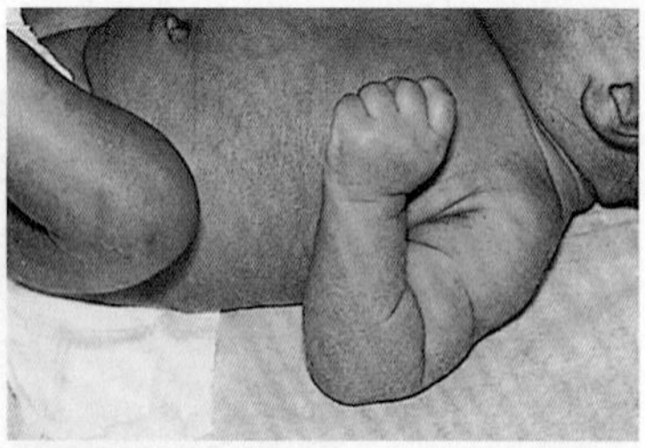

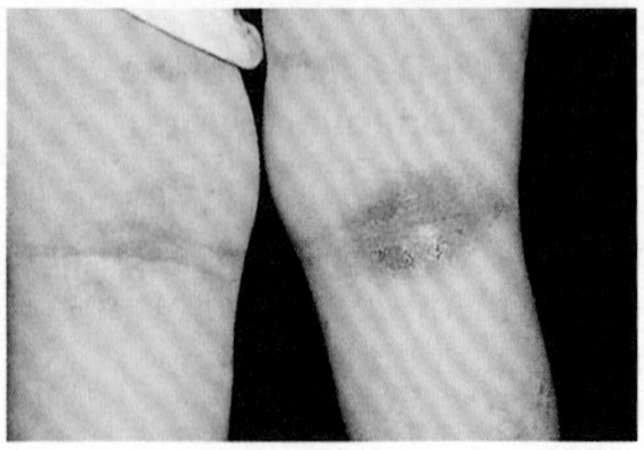

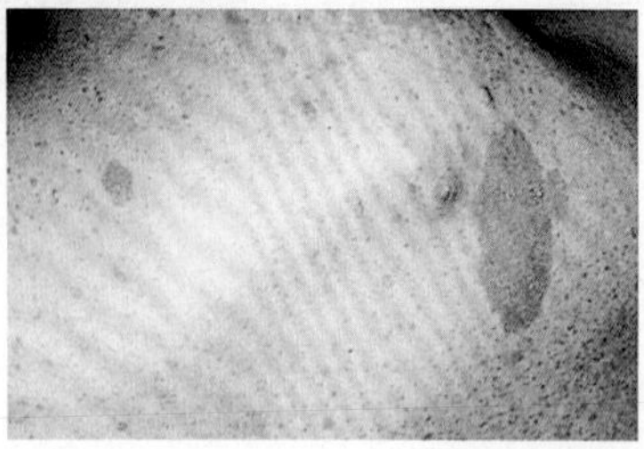

Neurofibromatosis

Characteristic features include more than five café-au-lait spots. Later findings include axillary freckling, neurofibromas, and Lish nodules (not shown).

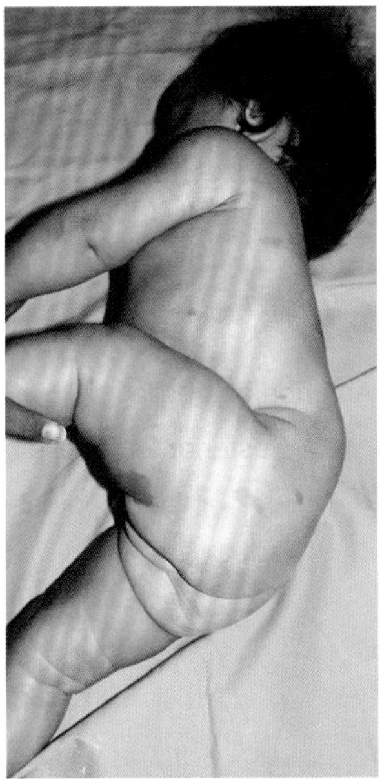

Diaper Region

Candidal Diaper Dermatitis

This bright red rash involves the intertriginous folds, with small "satellite lesions" along the edges.

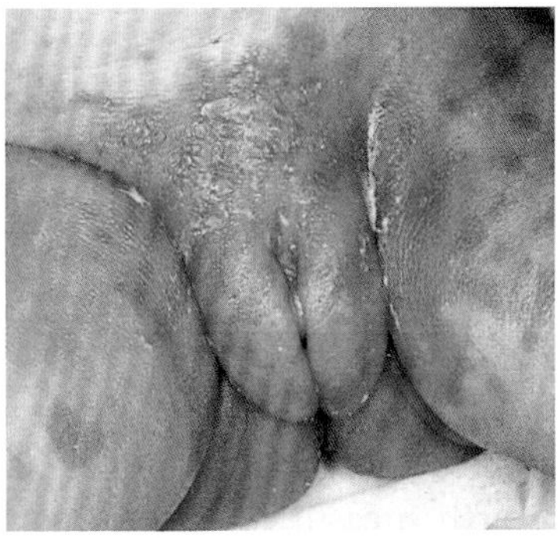

Contact Diaper Dermatitis

This irritant rash is secondary to diarrhea or irritation and is noted along contact areas (here, the area touching the diaper).

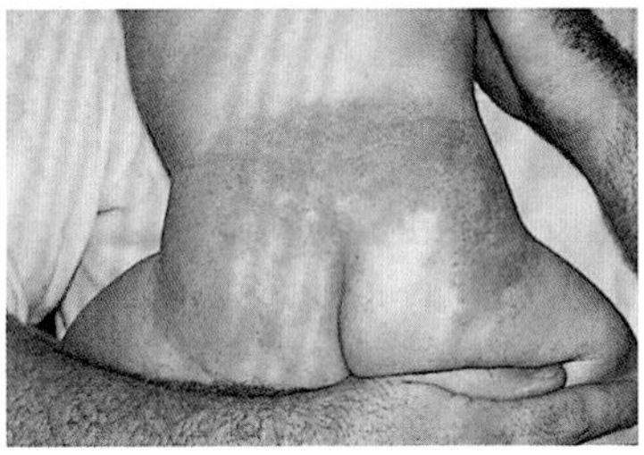

Impetigo

This infection is due to bacteria and can appear bullous or crusty and yellowed with some pus.

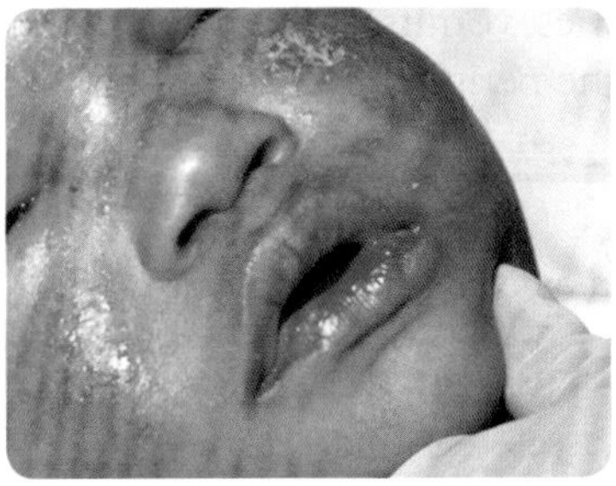

The Head

A newborn's head accounts for one fourth of the body length and one third of the body weight; these proportions change so that by adulthood, the head accounts for one eighth of the body length and about one tenth of the body weight.

Sutures and Fontanelles

Membranous tissue spaces called sutures separate the bones of the skull from one another. The areas where the major sutures intersect in the anterior and posterior portions of the skull are known as *fontanelles.* Examine the *sutures* and *fontanelles* carefully (Fig. 23-17).

An enlarged posterior fontanelle may be present in *congenital hypothyroidism.*

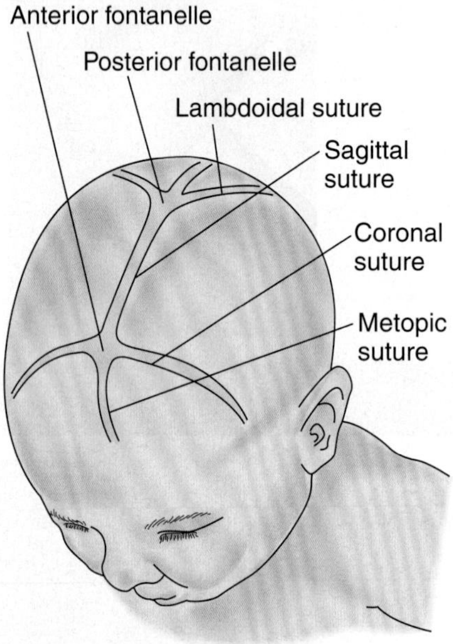

FIGURE 23-17 Locations of infant fontanelles.

On palpation, the sutures feel like ridges and the fontanelles like soft concavities. The *anterior fontanelle* at birth measures 4 to 6 cm in diameter and usually closes between 4 and 26 months of age (90% between 7 and 19 months). The *posterior fontanelle* measures 1 to 2 cm at birth and usually closes by 2 months. Table 23-5 outlines abnormalities of the head.

A bulging, tense fontanelle is observed in infants with *increased intracranial pressure,* which may be caused by *central nervous system infections, neoplastic disease,* or **hydrocephalus** (obstruction of the circulation of cerebrospinal fluid within the ventricles of the brain).

Carefully examine the fontanelle because its fullness reflects *intracranial pressure.* Palpate the fontanelle while the baby is sitting quietly or being held upright. Experienced pediatric nurses often palpate the fontanelles at the beginning of the examination. In normal infants, the anterior fontanelle is soft and flat. Increased intracranial pressure produces a bulging, full anterior fontanelle and is seen when a baby cries, vomits, or has underlying pathology. Pulsations of the fontanelle reflect the peripheral pulse and are normal.

CLINICAL TIP
A depressed anterior fontanelle may be a sign of *dehydration.*

Inspect the scalp veins carefully to assess for dilatation.

Dilated scalp veins are indicative of long-standing *increased intracranial pressure.*

TABLE 23-5 Abnormalities of the Head

Hydrocephalus

In hydrocephaly, the anterior fontanelle is bulging, and the eyes may be deviated downward, revealing the upper scleras and creating the *setting sun* sign, as shown here. The setting sun sign is also seen briefly in some normal newborns. (Figure reprinted with permission from Fleisher, G. R., Ludwig, S., Baskin, M. N. [2004]. *Atlas of Pediatric Emergency Medicine*. Lippincott Williams & Wilkins.)

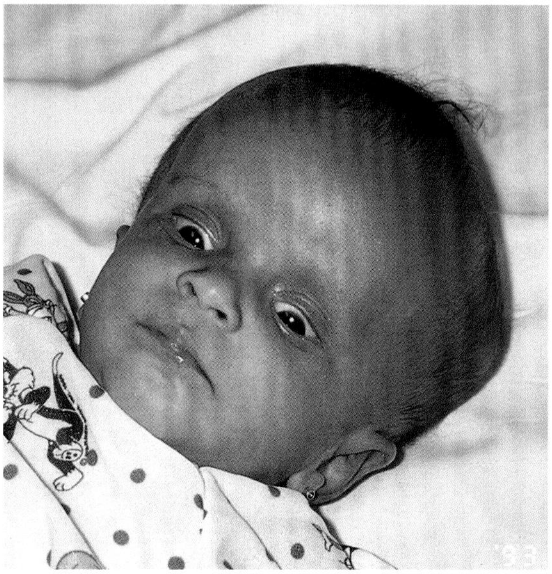

Craniosynostosis

Craniosynostosis is a condition of premature closure of one or more sutures of the skull. This results in an abnormal growth and shape of the skull because growth will occur across sutures that are not affected but not across sutures that are affected. The figures demonstrate different skull shapes associated with the various names of craniosynostosis. The prematurely closed suture line is noted by the absence of a suture line in each figure. Scaphocephaly and frontal plagiocephaly are the most common forms of craniosynostosis. The *blue shading* shows areas of maximal flattening. The *red arrows* show the direction of continued growth across the sutures, which is normal.

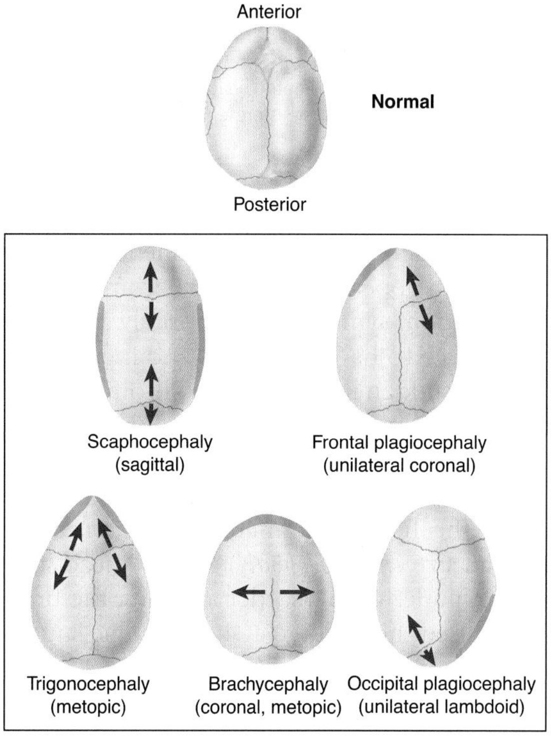

Reprinted with permission from Fleisher, G. R., Ludwig, S., & Baskin, M. N. (2004). *Atlas of pediatric emergency medicine*. Lippincott Williams & Wilkins.

Skull Symmetry and Head Circumference

Assess skull symmetry. Careful inspection of the skull from the front or back of the infant helps you assess its symmetry (Fig. 23-18).

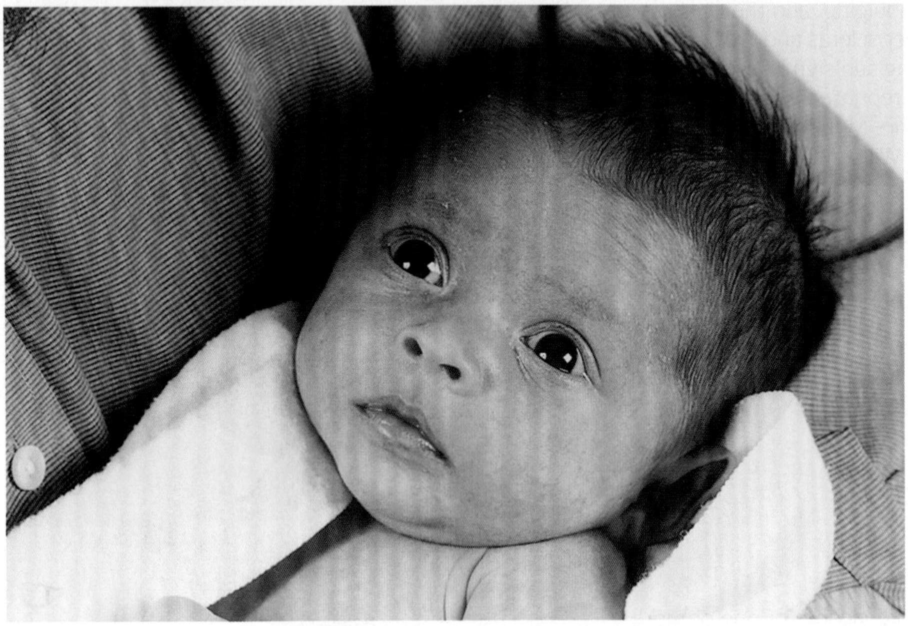

FIGURE 23-18 Look for asymmetric head swelling, which after the newborn period, may be due to trauma from a fall or abuse. None is present in this patient.

Asymmetry of the cranial vault (**plagiocephaly**) occurs when an infant lies mostly on one side, resulting in a flattening of the parieto-occipital region on the dependent side and a prominence of the frontal region on the opposite side. It disappears as the baby becomes more active and spends less time in one position; symmetry is almost always restored. Interestingly, the current guidance to have newborns and infants sleep on their backs to reduce the risk for sudden infant death syndrome (SIDS) has resulted in more cases of plagiocephaly. This condition can be prevented by frequent repositioning (providing "tummy time") when the infant is awake.

Plagiocephaly may also reflect pathology such as *torticollis* from injury to the sternocleidomastoid muscle at birth or *lack of stimulation* of the infant.

Measure the head circumference (see Fig. 23-13) to detect abnormally large head size (*macrocephaly*) or small head size (*microcephaly*), which may signify an underlying disorder affecting the brain. Palpate along the suture lines. A raised, bony ridge at a suture line suggests craniosynostosis.

Premature closure of cranial sutures causes *craniosynostosis* (see Table 23-5, "Abnormalities of the Head"), with an abnormally shaped skull. *Sagittal suture* synostosis causes a narrow head from lack of growth of the parietal bones.

Palpate the infant's skull with care. The cranial bones usually appear "soft" or pliable; they will normally become firmer with increasing age.

In *craniotabes,* the cranial bones feel springy. Craniotabes can result from increased intracranial pressure, as with *hydrocephaly;* metabolic disturbances such as *rickets;* and infection such as *congenital syphilis.*

Facial Symmetry

Check the *face* of infants for symmetry. In utero positioning may result in transient facial asymmetries. If the head is flexed on the sternum, a shortened chin (*micrognathia*) may result.

Micrognathia may also be part of a syndrome such as *Pierre Robin syndrome.*

Examine the face for an overall impression of the *facies;* it is helpful to compare with the face of the parents. An abnormal-appearing facies can identify specific syndromes (Table 23-6).

A child with abnormal shape or length of palpebral fissures, upslanting is present in Down syndrome, downslanting in Noonan syndrome, and shortness with fetal alcohol effects.

TABLE 23-6 Diagnostic Facies in Infancy and Childhood

Fetal Alcohol Syndrome

Babies born to people with chronic alcoholism are at increased risk for growth deficiency, microcephaly, and intellectual disability. Facial characteristics include short palpebral fissures, a wide and flattened philtrum (the vertical groove in the midline of the upper lip), and thin lips.

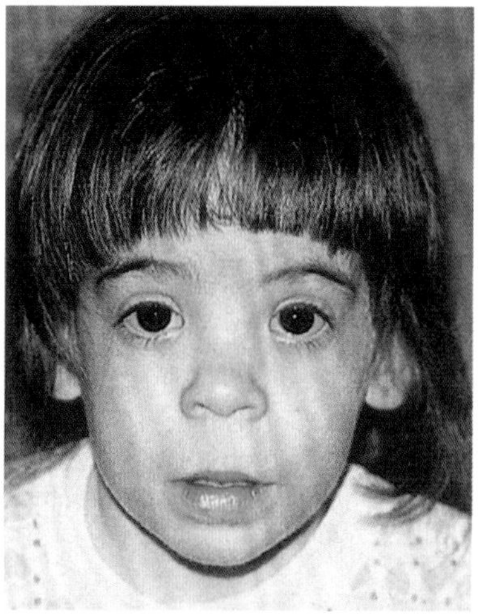

Congenital Hypothyroidism

The child with congenital hypothyroidism (*cretinism*) has coarse facial features, a low-set hair line, sparse eyebrows, and an enlarged tongue. Associated features include a hoarse cry, umbilical hernia, dry and cold extremities, myxedema, mottled skin, and intellectual disability. Most infants with congenital hypothyroidism have no physical stigmata; this has led to screening of all newborns in the United States and most other developed countries for congenital hypothyroidism.

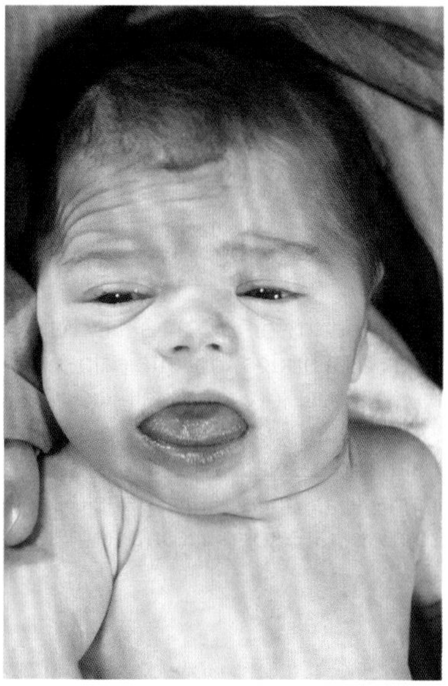

(*continued*)

TABLE 23-6 Diagnostic Facies in Infancy and Childhood *(Continued)*

Congenital Syphilis

In utero infection by *Treponema pallidum* usually occurs after the 16th wk of gestation and affects virtually all fetal organs. If it is not treated, the mortality rate is quite high. Signs of illness appear in survivors within the first month of life. Facial stigmata often include bulging of the frontal bones and nasal bridge depression (*saddle nose*), both from periostitis; rhinitis from weeping nasal mucosal lesions (*snuffles*); and a circumoral rash. Mucocutaneous inflammation and fissuring of the mouth and lips (*rhagades*), not shown here, may also occur as stigmata of congenital syphilis, as may craniotabes tibial periostitis (*saber shins*) and dental dysplasia (*Hutchinson teeth*—see Table 12-7).

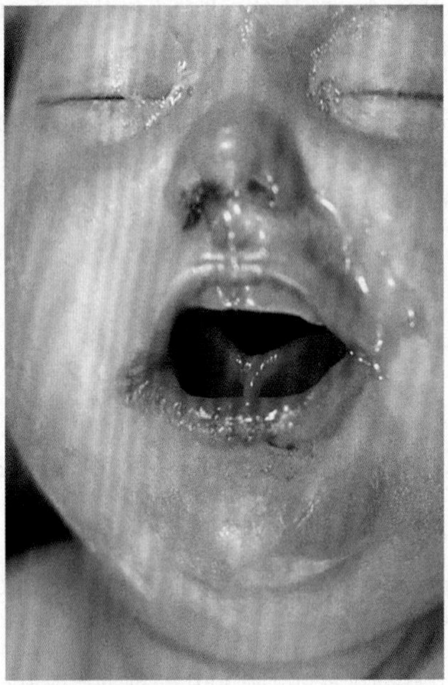

Facial Nerve Palsy

Peripheral (lower motor neuron) paralysis of the facial nerve may be from (1) an injury to the nerve from pressure during labor and birth, (2) inflammation of the middle ear branch of the nerve during episodes of acute or chronic otitis media, or (3) unknown causes (Bell palsy). The nasolabial fold on the affected left side is flattened, and the eye does not close. This is accentuated during crying, as shown here. Full recovery occurs in ≥90% of those affected.

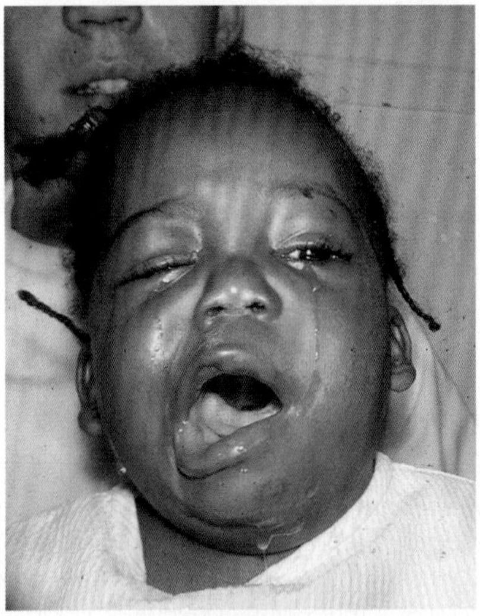

Down Syndrome

The child with Down syndrome (trisomy 21) usually has a small, rounded head; a flattened nasal bridge; oblique palpebral fissures; prominent epicanthal folds; small, low-set, shell-like ears; and a relatively large tongue. Associated features include generalized hypotonia, transverse palmar creases (*simian lines*), shortening and incurving of the fifth fingers (*clinodactyly*), Brushfield spots (see Table 23-7), and mild to moderate cognitive impairment.

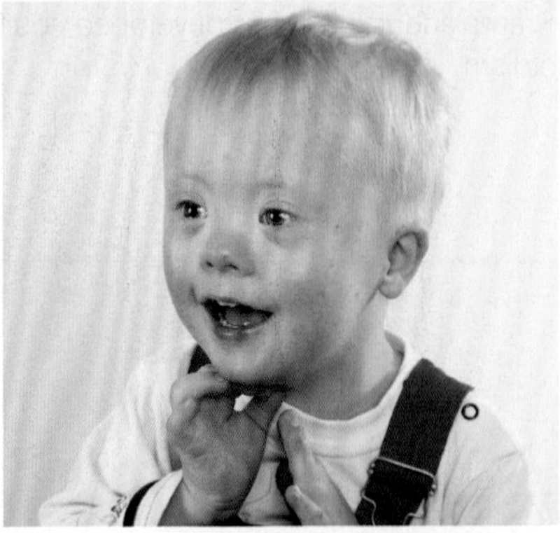

Battered Child Syndrome

The child who has been physically abused (battered) may have old *and* fresh bruises on the head and face and may either look sad and forlorn or be actively seeking to please. Other stigmata include bruises in areas (axilla and groin) not usually subject to injury rather than the bony prominences; x-ray evidence of fractures of the skull, ribs, and long bones in various stages of healing; and skin lesions that are morphologically similar to implements used to inflict trauma (hand, belt buckle, strap, rope, coat hanger, or lit cigarette). Of note, it is more common among abused children to note bruises on protected areas and not on bony prominences.

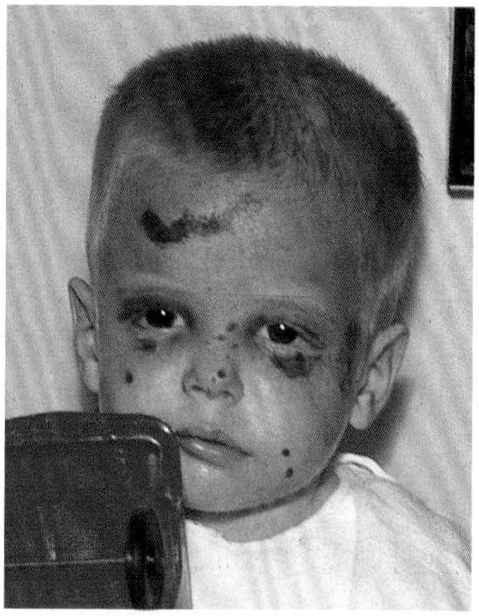

Perennial Allergic Rhinitis

The child suffering from perennial allergic rhinitis has an open mouth (cannot breathe through the nose) and edema and discoloration of the lower orbitopalpebral grooves ("allergic shiners"). Such a child may often push the nose upward and backward with a hand ("allergic salute") and to grimace (wrinkle the nose and mouth) to relieve nasal itching and obstruction. (Photograph reproduced with permission from Marks, M. B. [1966]. Allergic shiners: dark circles under the eyes in children. *Clinical Pediatrics*, *5*, 656.)

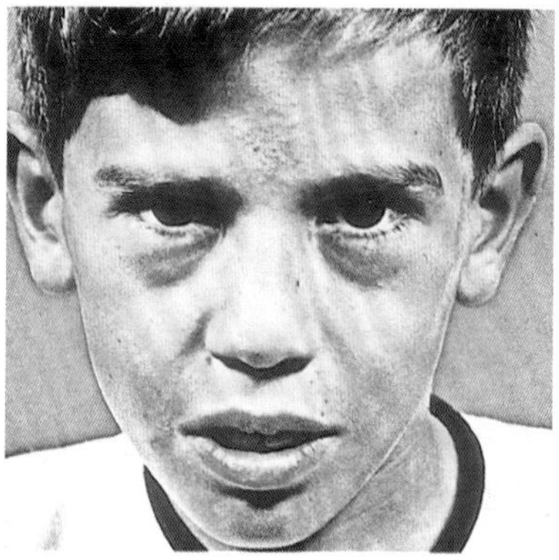

Hyperthyroidism

Thyrotoxicosis (*Graves disease*) occurs in approximately two per 1,000 children younger than 10 y. Affected children exhibit hypermetabolism tachycardia and accelerated linear growth. Facial characteristics shown in this 6-y-old girl are "staring" eyes (not true exophthalmos, which is rare in children) and an enlarged thyroid gland (*goiter*). See Table 10-4.

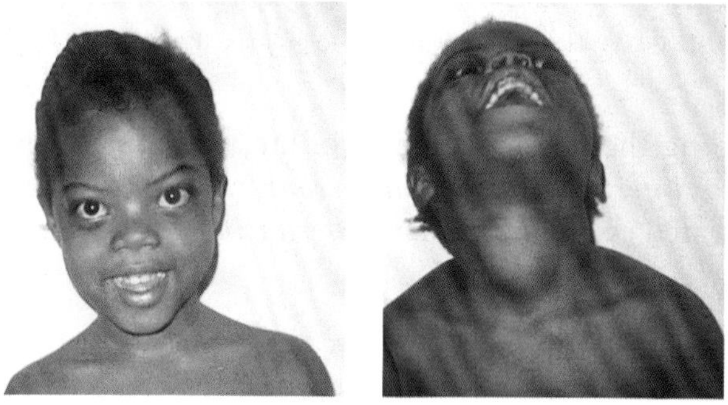

The Eyes

Inspection

Bright light causes infants to blink, so use subdued lighting. If you awaken the baby gently, turn down the lights, and support the baby in a sitting position, you will often find that the eyes open.

To examine the eyes of infants and young children, use some tricks to encourage cooperation. Small colorful toys are useful as fixation devices in examining the eyes.

Newborns may look at your face and follow a bright light if you catch them during an alert period. By 2 months, most infants can follow an object.

Examine infants for *eye movements.* Hold the baby upright, supporting the head (Fig. 23-19). Rotate yourself with the baby slowly in one direction. This usually causes the baby's eyes to open, allowing you to examine the sclerae, pupils, irises, and extraocular movements. The baby's eyes gaze in the direction you are turning. When the rotation stops, the eyes look in the opposite direction after a few nystagmoid movements.

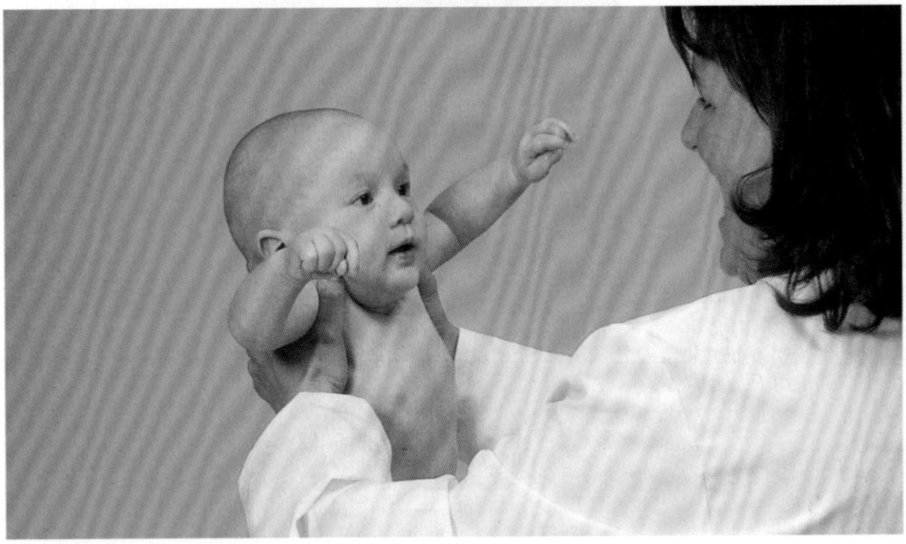

FIGURE 23-19 Hold the baby upright to examine the eyes.

Nystagmus (wandering or shaking eye movements) persisting after a few days after birth or persisting after the maneuver described may indicate *poor vision* or *central nervous system disease.*

During the first few months of life, some infants have intermittent crossed eyes (*intermittent alternating convergent strabismus,* or *esotropia*) or laterally deviated eyes (*intermittent alternating divergent strabismus,* or *exotropia*).

Alternating convergent or divergent *strabismus* persisting beyond 3 months or persistent strabismus of any type may indicate *ocular motor weakness* or another abnormality in the visual system.

Observe pupillary reactions by response to light or by covering each eye with your hand and then uncovering it. They should be equal in size and reaction to light.

Inspect the irises carefully for abnormalities (Table 23-7).

Brushfield spots (seen with an ophthalmoscope) are a ring of white specks in the iris. Although sometimes present in normal children, these strongly suggest *Down syndrome.*

TABLE 23-7 Abnormalities of the Eyes, Ears, and Mouth

Eye Abnormalities

Brushfield Spots

These abnormal speckling spots on the iris suggest Down syndrome.

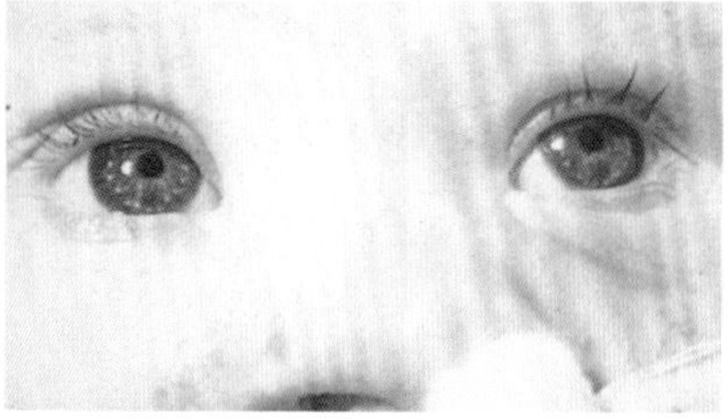

Strabismus

Strabismus, or misalignment of the eyes, can lead to visual impairment. Esotropia, shown here, is an inward deviation.

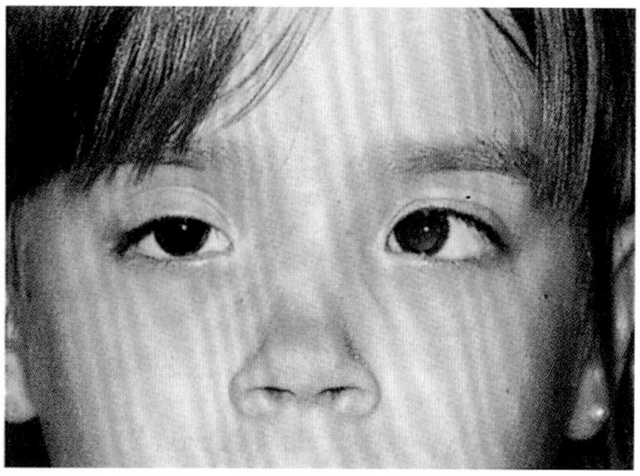

Ear Abnormalities

Otitis Media

Otitis media is one of the most common conditions in young children. The spectrum of otitis media is shown here. **A.** Typical acute otitis media with a red, distorted, bulging tympanic membrane in a highly symptomatic child. **B.** Acute otitis media with bullae formation and fluid visible behind the tympanic membrane. **C.** Otitis media with effusion, showing a yellowish fluid behind a retracted and thickened tympanic membrane. Often, you can no longer visualize the normal landmarks such as the light reflex and handle of the malleus.

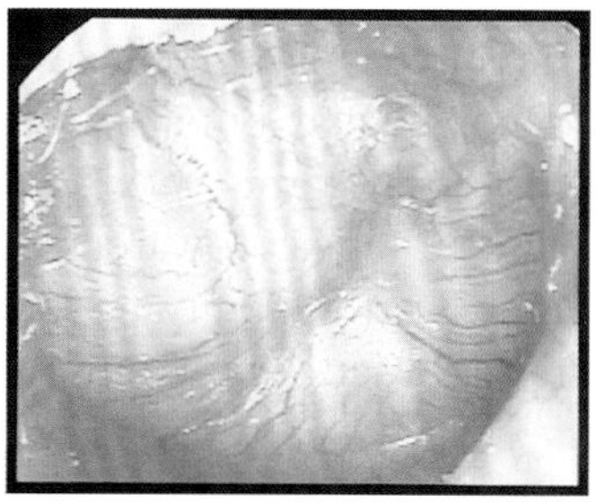

A

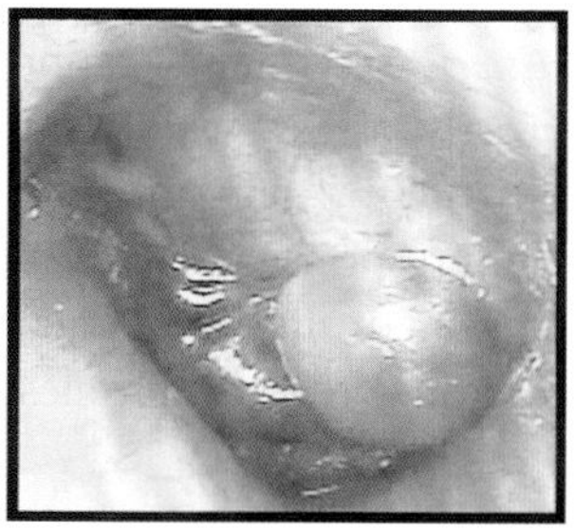

B

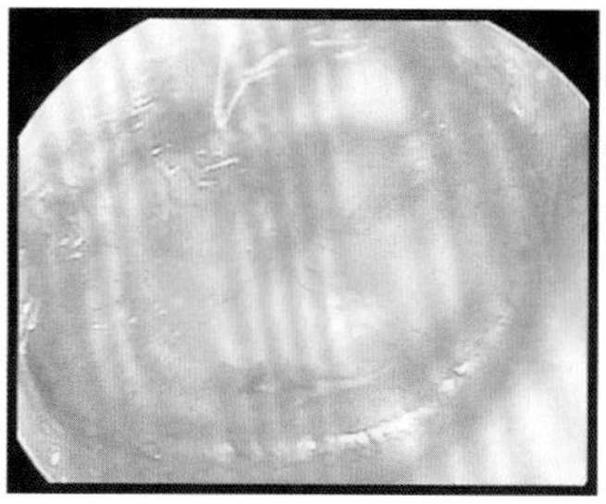

C

(continued)

TABLE 23-7 Abnormalities of the Eyes, Ears, and Mouth (*Continued*)

Mouth Abnormalities

Oral Candidiasis ("Thrush")

This infection is common in infants. The white plaques do not rub off.

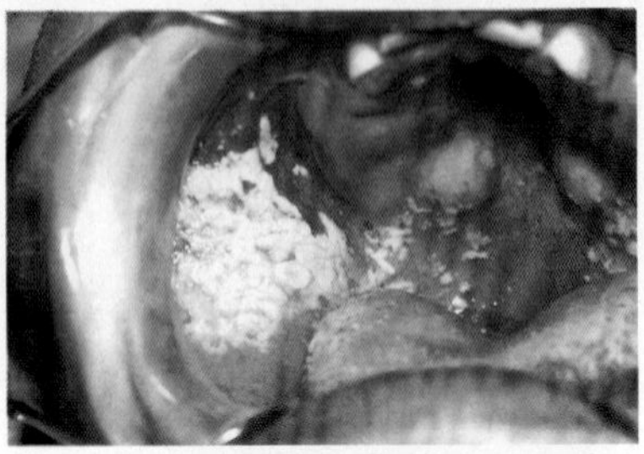

Herpetic Stomatitis

Tender ulcerations on the oral mucosa are surrounded by erythema.

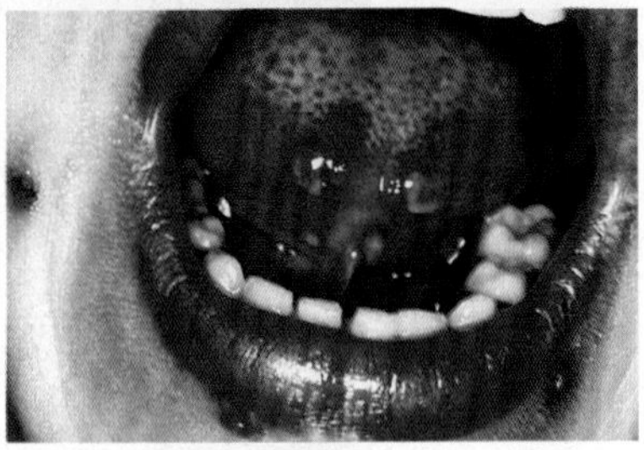

Source of photos: *Otitis Media*—Courtesy of Alejandro Hoberman, Children's Hospital of Pittsburgh, University of Pittsburgh.

Examine the *conjunctiva* for swelling or redness.

Visual acuity in infants cannot be measured. Visual reflexes can be used to indirectly assess vision: direct and consensual pupillary constriction in response to light, blinking in response to bright light (*optic blink reflex*), and blinking in response to quick movement of an object toward the eyes. During the first year of life, visual acuity sharpens as the ability to focus improves. Infants achieve the visual milestones in the order outlined in Table 23-8.

Persistent ocular discharge and tearing since birth may be from *dacryocystitis* (inflammation of the lacrimal sac) or *nasolacrimal duct obstruction.*

TABLE 23-8 Visual Milestones of Infancy

Age	Milestone
Birth	Blinks, may regard face
1 mo	Fixes on objects
1/2–2 mo	Coordinated eye movements
3 mo	Eyes converge, baby reaches toward a visual stimulus
12 mo	Acuity around 20/80

Source: Hyvarinen, L. (1994). Assessment of visually impaired infants. *Ophthalmology Clinics of North America*, *7*, 219.

Failure to progress along these visual developmental milestones may indicate *delayed visual maturation.*

Ophthalmoscopic Examination

For the *ophthalmoscopic examination*, with the infant awake and eyes open, examine the red retinal reflex by setting the ophthalmoscope at 0 diopters and viewing the pupil from about 10 in. Normally, a red or orange color is reflected from the fundus through the pupil.

Congenital glaucoma may cause cloudiness of the cornea. A dark light reflex can result from *cataracts, retinopathy of prematurity,* or other disorders. A white retinal reflex (*leukokoria*) is abnormal, and *cataract, retinal detachment, chorioretinitis,* or *retinoblastoma* should be suspected.

If history or examination findings indicate the need for a thorough ophthalmologic examination, refer the infant to a pediatric ophthalmologist.

The Ears

The physical examination of the ears of infants is important because many abnormalities can be detected, including structural problems, otitis media, and hearing loss. The goals are to determine the *position, shape,* and *features of the ear* and to detect abnormalities. Note ear position in relation to the eyes. An imaginary line drawn across the inner and outer canthi of the eyes should cross the auricle (the pinna of the ear); if the auricle is below this line, the infant has low-set ears. Draw this imaginary line across the face of the child in Figure 23-20; note that it crosses the auricle.

Small, deformed, or low-set auricles may indicate associated *congenital defects,* especially renal disease.

A small skin tab, cleft, or pit found just forward of the tragus represents a remnant of the *first branchial cleft* and usually has no significance.

The infant's ear canal is directed downward from outside; therefore, pull the auricle gently downward, not upward, for the best view of the eardrum. Once the tympanic membrane is visible, note that the light reflex is diffuse and does not become cone-shaped for several months.

Signs that an infant can hear are listed in Table 23-9.

TABLE 23-9 Signs that an Infant Can Hear

Age (Months)	Sign
0–2	Startle response and blink to a sudden noise Calming down with soothing voice or music
2–3	Change in body movements in response to sound Change in facial expression to familiar sounds
3–4	Turning eyes and head to sound
6–7	Turning to listen to voices and conversation Appropriate language development

In the absence of universal hearing screening many children with *hearing deficits* are not diagnosed until 2 y of age. Clues to hearing deficits include parental concern about hearing, delayed speech, and lack of developmental indicators of hearing.

The Nose and Sinuses

The most important component of the examination of the nose of infants is to test for patency of the nasal passages. You can do this by gently occluding each nostril alternately while holding the infant's mouth closed. This normally will not cause stress because most infants are nasal breathers. Indeed, some infants are *obligate nasal breathers* and have difficulty breathing through their mouths. Do not occlude both nares simultaneously—this will cause considerable distress.

The nasal passages in newborns may be obstructed in *choanal atresia*, a congenital disorder in which the back of the nasal passage (choana) is blocked by bone or membranes.

Inspect the nose to ensure that the nasal septum is midline.

The Mouth and Pharynx

Use both inspection with a tongue depressor and flashlight and palpation to inspect the mouth and pharynx. The newborn's mouth is **edentulous** (without teeth), and the alveolar mucosa is smooth with finely serrated borders. Occasionally, pearl-like retention cysts are seen along the alveolar ridges and are easily mistaken for teeth; they disappear within 1 or 2 months. Petechiae are commonly found on the soft palate after birth. Palpate the upper hard palate to make sure it is intact. *Epstein pearls,* tiny white or yellow rounded mucous retention cysts, are located along the posterior midline of the hard palate. They disappear within months.

Cysts may be noted on the tongue or mouth. Thyroglossal duct cysts may open under the tongue.

Rarely, *supernumerary teeth* are noted. These are usually misshapen and are shed within days but are removed to prevent aspiration.

Infants produce little saliva during the first 3 months. Older infants produce lots of saliva and drool frequently.

Inspect the tongue. The frenulum varies in tightness—sometimes it extends almost to the tip; and other times, it is short, limiting protrusion of the tongue (ankyloglossia or tongue tie).

Although unusual, a prominent, protruding tongue may signal *congenital hypothyroidism* or *Down syndrome.*

You will often see a whitish covering on the tongue. If this coating is from milk, it can be easily removed by scraping or wiping it away. Use a tongue depressor or your gloved finger to wipe away the coating.

Oral candidiasis (thrush) is common in infants. The white plaques are difficult to wipe away and have an erythematous raw base. See Table 23-7, "Abnormalities of the Eyes, Ears, and Mouth."

The pharynx of the infant is best seen while the baby is crying. You will likely have difficulty using a tongue depressor because it produces a strong gag reflex. Infants do not have prominent lymphoid tissue so you will probably not visualize the tonsils, which increase in size as children grow. Listen to the quality of the *infant's cry.* Normal infants have a lusty, strong cry. Table 23-10 lists some unusual types of infant cries.

A congenital fissure of the median line of the palate is a *cleft palate.*

Macroglossia is associated with several systemic conditions. If associated with hypoglycemia and omphalocele, the diagnosis is likely Beckwith–Wiedemann syndrome.

TABLE 23-10 Abnormal Infant Cries

Type	Possible Abnormality
Shrill or high-pitched	Increased intracranial pressure; also in newborns born to narcotic-addicted mothers
Hoarse	Hypocalcemic tetany or congenital hypothyroidism
Continuous inspiratory and expiratory stridor	Upper airway obstruction from various lesions (e.g., a polyp or hemangioma), a relatively small larynx (infantile laryngeal stridor), or a delay in the development of the cartilage in the tracheal rings (tracheomalacia)
Absence of cry	Severe illness, vocal cord paralysis, or profound brain damage

Inspiratory stridor beginning at birth suggests a congenital abnormality as described here. Stridor that appears following birth can be due to infections such as *croup, a foreign body, or gastroesophageal reflux.*

While there is a predictable pattern of tooth eruption, there is wide variation in the age at which teeth appear. A rule of thumb is that a child will have one tooth for each month of age between 6 and 26 months up to a maximum of 20 primary teeth.

The Neck

Palpate the *lymph nodes of the neck* (Fig. 23-20) and assess for any additional masses such as *congenital cysts*. Because the necks of infants are short, it is best to palpate the neck while infants are lying supine, whereas older children are best examined while sitting. Check the position of the thyroid cartilage and trachea.

Preauricular cysts and sinuses are common, pinhole-sized pits, usually located anterior to the helix of the ear. They are often bilateral and may occasionally be associated with *hearing deficits* and renal disorders.

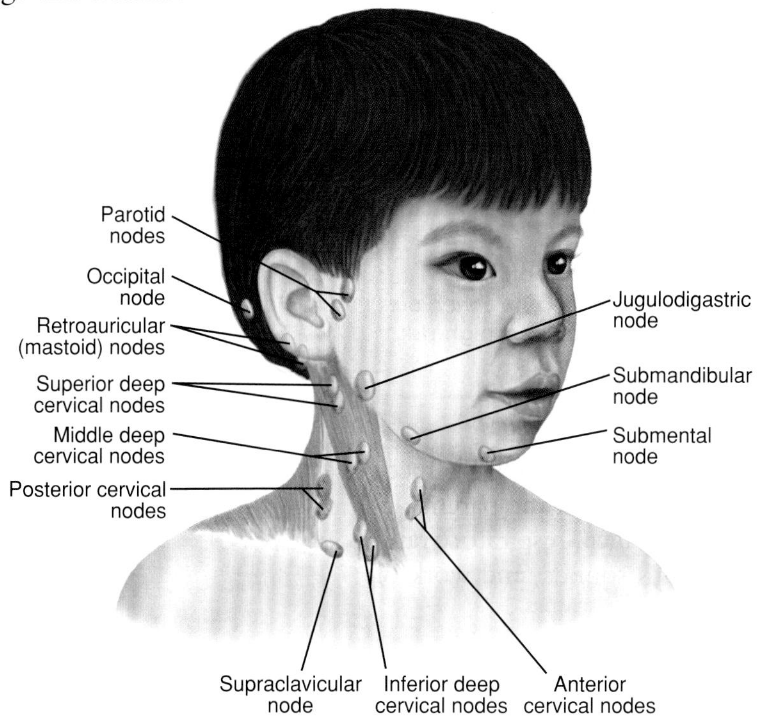

FIGURE 23-20 Lymph nodes of the neck.

Palpate the *clavicles* and look for evidence of a fracture. If present, you may feel a break in the contour of the bone, tenderness, and crepitus at the fracture site, and you may notice limited movement of the arm on the affected side.

The Thorax and Lungs

The infant's *thorax* is more rounded than those of older children and adults. The thin chest wall has little musculature; thus, lung and heart sounds are transmitted quite clearly. The bony and cartilaginous rib cage is soft and pliant. The tip of the xiphoid process often protrudes anteriorly, immediately beneath the skin.

Two types of chest wall abnormalities noted in childhood include **pectus excavatum** (Fig. 23-21A), or "funnel chest," and *pectus carinatum* (Fig. 23-21B), or "chicken breast deformity."

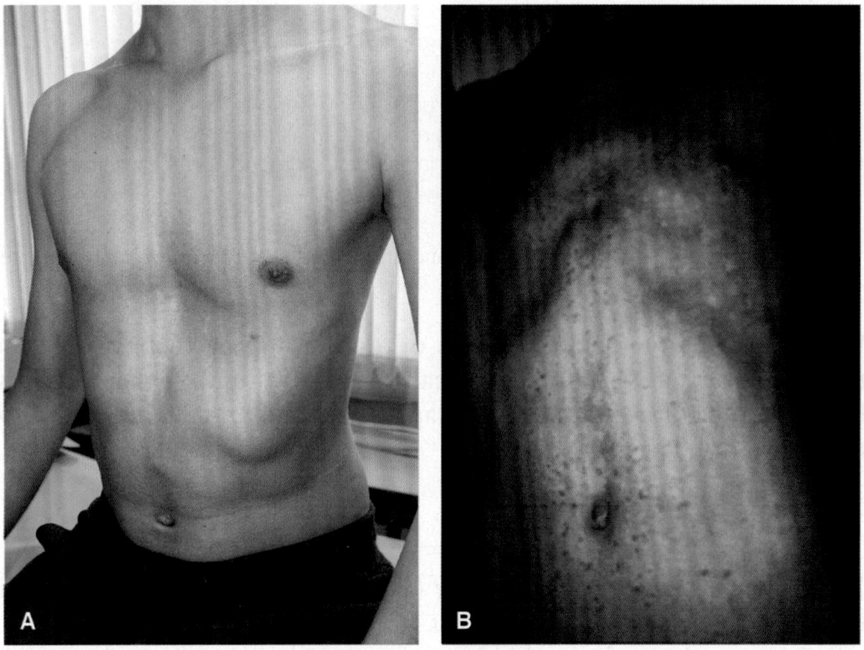

FIGURE 23-21 A. Pectus excavatum, a congenital chest wall deformity. (Douglas Olivares/Shutterstock) **B.** Pectus carinatum. (Reprinted with permission from Salimpour, R. R., Salimpour, P., & Salimpour, P. [2013]. *Photographic atlas of pediatric disorders and diagnosis*. Lippincott Williams & Wilkins.)

Inspection

Carefully assess respirations and breathing patterns.

CLINICAL TIP
Apnea is cessation of breathing for more than 20 seconds. It is often accompanied by bradycardia and may indicate *respiratory disease, central nervous system disease,* or rarely, a *cardiopulmonary condition.* Apnea may be a high-risk factor for *SIDS.*

Do not rush to the stethoscope. Instead, observe the infant carefully. Inspection is easiest when infants are not crying; thus, work with the parents to settle the child. On observation, note general appearance, respiratory rate, color, nasal component of breathing, audible breath sounds, and work of breathing, as described in Table 23-11.

TABLE 23-11 Observing Respiration—Before You Touch the Child

Type of Assessment	Specific Observable Pathology
General appearance	Inability to feed or smile Inconsolable
Respiratory rate	Tachypnea, apnea (see Table 13-5, "Abnormalities in Rate and Rhythm of Breathing")
Color	Pallor or cyanosis
Nasal component of breathing	Nasal flaring (enlargement of both nasal openings during inspiration)
Audible breath sounds	Grunting (repetitive, short expiratory sound) Wheezing (musical expiratory sound) Stridor (high-pitched, inspiratory noise) Obstruction (lack of breath sounds)
Work of breathing	Nasal flaring (excessive movement of nares) Grunting (expiratory noises) Retractions (chest indrawing): • Supraclavicular (soft tissue above clavicles) • Intercostal (indrawing of the skin between ribs) • Subcostal (just below the costal margin) Paradoxical (seesaw) breathing (abdomen moves outward while chest moves inward during inspiration)

Any of these abnormalities should raise concern about underlying respiratory pathology.

Lower respiratory infections, defined as infections below the vocal cords, are common in infants and include *bronchiolitis* and *pneumonia.*

Acute stridor is a potentially serious condition; causes include *laryngotracheobronchitis (croup), epiglottitis, bacterial tracheitis, foreign body,* or a *vascular ring.*

In infants, abnormal work of breathing plus abnormal findings on auscultation are the best findings for ruling in *pneumonia.* The best sign for ruling *out* pneumonia is the absence of tachypnea.

Because infants are obligate nasal breathers, observe their noses as they breathe. Look for *nasal flaring*. Observe breathing with the infant's mouth closed or during nursing or sucking on a bottle to assess for nasal patency. Listen to the sounds of breathing; note any *grunting, audible wheezing,* or *lack of breath sounds (obstruction). Nasal flaring, grunting, retractions, and wheezing are all signs of respiratory distress.*

Nasal flaring may be the result of *upper respiratory infections* with subsequent obstruction of their small nares, but it may also be caused by pneumonia or other serious respiratory infections.

Observe two aspects of the infant's breathing: *audible breath sounds* and *work of breathing*. These are particularly relevant in assessing both upper and lower respiratory illness.

In healthy infants, the ribs do not move much during quiet breathing. Any outward movement is produced by descent of the diaphragm, which compresses the abdominal contents and in turn shifts the lower ribs outward.

Obstructive respiratory disease in infants can result in the *Hoover sign,* or **paradoxical breathing.**

Asymmetric chest movement may indicate a space-occupying lesion. Pulmonary disease causes increased abdominal breathing and can result in *retractions (chest indrawing)*, an indicator of pulmonary disease before 2 years of age. **Retractions** are inward movement of the skin between the ribs during inspiration (Fig. 23-22).

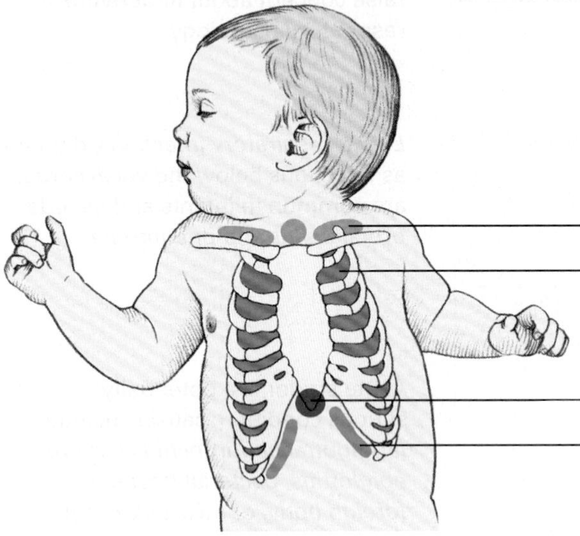

FIGURE 23-22 Locations of retractions.

Palpation

Assess tactile fremitus by *palpation*. Place your hand on the chest when the infant cries or makes noise. Place your hand or fingertips over each side of the chest and feel for symmetry in the transmitted vibrations. Percussion is not helpful in infants except in extreme instances. The infant's chest is hyperresonant throughout, and it is difficult to detect abnormalities on percussion.

Because of the excellent transmission of sounds throughout the chest, any abnormalities of tactile fremitus or on percussion suggest severe pathology, such as a large *pneumonic consolidation.*

Auscultation

After performing these maneuvers, it is time for *auscultation*. Infant breath sounds are louder and harsher than those of adults because the stethoscope is closer to the origin of the sounds. Also, it is often difficult to distinguish transmitted upper airway sounds from sounds originating in the chest. Table 23-12 has some useful hints for distinguishing the two. Upper airway sounds tend to be loud, transmitted symmetrically throughout the chest, and loudest as you move your stethoscope toward the neck. They are usually coarse inspiratory sounds. Lower airway sounds are loudest over the site of pathology, often asymmetric, and often occur during expiration.

Biphasic sounds (wheezing) imply severe obstruction from intrathoracic airway narrowing or severe obstruction from extrathoracic airway narrowing.

Expiratory sounds usually arise from an intrathoracic source, while inspiratory sounds typically arise from an extrathoracic airway such as the trachea. During expiration, the diameter of the intrathoracic airways decreases because radial forces from the surrounding lung do not hold the airways open as occurs during inspiration. Higher flow rates during inspiration produce turbulent flow, resulting in appreciable sounds.

TABLE 23-12 Distinguishing Upper Airway from Lower Airway Sounds in Infants

Technique	Upper Airway	Lower Airway
Compare sounds from nose/stethoscope	Same sounds	Often different sounds
Listen to harshness of sounds	Harsh and loud	Variable
Note symmetry (left/right)	Symmetric	Often asymmetric
Compare sounds at different locations (higher or lower)	Sounds louder as stethoscope is moved up chest	Often sounds louder lower in chest toward abdomen
Inspiratory vs. expiratory	Almost always inspiratory	Often has expiratory phase

Diminished breath sounds in one side of the chest suggest unilateral lesions (e.g., *congenital diaphragmatic hernia or pneumothorax*).

The characteristics of the *breath sounds,* such as vesicular and bronchovesicular, and of the adventitious lung sounds, such as crackles, wheezes, and rhonchi, are the same as those for adults, except that they may be more difficult to distinguish in infants and often occur together. Wheezes and rhonchi are common in infants. *Wheezes,* often audible without the stethoscope, occur more frequently because of the smaller size of the tracheobronchial tree. *Rhonchi* reflect obstruction of larger airways, or bronchi. *Crackles* (rales) are discontinuous sounds (see Chapter 13) near the end of inspiration; they are usually caused by lung disorders and are far less likely to represent cardiac failure in infants than in adults. They tend to be harsher than in adults.

Wheezes in infants occur commonly from *asthma* or *bronchiolitis.*

Crackles (rales) can be heard with *pneumonia* and *bronchiolitis.*

Upper respiratory infections are not serious in infants but can produce loud inspiratory sounds that are transmitted to the chest.

The Heart

Inspection

Before examining the heart itself, observe the infant carefully for any cyanosis. It is important to detect *central cyanosis* because it is always abnormal and has many congenital cardiac abnormalities (Table 23-13), as well as respiratory diseases, present with cyanosis.

Central cyanosis without acute respiratory symptoms suggests cardiac disease.

Recognizing minimal degrees of cyanosis requires care. Look at the tongue, or at the conjunctivae, in addition to assessing skin color. A true strawberry pink is normal, whereas any hint of raspberry red suggests desaturation and requires urgent evaluation.

TABLE 23-13 Congenital Heart Murmurs

Some heart murmurs reflect underlying heart disease. If you understand their physiologic causes, you will more readily be able to identify and distinguish them from innocent heart murmurs. Obstructive lesions result when blood flows through undersized valves. Because this problem does not depend on the drop in pulmonary vascular resistance following birth, these murmurs are audible at birth. Defects with left-to-right shunts, on the other hand, depend on the drop in pulmonary vascular resistance that occurs shortly after birth. High-pressured shunts such as ventricular septal defect, patent ductus arteriosus, and persistent truncus arteriosus are not heard until 1 wk or more after birth. Low-pressured left-to-right shunts, such as atrial septal defects, may not be heard until 1 y or more. Many children with congenital cardiac defects have combinations of defects or variations of abnormalities, so findings on cardiac examination may not follow these classic patterns. This table shows a limited selection of the more common murmurs, starting with murmurs that appear in the newborn period.

Congenital Defect and Mechanism	Characteristics of the Murmur	Associated Findings
Pulmonary Valve Stenosis		
Usually a normal valve annulus with fusion of some or most of the valve leaflets, restricting flow across the valve *Mild* 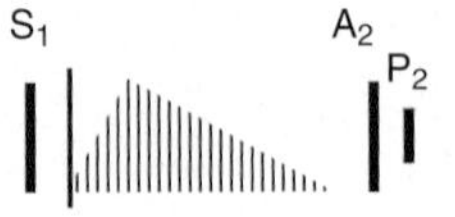 *Severe* 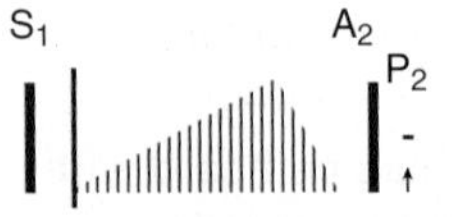	*Location.* Upper left sternal border *Radiation.* In mild degrees of stenosis, the murmur may be heard over the course of the pulmonary arteries in the lung fields. *Intensity.* Increases in intensity and duration as the degree of obstruction increases *Quality.* Ejection, peaking later in systole as the obstruction increases	Usually a prominent ejection click in early systole Pulmonary component of the second sounds at the base (P_2) becomes delayed and softer, disappearing as obstruction increases. Inspiration may increase murmur; expiration may increase click. Growth is usually normal. Newborns with severe stenosis may be cyanotic from right-to-left atrial shunting and rapidly develop heart failure as the ductus arteriosus closes.
Aortic Valve Stenosis		
Usually a bicuspid valve with progressive obstruction, but may occur as a result of a dysplastic valve or damage from rheumatic fever or degenerative disease 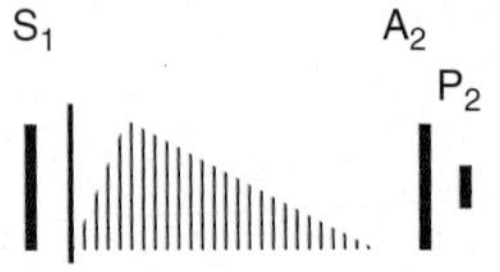	*Location.* Midsternum, upper right sternal border *Radiation.* To the carotid arteries and suprasternal notch; may also be a thrill *Intensity.* Varies, louder with increasingly severe obstruction *Quality.* An ejection, often harsh, systolic murmur	May be an associated ejection click The aortic closure sound may be increased in intensity. There may be a diastolic murmur of aortic valve regurgitation (not shown in the diagram). Newborns with severe stenosis may have weak or absent pulses and severe congestive heart failure. May not be audible until adulthood even though the valve is congenitally abnormal
Tetralogy of Fallot		
Complex defect with ventricular septal defect, infundibular and usually valvular right ventricular outflow obstruction, malrotation of the aorta, and right-to-left shunting at ventricular septal level *With Pulmonic Stenosis* 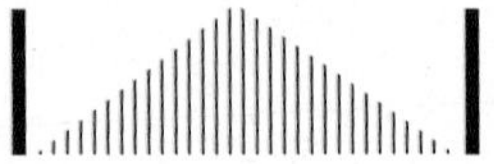 *With Pulmonic Atresia* 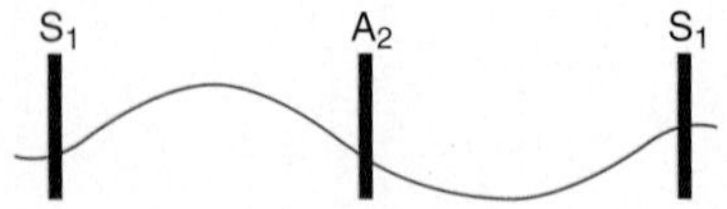	*General.* Variable cyanosis, increasing with activity *Location.* Mid-to-upper left sternal border. If there is pulmonary atresia, there is the continuous murmur of ductus arteriosus flow at upper left sternal border or in the back. *Radiation.* Little, to upper left sternal border, occasionally to lung fields *Intensity.* Usually grade III–IV *Quality.* Mid-peaking, systolic ejection murmur	Normal pulses The pulmonary closure sound is usually not heard. May have abrupt hypercyanotic spells with sudden increase in cyanosis, air hunger, altered level of awareness Failure to gain weight with persistent and increasingly severe cyanosis Long-term persistence of cyanosis accompanied by clubbing of fingers and toes Persistent hypoxemia leads to polycythemia, which will accentuate the cyanosis.

Congenital Defect and Mechanism	Characteristics of the Murmur	Associated Findings
Transposition of the Great Arteries A severe defect with failure of rotation of the great vessels, leaving the aorta to arise from the right ventricle and the pulmonary artery from the left ventricle	*General.* Intense generalized cyanosis *Location.* No characteristic murmur; if present, it may reflect an associated defect such as a ventricular septal defect. *Radiation and Quality.* Depends on associated abnormalities	Single loud second sound of the anterior aortic valve Frequent rapid development of congestive heart failure Frequent associated defects as described at the left
Ventricular Septal Defect (VSD) Blood going from a high-pressured left ventricle through a defect in the septum to the lower-pressured right ventricle creates turbulence, usually throughout systole.[a] 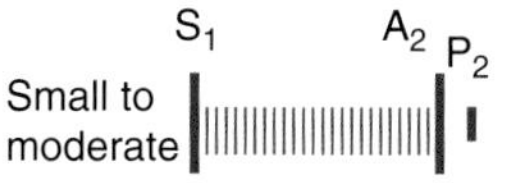	*Location.* Lower left sternal border *Radiation.* Little *Intensity.* Variable, only partially determined by the size of the shunt. Small shunts with a high-pressure gradient may have very loud murmurs. Large defects with elevated pulmonary vascular resistance may have no murmur. Grade II–IV/VI with a thrill if grade IV/VI or higher *Quality.* Pansystolic, usually harsh, may obscure S_1 and S_2 if loud enough	With large shunts, there may be a low-pitched middiastolic murmur of relative mitral stenosis at the apex. As pulmonary artery pressure increases, the pulmonic component of the second sounds at the base increases in intensity. When pulmonary artery pressure equals aortic pressure, there may be no murmur, and P_2 will be very loud. In low-volume shunts, growth is normal. In larger shunts, heart failure may occur by 6–8 wk. Poor weight gain, poor feeding. Associated defects are frequent.
Patent Ductus Arteriosus Continuous flow from aorta to pulmonary artery throughout the cardiac cycle when ductus arteriosus does not close after birth[a] 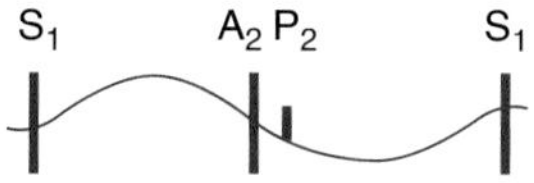	*Location.* Upper left sternal border and to left *Radiation.* Sometimes to the back *Intensity.* Varies depending on size of the shunt, usually grade II–III/VI *Quality.* A rather hollow, sometimes machinery-like murmur that is continuous throughout the cardiac cycle, although occasionally almost inaudible in late diastole, uninterrupted by the heart sounds, louder in systole	Full to bounding pulses Noticed at birth in the premature infant who may have bounding pulses, a hyperdynamic precordium, and an atypical murmur Noticed later in the full-term infant as pulmonary vascular resistance falls May develop heart failure at 4–6 wk if large shunt Poor weight gain related to size of shunt Pulmonary hypertension affects murmur as above.
Atrial Septal Defect Left-to-right shunt through an opening in the atrial septum, possible at various levels 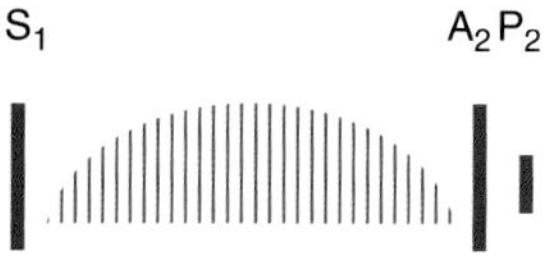	*Location.* Upper left sternal border *Radiation.* To the back *Intensity.* Variable, usually grade II–III/VI *Quality.* Ejection but without the harsh quality	Widely split second sounds throughout all phases of respiration, normal intensity Usually not heard until after age of 1 y Gradual decrease in weight gain as shunt increases Decreased exercise tolerance, subtle, not dramatic Heart failure is rare.

[a]Small to moderate size.

The distribution of the cyanosis should be evaluated (Table 23-14). An oximetry reading will confirm desaturation.

TABLE 23-14 Cyanosis in Children

It is important to recognize cyanosis. The best location to assess for cyanosis is the mucous membranes. Cyanosis has "raspberry" color, while normal mucous membranes should have a "strawberry" color. Try to identify the cyanosis in these photographs before reading the descriptions.

Generalized Cyanosis

This patient has total anomalous pulmonary venous return and an oxygen saturation level of 80%. (*Generalized Cyanosis*—Bickley, L. S., Szilagyi, P. G., Hoffman, R. M., & Soriano, R. P. [2020]. *Bates' guide to physical examination and history taking* [13th ed.]. Wolters Kluwer.)

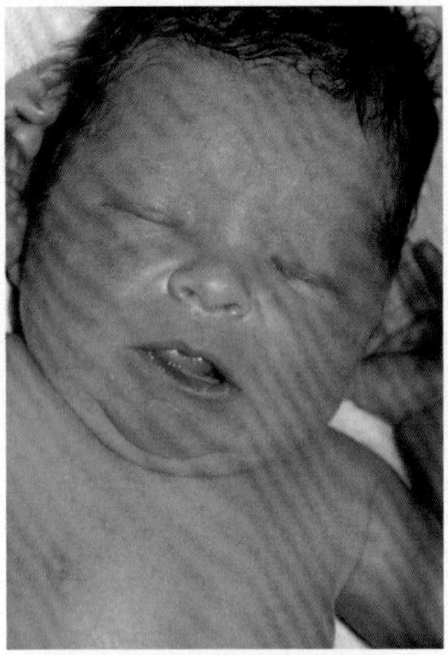

Perioral Cyanosis

This patient has mild cyanosis above the lips, but the mucous membranes remain pink.

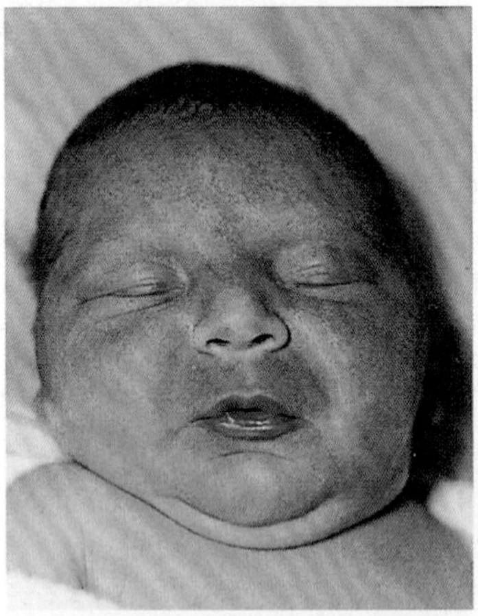

Bluish Lips, Giving Appearance of Cyanosis

Normal pigment deposition in the vermilion border of the lips gives them a bluish hue, but the mucous membranes are pink.

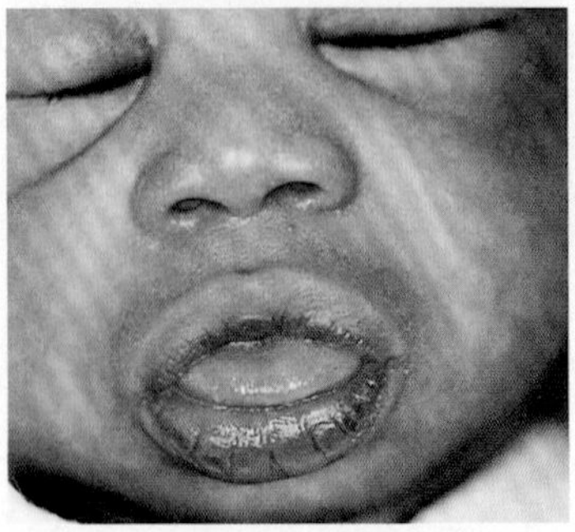

Acrocyanosis

Acrocyanosis commonly appears on the feet and hands of babies shortly after birth. This infant is a 32-wk newborn.

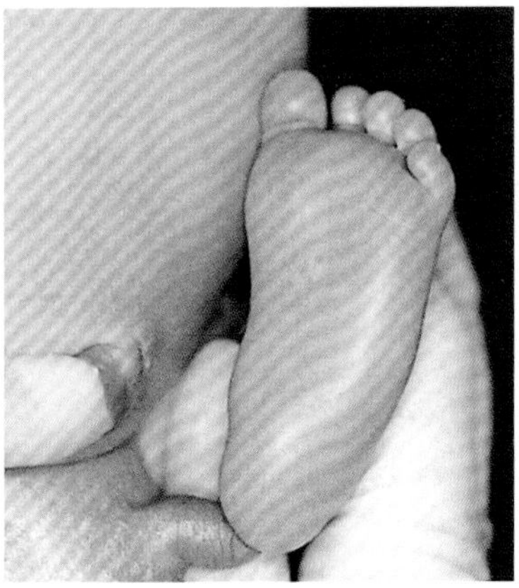

Source of photos: Fletcher, M. (1998). *Physical diagnosis in neonatology*. Lippincott-Raven.

Observe the infant for *general signs of health*. The infant's nutritional status, responsiveness, happiness, and irritability and fatigue are all clues that may be useful in evaluating cardiac disease. Note that noncardiac findings can be present in infants with cardiac disease (Box 23-3).

Tachypnea, tachycardia, and hepatomegaly in infants suggest *congestive heart failure*.

BOX 23-3 COMMON NONCARDIAC FINDINGS IN INFANTS WITH CARDIAC DISEASE

- Poor feeding
- Failure to thrive
- Irritability
- Tachypnea
- Hepatomegaly
- Clubbing
- Poor overall appearance
- Weakness
- Fatigue

Observe the respiratory rate and pattern to help distinguish the degree of illness and cardiac versus pulmonary diseases. An increase in respiratory effort is expected from pulmonary diseases; while in cardiac disease, there may be tachypnea without increased work of breathing (called "peaceful tachypnea") until congestive heart failure becomes significant.

A diffuse bulge outward of the left side of the chest suggests long-standing *cardiomegaly* (an enlarged heart).

Palpation

Pulses

The major branches of the aorta can be assessed by evaluation of the *peripheral pulses*. In neonates and infants, the brachial artery pulse in the antecubital fossa is easier to feel than the radial artery pulse at the wrist. Both temporal arteries should be felt just in front of the ear.

Palpate femoral pulses. They lie in the midline just below the inguinal crease between the iliac crest and the symphysis pubis. Take your time and search for femoral pulses; they are difficult to detect in chubby, squirming infants. If the infant's thighs are flexed on the abdomen first, this may overcome the reflex flexion that occurs when you then extend the legs.

The absence or diminution of femoral pulses is indicative of *coarctation of the aorta*. If femoral pulses cannot be detected, measure blood pressures of the lower and upper extremities. Normally the blood pressure in the lower extremity is slightly higher than in the upper extremities. If they are equal or lower in the legs, coarctation is likely to be present.

Palpate the dorsalis pedis and posterior tibial pulses (Fig. 23-23), which may be difficult to feel unless there is an abnormality involving aortic runoff. Normal pulses should have a sharp rise and should be firm and well localized.

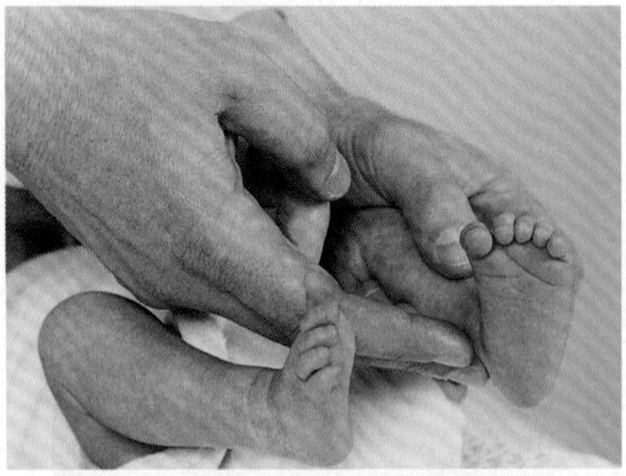

FIGURE 23-23 Palpating the posterior tibial pulse.

A weak or *thready,* difficult-to-feel pulse may reflect *myocardial dysfunction* and *congestive heart failure,* particularly if associated with an unusual degree of tachycardia.

As discussed in the "Blood Pressure" section, carefully measure the *blood pressure* of infants and children as part of the cardiac examination.

Apical Impulse

The apical impulse is not always palpable in infants and is affected by respiratory patterns, a full stomach, and the infant's positioning. It is usually an interspace higher than in adults during the first few years of life because the heart lies more horizontally within the chest.

A *"rolling" heave* at the left sternal border suggests an *increase in right ventricular work,* whereas the same kind of motion closer to the apex suggests the same thing for the left ventricle.

Chest Wall

Palpation of the chest wall will allow you to assess volume changes within the heart. For example, a hyperdynamic precordium reflects a big volume change.

Thrills

Thrills are palpable when turbulence within the heart or great vessels is transmitted to the surface. Knowledge of the structures of the precordium helps pinpoint the origin of the thrill. Thrills are easiest to feel with your palm or the base of your fingers rather than your fingertips. Thrills have a somewhat rough, vibrating quality. Figure 23-24 shows locations of thrills from various cardiac abnormalities that occur in infants and children.

Visible and palpable chest pulsations suggest a hyperdynamic state from either increased metabolic rate or inefficient pumping as a result of an underlying cardiac defect.

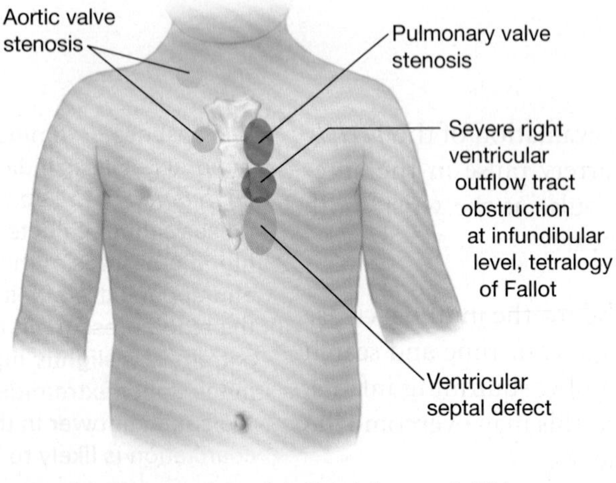

FIGURE 23-24 Locations of thrills in infants and children.

Auscultation

The *heart rhythm* can be evaluated more easily in infants by listening to the heart than by feeling the peripheral pulses; in older children, it can be done either way. Infants and children commonly have a normal sinus arrhythmia with the heart rate increasing on inspiration and decreasing on expiration, sometimes quite abruptly. This normal finding can be identified by its repetitive nature and its correlation with respiration.

The most common dysrhythmia in infants is *PSVT,* or *paroxysmal atrial tachycardia (PAT)*. It can occur at any age, including in utero. It is remarkably well tolerated by some infants and children and is found on examination. The child may look perfectly healthy or may be mildly pale or have tachypnea. The heart rate is sustained and regular at around 240 beats per minute or more. Some children, particularly neonates, may appear very ill. In older children, this dysrhythmia is more likely to be truly paroxysmal, with episodes of varying duration and frequency.

See Table 23-2, "Abnormalities in Heart Rhythm and Blood Pressure."

Many infants and some older children have premature atrial or ventricular beats that are often appreciated as "skipped" beats.

Heart Sounds

Heart sounds are challenging to assess in infants because they are rapid and often obscured by respiratory or other sounds. Nevertheless, evaluate the S_1 and S_2 heart sounds carefully and systematically. They are normally crisp. You can usually hear the second sound (S_2) at the base separately, but they should fuse into a single sound in deep expiration. In the neonate, you should be able to detect a split S_2 if you examine the infant when the infant is completely quiet or asleep. Detecting this split eliminates many, but not all, of the more serious congenital cardiac defects.

Distant heart tones suggest *pericardial effusion;* mushy, less distinct heart sounds suggest *myocardial dysfunction.*

In addition to trying to detect splitting of the S_2, listen for the intensity of A_2 and P_2 (Fig. 23-25). The aortic, or first component of the second sound at the base, is normally louder than the pulmonic, or second component.

A louder-than-normal pulmonic component, particularly when louder than the aortic sound, suggests *pulmonary hypertension.*

Persistent splitting of S_2 may indicate a right ventricular volume load such as *atrial septal defect, anomalies of pulmonary venous return,* or *chronic anemia.*

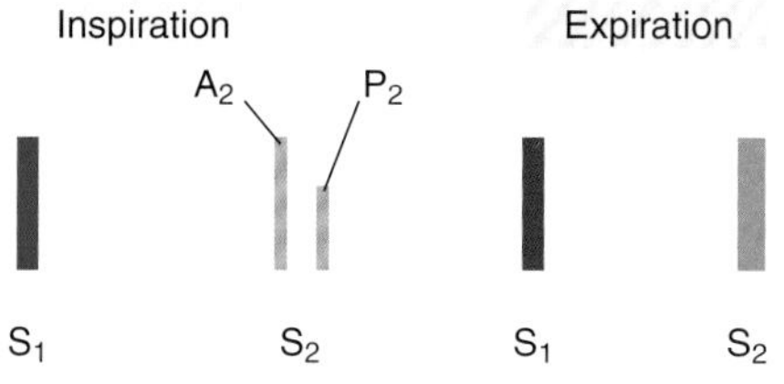

FIGURE 23-25 Split S_2 on inspiration.

A *third heart sound may be detected*. It is low-pitched, early diastolic sounds best heard at the lower left sternal border, or apex. These are frequently heard in children and are normal (Fig. 23-26). They reflect rapid ventricular filling.

The third heart sound (S_3) should be differentiated from the higher-intensity third heart sound gallop, which is a sign of underlying pathology.

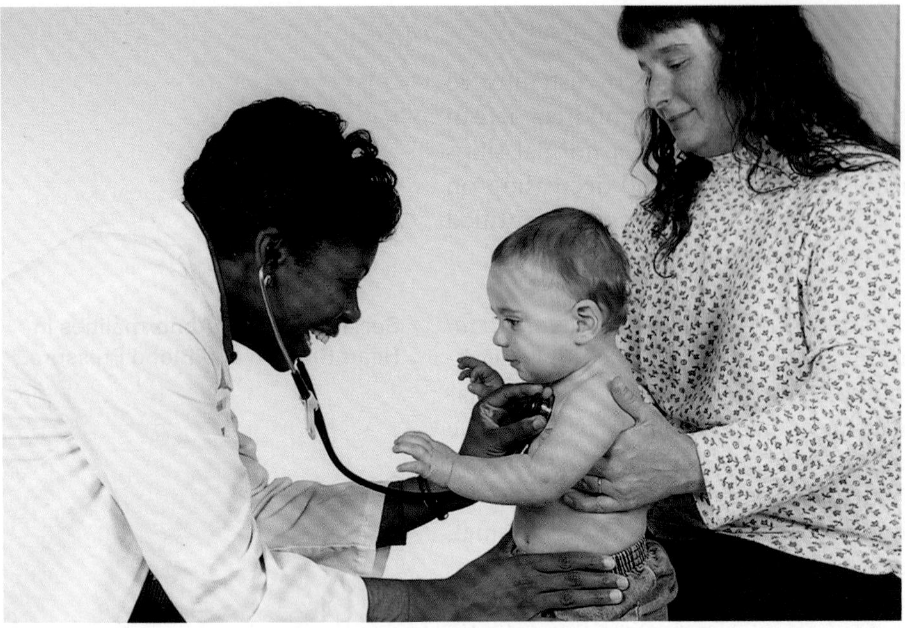

FIGURE 23-26 Listen to the infant's heart while the baby is sitting on the parent's lap. This may help keep the infant calm and quiet.

Fourth heart sounds (S_4), which are not often heard in children, are low-frequency, late diastolic sounds, occurring just before the first heart sound.

Fourth heart sounds represent decreased ventricular compliance, suggesting *congestive heart failure.*

Heart Murmurs

One of the most challenging aspects of cardiac examination in children is the evaluation of *heart murmurs.* A major challenge is distinguishing common benign murmurs from unusual or pathologic ones. Characterize heart murmurs in infants and children by noting their specific location (e.g., left upper sternal border, not just left sternal border), timing, intensity, and quality.

See Table 23-13, "Congenital Heart Murmurs."

An important rule of thumb is that, by definition, *benign murmurs in children have no associated abnormal findings.* Many (but not all) children with serious cardiac malformations have signs and symptoms other than a heart murmur obtainable on careful history or examination. Many have other noncardiac signs and symptoms, including evidence of genetic defects that may offer helpful diagnostic clues.

Any of the *noncardiac findings* (see Box 23-3) that frequently accompany cardiac disease in children markedly raises the possibility that a murmur is pathologic (Box 23-4).

Many children will have one or more *functional, or benign, heart murmurs* before reaching adulthood (Frank & Jacobe, 2011; Gessner, 1997; Wierwille, 2011). It is important to identify functional murmurs by their specific qualities rather than by their intensity.

BOX 23-4 PHYSIOLOGIC BASIS FOR SOME PATHOLOGIC HEART MURMURS

Change in Pulmonary Vascular Resistance

Heart murmurs that are dependent on a postnatal drop in pulmonary vascular resistance, allowing turbulent flow from the high-pressure systemic circuit to the lower-pressure pulmonary circuit, are not audible until such a drop has occurred. Therefore, except in premature infants, murmurs of a *ventricular septal defect* or *patent ductus arteriosus* are not heard in the first few days of life and usually become audible after a week to 10 days.

Obstructive Lesions

Obstructive lesions, such as *pulmonic and aortic stenosis,* are caused by normal blood flow through two small valves. They are not dependent on a drop in pulmonary vascular resistance. They are audible at birth.

Pressure Gradient Differences

Murmurs of *atrioventricular valve regurgitation* are audible at birth because of the high-pressure gradient between the ventricle and its atrium.

Changes Associated with Growth of Children

Some murmurs do not follow the rules above but become audible because of alterations in normal blood flow that occurs with growth. For example, even though it is an obstructive defect, *aortic stenosis* may not be audible until considerable growth has occurred and indeed is frequently not heard until adulthood though a congenitally abnormal valve is responsible. Similarly, the pulmonary flow murmur of an *atrial septal defect* may not be heard for a year or more because right ventricular compliance gradually increases and the shunt becomes larger, eventually producing a murmur caused by too much blood flow across a normal pulmonic valve.

A newborn with a heart murmur and central cyanosis likely has congenital heart disease and requires urgent cardiac evaluation.

When any murmur in a child is detected, note all of the signs and symptoms described in Chapter 14 to help you distinguish *pathologic murmurs* from the benign murmurs.

The Breasts

The breasts of the infant should be undeveloped and flush with the chest wall. Residual enlargement from maternal estrogen may last for several months after birth. The breasts may also be engorged with a white liquid, sometimes colloquially called "witch's milk," which may last 1 or 2 weeks.

In *premature thelarche* (onset of secondary breast development), breast development occurs, most often between 6 months and 2 years. Other signs of puberty or hormonal abnormalities are not present.

The Abdomen

Inspection

Inspect the abdomen with the infant lying supine (and optimally asleep). The infant's abdomen is protuberant as a result of poorly developed abdominal musculature. Abdominal wall blood vessels and intestinal peristalsis are easily noticed.

Inspect the area around the umbilicus for redness or swelling. *Umbilical hernias* are detectable by a few weeks of age. Most disappear by 1 year, nearly all by 5 years.

Umbilical hernias in infants are caused by a defect in the abdominal wall and can be up to 6 cm in diameter and quite protuberant with intra-abdominal pressure.

In some normal infants, a **diastasis recti** may be noticed. This involves separation of the two rectus abdominis muscles, causing a midline ridge, most apparent when the infant contracts the abdominal muscles. A benign condition in most cases, it resolves during early childhood.

Auscultation

Auscultation of a quiet infant's abdomen is easy. Do not be surprised if you hear an orchestra of musical tinkling bowel sounds upon placement of your stethoscope on the infant's abdomen.

An increase in pitch or frequency of bowel sounds is heard with *gastroenteritis* or rarely with *intestinal obstruction.*

Percussion and Palpation

The infant's abdomen can be percussed as an adult's, but be prepared to note greater tympanitic sounds because of the infant's propensity to swallow air. Percussion is useful for determining the size of organs and abdominal masses.

A silent, tympanic, distended, and tender abdomen suggests *peritonitis.*

It is easy to *palpate* an infant's abdomen because infants like being touched. A useful technique to relax the infant, shown in Figure 23-27, is to hold the legs flexed at the knees and hips with one hand and palpate the abdomen with the other. A pacifier may be used to quiet the infant in this position.

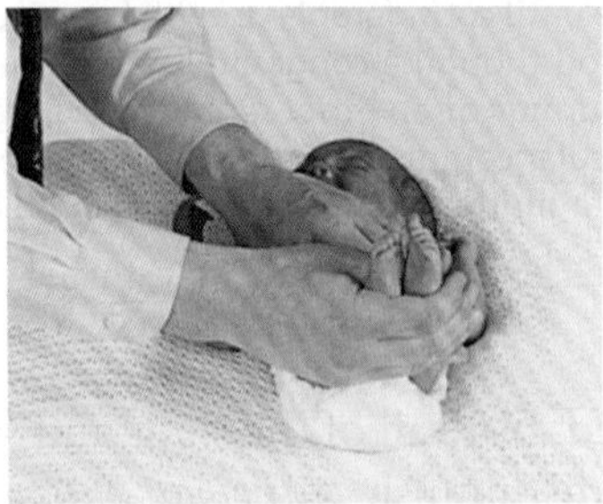

FIGURE 23-27 Palpating the infant's abdomen.

Start gently palpating the liver of infants low in the abdomen, moving upward with your fingers. This technique helps you avoid missing an extremely enlarged liver that extends down into the pelvis. With a careful examination, you can feel the liver edge in most infants 1 to 2 cm below the right costal margin.

An enlarged, tender liver may be due to *congestive heart failure* or to *storage diseases.* Among newborns, causes of hepatomegaly include *hepatitis, storage diseases, vascular congestion,* and *biliary obstruction.*

One technique for assessing liver size in infants is simultaneous percussion and auscultation. Percuss and simultaneously auscultate, noting a change in sound as you percuss over the liver or beyond it.

The *spleen,* like the liver, is felt easily in most infants. It is also soft with a sharp edge, and it projects downward like a tongue from under the left costal margin. The spleen is moveable and rarely extends more than 1 to 2 cm below the left costal margin.

Several diseases can cause splenomegaly, including *infections, hemolytic anemias, infiltrative disorders, inflammatory* or *autoimmune diseases,* and *portal hypertension.*

Palpate the *other abdominal structures.* You will commonly note pulsations in the epigastrium caused by the aorta. This is felt on deep palpation to the left of the midline.

Abnormal abdominal masses in infants can be associated with the kidney (e.g., *hydronephrosis*), bladder (e.g., *urethral obstruction*) or bowel (e.g., *Hirschsprung disease, intussusception*), and tumors.

The kidneys of infants may be palpated by carefully placing the fingers of one hand on the abdomen in front of the kidney and those of the other hand on the back behind the kidney. The descending colon is a sausage-like mass in the left lower quadrant.

In *pyloric stenosis* (narrowing of the pyloric valve), deep palpation in the right upper quadrant or midline can reveal an "olive," or a 2-cm firm pyloric mass. While feeding, some infants with this condition will have visible peristaltic waves pass across the abdomen followed by projectile vomiting. Infants with this condition tend to present at about 4 to 6 weeks of age.

Once the normal structures in the infant's abdomen have been identified, use palpation to identify abnormal masses.

Male Genitalia

Inspect the male genitalia with the infant supine, noting the appearance of the penis, testes, and scrotum. The *foreskin* completely covers the *glans penis.* It is nonretractable at birth, though you may be able to retract it enough to visualize the external urethral meatus. The foreskin gradually loosens over months to years and becomes retractable.

Circumcision is the removal of the foreskin from the human penis. While the AAP states that the health benefits of newborn male circumcision (e.g., reduced risks of HIV and STIs) outweigh the risks, it also notes that the benefits are not great enough to recommend universal newborn circumcision and therefore recommends that the final decision be deferred to parents based on their religious, ethical, and cultural beliefs (AAP, 2012).

Inspect the *shaft of the penis,* noting any abnormalities on the ventral surface. Make sure the penis appears straight. Table 23-15 illustrates abnormalities that may be found in the male infant's genitourinary system.

Hypospadias refers to an abnormal location of the urethral orifice at some point along the ventral surface of the glans or shaft of the penis. The foreskin is incompletely formed ventrally.

A fixed, downward curving of the penis is a *chordee;* this may accompany a hypospadias.

Inspect the *scrotum,* noting rugae (ridges of skin), which should be present by 40 weeks of gestation. Palpate the testes in the scrotal sacs, proceeding downward from the external inguinal ring to the scrotum. If you feel a testis up in the inguinal canal, gently milk it downward into the scrotum. The newborn's testes should be about 10 mm in width and 15 mm in length and should lie in the scrotal sacs most of the time. If an infant's testicle has not descended by 6 months, referral to a specialist is indicated.

In newborns with an *undescended testicle* (*cryptorchidism*), the scrotum often appears underdeveloped and tight, and palpation reveals an absence of scrotal contents (see Table 23-15, "The Genitourinary System").

Examine the testes for swelling within the scrotal sac and over the inguinal ring. If you detect swelling in the scrotal sac, try to differentiate it from the testis. Note whether the size changes when the infant increases abdominal pressure by crying. Two common scrotal masses in newborns are *hydroceles* and *inguinal hernias;* both frequently coexist, and are more common on the right side. See Table 21-7, "Abnormalities of the Penis and Scrotum."

TABLE 23-15 The Male Genitourinary System

Hypospadias

Hypospadias is the most common congenital penile abnormality. The urethral meatus opens abnormally on the ventral surface of the penis. One form is shown above; more severe forms involve openings on the lower shaft or scrotum.

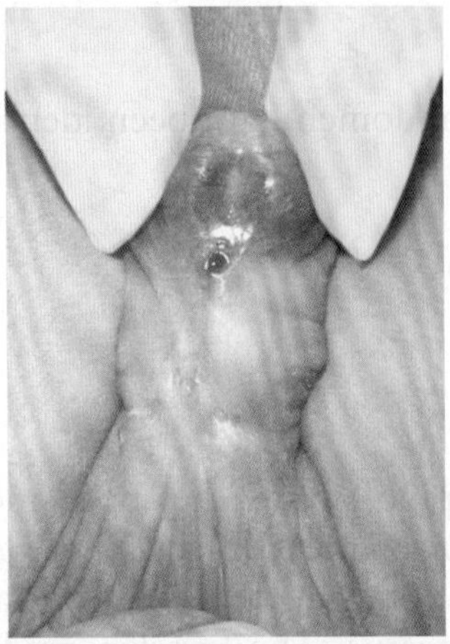

Undescended Testicle

You should distinguish between undescended testes, shown above (with testes in the inguinal canals), from highly retractile testes from an active cremasteric reflex.

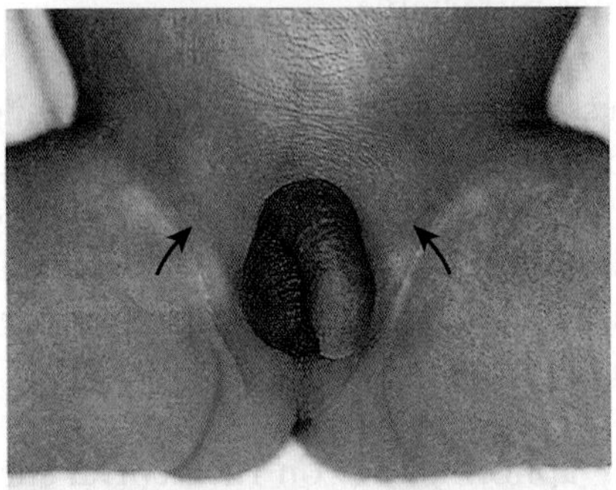

Sources of photos: *Hypospadias*—Courtesy of Warren Snodgrass, MD, UT-Southwestern Medical Center at Dallas; *Undescended Testicle*—Fletcher, M. (1998). *Physical diagnosis in neonatology*. Lippincott-Raven.

Hydroceles (accumulation of serous fluid in a sac, Fig. 23-28) overlie the testes and the spermatic cord, are not reducible, and can be transilluminated. During transillumination of the scrotum, the light will pass through the clear fluid of the hydrocele causing the scrotum to appear red. Most hydroceles resolve by 18 months. Hernias are separate from the testes, are usually reducible, and often do not transilluminate. They do not resolve.

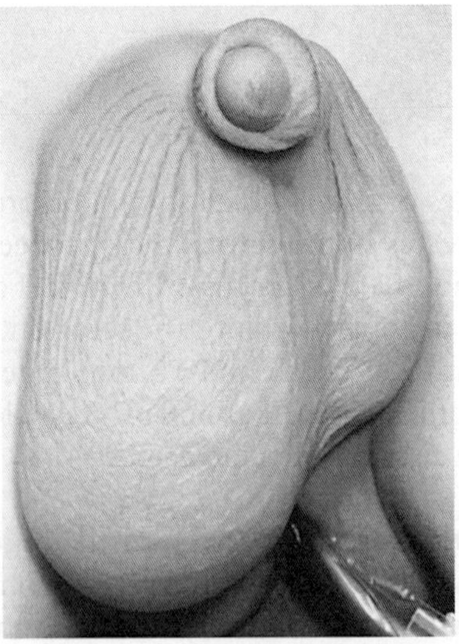

FIGURE 23-28 Hydrocele is present in the right scrotum. (Reprinted with permission from Fleisher, G. R., Ludwig, S., & Baskin, M. N. [2004]. *Atlas of pediatric emergency medicine*. Lippincott Williams & Wilkins, Fig. 9.3.)

Female Genitalia

In the infant female, the labia majora and minora have a dull pink color in light-skinned infants and may be hyperpigmented in dark-skinned infants.

Ambiguous genitalia, involving masculinization of the female external genitalia, is a rare condition caused by endocrine disorders such as *congenital adrenal hyperplasia.*

Examine the female genitalia with the infant supine (Fig. 23-29).

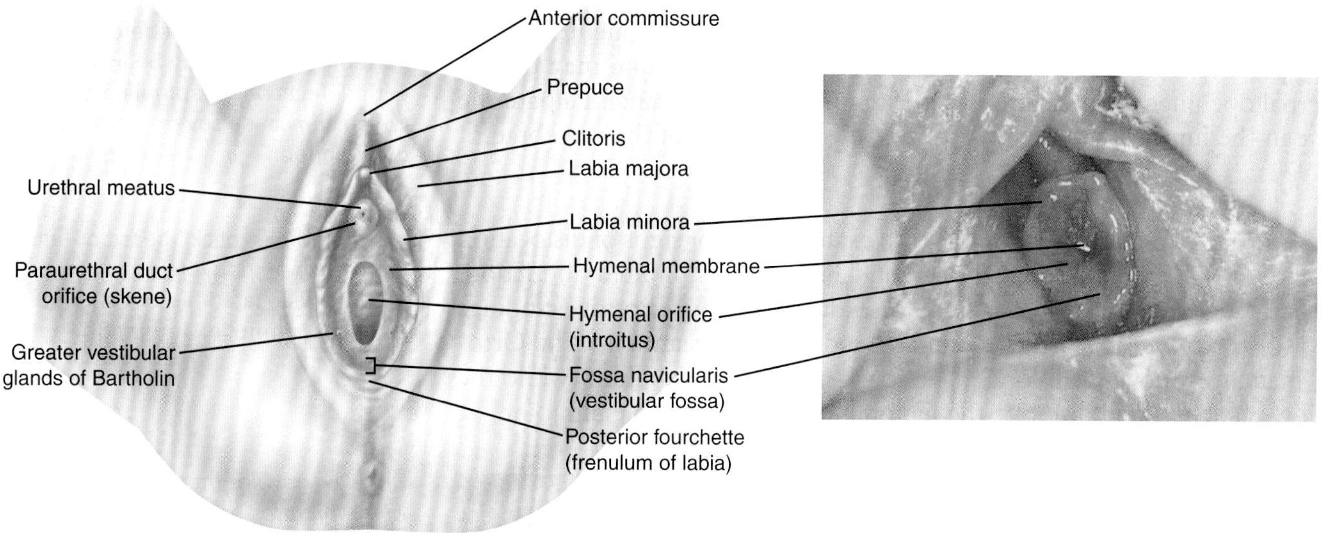

FIGURE 23-29 Anatomy of the female genitalia of an infant.

Examine the different structures systematically, including the size of the clitoris, the color and size of the labia majora, and any rashes, bruises, or external lesions. Next, separate the labia majora at their midpoint with the thumb of each hand for young infants. Infants will not mind the examination because they are used to having their diapers changed and their bodies washed.

Labial adhesions occur not infrequently, tend to be paper thin, and often disappear without treatment.

Inspect the urethral orifice and the labia minora. Inspect the hymen, which in infants is a thickened, avascular structure with a central orifice, covering the vaginal opening. You should note a vaginal opening, though the hymen is thickened. Note any discharge.

An imperforate hymen may be noted at birth. Refer the infant to a pediatrician or nurse practitioner if found.

Rectal Examination

The rectal examination is generally not performed for infants or children unless there is question of patency of the anus or an abdominal mass. Refer the patient to the pediatrician or pediatric nurse practitioner if an imperforate anus is found.

The Musculoskeletal System

Enormous changes in the musculoskeletal system occur during infancy. Much of the examination of the infant focuses on detection of congenital abnormalities, particularly in the hands, spine, hips, legs, and feet. With a little practice, you will be able to combine the musculoskeletal examination with the neurologic and developmental examination.

Careful inspection can reveal gross deformities such as dwarfism, congenital abnormalities of the extremities or digits, and annular bands that constrict an extremity.

Palpate along the *clavicle*, noting any lumps, tenderness, or crepitus; these may indicate a fracture.

Inspect the *spine* carefully. Subtle abnormalities such as pigmented spots, hairy patches, or deep pits within 1 cm or so of the midline may overlie external openings of sinus tracts that extend to the spinal canal. Palpate the spine in the lumbosacral region, noting any deformities of the vertebrae.

Spina bifida occulta (a defect of the vertebral bodies) may be associated with defects of the spinal cord, which can cause severe neurologic dysfunction.

Examine the infant's *hips* carefully at each examination for signs of dislocation (Yang et al., 2019). Positive Ortolani and Barlow tests, limited abduction, and leg-length discrepancy are signs of a dislocated hip. Positive findings need to be referred for further evaluation and possible treatment. The Ortolani maneuver moves a dislocated hip back into the acetabulum, while the Barlow maneuver will dislocate the femoral head in an unstable hip joint.

A soft audible "click" heard or felt with these maneuvers does not prove a dislocated hip but should prompt a careful examination.

Make sure the baby is relaxed. For the *Ortolani test* (Fig. 23-30), place the baby supine with the legs pointing toward you. Flex the legs to form right angles at the hips and knees, placing your index fingers over the greater trochanter of each femur and your thumbs over the lesser trochanters. Abduct both hips until the lateral aspect of each knee touches the examining table.

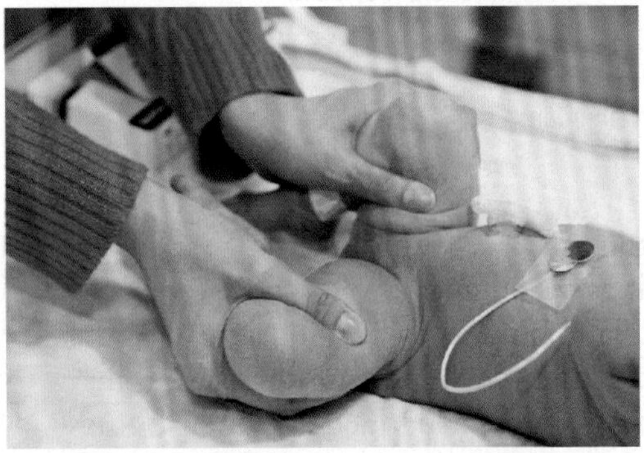

FIGURE 23-30 Adduction of the legs in the Ortolani test.

Signs of *developmental dysplasia of the hip are* any limitation of abduction in either or both hips and feeling a "clunk" as the femoral head, which lies posterior to the acetabulum, enters the acetabulum. A palpable movement of the femoral head back into place constitutes a *positive Ortolani sign.*

For the *Barlow test* (Fig. 23-31), position the infant as you did with the Ortolani test, supine with legs flexed 90 degrees at the hips and knees with your fingers along the femur. Adduct the thighs and apply gentle downward pressure and feel for a "clunk" as the femoral head slips over the rim of the acetabulum.

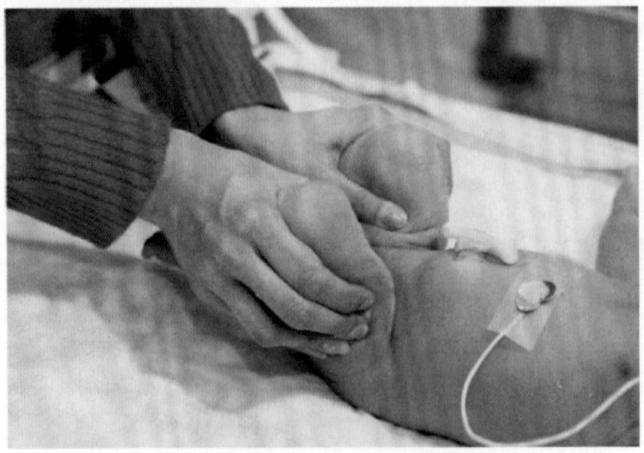

FIGURE 23-31 Abduction of the legs in the Barlow test.

Dislocation of the femur head during the Barlow test is a sign of developmental dysplasia of the hip.

CLINICAL TIP
Developmental dysplasia is important to detect as early appropriate treatment has excellent outcomes.

Femoral shortening may also be seen with hip dysplasia. *The Galeazzi* or *Allis test will show femoral shortening* (Fig. 23-32). With the child lying supine on a firm flat table or surface, flex the hips and knees and place the feet flat on the table near the buttocks. With the knees together, check the height of the knees, which should be even. If the knee height is uneven, the shorter knee will indicate the leg with hip dysplasia.

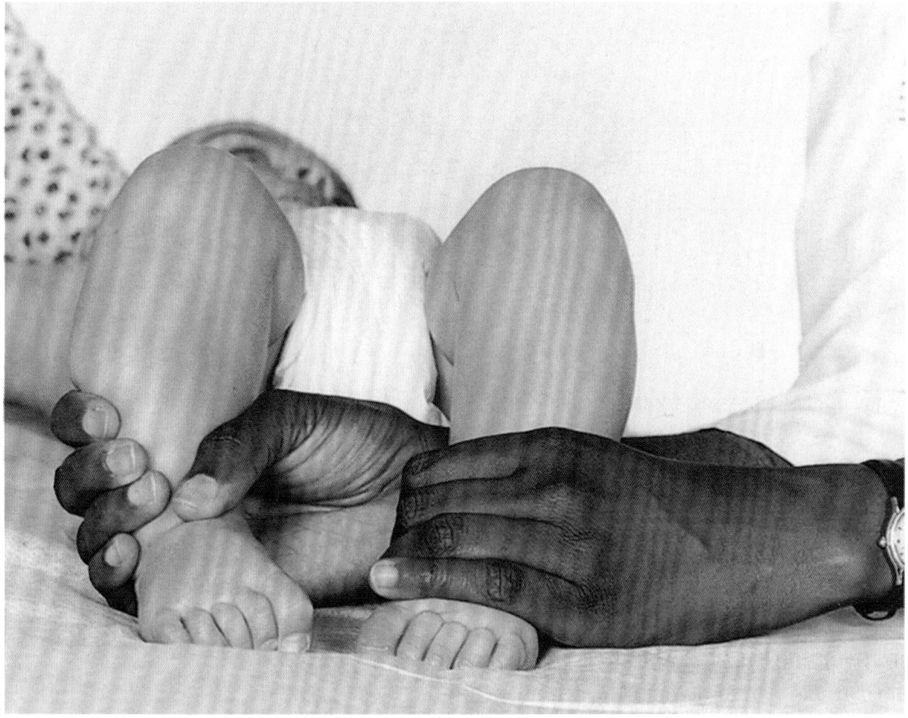

FIGURE 23-32 Checking femoral shortening with the Allis test.

In addition to examining the hips, it is important to examine an infant's *legs and feet* to detect developmental abnormalities. Assess symmetry, bowing, and torsion of the legs. There should be no discrepancy in leg length. It is common for normal infants to have asymmetric thigh skin folds, but if you do detect asymmetry, make sure you perform the instability tests because dislocated hips are commonly associated with this finding.

Most infants are *bowlegged,* reflecting their curled-up intrauterine position.

Severe bowing of the knees can be normal, but it can also be due to *rickets* or *Blount disease.* The most common cause of bowing is **tibial torsion** (an **inward twisting of the shin bones, which** causes the child's feet to turn inward).

Some infants without hip dysplasia exhibit twisting or *torsion of the tibia* inwardly or outwardly on its longitudinal axis. Parents may be concerned about a toeing in or toeing out of the foot and an awkward gait, all of which are usually normal. Tibial torsion corrects itself during the second year of life after months of weight bearing.

Pathologic tibial torsion occurs only in association with *deformities of the feet or hips.*

Now examine the feet. At birth, the feet may appear deformed from retaining their intrauterine positioning, often turned inward as shown in Figure 23-33. You should be able to correct the feet to the neutral (see Fig. 23-33A) and even to an overcorrected position (see Fig. 23-33B). You can also scratch or stroke along the outer edge to see if the foot assumes a normal position.

True *deformities of the feet* do not return to the neutral position even with manipulation.

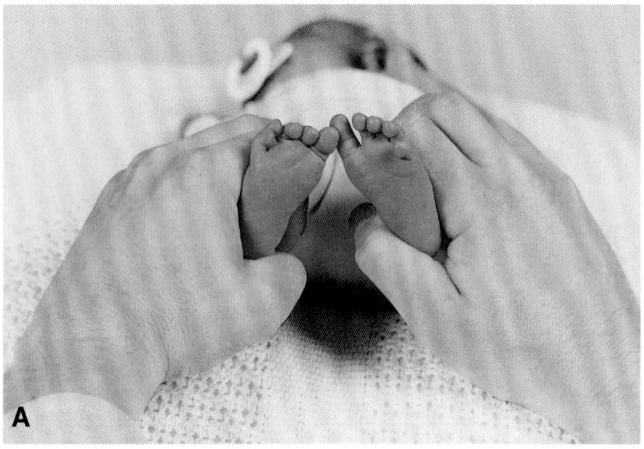

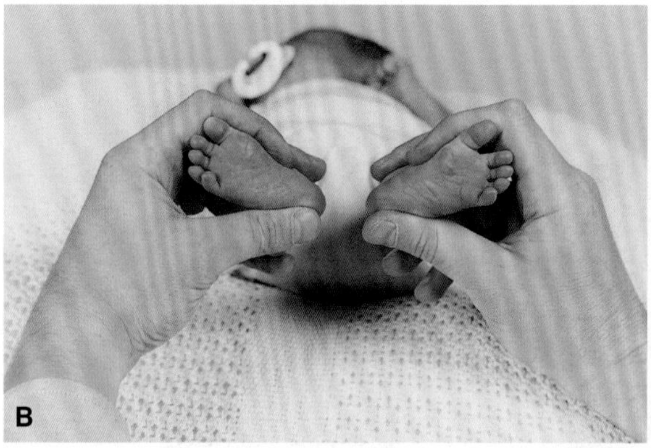

FIGURE 23-33 **A.** Assessing foot alignment in a neutral position. **B.** Assess foot alignment with the feet overcorrected.

The infant's foot appears flat because of a plantar fat pad. There is often inversion of the foot, elevating the outer margin. Other babies will have adduction of the forefoot without inversion, called **metatarsus adductus**, (metatarsal bones turned toward the midline, "pigeon-toed"), which requires close follow-up. Still others will have adduction of the entire foot. Finally, most toddlers have some pronation during early stages of weight bearing with eversion of the foot. In all of these normal variants, the abnormal position can be easily overcorrected past midline. They all tend to resolve within 1 or 2 years. See Table 23-16, "Common Musculoskeletal Findings in Young Children."

The most common severe congenital foot deformity is **talipes equinovarus** (talipes calcaneovalgus), or *clubfoot.*

The Nervous System

The examination of the nervous system in infants includes techniques that are highly specific to this particular age. Further, unlike many neurologic abnormalities in adults that produce asymmetric localized findings, neurologic abnormalities in infants often present as developmental abnormalities such as failure to do age-appropriate tasks. Therefore, the neurologic and developmental examinations need to proceed hand in hand. Finding a developmental abnormality should prompt you to pay particular attention to the neurologic examination.

TABLE 23-16 Common Musculoskeletal Findings in Young Children

Flat feet or *pes planus* from laxity of the soft-tissue structures of the foot

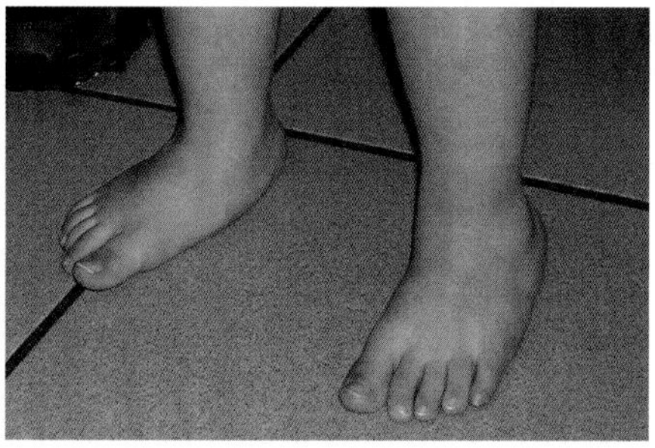

Inversion of the foot (*pes varus*)

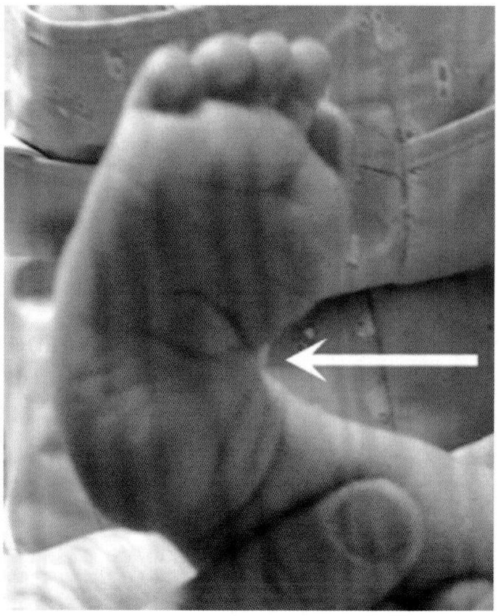

Metatarsus adductus in a child. The convex ("C") shape of the child's right foot suggests metatarsus adductus

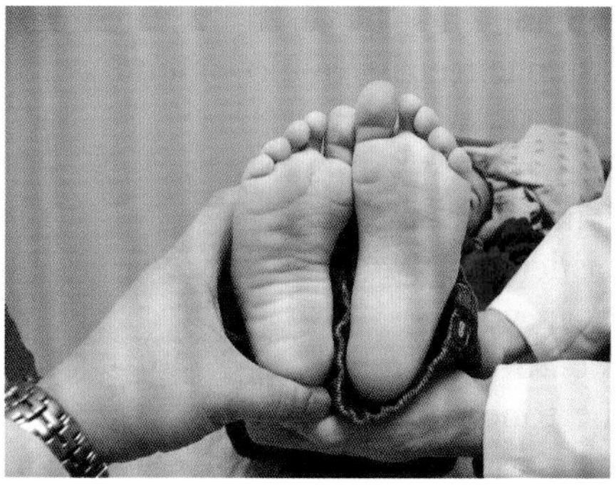

Pronation in a toddler. **A.** When viewed from behind, the hindfoot is everted. **B.** When viewed from the front, the forefoot is everted and abducted

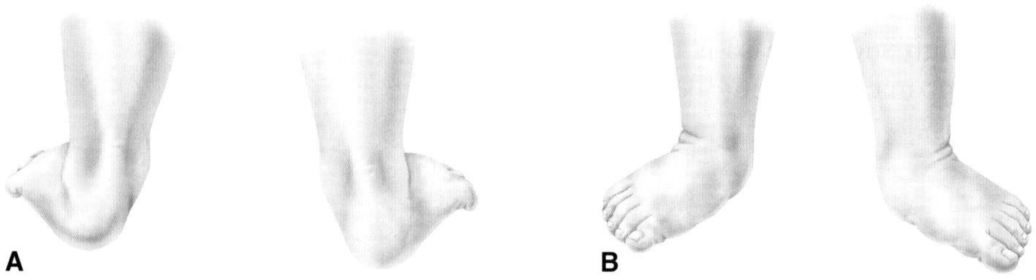

CLINICAL TIP
Signs of severe neurologic disease in infants include *extreme irritability, persistent asymmetry of posture, persistent extension of extremities, constant turning of the head to one side, marked extension of the head, neck, and extremities (opisthotonos), severe flaccidity, limited response to pain, and sometimes seizures.*

The neurologic screening examination of all infants should include assessment of mental status; gross and fine motor function, tone, cry, and deep tendon reflexes; and primitive reflexes. More detailed examinations of cranial nerve function and sensory function are indicated if you suspect any abnormalities from the history or screening.

The neurologic examination can reveal extensive disease but will not pinpoint specific functional deficits or minute lesions.

Subtle neonatal behaviors such as fine tremors, irritability, and poor self-regulation may indicate *withdrawal from nicotine* if the mother smoked during pregnancy.

Mental Status

Infants should appear alert when awake, regard faces, and attend to their parents' voices. The infant should display mental activity appropriate for their age.

Persistent irritability in the newborn may be a sign of *neurologic insult* or may reflect a variety of *metabolic, infectious,* or other *constitutional abnormalities,* or environmental conditions such as *drug withdrawal.*

Motor Function and Tone

Assess the *motor tone* of infants, first by carefully watching their position at rest and testing their resistance to passive movement.

Further assess *tone* as you move each major joint through its range of motion, noting any spasticity or flaccidity. Hold the baby in your hands, as shown in Figure 23-34, to determine whether the tone is normal, increased, or decreased. Either increased or decreased tone may indicate intracranial disease, though such disease is usually accompanied by a number of other signs.

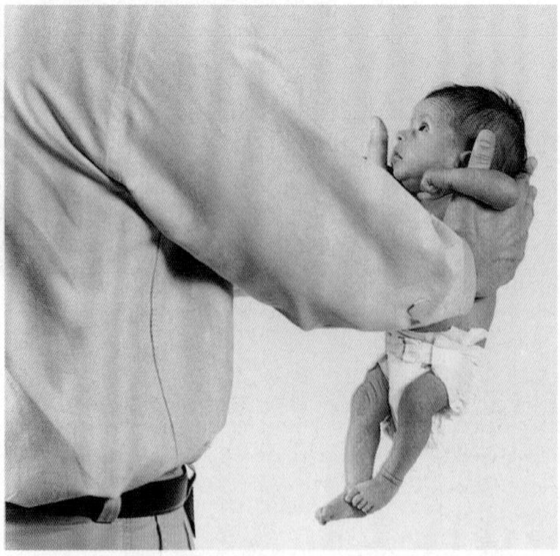

FIGURE 23-34 Assessing motor tone in the infant.

Infants with *hypotonia* often lie in a frog-leg position, with arms flexed and hands near the ears. Hypotonia can be caused by a variety of *central nervous system abnormalities* and *disorders of the motor unit.*

Sensory Function

The *sensory function* of the infant can be tested in only a limited way. Test for pain sensation by flicking the infant's palm or sole with your finger. Observe for withdrawal, arousal, and change in facial expression. Do not use a pin to test for pain.

If changes in facial expression or cry follow a painful stimulus but no withdrawal occurs, weakness or *paralysis* may be present.

Cranial Nerves

The *cranial nerves* of the infant can be tested, but this requires methods that differ from those used for the older child or adult. Table 23-17 provides useful strategies.

TABLE 23-17 Strategies to Assess Cranial Nerves in Newborns and Infants

Cranial Nerve	Function	Strategy
I	Olfactory	Difficult to test.
II	Visual acuity	Have the baby regard your face and look for facial response and tracking.
II, III	Response to light	Darken the room; raise the baby to sitting position to open the eyes. Use light and test for the *optic blink reflex* (blinking in response to light). Use the otoscope light (without speculum) to assess pupillary responses.
III, IV, VI	Extraocular movements	Observe how well the baby tracks your smiling face (or a bright light) and whether the eyes move together.
V	Motor	Test rooting reflex by stroking the infant's cheek. Test sucking reflex by watching the baby suck a breast, bottle, or pacifier, observing the strength of the suck.
VII	Facial	Observe the baby crying and smiling; note symmetry of the face and forehead.
VIII	Acoustic	Test acoustic blink reflex of both eyes in response to loud noise (blinking). Observe tracking in response to sound.

(continued)

Abnormalities in the cranial nerves suggest an intracranial lesion such as hemorrhage or a congenital malformation.

Congenital facial nerve palsy can result from birth trauma or developmental defects.

Dysphagia, or difficulty in swallowing, can occasionally be due to injury to CNs IX, X, and XII.

TABLE 23-17 Strategies to Assess Cranial Nerves in Newborns and Infants (*Continued*)

Cranial Nerve	Function	Strategy
IX, X	Swallow Gag	Observe coordination during swallowing. Test for gag reflex.
XI	Spinal accessory	Observe symmetry of shoulders.
XII	Hypoglossal	Observe coordination of sucking, swallowing, and tongue thrusting. Pinch the nostrils; observe reflex opening of the mouth with the tip of the tongue to the midline.

Deep Tendon Reflexes

The *deep tendon reflexes* are variable in infants because the corticospinal pathways are not fully developed. Thus, their exaggerated presence or absence has little diagnostic significance, unless this response is different from results of previous testing, extreme responses are observed, or responses are very asymmetric.

A progressive increase in deep tendon reflexes during the first year of life may indicate central nervous system disease such as *cerebral palsy,* especially if it is coupled with increased tone.

Use the same techniques to elicit deep tendon reflexes as you would for an adult. You can substitute your index or middle finger for the reflex hammer, as shown in Figure 23-35.

As in adults, asymmetric reflexes suggest a lesion of the peripheral nerves or spinal segment.

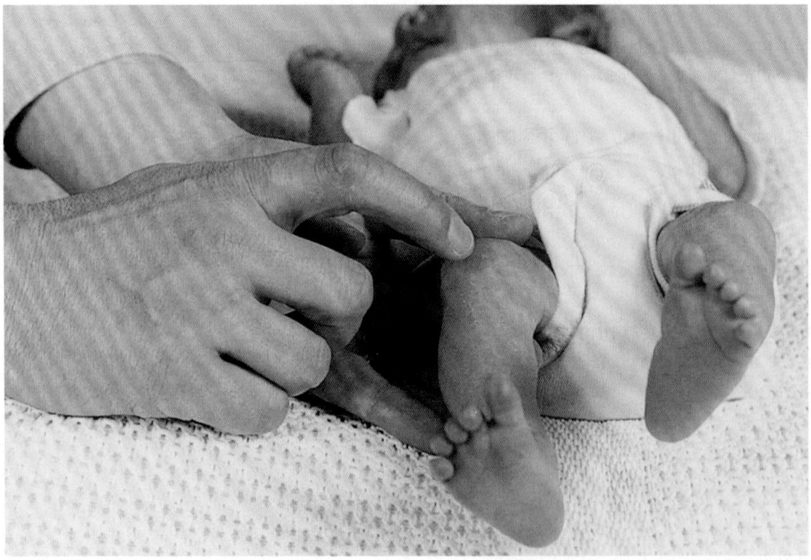

FIGURE 23-35 The examiner uses a finger to assess the infant's deep tendon reflexes.

The triceps, brachioradialis, and abdominal reflexes are difficult to elicit before 6 months of age. The *anal reflex* is present at birth and is important to elicit if a spinal cord lesion is suspected. This reflex is a contraction of the external anal sphincter when the examiner touches the skin near the anus.

An absent anal reflex suggests loss of innervation of the external sphincter muscle caused by a spinal cord abnormality such as a congenital anomaly (e.g., *spina bifida*), *tumor,* or *injury.*

In newborns, a **Babinski response** to plantar stimulation (dorsiflexion of big toe and fanning of other toes) can be elicited and may persist for several months. In order to best elicit the ankle reflex of an infant, grasp the infant's malleoli with one hand and quickly dorsiflex the ankle (Fig. 23-36). Do not be surprised if you note rapid, rhythmic plantar flexion of the newborn's foot (*ankle clonus*) in response to this maneuver. Up to 10 beats are normal in newborns and young infants; this is *unsustained ankle clonus.*

When the contractions are continuous (*sustained ankle clonus*), *central nervous system disease* should be suspected.

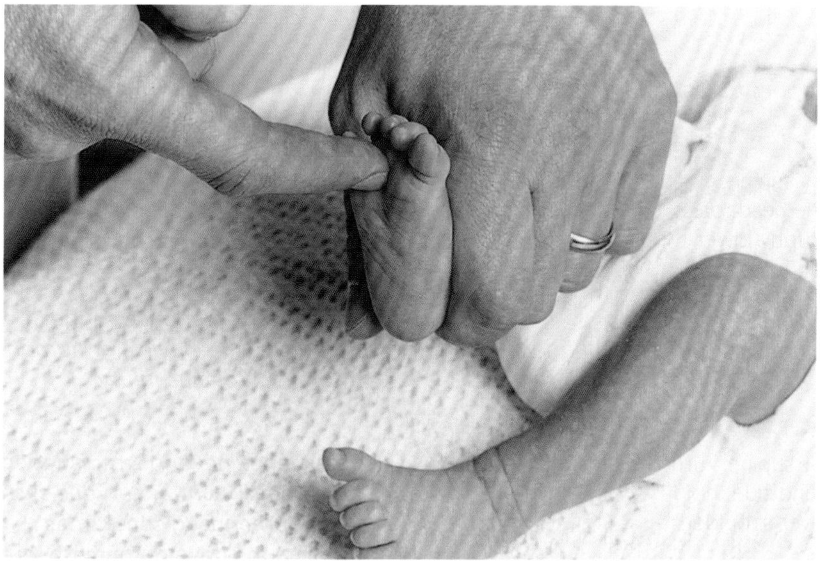

FIGURE 23-36 Testing the Babinski response.

Primitive Reflexes

Evaluate the infant's developing central nervous system by assessing *infantile automatisms,* called *primitive reflexes.* These develop during gestation, are generally demonstrable at birth, and disappear at defined ages. Abnormalities in these primitive reflexes suggest neurologic disease and merit more intensive investigation. The most important primitive reflexes are illustrated in Table 23-18.

A *neurologic* or *developmental abnormality* is suspected if primitive reflexes are

- Absent at appropriate age
- Present longer than normal
- Asymmetric
- Associated with posturing or twitching

Development

Refer to the developmental milestones in Figure 23-9, or use a validated developmental assessment tool to learn which age-specific developmental tasks to evaluate. Through observation and play with the infant, you can do both a developmental screening examination and an assessment for gross

TABLE 23-18 Primitive Reflexes

Primitive Reflex	Maneuver	Ages	
Palmar grasp reflex 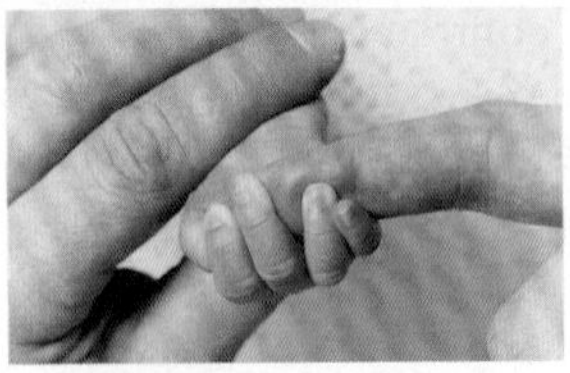	Place your fingers into the baby's hands and press against the palmar surfaces. The baby will flex all fingers to grasp your fingers.	Birth to 3–4 mo	Persistence of a palmar grasp reflex beyond 4 mo suggests *pyramidal tract dysfunction.* Persistence of a clenched hand beyond 2 mo suggests *central nervous system damage*, especially if fingers overlap thumb.
Plantar grasp reflex 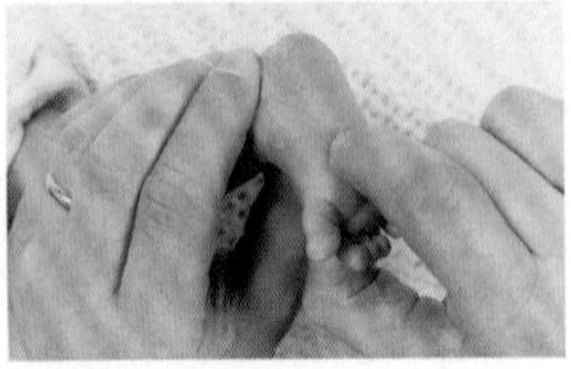	Touch the sole at the base of the toes. The toes will curl.	Birth to 6–8 mo	Persistence of a plantar grasp reflex beyond 8 mo suggests *pyramidal tract dysfunction.*
Moro reflex (startle reflex) 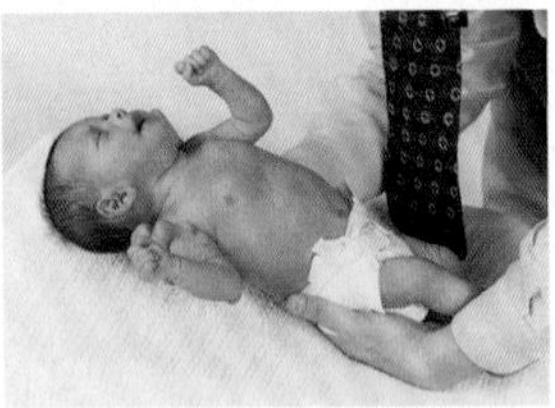	Hold the baby supine, supporting the head, back, and legs. Abruptly lower the entire body about 2 ft. The arms will abduct and extend, hands will open, and legs flex. The baby may cry.	Birth to 4 mo	Persistence beyond 4 mo suggests *neurologic disease* (e.g., *cerebral palsy*); beyond 6 mo strongly suggests it. Asymmetric response suggests *fracture of the clavicle or humerus or brachial plexus injury.*
Asymmetric tonic neck reflex 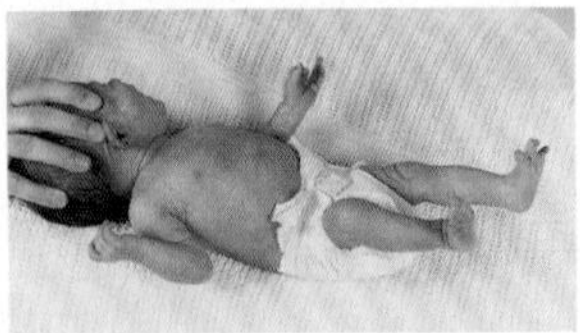	With the baby supine, turn the head to one side, holding the jaw over shoulder. The arm and leg on the side to which head is turned will extend while the opposite arm and leg will flex. Repeat on other side.	Birth to 2 mo	Persistence beyond 2 mo suggests *asymmetric central nervous system development* and sometimes predicts the development of *cerebral palsy.*
Positive support reflex 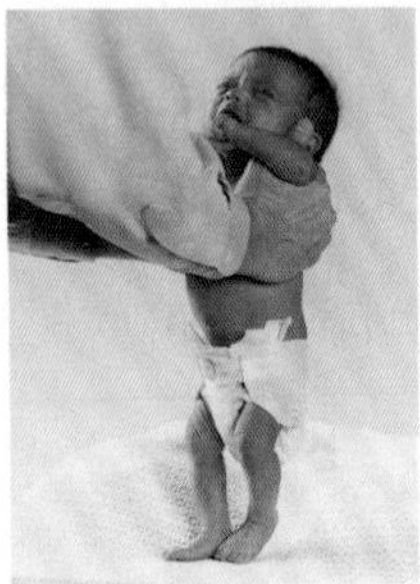	Hold the baby around the trunk and lower until the feet touch a flat surface. The hips, knees, and ankles extend; the baby stands up, partially bearing weight, and sagging after 20–30 sec.	Birth or 2 mo until 6 mo	Lack of reflex suggests *hypotonia or flaccidity.* Fixed extension and adduction of legs (scissoring) suggests *spasticity from neurologic disease, such as cerebral palsy.*

Primitive Reflex	Maneuver	Ages	
Rooting reflex 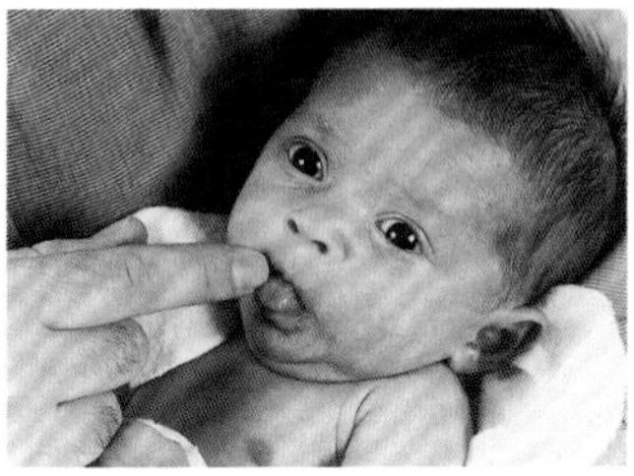	Stroke the perioral skin at the corners of the mouth. The mouth will open, and the baby will turn the head toward the stimulated side and suck.	Birth to 3–4 mo	Absence of rooting indicates *severe generalized or central nervous system disease.*
Trunk incurvation (Galant) reflex 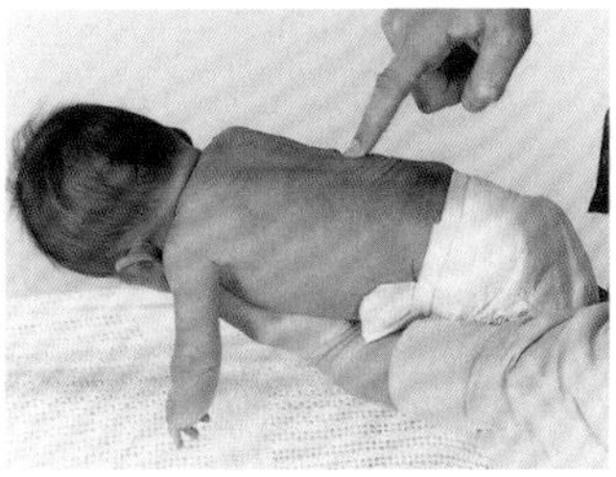	Support the baby prone with one hand, and stroke one side of the back 1 cm from midline from shoulder to buttocks. The spine will curve toward the stimulated side.	Birth to 2 mo	Absence of trunk incurvation suggests a *transverse spinal cord lesion or injury.* Persistence may indicate *delayed development.*
Stepping reflex 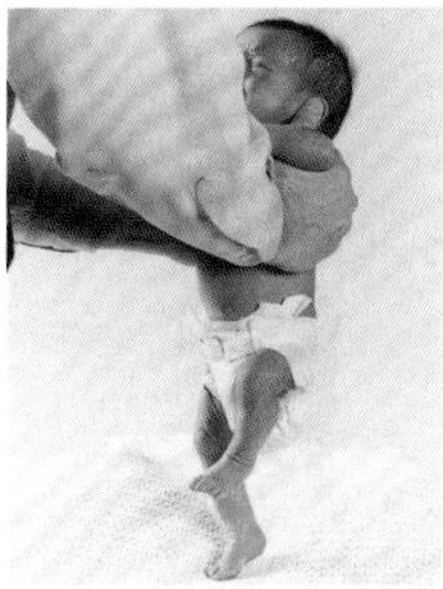	Hold the baby upright from behind as in the positive support reflex test. Have one sole touch the tabletop. The hip and knee of that foot will flex, and the other foot will step forward. Alternate stepping will occur.	Birth (best after 4 days); variable age to disappear	Absence of stepping may indicate *paralysis.* Babies born by breech delivery may not have stepping reflex.
Landau reflex 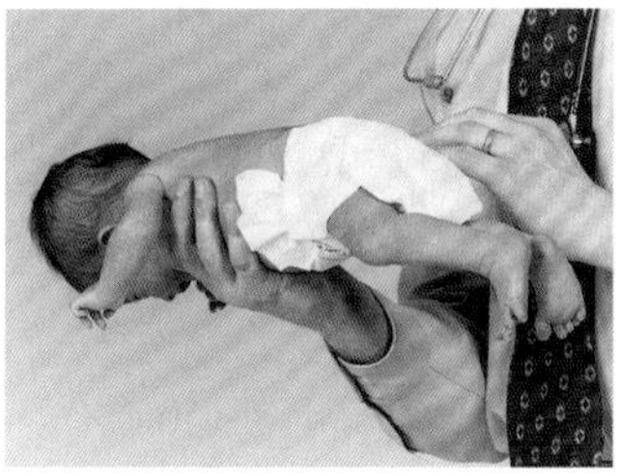	Suspend the baby prone with one hand. The head will lift up, and the spine will straighten.	Birth to 6 mo	Persistence may indicate *delayed development.*
Parachute reflex 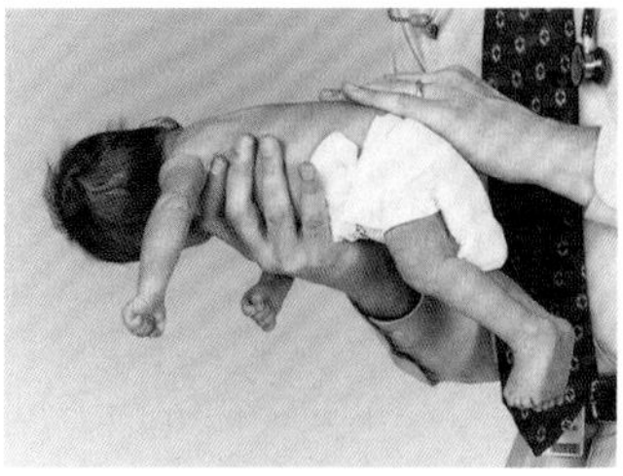	Suspend the baby prone and slowly lower the head toward a surface. The arms and legs will extend in a protective fashion.	4–6 mo and does not disappear	Delay in appearance may predict future *delays in voluntary motor development.*

and fine motor achievement. Specifically, look for *weakness* by observing sitting, standing, and transitions. Note *station,* or the posture of sitting or standing. Carefully observe the *gait* of the toddler, including balance and fluidity of movements. Fine motor development can be assessed in a similar way, combining the neurologic and developmental examination. Key milestones include the development of the pincer grasp, ability to manipulate objects with the hands, and more precise tasks, such as building a tower of cubes or scribbling. Fine and gross motor development progresses in a proximal to distal direction.

Assess the infant's cognitive and social-emotional development as you proceed with the comprehensive neurologic and developmental examination. Some neurologic abnormalities produce deficits or slowing in cognitive and social development. As stated, infants who have developmental delays may have abnormalities on the neurologic examination because much of the examination is based on age-specific norms.

Developmental delays across more than one domain (e.g., motor as well as cognitive) suggests more severe disease.

Health Promotion and Counseling

The AAP and an expert group called Bright Futures (AAP, 2020; Hagan et al., 2017) recommend health supervision visits (also called "well baby visits") for infants and their parents when infants reach the following ages: birth, at 3 to 5 days, by 1 month, and at 2, 4, 6, 9, and 12 months. This is called the *infant periodicity schedule*. Health supervision visits provide opportunities to answer questions for parents, assess the infant's growth and development, perform a comprehensive physical examination, and provide anticipatory guidance (Fig. 23-37). Age-appropriate anticipatory guidance includes healthy habits and behaviors, social competence of caregivers, parenting techniques, family relationships, and community interactions.

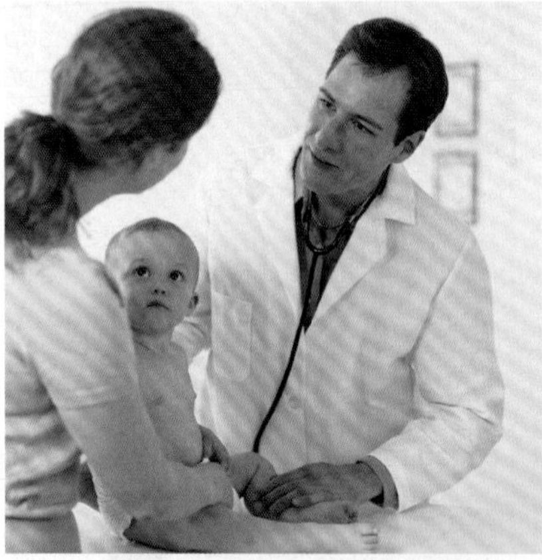

FIGURE 23-37 A parent and nurse discuss the infant's growth and health during the health supervision visit.

Regular visits provide an opportunity to plot a course for health and successful development. That infants are generally well during these visits enhances the quality of the experience. Parents are usually receptive to suggestions about health promotion which can have major, long-term influences on the child and family. Strong interviewing skills are necessary as you discuss strategies to optimize the health and well-being of infants.

Review the critical components of a health supervision visit for a 6-month-old in Box 23-5. Adjust this content to the appropriate developmental level of the infant.

BOX 23-5 COMPONENTS OF A HEALTH SUPERVISION VISIT FOR A 6-MONTH-OLD

Discussions with Parents

- Address parents' concerns and questions.
- Provide advice.
- Obtain a social history.
- Assess development, nutrition, sleep, elimination, safety, oral health, family relationships, stressors, parenting beliefs, and community factors.

Developmental Assessment

- Use a standardized developmental instrument to measure milestones yourself, for example, the Denver II.
- Alternately, review and discuss with the parents their responses to the ASQ-3, SWYC, or PEDS questionnaires.
- Assess milestones by history.
- Measure milestones by examination.

Physical Examination

Perform a careful examination, including growth parameters with percentiles for age.

Screening Tests

- Vision and hearing by examination
- Possibly hematocrit and lead if at high risk
- Social risk factors

Immunizations

See the CDC schedule at http://www.cdc.gov/vaccines/schedules/index.html.

Anticipatory Guidance

- Healthy habits and behaviors
  - Injury and illness prevention
    - Use infant car seat
    - Watch for rolling
    - Avoid poisons and tobacco, vaping, and e-cigarette exposure
    - "Back to sleep" position
  - Nutrition
    - Breast-feeding or bottle
    - Solids
    - No juice
    - Preventing choking and overfeeding
  - Oral health
    - No bottle in bed
    - Fluoride
    - Brushing teeth

CLINICAL TIP

Leaving a baby or toddler with a bottle of milk in the crib at night can cause "baby bottle syndrome." The milk bathes the child's teeth causing accelerated decay as the milk converts to lactic acid during the night. This is the biggest dental problem for very small children.

- Parent–infant interaction: Promoting development (e.g., play, reading, music, talking)
- Family relationships
  - Time for oneself
  - Babysitters
  - Support system
- Community interactions: Child care and resources

The AAP recommends against the use of baby walkers, due to the many injuries sustained by children in walkers even when the child is under adult supervision (HealthyChildren.org, 2018).

ASSESSING YOUNG AND SCHOOL-AGED CHILDREN

Development

Early Childhood: 1 to 4 Years

Physical Development

After infancy, the rate of physical growth slows by approximately half. After 2 years, toddlers gain about 2 to 3 kg (4.5 to 6.5 lb) and grow 5 cm (2 in) per year. Physical changes are impressive. Chubby, clumsy toddlers transform into leaner, more muscular preschoolers (Fig. 23-38).

Gross motor skills also develop quickly. Almost all children walk by 15 months, run well by 2 years, and pedal a tricycle and jump by 4 years. Fine motor skills develop through neurologic maturation and environmental manipulation. The 18-month-old who scribbles becomes a 2-year-old who draws lines and then a 4-year-old who makes circles.

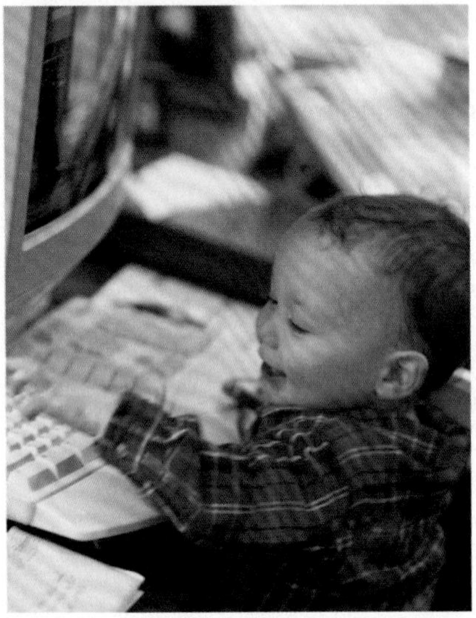

FIGURE 23-38 The toddler begins to develop fine motor control.

Cognitive and Language Development

Toddlers move from sensorimotor learning (through touching and looking) to symbolic thinking, solving simple problems, remembering songs, and engaging in imitative play. Language develops with extraordinary speed. An 18-month-old with 10 to 20 words becomes a 2-year-old with three-word sentences and then a 3-year-old who converses well. By 4 years, preschoolers form complex sentences. They remain preoperational, however, without sustained logical thought processes.

Social and Emotional Development

New intellectual pursuits are surpassed only by an emerging drive for independence. Because toddlers are impulsive, temper tantrums are common. Self-regulation is an important developmental task with wide range of normal behavior (Fig. 23-39).

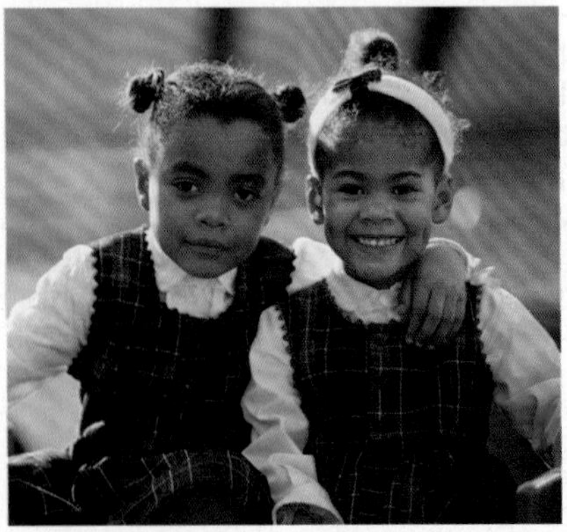

FIGURE 23-39 Preschoolers begin developing friendships with peers.

Middle Childhood: 5 to 10 Years

Middle childhood is an active period of growth and development (Fig. 23-40). Goal-directed exploration (Fig. 23-41), increased physical and cognitive abilities, and achievements by trial and error mark this stage. The physical examination is more straightforward during this age period, but always consider the developmental stages and tasks that school-aged children are facing (Table 23-19).

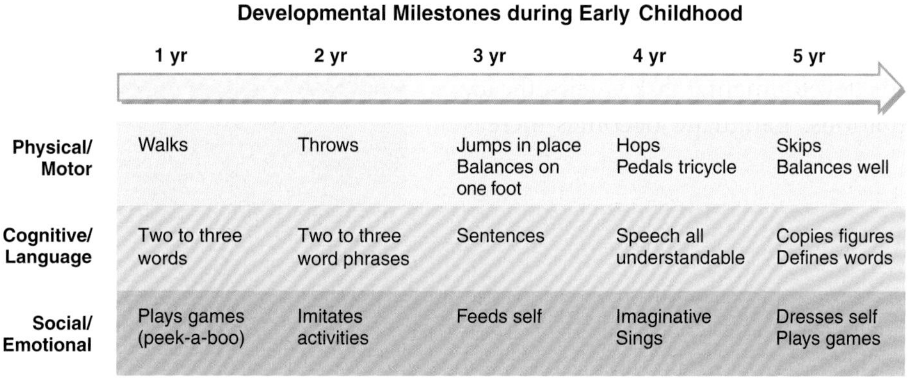
Developmental Milestones during Early Childhood
1 yr
2 yr
3 yr
4 yr
5 yr
Physical/ Motor
Walks
Throws
Jumps in place Balances on one foot
Hops Pedals tricycle
Skips Balances well
Cognitive/ Language
Two to three words
Two to three word phrases
Sentences
Speech all understandable
Copies figures Defines words
Social/ Emotional
Plays games (peek-a-boo)
Imitates activities
Feeds self
Imaginative Sings
Dresses self Plays games

FIGURE 23-40 Developmental milestones during early childhood.

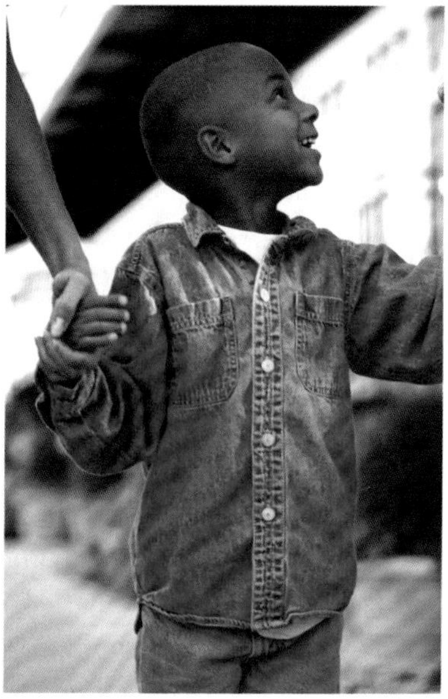

FIGURE 23-41 Children enjoy exploring new environments.

TABLE 23-19 Developmental Tasks during Middle Childhood

Task	Characteristic	Health Care Needs
Physical	Enhanced strength and coordination Competence in various tasks and activities	Screening for strengths, assessing problems Involving parents Support for disabilities Anticipatory guidance: safety, exercise, nutrition, sleep
Cognitive	"Concrete operational": focus on the present Achievement of knowledge and skills, self-efficacy	Emphasis on short-term consequences Support; screening for skills and school performance
Social	Achieving good "fit" with family, friends, school Sustained self-esteem Evolving self-identity	Assessment, support, advice about interactions Support, emphasis on strengths Understanding, advice, support

Physical Development

Children grow steadily but more slowly. Nevertheless, strength and coordination improve dramatically with more participation in activities (Fig. 23-42). This is also when children with physical disabilities or chronic illnesses become more aware of their limitations.

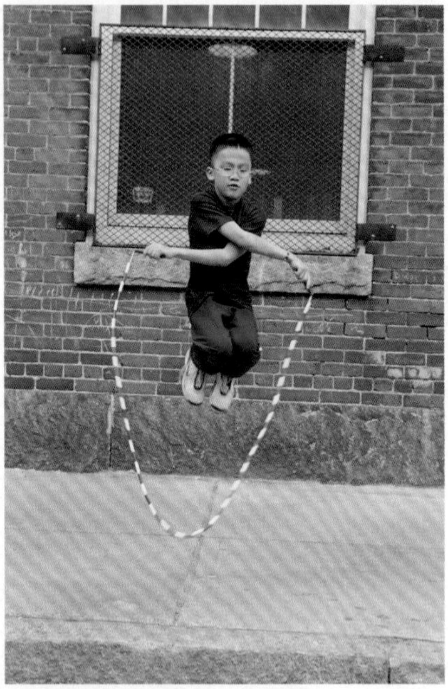

FIGURE 23-42 Motor skills and coordination improve during middle childhood.

Cognitive and Language Development

Children become "concrete operational"—capable of limited logic and more complex learning. They remain rooted in the present, with little ability to understand consequences or abstractions. School, family, and environment greatly influence learning. A major developmental task is self-efficacy, or the ability to thrive in different situations. Language becomes increasingly complex.

Social and Emotional Development

Children become progressively more independent, initiating activities and enjoying accomplishments. Achievements are critical for self-esteem and developing a "fit" within major social structures—family, school, and peer activity groups. Guilt and poor self-esteem also may emerge. Family and environment contribute enormously to the child's self-image. Moral development remains simple and concrete, with a clear sense of "right and wrong."

The Health History

An important and unique aspect of examining children is that parents are usually watching and taking part in the interaction, providing you the opportunity to observe the parent–child interaction. Note whether the child displays age-appropriate behaviors. Assess the "goodness of fit," the degree of match between a child's temperament and the parent's style of parenting. Although some abnormal interactions may result from the unnatural setting of the examination room, others may be a consequence of interactional problems. Careful *observation* of the child's interactions with parents and the child's unstructured play in the examination room can reveal *abnormalities in physical, cognitive, and social development or issues with parent–child relationship* (Box 23-6).

The health history of the child is similar to the infant health history updated for the child's developmental level. A complete history and prior health care information would be obtained if the child is a new patient. Otherwise, the history is continuously updated at each visit.

Normal toddlers are occasionally scared of or angry at the examiner. Often, they are uncooperative. Most eventually warm up to you. If this behavior continues or is not developmentally appropriate, there may be an *underlying behavioral or developmental abnormality.* Older, school-aged children have more self-control and prior experience with nurses and are generally cooperative with the examination. You can detect a surprising amount by using observation.

BOX 23-6 ABNORMALITIES DETECTED WHILE OBSERVING PLAY

Behavioral Problems[a]

- Poor parent–child interactions
- Sibling rivalry
- Inappropriate parental discipline
- "Difficult temperament"

Developmental Delay

- Gross motor delay
- Fine motor delay
- Language delay (expressive, receptive)
- Delay in social or emotional tasks (may use an age-appropriate developmental screening test)

Social or Environmental Problems

- Parental problem (e.g., stress, depression)
- Risk for abuse or neglect

Neurologic Problems

- Weakness
- Abnormal posture
- Spasticity
- Clumsiness
- Attentional problems and hyperactivity
- Autistic features
- Musculoskeletal abnormalities

[a]Note: The child's behavior during the visit may not represent typical behavior, but your observations may serve as a springboard for discussion with parents.

Assessing Younger Children

One challenge in examining children in this age group is avoiding a physical struggle, a crying child, or a distraught parent.

The child should remain dressed during the interview to minimize the child's apprehension. It also allows you to interact more naturally and observe the child playing, interacting with the parents, and undressing and dressing.

Toddlers who are 9 to 15 months may have *stranger anxiety,* a fear of strangers that is developmentally normal. It signals the toddler's growing awareness that the stranger is "new." You should not approach these toddlers quickly. Play can help the child warm up to you. Make sure they remain solidly in their parent's lap throughout much of the examination and that the parent remains close when the child is on the examination table.

Table 23-20 includes useful tips for examining young children.

Engage children in age-appropriate conversation. Ask simple questions about their illness or toys. Compliment their appearance or behavior, tell a story, or play a simple game to "break the ice." If a child is shy, turn your attention to the parent to allow the child to warm up gradually.

TABLE 23-20 Some Tips for Examining Young Children (1- to 4-Year-Olds)

Useful Strategies for Examination	Useful Toys and Aids
Examine a child sitting on the parent's lap. Try to be at the child's eye level.	"Blow out" the otoscope light.
First examine the child's toy or teddy bear, then the child.	"Beep" the stethoscope on your nose.
Let the child do some of the examination (e.g., move the stethoscope). Then go back and "get the places we missed."	Make tongue-depressor puppets.
Ask the toddler who keeps pushing you away to "hold your hand." Then have the toddler "help you" with the examination.	Use the child's own toys for play.
Some toddlers believe that if they cannot see you, then you are not there. Perform the examination while the child stands on the parent's lap, facing the parent.	Jingle your keys to test for hearing.
If 2-y-olds are holding something in each hand (such as tongue depressors), it is more difficult for them to fight or resist.	Shine the otoscope through the tip of your finger (or the child's finger) to show it doesn't hurt, "lighting it up," and then examine the child's ears with it.
	Use age-appropriate toys and books.

With certain exceptions, physical examination does not require use of the examining table—it can be done on the floor or with the child in a parent's lap. The key is to engage the child's cooperation. For young children who resist undressing, expose only the body part being examined. When examining siblings, begin with the oldest child, who is more likely to cooperate and set a good example. Approach the child pleasantly. Explain each step as you perform it. Continue conversing with the family to provide distraction.

Plan the examination to start with the least distressing procedures and end with the most distressing (usually involving the throat and ears). Begin with parts that can be done with the child sitting, such as examining the eyes or palpating the neck. Lying down may make a child feel vulnerable, so change positions with care. Once a child is supine, start with the abdomen, saving the throat and ears or genitalia for last. A parent's help may be needed to hold the child for examination of the ears or throat; however, use of formal restraints is inappropriate. Patience, distraction, play, flexibility in the order of the examination, and a caring but firm and gentle approach are all key to successfully examining the young child (Box 23-7).

BOX 23-7 MORE TIPS FOR EXAMINING THE YOUNG CHILD

- Use a reassuring voice throughout the examination.
- Let the child see and touch the examination tools you will be using.
- Avoid asking permission to examine a body part because you will do the examination anyway. Instead, ask the child which ear or which part of the body they would like you to examine "first."
- Examine the child in the parent's lap. Let the parent undress the child.
- If unable to console the child, give the child a short break.
- Make a game out of the examination. For example, say, "Let's see how big your tongue is!" or for the lung examination, ask them to "blow out the light" using a penlight.

Reassure parents that resistance to examination is developmentally appropriate. Some embarrassed parents scold the child, compounding the problem. Involve parents in the examination. Learn which techniques and approaches work best and are most comfortable for you.

Assessing Older Children

Many children at this age are modest. Providing gowns and leaving underwear in place as long as possible are wise approaches (Fig. 23-43). Suggest that children disrobe behind a curtain. Consider leaving the room while they change with their parents' help. Some children may prefer opposite-sex siblings to leave, but most prefer a parent of either sex to remain in the room. Parents of children younger than 11 years should stay with them.

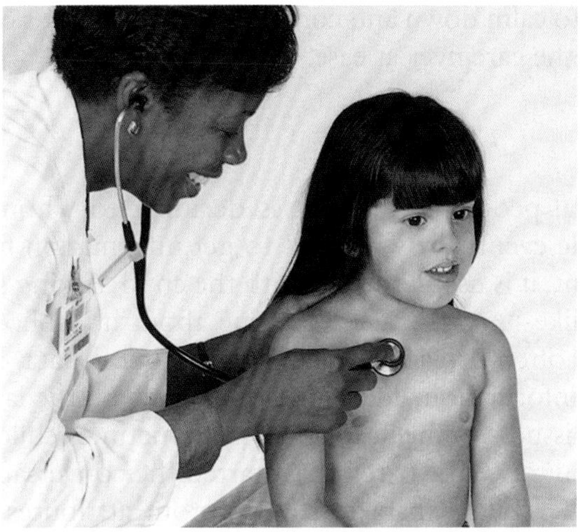

FIGURE 23-43 Listening to a child's heart sounds.

Children usually are accompanied by a parent or caregiver. Even when alone, they are often seeking health care at the request of their parents—indeed, the parent is usually sitting in the waiting room. When interviewing a child, you need to consider the needs and perspectives of both the child and the caregivers (Fig. 23-44).

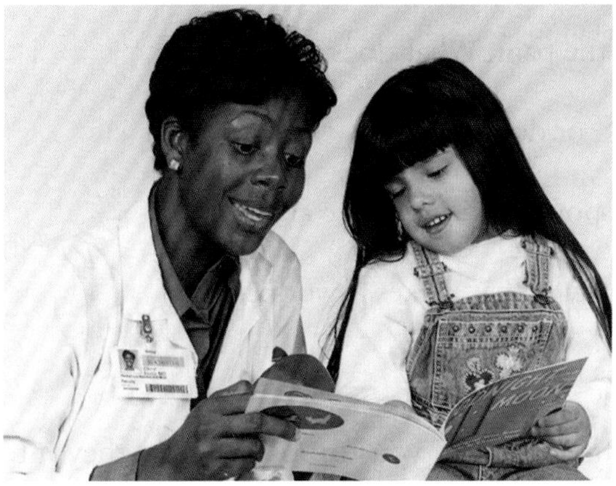

FIGURE 23-44 Reading a picture book about the physical examination can reassure the child about what will happen.

Establishing Rapport

Begin the interview by greeting and establishing rapport with each person present. Refer to the child by name rather than by "him" or "her." Clarify the role or relationship of all of the adults and children. "Please help me by telling me Jimmy's relationship to everyone here." Ask how caregivers would like to be addressed. When the family structure is not immediately clear, you may avoid embarrassment by asking directly about other members. "Who else lives in the home?" Do not assume that just because parents are separated, only one parent is actively involved in the child's life. Families come in many varieties; these include traditional families, single parents, separated/divorced parents, blended, same-sex parents, kinship families, foster families, and adoptive families.

Use your personal experiences with children to guide how you interact in a health care setting. To establish rapport, meet children on their own levels. Eye contact on their level, participating in playful engagement, and talking about what interests them are always good strategies. Ask children about their clothes, one of their toys, what books or TV shows they like, or their adult companion in an enthusiastic but gentle style. Spending time at the beginning of the interview to calm down and connect with an anxious child can put both the child and the caregiver at ease.

Working with Families

One challenge when several people are present is deciding to whom to direct your questions. While eventually you need to get information from both the child and the parent, it is useful to start with the child. Asking simple open-ended questions like "Are you sick? Tell me about it," followed by more specific questions often provides much of the clinical data. The parents can then verify the information, add details that give you the larger context, and identify other issues you need to address. Sometimes children are embarrassed to begin, but once the parent has started the conversation, direct questions back to the child. Characterize symptom attributes the same way you do with adults. For example:

- I heard that you are getting stomachaches. Tell me about them.
- Show me where you get the pain. What does it feel like?
- Is it sharp like a pin prick, or does it ache?
- Does it stay in the same spot, or does it move around?
- What helps make it go away? What makes it worse?
- What do you think causes it?

The presence of family members allows you to observe how they interact with the child. A child may be able to sit still or may get restless and start fidgeting. Watch how the parents set limits or fail to set limits when needed.

Physical Examination of Young and School-Aged Children

The order of the examination now begins to follow that used for adults. Examine painful areas last, and forewarn children about areas you are going to examine. If a child resists part of the examination, you can return to it at the end.

General Survey and Vital Signs

Somatic Growth

Height

After 2 years of age, children can be measured standing up provided they can stand up straight and remain still. Prior to measurement, shoes, hats, and hair ornaments are removed. A measuring device, such as a stadiometer, which is mounted on the wall is used. The child stands with the back of the head, shoulders, buttocks, heels, and feet together against the wall. The patient is looking straight ahead and the head plate is at a right angle (Fig. 23-45). Stand-up weight scales with a height attachment are not accurate.

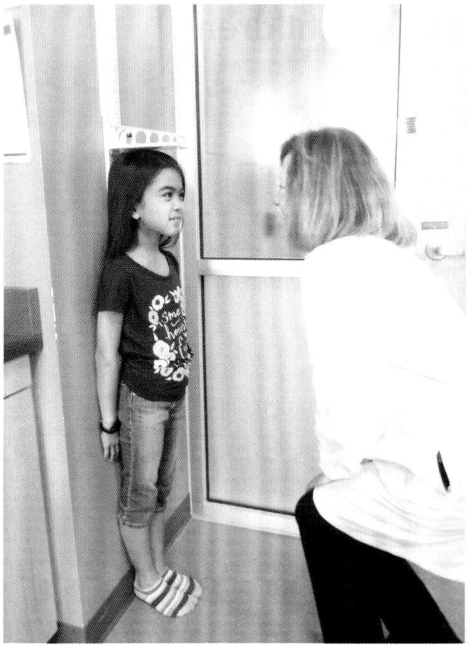

FIGURE 23-45 Measuring a child's height with a stadiometer against a wall.

A rule of thumb regarding height is that after age 2, children should grow at least 5 cm (2 in) per year. *During puberty, growth velocity increases.*

Short stature, defined as height less than the 5th percentile, can be a normal variant or caused by endocrine or other diseases. Normal variants include *familial short stature* and *constitutional delay.* Chronic diseases include *growth hormone deficiency,* other endocrine diseases, *gastrointestinal disease, renal* or *metabolic disease,* and *genetic syndromes.*

Most children with exogenous obesity are also tall for their age. Children with endocrine causes of obesity tend to be short.

Weight

Young children who can stand and school-aged children should be weighed in a gown (or in clothing without shoes) on a stand-up scale. Although initially nervous, most young children can be coaxed onto such scales. Use the same scale if possible for each visit.

Young children can have inadequate weight and height gain if caloric intake is insufficient. Etiologies of failure to thrive include *psychosocial, interactional, gastrointestinal, and endocrine disorders.*

Head Circumference

In general, head circumference is measured until the child reaches 24 months. Afterward, head circumference measurement may be helpful if you suspect a genetic or central nervous system disorder.

Body Mass Index for Age

Age- and sex-specific charts are now available to assess BMI in children (see Table 23-21 for interpreting a child's BMI). BMI in children is associated with body fat and related to subsequent health risks for obesity. BMI measurements are helpful for early detection of obesity in children older than 2 years. Obesity is now a major childhood epidemic, and it often begins before 6 to 8 years. Consequences of childhood obesity include hypertension, diabetes, metabolic syndrome, and poor self-esteem. Childhood obesity often leads to adult obesity and shortened lifespan. It is helpful to give parents their child's BMI results together with information about the impact of healthy eating and physical activity.

Childhood obesity is a significant epidemic. "An estimated 18.5% of U.S. children and adolescents aged 2 to 19 years have obesity, including 5.6% with severe obesity, and another 16.6% are overweight (Hales et al., 2018)." Long-term morbidity from childhood obesity spans many organ systems, including cardiovascular, endocrine, renal, musculoskeletal, gastrointestinal, and psychological systems. Prevention, early detection, and aggressive management are needed.

TABLE 23-21 Interpreting BMI in Children

Group	BMI for Age
Underweight	<5th percentile
Healthy weight	5th to ≤85th percentile
Overweight	85th to ≤95th percentile
Obesity	≥95th percentile
Severe obesity	≥120% of the 95th percentile

Source: Ogden, C. L., & Flegal, K. M. (2010). *Changes in terminology for childhood overweight and obesity*. National health statistics reports; no 25. National Center for Health Statistics.

Vital Signs

Blood Pressure

Hypertension during childhood is more common than previously thought, and it is important to recognize, confirm, and appropriately manage it. Children have elevated blood pressure during exercise, crying, and anxiety. Although young children may be anxious at first, when the procedure is explained and demonstrated beforehand, most children are cooperative. If the blood pressure is initially elevated, you can perform blood pressure readings again at the end of the examination; one trick is to leave the cuff on the arm (deflated) and repeat the reading later. Elevated readings must always be confirmed by subsequent measurements.

A common cause of apparent hypertension is anxiety or "white coat hypertension." The most frequent "cause" of an elevated blood pressure in children is an *improperly performed examination,* often due to an incorrect cuff size.

A proper cuff size is essential for accurate determination of blood pressure in children (Fig. 23-46). Select the blood pressure cuff as you would for adults. It should be wide enough to cover two thirds of the upper arm or leg. A cuff that is too narrow falsely elevates the blood pressure reading, whereas a wider cuff lowers it and may interfere with proper placement of the stethoscope diaphragm over the artery.

In children, as in adults, systolic blood pressure readings from the thigh are approximately 10 mm Hg higher than those from the upper arm. If they are the same or lower, coarctation of the aorta (a congenital malformation resulting in narrowing of the aorta, usually near the ductus arteriosus, which restricts blood flow to the lower body) should be suspected.

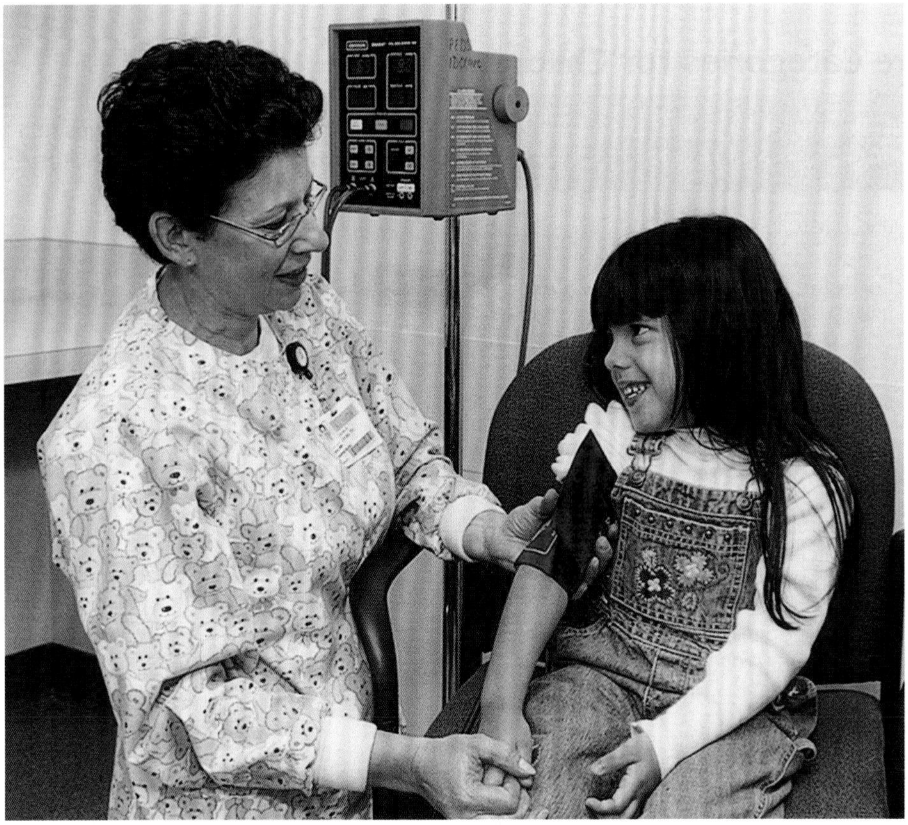

FIGURE 23-46 Using the correct cuff size when taking the child's blood pressure is important.

With children, as with adults, *the first Korotkoff sound indicates systolic pressure and* the point at which the Korotkoff sounds disappear constitutes the diastolic pressure. If the sounds continue to be heard to 0, record three numbers, the first Korotkoff sound, (where the sound softens) and 0 (e.g., 98/62/0). At times, especially among young children with baby fat, the Korotkoff sounds are not easily heard. In such instances, use palpation to determine the systolic blood pressure, remembering that the systolic pressure is approximately 10 mm Hg lower by palpation than by auscultation.

An electronic sphygmomanometer can be used if the Korotkoff sounds are inaudible. The child's limb must be still during the measurement. Gentle restraint may be necessary to prevent movement.

Transient hypertension in children can be caused by some common childhood medications, including those to treat asthma (e.g., prednisone) and attention-deficit/hyperactivity disorder (ADHD; e.g., Ritalin).

In 2004, the National Heart, Lung, and Blood Institute's National High Blood Pressure Working Group on Hypertension Control in Children and Adolescents defined normal, high–normal, and high blood pressure as outlined in Table 23-22, with measurements on at least three separate occasions (Hales et al., 2018).

Causes of *sustained hypertension* (Ingelfinger, 2014) in childhood include renal parenchymal or artery disease, coarctation of the aorta, and primary hypertension. Obesity is highly associated with hypertension in childhood.

TABLE 23-22 Blood Pressure Categories for Children

Blood Pressure Category	Average Systolic and/or Diastolic Blood Pressure for Age, Sex, and Height
Normal[a]	Both systolic and diastolic <90th percentile
Elevated	Systolic blood pressure and/or diastolic blood pressure ≥90th but <95th percentile (whichever is lower)
Hypertension	
Stage 1	Systolic blood pressure and/or diastolic blood pressure ≥95th percentile to <95th percentile plus 12 mm Hg or 130/80 to 139/89 mm Hg (whichever is lower)
Stage 2	Systolic blood pressure and/or diastolic blood pressure P ≥95th percentile plus 12 mm Hg or ≥140/90 mm Hg (whichever is lower)

[a]Refer to standard blood pressure tables based on age.
Source: Benenson, I., Frederick, A., Waldron, F. A., & Porter, S. (2020). Pediatric hypertension: A guideline update. *The Nurse Practitioner*, *45*(5), 16–23.

See Table 23-2, "Abnormalities in Heart Rhythm and Blood Pressure."

The epidemic of childhood obesity has also resulted in a rising prevalence of childhood hypertension (Benenson et al., 2020). Children who have hypertension should be evaluated extensively to determine the cause. For infants and young children, a specific cause can usually be found. An increasing proportion of older children and adolescents, however, have essential or primary hypertension. In all cases, it is important to repeat measurements to reduce the possibility that the elevation reflects anxiety. Sometimes repeating measurements in school is a way to obtain readings in a more relaxed environment. Hypertension and obesity often coexist in children.

It is important to not *falsely label* a child or adolescent as having hypertension because of the stigma of labeling, potential limitations to activities, and possible side effects of treatment.

Pulse

Average heart rates and normal ranges are shown in Table 23-23. Measure the heart rate over a 60-second interval.

TABLE 23-23 Average Heart Rate of Children at Rest

Age (Years)	Average Rate (Median)	Range (1st to 99th Percentile)
1–2	115–125	80–160
2–6	95–115	62–145
6–10	85–95	52–125

Source: Fleming, S., Thompson, M., Stevens, R., Heneghan, C., Plüddemann, A., Maconochie, I., Tarassenko, L., & Mant, D. (2011). Normal ranges of heart rate and respiratory rate in children from birth to 18 years of age: A systematic review of observational studies. *Lancet*, *377*(9770), 1011–1018.

Sinus bradycardia is a heart rate less than 100 beats per min in infants and toddlers and less than 60 beats per min in children 3–9 y.

Respiratory Rate

The rate of respirations per minute ranges from 20 to 40 during early childhood and 15 to 25 during late childhood, reaching adult levels at around 15 years of age (Fleming et al., 2011).

CLINICAL TIP
Children with respiratory diseases such as bronchiolitis or *pneumonia* have rapid respirations (up to 80 to 90/min) but *also* increased work of breathing such as grunting, nasal flaring, or use of accessory muscles.

For young children, observe the movements of the chest wall for two 30-second intervals or over 1 minute, preferably before stimulating them. Direct auscultation of the chest or placing the stethoscope in front of the mouth is also useful for counting respirations, but the measurement may be falsely elevated if the child becomes agitated. For older children, use the same technique as that used for adults.

The commonly accepted cutoff for tachypnea in children older than 1 year is a respiratory rate greater than 40 breaths per minute.

The best single physical finding for ruling out *pneumonia* is an absence of tachypnea.

Temperature

In children, auditory canal or temporal artery temperature recordings are preferable because they can be obtained quickly with essentially no discomfort.

CLINICAL TIP
Young children with infections can have extremely high fevers (up to 104°F or 40°C). Children younger than 3 years, who appear very ill with a fever, should be evaluated for possible sepsis, urinary tract infection, pneumonia, or other infectious etiology.

The Skin

After a child's first year of life, the techniques of examination are the same as those for the adult (see Chapter 9).

CLINICAL TIP
Infants and children who are unconscious, immobile, restrained, or have a medical device placed can develop hospital-acquired pressure injuries. The Braden QD Scale, a revision of the Braden Scale (see Chapter 9), is a pediatric-specific risk assessment tool that can be used for newborn to teenage patients. The tool is available at: http://www.marthaaqcurley.com/braden-qd.html. It is free to reproduce and use without modification for research or clinical practice (Chamblee et al., 2018).

See Table 23-24, "Warts, Lesions that Resemble Warts, and Other Raised Lesions," and Table 23-25, "Common Skin Lesions during Childhood."

TABLE 23-24 Warts, Lesions that Resemble Warts, and Other Raised Lesions

Verruca Vulgaris

Dry, rough warts on hands

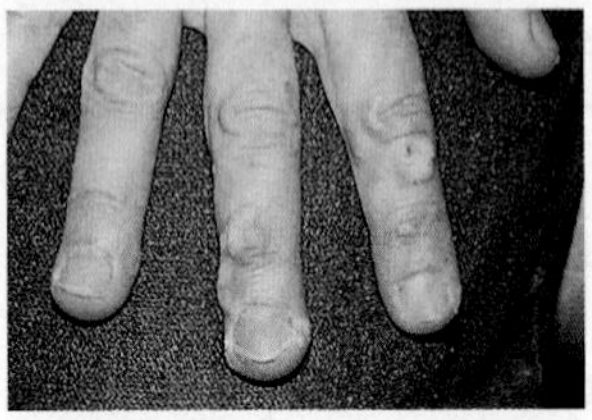

Verruca Plana

Small, flat warts

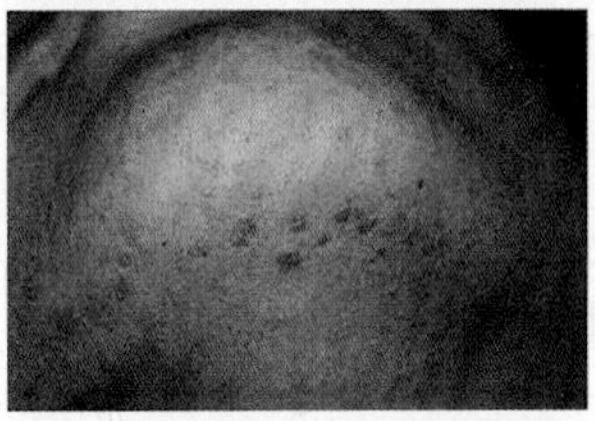

Plantar Warts

Tender warts on feet

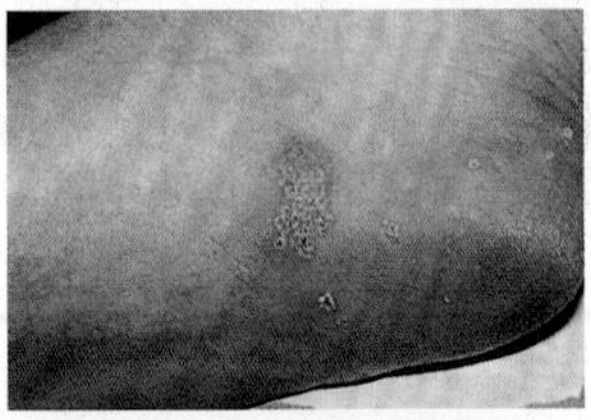

Molluscum Contagiosum

Dome-shaped, fleshy lesions

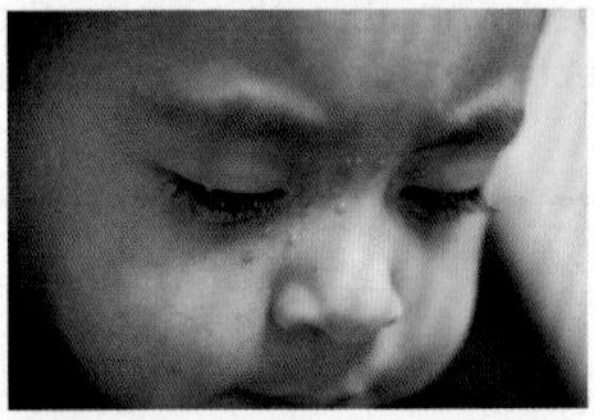

Adolescent Acne

Acne in adolescents involves open comedones (blackheads) and closed comedones (white-heads) shown on top, and inflamed pustules (on bottom)

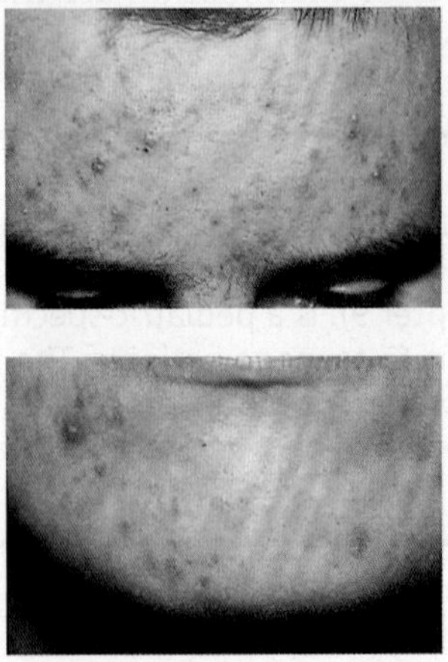

TABLE 23-25 Common Skin Lesions during Childhood

Insect Bites

Intensely pruritic, red, distinct papules characterize these lesions.

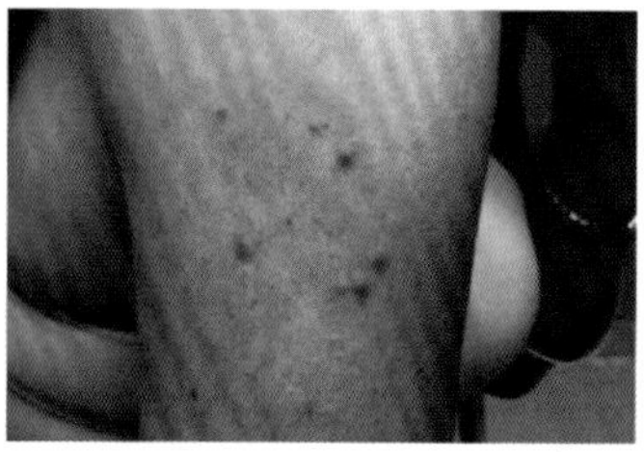

Urticaria (Hives)

This pruritic, allergic sensitivity reaction changes shape quickly.

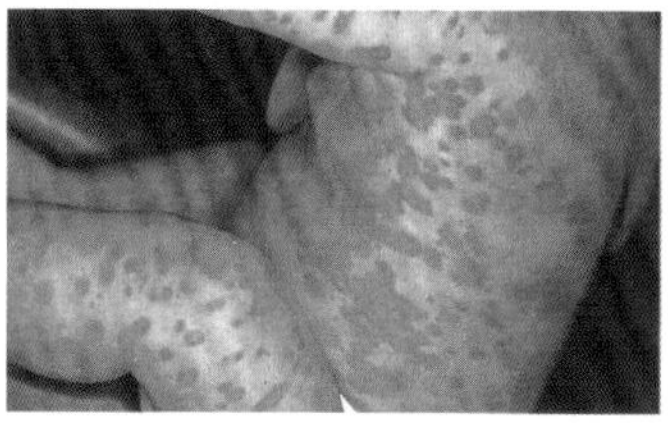

Tinea Capitis

Scaling, crusting, and hair loss are seen in the scalp, along with a painful plaque (kerion) and occipital lymph node (*arrow*).

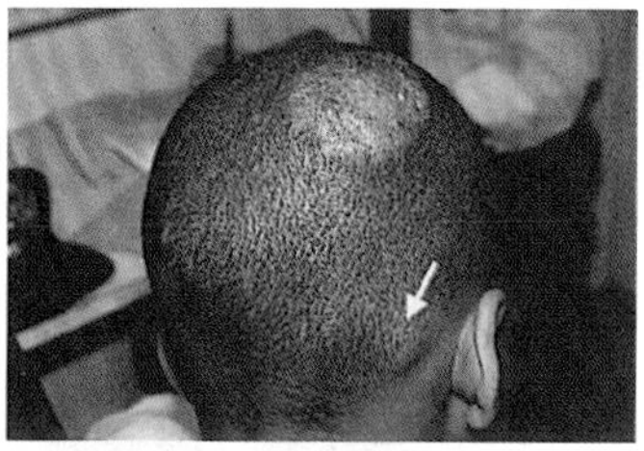

Tinea Corporis

This annular lesion has central clearing and papules along the border.

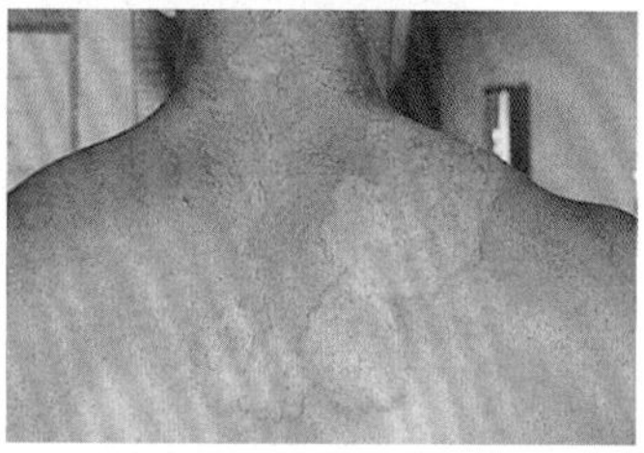

Scabies

Intensely itchy papules and vesicles, sometimes burrows, most often on extremities.

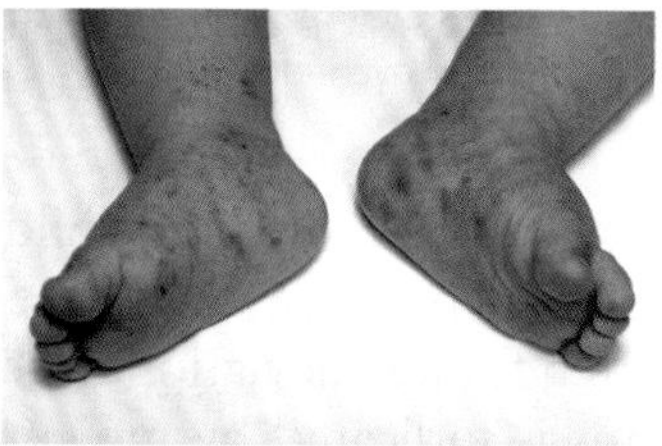

Pityriasis Rosea

Oval lesions on trunk, in older children, often in a pine tree pattern, sometimes a herald patch (a large patch that appears first).

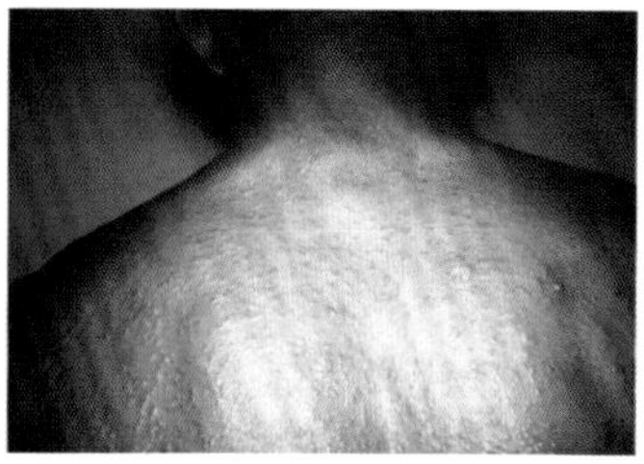

Source of photos: *Insect bites*—Schalock, P. C., Hsu, J. T. S., Arndt, K. A. (2010). *Lippincott's primary care dermatology*. Lippincott Williams & Wilkins; *Tinea Capitis, and Tinea Corporis*—Goodheart, H. (1999). *A photoguide of common skin disorders*. Williams & Wilkins.

The Head

In examining the head and neck, tailor your examination to the child's stage of growth and development.

Even before touching the child, carefully observe the shape of the head, its symmetry, and the presence of abnormal facies. Abnormal facies may not be apparent until later in childhood; therefore, carefully examine the face as well as the head of all children.

See Table 23-6, "Diagnostic Facies in infancy and Childhood."

The Eyes

The two most important components of the eye examination for young children are to determine whether the gaze is conjugate or symmetric and to test visual acuity in each eye.

Strabismus in children requires treatment by an ophthalmologist.

Conjugate Gaze

Use the methods described in Chapter 11 for adults to assess *conjugate gaze*, or the *position and alignment of the eyes*, and the function of the extraocular muscles. The corneal light reflex test (Fig. 23-47) and the cover-uncover test (Fig. 23-48) are particularly useful in young children.

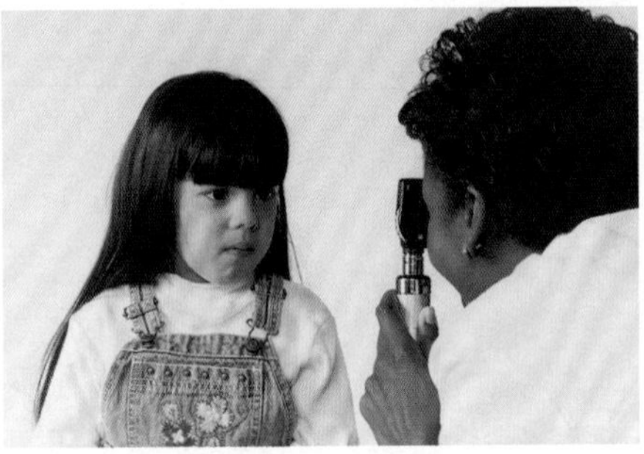

FIGURE 23-47 Testing conjugate gaze with the corneal light reflex test.

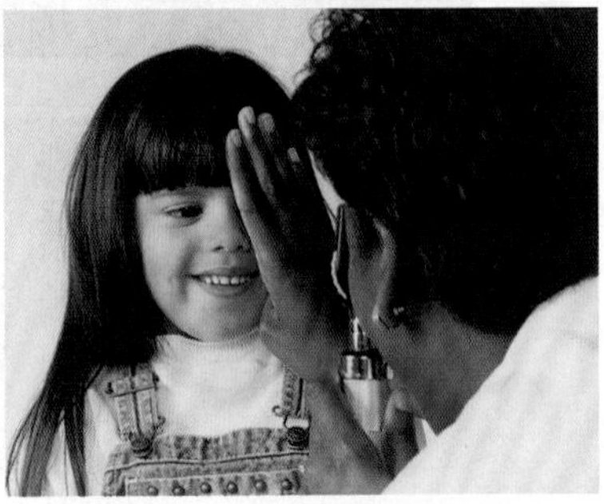

FIGURE 23-48 Testing conjugate gaze with the cover-uncover test.

Perform the cover-uncover test as a game by having the young child watch your nose or tell you if you are smiling or not while you cover one of the child's eyes. When you uncover the eye, watch for any deviation of that eye. Repeat for the other eye. Latent strabismus is indicated by movement of either eye when uncovered.

CLINICAL TIP
Both *ocular strabismus* and *anisometropia* (eyes with significantly different refractive errors) can result in amblyopia, or reduced vision in an otherwise normal eye. *Amblyopia* can lead to a "lazy eye," with permanently reduced visual acuity if not corrected early (generally by 6 years).

Visual Acuity

It may not be possible to measure the visual acuity of children younger than 3 years who cannot identify pictures on an eye chart. For these children, the simplest examination is to assess for fixation preference by alternately covering one eye; the child with normal vision will not object, but a child with poor vision in one eye will object to having the good eye covered. In all tests of visual acuity, it is important that both eyes show the same result. If you or the parent have any doubts about visual acuity, it is wise to refer to an optometrist or ophthalmologist because this aspect of the physical examination is insensitive.

Reduced visual acuity is more likely among children who were born prematurely and among those with other neurologic or developmental disorders.

Expected visual acuity by age is outlined in Table 23-26.

TABLE 23-26 Expected Visual Acuity

Age	Acuity
3 mo	Eyes converge, baby reaches for object
12 mo	~20/200
Younger than 4 y	20/40
4 y and older	20/30

Any difference in visual acuity between the eyes (e.g., 20/20 on the left and 20/30 on the right) is abnormal by age 5 y, and the patient should be referred to an ophthalmologist.

Visual acuity in children 4 years and older can usually be formally tested using an eye chart with one of a variety of optotypes (characters or symbols). A child who does not know letters or numbers can be reliably tested using pictures, symbols, or the "E" chart. Using the "E" chart, most children will cooperate by telling you in which direction the "E" is pointing.

The most common visual disorder of childhood is *myopia* (abnormalities in near vision), which can be easily detected using this examination technique. Myopia can lead to reading difficulties, headaches, and school problems, as well as double vision.

Visual Fields

The *visual fields* can be examined in infants and young children with the child sitting on the parent's lap. One eye should be tested at a time with the other eye covered (Fig. 23-49). Hold the child's head in the midline while bringing an object such as a toy into the field of vision from behind the child. The overall method is the same as that for adults, except that you will have to make this into a game for your patient (Fig. 23-50).

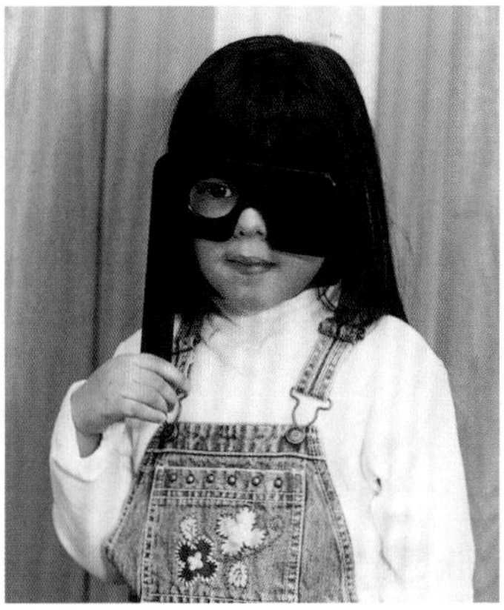

FIGURE 23-49 Have the child "help" with the visual field examination by holding the eye occluder.

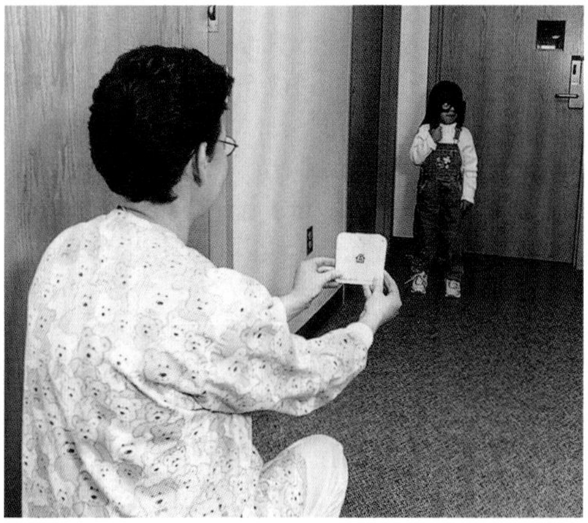

FIGURE 23-50 The nurse asks the child to identify a toy to assess vision.

The Ears

Examining the *ear canal and drum* can be difficult in young children who are sensitive and fearful because they cannot observe the procedure. If the child is not too fearful, examine the ears with the child sitting on a parent's lap. Make a game out of the otoscopic examination, or talk playfully to allay fears during the examination. It may help to place the otoscopic speculum gently into the external auditory canal of one ear and then withdraw it so the child gets used to the procedure before the actual examination. Unfortunately, many young children need to be briefly restrained during this examination, which is why you may want to leave it for the end.

Ask the parent for a preference regarding the positioning of the child for the examination. There are two common positions—the child lying down and restrained, and the child sitting in the parent's lap. If the child is held supine, have the parent hold the arms either extended or close to the sides to limit motions. Hold the head and retract the tragus with one hand while you hold the otoscope with your other hand. If the child is on the parent's lap, the child's legs should be between the parent's legs. The parent could help by placing one arm around the child's body and using the second arm to steady the head (with the parent's hand on the child's forehead). Tips for examining the child's ears are listed in Box 23-8.

BOX 23-8 TIPS FOR CONDUCTING THE OTOSCOPIC EXAMINATION

- Use the best angle of the otoscope.
- Use the largest possible speculum. A larger speculum allows you to better visualize the tympanic membrane and is less painful since it is not inserted as far as a smaller speculum.
- Do not apply too much pressure, which will cause the child to cry.
- Insert the speculum 1/4 to 1/2 in into the canal.
- First find the landmarks. Be careful, as sometimes the ear canal resembles the tympanic membrane.
- Note whether the tympanic membrane is abnormal.

Tympanic Membranes

Until approximately 3 years, the external auditory canal is directed downward similar to infants and the auricle must be pulled downward and backward to afford the best view. After about 3 years, the ear canal assumes an adult-like slope and the auricle is pulled upward and backward. Steady the child's head with one hand (your left hand if you are right-handed), and with that same hand pull on the auricle. With your other hand, position the otoscope.

There are two ways to hold the otoscope:

- The first is with the otoscope handle pointing upward or laterally while you pull on the auricle (Fig. 23-51). Hold the lateral aspect of your hand that has the otoscope against the child's head to provide a buffer against sudden movements by the patient.

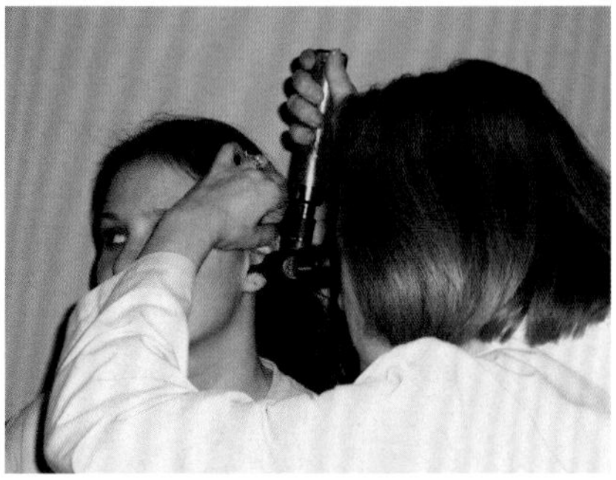

FIGURE 23-51 Holding the otoscope with the handle up.

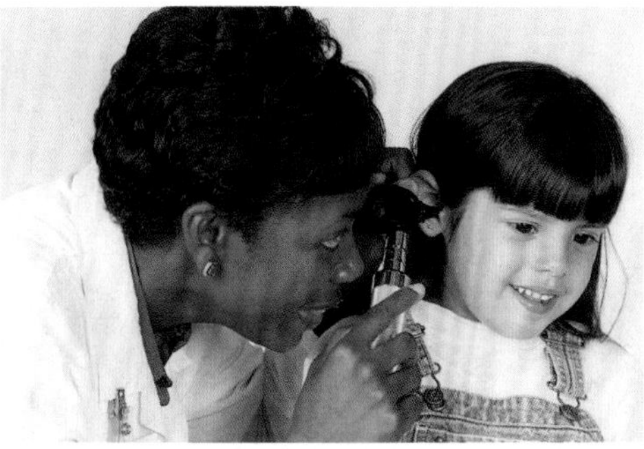

FIGURE 23-52 Holding the otoscope with the handle down.

- The second technique may be used because of the different angle of the auditory canal in children. Hold the otoscope with the handle pointing down toward the child's feet while you pull on the auricle (Fig. 23-52). Hold the head and pull up on the auricle with one hand while you hold the otoscope with the other hand.

Acute otitis media is a common condition of childhood. A symptomatic child typically has a red, bulging tympanic membrane with a dull or absent light reflex. Purulent material may also be seen behind the tympanic membrane. See Table 23-7, "Abnormalities of the Eyes, Ears, and Mouth." The most useful symptom in making the diagnosis is ear pain if combined with the above signs (Paul & Moreno, 2020).

Gently move and pull on the *auricle* before or during your otoscopic examination. Carefully inspect the area behind the auricle, over the mastoid bone.

CLINICAL TIP

With *otitis externa* (but not otitis media), movement of the auricle elicits pain.

With acute *mastoiditis,* the auricle may protrude forward and outward, and the area over the mastoid bone is red, swollen, and tender.

Formal Hearing Testing

Although formal hearing testing is necessary for accurate detection of hearing deficits in young children, you can grossly test for hearing by using the whispered voice test. To do this, stand behind the child (so that the child cannot read your lips), cover one of the child's ear canals, and rub the tragus, using a circular motion. Whisper letters, numbers, or a word, and have the child repeat it; then test the other ear.

Younger children who fail these screening maneuvers or who have speech delays should have audiometric testing. These children may have *hearing deficits* or central auditory processing disorders.

The AAP recommends that *all children older than 4 years have a full-scale acoustic screening test using standardized equipment* (Fig. 23-53) (AAP, 2020). Even though a normal hearing screen at birth is reassuring, some hearing loss is acquired as children age and hearing loss can dramatically affect a child's language and development.

Up to 15% of school-aged children have at least mild hearing loss, emphasizing the importance of screening for hearing prior to school age (CDC, 2020b).

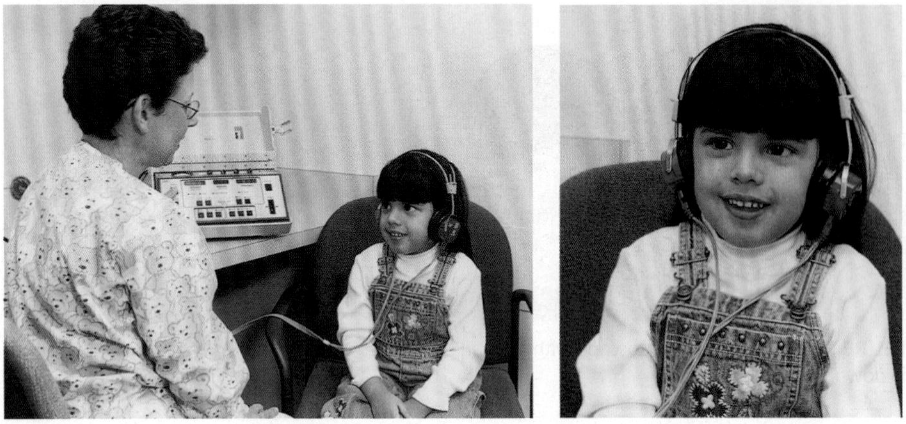

FIGURE 23-53 The child wears earphones to block extraneous sounds during the audiometry examination.

The Nose and Sinuses

Inspect the anterior portion of the nose by using a large speculum on your otoscope (Fig. 23-54). Inspect the nasal mucous membranes, noting their color and condition. Look for nasal septal deviation and the presence of polyps.

Nasal polyps are flesh-colored growths inside the nares. They are generally isolated findings but in some cases are present as part of a syndrome.

Children with purulent rhinorrhea (generally unilateral) for more than 10 days and also headache, sore throat, and tenderness over the sinuses may have *sinusitis.*

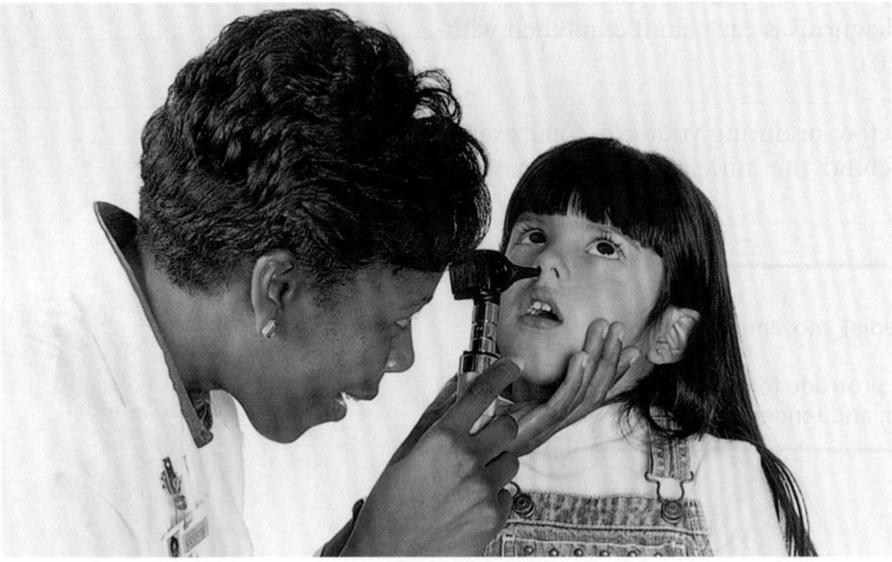

FIGURE 23-54 The nurse uses an otoscope to examine the child's interior nose and sinuses.

CLINICAL TIP

Pale, boggy nasal mucous membranes are found in children with *chronic (perennial) allergic rhinitis.* Purulent rhinitis is common in viral infections but may also be a symptom of *sinusitis.* Foul-smelling, purulent, unilateral discharge from the nose may be due to a *foreign body* in the nose. This is particularly common among young preschool children, who tend to stick objects into any body orifice.

Sinuses develop at varying ages. The sinuses of older children can be palpated or percussed as in adults, looking for tenderness.

The Mouth and Pharynx

For anxious or young children, it is wise to leave this part of the examination until the end, because it may require parental assistance. The young, cooperative child may be more comfortable sitting in the parent's lap.

Box 23-9 includes some tricks to getting children to open their mouths. The child who can say "ahhh" will usually offer a sufficient (albeit brief) view of the posterior pharynx so that a tongue blade is unnecessary (Fig. 23-55). Healthy children are more likely to cooperate with this examination than sick children, especially if the sick child sees the tongue blade or has had previous experience with throat cultures.

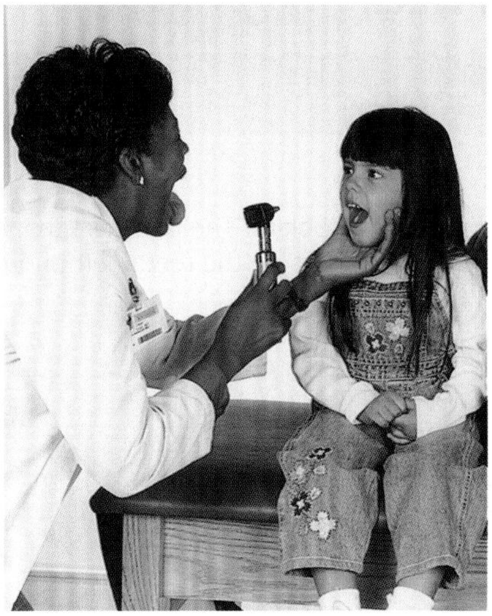

FIGURE 23-55 The nurse uses an otoscope to illuminate the child's mouth and pharynx.

If you need to use the tongue depressor, push down and pull slightly forward toward yourself while the child says "ahhh," being careful not to place the blade too far posteriorly, eliciting a gag reflex.

BOX 23-9 HOW TO GET CHILDREN TO OPEN THEIR MOUTHS

- Ask the child to say "ahhh," and turn it into a game.
  - "Now let's see what's in your mouth."
  - "Can you stick out your *whole tongue*?"
  - "I bet you can't open your mouth *really wide*!"
  - "Let me see the inside of your teeth."
- Don't show a tongue depressor unless necessary.
- Demonstrate first on an older sibling (or even the parent).
- Offer enthusiastic praise for opening their mouths a little, and encourage them to open even wider.

Examine the *teeth* for the timing and sequence of eruption, number, character, condition, and position. Abnormalities of the enamel may reflect local or general disease.

Dental caries are the most common health problem in children. They are particularly prevalent in impoverished populations and can cause both short-term and long-term problems (NIH. National Institute of Dental and Craniofacial Research, 2018). Caries are highly treatable, but require a dental visit.

Carefully inspect the upper teeth. This is a common location for *nursing bottle caries.* The technique, called "lift the lip," can facilitate visualization of dental caries. Gently raise the child's upper lip with your gloved thumb to visualize the outside of the upper teeth. Visualize the inside of the upper teeth by having the child look up at the ceiling with the mouth wide open.

Dental caries are caused by bacterial activity. Caries are more likely among young children who are put to bed nursing from a bottle, allowing formula to pool around the teeth ("baby bottle syndrome").

Table 23-27 includes abnormalities of the teeth as well as the pharynx and neck.

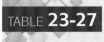

TABLE 23-27 Abnormalities of the Teeth, Pharynx, and Neck

Dental Abnormalities

Dental Caries

Dental caries are a major global health and pediatric problem. The photographs below show different characteristics of caries. White spots on the teeth (left photo) often reflect early caries.

Nursing-bottle caries

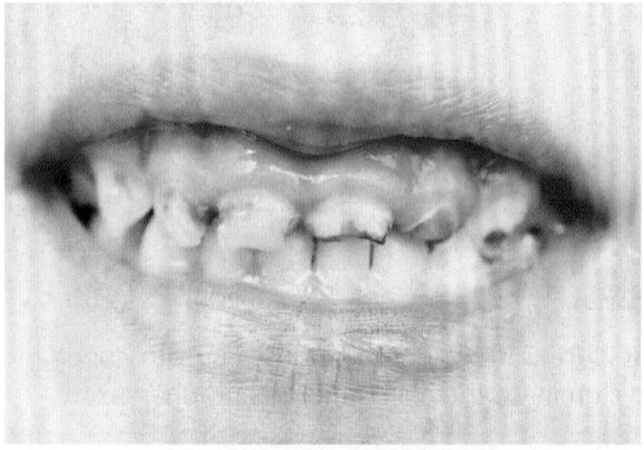

Severe erosion

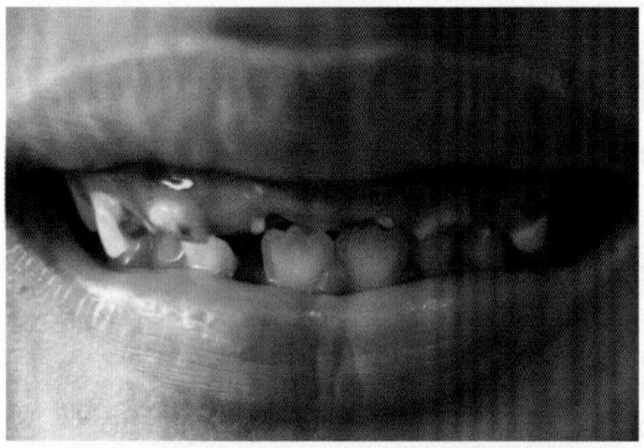

Staining of the Teeth

Various causes can lead to staining of the teeth of children, including intrinsic stains such as tetracycline (right) or extrinsic stains such as poor oral hygiene (not shown). Extrinsic stains can be removed.

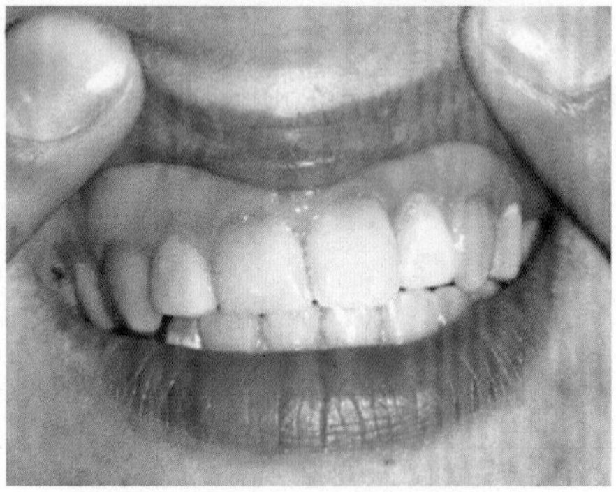

Staining of the teeth may be intrinsic or extrinsic. Intrinsic stains discolor the deeper layers of enamel and even the dentin of the tooth during development. Excessive fluoride intake can cause intrinsic staining. Rarely seen today, tetracycline use before 8 y of age may also cause intrinsic staining. Iron preparation (black stain) is an example of AN extrinsic stain. Extrinsic stains can be polished off; intrinsic stains cannot.

Streptococcal Pharyngitis ("Strep Throat")

This common childhood infection has a classic presentation of erythema of the posterior pharynx and palatal petechiae (*top*). A foul-smelling exudate (*bottom*) is also commonly noted.

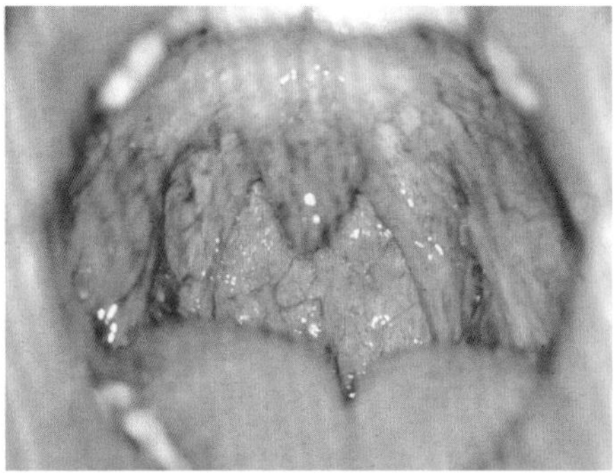

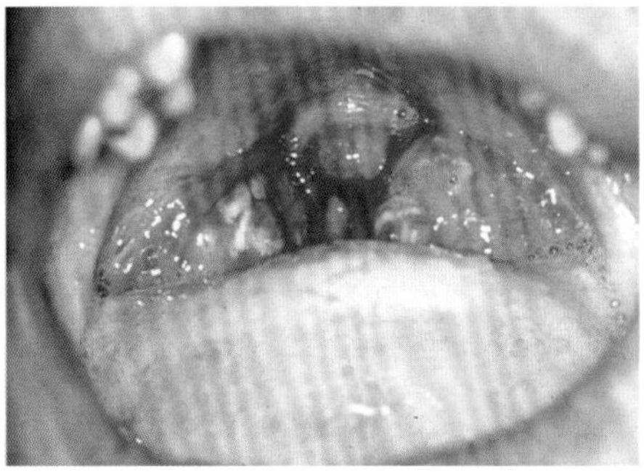

Lymphadenopathy

Enlarged and tender cervical lymph nodes are common in children. The most likely causes are viral and bacterial infections. Lymph node enlargement can be bilateral, as shown here.

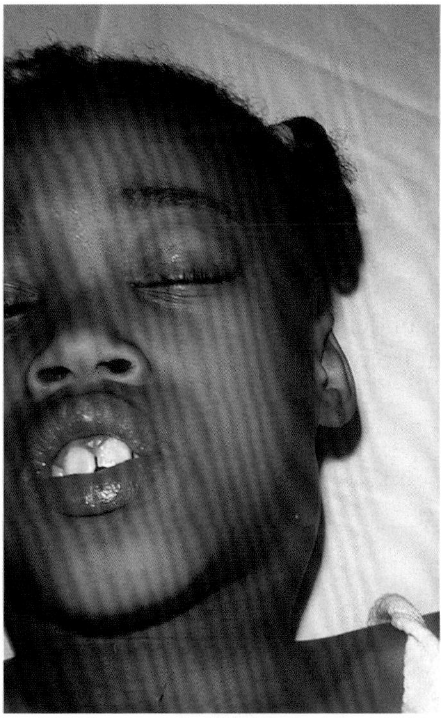

Sources of photos: *Nursing-bottle caries*—Arctic Ice/Shutterstock; *Severe erosion*—phungatanee/Shutterstock; *Staining of the Teeth*—Delong, N., & Burkhart, N. W. (2012). *General and oral pathology for the dental hygienist* (2nd ed.). Wolters Kluwer; *Streptococcal pharyngitis*—The Wellcome Trust, National Medical Slide Bank, London, UK; *Lymphadenopathy*—Fleisher, G. R., Ludwig, W., & Baskin, M. N. (2004). *Atlas of pediatric emergency medicine*. Lippincott Williams & Wilkins.

Table 23-28 outlines the common pattern of tooth eruption. In general, lower teeth erupt earlier than upper teeth.

TABLE 23-28 Tooth Types and Age of Eruption

	Approximate Age of Eruption	
Tooth Type	**Primary (Months)**	**Permanent (Years)**
Central incisor	6–12	6–8
Lateral incisor	9–16	7–9
Cuspids	16–23	9–12
First bicuspids	—	10–12
Second bicuspids	—	10–12
First molars	13–19	6–7
Second molars	23–33	11–13
Third molars	—	17–21

Source: American Dental Association (ADA). (n.d.). Eruption charts. https://www.mouthhealthy.org/en/az-topics/e/eruption-charts#main-content

Look for abnormalities of the position of the teeth. These include malocclusion, maxillary protrusion (*overbite*), and mandibular protrusion (*underbite*). You can demonstrate the latter two by asking the child to bite down hard while either you or the child parts the lips. Observe the true bite. In normal positioning, the lower teeth are contained within the arch formed by the upper teeth.

Malocclusion and misalignment of teeth can be from thumb sucking, a hereditary condition, or premature loss of primary teeth.

Carefully inspect the *tongue,* including the underside. Most children will happily stick their tongue out at you, move it from side to side, and demonstrate its color (Fig. 23-56).

Common abnormalities include *coated tongue* in viral infections, and *strawberry tongue,* found in scarlet fever.

Some young children have a tight frenulum. Children who are severely "tongue-tied" might have a speech impediment. Have the child touch the tongue to the roof of the mouth to diagnose this condition, which often does not require treatment unless it interferes with eating or speech.

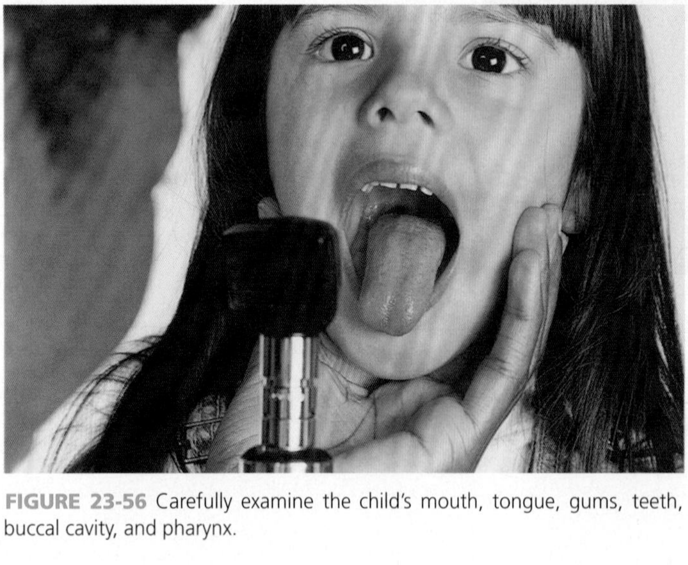

FIGURE 23-56 Carefully examine the child's mouth, tongue, gums, teeth, buccal cavity, and pharynx.

Note the size, position, symmetry, and appearance of the *tonsils*. The peak growth of tonsillar tissue is between 8 and 16 years. The size of the tonsils varies considerably in children and is often categorized on a scale of 1+ to 4+, with 1+ being easy visibility of the gap between the tonsils, and 4+ being tonsils that touch in the midline with the mouth wide open. The tonsils in children often appear more obstructive than they really are.

CLINICAL TIP

Streptococcal pharyngitis typically produces a strawberry tongue, white or yellow exudates on the tonsils or posterior pharynx, a beefy-red uvula, and palatal petechiae. See Table 23-27, "Abnormalities of the Teeth, Pharynx, and Neck." Together with these signs, the most helpful historical information is exposure to strep throat infection within 2 weeks.

Tonsils in children usually have deep crypts on their surfaces, which often have white concretions or food particles protruding from their depths. This does not indicate disease.

A *peritonsillar abscess* is suggested by erythema and asymmetric enlargement of one of the tonsils and lateral displacement of the uvula.

Look for clues of a submucosal cleft palate, such as notching of the posterior margin of the hard palate or a bifid *uvula*. Because the mucosa is intact, the underlying defect is easily missed, but needs referral to otolaryngology.

Rarely, you may encounter a child who has a sore throat and has difficulty swallowing saliva, and who is sitting up stiffly in a "tripod" position because of throat obstruction. Do not open this child's mouth because they may have acute epiglottitis.

CLINICAL TIP

Acute epiglottitis is now rare in the United States because of immunization against *Haemophilus influenzae* type B. *Suspected epiglottitis is* contraindication to examination of the throat because of potential gagging and laryngeal obstruction.

Note the quality of the child's voice. Certain abnormalities can change the pitch and quality of the voice:

- *Bacterial tracheitis* can cause airway obstruction.
- *Tonsillitis* can be caused by bacteria, such as *Streptococcus*, or viruses. The "rocks in the mouth" voice is accompanied by enlarged tonsils with exudates.
- The epidemic of childhood obesity has resulted in many children who snore and have *sleep apnea*.
- You may note an abnormal breath odor, which may help lead to a specific diagnosis.

Halitosis in a child can be caused by *upper respiratory, pharyngeal, or mouth infection; foreign body in the nose; dental disease; sinusitis; and gastroesophageal reflux* (among other causes).

The Neck

Beyond infancy, the techniques for examining the neck are the same as for adults. Lymphadenopathy is unusual during infancy but common during childhood. The child's lymphatic system reaches its zenith of growth at 12 years, and cervical or tonsillar lymph nodes reach their peak size between 8 and 16 years.

Lymphadenopathy is usually from viral or bacterial infections. See Table 23-27, "Abnormalities of the Teeth, Pharynx, and Neck."

The majority of enlarged lymph nodes in children are due to infections (mostly viral but also bacterial) and not to malignant disease, though the latter is a concern for many parents. It is important to differentiate normal lymph nodes from abnormal ones or from congenital cysts of the neck.

Malignancy is more likely if the node is greater than 2 cm, is hard, is fixed to the skin or underlying tissues (i.e., not mobile), or is accompanied by serious systemic signs such as weight loss.

Figure 23-30 demonstrates the typical anatomic locations of lymph nodes.

Check for *neck mobility*. It is important to ensure that the neck of all children is supple and easily mobile in all directions. This is particularly important when the patient is holding the head in an asymmetric manner and when central nervous system disease such as meningitis is suspected.

In young children with small necks, it may be difficult to differentiate low posterior cervical lymph nodes from *supraclavicular lymph nodes* (which are always abnormal and raise suspicion for malignancy).

In children, the presence of nuchal rigidity is a more reliable indicator of meningeal irritation than the *Brudzinski sign* or *Kernig sign*. To detect nuchal rigidity in older children, ask the child to sit with legs extended on the examining table. Normally, children should be able to sit upright and touch their chins to their chests. Younger children can be persuaded to flex their necks by having them follow a small toy or light beam. You also can test for nuchal rigidity with the child lying on the examining table, as shown in Figure 23-57. Nearly all children with nuchal rigidity will be extremely sick, irritable, and difficult to examine.

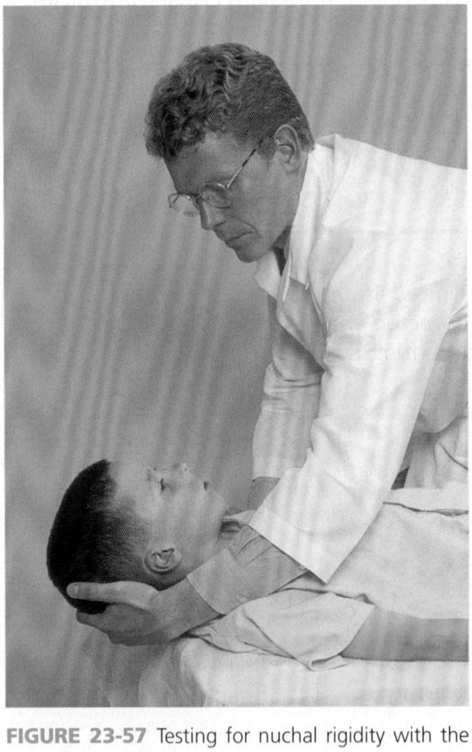

FIGURE 23-57 Testing for nuchal rigidity with the child lying on the table.

CLINICAL TIP

Nuchal rigidity is marked resistance to movement of the head in any direction. It suggests meningeal irritation due to *meningitis, bleeding, tumor,* or *other causes.* These children are extremely irritable and difficult to console and may have "paradoxical irritability"—increased irritability when being held.

When meningeal irritation is present, the child assumes the **tripod position** (Fig. 23-58) and is unable to assume a full upright position to perform the chin-to-chest maneuver.

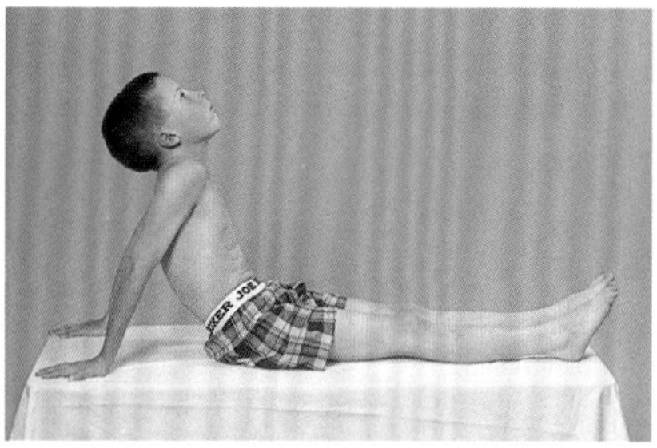

FIGURE 23-58 The tripod position seen with meningeal irritation and nuchal rigidity.

The Thorax and Lungs

As children age, lung examination becomes similar to that for adults. Cooperation is critical. Auscultation is usually easiest when a child barely notices (as when in a parent's lap). Let a toddler who seems fearful of the stethoscope play with it before touching the child's chest.

With upper airway obstruction such as *croup*, inspiration is prolonged and accompanied by other signs such as *stridor, cough, or rhonchi*. With lower airway obstruction such as *asthma*, expiration is prolonged and often accompanied by *wheezing*.

Assess the relative proportion of time spent on inspiration versus expiration. The normal ratio is about 1:1. Prolonged inspirations or expirations are a clue to disease location. Degree of prolongation and effort, or "work of breathing," are related to disease severity.

CLINICAL TIP

Pneumonia in young children is generally manifested by fever, tachypnea, dyspnea, and increased work of breathing.

Young children asked to "take deep breaths" often hold their breath, further complicating auscultation. It is easier to let preschoolers breathe normally. Demonstrate to older children how to take nice, quiet, deep breaths. Make it a game. To accomplish a forced expiratory maneuver, ask the child to blow out candles on an imaginary birthday cake (Fig. 23-59).

While *upper respiratory infections* due to viruses can cause young infants to appear quite ill, in children they present with the same signs as in adults, and children can appear well, without lower respiratory signs.

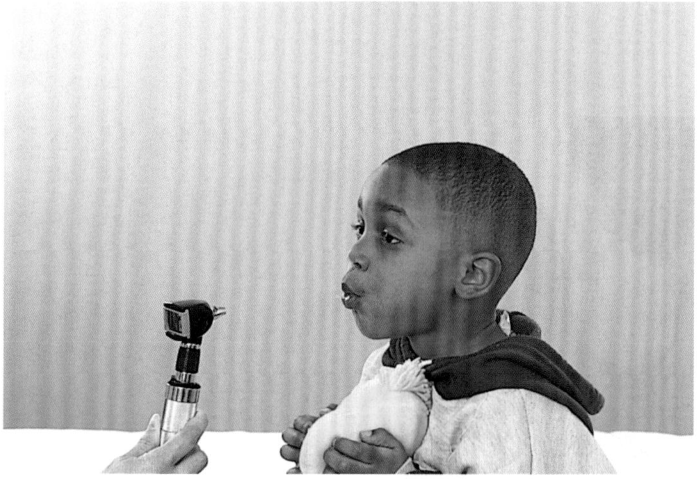

FIGURE 23-59 The stethoscope can be used as a "candle." Ask the child to "blow" out the light. The nurse can turn off the light when the child exhales effectively.

Childhood asthma is an extremely common condition throughout the world. Children with acute asthma present with varying severity and often have increased work of breathing. Expiratory wheezing and a prolonged expiratory phase, caused by reversible bronchospasm, may be heard without the stethoscope and are apparent on auscultation. Wheezes, often accompanied by inspiratory rhonchi, are most commonly caused by upper respiratory infections which can also trigger asthma attacks.

Children in respiratory distress may assume a "*tripod position*" in which they lean forward to optimize airway patency (Fig. 23-60). This same position can also be caused by pharyngeal obstruction.

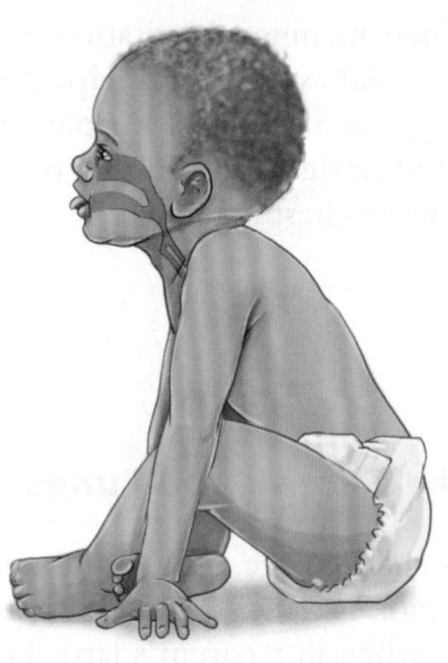

FIGURE 23-60 Characteristic posture of a child with acute epiglottitis: leaning forward on hands, in the "tripod" position; mouth open, tongue out, head forward, and tilted up in a sniffing position in an effort to relieve the acute airway obstruction secondary to swollen epiglottis. (Reprinted with permission from Hatfield, N. T., & Kincheloe, C. A. (2017). *Introductory maternity and pediatric nursing* (4th ed.). Wolters Kluwer.)

Older children will be cooperative for the respiratory examination and can even go through the maneuvers of assessing fremitus or listening to "E to A" changes (egophony) (see p. 382). As children grow, the evaluation by observation discussed on the previous page, such as assessing the work of breathing, nasal flaring, and grunting, becomes less helpful in assessing for respiratory pathology. Palpation, percussion, and auscultation achieve greater importance in a careful examination of the thorax and lungs.

The Heart

The examination of the heart and vascular systems in infants and children is similar to that in adults; however, a child's fearfulness or inability to cooperate may make the examination difficult while their desire to play will make the examination easier and more productive. Use your knowledge of the developmental stage of each child. A 2-year-old may be easiest to examine while standing or sitting on the parent's lap, facing their shoulder, or being held (Fig. 23-61). Give young children something to hold in each hand. They cannot figure out how to drop one object and therefore have no hand free to push you away. Endless chatter to small children will hold their attention and they will forget that you are examining them (Fig. 23-62). Let older children move the stethoscope themselves, going back to listen properly. Use your imagination to make the examination work.

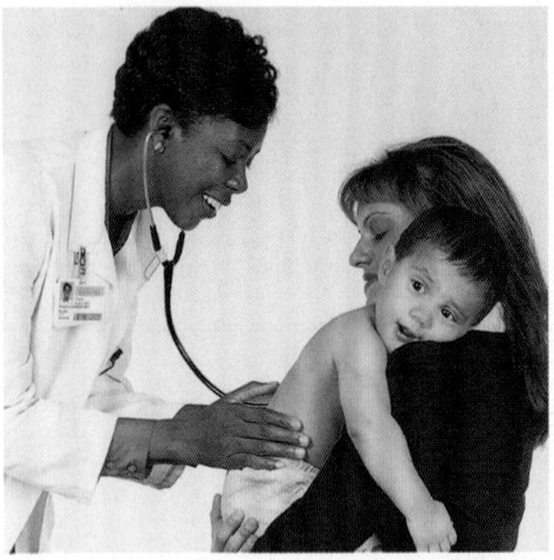

FIGURE 23-61 The nurse listens to an infant's heart while the parent holds him.

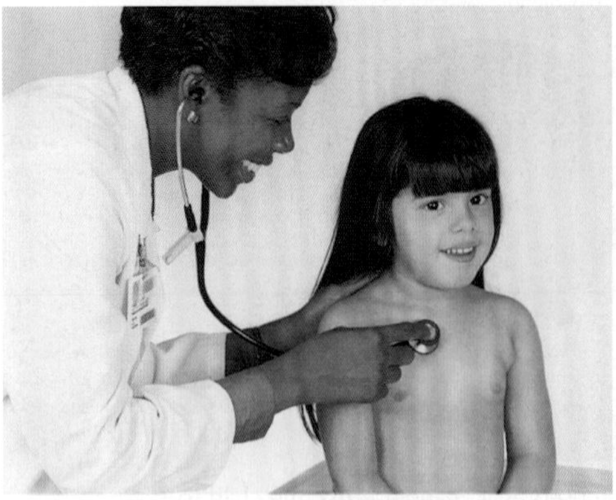

FIGURE 23-62 The nurse listens to the preschooler's heart.

Benign Murmurs

Preschool and school-aged children often have benign murmurs (Table 23-29). The most common (*Still murmur*) is a grade I–II/VI, musical, vibratory, early, and midsystolic murmur with multiple overtones located over the mid- or lower left sternal border; it may also be heard over the carotid arteries. Carotid artery compression will usually cause the precordial murmur to disappear. This murmur may be extremely variable and may be accentuated when cardiac output is increased, as occurs with fever or exercise.

TABLE 23-29 Location and Characteristics of Benign Heart Murmurs in Children

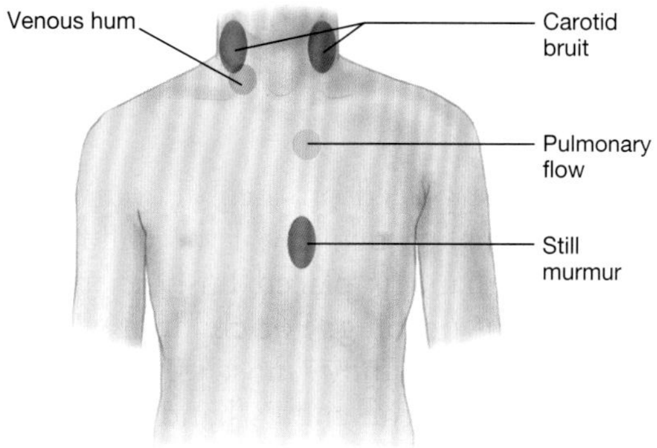

Typical Age	Name	Tonal Characteristics	Description and Location
Preschool or early school age	*Still murmur*	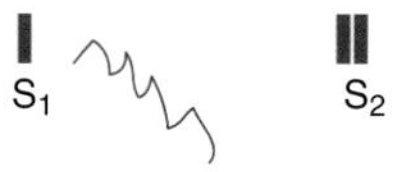	Grade I–II/VI, musical, vibratory Multiple overtones Early and midsystolic Mid/lower left sternal border Frequently also a carotid bruit
Preschool or early school age	*Venous hum*	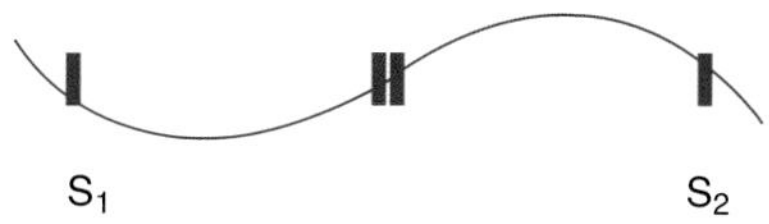	Soft, hollow, continuous Louder in diastole Under clavicle Can be eliminated by maneuvers
Preschool and later	*Carotid bruit*	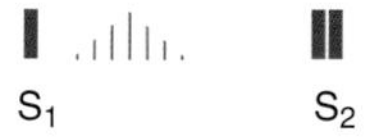	Early and midsystolic Usually louder on left Eliminated by carotid compression
Preschool and school age	*Pulmonary flow murmur*	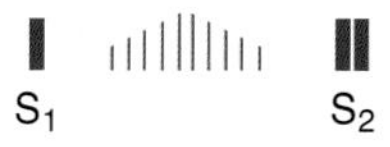	Grade II–III systolic ejection Loudest at pulmonary auscultation area Harsh, nonvibratory Intensity increases when in the supine position

In preschool or school-aged children, you may detect a *venous hum*. This is a soft, hollow, continuous sound, louder in diastole, heard just below the right clavicle. It can be completely eliminated by maneuvers that affect venous return, such as lying supine, changing head position, or jugular venous compression. It has the same quality as breath sounds and therefore is frequently overlooked.

Among young children, murmurs without the recognizable features of the two common benign sounds may signify underlying heart disease and should be evaluated thoroughly by a pediatric cardiologist.

Pathologic murmurs that signify cardiac disease can first appear after infancy and during childhood. Examples include aortic stenosis and mitral valve disease. See Table 23-13, "Congenital Heart Murmurs."

The Abdomen

Toddlers and young children commonly have protuberant abdomens most apparent when they are upright. The examination can follow the same order as for adults, except that the child may need to be distracted during the examination.

An exaggerated "potbelly appearance" may indicate malabsorption from *celiac disease, cystic fibrosis,* or *constipation* or *aerophagia.*

Most children are ticklish when a hand is first placed on their abdomens for *palpation*. This reaction tends to disappear, particularly if the child is distracted with conversation and the whole hand is placed flush on the abdominal surface for a few moments without probing. For children who are particularly sensitive and who tighten their abdominal muscles, start by placing the child's hand under yours. Eventually the child's hand can be removed and the abdomen freely palpated.

CLINICAL TIP

A common condition of childhood that can occasionally cause a protuberant abdomen is constipation. The abdomen is often tympanic on percussion, and stool is often felt on palpation.

Also try flexing the knees and hips to relax the child's abdominal wall, as shown in Figure 23-63. Palpate lightly in all areas, then deeply, leaving the site of potential pathology to the end.

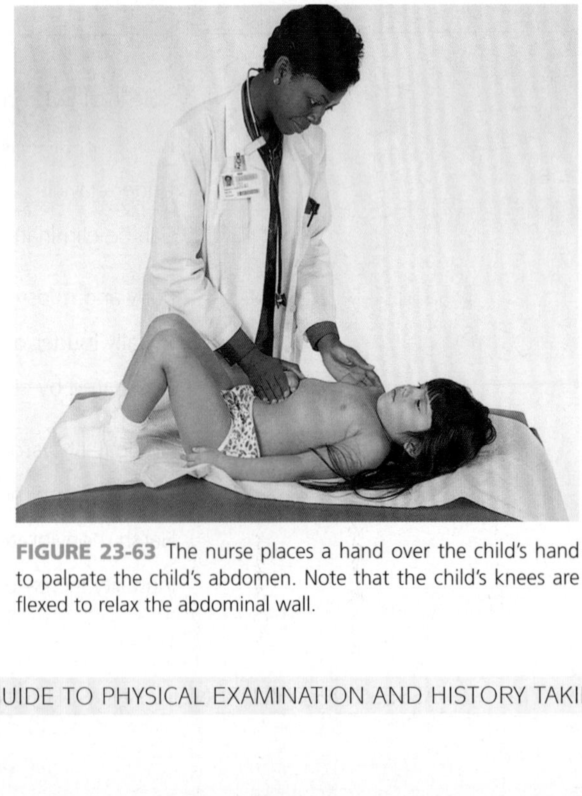

FIGURE 23-63 The nurse places a hand over the child's hand to palpate the child's abdomen. Note that the child's knees are flexed to relax the abdominal wall.

Many children present with abdominal pain from *acute gastroenteritis.* Despite pain, their physical examination is relatively normal except for increased bowel sounds on auscultation and mild tenderness on palpation.

When palpating for the liver borders, be aware of the normal liver span in relation to the child's age as outlined in Table 23-30.

Hepatomegaly in young children is unusual. It can be caused by *cystic fibrosis, protein malabsorption, parasites, fatty liver, and tumors.*

TABLE 23-30 Expected Liver Span of Children by Percussion

Age in Years	Mean Estimated Liver Span (cm) Males	Females
2	3.5	3.6
3	4.0	4.0
4	4.4	4.3
5	4.8	4.5
6	5.1	4.8
8	5.6	5.1
10	6.1	5.4

The *spleen,* like the liver, is felt easily in most children. It too is soft with a sharp edge, and it projects downward like a tongue from under the left costal margin. The spleen is moveable and rarely extends more than 1 cm to 2 cm below the costal margin.

Various diseases can cause splenomegaly, including *infections, hematologic disorders* such as *hemolytic anemias, infiltrative disorders,* and *inflammatory or autoimmune diseases,* as well as congestion from *portal hypertension.*

Palpate the *other abdominal structures.* You will commonly note pulsations in the epigastrium caused by the aorta. This is felt most easily to the left of the midline on deep palpation.

Palpating for abdominal tenderness in an older child is the same as for the adult; localization of tenderness may help you pinpoint the abdominal structures most likely to be causing the abdominal pain.

In a child with an acute abdominal pain, as in *acute appendicitis,* special techniques are helpful, such as checking for involuntary rigidity, rebound tenderness, a Rovsing sign, or a positive psoas or obturator sign (see the Chapter 16 section, "Assessing Possible Appendicitis") (McGee, 2018). *Gastroenteritis, constipation,* and *gastrointestinal obstruction* are other possible etiologies of acute abdominal pain.

Male Genitalia

The genital examination can be anxiety-provoking for the older child and adolescent (especially if you are of the opposite sex), for parents, and for you; however, if not performed, a significant finding may be missed.

Depending on the child's developmental stage, explain what parts of the body you will check and that this is part of the routine examination.

Inspect the penis. The size in prepubertal children has little significance unless it is abnormally large. In obese boys, the fat pad over the symphysis pubis may obscure the penis.

In *precocious puberty,* the penis and testes are enlarged, with signs of pubertal changes. This is caused by a variety of conditions associated with excess androgens, including *adrenal or pituitary tumors.* Other pubertal changes also occur.

There is an art to *palpation* of the young patient's scrotum and testes because many have an extremely active cremasteric reflex that may cause the testis to retract upward into the inguinal canal and thereby appear to be undescended. Examine the child when relaxed because anxiety stimulates the cremasteric reflex. With warm hands, palpate the lower abdomen, working your way downward toward the scrotum along the inguinal canal. This will minimize retraction of the testes into the canal.

A useful technique is to have the patient sit cross-legged on the examining table, as shown in Figure 23-64. You can also give him a balloon to inflate or an object to lift to increase intra-abdominal pressure. If you can detect the testis in the scrotum, it is descended even if it spends much time in the inguinal canal.

Cryptorchidism may be noted at this age. It requires surgical correction. It should be differentiated from a retractable testis. See Table 23-15, "The Male Genitourinary System."

The cremasteric reflex can be tested by scratching the medial aspect of the thigh. The testis on the side being scratched will move upward.

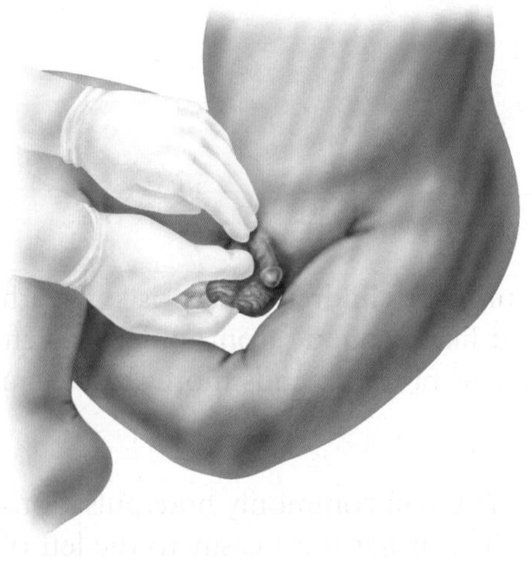

FIGURE 23-64 Examining the testis with the child sitting cross-legged.

CLINICAL TIP

A painful testicle requires rapid treatment; common causes include infection such as *epididymitis* or *orchitis, torsion of the testicle,* or *torsion of the appendix testis.*

Inguinal hernias in older boys present as they do in adult men with swelling in the inguinal canal, particularly following a Valsalva maneuver.

Female Genitalia

After infancy, the labia majora and minora flatten out, and the hymenal membrane becomes thin, translucent, and vascular, with the edges easily identified.

The appearance of pubic hair before 7 years should be considered *precocious puberty* and requires evaluation to determine the cause.

The genital examination is the same for all ages of children from late infancy until adolescence. Use a calm, gentle approach, including a developmentally appropriate explanation as you do the examination. A bright light source is essential. Most children can be examined in the supine, frog-leg position.

Rashes on the external genitals can be from various causes such as physical irritation, sweating, and candidal or bacterial infections.

If the child seems reluctant, it may be helpful to have the parent sit on the examination table with the child; alternatively, the examination may be performed while the child sits in the parent's lap. Do not use stirrups, as these may frighten the child. Figure 23-65 demonstrates a 5-year-old child sitting on her parent's lap with the parent holding her knees outstretched.

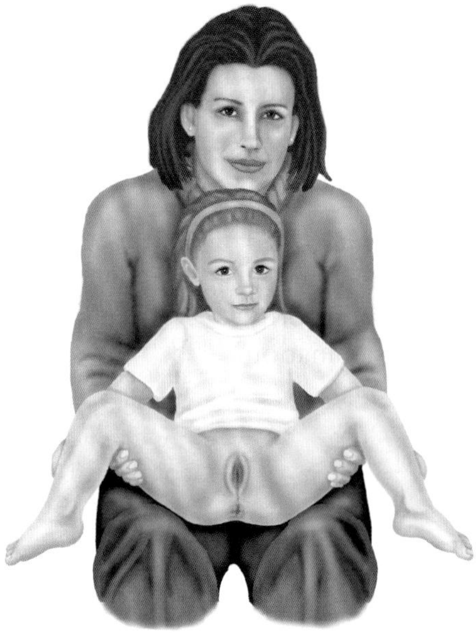

FIGURE 23-65 A parent holds the patient with her legs opened for the genital examination.

Examine the genitalia in an efficient and systematic manner. Inspect the external genitalia for pubic hair, the size of the clitoris, the color and size of the labia majora, and the presence of rashes, bruises, or other lesions.

Next, visualize the structures by separating the labia with your fingers as shown in Figure 23-66. *Labial adhesions,* or fusion of the labia minora, may be noted in prepubertal children and can obscure the vaginal and urethral orifices. They may be a normal variant.

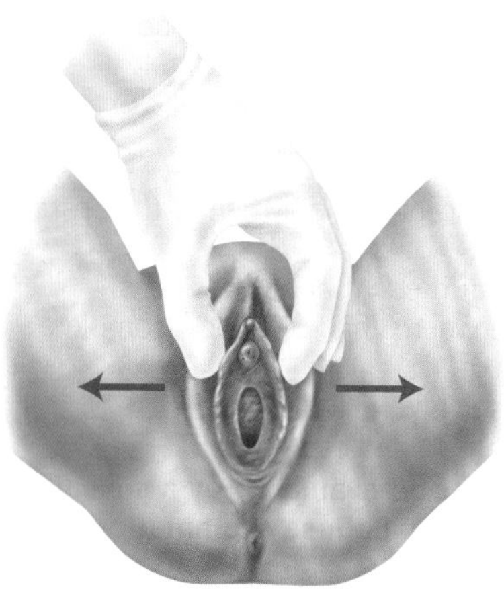

FIGURE 23-66 Gently spread the labia to inspect the external genitalia.

Purulent, profuse, malodorous, and blood-tinged discharge should be evaluated for the presence of *infiltration, foreign body,* or *trauma.*

CLINICAL TIP

A *vaginal discharge* in early childhood can be from *perineal irritation* (e.g., bubble baths or soaps), *foreign body, vaginitis,* or a *sexually transmitted infection* from sexual abuse.

Vaginal bleeding is always concerning. Etiologies include *vaginal irritation, accidental trauma, sexual abuse, foreign body,* and *tumors. Precocious puberty* from many causes can induce menses in a young girl.

Avoid touching the hymenal edges because the hymen is tender without the protective effects of hormones. Examine for discharge, labial adhesions, lesions, and hygiene. A thin, white discharge (leukorrhea) is often present. A speculum examination of the vagina and cervix is not necessary in a prepubertal child unless there is suspicion of severe trauma or foreign body. An experienced gynecologist or advanced practice nurse should perform the speculum examination.

Abrasions or signs of trauma of the external genitalia can be from benign causes such as masturbation, irritants, or accidental trauma, but they should also raise the possibility of *sexual abuse.*

The physical examination may reveal signs that suggest *sexual abuse,* and the examination is particularly important if there are suspicious clues in the history. Bear in mind that even with known abuse, the great majority of examinations will be unremarkable; thus, a normal genital examination does not rule out sexual abuse. See Table 23-31.

Sexual abuse is unfortunately too common throughout the world. Twenty percent of women and 5% to 10% of men recall a childhood sexual assault or sexual abuse incident; while many of these do not involve severe physical trauma, some do (National Center for Victims of Crimes, n.d.).

TABLE 23-31 Physical Signs of Sexual Abuse

Possible Indications

- Marked and immediate dilatation of the anus in knee-chest position, with no constipation, stool in the vault, or neurologic disorders
- Hymenal notch or cleft that extends greater than 50% of the inferior hymenal rim (confirmed in knee-chest position)
- Condyloma acuminata in a child older than 3 y
- Bruising, abrasions, lacerations, or bite marks of labia or perihymenal tissue
- Herpes of the anogenital area beyond the neonatal period
- Purulent or malodorous vaginal discharge in a young girl (culture and view all discharges under a microscope for evidence of a sexually transmitted disease)

Strong Indications

- Lacerations, ecchymoses, and newly healed scars of the hymen or the posterior fourchette
- No hymenal tissue from 3 to 9 o'clock (confirmed in various positions)
- Healed hymenal transections, especially between 3 and 9 o'clock (complete cleft)
- Perianal lacerations extending to external sphincter

A child with concerning physical signs must be evaluated by a sexual abuse expert for a complete history and sexual abuse examination.

Any physical sign must be evaluated in light of the entire history, other parts of the physical examination, and laboratory data.

Sexual abuse. Acute laceration.

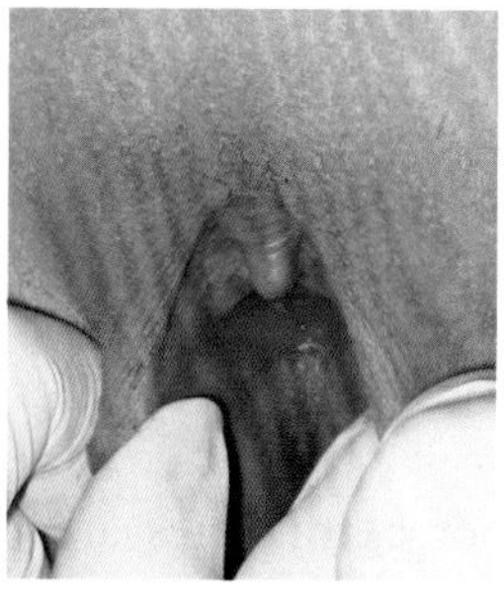

Sexual abuse, nonacute. Deep, wide posterior midline hymenal cleft extending to the vaginal wall (examined in prone knee chest position). Cleft represents healed complete hymenal tear or transection in a 15-year-old girl who disclosed multiple acts of penile vaginal penetration.

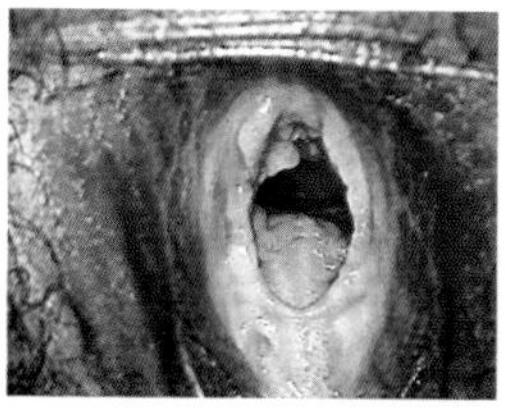

Sexual abuse, nonacute. Two deep, posterior midline hymenal clefts extending to the vaginal wall. Clefts represent healed complete hymenal tears or transections in a 11-year-old girl who described a single act of penile vaginal penetration accompanied by pain and bleeding 2 weeks previously.

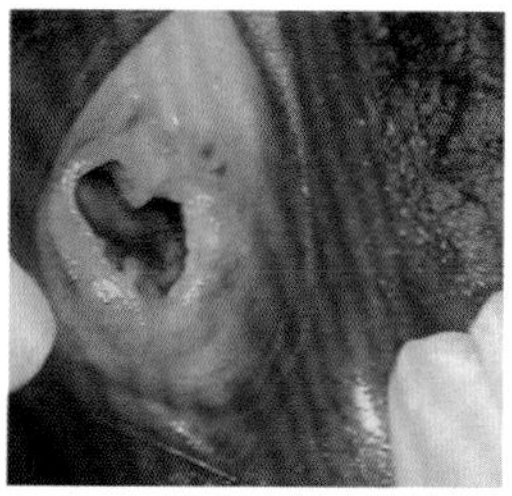

Genital warts. Multiple genital warts are seen in vaginal vestibule of 6-year-old girl who disclosed only digital penetration. Blood vessels in the irregular masses create the red stippling of the wart surface.

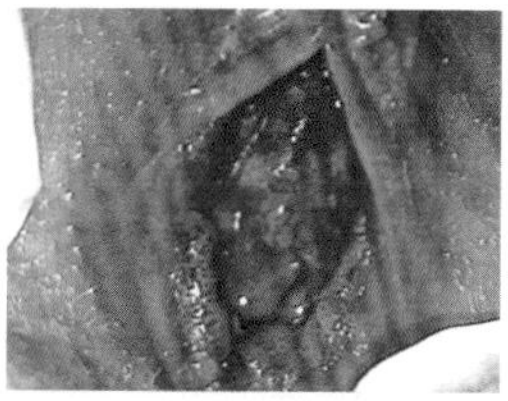

Lichen sclerosus et atrophicus. Characteristic subepidermal hemorrhages in a 4-year-old girl with a 3-week history of genital itching and intermittent dysuria. Note lesions extend over clitoral prepuce with fissuring due to friability in midline superior to clitoris. Lesions showed only slight improvement at follow-up weeks later.

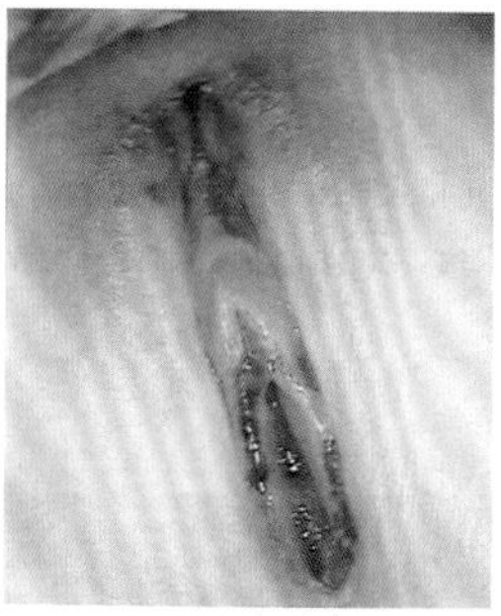

Perianal condylomata around the anus due to a human papillomavirus infection.

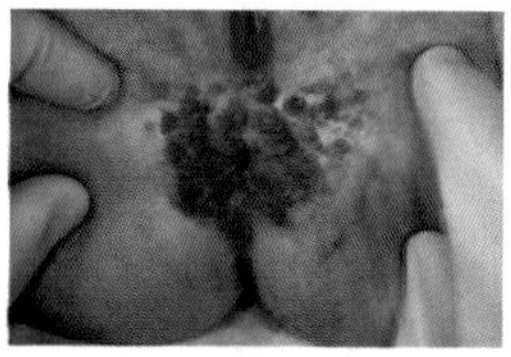

All photos except condylomata courtesy of Allan, R. De Jong, MD; *Condylomata*—Emans, S. J., Laufer, M. R., & DiVasta, A. D. (2019). *Goldstein's pediatric and adolescent gynecology* (7th ed.). Wolters Kluwer.

The Rectal Examination

The rectal examination is not routine. If intra-abdominal, pelvic, or perirectal disease is suspected, the child should be referred to an advanced care provider.

The Musculoskeletal System

In older children, abnormalities of the upper extremities are rare in the absence of injury.

Toddlers may acquire *nursemaid's elbow* or subluxation of the radial head from a tugging injury. They will hold their arms slightly flexed at the elbows but will resist using their arm.

The normal young child has increased lumbar concavity and decreased thoracic convexity compared with the adult and often has a protuberant abdomen.

Observe the child standing and walking barefoot. You can also ask the child to touch the toes, rise from sitting, run a short distance, and pick up objects. You will detect most abnormalities by watching carefully from both front and behind. To indirectly assess the child's gait pattern, you can also look at the soles of the shoes to see whether one side of the soles is worn down.

The most common lower extremity pathology in childhood is injury from accidents. Joint injuries, fractures, sprains, strains, and serious ligament injuries such as anterior cruciate ligament (ACL) tears of the knee are all too common in children.

CLINICAL TIP

The cause of *acute limp* in childhood is usually trauma or injury although infection of the bone, joint, or muscle should be considered. In an obese child, consider *slipped capital femoral epiphysis.*

Severe bowing of the legs (*genu varum*) may still be physiologic bowing that will spontaneously resolve. Extreme bowing or unilateral bowing may be from pathologic causes such as *rickets* or *tibia vara (Blount disease).*

During early infancy, there is a common and normal progression from bowleggedness (Fig. 23-67), which begins to disappear at about 18 months of age, often followed by transition toward knock-knees. The *knock-knee pattern* (Fig. 23-68) is usually maximal by age 3 to 4 and gradually corrects by age 9 or 10.

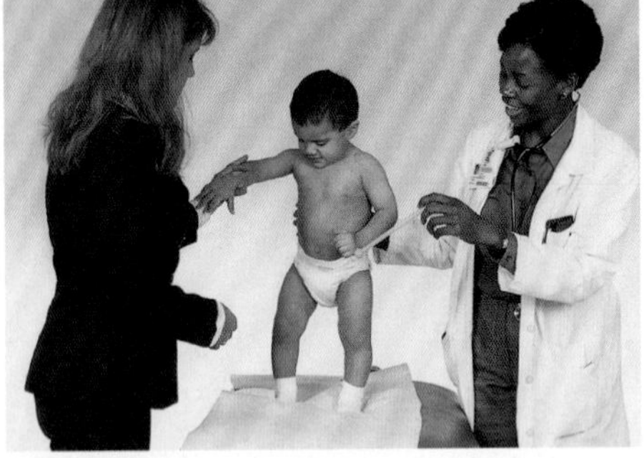

FIGURE 23-67 Toddler with bow legs.

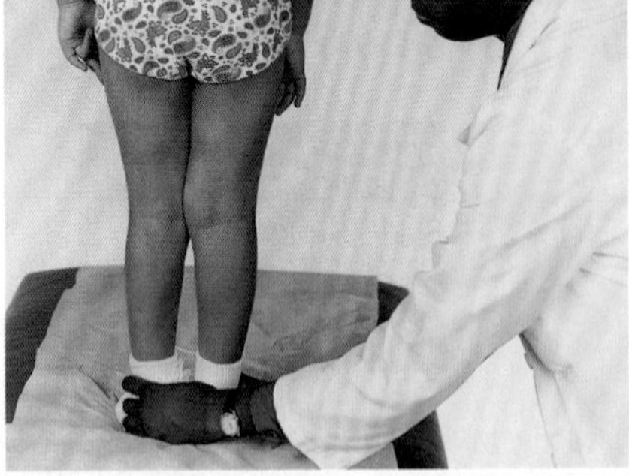

FIGURE 23-68 Preschooler with knock-knees.

Children may *toe in* when they begin to walk. This may increase up to 4 years of age and then gradually disappear by about 10 years of age.

Inspect any child who can stand for *scoliosis,* using techniques described under the "Assessing Adolescents" section. Also, have the child stand straight and place your hands horizontally over the iliac crests from behind. Small discrepancies can be appreciated. If such a discrepancy is noted and you suspect leg-length discrepancy, with one iliac crest higher than the other, a technique is to place a book under the shorter leg; this should eliminate the discrepancy.

Test for severe hip disease, with its associated weakness of the gluteus medius muscle. Observe from behind as the child shifts weight from one leg to the other. A pelvis that remains level when weight is shifted from one foot to the other is normal, or a *negative Trendelenburg sign* (Fig. 23-69A). An abnormal positive sign is seen in *severe hip disease;* that is, the pelvis tilts toward the unaffected hip during weight bearing on the affected side, a *positive Trendelenburg sign* (Fig. 23-69B).

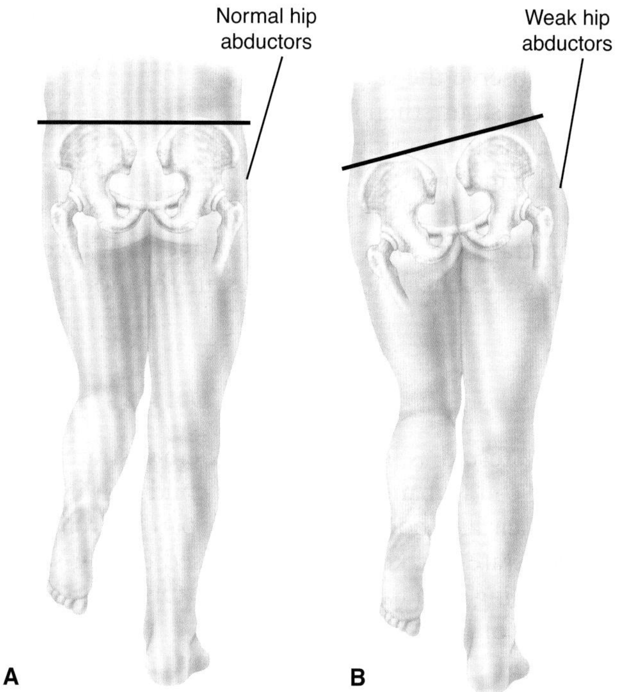

FIGURE 23-69 **A.** A negative Trendelenburg sign: The pelvis remains level when the child stands on one foot, a normal finding. **B.** A positive Trendelenburg sign: The child's pelvis tilts due to weakened abductor muscles in the affected hip.

The Nervous System

Beyond infancy, the neurologic examination includes the components evaluated in adults. Again, you should combine the neurologic and developmental assessment and will need to turn this into a game with the child to assess optimal development and neurologic performance.

Problems with social interaction, verbal and nonverbal communication, restricted interests, and repetitive behaviors could be signs of *autism.*

Sensation

The sensory examination can be performed using a cotton ball or cotton swab. This is best performed with the child's eyes closed. Do not use pin pricks, which may scare the child.

Gait, Strength, and Coordination

Observe the child's gait while the child is walking and optimally running. Note any asymmetries, weakness, undue tripping, or clumsiness. You can follow the developmental milestones to test for appropriate maneuvers such as heel-to-toe walking (Fig. 23-70), hopping, and jumping. Use a toy to test for coordination and strength of the upper extremities.

In children with uncoordinated gait, be sure to distinguish *orthopedic causes* such as positional deformities of the hip, knee, or foot from *neurologic abnormalities* such as *cerebral palsy, ataxia,* or *neuromuscular conditions.*

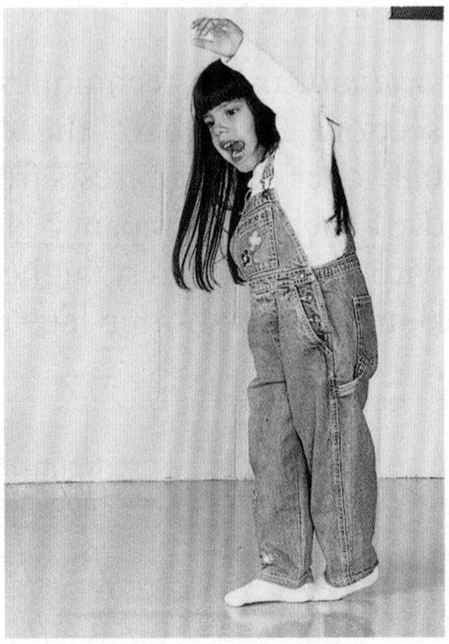

FIGURE 23-70 A preschooler walking heel to toe.

If you are concerned about the child's strength, have the child lie on the floor and then stand up, and closely observe the stages. Most normal children will first sit up, then flex the knees and extend the arms to the side to push off from the floor and stand up.

In certain forms of *muscular dystrophy* with weakness of the pelvic girdle muscles, children will rise to standing by rolling over prone and pushing off the floor with the arms while the legs remain extended (*Gower sign*).

Hand preference is demonstrated in most children by age 2. If a younger child has clear hand preference, check for weakness in the nonpreferred upper extremity.

Deep Tendon Reflexes

Deep tendon reflexes can be tested as in adults. First demonstrate the use of the reflex hammer on the child's hand to assure the child that it will not hurt. Children love to feel their legs bounce when their patellar reflexes are tested. The child must cooperate and keep the eyes closed during some of this examination because tensing will disrupt the results. One trick is to ask the child to pretend the arms or legs "are asleep."

Children with mild cerebral palsy may have both slightly *increased tone* and *hyperreflexia.*

Development

You can ask children older than 3 years to draw a picture, copy objects as seen in the DENVER II, and then discuss their pictures to test simultaneously for fine motor coordination, cognition, and language.

Among school-aged children, the best test for development is their school performance. You can obtain school records or psychological testing results, obviating the need for the clinician to formally test an older child's development.

Cerebellar Function

The cerebellar examination can be tested using finger-to-nose (Fig. 23-71) and rapid alternating movements of the hands or fingers. The younger child may be slower than an adult when performing the rapid alternating movements. Children enjoy this game. Children older than 5 years should be able to tell right from left, so you can assign them right–left discrimination tasks, as is done in the adult patient.

Distinguish between isolated delays in one aspect of development (e.g., coordination or language) and more generalized delays that occur in several components. The latter is more likely to reflect global neurologic disorders such as *cognitive disabilities* that can be caused by many etiologies.

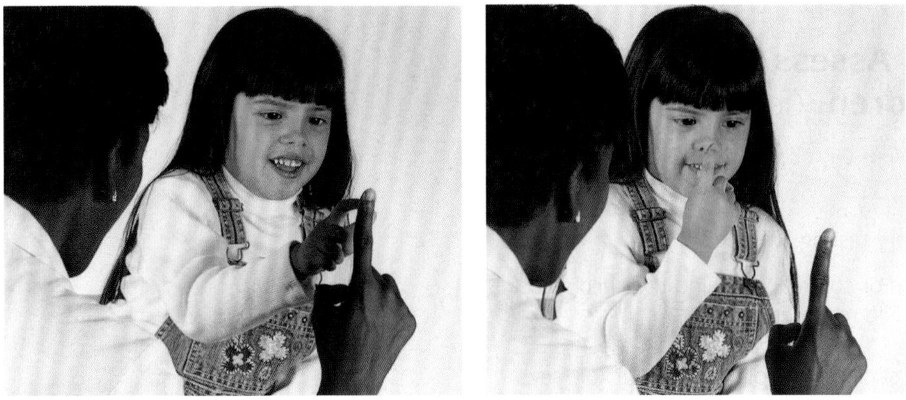

FIGURE 23-71 A child performs the finger-to-nose test with the nurse.

Some children with *ADHD* will have great difficulty cooperating with your neurologic and developmental examination because of problems focusing. These children often have high energy levels, cannot stay still for extended periods, and have a history of difficulty in school or structured situations. However, other conditions may have similar symptoms so a complete history and physical examination is warranted.

Cranial Nerves

The cranial nerves can be assessed well using developmentally appropriate strategies as outlined in Table 23-32.

Localizing neurologic signs are rare in children but can be caused by trauma, brain tumor, intracranial bleed, or infection.

Children with meningitis, encephalitis, or cerebral abscess can have abnormalities of cranial nerves although they also have altered consciousness and other signs.

TABLE 23-32 Strategies to Assess Cranial Nerves in Young Children

Cranial Nerve	Strategy
I (Olfactory)	Testable in older children.
II (Visual acuity)	Use Snellen chart after age 3 y. Test visual fields as for an adult. A parent may need to hold the child's head.
III, IV, VI (Extraocular movements)	Have the child track a light or an object (a toy is preferable). A parent may need to hold the child's head steady.
V (Motor)	Play a game with a soft cotton ball to test sensation. Have the child clench the teeth and chew or swallow some food.
VII (Facial)	Have the child "make faces" or imitate you as you make faces (including moving your eyebrows), and observe symmetry and facial movements.

(continued)

TABLE 23-32 **Strategies to Assess Cranial Nerves in Young Children** *(Continued)*

Cranial Nerve	Strategy
VIII (Acoustic)	Perform auditory testing after age 4 y. Whisper a word or command behind the child's back and have the child repeat it.
IX, X (Swallow and gag)	Have the child stick the "whole tongue out" or "say 'ah.'" Observe movement of the uvula and soft palate. Test the gag reflex.
XI (Spinal accessory)	Have the child push your hand away with their head. Have the child shrug their shoulders while you push down with your hands to "see how strong you are."
XII (Hypoglossal)	Ask the child to "stick out your tongue all the way."

Monitoring for Delirium

Children can develop delirium. Seriously ill children should be monitored each shift for delirium, especially those in an intensive care unit environment and those who are mechanically ventilated. Children with developmental delay or a preexisting anxiety disorder are also more prone to delirium. There are five primary characteristics seen in children experiencing delirium: agitation, disorientation, hallucinations, inattention, and sleep–wake cycle disturbances. The Cornell Assessment of Pediatric Delirium (CAPD) can be used to assess children for delirium (Holly et al., 2018).

Health Promotion and Counseling

Children 1 to 4 Years

The AAP and Bright Futures periodicity schedules for children include health supervision visits at 12, 15, 18, and 24 months followed by annual visits when the child is 3 and 4 years old (Herman-Giddens et al., 2012). An additional visit at 30 months is also recommended to assess the child's development.

During these health supervision visits, nurses address concerns and questions from parents, evaluate the child's growth and development, perform a comprehensive physical examination, and provide anticipatory guidance about healthy habits and behaviors, social competence of caregivers, family relationships, and community interactions.

This is a critical age for preventing childhood obesity: many children begin their trajectory toward obesity between ages 3 and 4. It is also important to adequately assess the child's development. Standardized developmental screening instruments are increasingly being recommended to measure the different dimensions of a child's development. Similarly, it is important to differentiate normal (but potentially challenging) childhood behavior from abnormal behavioral or mental health problems (Fig. 23-72) (AAP, 2020).

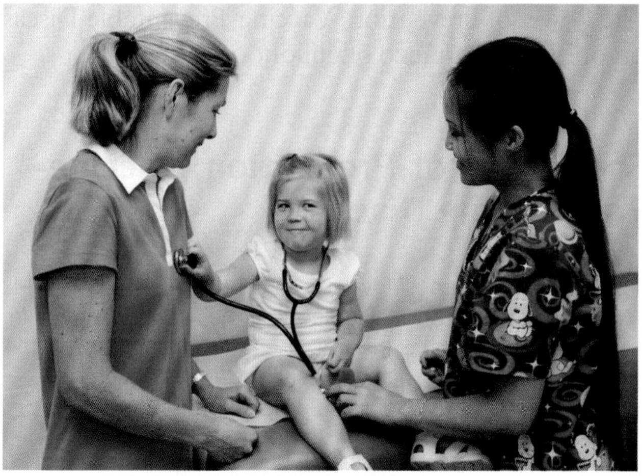

FIGURE 23-72 Allowing the child to try out medical instruments will decrease fear.

Box 23-10 summarizes the major components of a health supervision visit for a 3-year-old, stressing health promotion. You do not have to wait for a health supervision visit to address many of these health promotion issues; they can be addressed during other types of visits, even when the child is mildly ill.

BOX 23-10 COMPONENTS OF A HEALTH SUPERVISION VISIT FOR A 3-YEAR-OLD

Discussions with Parents

- Address parent concerns.
- Provide advice.
- Assess child care, school, and social environments.
- Assess major topic areas: development, nutrition, safety, oral health, family relationships, and community.

Developmental Assessment

- Assess milestones: gross and fine motor skills, personal–social, language, and cognitive development.
- Use a validated developmental screening tool.

Physical Examination

Perform a careful examination, including growth parameters with percentiles for age.

Screening Tests

- Vision and hearing (formal testing at age 4)
- Hematocrit and lead (if high risk or at ages 1 to 3)
- Screen for social risk factors.

Immunizations

See schedule on the CDC website at http://www.cdc.gov/vaccines/schedules/hcp/child-adolescent.html.

Anticipatory Guidance

- Healthy habits and behaviors
  - Injury and illness prevention—Car seat, poisons, tobacco exposure, supervision of activities
  - Nutrition—Obesity assessment, healthy meals and snacks
  - Oral health—Brushing teeth, dentist visits
- Parent–infant interaction—Reading and fun times, child directed play, limiting screen time
- Family relationships—Activities, babysitters
- Community interaction—Child care, family resources

Source: American Academy of Pediatrics. (AAP). (2020). *Bright futures*. Retrieved March, 2020, from https://brightfutures.aap.org/materials-and-tools/guidelines-and-pocket-guide/Pages/default.aspx

See Table 23-33, "The Power of Prevention: Vaccine-Preventable Diseases" for more information on the importance of childhood vaccines.

TABLE 23-33 The Power of Prevention: Vaccine-Preventable Diseases

This table shows photographs of children with vaccine-preventable diseases. Childhood vaccines have been named the single most important medical intervention in the world in terms of influence on public health. Because of vaccinations, we hope you will never see many of these conditions, but you should be able to identify them. Try to identify the diseases before reading the descriptions.

Polio

The deformed leg of this child is from polio

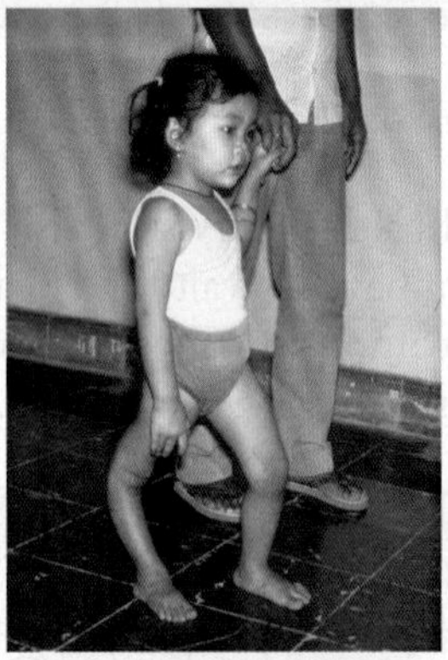

Measles

Characteristic rash of measles in the presence of a child who also has coryza, conjunctivitis, fever, and this diffuse rash

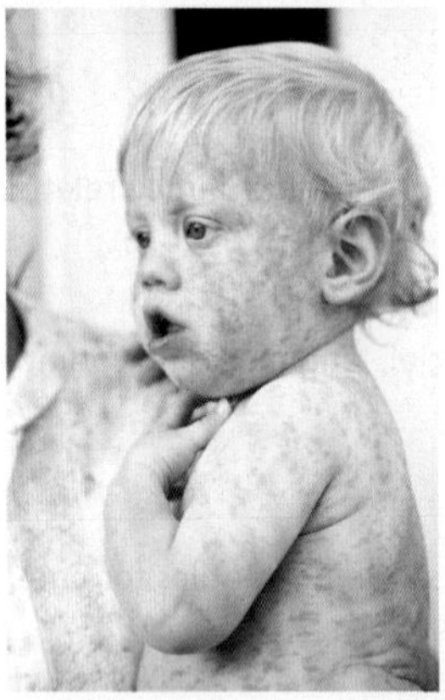

Rubella

Rubella rash on a child's back

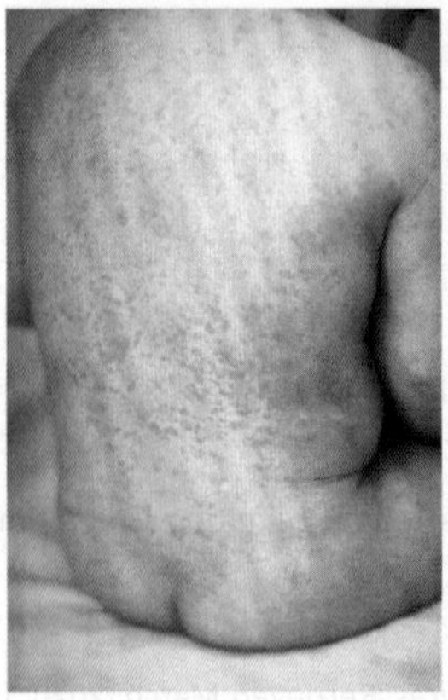

Tetanus

Rigid newborn with neonatal tetanus

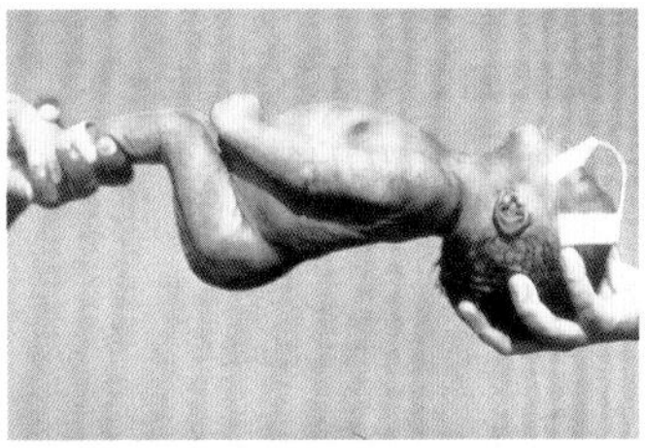

Haemophilus Influenzae Type b

Periorbital cellulitis from this invasive bacterial disease

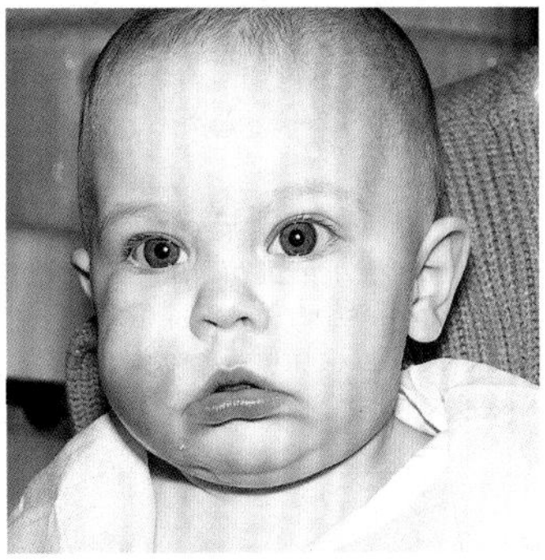

Meningitis

Nuchal rigidity

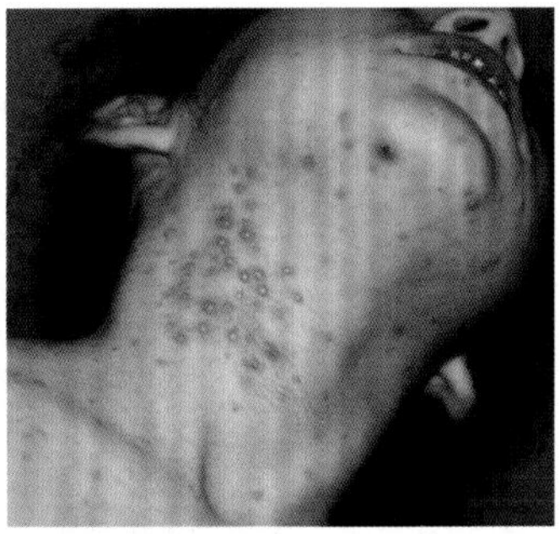

Varicella

An infant with a severe form of varicella

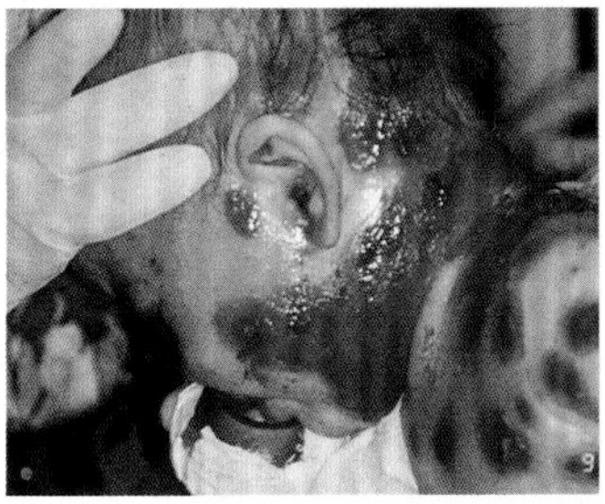

Pertussis

Paroxysmal cough with a "whoop" at the end

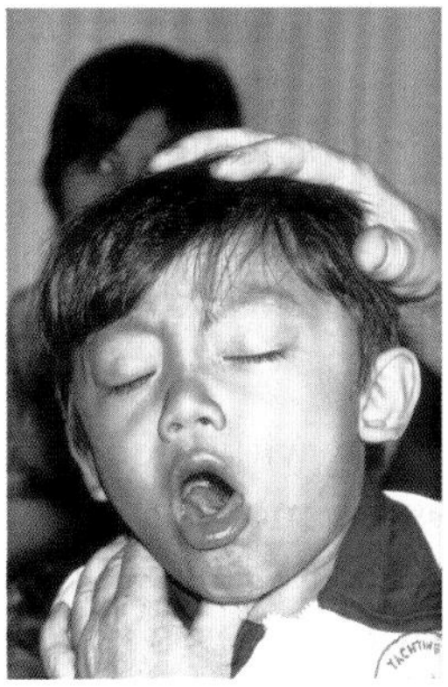

(continued)

TABLE 23-33 The Power of Prevention: Vaccine-Preventable Diseases *(Continued)*

Cervical Cancer

Largely prevented through vaccination with human papillomavirus vaccine

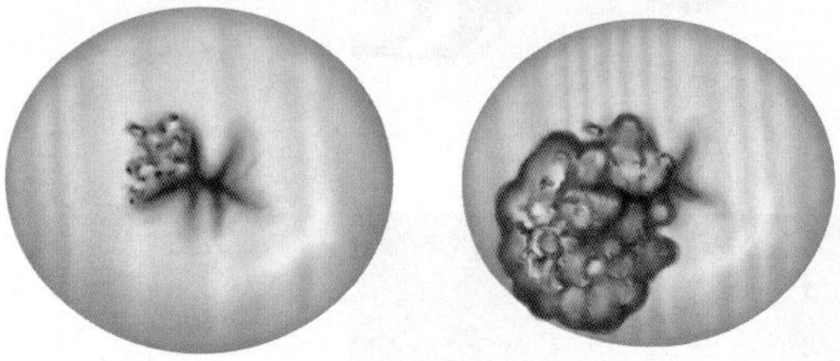

Sources of photos: *Polio*—Centers for Disease Control and Prevention; *Haemophilus influenzae*—Fleisher, G. R., Ludwig, W., & Baskin, M. N., (2004). *Atlas of pediatric emergency medicine*. Lippincott Williams & Wilkins; *Varicella*—Courtesy of Barbara Watson, MD, Albert Einstein Medical Center and Division of Disease Control, Philadelphia, Department of Health; all others courtesy of Centers for Disease Control and Prevention.

Children 5 to 10 Years

The AAP and Bright Futures periodicity schedules for children recommend annual health supervision visits during this period (AAP, 2020). As for earlier ages, these visits present opportunities to assess the child's physical, mental, and developmental health; the parent–child relationship; and the child's relationships with peers and school performance (Fig. 23-73). Once again, health promotion should be incorporated into all interactions with children and families; take advantage of any opportunity to promote optimal health and development and to enhance the child's involvement in normalizing activities.

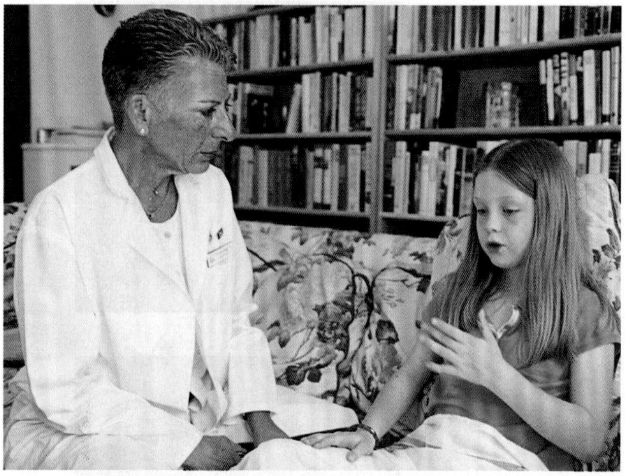

FIGURE 23-73 Anticipatory guidance discussions with the child should be done in a comfortable environment, not with the child undressed on an examination table.

In addition to discussing issues of health, safety, development, and anticipatory guidance with parents, include the child in these conversations, using age-appropriate language and concepts. For example, the child's major environment beyond the family involves school. Discuss the child's experience and perceptions of school, interactions with peers, as well as other cognitive and social activities. During these discussions, focus on healthy habits such as good nutrition, exercise, reading, stimulating activities, healthy sleep hygiene, screen time, and safety.

School-aged children often begin participating in organized sports. Anticipatory guidance should include the appropriate safety equipment for sports the child plays. Parents should learn the signs and symptoms for concussions if the child plays a sport with increased risk of head injuries.

About 15% to 18% of children in the United States live with a chronic health condition, defined as health problems that last over 3 months, affecting the patient's normal activities, and requiring multiple hospitalizations, home health care, and/or extensive medical care (CS Mott Children's Hospital. Michigan Medicine, n.d.). One in six U.S. children aged 2 to 8 years

(17.4%) had a diagnosed mental, behavioral, or developmental disorder in a 2016 survey. Diagnoses of depression and anxiety are more common with increased age (CDC, 2020a).

These children should be seen more frequently for monitoring, disease management, and preventive care. Some behaviors that become established at this age can lead to or exacerbate chronic conditions such as obesity or eating disorders. Therefore, health promotion is critical to optimize healthy habits and minimize unhealthy ones. Helping families and children with chronic diseases deal most effectively with these disorders is a key part of health promotion. For all children, the well-being of the family is critical to the child's health; thus, health promotion involves assessing and promoting the family's overall health.

The specific components of the health supervision visit for older children are the same as the components for younger children, shown in Box 23-10. "Components of a Health Supervision Visit for a 3-Year-Old." Emphasize school performance and experiences as well as appropriate and safe sports and activities and healthy peer relationships.

ASSESSING ADOLESCENTS

Development

Adolescence can be divided into three stages: early, middle, and late. Your interview and examination techniques will vary widely depending on the adolescent's physical (Fig. 23-74), cognitive, and social-emotional levels of development.

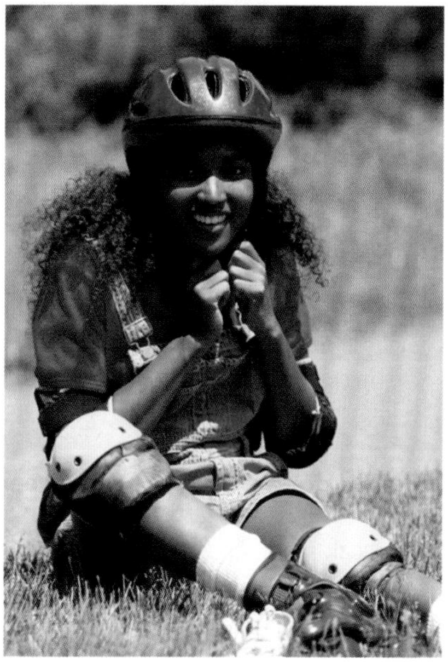

FIGURE 23-74 Adolescents enjoy competitive sports. Encourage them to use appropriate safety equipment.

Physical Development

Adolescence is the period of transition from childhood to adulthood. The physical transformation generally occurs over a period of years, beginning at an average age of 10 in girls and 11 in boys. On average, girls end pubertal development with a growth spurt by age 14 and boys by age 16. The age of onset and duration of puberty vary widely, although the stages follow the same sequence in all adolescents. Early adolescents are preoccupied with these physical changes.

Cognitive Development

Although less obvious, cognitive changes during adolescence are as dramatic as changes in physique. Most adolescents progress from concrete to formal operational thinking, acquiring an ability to reason logically and abstractly and to consider future implications of current actions. Although the interview and examination resemble those of adults, keep in mind the wide variability in cognitive development of adolescents and their often erratic and still limited ability to see beyond simple solutions. Moral thinking becomes sophisticated, with lots of time spent on debating issues. Recent evidence shows that brain development (especially in the right prefrontal cortex) probably continues well into the 20s.

Social and Emotional Development

Adolescence is a tumultuous time, marked by the transition from family-dominated influences to increasing autonomy and peer influence (Fig. 23-75). The struggle for identity, independence, and eventually intimacy leads to much stress, many health-related problems, and, often, high-risk behaviors. This struggle also provides you with an important opportunity for health promotion.

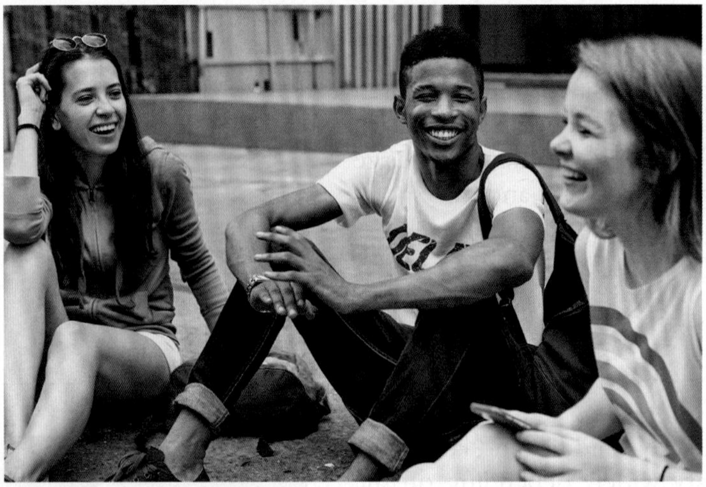

FIGURE 23-75 In adolescence, peers are increasingly important. (Rawpixel.com/Shutterstock)

Table 23-34 outlines the developmental tasks of adolescence.

TABLE 23-34 Developmental Tasks of Adolescence

Task	Characteristic	Health Care Approaches
Early Adolescence (10- to 14-Year-Olds)		
Physical	Puberty (F: 10–14; M: 11–16) variable	Confidentiality; privacy
Cognitive	Concrete operational	Emphasis on short term
Social identity	"Am I normal?" Peers increasingly important.	Reassurance and positive attitude
Independence	Ambivalence (family, self, peers)	Support for growing autonomy

Task	Characteristic	Health Care Approaches
Middle Adolescence (15- to 16-Year-Olds)		
Physical	Females more comfortable, males awkward	Support if patient varies from medical norms
Cognitive	Transition; many ideas, often highly emotional thinker	Problem solving, decision making, increased responsibility
Social identity	"Who am I?" Much introspection; global issues	Nonjudgmental acceptance
Independence	Limit testing; "experimental" behaviors; dating	Consistency; limit setting
Late Adolescence (17- to 20-Year-Olds)		
Physical	Adult appearance	Minimal unless chronic illness present
Cognitive	Formal operational (for many but not all 17- to 20-y-olds)	Approach as an adult
Social identity	Role with respect to others; sexuality; future	Encouragement of identity to allow growth, safety, and healthy decision making
Independence	Separation from family; toward real independence	Support, anticipatory guidance

The Health History

A complete history and prior health care information is obtained if the adolescent is a new patient. Otherwise, the history is continuously updated at each visit as with the child's history. The key to successfully examining adolescents is a comfortable, confidential environment (Fig. 23-76). This makes the examination more relaxed and informative. Consider the teen's cognitive and social development when considering issues of privacy, parental involvement, and confidentiality.

Like most people, adolescents usually respond positively to anyone demonstrating a genuine interest in them. Show such interest early and then sustain the connection for effective communication.

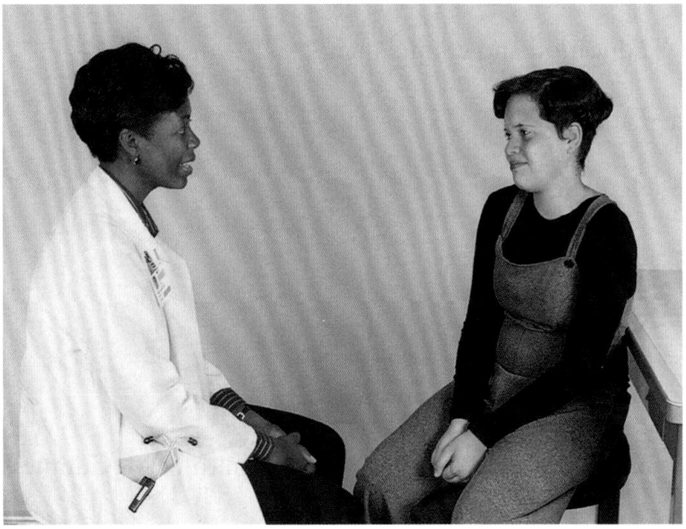

FIGURE 23-76 Interview the teen patient in privacy and sit at the same level to facilitate conversation.

Adolescents are more likely to open up when the interview focuses on them rather than on their problems. In contrast to most other interviews, *start with specific questions* to build trust and rapport and get the conversation going. The nurse may have to do more talking than usual at the beginning. A good way to start is to chat informally about friends, school, hobbies, and family. Using silence in an attempt to get adolescents to talk or asking about feelings directly is usually not productive.

It is particularly important to use summarization and transitional statements and to explain what will happen during the physical examination. The physical examination can also be an opportunity to engage young people. Once rapport is established, return to more open-ended questions. At that point, make sure to ask what concerns or questions the adolescent may have. Because adolescents are often reluctant to ask their most important questions (which are sometimes about sensitive topics), ask if the adolescent has anything else to discuss. A useful phrase to use is "tell me what other questions you have." Another option is to use the phrase, "Other kids your age often have questions about…"

Adolescent behavior is related to developmental stage and not necessarily to chronologic age or physical maturation. Age and appearance may fool you into assuming they are functioning on a more future-oriented and realistic level. This is particularly true regarding "early bloomers," who look older than their age. The reverse can also be true, especially in teens with delayed puberty or chronic illness.

Risky behaviors in adolescence may have long-term consequences. The HEEADSSS psychosocial assessment tool is an effective way to engage the adolescent in discussion of potentially risky behaviors. The acronym stands for:

- ***H***ome
- ***E***ducation and employment
- ***E***ating
- ***A***ctivities
- ***D***rugs and alcohol
- ***S***exuality
- ***S***uicide depression and self-harm
- ***S***afety from injury and violence (Smith & McGuinness, 2017)

Issues of *confidentiality* are important in adolescence. Explain to both parents and adolescents that the best health care allows adolescents some degree of independence and confidentiality. It helps if the nurse starts asking the parent to leave the room for part of the interview when the child is age 10 or 11 years. This prepares both parents and teens for future visits when the patient spends time alone with the nurse.

Before the parent leaves, obtain relevant medical history, such as certain elements of past history, and clarify the parent's agenda for the visit. Also discuss the need for confidentiality. Explain that the purpose of confidentiality is to improve health care, not to keep secrets. Adolescents need to know that you will hold in confidence what they discuss. However, never make confidentiality unlimited. Always state explicitly that you will act on information if concerned about safety. For instance, "I will not tell your parents what we talk about unless you give me permission or I am concerned about your safety. For example, if you were to talk to me about hurting yourself or someone else or you are being hurt or bullied, I may need to discuss it with others."

The goal is to help adolescents bring their concerns or questions to their parents. Encourage adolescents to discuss sensitive issues with their parents and offer to be present or help. Although young people may believe that their parents will react negatively, you may be able to promote more open dialogue. Occasionally you will encounter a parent who is rigid and punitive. It is important to carefully assess the parent's perspective prior to further discussion, and to obtain the explicit consent of the young person.

As in middle childhood, modesty is important. The patient should remain dressed until the examination begins, and should have privacy while putting on a gown. Not all adolescents are willing to don a gown so partially uncovering as the examination proceeds to preserve the patient's modesty is important. Most adolescents older than 13 years prefer to be examined without a parent in the room, but this depends on the patient's developmental level, familiarity with the examiner, relationship with the parent, and cultural and medical issues. For younger adolescents, ask the adolescent and parent their preferences. It is advisable to have a chaperone in the room when examining a female patient's breasts or genitalia of both sexes.

The sequence and content of the physical examination of the adolescent are similar to those in the adult. Keep in mind, however, particular issues unique to adolescents, such as puberty, growth, development, family and peer relationships, sexuality, healthy decision making, and high-risk behaviors (Fig. 23-77).

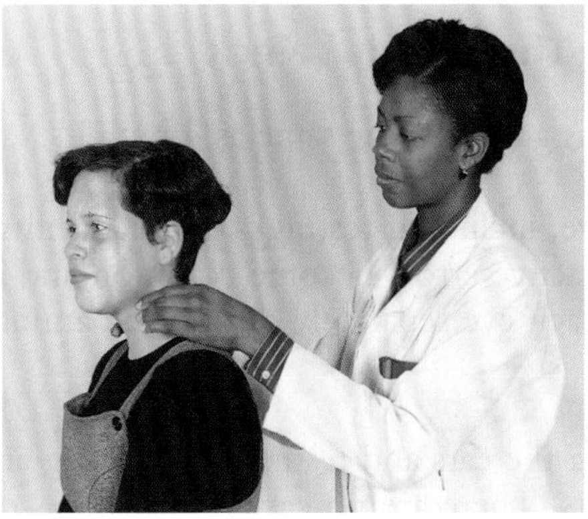

FIGURE 23-77 Put the adolescent at ease by explaining the examinations and reasons for performing them.

Physical Examination of the Adolescent

General Survey and Vital Signs

Somatic Growth

Adolescents should wear gowns to be weighed, or have them remove their shoes and heavy clothing. This is particularly important for adolescent girls being evaluated for underweight problems. Ideally, serial weights (and heights) should use the same scale.

Both obesity and eating disorders (anorexia and bulimia) among adolescents are major public health problems, requiring frequent assessments of weight, monitoring for complications, and promoting healthy choices and self-concept.

Vital Signs

Ongoing evaluations of blood pressure are important for adolescents. The average heart rate from age 10 to 14 years is 85 beats per minute with a range of 55 to 115 beats per minute considered normal. Average heart rate for those 15 years and older is 60 to 100 beats per minute.

Causes of sustained hypertension for this age group include *primary hypertension, renal parenchymal disease,* and *drug use.*

The Skin

Examine the adolescent's skin carefully. Many teens will have concerns about various skin lesions, such as acne, dimples, blemishes, stretch marks, and moles. Stretch marks have become more common with the epidemic of obesity.

Adolescent acne, a common skin condition, tends to resolve eventually but often benefits from proper treatment. It generally begins during middle to late puberty.

Many adolescents spend considerable time in the sun and at tanning salons. You may detect this during a comprehensive health history or by noticing signs of tanning during the physical examination. This is a good opportunity to counsel adolescents about the dangers of excessive ultraviolet exposure, the need for sunscreen, and the risks of tanning salons.

Moles or benign nevi may appear during adolescence. Their characteristics differentiate them from atypical nevi, discussed in Chapter 9, "The Integumentary System."

Counsel older adolescents to begin performing a regular self-examination of the skin, as discussed in Chapter 9.

The Head, Ears, Eyes, Nose, Throat, and Neck

The examination of these body parts is generally the same as for adults.

The methods used to examine the eye, including testing for visual acuity, are the same as those for adults. Refractive errors become common and it is important to test visual acuity of each eye separately during the annual health supervision visit.

An adolescent with persistent fever, tonsillar pharyngitis, and cervical lymphadenopathy may have *infectious mononucleosis.*

The ease and techniques of examining the ears and testing the hearing are similar to the methods used for adults. There are no ear abnormalities or variations of normal unique to this age group.

The Heart

The technique and sequence of examination are the same as those for adults. Murmurs are a continued cardiovascular issue for evaluation.

The *benign pulmonary flow murmur* is a grade I–II/VI soft, nonharsh murmur, beginning after the first sound and ending before the second sound (Table 23-35). An adolescent with a benign pulmonary ejection murmur will have normal intensity and normally split second heart sounds.

A pulmonary flow murmur accompanied by a fixed split-second heart sound suggests right-heart volume load such as an *atrial septal defect*. See Table 23-13, "Congenital Heart Murmurs."

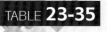

TABLE 23-35 Location and Characteristics of Benign Heart Murmurs in Adolescents

Location

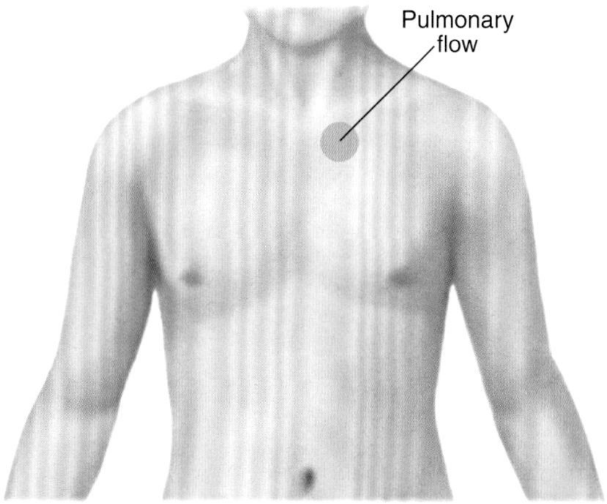

Typical Age	Name	Tonal Characteristics	Description and Location
Adolescence and later	*Pulmonary flow murmur*		Grade I–II/VI soft, nonharsh Upper left sternal border Normal P_2

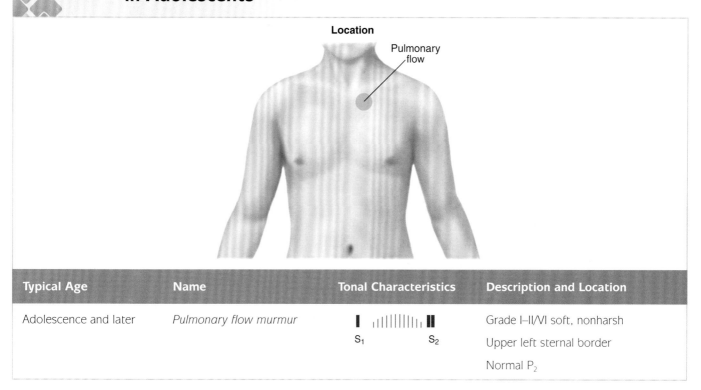

The Breasts

Physical changes in a young girl's breasts are one of the first signs of puberty. As in most developmental changes, there is a systematic progression. Generally, over a 4-year period, the breasts progress through five stages, called Tanner stages or **Tanner sexual maturity rating** (SMR) stages, as shown in Table 23-36. Breast buds in the preadolescent enlarge, changing the contour of the breasts and areola (the areola also darkens in color). These stages are accompanied by the development of pubic hair and other secondary sexual characteristics, as discussed in the later "Female Genitalia" section. Menarche usually occurs when a girl is in breast stage 3 or 4, and by then she has passed her peak growth spurt (Fig. 23-78).

TABLE 23-36 Sexual Maturity Ratings in Girls: Breasts

Stage 1	Preadolescents: only a small elevated nipple	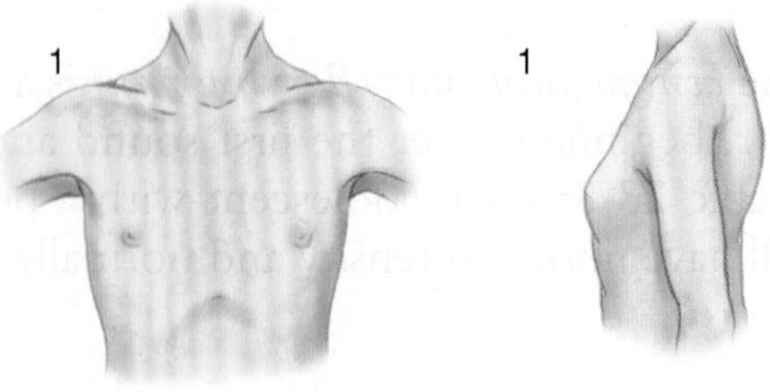
Stage 2	The breast bud stage: a small mound of breast and nipple develops: the areola widens	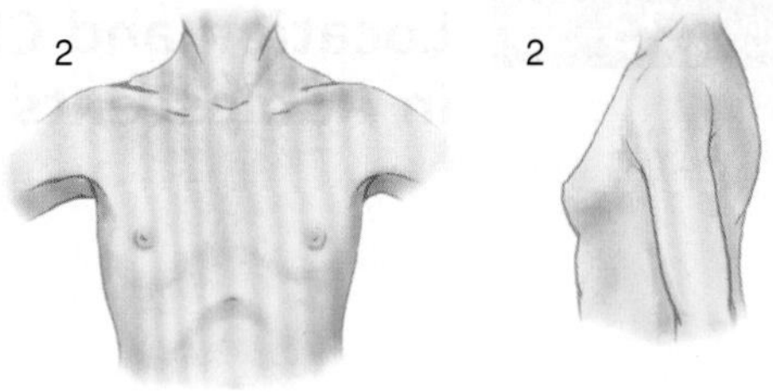
Stage 3	The breast and areola enlarge: the nipple is flush with the breast surface	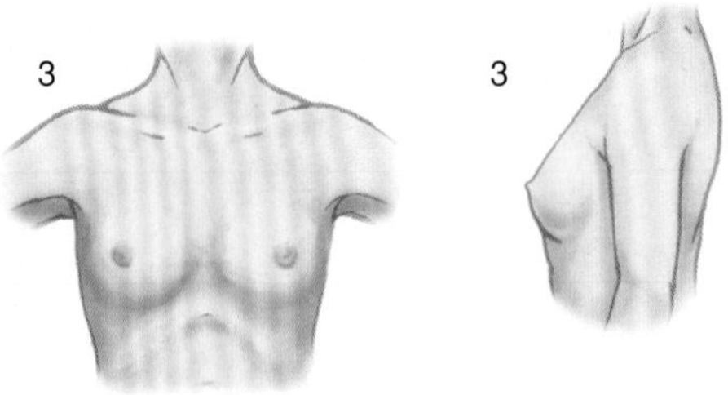
Stage 4	The areola and nipple form a secondary mound over the breast	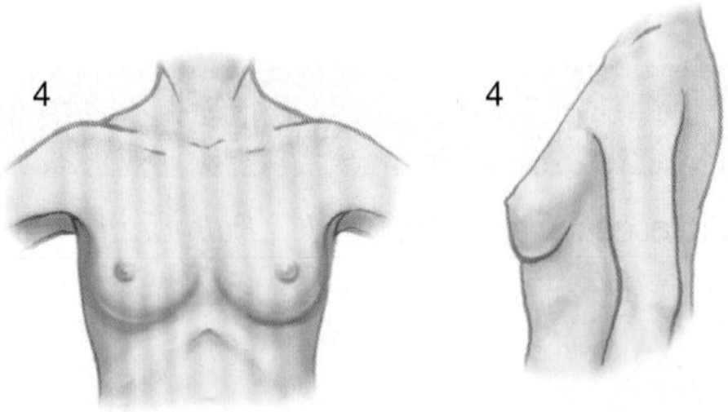
Stage 5	Mature breast: only the nipple protrudes; the areola is flush with the breast contour (the areola may continue as a secondary mound in some women)	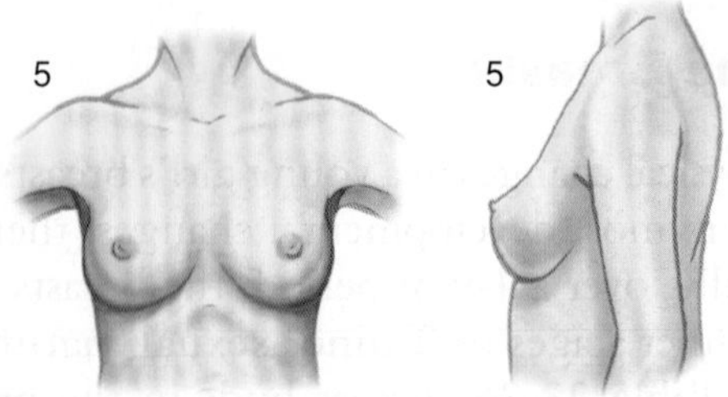

Data from Tanner, J. M. (1962). *Growth at adolescence* (2nd ed.). Blackwell Scientific Publications; Reprinted with permission from Kyle, T., & Carman, S. (2020). *Essentials of pediatric nursing* (4th ed.). Wolters Kluwer.

Pubertal Change	Age
Height spurt	9.5 to 16.5 years
Menarche	10.0 to 16.5 years
Breasts	
Stage 2	11 to 12 years
Stage 3	12 to 13 years
Stage 4	13 to 15 years
Stage 5	Older than 15 years
Pubic hair	**7 to 14 years**

FIGURE 23-78 Pubertal changes in female adolescents; the numbers indicate the ranges in age within which certain changes occur (Data from Marshall, W. A., & Tanner, J. M. (1970). Variations in the pattern of pubertal changes in boys. *Archives of disease in childhood*, *45*(239), 22.)

For years, the normal range for onset of breast development (**thelarche**) and pubic hair was 8 to 13 years (average, 11 years) with earlier onset considered abnormal (Biro et al., 2010; Biro et al., 2013; Herman-Giddens et al., 1997). Some studies suggest that the *lower age cutoff should be 7 years for White girls and 6 years for African American and Hispanic girls.* Breast development varies by age, race, and ethnicity (Biro et al., 2010). Breasts develop at different rates in approximately 10% of girls with resultant asymmetry of size or Tanner stage. Reassurance that this generally resolves is helpful to the patient.

Masses or nodules in the breasts of adolescent girls should be examined carefully. They are usually *benign fibroadenomas* or *cysts;* less likely etiologies include *abscesses* or *lipomas.* Breast carcinoma is extremely rare in adolescence and nearly always occurs in families with a strong history of the disease (ACOG Committee on Adolescent Health Care, 2006).

Breast asymmetry is common in adolescents, particularly when adolescents are between Tanner stages 2 and 4. This is nearly always a benign condition.

Older adolescent girls should undergo a comprehensive breast examination with an explanation of the anatomy of the breast, how the normal breast feels when palpated, and the normal changes the breast goes through during the menstrual cycle. The nurse can guide the adolescent through self-palpation in order to learn how her breast feels. The nurse can explain that regular self-breast examinations may discover a potentially cancerous node, but that self-examinations have not been shown to reduce breast cancer mortality. See Chapter 15 for more information on self-examinations and how to perform them. A second person (parent or health care provider) should be present during the examination.

Breasts in boys consist of a small nipple and areola. During puberty, about one third of boys develop a breast bud 2 cm or more in diameter, usually in one breast. Obese boys may develop substantial breast tissue.

Many adolescent boys develop gynecomastia (enlarged breasts) on one or both sides. Although usually slight, it can be embarrassing. It generally resolves in a few years.

The Abdomen

Techniques of abdominal examination are the same as for adults. The size of the liver approaches the adult size as the teen progresses through puberty, and is related to the adolescent's overall height.

Hepatomegaly in teens may be from *infections* such as *hepatitis* or infectious *mononucleosis, inflammatory bowel disease,* or *tumors.*

Male Genitalia

The genital examination of the adolescent boy proceeds like the examination of the adult male. Be aware of the embarrassment many boys experience during this examination.

Important anatomic changes in the male genitalia accompany puberty and help to define its progress. The first reliable sign of puberty, starting between ages 9 and 13.5 years, is an increase in the size of the testes. Next, pubic hair appears, along with progressive enlargement of the penis. The complete change from preadolescent to adult anatomy requires about 3 years with a range of 1.8 to 5 years (Herman-Giddens et al., 2012).

Delayed puberty is suspected in boys who have no signs of pubertal development by 14 years of age.

When examining the adolescent male, assign a sexual maturity rating. The five stages of sexual development, first described by Tanner, are outlined and illustrated in Table 23-37. These involve changes in the penis, testes, and scrotum. In addition, in about 80% of men, pubic hair spreads farther up the abdomen in a triangular pattern pointing toward the umbilicus; this phase is not completed until the 20s.

The most common cause of delayed puberty in males is *constitutional delay,* frequently a familial condition involving delayed bone and physical maturation but normal hormonal levels.

TABLE 23-37 Sexual Maturity Ratings in Boys

In assigning SMRs in boys, observe each of the three characteristics separately because they may develop at different rates. Record two separate ratings: pubic hair and genital. If the penis and testes differ in their stages, average the two into a single figure for the genital rating.

	Pubic Hair	Penis	Testes and Scrotum	
Stage 1	Preadolescent—no pubic hair except for the fine body hair (vellus hair) similar to that on the abdomen	Preadolescent—same size and proportions as in childhood	Preadolescent—same size and proportions as in childhood	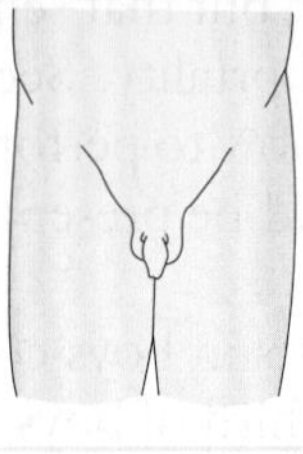
Stage 2	Sparse growth of long, slightly pigmented, downy hair, straight or only slightly curled, chiefly at the base of the penis	Slight or no enlargement	Testes larger; scrotum larger, somewhat reddened and altered in texture	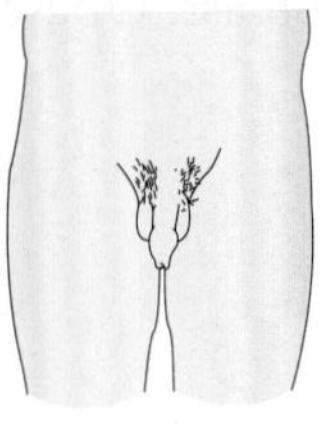

	Pubic Hair	Penis	Testes and Scrotum	
Stage 3	Darker, coarser, curlier hair spreading sparsely over the pubic symphysis	Larger, especially in length	Further enlarged	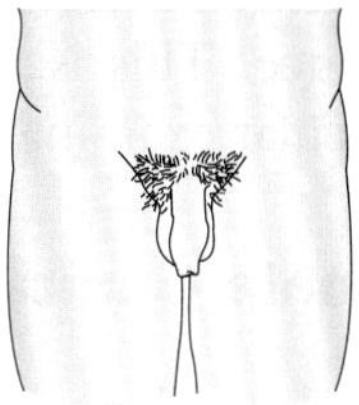
Stage 4	Coarse and curly hair, as in the adult; area covered greater than in stage 3 but not as great as in the adult and not yet including the thighs	Further enlarged in length and breadth, with development of the glans	Further enlarged; scrotal skin darkened	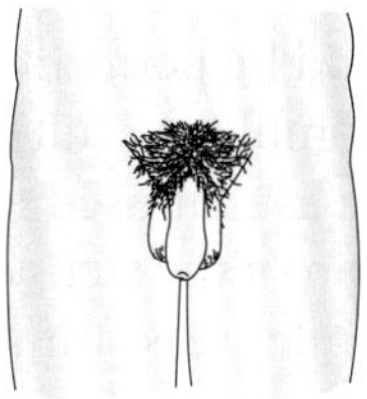
Stage 5	Hair adult in quantity and quality, spread to the medial surfaces of the thighs but not up over the abdomen	Adult in size and shape	Adult in size and shape	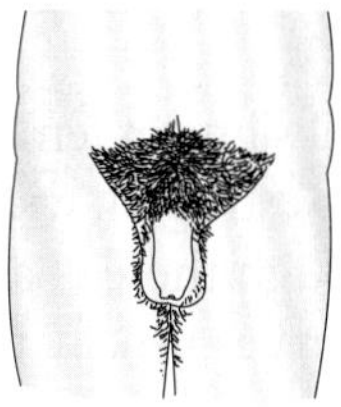

Data from Tanner, J. M. (1962). *Growth at adolescence* (2nd ed.). Blackwell Scientific Publications; Drawings reprinted with permission from Marino, B., & Fine, S. (2019). *Blueprints: Pediatrics* (7th ed.). Wolters Kluwer.

An important developmental principle is that physical pubertal changes progress along a well-established sequence (Fig. 23-79). Although age ranges for start and completion are wide, the sequence for each boy is nevertheless the same. This is helpful in counseling anxious adolescents about current and future maturation and the wide range of normal for puberty. It is also helpful for detecting abnormal physical changes.

Pubertal Change	Age
Height spurt	10 to 17.5 years
Penis	10.5 to 16.5 years
Testis	9 to 17 years
Genital	
Stage 2	11.5 to 12.5 years
Stage 3	12.5 to 13.5 years
Stage 4	13.5 to 15 years
Stage 5	Older than 15 years
Pubic hair	9 to 16 years

FIGURE 23-79 Pubertal changes in male adolescents; the numbers indicate the ranges in age within which certain changes occur. (Data from Marshall, W. A., & Tanner, J. M. [1970]. Variations in the patterns of pubertal changes in boys. *Archives of disease in childhood*, *45*(239), 22.)

Observe the penis for sores and discharge as you would in an adult male.

Although nocturnal or daytime ejaculation tends to begin around sexual maturity rating 3, a finding on either history or physical examination of penile discharge may indicate a *sexually transmitted infection.*

In uncircumcised males, the foreskin should be easily retractable by adolescence. This is also an opportunity to discuss normal hygiene. Discuss testicular examination in older boys by age 18.

Female Genitalia

The external examination of adolescent female genitalia proceeds in the same manner as for school-age children. An adolescent's first pelvic examination should be performed by an experienced health care provider. If it is necessary to complete a full pelvic examination on an adolescent, the technique is the same as that used for an adult, including the rectal examination. A full explanation of the steps of the examination, demonstration of the instruments, and a gentle, reassuring approach are necessary because the adolescent is usually quite anxious (American College of Obstetricians and Gynecologists, 2006). A parent or another health care provider must be present.

Vaginal discharge in a young adolescent should be treated as in the adult. Causes include *physiologic leukorrhea, sexually transmitted infections* from consensual sexual activity or *sexual abuse, bacterial vaginosis, foreign body,* and *external irritants.*

Initial signs of female puberty are hymenal thickening and redundancy secondary to estrogen, widening of the hips, and beginning of a growth spurt in height, although these changes are difficult to detect. The first easily detectable sign of puberty is usually the appearance of breast buds, though pubic hair sometimes appears earlier. The average age of the appearance of pubic hair has decreased in recent years, and current consensus is that the appearance of pubic hair as early as 7 years can be normal, particularly in dark-skinned girls who develop secondary sexual characteristics at an earlier age (Kaplowitz & Bloch, 2016).

Pubertal development prior to the normal age ranges may signify *precocious puberty,* which has a variety of endocrine and central nervous system causes.

Assign a sexual maturity rating to every female regardless of chronologic age. The assessment of sexual maturity in girls is based on both growth of pubic hair and the development of breasts. Counsel girls about this sequence and their current stage. The assessment (Tanner staging) of pubic hair growth is shown in Table 23-38. See Table 23-36 for breast development assessment.

Although there is a wide variation in the age of onset and completion of puberty, remember that the stages occur in a predictable sequence, as shown in Figure 23-78.

Obesity in females can be associated with early onset of puberty.

Amenorrhea in adolescence can be primary (no menarche by age 16) or secondary (cessation of menses in an adolescent who had previously menstruated). While primary amenorrhea is usually due to anatomic or genetic causes, secondary amenorrhea can be due to a variety of etiologies such as *stress, excessive exercise, eating disorders, and pregnancy.*

Delayed puberty (no breasts or pubic hair development by age 12) is usually caused by inadequate gonadotropin secretion from the anterior pituitary due to defective hypothalamic GnRH production. A common cause is anorexia nervosa.

Delayed puberty in an adolescent female below the 3rd percentile in height may be from Turner syndrome or chronic disease. The two most common causes of delayed sexual development in an extremely thin adolescent girl are anorexia nervosa and chronic disease.

TABLE 23-38 Sexual Maturity Ratings in Girls: Pubic Hair

Stage 1	Preadolescent—no pubic hair except for the fine body hair (vellus hair) similar to that on the abdomen	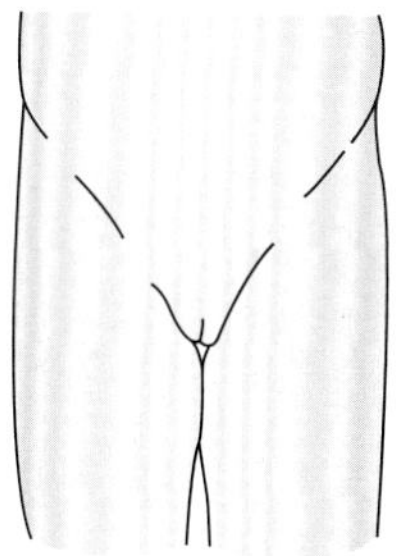
Stage 2	Sparse growth of long, slightly pigmented, downy hair, straight or only slightly curled, chiefly along the labia	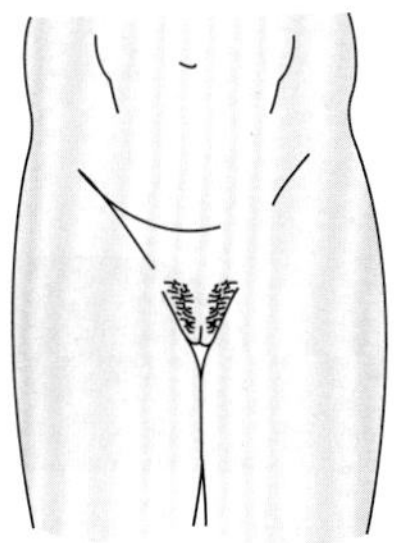
Stage 3	Darker, coarser, curlier hair, spreading sparsely over the pubic symphysis	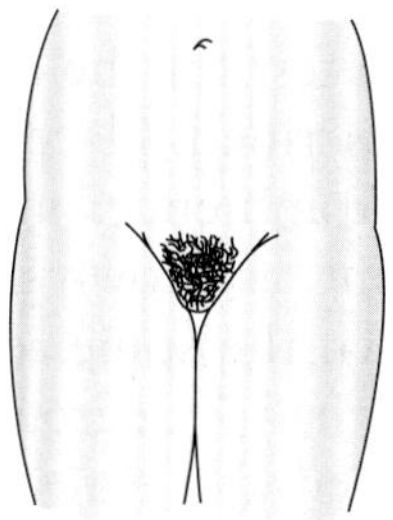
Stage 4	Coarse and curly hair as in adults; area covered greater than in stage 3 but not as great as in the adult and not yet including the thighs	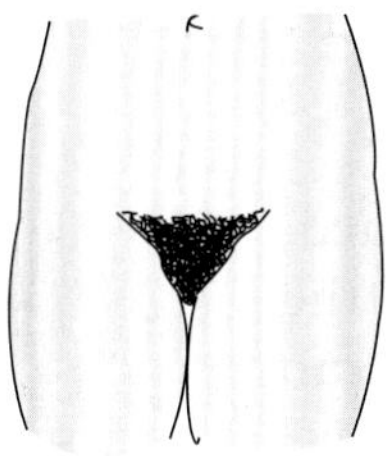
Stage 5	Hair adult in quantity and quality, spread on the medial surfaces of the thighs but not up over the abdomen	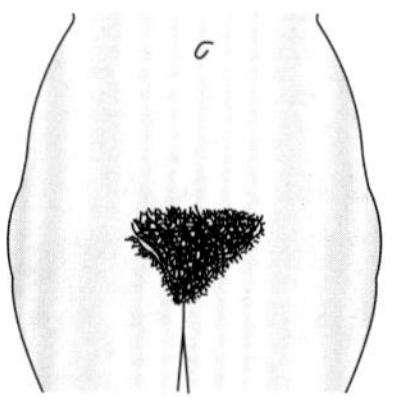

Data from Tanner, J. M. (1962). *Growth at adolescence* (2nd ed.). Blackwell Scientific Publications; Drawings reprinted with permission from Marino, B., & Fine, S. (2019). *Blueprints: Pediatrics* (7th ed.). Wolters Kluwer.

The Musculoskeletal System

Evaluations for **scoliosis** (lateral curvature of the spine) and screening for participation in sports remain common components of examination in adolescents. Other segments of the musculoskeletal examination are the same as for adults.

Assessing for Scoliosis

First, examine the patient standing, assessing symmetry of shoulders, scapula, and hips. Then have the patient bend forward with the knees straight and head hanging straight down between extended arms (Adams forward bend test). Next evaluate any asymmetry in positioning. Scoliosis in a young child is unusual and abnormal; mild scoliosis in an older child is not uncommon. Scoliosis appears as an asymmetrical rise in the thoracic region (as shown in Fig. 23-80), lumbar region, or both.

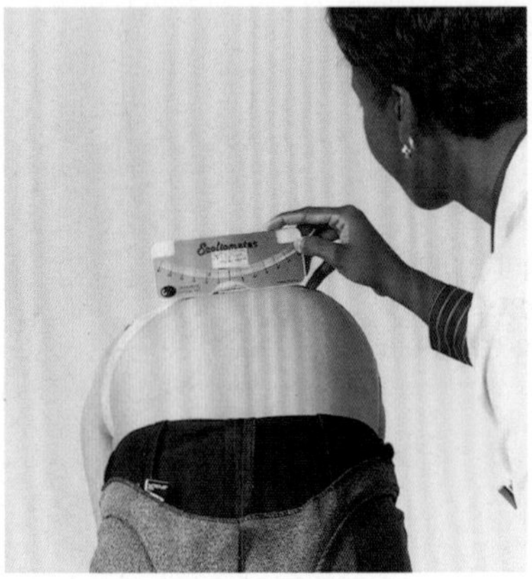

FIGURE 23-80 Measure and record the degree of scoliosis with a scoliometer.

If scoliosis is detected, use a scoliometer to test for the degree of scoliosis. Have the teen bend forward again as described. Place the scoliometer over the spine at a point of maximum prominence, making sure that the spine is parallel to the floor at that point, as shown in Fig. 23-80. If needed, move the scoliometer up and down the spine to find the point of maximal prominence. An angle greater than 7 degrees on the scoliometer is a reason for concern and often used as a threshold for referral to a specialist. Of note, the sensitivity and specificity of both the Adams forward bend test and scoliometer vary greatly according to the skill and experience of the examiner.

Several types of *scoliosis* may present during childhood. Idiopathic scoliosis (75% of cases), seen mostly in girls, is usually detected in early adolescence. As seen in the patient in Figure 23-80, the right hemithorax is generally prominent. Scoliosis is more common among children and adolescents with neurologic or musculoskeletal abnormalities.

A *plumb line,* a string with a weight attached, can also be used to assess symmetry of the back (Fig. 23-81). Place the top of the plumb line at C7 and have the patient stand straight. The plumb line should extend to the gluteal crease (not seen here).

Apparent scoliosis, including an abnormal plumb line test, can be caused by a *leg-length discrepancy.*

The remainder of the musculoskeletal examination is similar to that for adults, except for the sports preparticipation screening examination described in the next section.

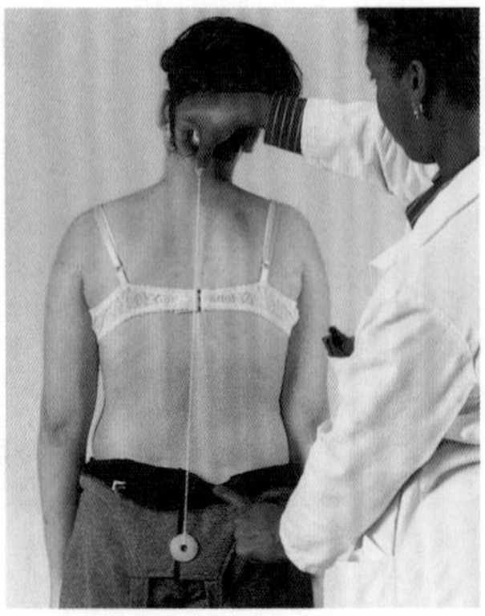

FIGURE 23-81 Assessing scoliosis with a plumb line.

The Sports Preparticipation Screening Evaluation

More than 25 million children and adolescents in the United States and several other countries participate in organized sports and often require medical clearance. Start the evaluation with a thorough medical history, focusing on cardiovascular risk factors, prior surgeries, prior injuries including concussions, other medical problems, and a family history. The complete history is the most sensitive and specific part of the evaluation for detection of risk factors or abnormalities that would preclude participation in sports. The preparticipation physical evaluation is often the only time a healthy adolescent will see a medical professional, so it is important to include some screening questions and anticipatory guidance (see the discussion in the "Health Promotion and Counseling" section). Finally, perform a general physical with special attention to the heart and lungs and vision and hearing screenings. Include a focused, thorough musculoskeletal examination, looking for weakness, limited range of motion, and evidence of previous injury.

Important risk factors for sudden cardiovascular death during sports include episodes of *dizziness or palpitations, prior syncope* (particularly if associated with exercise), or family history of *sudden death* or cardiomyopathy in young or middle-aged relatives.

During the preparticipation sports physical, assess carefully for *cardiac murmurs* and *wheezing* in the lungs. Also, if the adolescent has had head injuries or a concussion, perform a careful, focused neurologic examination (Halstead et al., 2018). A child or adolescent should not participate in sports until all signs and symptoms of a concussion have subsided.

The Nervous System

The neurologic examination of the adolescent and the adult is the same. Still, assess the adolescent's developmental achievement according to age-specific milestones, as described in Table 23-34.

Health Promotion and Counseling

The AAP recommends annual health supervision visits for adolescents (AAP, 2020). Because adolescents tend to be seen less frequently than do younger children for any health care visit, be sure to include health promotion during all health encounters with youth. In addition, adolescents with chronic problems or high-risk behaviors may require additional visits for health promotion and anticipatory guidance.

Most chronic diseases of adults have their antecedents in childhood or adolescence. For example, obesity, cardiovascular disease, addiction (to drugs, tobacco, or alcohol), and depression are all influenced by childhood and teen experiences and by behaviors established during adolescence. More specifically, most obese adults were obese as adolescents or had abnormal indicators such as elevated BMI scores. Almost all adults who are addicted to tobacco began their tobacco habits before 18 years. Therefore, a major component of health promotion for adolescents includes discussions about health behaviors or habits. Effective health promotion can help patients develop healthy habits and lifestyles and avoid several chronic health problems.

Because some health promotion topics involve confidential issues such as mental health, addiction, sexual behavior, and eating disorders, speak to adolescents (particularly older teens) privately during part of a visit that involves health supervision. Box 23-11 outlines components of the adolescent health supervision visit.

BOX 23-11 COMPONENTS OF A HEALTH SUPERVISION VISIT FOR ADOLESCENTS 11 TO 18 YEARS

Discussions with Parents

- Address parent concerns.
- Provide advice about supervision, encouraging progressively responsible decision making.
- Discuss school, activities, and social interactions.
- Discuss patient's behaviors, habits, and mental health.

Discussions with Adolescent

- Social and emotional development—Mental health, friends, family, bullying
- Physical development—Puberty, self-concept
- Behaviors and habits—Nutrition, exercise, TV, video games or computer screen time, tobacco use/vaping, drugs/alcohol, sleep
- Relationships and sexuality—Dating, sexual activity, sexual orientation, forced sex, human papillomavirus vaccination, contraception and sexually transmitted infection prevention, testing and treatment (Santa Maria et al., 2017)
- Family functioning—Relations with parents and siblings
- School performance—Activities, strengths, goals

Physical Examination

Perform a careful examination; note growth parameters and sexual maturity ratings.

Screening Tests

- Vision and hearing
- Blood pressure
- Consider hematocrit (especially in females)
- Assess emotional health and risk factors

Immunizations

See schedule on the CDC website at http://www.cdc.gov/vaccines/schedules/index.html.

Anticipatory Guidance—Teen

- Promote healthy habits and behaviors:
  - Injury and illness prevention—Seat belts, drunk driving, helmets, sun, weapons
  - Nutrition—Healthy meals and snacks, healthy weight
  - Oral health—Dentist visits, brushing and flossing
  - Physical activity and screen time
- Sexuality:
  - Ensure confidentiality
  - Sexual behaviors
  - Safer sex practices
  - Contraception if needed
- High-risk behaviors:
  - Prevention strategies
  - Parent–teen interactions
  - Peer interactions
  - Communication and rules
- Social achievement:
  - Activities
  - School
  - Future
- Community interaction: Resources, involvement

Anticipatory Guidance—Parent

- Positive interactions
- Support
- Safety
- Limit setting
- Family values
- Modeling behaviors
- Increased responsibility

RECORDING YOUR FINDINGS

Note the wording modifications necessary to accommodate reports from the small child's parent, rather than from the child, in the sample record in Box 23-12.

BOX 23-12 RECORDING THE EXAMINATION: THE PEDIATRIC PATIENT

3/11/21
Brian is an active, 26-month-old boy accompanied by his mother who is concerned about his development and behavior.

Referral. None.

Source and Reliability. Mother (Mom), reliable.

Chief Complaint. Slow development and difficult behavior.

Present Illness. Brian appears to be developing more slowly than his older sister did. He uses only single words and simple phrases, rarely combines words, and appears frustrated with not being able to communicate. People understand approximately 25% of his speech. Physical development seems appropriate for his age; he can throw a ball, kick, scribble, and dress himself well. He has had no head trauma, chronic illnesses, seizures, or regression in his milestones.

Mother also is concerned about his behavior. Brian is extremely stubborn, frequently has tantrums, gets angry easily (especially with his older sister), throws objects, bites, and physically strikes others when he doesn't get his way. His behavior seems worse around Mother, who report that he is "fine" at his child care center. He moves from one activity to another with an inability to sit still to read or play a game. Of note, he is sometimes affectionate and cuddly. He does make eye contact and plays normally with toys. He has no unusual movements.

Brian is a picky eater who eats a large quantity of junk food and little else. He will not eat fruits or vegetables and drinks enormous quantities of juice and soda. His parents have tried everything to get him to eat healthy food without success.

The family has been under substantial stress during the past year because Brian's father has been unemployed. Although Brian now has Medicaid insurance, the parents are uninsured.

Brian's sleep pattern appears normal for his age.

Medications. One multivitamin daily.

Past History

Pregnancy. Uneventful. Mother reduced tobacco intake to a half-pack a day and drank a glass of wine once a month. She denies use of other drugs or any infections.

Newborn Period. Born vaginally at 40 weeks; left the hospital in 2 days. Birth weight 2.5 kg (5 lb, 8 oz). Mother does not know why Brian was small at birth.

Illnesses. Only minor illnesses; no hospitalizations.

Accidents. Required sutures last year for a facial laceration secondary to a fall on the road. He did not lose consciousness and had no sequelae.

Preventive Care. Regular preventive check-ups. Six months ago, his regular physician said that Brian was a bit behind on some developmental milestones and suggested a child care center and increased parental attention to reading, speaking, playing, and stimulation. Immunizations up to date. Lead level was elevated mildly last year, and Mother reports he had "low blood." Physician recommended iron supplements and foods high in iron, but Brian won't eat these foods.

Family History

Family history of diabetes (maternal grandmother and paternal grandfather, both diagnosed after 60 years of age), hypertension (paternal grandfather). No family history of childhood developmental, psychiatric, or chronic illnesses.

Developmental History. Sat up at 6 months, crawled at 9 months, and walked at 13 months. First words ("mama" and "car") said at approximately 1 year.

Personal and Social History. Parents are married and live with the two children in a rented single family-house. Dad has not had a steady job for 1 year but has worked intermittently in construction. Mother works as a waitress part-time while Brian is in child care.

Mother reports having depression during Brian's first year and attended some counseling sessions but stopped because she could not pay for them or medications. She gets support from her mother who lives 30 minutes away, and many friends, some who babysit occasionally.

(continued)

BOX 23-12 RECORDING THE EXAMINATION: THE PEDIATRIC PATIENT (*Continued*)

Despite substantial family stress, Mother describes a loving and intact family. They try to eat dinner together daily, limit television, read to both children (though Brian won't sit still), and go to the nearby park regularly to play.

Environmental Exposures. Both parents smoke, though generally outside the house.

Safety. Mother reports this as a major concern; she feels she can barely leave Brian out of her sight without him getting into something. She fears he will run in front of a car, so the family is thinking of fencing in their small yard. Brian sits in his car seat most of the time; smoke detectors work in the home. Guns are locked; medications are in a cabinet in the parents' bedroom; childproof cabinet locks are on cabinets with cleaning supplies.

Review of Systems

General. Denies major illnesses.

Skin. Dry and itchy. Last year hydrocortisone prescribed which relieved the itching.

Head, Eyes, Ears, Nose, and Throat (HEENT). *Head:* Denies trauma. *Eyes:* Vision "fine." *Ears:* Multiple infections in the past year. Frequently ignores parents' requests; they can't tell if this is purposeful or if he can't hear well. *Nose:* Often runny; Mother wonders about allergies. *Mouth:* No dentist visit yet. Brushes teeth sometimes (a frequent source of dispute).

Neck. Denies lumps but glands in neck seem "large."

Respiratory. Frequent cough and whistle in chest. Mother cannot identify trigger; it tends to go away. He can run around all day without seeming to get tired.

Cardiovascular. No known heart disease. Murmur when younger, but it "went away."

Gastrointestinal. Appetite and eating habits described above. Daily bowel movements. In the process of toilet training and wears pull-ups at night and underwear during day.

Urinary. Good stream. Denies prior urinary tract infections.

Genital. Appropriate for age.

Musculoskeletal. He is active and never seems to get tired. Minor bumps and bruises occasionally; denies fractures and pain.

Neurologic. Walks and runs well; seems coordinated for age. Denies stiffness, seizures, or fainting. Mother says his memory seems great, but his attention span is "poor."

Psychiatric. Generally seems happy. Cries easily; bounces back and forth from trying to be independent to wanting cuddling and comforting.

Physical Examination

Active and energetic toddler. Plays with reflex hammer, pretending it is a truck. Appears closely bonded with his mother, looking at her occasionally for comfort. She seems concerned that Brian will break something. His face and clothes are clean.

Vital Signs. Ht 90 cm (90th percentile). Wt 16 kg (greater than 95th percentile). BMI 19.8 (greater than 95th percentile). Head circumference 50 cm (75th percentile). Blood pressure 108/58. Heart rate 90 and regular. Respiratory rate 30; varies with activity. Temperature (temporal artery) 37.5°C. No obvious pain.

Skin. Olive, visible bruises on anterior legs; patchy, dry skin over external surface of elbows; elastic, turgor less than 2 seconds.

HEENT. *Head:* Normocephalic; no lesions. *Eyes:* Difficult to examine due to movement. Symmetric with equal extraocular movements bilaterally. Pupils 4 to 5 mm and symmetrically reactive to light. Discs difficult to visualize; no hemorrhages noted. *Ears:* Auricle, no external lesions. External canals and tympanic membranes without exudate, cerumen, or foreign objects bilaterally. *Nose:* Nares equal; septum midline. *Mouth:* Several darkened teeth (inside surface of upper incisors). One cavity on upper right incisor. Tongue pink, midline, full range of motion. Cobblestoning of posterior pharynx; no exudates. Tonsils +3/4, pink. No allergic shiners.

Neck. Supple, midline trachea, thyroid not palpable.

Lymph Nodes. 0.5-cm tonsillar lymph nodes bilaterally. 0.5-cm inguinal nodes bilaterally. Palpable lymph nodes round, mobile, and nontender.

When the posterior pharynx is *bumpy,* like a cobblestone street, it may be described as being cobblestoned.

BOX 23-12 RECORDING THE EXAMINATION: THE PEDIATRIC PATIENT (*Continued*)

Lungs. Equal expansion. No tachypnea or dyspnea. Congestion audible, but seems to be upper airway (louder near mouth, symmetric). No rhonchi, rales, or wheezes. Clear to auscultation.

Cardiovascular. Apical impulse in fourth intercostal space medial to the midclavicular line. Positive S_1 and S_2, regular rhythm. No murmurs or abnormal heart sounds. Femoral pulses and dorsalis pedis pulses 2+ bilaterally.

Breasts. Minimal fat bilaterally.

Abdomen. Protuberant, soft; no masses or tenderness. Liver span 2 cm below right costal margin and not tender. Spleen and kidneys not palpable.

Genitalia. Tanner 1 circumcised penis; no pubic hair, lesions, or discharge. Testes descended, difficult to palpate because of active cremasteric reflex. Scrotum equal bilaterally.

Musculoskeletal. Full range of motion of upper and lower extremities and all joints bilaterally. Spine straight. Gait coordinated, wide-based.

Neurologic. *Mental Status:* Happy, cooperative, active child. *Developmental (DENVER II):* Gross motor—Jumps and throws objects. Fine motor—Imitates vertical line. Language—Does not combine words; single words only, three to four noted during examination. Personal–social—Washes face, brushes teeth, and puts on shirt. Overall—At level, except for language, which appears delayed. *Cranial Nerves:* Intact, although several difficult to elicit. *Cerebellar:* Gait age appropriate with steady balance and opposite arm swing. *Deep tendon reflexes (DTRs):* 2+ and symmetric throughout with plantar response bilaterally. *Sensory:* Deferred.

BIBLIOGRAPHY

CITATIONS

ACOG Committee on Adolescent Health Care. (2006). ACOG Committee Opinion no. 350, November 2006: Breast concerns in the adolescent. *Obstetrics and Gynecology, 108*(5), 1329–1336.

American Academy of Pediatrics. (AAP). (2012). Task force on circumcision, circumcision policy statement. *Pediatrics, 130*(3), 585–586.

American Academy of Pediatrics. (AAP). (2020). *Bright futures.* Retrieved March, 2020, from https://brightfutures.aap.org/materials-and-tools/guidelines-and-pocket-guide/Pages/default.aspx

American Academy of Pediatrics. (AAP). (2021). *Immunizations.* Retrieved February, 2021, from http://www2.aap.org/immunization/izschedule.html

American College of Obstetricians and Gynecologists. (2006). The initial reproductive health visit. ACOG Committee Opinion No. 811. *Obstetrics and Gynecology, 108*(5), 1329–1336.

American Dental Association (ADA). (n.d.). Eruption charts. https://www.mouthhealthy.org/en/az-topics/e/eruption-charts#main-content

Benenson, I., Frederick, A., Waldron, F. A., & Porter, S. (2020). Pediatric hypertension: A guideline update. *The Nurse Practitioner, 45*(5), 16–23.

Biro, F. M., Galvez, M. P., Greenspan, L. C., Succop, P. A., Vangeepuram, N., Pinney, S. M., Teitelbaum, S., Windham, G. C., Kushi, L. H., & Wolff, M. S. (2010). Pubertal assessment method and baseline characteristics in a mixed longitudinal study of girls. *Pediatrics, 126*(3), e583–590.

Biro, F. M., Greenspan, L. C., Galvez, M. P., Pinney, S. M., Teitelbaum, S., Windham, G. C., Deardorff, J., Herrick, R. L., Succop, P. A., Hiatt, R. A., Kushi, L. H., & Wolff, M. S. (2013). Onset of breast development in a longitudinal cohort. *Pediatrics, 132*, 1019–1927.

CDC. National Center for Health Statistics. (2010). *Growth charts: WHO growth charts.* Retrieved May 13, 2021, from https://www.cdc.gov/growthcharts/who_charts.htm#The%20WHO%20Growth%20Charts

CDC. National Center for Health Statistics. (2016). *CDC growth charts.* Retrieved May 13, 2021, from https://www.cdc.gov/growthcharts/cdc_charts.htm

Centers for Disease Control and Prevention (CDC). (2020a). *Children's mental health. Data and statistics on children's mental health.* Retrieved November 2, 2021, from https://www.cdc.gov/childrensmentalhealth/data.html

Centers for Disease Control and Prevention (CDC).(2020b). *Hearing loss in children. Data and statistics about hearing loss in children.* Retrieved June 8, 2021, from https://www.cdc.gov/ncbddd/hearingloss/data.html

Centers for Disease Control and Prevention (CDC). (2021). *Immunization schedules.* Retrieved February 12, 2021, from http://www.cdc.gov/vaccines/schedules/index.html

Chamblee, T. B., Pasek, T. A., Caillouette, C. N., Stellar, J. J., Quigley, S. M., & Curley, M. A. Q. (2018). How to predict pediatric pressure injury risk with the Braden QD Scale. *American Journal of Nursing, 118*(11), 34–43.

Christensen, D., & Zubler, J. (2020). From the CDC: Understanding autism spectrum disorder. *American Journal of Nursing, 120*(10), 30–37.

Colson, E. R., & Dworkin, P. H. (1997). Toddler development. *Pediatrics in Review, 18*(8), 255–259.

Copelan, J. (1995). Normal speech and development. *Pediatrics in Review, 18*, 91–100.

CS Mott Children's Hospital. Michigan Medicine. (n.d.). *Your child parenting guides and resources.* Retrieved May 16, 2021, from https://www.mottchildren.org/your-child

Dunlap, J. J., & Filipek, P. A. (2020). Autism spectrum disorder: The nurse's role. *American Journal of Nursing, 120*(11), 40–49.

Fleming, S., Thompson, M., Stevens, R., Heneghan, C., Plüddemann, A., Maconochie, I., Tarassenko, L., & Mant, D. (2011). Normal ranges of heart rate and respiratory rate in children from birth to 18 years of age: A systematic review of observational studies. *Lancet, 377*(9770), 1011–1018.

Frank, J. E., & Jacobe, K. M. (2011) Evaluation and management of heart murmurs in children. *American Family Physician, 84*, 793–800.

Freund, D., & Bolick, B. N. (2019). Assessing a child's pain. *American Journal of Nursing, 119*(5), 34–41.

Gessner, I. H. (1997). What makes a heart murmur innocent? *Pediatric Annals, 26*(2), 82–91.

Hagan, J. F., Shaw, J. S., & Duncan, P. M. (Eds.). (2017). *Bright futures: Guidelines for health supervision of infants, children and adolescents* (4th ed.). American Academy of Pediatrics.

Hales, C. M., Fryar, C. D., Carroll, M. D., Freedman, D. S., & Ogden, C. L. (2018). Trends in obesity and severe obesity prevalence in US youth and adults by sex and age, 2007–2008 to 2015–2016. *JAMA, 319*(16), 1723–1725.

Halstead, M. E., Walter, K. D., & Moffatt, K.; Council on Sports Medicine and Fitness. (2018). Sport-related concussion in children and adolescents. *Pediatrics, 142*(6), e20183074.

HealthyChildren.org. (2018). *Baby walkers: A dangerous choice.* Retrieved September 17, 2018, from https://www.healthychildren.org/English/safety-prevention/at-home/Pages/Baby-Walkers-A-Dangerous-Choice.aspx

Herman-Giddens, M. E., Slora, E. J., Wasserman, R. C., Bourdony, C. J., Bhapkar, M. V., Koch, G. G., & Hasemeier, C. M. (1997). Secondary sexual characteristics and menses in young girls seen in office practice: A study from the Pediatric Research in Office Settings Network. *Pediatrics, 99*(4), 505–512.

Herman-Giddens, M. E., Steffes, J., Harris, D., Slora, E., Hussey, M., Dowshen, S. A., Wasserman, R., Serwint, J. R., Smitherman, L., & Reiter, E. O. (2012). Secondary sexual characteristics in boys: Data from the Pediatric Research in Office Settings Network. *Pediatrics, 130*, e1058–e1068.

Holly, C., Porter, S., Echevarria, M., Dreker, M., & Ruzehaji, S. (2018). Recognizing delirium in hospitalized children: A systematic review of the evidence on risk factors and characteristics. *The American Journal of Nursing, 118*(4), 24–36.

Hyvarinen, L. (1994). Assessment of visually impaired infants. *Ophthalmology Clinics of North America, 7*, 219.

Ingelfinger, J. R. (2014). The child or adolescent with elevated blood pressure. *The New England Journal of Medicine, 370*, 2316–2325.

Johnson, C. P., & Blasco, P. A. (1997). Infant growth and development. *Pediatrics in Review, 18*(7), 224–242.

Kaplowitz, P., & Bloch, C.; Section on Endocrinology, American Academy of Pediatrics. (2016). Evaluation and referral of children with signs of early puberty. *Pediatrics, 137*(1), 2015–3732. https://doi-org/10.1542/peds.2015-3732

Marshall, W. A., & Tanner, J. M. (1969). Variations in pubertal changes in girls. *Arch Dis Child, 44*(235), 291–303.

Marshall, W. A., & Tanner, J. M. (1970). Variations in pubertal changes in boys. *Arch Dis Child, 45*(239), 13–23.

Matossian, D. (2018). Pediatric hypertension. *Pediatric Annals, 47*(12), e499–e503.

McGee, S. (2018). Chapter 52: Abdominal pain and tenderness. In *Evidence-based physical diagnosis* (4th ed.). Elsevier.

National Center for Victims of Crimes. (n.d.) *Child sexual abuse statistics.* Retrieved May 16, 2021, from https://victimsofcrime.org/child-sexual-abuse-statistics/

NIH. National Heart, Lung, and Blood Institute. (2005). *The fourth report on the diagnosis, evaluation, and treatment of high blood pressure in children and adolescents.* Retrieved May 16, 2021, from https://www.nhlbi.nih.gov/health-topics/fourth-report-on-diagnosis-evaluation-treatment-high-blood-pressure-in-children-and-adolescents

NIH. National Institute of Dental and Craniofacial Research. (2018). *Dental caries (tooth decay) in children age 2 to 11.* Retrieved July, 2018, fromhttps://www.nidcr.nih.gov/research/data-statistics/dental-caries/children#:~:text=–dental%20caries%20in%20primary%20baby%20teeth%20%28severity%29%201,with%20lower%20incomes%20have%20more%20untreated%20primary%20teeth

NIH. National Institute of Mental Health. (2018). *Autism spectrum disorder.* Retrieved March, 2018, from https://www.nimh.nih.gov/health/topics/autism-spectrum-disorders-asd/index.shtml

Ogden, C. L., & Flegal, K. M. (2010). *Changes in terminology for childhood overweight and obesity.* National health statistics reports; no 25. National Center for Health Statistics.

Paul, C. R., & Moreno, M. A. (2020). Acute otitis media. *JAMA Pediatrics, 174*(3), 308.

Perrin, E. C., & Sheldrick, R. C. (2013). *Development and implementation of developmental screening tools in primary care.* American Psychological Association. Retrieved November 12, 2020, from https://www.apa.org/pi/families/resources/primary-care/screening-tools

Quinn, B. L., Solodiuk, J. C., Morrill, D., & Mauskar, S. (2018). Pain in nonverbal children with medical complexity: A two year retrospective study. *American Journal of Nursing, 118*(8), 28–37.

Santa Maria, D., Guilamo-Ramos, V., Jemmott, L. S., Derouin, A., & Villarruel, A. (2017). Nurses on the front lines: Improving adolescent sexual and reproductive health across health care settings. *American Journal of Nursing, 117*(1), 42–51.

Smith, G. L., & McGuinness, T. M. (2017). Adolescent psychosocial assessment: The HEEADSSS. *Journal of Psychosocial Nursing and Mental Health Services, 55*(5), 24–27.

Wierwille, L. (2011). Pediatric heart murmurs: Evaluation and management in primary care. *Nurse Practitioner, 36*, 22–28; quiz 8–9.

Yang, S., Zusman, N., Lieberman, E., & Goldstein, R. Y. (2019). Developmental dysplasia of the hip. *Pediatrics, 143*(1), e20181147.

24 ASSESSING OLDER ADULTS

Written in collaboration with
Anne Bradley Mitchell, PhD, ANP-BC, FGSA

KEY TERMS

activities of daily living (ADLs)
delirium
drusen
dyspareunia
ectropion
entropion
ethnogeriatric
geriatric syndromes
gingivitis
instrumental activities of daily living (IADLs)
malodor
orthostatic hypotension
presbycusis
presbyopia
sarcopenia

Learning Objectives

The student will:

1. Recognize normal physiologic changes in the older adult.
2. Use the techniques that best facilitate the health history and physical examination of the older adult.
3. Identify focus areas during the health history specific to the older adult.
4. Use screening tools in the assessment of older adults.
5. Perform a health history on an older adult.
6. Perform a physical examination on an older adult.
7. Document findings from assessment of an older adult.
8. Address areas of health promotion and counseling specific to the older adult.

Older Americans now number more than 49 million, which is 15% of the population. That number is expected to reach 71 million by 2030 and 98 million by 2060, constituting more than 25% of the population (Centers for Disease Control [CDC], 2021). The current lifespan of Americans at birth is 77.48 years (Andrasfay & Goldman, 2021) with the biologic female life expectancy at 80.5 years and the biologic male expectancy at 75.1 years (Centers for Disease Control and Prevention, U.S. Department of Health and Human Services, 2021). The recent decrease is attributed to the COVID-19 pandemic which disproportionally affected Black and Hispanic/Latinx populations (Andrasfay & Goldman, 2021). Hence, the "demographic imperative" to societies worldwide is to maximize not only lifespan but also "health span," so that older adults maintain full function as long as possible, enjoying rich and active lives in their homes and communities (Fig. 24-1).

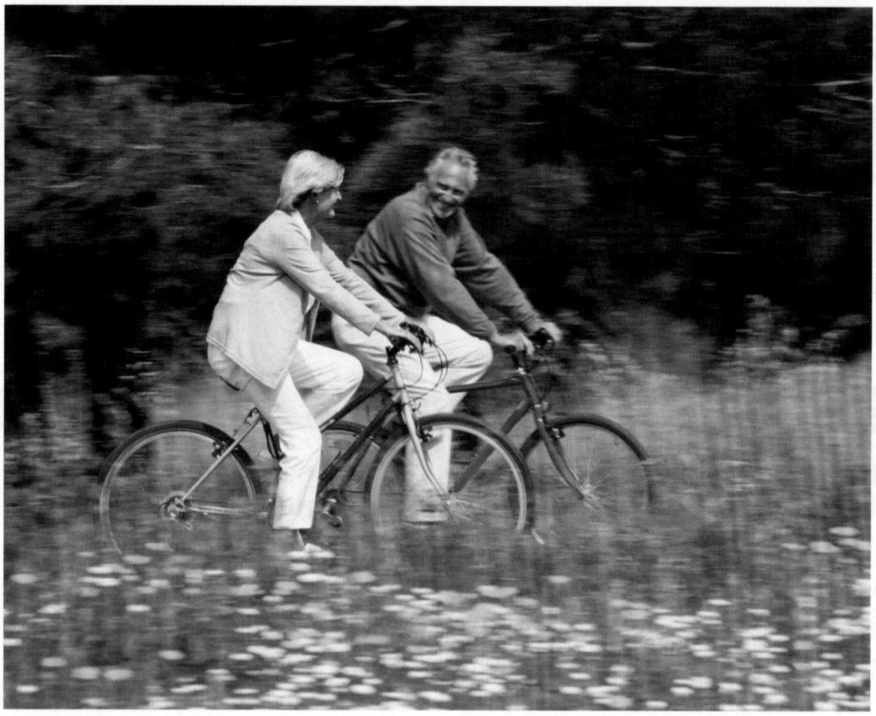

FIGURE 24-1 With an aging population, health promotion efforts should emphasize maintaining quality of life for as long as possible.

Although statistics group aging by decades, aging is hardly chronologic and measured by time in years, but rather it encompasses a wealth of wisdom and lived experience in addition to the complex interplay of health and illness. The aging population is highly heterogeneous—in disposition, social networks, level of physical activity, and biology. Frailty is one of society's common myths about aging; more than 95% of Americans older than 65 live in the general community, and only 5% reside in institutional facilities (Centers for Disease Control and Prevention, U.S. Department of Health and Human Services, 2021). For those over age 85, only 10% live in institutional facilities (Arias et al., 2021).

Self-reported health status and functional status supersede disability as measures of healthy aging. Among all cohorts over age 65, 78% rated their health as "good," "very good," or "excellent" (Arias et al., 2021). However, recent trends suggest that obesity may increase future levels of disability, especially in African American and Hispanic adults aged 60 to 69 years. Now 38% of adults aged 65 years and over are obese, compared to 22% from 1988 to 1994. Studies show that successful aging is not strictly medical, but rests on variables such as positive cognition and mental health, physical activity, and social networks (Ortman et al., 2020).

Terminology related to aging is in flux. This chapter uses the term "older adult"; however, evidence related to specific designations is lacking, so take the time to find out how your patient would like to be addressed and which terms they prefer. In 2017, several organizations advocated for the consistent, nonjudgmental term "older adult" in writing and reports about people over age 65. This chapter uses the term "older adult" to align with this directive (Federal Interagency Forum on Aging Related Statistics, 2016).

Assessing the older adult presents special opportunities and challenges. This chapter highlights only key points, as assessment of older adults encompasses much more than a single chapter can impart. Many of these challenges are quite different from those of the disease-oriented approach of history taking and physical examination for younger patients. The focus here is on healthy or "successful" aging; the need to understand and mobilize family, social, and community supports; the importance of functional assessment skills; and the opportunities for promoting the older adult's long-term health and safety. It is important to distinguish between normal aging changes and abnormalities commonly found in older people.

Promoting healthy aging leads to interactive goals in clinical care—"an informed active patient interacting with a prepared proactive team, resulting in high-quality satisfying encounters and improved outcomes" and a distinct set of clinical attitudes and skills (Bamia et al., 2017; Davy et al., 2015; Lundebjerg et al., 2017). Experts recommend "goal-oriented patient care" that is patient-centered, defined as "respectful of and responsive to individual patient preferences, needs, and values, and ensuring that patient values guide all clinical decisions" (Partnership for Health in Aging Workgroup on Interdisciplinary Team Training in Geriatrics, 2014). For older adults, this means focusing on the patient's "individual health goals within or across a variety of dimensions (e.g., symptoms; physical functional status, including mobility; and social and role functions) and to determine how these goals are being met" (Bodenheimer et al., 2002). This approach individualizes decision making and allows patients to express preferences about which health states are important and a priority, for example, choosing better symptom control over a longer lifespan. Goal-oriented care moves beyond prevention, disease-specific care processes, and condition-specific indicators, such as targets for glucose or blood pressure.

New paradigms also highlight the importance of shifting assessment to *geriatric syndromes* that fall outside traditional disease models but are strongly linked to **activities of daily living (ADLs)**. These syndromes are present in almost 50% of older adults (Institute of Medicine, 2011). Managing these conditions, such as cognitive impairment, falls, incontinence, low body mass index (BMI), dizziness, and impaired vision and hearing, presents both opportunities and challenges. The focus is on healthy or "successful" aging, including the need to understand and mobilize family, social, and community supports; the importance of skills directed to functional assessment, which can be considered a "sixth vital sign"; and the opportunities for promoting the older adult's long-term health and safety. Box 24-1 outlines specific nursing interventions to help a patient meet minimum geriatric competencies.

BOX 24-1 NURSING INTERVENTIONS TO MEET MINIMUM GERIATRIC COMPETENCIES

Medication Management

Explain any impacts of age-related changes on drug selection and dose based on knowledge of age-related changes in renal and hepatic function, body composition, and central nervous system sensitivity.

Identify medications, including anticholinergic, psychoactive, anticoagulant, analgesic, hypoglycemic, and cardiovascular drugs that should be avoided or used with caution in older adults and explain the potential problems associated with each.

Document a patient's complete medication list, including prescribed, herbal, and over-the-counter medications; and for each medication, provide the dose, frequency, indication, benefits, side effects, and an assessment of adherence.

Cognitive and Behavioral Disorders

Define and distinguish the clinical presentations of delirium, dementia, and depression.

Formulate a differential diagnosis and implement initial evaluation in a patient who exhibits cognitive impairment.

Urgently initiate a diagnostic workup to determine the root cause (etiology) of delirium in an older patient.

Perform and interpret a cognitive assessment in older patients for whom there are concerns regarding memory or function.

Develop an evaluation and nonpharmacologic management plan for patients exhibiting agitation, dementia, and/or delirium.

Self-Care Capacity

Assess and describe baseline and current functional abilities (i.e., instrumental activities of daily living, activities of daily living, and special senses) in an older patient by collecting historical data from multiple sources and performing a confirmatory physical examination.

Develop a preliminary management plan for patients presenting with functional deficits, including adaptive interventions and involvement of interdisciplinary team members, such as social work, nursing, rehabilitation, nutrition, and pharmacy.

Identify and assess safety risks in the home environment, and make recommendations to mitigate these.

Falls, Balance, and Gait Disorders

Ask all patients older than 65 years or their caregivers about falls in the last year, watch the patient rise from a chair and walk (or transfer), and then record and interpret the findings.

For a patient who has fallen, construct a differential diagnosis and evaluation plan that addresses the multiple etiologies identified by history, physical examination, and functional assessment.

Health Care Planning and Promotion

Define and differentiate among types of code status, health care proxies, and advanced directives in the site where one is training or working.

Accurately identify clinical situations in which life expectancy, functional status, patient preference, or goals of care should override standard recommendations for screening tests in older adults.

Use assessment tools for geriatrics and geriatric syndromes, including falls, delirium/cognitive impairment, and functional dependence in every patient. The Hartford Institute for Geriatric Nursing has a clinical website, "ConsultGeri," which provides access to many assessment tools at https://hign.org/consultgeri/try-this-series. Identify frail older patients, as they are most vulnerable to adverse outcomes and most benefit from a holistic geriatric approach.

BOX 24-1 NURSING INTERVENTIONS TO MEET MINIMUM GERIATRIC COMPETENCIES *(Continued)*

Accurately identify clinical situations in which life expectancy, functional status, patient preference, or goals of care should override standard recommendations for treatment in older adults.

Atypical Presentation of Disease

Identify at least three physiologic changes of aging for each organ system and their effects on the patient, including their contribution to balance and homeostenosis (the age-related narrowing of homeostatic reserve mechanisms).

As people age, they have a reduced ability to maintain homeostasis and have less functional reserve to cope with biologic stresses such as increasing their heart rate to cope with increased oxygen demand of heavy physical activity.

Generate a differential diagnosis based on recognition of the unique presentations of common conditions in older adults, including acute coronary syndrome, dehydration, urinary tract infection, acute abdomen, and pneumonia.

Palliative Care

Assess and provide initial management of pain and key nonpain symptoms based on the patient's goals of care.

Identify the psychological, social, and spiritual needs of patients with advanced illness as well as their family members and link these identified needs with the appropriate interdisciplinary team members.

Present palliative care (including hospice) as a positive, active treatment option for a patient with advanced disease.

Hospital Care for Older Adults

Identify potential hazards of hospitalization for all older adult patients (including immobility, delirium, medication side effects, malnutrition, pressure injuries, procedures, perioperative and postoperative periods, and hospital-acquired infections), and identify potential prevention strategies.

Explain the risks, indications, alternatives, and contraindications for indwelling (Foley) catheter use in the older adult patient.

Explain the risks, indications, alternatives, and contraindications for physical and pharmacologic restraint use.

Communicate the key components of a safe discharge plan (e.g., accurate medication list, plan for follow-up), including comparing/contrasting potential sites for discharge.

Conduct a surveillance examination of areas of the skin at high risk for pressure injuries and describe existing injuries.

Reprinted with permission from Leipzig, R. M., Granville, L., & Simpson, D. (2009). Keeping granny safe on July 1: A consensus on minimum geriatrics competencies for graduating medical students. *Academic Medicine*, *84*(5), 604–610. https://doi.org/10.1097/ACM.0b013e31819fab70.

ANATOMY AND PHYSIOLOGY

Primary aging reflects changes in physiologic reserves over time that are independent of changes from disease. These changes are likely to appear during periods of stress, such as exposure to fluctuating temperatures, dehydration, or even shock. In aging, decreased cutaneous vasoconstriction and sweat production can impair responses to heat; declines in thirst may delay recovery from dehydration; and the physiologic drops in maximum cardiac output, left ventricular filling, and maximum heart rate (HR) from aging may impair the response to shock.

At the same time, the aging population displays marked heterogeneity. Researchers have identified vast differences in how people age and have distinguished "usual" aging, with its complexity of diseases and impairments, from "optimal" aging. Optimal aging occurs in those who escape debilitating disease entirely and maintain healthy lives late into their 80s and 90s. Studies of centenarians show that genes account for approximately 20% to 30% probability of living to the age of 100. Importantly, healthy lifestyles also account for 20% to 30% (Carlson et al., 2015; Reuben & Tinetti, 2012). These findings provide evidence to promote modifiable lifestyle choices like optimal nutrition, strength training, and exercise. Promoting optimal function in older adults delays the depletion of physiologic reserves and the onset of frailty.

Vital Signs

Blood Pressure

In Western societies, systolic blood pressure (SBP) tends to rise with aging. The aorta and large arteries stiffen and become atherosclerotic. As the aorta becomes less distensible, a given stroke volume causes a greater rise in SBP; *systolic hypertension* with a *widened pulse pressure* (PP) often ensues. Diastolic blood pressure (DBP) stops rising at approximately the sixth decade. At the other extreme, some older adults develop a tendency toward **orthostatic hypotension** (postural hypotension), which is a sudden drop in blood pressure upon rising to a standing position.

Heart Rate and Rhythm

In older adults, resting HR remains unchanged, but pacemaker cells decline in the sinoatrial node and the maximal HR, which affects the response to exercise and physiologic stress (Sebastiani et al., 2014). Older adults are more likely to have abnormal heart rhythms such as atrial or ventricular ectopy. Asymptomatic rhythm changes are generally benign. However, some rhythm changes cause *syncope*, which is a temporary loss of consciousness.

Respiratory Rate and Temperature

Respiratory rate (RR) and temperature are unchanged in older adulthood, but changes in temperature regulation lead to a susceptibility to *hypothermia*.

Skin, Nails, and Hair

With age, the skin wrinkles, becomes lax, and loses turgor. The vascularity of the dermis decreases, causing lighter skin to look paler and opaque. Skin on the backs of the hands and forearms appears thin, fragile, loose, and transparent. There may be purple patches or macules, termed actinic purpura, that fade over time. These spots and patches come from blood that has leaked through poorly supported capillaries and spread within the dermis.

Nails lose luster with age and may yellow and thicken, especially on the toes.

Hair undergoes a series of changes. Scalp hair loses its pigment, changing hair color to gray. Hair loss on the scalp is genetically determined. As early as 20 years, a man's hairline may start to recede at the temples and then at the vertex (Fig. 24-2). In women, hair loss follows a similar but less severe pattern. In both sexes, the number of scalp hairs decreases in a generalized pattern, and the diameter of each hair gets smaller. Less familiar, but probably more clinically important, is normal hair loss elsewhere on the body: the trunk, pubic areas, axillae, and limbs. As women reach age 55, coarse facial hairs may appear on the chin and upper lip but do not increase further.

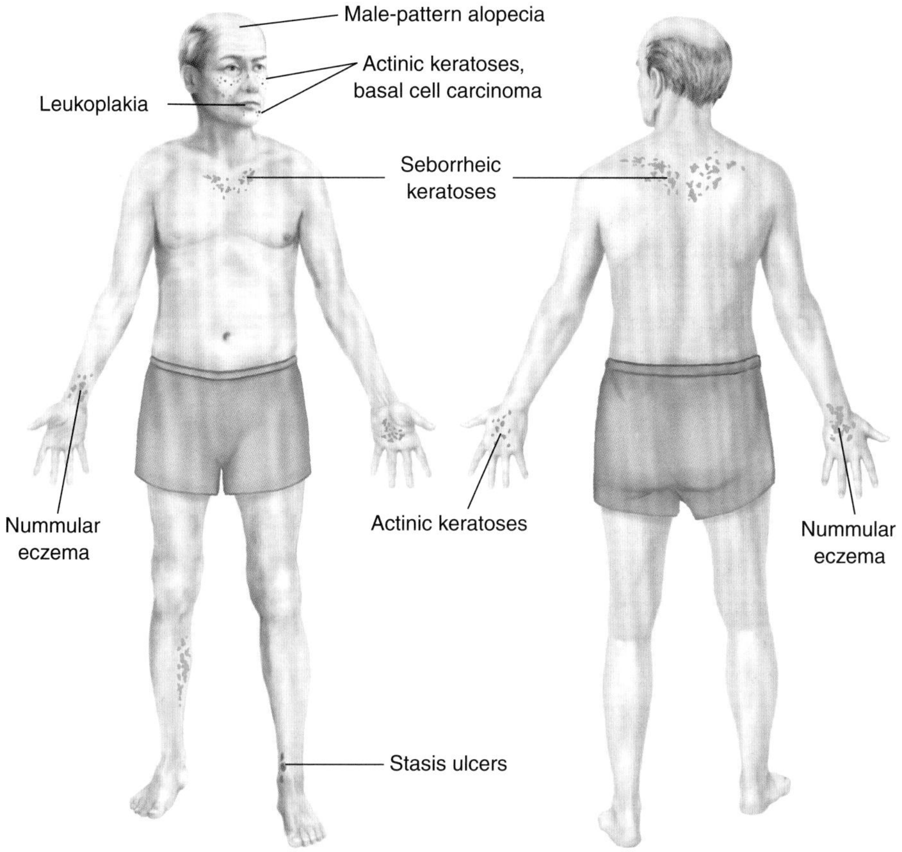

FIGURE 24-2 Potential integumentary changes in an older adult.

Head and Neck

Eyes and Visual Acuity

The eyes, ears, and mouth show more visible changes of aging. The fat that surrounds and cushions the eye within the bony orbit may atrophy, causing the eyeball to recede. The skin of the eyelids becomes wrinkled and may hang in looser folds. Fat may push the fascia of the eyelids forward, creating soft bulges, especially in the lower lids and the inner third of the upper lids. Because their eyes produce fewer lacrimal secretions, older patients may complain of dry eyes. The corneas lose some of their luster.

The pupils become smaller, which makes it more difficult to examine the ocular fundi. The pupils may also become slightly irregular but should continue to respond to light and show the near reaction.

Visual acuity remains fairly constant between 20 and 50 years. It diminishes gradually until approximately 70 years and then more rapidly. Nevertheless, most older adults retain good to adequate vision (20/20 to 20/70 as measured by standard charts). Near vision, however, begins to blur noticeably for virtually everyone. From childhood on, the lens gradually loses its elasticity, and the eye grows progressively less able to accommodate and focus on nearby objects. Ensuing **presbyopia** usually becomes noticeable during the 40s.

Up to 75% of those over age 65 are estimated to have visual problems that they do not disclose (Sebastiani et al., 2014). Aging affects the lenses and increases risk for *cataracts*, *glaucoma*, and *macular degeneration*. Thickening and yellowing of the lenses impair the passage of light to the retinas, requiring more light for reading and doing fine work. Cataracts affect 10% of patients in their 60s and 30% of people in their 80s. Because the lens continues to expand with aging, it may push the iris forward, narrowing the angle between iris and cornea and increasing the risk of *narrow-angle glaucoma*.

See Chapter 11, "The Eyes."

Hearing

Hearing acuity usually declines with age. Early losses, which start in young adulthood, involve primarily high-pitched sounds beyond the range of human speech that have relatively little functional significance. Gradually, loss extends to sounds in the middle and lower ranges. When a person fails to hear the higher tones of words but still hears the lower tones, words sound distorted and are difficult to understand, especially in noisy environments. Hearing loss associated with aging, known as **presbycusis**, becomes increasingly evident usually after 50 years.

Mouth, Teeth, and Lymph Nodes

Diminished salivary secretions and a decreased sense of taste accompany aging. Medications and various diseases may intensify these changes. Decreased olfaction and increased sensitivity to bitterness and saltiness also affect taste. Teeth may wear down, become abraded, or be lost to dental caries or periodontal disease. In patients without teeth, the lower portion of the face looks small and sunken, with accentuated "purse-string" wrinkles radiating from the mouth. Overclosure of the mouth may lead to maceration of the skin at the corners, a condition known as *angular cheilitis*. The bony ridges of the jaws that once surrounded the tooth sockets are gradually resorbed, especially in the lower jaw.

See Chapter 12, "Ear, Nose, Mouth, and Throat."

With aging, the cervical lymph nodes become less palpable. In contrast, the submandibular glands become easier to feel.

Thorax and Lungs

As people age, they lose lung capacity during exercise (Inglés et al., 2019). The chest wall becomes stiffer and harder to move, respiratory muscles may weaken, and the lungs lose some of their elastic recoil. Lung mass and the surface area for gas exchange decline, and residual volume increases as the alveoli enlarge. An increase in closing volumes of small airways predisposes older adults to atelectasis and risk of pneumonia. Diaphragmatic strength declines. The speed of breathing out with maximal effort gradually diminishes, and the cough becomes less effective. There is a decrease in arterial pO_2, but the O_2 saturation normally remains above 90%.

Skeletal changes associated with aging may accentuate the dorsal curve of the thoracic spine. Osteoporotic vertebral collapse produces *kyphosis*, which increases the anteroposterior diameter of the chest. The resulting "barrel chest," however, has little effect on function.

Cardiovascular System

Cardiovascular findings vary significantly with age. Aging also affects vascular sounds in the neck and adds to the significance of extra heart sounds like S_3 and S_4 and of murmurs.

Neck Vessels

Lengthening and tortuosity of the aorta and its branches occasionally result in kinking or buckling of the carotid artery low in the neck, especially on the right. The resulting pulsatile mass, occurring chiefly in women with hypertension, may be mistaken for a carotid aneurysm—which is a true dilation of the artery. A tortuous aorta occasionally raises the pressure in the jugular veins on the left side of the neck by impairing their drainage within the thorax.

In older adults, systolic bruits heard in the middle or upper portions of the carotid arteries indicate stenosis from atherosclerotic plaque. Cervical or carotid bruits in younger people are usually innocent.

Cardiac Output

Myocardial contraction is less responsive to stimulation from beta-adrenergic catecholamines. There is a modest drop in resting HR but a significant drop in the maximum HR during exercise. Though HR drops, stroke volume increases, so cardiac output is maintained. Diastolic dysfunction arises from decreased early diastolic filling and greater dependence on atrial contraction. There is increased myocardial stiffness, notably in the left ventricle, which also hypertrophies.

Risk of heart failure increases with loss of atrial contraction and onset of atrial fibrillation due to decreased ventricular filling.

Extra Heart Sounds—S_3 and S_4

A physiologic *third heart sound*, commonly heard in children and young adults, may persist as late as age 40, especially in women. After age 40, however, an S_3 strongly suggests heart failure from volume overload of the left ventricle in conditions such as heart failure and valvular heart disease (e.g., mitral regurgitation). In contrast, a *fourth heart sound* is seldom heard in young adults other than well-conditioned athletes. An S_4 can be heard in otherwise healthy older people but often suggests decreased ventricular compliance and impaired ventricular filling.

See Table 14-10, "Extra Heart Sounds in Diastole."

Cardiac Murmurs

Middle-aged and older adults commonly have a *systolic aortic murmur*. This murmur is detected in approximately one third of people at age 60 and in more than half of those reaching age 85. With aging, fibrotic changes thicken the bases of the aortic cusps. Calcification follows, resulting in audible vibrations. Turbulence produced by blood flow into a dilated aorta may further augment this murmur. In most older adults, the process of fibrosis and calcification, known as *aortic sclerosis*, does not impede blood flow. In some, the aortic valve leaflets become calcified and immobile, resulting in *aortic stenosis* and outflow obstruction. A brisk carotid upstroke can help distinguish aortic sclerosis from aortic stenosis, which has a delayed carotid upstroke, but clinically distinguishing these conditions is difficult. Both carry increased risk for cardiovascular morbidity and mortality.

Similar changes alter the mitral valve, approximately one decade later than the aortic valve. Calcification of the mitral valve annulus, or valve ring, impedes normal valve closure during systole, causing the systolic murmur of *mitral regurgitation*. This change in the configuration of the valve may become pathologic as volume overload increases in the left ventricle.

Peripheral Vascular System

The peripheral arteries tend to lengthen, become tortuous, and feel harder and less resilient. There is increased arterial stiffness and decreased endothelial function (Inglés et al., 2019). The trophic changes in skin, nails, and hair discussed earlier occur independently, though they may not accompany arterial disease. Although arterial and venous disorders, especially atherosclerosis, are more common in older adults, these are not normal changes of aging. Loss of arterial pulsations is not typical, however, and demands careful evaluation. Abdominal or back pain in older adults raises the important concern of possible abdominal aortic aneurysm, especially in men who smoke over age 65. Rarely, after age 50, but especially after age 70, the temporal arteries may develop giant cell, or temporal arteritis, leading to loss of vision in 15% of patients and headache and jaw claudication.

Breasts and Axillae

The normal adult female breast is soft, and may be granular, nodular, or lumpy. This uneven texture represents physiologic nodularity palpable throughout or only in parts of the breast. With aging, the female breasts tend to become smaller, more flaccid, and more pendulous as glandular tissue atrophies and is replaced by fatty tissue. The ducts surrounding the nipple may become more palpable as firm, stringy strands. Axillary hair diminishes. Males may develop gynecomastia or increased breast fullness due to obesity and hormonal changes.

Abdomen

During the middle and later years, the abdominal muscles tend to weaken, there is decreased activity of lipoprotein lipase, and fat may accumulate in the lower abdomen and near the hips even when the weight is stable. These changes often produce a softer, more protruding abdomen, which patients may interpret as fluid or evidence of disease. The change in abdominal fat distribution increases the risk of cardiovascular disease.

Aging can blunt the manifestations of acute abdominal disease. Pain may be less severe, fever is often less pronounced, and signs of peritoneal inflammation, such as muscular guarding and rebound tenderness, may be diminished or even absent.

See Chapter 15, "The Peripheral Vascular System and Lymphatic System."

Genitalia and Reproductive Organs

In women, ovarian function usually starts to diminish during the fifth decade; on average, menstrual periods cease between 48 and 55 years. As estrogen stimulation falls, many women experience hot flashes, sometimes for up to 5 years. Symptoms range from flushing, sweating, and palpitations to chills and anxiety. Sleep disruption and mood changes are common. Women may report vaginal dryness, urge incontinence, and **dyspareunia** (pain or difficulty with sex). Several vulvovaginal changes occur: pubic hair becomes sparse as well as gray, the labia and clitoris become smaller, the vagina narrows and shortens, and the vaginal mucosa becomes thin, pale, and dry with loss of lubrication. The uterus and ovaries diminish in size. Within 10 years after menopause, the ovaries are usually no longer palpable. The suspensory ligaments of the adnexa, uterus, and bladder may also relax. Sexuality and sexual interest are often unchanged, particularly when women are untroubled by partner issues, partner loss, or unusual work or life stress (Kane et al., 2018).

As men age, sexual interest appears to remain intact, though frequency of intercourse declines. Several physiologic changes accompany decreasing testosterone levels (Inglés et al., 2019). Erections become more dependent on tactile stimulation and less responsive to erotic cues. The penis decreases in size, and the testicles drop lower in the scrotum. Protracted illnesses, more so than aging, lead to decreased testicular size. Pubic hair may decrease and become gray. Erectile dysfunction, or the inability to have an erection, affects approximately 50% of older men but should not be considered a normal part of aging; it can be associated with an underlying disease. Vascular causes are the most common from both atherosclerotic arterial occlusive disease and corpora cavernosa venous leak. Chronic diseases such as diabetes, hypertension, dyslipidemia, and smoking, as well as medication side effects, all contribute to the prevalence of erectile dysfunction.

The prevalence of *urinary incontinence* increases with age in all genders. Incontinence may be related to decreased innervation and contractility of the detrusor muscle, loss of bladder capacity, changes in urinary flow rate, and the ability to inhibit voiding.

In women, injury to or weakening of the supporting muscles of the pelvic floor could exacerbate incontinence. This could potentially occur because of past vaginal childbirth(s) or surgery related to the reproductive system. Decreased production of estrogen after menopause can also exacerbate incontinence.

In men, there is androgen-dependent proliferation of prostate epithelial and stromal tissue, termed *benign prostatic hyperplasia (BPH)*, that begins in the third decade, continues to the seventh decade, then appears to plateau. Only half of men will have clinically significant enlargement, and of those, only half will report symptoms such as urinary hesitancy, dribbling, and incomplete emptying.

For everyone, the symptoms of urinary incontinence can often be traced to other causes like coexisting disease, use of medications, and lower urinary tract abnormalities (Morley & Tolsen, 2012a).

Musculoskeletal System

All adults lose cortical and trabecular bone mass as adulthood progresses, men more slowly and women more rapidly after menopause, leading to increased risk of fracture. Calcium resorption from bone rather than diet increases with aging as parathyroid hormone levels rise. Subtle losses in height begin soon after maturity; significant shortening is obvious by old age. Most loss of height occurs in the trunk and reflects thinning of the intervertebral discs and shortening or even collapse of the vertebral bodies from osteoporosis, leading to kyphosis and an increase in the anteroposterior diameter of the chest. Added flexion at the knees and hips also contributes to shortened stature. These changes cause the limbs of an older adult to look long in proportion to the trunk. With aging, there is a 30% to 50% decline in muscle mass in relation to body weight in both men and women, and ligaments lose some of their tensile strength. Range of motion diminishes, partly because of osteoarthritis. **Sarcopenia** is the loss of lean body mass and strength with aging (Morley & Tolsen, 2012b). The causes of muscle loss are multifactorial, including inflammatory and endocrine changes as well as sedentary lifestyles. There is substantial evidence that strength training in older adults can slow or reverse this process.

Mental Status Assessment and Nervous System

Aging affects all aspects of the nervous system, from mental status to motor and sensory function and reflexes. Brain volume, cortical brain cells, and intrinsic regional connecting networks decrease, and both microanatomic and biochemical changes have been identified (Hollingsworth & Wilt, 2014). Nevertheless, most older adults maintain their self-esteem and adapt well to their changing capacities and circumstances.

Mental Status

Although older adults generally perform well on mental status examinations, they may display select impairments, especially at advanced ages. Many older people complain about memory issues. This is usually from "benign forgetfulness," which can occur at any age. This term refers to difficulty recalling the names of people or objects or details of specific events. Identifying this as a common phenomenon can decrease fears of Alzheimer disease (AD). Older adults also retrieve and process data more slowly and take more time to learn new information. Their motor responses may slow and their ability to perform complex tasks may diminish.

Frequently, the nurse distinguishes these age-related changes in the nervous system from manifestations of mental disorders that are prevalent in older adults, such as *depression* and *dementia*. Differentiating these ailments may be difficult, because both mood disturbances and cognitive changes can alter the patient's ability to recognize or report symptoms. Older adults are also more susceptible to **delirium**, a transient state of confusion that has an underlying etiology. Common etiologies include presence of an infection, medication interactions, and changes in environment such as during a hospitalization. The nurse must be alert to complex presentations such as a delirium superimposed on an older adult with dementia. It is important to recognize these conditions promptly in order to delay functional decline. Recall that sensory and motor findings in older patients that are physiologic, such as the changes in hearing, vision, extraocular movements, and pupillary size, shape, and reactivity, are abnormal in younger adults. Differences in delirium and dementia are outlined in Table 24-1.

Review Chapter 19, "Mental Status and Mental Health Assessment."

TABLE 24-1 Delirium and Dementia

Delirium and dementia are common. They each affect multiple aspects of mental status and have many possible causes. Some clinical features and their effects on mental status are compared below.

	Delirium	Dementia
Onset	Acute	Insidious
Course	Fluctuating, with lucid intervals; worse at night	Slowly progressive
Duration	Hours to weeks	Months to years
Sleep/Wake cycle	Always disrupted	Sleep fragmented
General medical illness or drug toxicity	Either or both present	Often absent, especially in Alzheimer disease
Mental Status		
Level of consciousness	Disturbed; person less clearly aware of the environment and less able to focus, sustain, or shift attention	Usually normal until late in the course of the illness
Behavior	Activity often abnormally decreased (somnolence) or increased (agitation, hypervigilance)	Normal to slow; may become inappropriate
Speech	May be hesitant, slow or rapid, incoherent	Difficulty in finding words, aphasia
Mood	Fluctuating, labile, from fearful or irritable to normal or depressed	Often flat, depressed
Thought process	Disorganized, may be incoherent	Impoverished; speech gives little information
Thought content	Delusions common, often transient	Delusions may occur
Perceptions	Illusions, hallucinations, most often visual	Hallucinations may occur
Judgment	Impaired, often to a varying degree	Increasingly impaired over the course of the illness
Orientation	Usually disoriented, especially for time. A known place may seem unfamiliar	Fairly well maintained, but becomes impaired in the later stages of illness
Attention	Fluctuates with inattention; person easily distracted, unable to concentrate on selected tasks	Usually unaffected until late in the illness
Memory	Immediate and recent memory impaired	Recent memory and new learning especially impaired
Examples of Cause	Delirium tremens (due to withdrawal from alcohol) Infection Uremia Acute hepatic failure Acute cerebral vasculitis Atropine poisoning	*Reversible:* Vitamin B_{12} deficiency, thyroid disorders *Irreversible:* Alzheimer disease, vascular dementia (from multiple infarcts), dementia due to head trauma

Note: Delirium may be superimposed on dementia.

Emotional Concerns

Older adults experience the deaths of loved ones and friends, retirement from valued employment, diminution in income, and often growing social isolation in addition to physiologic changes and decreased physical capacity. Including the impact of these significant life events in the assessment of mood and affect and addressing these issues may improve the patient's quality of life (Fig. 24-3).

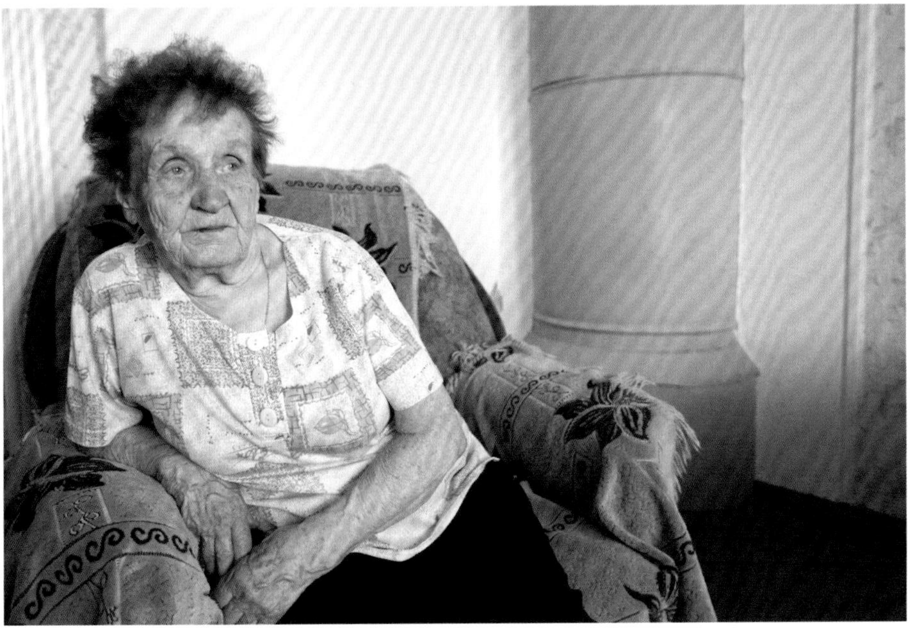

FIGURE 24-3 Lifestyle changes in older adulthood indicate the need for careful assessment of mood and affect.

Motor System

Changes in the motor system are common with aging. Older adults move and react with less speed and agility, and skeletal muscles decrease in bulk. The hands of an older patient often look thin and bony as a result of atrophy of the interosseous muscles that leaves concavities or grooves. Muscle wasting tends to appear between the thumb and the hand (the first and second metacarpals), then affect the other metacarpals. It may also flatten the thenar and hypothenar eminences of the palms. Arm and leg muscles can also show signs of atrophy, exaggerating the apparent size of adjacent joints. Muscle strength, though diminished, is relatively well maintained.

Occasionally, older adults develop a benign essential tremor in the head, jaw, lips, or hands that may be confused with Parkinsonism. Unlike Parkinsonian tremors, however, essential tremors are slightly faster and disappear at rest, and there is no associated muscle rigidity.

See Chapter 20, "The Nervous System," Table 20-10, "Abnormalities of Gait and Posture."

Vibratory and Position Sense, Reflexes

Aging can also affect vibratory and position sense and reflexes. Older adults frequently lose some or all vibration sense in the feet and ankles (but not in the fingers or over the shins). Less commonly, position sense may diminish or disappear. The gag reflex may be diminished or absent. Abdominal reflexes may diminish or disappear. Ankle reflexes may be symmetrically decreased or absent, even when reinforced. Less commonly, knee reflexes are similarly affected. Partly because of musculoskeletal changes in the feet, the plantar responses become less obvious and more difficult to interpret. If there are associated neurologic findings, or if atrophy and reflex changes are asymmetric, search for an explanation other than aging.

THE HEALTH HISTORY

Approach to the Older Adult Patient

Modify your usual approach when obtaining the health history and interviewing older adults. As with all patients, the nurse's demeanor should convey respect, patience, and cultural awareness. Inquire about issues regarding privacy such as "Would you like a friend or family member to be present during the interview?" or "May I share information about your examination with your family or friend?" Be sure to address patients according to their preference.

Adjust the Environment

First, take the time to adjust the environment of the office, hospital, or nursing home to put your patient at ease. Recall the older adult's physiologic changes in temperature regulation, and make sure the office is neither too cool nor too warm. Brighter lighting helps compensate for changes in the lens and allows the older patient to see your facial expressions and gestures more clearly. Ensure the patient is not facing a window, as the glare may also impair the ability to see well. The nurse should face the patient directly and sit at eye level (Fig. 24-4). Focusing on personal electronic devices or turning away from the patient to search the electronic medical record should be avoided.

More than 50% of older adults have hearing deficits, especially for higher-frequency tones, so choose a quiet room that is free of distractions or noise. Turn off the radio or television before you start the conversation. If appropriate, consider using a "pocket talker," a small, portable microphone that amplifies your voice and connects to an earpiece inserted by the patient. Speak in low tones, and make sure the patient is using glasses, hearing aids, and dentures when needed to assist with communication. Patients with quadriceps weakness benefit from chairs with higher seating and sturdy arms to help raise themselves as well as wide stools with handrails leading up to the examining table.

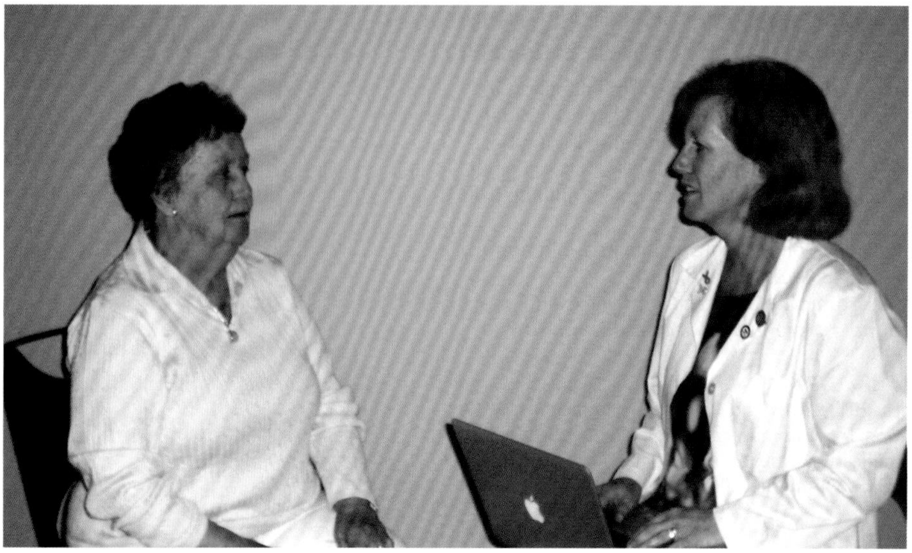

FIGURE 24-4 The nurse should face the patient and sit at eye level.

Shape the Content and Pace of the Visit

With older adults, rethink the traditional format of the visit. Older patients often measure their lives in terms of years left rather than years lived. They may reminisce about the past and reflect on previous experiences. By listening to these life reviews, a nurse gains important insights and an understanding of the individual, facilitating support of patients as they work through painful feelings or recapture joys and accomplishments.

At the same time, it is important to balance the need to assess complex problems with the patient's endurance and possible fatigue. To expand time for listening to the patient but prevent exhaustion, make ample use of brief screening tools (Demonet, 2012; Evans, 2015), information from home visits and the medical record, and reports from family members, caregivers, and allied health professionals. Consider dividing the initial assessment into two visits. Two or more shorter visits may be less fatiguing and more productive to allow more time to respond to questions, since explanations may be slow and lengthy.

See an outline of brief screening tools in Table 24-2.

Address Cultural Dimensions of Aging

Knowledge and skills about the cultural dimensions of aging are the cornerstone to improving health care for the rapidly growing number of older adults of diverse ethnic and racial backgrounds. In fact, the demographic imperative for older adults can be called the *ethnogeriatric imperative* (Yeo et al., 2017). The numbers of adults older than 65 not born in the U.S. is predicted to almost double from 13.2% to 25.8% from 2014 to 2060. Box 24-2 outlines projected demographic statistics of the aging American population.

BOX 24-2 GERIATRIC DIVERSITY: NOW AND IN 2060

- *Hispanic Americans* over the age of 65 years will increase in number from 4 million in 2017, or 8% of the older adult population, to 19.9 million in 2060, or 21% of the older adult population. *Non-Hispanic African American* older adults will increase in number from 4.5 million in 2017 (9%), to 12.1 million in 2060 (13%).
- *Non-Hispanic Asian Americans* older adults will increase in number from 2.2 million in 2017 (4%), to 7.9 million in 2060 (8%).
- *Non-Hispanic American Indian and/or Alaska Native* older adults will increase in number from 272,250 in 2017 (0.5%), to more than 648,000 in 2060 (0.7%).
- The older adult population is growing more ethnically and racially diverse and the population of *Non-Hispanic White* older adults is projected to decrease from 77% to 55% of the population.

Data from U.S. Census Bureau, Population Estimates, 2017, 2018 and Population Projections, 2017, 2018. Administration on Aging (AoA), Administration for Community Living, U.S. Department of Health and Human Services. 2018 Profile of Older Americans. Retrieved April 9, 2021, from https://acl.gov/sites/default/files/Aging%20and%20Disability%20in%20America/2018OlderAmericansProfile.pdf

The changing demographics of aging Americans only hint at how older adults of different ethnicities experience suffering, illness, and decisions about their health care. Cultural and socioeconomic attributes affect the epidemiology of illness and mental health, the process of acculturation in families, individual concerns about aging, choices about healers and when to pursue symptoms, the potential for misdiagnosis, and disparities in health outcomes (Rosen & Reuben, 2011). Culture, including spiritual beliefs, shapes views about the entire spectrum of aging: work and retirement, perceptions of health and illness, the utility of medications, use of health care proxies, and preferences about dying, to name just a few.

The CDC Health Disparities and Inequalities Report—United States, 2013 "highlights health disparities and inequalities across a wide range of diseases, behavioral risk factors, environmental exposures, social determinants, and health care access by sex, race and ethnicity, income, education, health literacy, disability status, and other social characteristics" (Jackson & Gracia, 2014; Yeo, 2009). Aging racial/ethnic minority populations have poorer health outcomes in cardiovascular disease, diabetes, cancer, asthma, and human immunodeficiency virus/acquired immunodeficiency syndrome (HIV/AIDS), as well as shorter lifespans (Centers for Disease Control and Prevention, 2020b). Despite advances in **ethnogeriatrics** (care for older adults from diverse populations) (August & Sorkin, 2010; Ng et al., 2014; Stanford School of Medicine, 2016), information on racial and ethnic disparities in later life regarding chronic disease, ADLs, and self-rated health status remains "limited and inconsistent," and guidelines for providing individualized, culturally appropriate care are sparse (Jackson & Gracia, 2014).

Improving competence in care for diverse older populations is a critical step in improving health outcomes. The *ETHNIC(S)* mnemonic helps clinicians escape the pitfalls of group-labeling by expanding individual history taking to include *explanation, treatment, healers, negotiate, intervention, collaborate, and spirituality* (Office of Minority Health, Department of Health & Human Services, 2020). This model may still miss important information about cultural identity, social supports, health literacy, and views about health care (Aggarwal et al., 2014). Experts recommend letting patients establish their cultural identity by exploring four key areas during the interview: the individual's cultural identity, cultural explanations of the individual's illness, cultural factors related to the psychosocial environment and levels of function, and cultural elements in the clinician–patient relationship. Test your "ethnogeriatric IQ" at the Stanford Geriatrics Education Center website and explore the Stanford curriculum in ethnogeriatrics (Aggarwal, 2010; Kobylarz et al., 2002). Learn to convey respect for older adults through culturally specific nonverbal communication. Direct eye contact or handshaking, for example, may not be culturally appropriate for every patient. Identify critical life experiences from the country of origin or migration history that affect the patient's outlook and psyche. Ask about family decision making, spiritual advisors, and traditional healers and practices. The Office of Minority Health in the Department of Health and Human Services has developed *Think Cultural Health*, a resource center to improve quality of care through cultural and linguistic competencies and continuing education programs (Ng et al., 2014).

Cultural values particularly affect decisions about the end of life. Community elders, family, and even an extended community group may make these decisions with or for the older patient. Such group decision making is quite different from the focus on individual autonomy and informed consent featured in contemporary American health care settings. Eliciting the stresses of migration and acculturation, using translators effectively, enlisting "patient navigators" from the family and community, and accessing culturally validated assessment tools like the Geriatric Depression Scale will help you provide empathic care of older adults.

See Chapter 3, "Interviewing and Communication," for a discussion on working with translators.

Elicit Symptoms from the Older Adult

Eliciting the history calls for an astute nurse: patients may accidentally or purposefully underreport symptoms, the presentation of acute illnesses may be different from patient to patient, common symptoms may mask a geriatric syndrome, and/or patients may have cognitive impairment.

Underreporting Symptoms

Older patients tend to give more positive ratings to their overall health than do younger adults, even when affected by disease and disability. It is best to start the visit with open-ended questions like "How can I help you today?" Older patients may be reluctant to report their symptoms. Some are afraid or embarrassed; others try to avoid medical expenses or the discomforts of diagnosis and treatment. Still others overlook their symptoms (e.g., pain), thinking them to be merely part of aging, or they may simply forget about them. To reduce the risk for late recognition of disease and delayed intervention, you may need to adopt more direct questions, use well-validated geriatric screening tools, and consult with family members and caregivers. Box 24-3 includes additional tips for effective communication with older adult patients.

BOX 24-3 TIPS FOR COMMUNICATING EFFECTIVELY WITH OLDER ADULTS

- Provide a well-lit, moderately warm setting with minimal background noise, a safe chair, and access to the examining table.
- Face the patient and speak in low tones; make sure the patient is using glasses, hearing devices, and dentures if needed.
- Adjust the pace and content of the interview to the stamina of the patient; consider two visits for initial evaluations.
- Allow time for open-ended questions and reminiscing; include family and caregivers when needed, especially if the patient has a cognitive impairment.
- Make use of brief screening instruments, the medical record, and reports from allied health professionals.
- Carefully assess symptoms, especially fatigue, loss of appetite, weight loss, incontinence, skin integrity, dizziness, falls, and pain, for clues to underlying disorders and geriatric disorders.
- Make sure written instructions are in large print and easy to read.

Acute illnesses present differently in older adults. Older patients with infections are less likely to have a fever. Older patients experiencing myocardial infarction are less likely to report chest pain; and symptoms have an atypical presentation, such as shortness of breath, palpitations, syncope, and confusion (Stanford Geriatrics Education Center, 2020). Older patients with hyperthyroidism or hypothyroidism have fewer symptoms and signs. One third of older adults with hyperthyroidism present with fatigue, weight loss, and tachycardia in lieu of the classic features of heat intolerance, sweating, and hyperreflexia (Samuels, 2000). Up to 35% present with atrial fibrillation. Hyperthyroidism increases the risk of osteoporosis; and in affected women, risk of hip and vertebral fractures increases threefold. In older adults, hypothyroidism is most commonly caused by autoimmune thyroiditis (*Hashimoto thyroiditis*); fatigue, weakness, constipation, dry skin, and cold intolerance are often attributed to other conditions, medication side effects, or aging.

CLINICAL TIP
In older adults, the prevalence of hyperthyroidism is 1% to 3% (Samuels, 2000).

Geriatric Syndromes

Managing an increasing number of interrelated conditions calls for recognizing the symptom clusters typical of different **geriatric syndromes**. A geriatric syndrome represents serious issues for older adults and is often related to functional decline. Geriatric syndromes impact quality of life, and nurses need to be aware of them. One symptom may relate to several others. It is especially important to be vigilant and recognize these syndromes because symptoms may cluster in patterns unfamiliar to the patient (Bhatia & Naik, 2013). It is important for nurses to obtain an accurate assessment using both subjective and objective information.

Geriatric syndromes have been found in more than half of adults over age 65 in contrast to the conventional search in younger patients for a "single unifying diagnosis" (Papaleontiou & Haymart, 2012).

SPICES is a mnemonic that focuses on frequent geriatric syndromes of the older adult:

- *S*leep disorders
- *P*roblems with eating or feeding
- *I*ncontinence
- *C*onfusion
- *E*vidence of falls
- *S*kin breakdown

Although not a comprehensive compilation, SPICES clearly directs attention to key areas for the nurse to begin assessing and planning for appropriate interventions (Fulmer, 2007; Koroukian et al., 2015; Strandberg et al., 2013).

CLINICAL TIP

The Hartford Institute of Geriatric Nursing has a comprehensive website with general assessment tools designed for nurses caring for older adults. The entire assessment series site can be accessed at http://consultgeri.org/tools/try-this-series. SPICES is the first issue in the series (Kagan, 2010).

Cognitive Impairment

A number of parameters affect assessment of health status. Evidence suggests that self-report continues to be reliable in older adults, especially for prevalence of chronic conditions (Fernández-Ruiz et al., 2013; Fulmer & Wallace, 2020; Mendonça et al., 2016; Montlahuc et al., 2011; Nurses Improving Care for Healthsystem Elders [NICHE], 2020). When compared with healthy peers, older adults with mild cognitive impairment provide sufficient history to reveal concurrent disorders. Use simple sentences with prompts to elicit necessary information. For patients with more severe impairments, confirm key symptoms with family members or caregivers in the patient's presence and with their consent. To avoid invalid assumptions, explore how older patients view themselves and their situations. Listen for their priorities and coping skills. These insights strengthen your partnerships with both patients and families as you evolve plans for care and treatment. Learn to recognize and avoid stereotypes that distort your appreciation of each patient as unique with a variety of life experiences.

Special Areas of Concern When Assessing Common or Concerning Symptoms

Symptoms in the older adult can have many meanings and interconnections, as seen in geriatric syndromes. Explore the meaning of these symptoms as you would with all patients, and for the older adults, place these symptoms in the context of the overall functional assessment of the ADLs. Several topics warrant special attention as you gather the health history (Box 24-4). Approach these areas with extra thoroughness and sensitivity, always with the goal of helping the older adult maintain optimal level of function and well-being.

BOX 24-4 COMMON TOPICS FOR HEALTH HISTORY OF THE OLDER ADULT PATIENT

- Functional assessment
- Activities of daily living
- Instrumental activities of daily living
- Medications
- Nutrition
- Pain (acute and persistent)
- Sexuality
- Urinary incontinence
- Smoking and alcohol use

Functional Assessment

The 10-Minute Geriatric Screener (Table 24-2) assesses for age-related changes that help older adults maintain optimal function. It covers the three important domains of geriatric assessment: physical, cognitive, and psychosocial function. Note that it addresses vision and hearing, key sensory modalities that can be followed with additional objective testing such as using an eye chart for vision, asking the patient about hearing, followed by the whisper test and more formal testing if indicated. It also includes questions about mobility, urinary incontinence (an often unreported problem), nutrition, memory, depression, and physical disabilities. All these components can affect social interaction and self-esteem in the elderly.

Activities of Daily Living

The daily activities of older adults, especially those with chronic illnesses, provide an important baseline for the future. First, ask about the capacity to perform *ADLs*, which consist of six basic self-care abilities. Then move on to higher-level functions, the **instrumental activities of daily living (IADLs)** (Table 24-3). Can the patient perform these activities independently, does the patient need some help, or is the patient entirely dependent on others?

Start with an open-ended request such as: "Tell me about your typical day" or "Tell me about your day yesterday." Then move to a greater level of detail. "You got up at 8 AM?" "How was getting out of bed?" "What did you do next?" Ask if activity levels have changed, who is available for help, and what helpers or caregivers do. Remember that assessing the patient's safety is a clinical priority.

TABLE 24-2 10-Minute Geriatric Screener

Problem	Screening Measure	Positive Screen
Vision	Ask: "Do you have difficulty driving, watching television, reading, or doing any of your daily activities because of your eyesight?" If yes, then: Test each eye with the Snellen chart while the patient wears corrective lenses (if applicable).	Yes to question and inability to read greater than 20/40 on Snellen chart
Hearing	Use audioscope set at 40 dB. Test hearing using 1,000 and 2,000 Hz.	Inability to hear 1,000 or 2,000 Hz in both ears or either of these frequencies in one ear
Leg mobility	Time the patient after asking: "Rise from the chair. Walk 20 ft briskly, turn, walk back to the chair, and sit down."	Unable to complete task in 15 sec
Urinary incontinence	Ask: "In the last year, have you ever been unable to hold your urine and gotten wet?" If yes, then ask: "Have you lost urine on at least six separate occasions?"	Yes to both questions
Nutrition/Weight loss	Ask: "Have you lost 10 lb over the past 6 mo without trying to do so?" Weigh the patient.	Yes to the question or weight <100 lb
Memory	Three-item recall	Unable to remember all three items after 1 min
Depression	Ask: "Do you often feel sad or depressed?"	Yes to the question
Physical disability	Six questions: "Are you unable to...: "Do strenuous activities like fast walking or bicycling?" "Do heavy work around the house like washing windows, walls, or floors?" "Go shopping for groceries or clothes?" "Get to places outside of walking distance?" "Bathe, either a sponge bath, tub bath, or shower?" "Dress, like putting on a shirt, buttoning and zipping, or putting on shoes?"	Yes to any of the questions

Source: Vogelsang, E. M. (2014). Self-rated health changes and oldest-old mortality. *Journals of Gerontology. Series B, Psychological Sciences and Social Sciences*, *69*(4), 612–621.

TABLE 24-3 Activities of Daily Living and Instrumental Activities of Daily Living

Physical Activities of Daily Living (ADLs)	Instrumental Activities of Daily Living (IADLs)
Bathing	Using the telephone
Dressing	Shopping
Toileting	Preparing food
Transferring	Housekeeping
Continence	Doing laundry
Feeding	Transportation, including driving
	Taking medicine
	Managing money

Source: Iecovich, E., & Biderman, A. (2013). Concordance between self-reported and physician-reported chronic co-morbidity among disabled older adults. *Canadian Journal on Aging = La Revue Canadienne Du Vieillissement*, *32*(3), 287–297; and Moore, A. A., & Siu, A. L. (1996). Screening for common problems in ambulatory elderly: Clinical confirmation of a screening instrument. *American Journal of Medicine*, *100*, 438–443.

Medications

The magnitude of adverse drug events leading to hospitalization and poor patient outcomes underscores the importance of a thorough medication history. Adults over the age of 65 receive approximately 30% of all prescriptions. Approximately 80% of adults over the age of 65 have at least one of six chronic conditions—arthritis, current asthma, cancer, cardiovascular disease, chronic obstructive pulmonary disease (COPD), or diabetes—and over 87% take at least one prescription drug each day while 36% take at least one over-the-counter medication (Katz et al., 1963; Lawton & Brody, 1969). Almost 40% take five or more prescription drugs daily. Older adults have more than 50% of all reported adverse drug reactions causing hospital admission, reflecting pharmacodynamic changes in the distribution, metabolism, and elimination of drugs that place them at increased risk. When discussing medications, remember:

- A thorough *medication history* includes name, dose, frequency, and the *patient's view* of the reason for taking each drug.
- Ask the patient to bring in all medication bottles and over-the-counter products to develop an accurate medication list.
- Explore all components of polypharmacy, a major cause of morbidity, including suboptimal prescribing, concurrent use of multiple drugs, underuse, inappropriate use, and nonadherence.
- Ask specifically about over-the-counter products; vitamin and nutritional supplements; and mood-altering drugs such as narcotics, benzodiazepines,

and recreational substances (Centers for Medicare & Medicaid Services, 2021).

- Assess medications for drug interactions.

- Be particularly careful when treating *insomnia*, estimated to occur in 40% of older adults. A *sleep history* provides information essential for diagnosis; a *sleep diary* may be especially helpful in uncovering the origins of poor sleep patterns (Qato et al., 2016). Increased exercise may be the best remedy. Experts on sleep disorders can be good resources for patients (Wang & Andrade, 2013).

Medications are the single most common modifiable risk factor associated with falls. Review strategies for avoiding polypharmacy (Bloom et al., 2009; Rodriguez et al., 2015). The nurse should apply the advisory that medication dosages for older adults should "start low and go slow." Nurses need to recognize the normal dosages for medications and consider consulting with the health care provider or pharmacist if a medication dosage appears high for an older adult given their age and overall health status. Learn about drug–drug interactions and consult the *Beers Criteria*, widely used by health care providers, educators, and policymakers. These criteria include listing hazardous drugs for older adults (Wooten, 2015). Risk factors for adverse drug reactions in hospitalized older adults are listed in Box 24-5.

BOX 24-5 HOSPITALIZED OLDER ADULTS: RISK FACTORS FOR ADVERSE DRUG REACTIONS

- More than four comorbid conditions
- Heart failure, renal failure, or liver disease
- Age 80 years or older
- Number of drugs, especially if eight or more
- Use of warfarin, insulins, oral antiplatelet agents, or oral hypoglycemic agents
- Previous adverse drug reaction
- Hyperlipidemia
- Raised white cell count
- Use of antidiabetic agents
- Length of stay 12 days or longer

Data from Onder, G., Petrovic, M., & Balamurugan, T. (2010). Less is more. Development and validation of a score to assess risk of adverse drug reactions among the in-hospital patients 65 years or older. *Archives of Internal Medicine, 170*, 1142.
Source: Wooten, J. M. (2015). Rules for improving pharmacotherapy in older adult patients: part 2 (rules 6–10). *Southern Medical Journal, 108*, 145–150.

Nutrition

Taking a diet history and using nutritional screening tools often reveal nutritional deficits. The prevalence of undernutrition increases with age, affecting up to 5% of older adults in the community, over 50% of nursing home residents, and up to 50% of older patients at hospital discharge (American Geriatrics Society, 2019b). Recent data suggest that only 30% to 40% meet recommended guidelines for daily intake of fruit and vegetables (Onder et al., 2010). Older adults with chronic diseases are particularly vulnerable, especially those with poor dentition, oral or gastrointestinal disorders, depression or other psychiatric illness, and drug regimens that affect appetite and oral secretions (American Geriatrics Society, 2018a). Nurses should screen for social isolation as this can also be a contributing factor for decreased nutritional intake (American Geriatrics Society, 2018a).

For underweight older adults, the serum albumin is an independent risk factor for all-cause mortality, though albumin does not have the specificity to be a true marker of malnutrition. Screening for vitamin D deficiency is recommended given its role in decreasing the risk of injury from falls (American Geriatrics Society, 2019b). Assess the average daily fluid intake. Older adults need to ingest approximately 30 mL/kg/d or 1 mL/kcal fluids. Dehydration is the most common fluid or electrolyte disturbance in older adults (American Geriatrics Society, 2019b). The Mini Nutritional Assessment (Fig. 24-5) has a short form with six questions to screen patients older than 65 for malnutrition or risk of malnutrition.

Acute and Persistent Pain

Pain and associated complaints account for 80% of clinician visits. Prevalence of pain may reach 25% to 50% in community-dwelling adults and 45% to 80% in nursing home residents (Morley, 2018). Pain usually arises from musculoskeletal complaints like back and joint pain (National Academies of Sciences, Engineering, & Medicine, 2020). Headache, neuralgias from diabetes and herpes zoster, nighttime leg pain, and cancer pain are also common. Older patients are less likely to report pain, leading to undue suffering, depression, social isolation, physical disability, and loss of function (Morley, 2018). The American Geriatrics Society favors the term "persistent pain," because "chronic pain" is associated with negative stereotypes (National Academies of Sciences, Engineering, & Medicine, 2020).

Accurate assessment of pain is the basis of effective treatment and is often complicated by psychological, social, and cultural influences (Morley, 2018). Inquire about pain *each time* you meet with an older patient. Assessing pain in older adults is challenging. Patients may be reluctant to report symptoms due to the misconception that pain is part of normal aging process, fears of additional testing, costs of care and medication, denial of disease, cognitive or verbal impairments, and/or barriers of trust, language, or cultural understanding. Patients may report multiple conditions that complicate assessment. Nonetheless, evidence shows that when patients do report pain, even those with mild to moderate cognitive impairment, self-report is reliable. Ask specifically, "Are you having any pain right now? How about during the past week?" Be alert for signs of untreated pain, such as use of the terms "burning," "discomfort," or "soreness"; depressed affect; and nonverbal change in posture or gait. Many multidimensional and unidimensional pain scales are available. Unidimensional scales such as the Visual Analogue Scale, graphic pictures, and the verbal 0–10 scale have all been validated and are easy to use (Morley, 2018). For patients with cognitive deficits, the PAINAD is a validated tool of five items: breathing, negative vocalization, facial expressions, body language, and consolability

Refer to the pain scale in Chapter 7, "General Survey Including Vital Signs and Pain."

Mini Nutritional Assessment MNA®

Nestlé NutritionInstitute

Last name: First name:

Sex: Age: Weight, kg: Height, cm: Date:

Complete the screen by filling in the boxes with the appropriate numbers. Total the numbers for the final screening score.

Screening

A Has food intake declined over the past 3 months due to loss of appetite, digestive problems, chewing or swallowing difficulties?

0 = severe decrease in food intake
1 = moderate decrease in food intake
2 = no decrease in food intake ☐

B Weight loss during the last 3 months

0 = weight loss greater than 3 kg (6.6 lbs)
1 = does not know
2 = weight loss between 1 and 3 kg (2.2 and 6.6 lbs)
3 = no weight loss ☐

C Mobility

0 = bed or chair bound
1 = able to get out of bed / chair but does not go out
2 = goes out ☐

D Has suffered psychological stress or acute disease in the past 3 months?

0 = yes 2 = no ☐

E Neuropsychological problems

0 = severe dementia or depression
1 = mild dementia
2 = no psychological problems ☐

F1 Body Mass Index (BMI) (weight in kg) / (height in m)^2

0 = BMI less than 19
1 = BMI 19 to less than 21
2 = BMI 21 to less than 23
3 = BMI 23 or greater ☐

IF BMI IS NOT AVAILABLE, REPLACE QUESTION F1 WITH QUESTION F2.
DO NOT ANSWER QUESTION F2 IF QUESTION F1 IS ALREADY COMPLETED.

F2 Calf circumference (CC) in cm

0 = CC less than 31
3 = CC 31 or greater ☐

Screening score (max. 14 points)

12 - 14 points: Normal nutritional status
8 - 11 points: At risk of malnutrition
0 - 7 points: Malnourished ☐☐

References

1. Vellas B, Villars H, Abellan G, *et al.* Overview of the MNA® - Its History and Challenges. *J Nutr Health Aging.* 2006;**10**:456-465.
2. Rubenstein LZ, Harker JO, Salva A, Guigoz Y, Vellas B. Screening for Undernutrition in Geriatric Practice: Developing the Short-Form Mini Nutritional Assessment (MNA-SF). *J. Geront.* 2001; **56A**: M366-377
3. Guigoz Y. The Mini-Nutritional Assessment (MNA®) Review of the Literature - What does it tell us? *J Nutr Health Aging.* 2006; **10**:466-487.
4. Kaiser MJ, Bauer JM, Ramsch C, et al. Validation of the Mini Nutritional Assessment Short-Form (MNA®-SF): A practical tool for identification of nutritional status. *J Nutr Health Aging.* 2009; **13**:782-788.

For more information: www.mna-elderly.com

FIGURE 24-5 The Mini Nutritional Assessment. (Reprinted with permission of the Nestlé Nutrition Institute. ® Société des Produits Nestlé SA, Trademark Owners. © Société des Produits Nestlé SA 1994, Revision 2009. Vellas, B., Villars, H., Abellan, G., Soto, M. E., Rolland, Y., Guigoz, Y., Morley, J. E., Chumlea, W., Salva, A., Rubenstein, L. Z., & Garry, P. (2006). Overview of the MNA® - Its history and challenges. *The Journal of Nutrition, Health and Aging, 10*, 456–465. Rubenstein, L. Z., Harker, J. O., Salva, A., Guigoz, Y., & Vellas, B. (2001). Screening for undernutrition in geriatric practice: Developing the Short-Form Mini Nutritional Assessment (MNA-SF). *The Journals of Gerontology, 56A*, M366–377. Guigoz, Y. (2006). The Mini-Nutritional Assessment (MNA®) Review of the Literature - What does it tell us? *The Journal of Nutrition, Health and Aging, 10*, 466–487. Kaiser, M. J., Bauer, J. M., Ramsch, C., Uter, W., Guigoz, Y., Cederholm, T., Thomas, D. R., Anthony, P., Charlton, K. E., Maggio, M., Tsai, A. C., Grathwohl, D., Vellas, B., Sieber, C. C.; MNA-International Group. (2009). Validation of the Mini Nutritional Assessment Short-Form (MNA®-SF): A practical tool for identification of nutritional status. *The Journal of Nutrition, Health and Aging, 13*, 782–788. For additional information: www.mna-elderly.com.)

(American Geriatrics Society Panel on the Pharmacologic Management of Persistent Pain in Older Persons, 2009). In addition, interview caregivers or family members for relevant history of patients with severe cognitive deficits.

It is important to distinguish acute pain from persistent pain (Table 24-4) and thoroughly investigate its cause. In older adults, confusion, restlessness, fatigue, or irritability often accompany conditions causing pain. Assessing pain includes evaluation of these related conditions as well as the effect of pain on quality of life, social interactions, and functional level. Consider multidisciplinary assessment in complex cases if the cause cannot be identified and risks of disability and comorbidity are high.

TABLE 24-4 Characteristics of Acute and Persistent Pain

Acute Pain	Persistent Pain
Distinct onset	Lasts more than 3 mo
Obvious pathology	Often associated with psychological or functional impairment
Short duration	Can fluctuate in character and intensity over time
Common causes: postsurgical, trauma, headache	Common causes: arthritis, cancer, claudication, leg cramps, neuropathy, radiculopathy

Be familiar with the many modalities of pain relief, ranging from analgesics to numerous nonpharmacologic therapies, especially those that actively engage patients in their treatment plan and build self-reliance. Older adult patient education about pain has led to decreased reported pain and improved mobility (National Academies of Sciences, Engineering, & Medicine, 2020). Relaxation techniques, tai chi, acupuncture, massage, cognitive behavioral therapy, and biofeedback can reduce the use of medications and lessen the burden of polypharmacy and potential drug interactions in older adults (American Geriatrics Society Panel on the Pharmacologic Management of Persistent Pain in Older Persons, 2009).

See the 10-Minute Geriatric Screener in Table 24-2 for functional assessment.

Sexuality

Sex continues throughout the lifespan, and issues should be addressed as patients may have valid concerns requiring attention (Ali et al., 2018). The physical assessment section will address changes that occur with aging, including pain or medical conditions that may deter sexual responses such as diabetes or heart conditions. Suggestions to alleviate pain might be changes in positions, use of lubrication, heat application, and warm baths. Be sensitive to the sexual preferences of older adults, and guide them as needed to appropriate resources, including those that address the needs of the LGBTQIA community (Herr, 2011).

The PLISS IT Model has been used to initiate the discussion of sex (Smyth, 2018):

- **P**: Obtaining *p*ermission from the client to initiate sexual discussion
- **LI**: Providing the *l*imited *i*nformation needed to function sexually
- **SS**: Giving *s*pecific *s*uggestions for the individual to proceed with sexual relations
- **IT**: Providing *i*ntensive *t*herapy surrounding the issues of sexuality for that client

Urinary Incontinence

Urinary incontinence is more common among biologic females with up to one in three reporting incontinence and one in five biologic males reporting incontinence. It is estimated that over 60% of older adults in long-term care have urinary or stool incontinence (SAGE, 2020). Urinary incontinence may be related to physiologic changes of aging such as detrusor muscle weakness or the effects of BPH. Urinary incontinence is grouped into five types of incontinence: stress, overflow, urge, mixed, and functional (Annon, 1996).

During the health history, ask further questions using "OLD CART."

- *Onset:* When did the incontinence/leaking begin?
  Has it occurred before?
  How often does it occur?
  Does it occur when something else happens (e.g., sneezing, laughing, jumping)?
- *Location:* Where are you when this occurs?
- *Duration:* Does it last all day?
  Occasionally?
  Is there a pattern?
- *Characteristic symptoms:* Describe the urine (color, odor, amount, and times per day).
- *Associated manifestations:* What else is occurring? (Use the mnemonic "DRIP" that follows.) How is this affecting the quality of life?
- *Relieving factors:* Does changing the amount, type, or timing of fluid intake influence the incontinence?
- *Treatment:* Have you seen anyone for this?
  What have you done to try to improve this? Bladder training? Kegel exercises?

Nurses need to assess for transient causes of incontinence and be aware that up to 36% of older adults may develop urinary incontinence during an acute hospitalization (Annon, 1996). The "DRIP" mnemonic helps students assess potential causes of transient incontinence (Testa, 2015):

- D: Delirium
- R: Restricted mobility, retention
- I: Infection, inflammation, impaction
- P: Polyuria, pharmaceuticals

Smoking and Alcohol

Smoking is harmful at all ages. At each visit, screen older adults for their smoking habits, and assess their willingness to quit (Dowling-Castronovo & Bradway, 2017). The commitment to stop smoking may take time, but quitting is crucial for reducing risk of heart disease, pulmonary disease, malignancy, and loss of daily function.

Nurses should ask older adults about their alcohol consumption habits when obtaining the social health history. Screening for unhealthy alcohol use should occur annually in healthy older adults and when there is objective data that would indicate a suspicion (Kane et al., 2018). Recommended limits for consumption of *alcohol* are lower for adults older than 65 due to physiologic changes that alter alcohol metabolism, frequent comorbid illness, and risk of drug interactions. Older adults should have *no more than three drinks on any one day or seven drinks a week* (Centers for Disease Control and Prevention, 2020a).

More than 65% of adults over age 65 drink alcohol, and about 19% are considered at risk for excessive alcohol use. From 10% to 15% of older patients in primary care practices and up to 38% of hospitalized older adults are reported to have problematic alcohol consumption (US Preventive Services Task Force [USPSTF], 2018b).

Despite the high prevalence of alcohol use disorder, rates of detection and treatment are low. Screening all older adults for harmful alcohol use is especially important due to adverse interactions with most medications and exacerbation of comorbid illnesses, including cirrhosis, gastrointestinal bleeding or reflux disease, gout, hypertension, diabetes, insomnia, gait disorders, and depression in up to 30% of older patients (National Institute on Aging, 2020). Watch for clues of excess alcohol consumption, listed in Box 24-6, especially in older adults who present with recent bereavement or loss, pain, disability, depression, or a family history of alcohol disorders (USPSTF, 2018b).

BOX 24-6 DETECTING ALCOHOL USE DISORDERS IN OLDER ADULTS: CLINICAL CLUES

- Memory loss, cognitive impairment
- Depression, anxiety
- Neglect in hygiene, appearance
- Poor appetite, nutritional deficits
- Sleep disruption
- Hypertension refractory to therapy
- Blood glucose control issues
- Seizures refractory to therapy
- Impaired balance and gait, falls
- Recurrent gastritis or esophagitis
- Difficulty managing warfarin dosing
- Use of other addictive substances such as sedatives or narcotic analgesics, illicit drugs, nicotine

The AUDIT-C is used to determine risky drinking and has been shown to perform as well as the full AUDIT and notably better than self-reporting (Naegle, 2018). Although symptoms and signs are more subtle in older adults, making early detection more difficult, the AUDIT-C is sensitive and specific in this age group. Refer to the AUDIT-C test, Figure 4-3, in Chapter 4, "The Health History."

The AUDIT-C is scored on a scale of 0 to 12 (scores of 0 reflect no alcohol use). In men, a score of 4 or more is considered positive; in women, a score of 3 or more is considered positive. Generally, the higher the AUDIT-C score, the more likely it is that the patient's drinking is affecting their health and safety.

PHYSICAL EXAMINATION OF THE OLDER ADULT

General Survey

As the patient enters the room, how does the patient walk to the chair? Move onto the examining table? Are there changes in posture or involuntary movements? Note the patient's hygiene and dress. Assess the patient's apparent state of health, degree of vitality, and mood and affect. As you talk with the patient, decide if screening for cognitive changes is needed.

See the "Nervous System and Mental Status" section for a brief and well-validated screening tool for dementia (Bommersbach et al., 2015; Bradley et al., 2007). The Saint Louis University Mental Status (SLUMS) examination is another well-validated tool (Montreal Cognitive Assessment, 2015).

CLINICAL TIP

Undernutrition, slowed motor performance, loss of muscle mass, or weakness suggests frailty.

Kyphosis or abnormal gait can impair balance and increase risk of falls.

Flat or impoverished affect is seen in *depression, Parkinson disease,* or Alzheimer disease.

Vital Signs

Measure blood pressure using recommended techniques, checking for increased SBP and widened PP, defined as SBP minus DBP. With aging, SBP and peripheral vascular resistance increase, while DBP decreases. For adults aged 60 and older, the Eighth Joint National Committee (JNC8) recommends blood pressure targets of 150/90 mm Hg or lower but notes that if treatment results in SBP lower than 140 and is "well tolerated and without adverse effects to health or quality of life, treatment does not need to be adjusted" (Liew et al., 2015). However, in the "oldest old," those aged 80 years and older, other experts cite studies showing that blood pressure targets of 140 to less than 150/70 to 80 appear optimal for notable reductions in stroke, cardiovascular events, and all-cause mortality (James et al., 2014; Krakoff et al., 2014; Tariq, 2006).

Isolated systolic hypertension that is defined as a systolic pressure of 140 mm Hg or higher and a diastolic pressure lower than 90 mm Hg accounts for approximately 60% of hypertension in older adults (Benetos et al., 2015). This isolated hypertension increases the risk of stroke, renal failure, and heart disease.

Assess the patient for orthostatic hypotension, defined as a drop in SBP of 20 mm Hg or more and/or DBP of 10 mm Hg or more within 3 minutes of standing. Measure blood pressure and HR in two positions: supine after the patient rests for up to 10 minutes, then within 3 minutes after standing up (Bangalore et al., 2014).

Orthostatic hypotension occurs in 20% of older adults and in up to 50% of frail nursing home residents, especially when they first stand up. Symptoms include lightheadedness, weakness, unsteadiness, visual blurring, and in 20% to 30% of patients, syncope. Causes include medications, autonomic disorders, diabetes, prolonged bed rest, volume depletion, amyloidosis, postprandial state, and cardiovascular disorders (Jones, 2017).

Measure HR, RR, and temperature. The apical HR often yields better detection of arrhythmias in older patients than does the radial pulse. Use thermometers accurate for lower temperatures. Obtain oxygen saturation using a pulse oximeter.

RR of 25 or more breaths per minute may indicate lower respiratory infection, heart failure, or COPD exacerbation.

Hypothermia is more common in older adults.

Weight and height are especially important in the older adult population and necessary for calculation of the BMI. Weight is also a key clinical measure for patients with heart failure and chronic kidney disease. Weight should be measured at every visit, preferably with footwear removed. Use a stadiometer to obtain an accurate height measurement. Documented height should not be based on self-report by an older adult since adults lose on average 2 to 3 in of height, beginning in the seventh decade. Inaccurate height will result in an incorrectly calculated BMI (Mol et al., 2019).

Low weight is a key indicator of poor nutrition, seen in depression, alcoholism, cognitive impairment, malignancy, chronic organ failure (cardiac, renal, pulmonary), medication use, social isolation, poor dentition, and poverty. Rapidly increasing daily weights occur in fluid overload.

Skin

Note physiologic changes of aging, such as thinning, loss of elastic tissue and turgor, and wrinkling. Skin may be dry, flaky, rough, and often itchy (*asteatosis*), with a latticework of shallow fissures that creates a mosaic of small polygons, especially on the legs.

Observe any patchy changes in color. Check the extensor surface of the hands and forearms for white depigmented patches, or *pseudoscars*, and for well-demarcated vividly purple macules or patches, *actinic purpura* (Fig. 24-6), that may fade after several weeks.

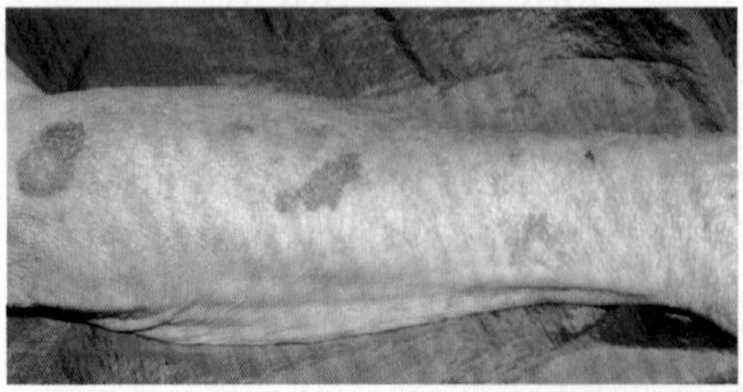

FIGURE 24-6 Actinic purpura.

Look for changes from sun exposure. Areas of skin may appear weather-beaten, thickened, yellowed, and deeply furrowed; there may be *solar or actinic lentigines*, or "liver spots," and *actinic keratoses*, superficial flattened papules covered by a dry scale.

CLINICAL TIP
Distinguish such sun-exposure lesions from a *basal cell carcinoma*, a translucent nodule that spreads and leaves a depressed center with a firm elevated border, and from a *squamous cell carcinoma*, a firm reddish-appearing lesion often emerging in a sun-exposed area. A dark-raised asymmetric lesion with irregular borders may be a *melanoma*. See Table 9-13, "Skin Tumors," and Table 9-14, "Benign and Malignant Nevi."

Inspect for the benign lesions of aging, namely, comedones, or blackheads, on the cheeks or around the eyes; *cherry angiomas*, which often appear early in adulthood; and *seborrheic keratoses*, raised yellowish lesions that feel greasy and velvety or warty.

CLINICAL TIP
Vesicular lesions occurring in a dermatomal distribution are suspicious for *herpes zoster* from reactivation of latent varicella-zoster virus in the dorsal root ganglia. Risk increases with age and impaired cell-mediated immunity (Cawley, 2017; Perlmuter et al., 2013).

In older bed-bound patients, especially when emaciated or neurologically impaired, inspect the skin thoroughly for damage or ulceration on the sacral and perianal areas, the lower back, heels, and elbows where pressure injuries commonly occur.

Pressure injuries may develop from obliteration of arteriolar and capillary blood flow to the skin or from shear force during movement across sheets or when lifted upright incorrectly. See Table 9-10, "Pressure Injuries."

Head and Neck

Perform a thorough evaluation of the head and neck.

See Chapter 10, "The Head and Neck."

Inspect the eyelids, the bony orbit, and the eye. The eye may appear recessed from atrophy of fat in the surrounding tissues. Observe any *senile ptosis* arising from weakening of the levator palpebrae, relaxation of the skin, and increased weight of the upper eyelid. Check the lower lids for **ectropion** (eyelid turns outward) or **entropion** (eyelid turns in). Note yellowing of the sclera, and *arcus senilis* which is a benign whitish ring around the limbus.

See Table 11-3, "Variations and Abnormalities of the Eyelids" and Table 11-4, "Lumps and Swelling in and around the Eyes."

Test visual acuity with correction in each eye, using a pocket Snellen chart or wall-mounted chart. Note any presbyopia, the loss of near vision arising from decreased elasticity of the lens related to aging.

One in four adults experiences some form of visual loss by age 80 (Lal et al., 2015).

Test pupillary constriction to light, both the direct and consensual response and during the near response. Then swing the light beam several times between the right and left eyes. Test the six directions of gaze. Except for possible impairment in upward gaze, extraocular movements should remain intact.

CLINICAL TIP
If the pupil dilates as the light swings over, a relative afferent pupillary defect is present, which is suspicious for optic nerve disease. Refer the patient to an ophthalmologist.

Using your ophthalmoscope, carefully examine the lenses and fundi.

The prevalence of cataracts, glaucoma, and macular degeneration all increase with age.

Using the ophthalmoscope beam, check at 1 to 2 ft for a red reflex. With the ophthalmoscope lens at +10 diopters, inspect each lens close to the eye for opacities. Do not depend on the flashlight alone because the lens may look clear superficially.

A red reflex is not seen with *cataracts*. At +10 diopters, a cataract appears white (Wilson, 2011). Cataracts are the world's leading cause of blindness. Risk factors include cigarette smoking, exposure to UVB light, high alcohol intake, diabetes, medications (including steroids), and trauma. See Table 11-5, "Opacities of the Cornea and Lens."

In older adults, the fundi lose their youthful shine and light reflections, and the arteries look narrowed, paler, straighter, and less brilliant. Assess the cup-to-disc ratio, usually 1:2 or less.

Retinal microvascular disease is linked to cerebral microvascular changes and cognitive impairment (Borooah et al., 2015; Pelletier et al., 2016).

CLINICAL TIP
An increased cup-to-disc ratio suggests *primary open-angle glaucoma (POAG)* caused by irreversible optic neuropathy and leading to loss of peripheral and central vision and blindness. Prevalence of POAG is four to five times higher in African Americans and Hispanics, though older, non-Hispanic White women are the highest in number affected (Liew et al., 2014; Wang et al., 2011).

Inspect the fundi for colloid bodies causing alterations in pigmentation, called **drusen** (Fig. 24-7).

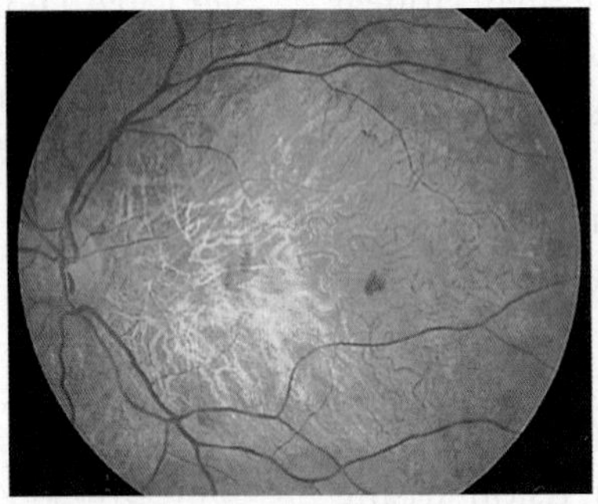

FIGURE 24-7 The fundus exhibiting drusen.

CLINICAL TIP
Macular degeneration causes poor central vision and blindness (Vajaranant et al., 2012). Types include *dry atrophic* (more common but less severe) and *wet exudative*, or neovascular. Drusen may be hard and sharply defined, or soft and confluent with altered pigmentation.

Test hearing by occluding one ear and using the whispered voice technique or an audioscope. Be sure to inspect the ear canals for cerumen, because removal of the cerumen can quickly improve hearing.

Ask if hearing loss is noticeable and if the answer is yes, proceed to audiometry testing. For those who do not notice a hearing loss, check acuity using the whispered voice test. For older adults who cannot discern pitch and frequency in the audiometer, refer to an audiologist. Recognize that this is a common finding as it is estimated that one in four older adults over age 70 may have a hearing impairment (Weinreb et al., 2014).

Examine the oral cavity for odor, appearance of the gingival mucosa, any caries, mobility of the teeth, and quantity of saliva. Inspect closely for lesions on any of the mucosal surfaces. Ask the patient to remove any dentures to check the gums for sores.

Malodor (an unpleasant smell) may occur with poor oral hygiene, periodontitis, or caries. **Gingivitis** (inflammation of the gums) accompanies periodontal disease. Dental plaque and cavitation may cause caries. For increased tooth mobility from abscesses or advanced caries, consider a referral to a dentist for tooth removal to prevent aspiration. Decreased salivation results from medications, radiation, Sjögren syndrome, or dehydration. Oral tumors can cause lesions, usually on the lateral margins of the tongue and floor of the mouth (McCabe, 2018; Ratnapriya & Chew, 2013). Older adults are retaining more of their natural teeth than in the past generations, but nurses need to be aware that disparities exist among those with limited resources (Friedman et al., 2014). A thorough oral inspection in conjunction with oral hygiene such as brushing and flossing are important interventions.

Continue with your usual examination of the thyroid gland and lymph nodes. In older adults common causes of hyperthyroidism are *Graves disease* and *toxic multinodular goiter*. Causes of hypothyroidism include autoimmune thyroiditis, followed by drugs, neck radiotherapy, thyroidectomy, radioiodine ablation, or deficiency in dietary iodine (Yellowitz & Schneiderman, 2014).

Thorax and Lungs

Complete the usual examination, observing for subtle signs of changes in pulmonary function.

Nurses can refer older adults for objective testing with spirometry, which most tolerate well (Griffin et al., 2019).

CLINICAL TIP

Increased anteroposterior diameter, purse-lipped breathing, and dyspnea with talking or minimal exertion suggest *COPD.* There is considerable overlap of asthma and COPD in older adults, heralded by nonspecific symptoms like dyspnea, cough, wheezing, and nocturnal onset.

Cardiovascular System

Review the findings from blood pressure and HR measurements.

Isolated systolic hypertension and a widened PP are cardiac risk factors, prompting a search for *left ventricular hypertrophy* (LVH).

Begin by inspecting the jugular venous pressure (JVP). Palpate the carotid upstrokes and auscultate for carotid bruits.

Carotid bruits can occur in *aortic stenosis*. The presence of bruits from *carotid stenosis* increases risk of ipsilateral stroke.

A *tortuous atherosclerotic aorta* can raise pressure in the left jugular veins by impairing emptying into the right atrium. It may also cause kinking of the carotid artery low in the neck on the right, chiefly in women with hypertension, which can be mistaken for a carotid aneurysm.

Assess the point of maximum impulse (PMI) or apical impulse, and auscultate for S_1 and S_2. Listen also for the extra sounds of S_3 and S_4. A sustained PMI is present in LVH; a diffuse PMI and an S_3 signal left ventricular dilatation from heart failure or cardiomyopathy; and an S_3 signals left ventricular dilatation from heart failure or cardiomyopathy. An S_4 often accompanies hypertension (Gambert & Steven, 2021).

Beginning in the second right interspace, listen for cardiac murmurs in all areas of auscultation (see Chapter 14, "The Cardiovascular System"). Describe the timing, shape, location of maximal intensity, radiation, intensity, pitch, and quality of each murmur you detect.

CLINICAL TIP

A systolic crescendo–decrescendo murmur in the second right interspace suggests *aortic sclerosis or aortic stenosis.* Both are associated with an increased risk of cardiovascular disease and death (Gibson et al., 2010; Goldberg, 2010).

A harsh holosystolic murmur at the apex radiating to the axilla suggests *mitral regurgitation*, the most common murmur in older adults.

Breasts and Axillae

Palpate the breasts carefully for lumps or masses. Include palpation of the tail of Spence that extends into the axilla. Examine the axillae for lymphadenopathy. Note any scaly, vesicular ulcerated lesions on or near the nipple.

CLINICAL TIP

Any lumps or masses in older women, and more rarely, in older men, mandate further investigation for possible breast cancer.

Paget disease with eczematoid scaling of the nipple is uncommon, but peaks between the ages of 50 and 60 years; this finding would be rare in the examination of an older adult (Coffey et al., 2014).

Abdomen

Inspect the abdomen for masses or visible pulsations. Auscultate for bruits over the aorta, and the renal and femoral arteries. Palpate to the right and left of the midline for aortic pulsations. Try to assess the width of the aorta by pressing more deeply with one hand on each of its lateral margins (see Chapter 16, "The Gastrointestinal and Renal Systems").

Abdominal bruits are suspicious for atherosclerotic vascular disease.

CLINICAL TIP
A widened aorta of 3 cm or greater and pulsatile mass are found in *abdominal aortic aneurysm,* especially in older male smokers. This finding requires a referral to a health care provider with a vascular specialty. The presence of an abdominal aortic aneurysm increases with age and is more common in males. This finding is common enough that a one-time ultrasound screening is recommended for males aged 65 to 75 who have a history of smoking, though screening is not recommended for females (Manning, 2013).

Peripheral Vascular System

Carefully palpate the brachial, radial, femoral, popliteal, posterior tibialis, and pedal pulses. Diminished or absent pulses are present in *peripheral arterial disease (PAD).* Confirm your findings with an office ankle–brachial index (ABI); if it is less than 0.9, the patient has PAD. ABI has a sensitivity of 70% and specificity of 90%. In patients with PAD, 30% to 60% report no leg symptoms (Sandoval-Leon et al., 2013).

See Chapter 15, "The Peripheral Vascular System and Lymphatic System."

Female Genitalia

Inspect for changes related to menopause such as thinning of the skin, atrophy of the labia, and loss of pubic hair. Note redness, discharge, lesions, prolapsed uterus, or mutilation. A prolapsed organ into the vaginal vault is best observed when the patient is standing up. The nurse must consider patient safety at all times. Postmenopausal bleeding or any new discharge are reasons for a nurse to refer the older female to a gynecologist (USPSTF, 2019).

CLINICAL TIP
Erythema with satellite lesions results from *Candida* infection; erythema with ulceration or a necrotic center is suspicious for *vulvar carcinoma.* Multifocal reddened lesions with white scaling plaques occur in extramammary *Paget disease,* a form of intraepithelial adenocarcinoma (McDermott, 2015).

Male Genitalia

Examine the penis, retracting the foreskin if present. Examine the scrotum, testes, and epididymis. Note erythema, lesions, discharge, lumps, or pain on palpation. Normal changes of aging include decreased bilateral testicular size. Older men are susceptible to epididymitis due to enlarged prostate (Perkins & King, 2012).

Findings include smegma, penile cancer, epididymitis, and scrotal hydroceles.

Musculoskeletal System

The evaluation of this system begins with leg mobility testing during the *10-Minute Geriatric Screener* (see Table 24-2) at the onset of the visit. Leg mobility is routinely tested by the "*Timed Get Up and Go,*" or *TUG test* for gait and balance, an excellent screen for risk of falling (Box 24-7). Ask the patient to get up from a chair, walk 10 ft, turn, and return to the chair. Older adults should complete this test in 10 seconds.

BOX 24-7 TIMED GET UP AND GO TEST

Performed with patient wearing regular footwear, using usual walking aid if needed, and sitting back in a chair with armrest.

On the word, "Go," the patient is asked to:

1. Stand up from the arm chair
2. Walk 3 m (in a line)
3. Turn
4. Walk back to chair
5. Sit down

Time the second effort.

Observe patient for postural stability, steppage, stride length, and sway.

Scoring:

- **Normal:** completes task in less than 10 seconds
- **Abnormal:** completes task in more than 20 seconds

Low scores correlate with good functional independence; high scores correlate with poor functional independence and higher risk of falls.

Data from Get-up and Go Test. In: Mathias, S., Nayak, U. S. L., & Isaacs, B. (1986). Balance in elderly patient: The "get-up and go" test. *Archives of Physical Medicine and Rehabilitation, 67*, 387–389; Podsiadlo, D., & Richardson, S. (1991). The timed "Up & Go": A test of basic functional mobility for frail elderly persons. *Journal of the American Geriatrics Society, 39*, 142–148; Borson, S., Scanlan, J. M., Chen, P. J., & Ganguli, M. (2003). The Mini-Cog as a screen for dementia: Validation in a population-based sample. *Journal of the American Geriatrics Society, 51*, 1451–1454; Kaufman, J. M., Lapauw, B., Mahmoud, A., T'Sjoen, G., & Huhtaniemi, I. T. (2019). Aging and the male reproductive system. *Endocrine Reviews, 40*(4), 906–972. https://doi.org/10.1210/er.2018-00178; and Miller, K. L., & Baraldi, C. A. (2012). Geriatric gynecology: Promoting health and avoiding harm. *American Journal of Obstetrics and Gynecology, 207*, 355–367.

If the patient has joint deformities, deficits in mobility, pain with movement, or a delayed "get up and go," perform a more thorough examination of individual joints and a more comprehensive neurologic examination.

Assess for degenerative joint changes in *osteoarthritis* and joint inflammation from *rheumatoid* or *gouty arthritis*.

See Chapter 18, "The Musculoskeletal System."

Nervous System and Mental Status

As with the musculoskeletal examination, begin your evaluation of the nervous system with the *10-Minute Geriatric Screener* (see Table 24-2). Carefully assess memory and affect.

Learn to distinguish delirium from depression and dementia (see Table 24-1).

Search carefully for underlying causes. The Mini-Cog screening for cognitive impairment in older adults (Figs. 24-8 and 24-9) is available at: http://www.mini-cog.com

Mini-Cog™ [111–117]

Instructions for Administration & Scoring

ID: __________ Date: ____________________

Step 1: Three Word Registration

Look directly at person and say, "Please listen carefully. I am going to say three words that I want you to repeat back to me now and try to remember. The words are [select a list of words from the versions below]. Please say them for me now." If the person is unable to repeat the words after three attempts, move on to Step 2 (clock drawing).

The following and other word lists have been used in one or more clinical studies.[1-3] For repeated administrations, use of an alternative word list is recommended.

Version 1	Version 2	Version 3	Version 4	Version 5	Version 6
Banana	Leader	Village	River	Captain	Daughter
Sunrise	Season	Kitchen	Nation	Garden	Heaven
Chair	Table	Baby	Finger	Picture	Mountain

Step 2: Clock Drawing

Say: "Next, I want you to draw a clock for me. First, put in all of the numbers where they go." When that is completed, say: "Now, set the hands to 10 past 11."

Use preprinted circle (see next page) for this exercise. Repeat instructions as needed as this is not a memory test. Move to Step 3 if the clock is not complete within three minutes.

Step 3: Three Word Recall

Ask the person to recall the three words you stated in Step 1. Say: "What were the three words I asked you to remember?" Record the word list version number and the person's answers below.

Word List Version: _____ Person's Answers: ______________ ______________ ______________

Scoring

Word Recall: _____ (0-3 points)	1 point for each word spontaneously recalled without cueing.
Clock Draw: _____ (0 or 2 points)	Normal clock = 2 points. A normal clock has all numbers placed in the correct sequence and approximately correct position (e.g., 12, 3, 6 and 9 are in anchor positions) with no missing or duplicate numbers. Hands are pointing to the 11 and 2 (11:10). Hand length is not scored. Inability or refusal to draw a clock (abnormal) = 0 points.
Total Score: _____ (0-5 points)	Total score = Word Recall score + Clock Draw score. A cut point of <3 on the Mini-Cog™ has been validated for dementia screening, but many individuals with clinically meaningful cognitive impairment will score higher. When greater sensitivity is desired, a cut point of <4 is recommended as it may indicate a need for further evaluation of cognitive status.

FIGURE 24-8 The Mini-Cog screening tool for cognitive impairment. (Mini-Cog™ © S. Borson. All rights reserved. Reprinted with permission of the author solely for clinical and eductional purposes. May not be modified or used for commercial, marketing, or research purposes without permission of the author [soob@uw.edu].)

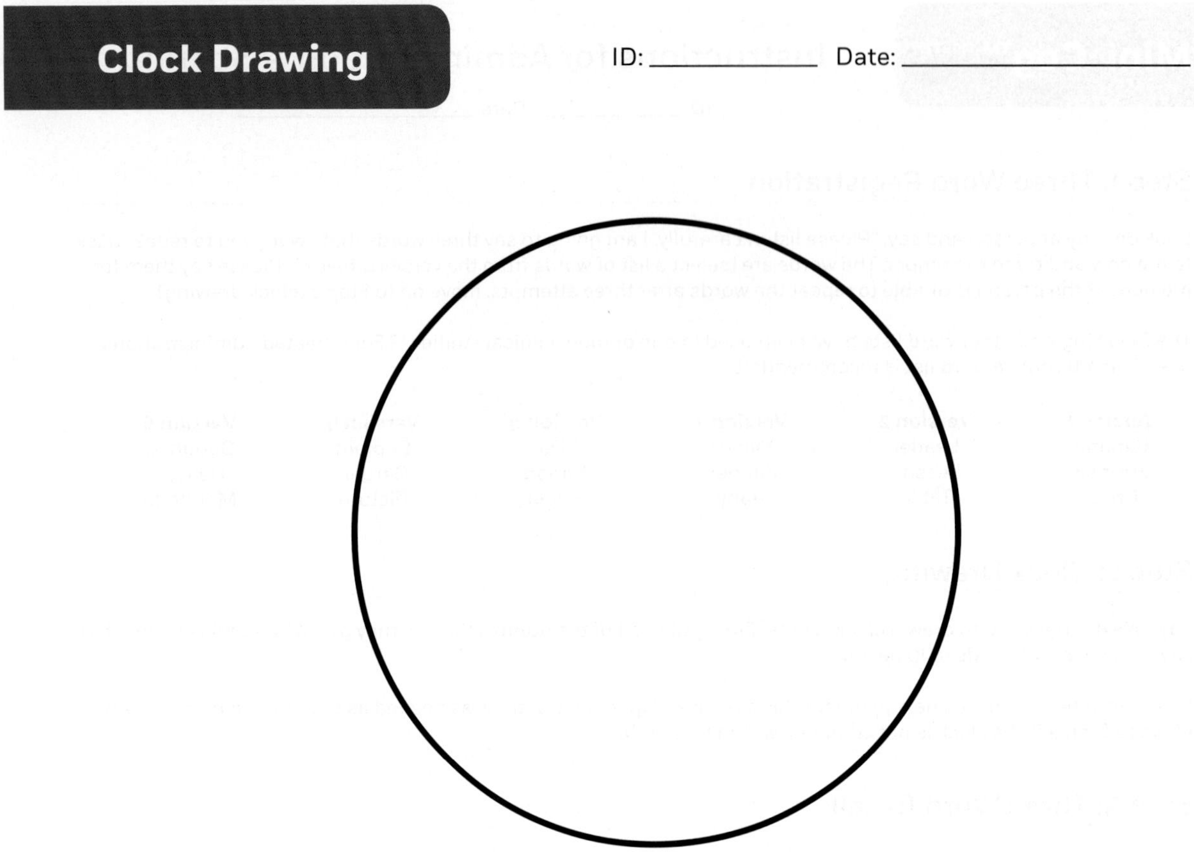
Clock Drawing ID:__________ Date:__________

Mini-Cog™ © S. Borson. All rights reserved. Reprinted with permission of the author solely for clinical and educational purposes. May not be modified or used for commercial, marketing, or research purposes without permission of the author (soob@uw.edu).
v. 01.19.16

FIGURE 24-9 A clock drawing exercise from the Mini-Cog screening tool. (Palsetia, 2018) (Mini-Cog™ © S. Borson. All rights reserved. Reprinted with permission of the author solely for clinical and eductional purposes. May not be modified or used for commercial, marketing, or research purposes without permission of the author [soob@uw.edu]).

The Montreal Cognitive Assessment (MOCA) is another screening option (Fig. 24-10). To ensure fidelity to the MOCA instrument, the creators require that clinicians now complete training to use it. Access it at https://www.mocatest.org/

The Saint Louis University Mental Status (SLUMS) is another cognitive screening tool that is widely used (Fig. 24-11). The SLUMS is an 11-item instrument that tests for cognitive function in eight domains. It is scored on a scale of 0 to 30, and the interpretation of the score is based on formal education of completion or noncompletion at the high school level (Tsoi et al., 2015).

Pay close attention to gait and balance, particularly standing balance; timed 10-ft walk; stride characteristics including width, pace, and length of stride; and careful turning. A recent study of neurologic versus nonneurologic (primarily hip and knee orthopedic) gait disorders showed that neurologic disorders like Parkinson, sensory ataxia, spastic, higher-level gait, and, particularly, multiple neurologic gait disorders tripled the risk for recurrent

Abnormalities of gait and balance, especially widening of the base, slowing and lengthening of stride, and difficulty turning, are correlated with risk for falls (Lewis, 2015; Mahlknecht et al., 2013).

NAME :
Education :   Date of birth :
Sex :   DATE :

MONTREAL COGNITIVE ASSESSMENT (MOCA)
Version 7.1 Original Version

VISUOSPATIAL / EXECUTIVE — POINTS

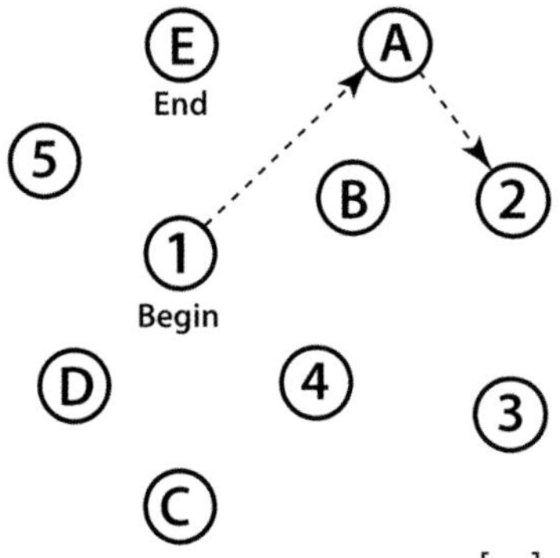

[ ]

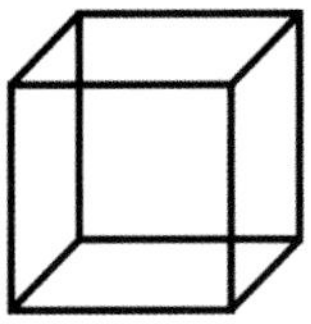

Copy cube

[ ]

Draw CLOCK (Ten past eleven)
(3 points)

[ ] Contour   [ ] Numbers   [ ] Hands

___/5

NAMING

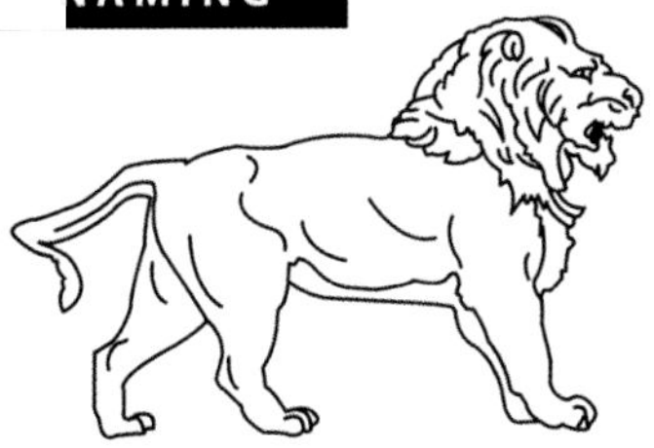

[ ]

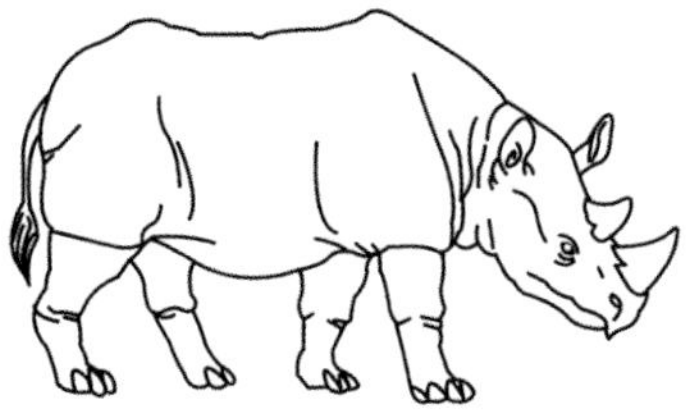

[ ]

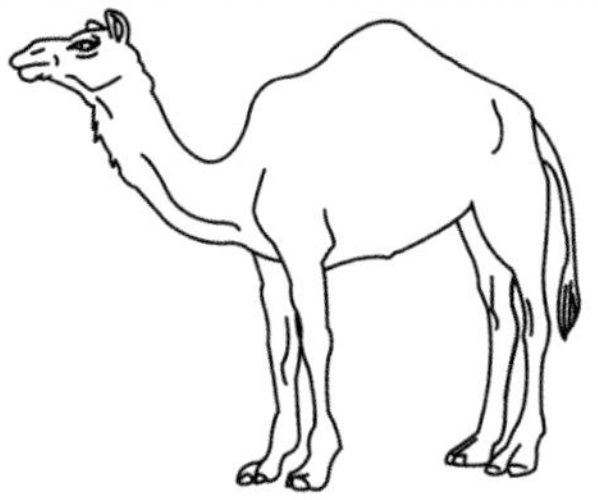

[ ]

___/3

MEMORY

Read list of words, subject must repeat them. Do 2 trials, even if 1st trial is successful. Do a recall after 5 minutes.

	FACE	VELVET	CHURCH	DAISY	RED
1st trial					
2nd trial					

No points

ATTENTION

Read list of digits (1 digit/ sec.).
Subject has to repeat them in the forward order [ ] 2 1 8 5 4
Subject has to repeat them in the backward order [ ] 7 4 2
___/2

Read list of letters. The subject must tap with his hand at each letter A. No points if ≥ 2 errors
[ ] F B A C M N A A J K L B A F A K D E A A A J A M O F A A B
___/1

Serial 7 subtraction starting at 100 [ ] 93 [ ] 86 [ ] 79 [ ] 72 [ ] 65
4 or 5 correct subtractions: **3 pts**, 2 or 3 correct: **2 pts**, 1 correct: **1 pt**, 0 correct: **0 pt**
___/3

LANGUAGE

Repeat : I only know that John is the one to help today. [ ]
The cat always hid under the couch when dogs were in the room. [ ]
___/2

Fluency / Name maximum number of words in one minute that begin with the letter F [ ] ____ (N ≥ 11 words)
___/1

ABSTRACTION

Similarity between e.g. banana - orange = fruit [ ] train – bicycle [ ] watch - ruler
___/2

DELAYED RECALL

Has to recall words	FACE	VELVET	CHURCH	DAISY	RED	Points for UNCUED recall only
WITH NO CUE	[ ]	[ ]	[ ]	[ ]	[ ]	
Optional: Category cue						
Optional: Multiple choice cue						

___/5

ORIENTATION

[ ] Date [ ] Month [ ] Year [ ] Day [ ] Place [ ] City
___/6

© Z.Nasreddine MD   **www.mocatest.org**   Normal ≥26 / 30   TOTAL ___/30
Add 1 point if ≤ 12 yr edu

Administered by: ____________________

FIGURE 24-10 The Montreal Cognitive Assessment. (Copyright Z. Nasreddine, MD. Reproduced with permission. Copies are available at www.mocatest.org.)

VAMC
SLUMS EXAMINATION

Questions about this assessment tool? E-mail aging@slu.edu

Name____________________ Age__________

Is the patient alert?__________ Level of education__________

__/1 (1) **1. What day of the week is it?**

__/1 (1) **2. What is the year?**

__/1 (1) **3. What state are we in?**

4. Please remember these five objects. I will ask you what they are later.

Apple Pen Tie House Car

5. You have $100 and you go to the store and buy a dozen apples for $3 and a tricycle for $20.

(1) **How much did you spend?**

__/3 (2) **How much do you have left?**

6. Please name as many animals as you can in one minute.

__/3 (0) 0-4 animals (1) 5-9 animals (2) 10-14 animals (3) 15+ animals

__/5 **7. What were the five objects I asked you to remember? 1 point for each one correct.**

8. I am going to give you a series of numbers and I would like you to give them to me backwards. For example, if I say 42, you would say 24.

__/2 (0) 87 (1) 648 (1) 8537

9. This is a clock face. Please put in the hour markers and the time at ten minutes to eleven o'clock.

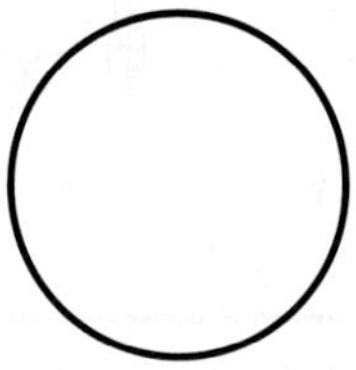

(2) Hour markers okay

__/4 (2) Time correct

(1) **10. Please place an X in the triangle.**

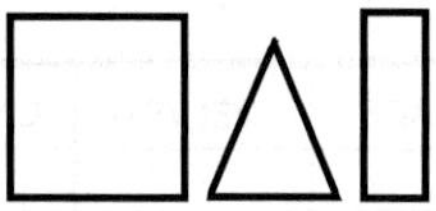

__/2 (1) **Which of the above figures is largest?**

11. I am going to tell you a story. Please listen carefully because afterwards, I'm going to ask you some questions about it.

Jill was a very successful stockbroker. She made a lot of money on the stock market. She then met Jack, a devastatingly handsome man. She married him and had three children. They lived in Chicago. She then stopped work and stayed at home to bring up her children. When they were teenagers, she went back to work. She and Jack lived happily ever after.

(2) **What was the female's name?** (2) **What work did she do?**

__/8 (2) **When did she go back to work?** (2) **What state did she live in?**

______ **TOTAL SCORE**

SCORING		
HIGH SCHOOL EDUCATION		LESS THAN HIGH SCHOOL EDUCATION
27-30	NORMAL	25-30
21-26	MILD NEUROCOGNITIVE DISORDER	20-24
1-20	DEMENTIA	1-19

CLINICIAN'S SIGNATURE ________ DATE ________ TIME ________

SH Tariq, N Tumosa, JT Chibnall, HM Perry III, and JE Morley. The Saint Louis University Mental Status (SLUMS) Examination for detecting mild cognitive impairment and dementia is more sensitive than the Mini-Mental Status Examination (MMSE) - A pilot study. *Am J Geriatr Psych* 14:900-10, 2006.

FIGURE 24-11 The Veterans Administration Medical Center (VAMC) Saint Louis University Mental Status assessment tool. (Reprinted from Tariq, S. H.,Tumosa, N., Chibnall, J. T., Perry III, H. M., & Morley, J. E. *The American Journal of Geriatric Psychiatry, 14*(11), 900–910. The Saint Louis University Mental Status (SLUMS) Examination for detecting mild cognitive impairment and dementia is more sensitive than the Mini-Mental Status Examination (MMSE) - A pilot study, 900–910. Copyright 2006. https://doi.org/10.1097/01.JGP.0000221510.33817.86.)

falls (St. Louis University Mental Status, 2020). Investigators are looking at the neurobiology of gait disorders as markers of preclinical dementia and other neurologic conditions that may lead to earlier diagnosis and new preventive strategies (Feliciano et al., 2013).

When gait abnormalities are detected, pursue a more detailed neurologic examination (Stevens & Phelan, 2013; Tinetti & Kumar, 2010). Distinguishing neurologic changes of aging from abnormal findings is challenging since neurologic abnormalities without identifiable disease are common in the older population and increase with age, occurring in up to 50% of older adults (Jankovic, 2015). Examples of age-related abnormalities include unequal pupil size, decreased arm swing and spontaneous movements, increased leg rigidity and abnormal gait, presence of the snout and grasp reflexes, decreased deep tendon reflexes, and decreased toe vibratory sense (Jankovic, 2015).

Examine for evidence of ***T***remor, ***R***igidity, ***A***kinesia, and ***P***ostural instability, or "TRAP," which are several of the most common features of Parkinson disease (Lam, 2011). Also look for bradykinesia, the most characteristic clinical sign, and micrographia (abnormally small or cramped handwriting), shuffling "freezing" gait, difficulty rising from a chair, and a stone-like face that does not demonstrate emotion.

Essential tremor is bilateral and symmetric, with a positive family history and commonly diminished by alcohol (Erro & Stamelou, 2018). Essential tremors occur with purposeful movement, and this can be differentiated from Parkinsonian tremors that occur at rest.

Persistent blinking after tapping on the forehead, and difficulty walking heel-to-toe in *Parkinson disease* are also more common.

These findings are seen in *Parkinson disease,* found in approximately 60,000 new cases a year and affecting about 1 million people in the United States (Nair & Sabbagh, 2015). Tremor is of slow frequency and occurs at rest, with a "pill-rolling" quality. It is aggravated by stress and inhibited during sleep or movement. Prodromal nonmotor symptoms including depression, rapid eye movement behavior disorder, and daytime sleepiness (Lam, 2011).

In summary, the assessment of the older adult does not follow the traditional format of the history and physical examination. It calls for enhanced techniques of interviewing, special emphasis on daily function and key topics related to older adult health, and a focus on functional assessment during the physical examination.

RECORDING YOUR FINDINGS

As you read through the physical examination in Box 24-8, you will notice some atypical findings. Try to test yourself, and see if you can interpret these findings in the context of all you have learned about the examination of the older adult.

BOX 24-8 RECORDING THE PHYSICAL EXAMINATION—THE OLDER ADULT

Mr. J, an 82-year-old man appears healthy but overweight with positive muscle bulk and tone. He is alert and interactive with recall of his life history. Accompanied by his son.

Vital Signs

Ht (without shoes) 5′10″ (178 cm). Wt (dressed) 195 lb. BMI 28. BP 145/88 right arm, supine; 154/94 left arm, supine. Orthostatic BP without changes. HR 98, regular. RR 18, regular. Temperature (oral) 98.6°F.

10-Minute Geriatric Screener

Vision. Patient reports difficulty reading. Visual acuity 20/60 (R eye), 20/40 (L eye) on Snellen chart with glasses.

Needs further evaluation for glasses

Hearing. Whisper test R with difficulty, L with increased difficulty, third attempt. Cannot hear 1,000 or 2,000 Hz with audioscope in either ear.

Needs further evaluation for hearing

Leg Mobility. Can walk 10 ft briskly, turn, walk back to chair, and sit down in 9 seconds.

Urinary Incontinence. Has lost urine and gotten wet on 20 separate days in the past 2 months.

Needs further evaluation for incontinence, including "DRIP" assessment, referral for prostate examination, bladder scan, and postvoid residual, which is normally ≤50 mL (requires bladder catheterization)

Nutrition. Has lost 15 lb over the past 6 months without trying.

Needs nutritional screen

Memory. Can remember three items after 1 minute.

Depression. Does not often feel sad or depressed.

Physical Disability. Can walk fast but cannot ride a bicycle (never learned). Can do moderate but not heavy work around the house. Can go shopping for groceries or clothes. Can go to places out of walking distance (son drives). Can bathe each day without difficulty. Can dress independently, including buttoning, zippering, and tying shoes.

Consider exercise regimen with strength and balance

Physical Examination

Skin, Hair, Nails. Tan, warm and moist. 1.5 cm solar lentigo above R eyebrow. Gray hair thinning at crown, dry with moderate amount of flakes; gray hairs evenly distributed over body. Nails without clubbing or cyanosis, slightly yellow and thick.

Head, Eyes, Ears, Nose, Throat (HEENT). Scalp without lesions. Skull NC/AT (normocephalic/atraumatic).

Eyes—symmetrical, lids—close BL, no ptosis or edema, conjunctiva pink, sclera muddy, iris brown. Lacrimal apparatus moist without additional drainage PERRLA (pupils equal, round, reactive to light and accommodation), 2 mm constricting to 1 mm BL. EOMs (extraocular movements) intact. Disc margins sharp, without hemorrhages or exudates. Mild arteriolar narrowing. Snellen with corrective glasses on 20/60 (R eye), 20/40 (L eye).

Ears—pinna without lumps, lesions, or tenderness; TMs (tympanic membranes) with cone of light, minimal tan, sticky cerumen BL. Weber midline, AC ≥ BC, whisper test R with difficulty, L, third attempt.

Nose—patent BL, mucosa and turbinates pink. No odor, frontal or maxillary sinus tenderness, exudates, polyps or bleeding. Septum midline.

Lips—pink, moist, without lesions or ulcerations. Oral mucosa pink, moist, without lesions or bleeding. Dentition fair, some loose teeth. Caries present. Tongue midline, slight beefy redness, no lesions. Uvula midline. Pharynx without exudates.

Neck. Supple. Trachea midline. Thyroid lobes slightly enlarged, no nodules.

Lymph Nodes. No preauricular, postauricular, occipital, tonsillar, submandibular, submental, superficial, posterior cervical, deep cervical chain, supraclavicular, cervical, axillary, epitrochlear, or inguinal lymph nodes.

BOX 24-8 RECORDING THE PHYSICAL EXAMINATION—THE OLDER ADULT (*Continued*)

Thorax and Lungs. A&P (anterior and posterior) thorax symmetric without retraction. Mild kyphosis. No tenderness, crepitus or lesions. Positive tactile fremitus. Lungs resonant throughout. Equal expansion. Diaphragmatic excursion descends 4 cm BL (bilateral). Vesicular breath sounds in all fields. No adventitious sounds.

Cardiovascular. R JVP 2 cm at 30 degrees. Carotid upstrokes brisk, without bruits. PMI 2 cm in diameter, tapping, in the fifth ICS L MCL (intercostal space, left, midclavicular line). II/VI harsh holosystolic murmur at the apex, radiating to the axilla. No S_3, S_4, or other murmurs.

Abdomen. Protuberant, symmetric without lesions, peristalsis, pulsations or increased vasculature. Active bowel sounds, no aortic, renal or iliac bruits. Soft, nontender. No masses or hepatosplenomegaly. Liver span 7 cm in R MCL; edge smooth and palpable. No CVAT (costal vertebral angle tenderness).

Genitourinary. Circumcised male. No penile lesions. Testes descended BL, smooth without masses or tenderness.

Extremities. Upper and lower—warm, without edema, bruising, pain, or increased vascularity.

Peripheral Vascular. BL radial, brachial, femoral, popliteal, dorsalis pedis, and posterior tibial pulses 2+ and symmetric.

Musculoskeletal. Mild degenerative changes in spine and at the knees, with quadriceps wasting. FROM in all joints. Motor: Decreased quadriceps bulk. Tone intact. Strength 4/5 throughout.

Neurologic. O×4 (person, place, time, situation), dressed appropriately for the weather, good spirits. MOCA score 27. Cranial nerves II–XII intact. BL RAMs, finger-to-nose sequence intact. Gait with widened base. Sensation intact to pinprick, light touch, position, and vibration (upper/lower extremities intact). Romberg negative. BL biceps, triceps, brachioradialis, knee, and ankle reflexes 2+ and symmetric, with plantar response.

HEALTH PROMOTION AND COUNSELING

Important topics for health promotion and counseling of the older adult include:

- When to screen
- Vision and hearing
- Exercise
- Safety, including fall assessment
- Immunizations
- Cancer screening
- Depression
- Dementia, mild cognitive impairment, and cognitive decline
- Older adult mistreatment and abuse
- Advanced directives and palliative care

When to Screen

As more adults live into their 80s and beyond, decisions about screening become more complex, and the evidence base for screening decisions becomes more limited (International Tremor Foundation, 2010; Parkinson's Disease Foundation, 2020). The aging population is physiologically heterogeneous, many with numerous chronic diseases but also many with delayed or absent disability. Moreover, level of function in "successful aging" does not always parallel the number of chronic ailments, and there are substantial regional gaps in availability and use of preventive services (International Tremor Foundation, 2010). Although there is relative consensus about immunization recommendations and falls prevention, screening for specific disease states remains more controversial. In general, individual screening decisions should be based on each older adult's health and functional status, including presence of comorbidities rather than age alone, life expectancy versus the course of the disease, and most importantly, patient preferences (International Tremor Foundation, 2010).

The American Geriatrics Society recommends a six-step approach to screening decisions (International Tremor Foundation, 2010):

1. Condition being screened for must be serious and prevalent in the population tested.
2. Disease should have an asymptomatic phase that can be detected by screening.
3. Screening must be safe, sensitive, and specific.
4. Effective treatment available early in the disease course results in lower morbidity and mortality than treatment after symptoms develop.
5. Screening costs should be acceptable.
6. Ideally, screening should have been found effective in a randomized controlled trial.

If life expectancy is short, give priority to treatment that benefits the patient in the time that remains. Consider deferring screening if it overburdens the older adults who have multiple medical problems, shortened life expectancy, or dementia. Tests that help with prognosis and planning may still be warranted even if the patient does not want to pursue treatment (Gestuvo, 2012).

Vision and Hearing

Screening for age-related changes in *vision* and *hearing* is important in helping older adults maintain optimal function as they are vital sensory modalities for daily living. They are key items in the 10-Minute Geriatric Screener (see Table 24-2).

- Test *vision* objectively using an eye chart.

- Asking the patient about any *hearing* loss is effective for screening, then proceed to the whisper test and more formal testing if indicated. Among adults aged 65 to 69 years, 1% have visual impairment, increasing to 17% of those over age 80 years. About a third of adults over age 65 years have hearing loss, increasing to 80% in those over age 80 years.

See Chapter 12, "Ear, Nose, Mouth, and Throat," for techniques for assessing hearing.

Exercise

Exercise is one of the most effective ways to promote healthy aging. Abundant literature documents the many benefits of physical activity in older adults, even in those who are frail (American Geriatrics Society, 2020; Eckstrom et al., 2013; Hötting & Röder, 2013). These include a "decrease in all-cause mortality; reduced risk of functional limitation and role limitation, falls, hypertension, diabetes, colorectal cancer, and breast cancer; and improvement in cognitive function, physical function, quality of life, gait speed, balance, and performance of activities of daily living" as well as preservation of cognition (Buchman et al., 2012).

Recommendations emphasize combining aerobic exercise with graded resistance training in major muscle groups to increase strength. Guidelines from the Centers for Disease Control and Prevention (CDC) are listed in Box 24-9. The CDC website provides information on higher targets for exercise and explanations of aerobic and strength training. For help with exercise plans, consult the exercise in medicine program of the American College of Sports Medicine (Lee et al., 2015). The many benefits of individualized, supervised exercise plans usually outweigh the risks of joint pain, falls, and cardiac events. Physical activity needs to be planned with the older adult, and an effective plan is one that the person is at least 70% confident that they can engage fully (Chou et al., 2012).

BOX 24-9 EXERCISE RECOMMENDATIONS FOR OLDER ADULTS

Adults need at least:

- 2 hours and 30 minutes (150 minutes) of moderate-intensity aerobic activity (i.e., brisk walking) every week *and*
- muscle-strengthening activities on 2 or more days a week that work all major muscle groups (legs, hips, back, abdomen, chest, shoulders, and arms).

OR

- 1 hour and 15 minutes (75 minutes) of vigorous-intensity aerobic activity (i.e., jogging or running) every week *and*
- muscle-strengthening activities on 2 or more days a week that work all major muscle groups (legs, hips, back, abdomen, chest, shoulders, and arms).

OR

- an equivalent mix of moderate- and vigorous-intensity aerobic activity *and*
- muscle-strengthening activities on 2 or more days a week that work all major muscle groups (i.e., legs, hips, back, abdomen, chest, shoulders, and arms).

Data from U.S. Department of Health and Human Services. (2018). *Physical activity guidelines for Americans* (2nd ed.). U.S. Department of Health and Human Services, Chapter 5: Active Older Adults. Retrieved November 1, 2020, from https://health.gov/sites/default/files/2019-09/Physical_Activity_Guidelines_2nd_edition.pdf#page=68; and American College of Sports Medicine. (2021). Health care providers action guide: How to implement exercise is medicine in your practice. Retrieved May 24, 2021, from https://www.exerciseismedicine.org/support_page.php/provider-action-guide/

Safety, Including Fall Risk Assessment

Falls are the most common cause of both fatal and nonfatal injuries in adults over 65 years of age. They are costly in terms of financially, physically, emotionally, and socially. Nonfatal fall injuries incur costs about $50 billion and fatal falls incur costs of $754 million (Crookham, 2013). Many have hip fractures and traumatic brain injuries that impact daily function and independence. Emergency room visits and deaths are most likely to involve yard and garden equipment, ladders and step stools, personal use items like hair dryers and flammable clothing, and bathroom and sports injuries. Encourage older adults to adopt corrective measures (Box 24-10) for poor lighting, chairs at awkward heights, slippery or irregular surfaces, and environmental hazards.

BOX 24-10 HOME SAFETY TIPS FOR OLDER ADULTS

- Install bright lighting and lightweight curtains or shades.
- Install handrails and lights on all staircases. Pathways and walkways should be well-lit.
- Remove items that cause tripping like papers, books, clothes, and shoes from stairs and walkways.
- Remove or secure small throw rugs and other rugs with double-sided tape.
- Wear shoes both inside and outside the house. Avoid bare feet and wearing slippers.
- Store medications safely.
- Keep commonly used items in cabinets that are easy to reach without using a step stool.
- Install grab bars and nonslip mats or safety strips in baths and showers.
- Repair faulty plugs and electrical cords.
- Install carbon monoxide and smoke alarms and have a plan for escaping fire.
- Secure all firearms.
- Have a medical alert device/system for emergency contacts or easy access to 911.

Source: U.S. Department of Health and Human Services. (2018). Chapter 5. Active older adults. In: *Physical activity guidelines for Americans* (2nd ed.). U.S. Department of Health and Human Services. https://health.gov/sites/default/files/2019-09/Physical_Activity_Guidelines_2nd_edition.pdf#page=68

Evidence links falls to morbidity and mortality in our older population. Each year, approximately 35% to 40% of healthy community-dwelling older adults experience falls. Incidence rates in nursing homes and hospitals are almost three times higher with related injuries in approximately 25% of patients. Loss of confidence from fear of falling and postfall anxiety further impair full recovery (Centers for Disease Control and Prevention, 2021).

Fall-related assessments should include details about the how the fall occurred, especially from witnesses, and identification of risk factors, medical comorbidities, medications, functional status, and environmental risks—coupled with interventions for prevention (Centers for Disease Control and Prevention, 2021). Gait velocity is also emerging as a significant predictor of falls and related adverse events (Florence et al., 2018). The Hendrich II Fall Risk Model tool (Fig. 24-12) is able to screen for those at risk of falling (Schoene et al., 2019). Effective single interventions include gait and balance training and exercise to strengthen muscles, reduction of home hazards, discontinuation of psychotropic medications, and multifactorial assessment with targeted interventions. Additional useful strategies include addressing change in postural blood pressure, attention to concurrent acute illness, reduction in medications to fewer than four, detection of sensory neuropathy and impairment of proprioception, investigation of any episodes of syncope, patient and family education, treatment of osteoporosis, and possible use of hip protectors.

Hendrich II Fall Risk Model ™

RISK FACTOR	RISK POINTS	SCORE
Confusion/Disorientation/Impulsivity	4	
Symptomatic Depression	2	
Altered Elimination	1	
Dizziness/Vertigo	1	
Gender (Male)	1	
Any Administered Antiepileptics (anticonvulsants): (Carbamazepine, Divalproex Sodium, Ethotoin, Ethosuximide, Felbamate, Fosphenytoin, Gabapentin, Lamotrigine, Mephenytoin, Methsuximide, Phenobarbital, Phenytoin, Primidone, Topiramate, Trimethadione, Valproic Acid)[1]	2	
Any Administered Benzodiazepines:[2] (Alprazolam, Chloridiazepoxide, Clonazepam, Clorazepate Dipotassium, Diazepam, Flurazepam, Halazepam[3], Lorazepam, Midazolam, Oxazepam, Temazepam, Triazolam)	1	
Get-Up-and-Go Test: "Rising from a Chair" If unable to assess, monitor for change in activity level, assess other risk factors, document both on patient chart with date and time.		
Ability to rise in single movement - No loss of balance with steps	0	
Pushes up, successful in one attempt	1	
Multiple attempts but successful	3	
Unable to rise without assistance during test If unable to assess, document this on the patient chart with the date and time.	4	
(A score of 5 or greater = High Risk)	TOTAL SCORE	

On-going Medication Review Updates:

Levetiracetam (Keppra) was not assessed during the original research conducted to create the Hendrich Fall Risk Model. As an antieptileptic, levetiracetam does have a side effect of somnolence and dizziness which contributes to its fall risk and should be scored (effective June 2010).

The study did not include the effect of benzodiazepine-like drugs since they were not on the market at the time. However, due to their similarity in drug structure, mechanism of action and drug effects, they should also be scored (effective January 2010).

Halazepam was included in the study but is no longer available in the United States (effective June 2010).

Upright Fall Prevention Program

V2012.1

FIGURE 24-12 The Henrich II Fall Risk Model.

Immunizations

Vaccinations recommended for older adults include for influenza; for pneumonia, both the pneumococcal conjugate vaccine (PCV13) and 23 valent pneumococcal polysaccharide vaccine (PPSV23) (PPSV23 is administered 1 year following PCV13); for herpes zoster (shingles); and for tetanus/diphtheria and pertussis (Tdap and Td). Older adults who serve as caregivers for young children should have the Tdap vaccination to protect against contracting pertussis. If an older adult has not had a Tdap vaccine in the past, they require a one-time dose. Additional information related to the COVID-19 vaccination recommendation is also available. The immunization schedule is updated annually. For the most up-to-date recommendations, consult the latest guidelines and contraindications provided by the CDC at

See also Chapter 13, "The Respiratory System."

http://www.cdc.gov/vaccines/schedules/hcp/adult.html (Hoffman, 2018). Provide information on acquiring immunizations to all older adults, especially encouraging Hispanic and African American older adults whose overall immunization rates remain low (Henrich, 2020).

Cancer Screening

Cancer screening recommendations for older adults remain controversial. The American Geriatrics Society states "It is important to consider a patient's remaining life expectancy, comorbidities, risk of disease, preferences, and cognitive and functional status when deciding which preventive health measures to offer. If the natural history of the disease is greater than the individual's remaining expected lifespan, screening is not indicated" (Centers for Disease Control and Prevention, 2021).

Older adults need to know that there are potential risks with specific screening such as a colonoscopy, and that consideration should focus on what is important to the patient and their family. Recent, more complex published frameworks include "weighing quantitative information, such as risk of cancer death and likelihood of beneficial and adverse screening outcomes, as well as qualitative factors, such as individual patients' values and preferences" (Centers for Disease Control and Prevention, 2021). The current recommendations of the USPSTF target straightforward age cutoffs and are summarized in Box 24-11 (Moran et al., 2017).

BOX 24-11 USPSTF SCREENING RECOMMENDATIONS FOR OLDER ADULTS

- Breast cancer (2016): Recommends mammography every 2 years for women aged 50 to 74 and cites insufficient evidence for screening women aged 75 years or older.
- Cervical cancer (2018): Recommends against routine screening for women over age 65 if they have had adequate recent screening with normal Papanicolaou (Pap) smears and are not otherwise at high risk for cervical cancer based on fair evidence. Certain considerations may also support screening in women older than 65 years who are otherwise at high risk (e.g., patients with a history of high-grade precancerous lesions or cervical cancer, in utero exposure to diethylstilbestrol, a compromised immune system).
- Colorectal cancer (2016): Recommends screening with colonoscopy every 10 years, sigmoidoscopy every 5 years with high-sensitivity fecal occult blood tests (FOBTs) every 3 years, or FOBTs every year beginning at age 50 through age 75. The decision to screen for colorectal cancer in adults aged 76 to 85 should be an individual one, taking into account the patient's overall health and prior screening history. Adults in this age group who have never been screened for colorectal cancer are more likely to benefit.
- Prostate cancer (2018): For men aged 55 to 69, the decision to undergo periodic prostate-specific antigen (PSA)-based screening for prostate cancer should be an individual one. Before deciding whether to be screened, men should have an opportunity to discuss the potential benefits and harms of screening with their clinician and to incorporate their values and preferences in the decision. The USPSTF recommends against PSA-based screening for prostate cancer in men 70 years and older.
- Lung cancer (2013): For adults aged 55 to 80 with a 30-pack/year smoking history, and those who currently smoke or have quit within the past 15 years, annual screening with low-dose computed tomography is recommended. Screening should be discontinued once a person has not smoked for 15 years or develops a health problem that substantially limits life expectancy or the ability or willingness to have curative lung surgery. Recommendations are to stop at ages 75 to 80.
- Skin cancer (2016): States that evidence is insufficient to balance the benefits and harms of whole-body skin examination.

Data from https://www.uspreventiveservicestaskforce.org/uspstf/recommendation-topics/uspstf-and-b-recommendations

HPV testing has been added to screen women for infections that increase the chance of getting Cerv. Ca. Women with negative HPV have less risk and longer screening test intervals.

Depression

See Chapter 19, "Mental Status and Mental Health Assessment."

Depression affects up to 2 million older adults in the United States, and it is often unreported and undertreated; 42% of surveyed older adults responded that depression is a normal phenomenon of aging (Walter & Covinsky, 2001). Prevalence rises in those with multiple comorbidities and hospitalizations. Screening for the general adult population, with services in place for diagnosis, treatment, and follow-up, is now recommended by the USPSTF (2016) and requires only one or two questions. The single screening question, "Do you often feel sad or depressed?" has a sensitivity of 69% and specificity of 90%. Two screening questions are 100% sensitive and 77% specific:

- "Over the past 2 weeks, have you felt down, depressed, or hopeless?" (screens for depressed mood)
- "Over the past 2 weeks, have you felt little interest or pleasure in doing things?" (screens for anhedonia)

Positive responses should prompt further investigation with scales such as the Geriatric Depression Scale or the nine-item Patient Health Questionnaire (PHQ-9) (Siu, 2016; Taylor, 2014). Depressed men over age 65 are at increased risk for suicide and require particularly careful evaluation. Effective treatment for older adults both reduces morbidity and extends life. Treatment may include exercise, supportive and group therapy, and/or medication (Walter & Covinsky, 2001).

Dementia, Mild Cognitive Impairment, and Cognitive Decline

Dementia is "an acquired condition that is characterized by a decline in at least two cognitive domains (e.g., loss of memory, attention, language, or visuospatial or executive functioning) that is severe enough to affect social or occupational functioning." Affected patients may also exhibit behavioral and psychological symptoms. In the *Diagnostic and Statistical Manual of Mental Disorders 5* (*DSM-5*), dementia is classified as a "major neurocognitive disorder" (Maurer, 2012). The major dementia syndromes include Alzheimer's Disease (AD), vascular dementia, frontotemporal dementia, dementia with Lewy bodies, Parkinson disease with dementia, and dementia of mixed etiology. AD, the predominant form, affects 11% of Americans over the age of 65, or roughly 5.1 million people; more than two thirds are women (Kroenke et al., 2001). By 2050, the prevalence is estimated to increase to 13.8 million cases. A nurse needs to be aware of the overall prevalence of dementia, though current evidence is insufficient to assess the balance of benefits and harms of screening for cognitive impairment in older adults (American Psychiatric Association, 2013). Risk factors include advancing age, family history, and the gene mutation apolipoprotein E (APOE) ε4. Risk of AD more than doubles in first-degree relatives. Risk doubles in the presence of one APOE ε4 allele and increases fivefold or more in the presence of two alleles, although only 2% of the population carries these genes (Alzheimer's Association, 2020).

The diagnosis of AD is challenging because the mechanisms of disease are still under intense investigation; the absence of a consistent and uniformly applied definition of disease hampers investigation of risk factors; between 60% and 90% of patients with AD have coexisting ischemic disease; and distinguishing *age-related cognitive decline* from *mild cognitive impairment* and AD can be subtle. In addition, delirium and depression can further complicate a diagnosis of dementia, and conversely delirium is difficult to determine in an older adult who has dementia (Blass & Rabins, 2014; USPSTF, 2020). Once you identify cognitive changes, the steps in Box 24-12 are helpful for planning patient care.

See Table 24-1, "Delirium and Dementia."

BOX 24-12 CARING FOR PATIENTS WITH ALTERED COGNITION

- Obtain collateral information from family members and caregivers.
- Consider formal neuropsychological testing.
- Investigate contributing factors such as medications; metabolic abnormalities; depression; delirium; and other medical and psychiatric conditions, including vascular risk from diabetes and hypertension.
- Counsel families about the challenges for caregivers. The NIH Senior Health website at http://nihseniorhealth.gov/alzheimerscare/afterthediagnosis/01.html details resources for caregiving help designed specifically for caregivers (Marcantonio, 2011). Review household safety measures that were noted in Box 24-11.
- Learn the laws about reporting *drivers with dementia* in your state. The American Geriatrics Society has developed a tool kit regarding the screening of older adults and for driving and how to speak with older adults and their caregivers about when to screen and how to screen (Inouye, 2018). There is not one specific algorithm for driving safety and driving cessation as underlying quantitative evidence linking assessment to road safety is limited. A 2013 Cochrane review details the pitfalls of disqualifying impaired drivers, which can lead to depression and social withdrawal if disqualification is premature (National Institutes of Health, 2018). The review concludes that for drivers with dementia, there is no good evidence that neuropsychological or on-road assessment will maintain mobility and improve safety. The authors call for more research to develop assessment tools "that can reliably identify unsafe drivers with dementia in an office setting" and determine what changes in function provide a threshold for disqualification, as no single validated test is available.
- Encourage patient and family discussion of appointing a health care proxy and arranging for power of attorney, health care power of attorney, and advance directives while the patient can still contribute to active decision making.

Older Adult Mistreatment and Abuse

Screen vulnerable older adults for possible *older adult mistreatment*, which includes physical abuse, psychological abuse, neglect, exploitation, and abandonment. Prevalence ranges from 5% to 10%, depending on the population studied, and is even higher among older adults with depression and dementia (American Geriatrics Society, 2019a; Martin et al., 2013). Many cases are undetected due to the patient's fear of reprisal, physical or cognitive inability to report, and unwillingness to expose the abuser; 80% to 90% of perpetrators are family members. Self-neglect, or the behavior of an older adult that threatens their own health and safety, is also a growing national concern and represents more than 50% of adult protective service referrals. Although several screening instruments are available, no valid reliable screening tools to identify abuse of vulnerable and/or older adults in the primary care setting are validated and therefore cited insufficient evidence for recommending screening is missing (Wang et al., 2015). Consequently, a careful history and high index of suspicion are important. Assess for physical signs, such as bruising, black eyes, fractures, bleeding, lacerations, or burns, and other signs such as a change in behavior, odor, the caregiver refusing to allow assessment of older adult alone, or use of restraints. If mistreatment is suspected, Adult Protective Services should be consulted. Reporting requirements vary for each state. If the nurse suspects that an older adult is in immediate danger, actions must focus on removing the older adult from their current setting (Wang et al., 2015).

Advance Directives and Palliative Care

Many older patients are interested in discussing end-of-life decisions and would like providers to initiate these discussions *before* the onset of serious illness (Acierno et al., 2010). *Advance care planning* involves several tasks: providing information, clarifying the patient's preferences, and identifying the surrogate decision maker. Patients trust nurses when having this conversation (USPSTF, 2018a). A nurse can begin this discussion by linking these decisions to a current illness or experiences with relatives or friends. Ask the patient about "do not resuscitate" orders specifying life support measures "if the heart or lungs were to stop or give out." Provide explanations with health literacy in mind, and ensure that the patient understands the terminology. Direct older adults and their family members to the National Institute on Aging website at https://www.nia.nih.gov/health/advance-care-planning-healthcare-directives (O'Sullivan et al., 2015). Also encourage the patient to designate in writing a health care proxy or durable power of attorney for health care, "someone who can make decisions reflecting your wishes in case of confusion or emergency."

Roughly half of hospitalized older adults require surrogate decision making within 48 hours of admission. Common topics include life-sustaining care, surgeries and procedures, and discharge planning (Kim et al., 2017). Conversations about life care choices help patients and their families prepare openly and in advance for a peaceful death. For the older adult, providing these discussions during office visits rather than in the stressful environment of the emergency department or intensive care unit is beneficial.

Experts note that *advance care directives* can be more flexible, depending on the situation. These directives "may range from general statements of values to such specific orders as [do not resuscitate], do not intubate, do not hospitalize, do not provide artificial hydration or nutrition, or do not administer antibiotics. Different situations, including different stages of health and illness, demand different types of advanced care directives and thus require both different conversations and different training in leading such discussions" (National Institute of Aging, 2018). Moreover, always consult competent patients first about their current options because their decisions supersede prior written instructions or the wishes of family members.

See also the Chapter 3 section, "Death and the Dying Patient."

For patients with advanced or terminal illnesses, include the review of advance directives in an overall plan for *palliative care*. Educate the patient and family that terminal illnesses do not refer only to cancer, but rather include a range of chronic disease states such as COPD, heart failure, and end-stage renal disease. Palliative care encompasses the alleviation of pain and suffering and the promotion of optimal quality of life across all phases of treatment, including curative interventions and rehabilitation. Its goals are "to consider the physical, mental, spiritual, and social well-being of patients and their families in order to maintain hope while ensuring patient dignity and respecting autonomy" both for patients with serious illnesses and for patients considering hospice care at the end of life (National Institute of Aging, 2018). To ease patient and family distress, use good communication skills: make good eye contact; ask open-ended questions; respond to anxiety, depression, or changes in the patient's affect; show empathy; and be sure to consult caregivers.

Nurses interact with older adults across a variety of settings from the acute care to home care to the assistive care continuum to long-term care. Nurses need to apply the person-centered approach with each encounter to obtain a thorough health history, physical assessment, functional assessment, screening for abuse, counseling on health promotion, and the patient's desires and goals for health care. Approach each older adult client in an individualized manner and obtain the history and perform physical and functional assessments spaced in a manner that will not tire or frustrate the patient. Consult the family as needed to interpret the older adult's desires as needed. Older adults present a unique challenge among populations for the nurse to perform a comprehensive geriatric assessment. This chapter on the unique needs for assessing older adults serves as a guide for the nurse to consider the many assessments and screening opportunities to offer the optimum quality of life for the older adult and their family.

BIBLIOGRAPHY

CITATIONS

Acierno, R., Hernandez, M. A., Amstadter, A. B., Resnick, H. S., Steve, K., Muzzy, W., & Kilpatrick, D. G. (2010). Prevalence and correlates of emotional, physical, sexual, and financial abuse and potential neglect in the United States: The National Elder Mistreatment Study. *American Journal of Public Health, 100*, 292–297.

Aggarwal, N. K. (2010). Reassessing cultural evaluations in geriatrics: Insights from cultural psychiatry. *Journal of the American Geriatrics Society, 58*(11), 2191–2196.

Aggarwal, N. K., Glass, A., Tirado, A., Boiler, M., Nicasio, A., Alegría, M., Wall, M., & Lewis-Fernández, R. (2014). The development of the DSM-5 Cultural Formulation Interview-Fidelity Instrument (CFI-FI): A pilot study. *Journal of Health Care for the Poor and Underserved, 25*(3), 1397–1417.

Ali, A., Arif, A. W., Bhan, C., Kumar, D., Malik, M. B., Sayyed, Z., Akhtar, K. H., & Ahmad, M. Q. (2018). Managing chronic pain in the elderly: An overview of the recent therapeutic advancements. *Cureus, 10*(9), e3293. https://doi.org/10.7759/cureus.3293

Alzheimer's Association. (2021). Alzheimer's disease: Facts and figures special report. Race, ethnicity and Alzheimer's in America. Retrieved May 24, 2021, from https://www.alz.org/media/Documents/alzheimers-facts-and-figures.pdf

American College of Sports Medicine. (2021). Health care providers action guide: How to implement exercise is medicine in your practice. Retrieved May 24, 2021, from https://www.exerciseismedicine.org/support_page.php/provider-action-guide/

American Geriatrics Society Panel on the Pharmacologic Management of Persistent Pain in Older Persons. (2009). Pharmacologic management of persistent pain in older persons. *Journal of the American Geriatrics Society, 57*, 1331–1346.

American Geriatrics Society. (2018a). GeriatricsCareOnline.org: Nutrition and weight. https://geriatricscareonline.org/FullText/B007/B007_CH017?parent_product_id=B007_PART001

American Geriatrics Society. (2019a). American Geriatrics Society 2019 Updated AGS Beers Criteria® for potentially inappropriate medication use in older adults. *Journal of the American Geriatrics Society, 67*(4), 674–694. https://doi.org/10.1111/jgs.15767

American Geriatrics Society. (2019b). *Clinician's guide to counseling older adults and driving* (4th ed.). American Geriatrics Society.

American Geriatrics Society. (2020). Geriatric evaluation and management tools: Screening and prevention 2018. Retrieved November 1, 2020, from https://geriatricscareonline.org/ProductAbstract/ags-geriatrics-evaluation-and-management-tools-gems-app/B025/

American Psychiatric Association. (2013). *Neurocognitive disorders, in diagnostic and statistical manual of mental disorders* (5th ed., p. 602). American Psychiatric Publishing.

Andrasfay, T., & Goldman, N. (2021). Reductions in 2020 US life expectancy due to COVID-19 and the disproportionate impact on the Black and Latino populations. *Proceedings of the National Academy of Sciences*, *118*(5), e2014746118. https://doi.org/10.1073/pnas.2014746118

Annon, J. (1996). The PLISSIT model: A proposed conceptual scheme for the behavioral treatment of sexual problems. *The Journal of Sex Education and Therapy*, *2*(2), 1–15.

Arias, E., Tejada-Vera, B., & Ahmad, F. (2021). Provisional life expectancy estimates for January through June, 2020. Vital Statistics Rapid Release; no 10. National Center for Health Statistics. https://dx.doi.org/10.15620/cdc:100392

August, K. J., & Sorkin, D. H. (2010). Racial and ethnic disparities in indicators of physical health status: Do they still exist throughout late life? *Journal of the American Geriatrics Society*, *58*, 2009–2015.

Bamia, C., Orfanos, P., Juerges, H., Schöttker, B., Brenner, H., Lorbeer, R., Aadahl, M., Matthews, C. E., Klinaki, E., Katsoulis, M., Lagiou, P., Bueno-de-Mesquita, H. B. A., Eriksson, S., Mons, U., Saum, K. U., Kubinova, R., Pajak, A., Tamosiunas, A., Malyutina, S.,...Trichopoulos, D. (2017). Self-rated health and all-cause and cause-specific mortality of older adults: Individual data meta-analysis of prospective cohort studies in the CHANCES Consortium. *Maturitas*, *103*, 37–44. https://doi.org/10.1016/j.maturitas.2017.06.023

Bangalore, S., Gong, Y., Cooper-DeHoff, R. M., Pepine, C. J., & Messerli, F. H. (2014). 2014 Eighth Joint National Committee panel recommendation for blood pressure targets revisited: Results from the INVEST study. *Journal of the American College of Cardiology*, *64*(8), 784–793.

Benetos, A., Rossignol, P., Cherubini, A., Joly, L., Grodzicki, T., Rajkumar, C., Strandberg, T. E., & Petrovic, M. (2015). Polypharmacy in the aging patient: Management of hypertension in octogenarians. *The Journal of the American Medical Association*, *314*(2), 170–180.

Bhatia, L. C., & Naik, R. H. (2013). Clinical profile of acute myocardial infarction in elderly patients. *Journal of Cardiovascular Disease Research*, *4*(2), 107–111.

Blass, D. M., & Rabins, P. V. (2014). In the clinic. Dementia. *Annals of Internal Medicine*, *161*, ITC1; quiz ITC16.

Bloom, H. G., Ahmed, I., Alessi, C. A., Ancoli-Israel, S., Buysse, D. J., Kryger, M. H., Phillips, B. A., Thorpy, M. J., Vitiello, M. V., & Zee, P. C. (2009). Evidence-based recommendations for the assessment and management of sleep disorders in older persons. *Journal of the American Geriatrics Society*, *57*(5), 761–789.

Bodenheimer, T., Wagner, E. H., & Brumbach, K. (2002). Improving primary care for patients with chronic illness. *The Journal of the American Medical Association*, *288*(14), 1775–1779.

Bommersbach, T. J., Lapid, M. I., Rummans, T. A., & Morse, R. M. (2015). Geriatric alcohol use disorder: A review for primary care physicians. *Mayo Clinic Proceedings*, *90*, 659–666.

Borooah, S., Dhillon, A., & Dhillon, B. (2015). Gradual loss of vision in adults. *BMJ (Clinical Research Ed.)*, *350*, h2093.

Borson, S., Scanlan, J. M., Chen, P. J., & Ganguli, M. (2003). The Mini-Cog as a screen for dementia: Validation in a population-based sample. *Journal of the American Geriatrics Society*, *51*, 1451–1454.

Bradley, K. A., DeBenedetti, A. F., Volk, R. J., Williams, E. C., Frank, D., & Kivlahan, D. R. (2007). AUDIT-C as a brief screen for alcohol misuse in primary care. *Alcoholism, Clinical and Experimental Research*, *31*(7), 1208–1217.

Buchman, A. S., Boyle, P. A., Yu, L., Shah, R. C., Wilson, R. S., & Bennett, D. A. (2012). Total daily physical activity and the risk of AD and cognitive decline in older adults. *Neurology*, *78*, 1323–1329.

Carlson, C., Merel, S. E., & Yukawa, M. (2015). Geriatric syndromes and geriatric assessment for the generalist. *Medical Clinics of North America*, *99*(2), 263–279.

Cawley, M. (2017). Reporting error in weight and height among older adults: Implications for estimating healthcare costs. *The Journal of the Economics of Ageing*, *9*, 122–44. https://doi.org/10.1016/j.jeoa.2016.10.001

Centers for Disease Control (CDC). (2021). Promoting health for older adults. National Center for Chronic Disease Prevention and Health Promotion (NCCDPHP). Retrieved April 9, 2021, from https://www.cdc.gov/chronicdisease/resources/publications/factsheets/promoting-health-for-older-adults.htm

Centers for Disease Control and Prevention. (2021). Preventing falls in older adults. Updated March 3, 2021. Retrieved May 25, 2021, from https://www.cdc.gov/falls/index.html

Centers for Disease Control and Prevention. (2020a). Current cigarette smoking among U.S. adults aged 18 years and older 2018. Retrieved October 25, 2020, from https://www.cdc.gov/tobacco/campaign/tips/resources/data/cigarette-smoking-in-united-states.html

Centers for Disease Control and Prevention. (2020b). CDC Health disparities and inequalities report (CHDIR). Retrieved November 5, 2020, from http://www.cdc.gov/minorityhealth/CHDIReport.html

Centers for Disease Control and Prevention. (2021). Vaccine information statements. Updated February 12, 2021. Retrieved May 25, 2021, from https://www.cdc.gov/vaccines/schedules/hcp/imz/adult.html

Centers for Medicare & Medicaid Services. (2021). *Chronic conditions charts.* Updated January 15, 2021. Retrieved May 25, 2021, from https://www.cms.gov/Research-Statistics-Data-and-Systems/Statistics-Trends-and-Reports/Chronic-Conditions/CC_Main

Chou, C. H., Hwang, C. L., & Wu, Y. T. (2012). Effect of exercise on physical function, daily living activities, and quality of life in the frail older adults: A meta-analysis. *Archives of Physical Medicine and Rehabilitation*, *93*, 237.

Coffey, S., Cox, B., & Williams, M. J. (2014). The prevalence, incidence, progression, and risks of aortic valve sclerosis: A systematic review and meta-analysis. *Journal of the American College of Cardiology*, *63*, 2852–2861.

Crookham, J. (2013). A guide to exercise prescription. *Primary Care*, *40*, 801–820.

Davy, C., Bleasel, J., Liu, H., Tchan, M., Ponniah, S., & Brown, A. (2015). Effectiveness of chronic care models: Opportunities for improving healthcare practice and health outcomes: A systematic review. *BMC Health Services Research, 15*, 194.

Demonet, J. F., & Celsis, P. (2012). Chapter 5: Aging of the brain. In: B. J. Vellas (Ed.), *Pathy's principles and practice of geriatric medicine* (5th ed., pp. 49). John Wiley & Sons, Inc.

Dowling-Castronovo, A., & Bradway, C. (2017). Urinary incontinence. In M. Boltz (Ed.), *Evidence-based geriatric nursing protocols for best practice* (5th ed., pp. 343–362). Springer Publishing Company, LLC.

Eckstrom, K., Feeny, D. H., Walter, L. C., Perdue, L. A., & Whitlock, E. P. (2013). Individualizing cancer screening in older adults: A narrative review and framework for future research. *Journal of General Internal Medicine, 28*, 292–298.

Erro, R. & Stamelou, M. (2018). Chapter 3. The motor syndromes of Parkinson's disease. In K. Bhatia (Ed.), *Parkinson's disease* (pp. 25–32). Academic Press.

Evans, W. J. (2015). Sarcopenia should reflect the contribution of age-associated changes in skeletal muscle to risk of morbidity and mortality in elderly people. *Journal of the American Medical Directors Association, 16*(7), 546–547.

Federal Interagency Forum on Aging Related Statistics. (2016). *Older Americans 2016, Key Indicators of Well Being*. See Indicators 17, Chronic Health Conditions (p. 28); 19, Respondent Assessed Health Statistics (p. 30); 22, Functional Limitations (p. 34); and 27, Obesity (p. 42). Federal Interagency Forum on Aging-Related Statistics. U.S. Government Printing Office. Retrieved October 13, 2020, from https://agingstats.gov/docs/LatestReport/Older-Americans-2016-Key-Indicators-of-WellBeing.pdf

Feliciano, L., Horning, S. M., Klebe, K. J., Anderson, S. L., Cornwell, R. E., & Davis, H. P. (2013). Utility of the SLUMS as a cognitive screening tool among a nonveteran sample of older adults. *American Journal of Geriatric Psychiatry, 21*(7), 623–630. https://doi.org/10.1016/j.jagp.2013.01.024

Fernández-Ruiz, M., Guerra-Vales, J. M., Trincado, R., Fernández, R., Medrano, M. J., Villarejo, A., Benito-León, J., & Bermejo-Pareja, F. (2013). The ability of self-rated health to predict mortality among community-dwelling elderly individuals differs according to the specific cause of death: Data from the NEDICES cohort. *Gerontology, 59*(4), 368–377.

Florence, C. S., Bergen, G., Atherly, A., Burns, E. R., Stevens, J. A., & Drake, C. (2018). Medical costs of fatal and nonfatal falls in older adults. *Journal of the American Geriatrics Society*. https://doi.org/10.1111/jgs.15304external icon

Friedman, P. K., Kaufman, L. B., & Karpas, S. L. (2014). Oral health disparity in older adults: Dental decay and tooth loss. *Dental Clinics of North America, 58*, 757–770.

Fulmer, T. (2007). How to try this: Fulmer SPICES. *The American Journal of Nursing, 107*(10), 40–48.

Fulmer, T., & Wallace, M. (2020). Fulmer SPICES: An overall assessment tool for Older Adults Hartford Institute of Geriatric Nursing Assessment Series. Revision 2019. Retrieved October 17, 2020, from https://hign.org/sites/default/files/2020-06/Try_This_General_Assessment_1.pdf

Gambert, & Steven, R. (2021). Thyroid, parathyroid, & adrenal gland disorders. In L. C. Walter (Ed.), *Current diagnosis and treatment geriatrics* (3rd ed.). McGraw-Hill. https://accessmedicine-mhmedical-com.proxy1.lib.tju.edu/content.aspx?bookid=2984&sectionid=250021240

Gestuvo, M. K. (2012). Health maintenance in older adults: Combining evidence and individual preferences. *The Mount Sinai Journal of Medicine, 79*, 560–578.

Gibson, P. G., McDonald, V. M., & Marks, G. B. (2010). Asthma in older adults. *Lancet, 376*, 803.

Goldberg, L. R. (2010). In the clinic. Heart failure. *Annals of Internal Medicine, 152*, ITC61–15; quiz ITC616.

Griffin, S. O., Griffin, P. M., Li, C. H., Bailey, W. D., Brunson, D., & Jones, J. A. (2019). Changes in older adults' oral health and disparities: 1999 to 2004 and 2011 to 2016. *Journal of the American Geriatrics Society, 67*(6), 1152–1157. https://doi.org/10.1111/jgs.15777

Henrich, A. (2020). Fall risk assessment for older adults: The Henrich II Fall Risk Model. Retrieved November 9, 2020, from https://hign.org/consultgeri/try-this-series/fall-risk-assessment-older-adults-hendrich-ii-fall-risk-model

Herr, K. (2011). Pain assessment strategies in older patients. *Journal of Pain, 12*(3), S3–S13. https://doi.org/10.1016/j.jpain.2010.11.011

Hoffman, H. (2018). Underreporting of fall injuries of older adults: Implications for wellness visit fall risk screening: Accuracy of self-reported fall injuries. *Journal of the American Geriatrics Society, 66*(6), 1195–200. https://doi.org/10.1111/jgs.15360

Hollingsworth, J. M., & Wilt, T. J. (2014). Lower urinary tract symptoms in men. *BMJ (Clinical Research Ed.), 14*(349), g4474. https://doi.org/10.1136/bmj.g4474

Hötting, K., & Röder B. (2013). Beneficial effects of physical exercise on neuroplasticity and cognition. *Neuroscience and Biobehavioral Reviews, 37*(9 Pt B), 2243–2257.

Iecovich, E., & Biderman, A. (2013). Concordance between self-reported and physician-reported chronic co-morbidity among disabled older adults. *Canadian Journal on Aging = La Revue Canadienne Du Vieillissement, 32*(3), 287–297.

Inglés, M., Mas-Bargues, C., Berna-Erro, A., Matheu, A., Sanchís, P., Avellana, J. A., Borrás, C., & Viña, J. (2019). Centenarians overexpress pluripotency-related genes. *The Journals of Gerontology: Series A, 74*(9), 1391–1395. https://doi.org/10.1093/gerona/gly168

Inouye, S. (2018). Delirium-A framework to improve acute care for older persons: Delirium and improving care for elders. *Journal of the American Geriatrics Society, 66*(3), 446–451. https://doi.org/10.1111/jgs.15296

Institute of Medicine. (2011). *Crossing the quality chasm: A new health system for the 21st century*. National Academy Press.

International Tremor Foundation. (2010). ET vs Parkinson's disease. Retrieved from https://essentialtremor.org/wp-content/uploads/2013/07/ETvsPD092012.pdf

Jackson, C. S., & Gracia, J. N. (2014). Addressing health and health-care disparities: The role of a diverse workforce and the social determinants of health. *Public Health Reports, 129*, 57–61.

James, P. A., Oparil, S., Carter, B. L., Cushman, W. C., Handler, J., Lackland, D. T., LeFevre, M. L., MacKenzie, T. D., Ogedegbe, O., Smith, S. C., Jr, Svetkey, L. P., Taler, S. J., Townsend, R. R., Wright, J. T., Jr, Narva, A. S., & Ortiz, E. (2014). 2014 evidence-based guidelines for the management of high blood pressure in adults: Report from the panel members appointed to the Eighth Joint National

Committee (JNC8). *The Journal of the American Medical Association, 311*(5), 507–520.

Jankovic, J. (2015). Gait disorders. *Neurologic Clinics, 33*, 249–268.

Jones, D. (2017). Optimal treated blood pressure for patients with isolated systolic hypertension. *Hypertension, 69*(2), 200–201. https://doi.org/10.1161/HYPERTENSIONAHA.116.08705

Kagan, S. H. (2010). Geriatric syndromes in practice: Delirium is not the only thing. *Geriatric Nursing, 31*(4), 299–304.

Kane, E. L., Ouslander, J. G., Resnick, B., & Malone, M. L. (2018). Chapter 8, Incontinence. In *Essentials of clinical geriatrics* (8th ed.). McGraw Hill Medical.

Kane, E. L., Ouslander, J. G., Resnick, B., & Malone, M. L. (2018). Chapter 3, Evaluating the geriatric patient. In *Essentials of clinical geriatrics* (8th ed.). McGraw Hill Medical.

Katz, S., Ford, A. B., Moskowitz, R. W., Jackson, B. A., & Jaffe, M. W. (1963). Studies of illness in the aged: The index of ADL: A standardized measure of biological and psychosocial function. *The Journal of the American Medical Association, 185*(12), 914–919. https://doi.org/10.1001/jama.1963.03060120024016

Kaufman, J. M., Lapauw, B., Mahmoud, A., T'Sjoen, G., & Huhtaniemi, I. T. (2019). Aging and the male reproductive system. *Endocrine Reviews, 40*(4), 906–972. https://doi.org/10.1210/er.2018-00178

Kim, H., Deatrick, J. A., & Ulrich, C. M. (2017). Ethical frameworks for surrogates' end-of-life planning experiences: A qualitative systematic review. *Nursing Ethics, 24*(1), 46–69. https://doi.org/10.1177/0969733016638145

Kobylarz, F. A., Heath, J. M., & Lide, R. C. (2002). The ETHNIC(S) mnemonic: A clinical tool for ethnogeriatric education. *Journal of the American Geriatrics Society, 50*(9), 1852–1859.

Koroukian, S. M., Warner, D. F., Owusu, C., & Given, C. W. (2015). Multimorbidity redefined: Prospective health outcomes and the cumulative effect of co-occurring conditions. *Preventing Chronic Disease, 12*, E55.

Krakoff, L. R., Gillespie, R. L., Ferdinand, K. C., Fergus, I. V., Akinboboye, O., Williams, K. A., Walsh, M. N., Bairey Merz, C. N., & Pepine, C. J. (2014). 2014 hypertension recommendations from the Eighth Joint National Committee panel members raise concerns for elderly black and female populations. *Journal of the American College of Cardiology, 64*(4), 394–402.

Kroenke, K., Spitzer, R. L., & Williams, J. B. (2001). The PHQ-9: Validity of a brief depression severity measure. *Journal of General Internal Medicine, 16*(9), 606–613. https://doi.org/10.1046/j.1525-1497.2001.016009606.x

Lal, H., Cunningham, A., Olivier, G., Chlibek, R., Diez-Domingo, J., Hwang, S. J., Levin, M. J., McElhaney, J. E., Poder, A., Puig-Barberà, J., Vesikari, T., Watanabe, D., Weckx, L., Zahaf, T., Heineman, T. C., & ZOE-50 Study Group. (2015). Efficacy of an adjuvanted herpes zoster subunit vaccine in older adults. *The New England Journal of Medicine, 372*(22), 2087–2096.

Lam, R. (2011). Office management of gait disorders in the elderly. *Canadian Family Physician, 57*, 765–770.

Lawton, M. P., & Brody, E. M. (1969). Assessment of older people: Self-maintaining and instrumental activities of daily living. *The Gerontologist, 9*(3), 179–186.

Lee, L., Heckman, G., & Mohar, F. J. (2015). Frailty: Identifying elderly patients at high risk of poor outcomes. *Canadian Family Physician, 61*, 227–231.

Lewis, S. J. (2015). Neurological update: Emerging issues in gait disorders. *Journal of Neurology, 262*, 1590–1595.

Liew, G., Baker, M. L., Wong, T. Y., Hand, P. J., Wang, J. J., Mitchell, P., De Silva, D. A., Wong, M. C., Rochtchina, E., Lindley, R. I., Wardlaw, J. M., Hankey, G. J., & Multi-Centre Retinal Stroke Study Group. (2014). Differing associations of white matter lesions and lacunar infarction with retinal microvascular signs. *International Journal of Stroke, 9*(7), 921–925.

Liew, T. M., Feng, L., Gao, Q., Ng, T. P., & Yap, P. (2015). Diagnostic utility of montreal cognitive assessment in the fifth edition of diagnostic and statistical manual of mental disorders: Major and mild neurocognitive disorders. *Journal of the American Medical Directors Association, 16*(2), 144–148.

Lundebjerg, N. E., Trucil, D. E., Hammond, E. C., & Applegate, W. B. (2017). When it comes to older adults, language matters: Journal of the American Geriatrics Society adopts modified American Medical Association Style. *Journal of the American Geriatrics Society, 65*(7), 1386–1388. https://doi.org/10.1111/jgs.14941

Mahlknecht, P., Kiechl, S., Bloem, B. R., Willeit, J., Scherfler, C., Gasperi, A., Rungger, G., Poewe, W., & Seppi, K. (2013). Prevalence and burden of gait disorders in elderly men and women aged 60–97 years: A population-based study. *PloS One, 8*(7), e69627.

Manning, M. J. (2013). Asymptomatic aortic stenosis in the elderly: A clinical review. *The Journal of the American Medical Association, 310*, 1490.

Marcantonio, E. R. (2011). In the clinic. Delirium. *Annals Of Internal Medicine, 154*, ITC6–1.

Martin, A. J., Marottoli, R., & O'Neill, D. (2013). Driving assessment for maintaining mobility and safety in drivers with dementia. *Cochrane Database of Systematic Reviews, 2013*, CD006222.

Mathias, S., Nayak, U. S., & Isaacs, B., (1986). Balance in elderly patients: The "get-up and go" test. *Archives of Physical Medicine and Rehabilitation, 67*, 387–389.

Maurer, D. M. (2012). Screening for depression. *American Family Physician, 85*, 139–144.

McCabe, D. (2018). Hearing screening in older adults. Hartford Try This Series. Retrieved November 13, 2020, from https://hign.org/consultgeri/try-this-series/hearing-screening-older-adults

McDermott, M. M. (2015). Lower extremity manifestations of peripheral artery disease: The pathophysiologic and functional implications of leg ischemia. *Circulation Research, 116*, 1540–1550.

Mendonça, M. D., Alves, L., & Bugalho, P. (2016). From subjective cognitive complaints to dementia: Who is at risk? A systematic review. *American Journal of Alzheimers Disease and Other Dementias, 31*(2), 105–114.

Miller, K. L., & Baraldi, C. A. (2012). Geriatric gynecology: Promoting health and avoiding harm. *American Journal of Obstetrics and Gynecology, 207*, 355–367.

Mol, A., Bui Hoang, P. T. S., Sharmin, S., Reijnierse, E. M., van Wezel, R. J. A., Meskers, C. G. M., & Maier, A. B. (2019). Orthostatic hypotension and falls in older adults: A systematic review and meta-analysis. *Journal of the American*

Medical Directors Association, *20*(5), 589–597.e5. https://doi.org/10.1016/j.jamda.2018.11.003

Montlahuc, C., Soumaré, A., Dufouil, C., Berr, C., Dartigues, J. F., Poncet, M., Tzourio, C., & Alpérovitch, A. (2011). Self-rated health and risk of incident dementia: A community-based elderly cohort, the 3C Study. *Neurology*, *77*(15), 1457–1464.

Montreal Cognitive Assessment. (2015). Retrieved January 20, 2016, from http://www.mocatest.org/

Moore, A. A., & Siu, A. L. (1996). Screening for common problems in ambulatory elderly: Clinical confirmation of a screening instrument. *American Journal of Medicine*, *100*, 438–443.

Moran, M. B., Chatterjee, J. S., Frank, L. B., Murphy, S. T., Zhao, N., Chen, N., & Ball-Rokeach, S. (2017). Individual, cultural and structural predictors of vaccine safety confidence and influenza vaccination among hispanic female subgroups. *Journal of Immigrant And Minority Health*, *19*(4), 790–800. https://doi.org/10.1007/s10903-016-0428-9

Morley, J. E. (2018). Defining undernutrition (malnutrition) in older persons. *Journal of Nutrition, Health and Aging*, *22*, 308–310. https://doi-org.proxy1.lib.tju.edu/10.1007/s12603-017-0991-3

Morley, J. E., & Tolsen, D. T. (2012a). Chapter 3: The physiology of aging. In B. J. Vellas, M. S. Pathy, & A. Sinclair (Eds.), *Pathy's principles and practice of geriatric medicine* (5th ed., pp. 33). John Wiley & Sons, Inc.

Morley, J. E., & Tolsen, D. T. (2012b). Chapter 9: Sexuality and aging. In B. J. Vellas, M. S. Pathy, & A. Sinclair (Eds.), *Pathy's principles and practice of geriatric medicine* (5th ed., pp. 93). John Wiley & Sons, Inc.

Naegle, M. (2018). Alcohol use screening and assessment for older adults consult. ConsultGeri: Try this series. Retrieved October 24, 2020, from https://hign.org/consultgeri/try-this-series/alcohol-use-screening-and-assessment-older-adults

Nair, A., & Sabbagh, M. N. (2015). Chapter 3. approach to the geriatric neurology patient: The neurologic examination, In *Geriatric neurology* (pp. 71–84). John Wiley & Sons, Inc.

National Academies of Sciences, Engineering, and Medicine. (2020). *Social isolation and loneliness in older adults: Opportunities for the health care system.* The National Academies Press. https://doi.org/10.17226/25663

National Institute on Aging. (2018). Advance care planning healthcare directives. Updated January 15, 2018. Retrieved November 13, 2020, from https://www.nia.nih.gov/health/advance-care-planning-healthcare-directives

National Institute on Aging. (2020). Facts about aging and alcohol. Retrieved November 9, 2020, from https://www.nia.nih.gov/health/facts-about-aging-and-alcohol

National Institutes of Health. (2018). Getting help with Alzheimer's caregiving. Updated January 15, 2018. Retrieved November 13, 2020, from https://www.nia.nih.gov/health/getting-help-alzheimers-caregiving

Ng, J. H., Bierman, A. S., Elliott, M. N., Wilson, R. L., Xia, C., & Scholle, S. H. (2014). Beyond black and white: Race/ethnicity and health status among older adults. *American Journal of Managed Care*, *20*(3), 239–248.

Nurses Improving Care for Healthsystem Elders (NICHE). (2020). Program at the Hartford Institute for Geriatric Nursing. Retrieved November 6, 2020, from https://nicheprogram.org/

Office of Minority Health, Department of Health and Human Services. (2020). Think cultural health. Retrieved November 6, 2020, from https://www.thinkculturalhealth.hhs.gov/index.asp

Onder, G., Petrovic, M., & Balamurugan, T. (2010). Less is more. Development and validation of a score to assess risk of adverse drug reactions among the in-hospital patients 65 years or older. *Archives of Internal Medicine*, *170*, 1142.

Ortman, J. M., Veloff, V., & Hogan, H. (2020). An aging nation: The older population in the United States: Population estimates and projections: Current population reports. Retrieved November 19, 2020, from https://www.census.gov/prod/2014pubs/p25-1140.pdf

O'Sullivan, R., Mailo, K., Angeles, R., & Agarwal, G. (2015). Advance directives: Survey of primary care patients. *Canadian Family Physician*, *61*(4), 353–356.

Palsetia, R. (2018). The clock drawing test versus mini-mental status examination as a screening tool for dementia: A clinical comparison. *Indian Journal of Psychological Medicine*, *40*(1), 1–10. https://doi.org/10.4103/IJPSYM.IJPSYM_244_17

Papaleontiou, M., & Haymart, M. R. (2012). Approach to and treatment of thyroid disorders in the elderly. *Medical Clinics of North America*, *96*, 297–310.

Parkinson's Disease Foundation. (2020). Statistics on Parkinson's. Retrieved October 26, 2020, from https://www.parkinson.org/Understanding-Parkinsons/Statistics

Partnership for Health in Aging Workgroup on Interdisciplinary Team Training in Geriatrics. (2014). Position statement on interdisciplinary team training in geriatrics: An essential component of quality health care for older adults. *Journal of the American Geriatrics Society*, *62*(5), 961–965.

Pelletier, A. L., Rojas-Roldan, L., & Coffin, J. (2016). Vision loss in older adults. *American Family Physician*, *94*(3), 219–226.

Perkins, K., King, M. (2012). Geriatric gynecology. *Emergency Medicine Clinics of North America*, *30*(4), 1007–19. https://doi.org/10.1016/j.emc.2012.08.011

Perlmuter, L. C., Sarda, G., Casavant, V., & Mosnaim, A. D. (2013). A review of the etiology, associated comorbidities, and treatment of orthostatic hypotension. *American Journal of Therapeutics*, *20*(3), 279–291.

Podsiadlo, D., & Richardson, S. (1991). The Timed "Up and Go": A test of basic functional mobility for frail elderly persons. *Journal of the American Geriatrics Society*, *39*, 142–148.

Qato, D. M., Wilder, J., Schumm, L. P., Gillet, V., & Alexander, G. C. (2016). Changes in prescription and over-the-counter medication and dietary supplement use among older adults in the United States, 2005 vs 2011. *JAMA Internal Medicine*, *176*(4), 473–482.

Ratnapriya, R., & Chew, E. Y. (2013). Age-related macular degeneration-clinical review and genetics update. *Clinical Genetics*, *84*, 160–166.

Reuben, D. B., & Tinetti, M. E. (2012). Goal-oriented patient care—an alternative health outcome paradigm. *The New England Journal of Medicine*, *366*(9), 777–779.

Rodriguez, J. C., Dzierzewski, J. M., & Alessi, C. A. (2015). Sleep problems in the elderly. *Medical Clinics of North America*, *99*, 431–439.

Rosen, S. L., & Reuben, D. B. (2011). Geriatric assessment tools. *The Mount Sinai Journal of Medicine*, *78*(4), 489–497.

SAGE. (2020). SAGE advocacy and services for LGBT elders. Retrieved May 25, 2021, from https://www.sageusa.org/

Saint Louis University. (2020). Saint Louis University Mental Status. Retrieved May 25, 2021, from https://www.slu.edu/medicine/internal-medicine/geriatric-medicine/aging-successfully/assessment-tools/mental-status-exam.php

Samuels, M. H. (2000). Hyperthyroidism in aging. [Updated 2018 March 21]. In: K. R. Feingold, B. Anawalt, & A. Boyce (Eds.), *Endotext [Internet]*. MDText.com, Inc. https://www.ncbi.nlm.nih.gov/books/NBK278986

Sandoval-Leon, A. C., Drews-Elger, K., Gomez-Fernandez, C. R., Yepes, M. M., & Lippman, M. E. (2013). Paget's disease of the nipple. *Breast Cancer Research and Treatment*, *141*(1), 1–12.

Schoene, D., Heller, C., Aung, Y. N., Sieber, C. C., Kemmler, W., & Freiberger, E. (2019). A systematic review on the influence of fear of falling on quality of life in older people: Is there a role for falls? *Clinical Interventions in Aging*, *14*, 701–719. https://doi.org/10.2147/CIA.S197857

Sebastiani, P., Bae, H., Sun, F. X., Andersen, S. L., Daw, E. W., Malovini, A., Kojima, T., Hirose, N., Schupf, N., Puca, A., & Perls, T. T. (2014). Meta analysis of genetic variants associated with human exceptional longevity. *Aging*, *5*(9), 653–661.

Siu, A. L., & U.S. Preventive Services Task Force (USPSTF). (2016). Screening for depression in adults: US Preventive Services Task Force recommendation statement. *The Journal of the American Medical Association*, *315*(4), 380–387. https://doi.org/10.1001/jama.2015.18392. Retrieved November 5, 2020, from https://www.uspreventiveservicestaskforce.org/uspstf/recommendation/depression-in-adults-screening

Smyth, C. (2018). Sexuality assessment for older adults. Retrieved October 22, 2020, from https://hign.org/sites/default/files/2020-06/Try_This_General_Assessment_10.pdf

Stanford Geriatrics Education Center. (2020). Test your ethnogeriatric IQ. Retrieved November 6, 2020, from https://sgec.stanford.edu/resources/training.html

Stanford School of Medicine. (2016). Ethnogeriatrics. Retrieved January 2016, from http://geriatrics.stanford.edu/

Stevens, J. A., & Phelan, E. A. (2013). Development of STEADI: A fall prevention resource for health care providers. *Health Promotion Practice*, *14*, 706–714.

Strandberg, T. E., Pitkälä, K. H., Tilvis, R. S., O'Neill, D., & Erkinjuntti, T. J. (2013). Geriatric syndromes—vascular disorders? *Annals of Medicine*, *45*(3), 265–273.

Tariq, T. (2006). Comparison of the Saint Louis University Mental Status Examination and the Mini-Mental State Examination for detecting dementia and mild neurocognitive disorder—A pilot study. *The American Journal of Geriatric Psychiatry*, *14*(11), 900–910. https://doi.org/10.1097/01.jgp.0000221510.33817.86

Taylor, W. D. (2014). Depression in the elderly. *The New England Journal of Medicine*, *371*, 1228.

Testa, A. (2015). Understanding urinary incontinence in adults. *Urologic Nursing*, *35*(2), 82–86. https://doi.org/10.7257/1053-816X.2015.35.2.82

Tinetti, M. E., & Kumar, C. (2010). The patient who falls: "It's always a trade-off". *The Journal of the American Medical Association*, *303*, 258–266.

Tsoi, K., Chan, J., Hirai, H. W., Wong, S. Y., & Kwok, T. C. (2015). Cognitive tests to detect dementia: A systematic review and meta-analysis. *JAMA Internal Medicine*, *175*(9), 1450–1458.

U.S. Department of Health and Human Services. (2018). Chapter 5. Active older adults. In: *Physical activity guidelines for Americans* (2nd ed.). U.S. Department of Health and Human Services. https://health.gov/sites/default/files/2019-09/Physical_Activity_Guidelines_2nd_edition.pdf#page=68

U.S. Preventive Services Task Force (USPSTF). (2016). Retrieved November 1, 2020, from https://www.uspreventiveservicestaskforce.org/uspstf/topic_search_results

U.S. Preventive Services Task Force (USPSTF). (2018a). Final recommendation statement. Intimate partner violence, elder abuse, and abuse of elderly and vulnerable Adults: screening. Retrieved November 5, 2020, from http://www.uspreventiveservicestaskforce.org/Page/Document/UpdateSummaryFinal/intimate-partner-violence-and-abuse-of-elderly-and-vulnerable-adults-screening?ds=1&s=elder abuse

U.S. Preventive Services Task Force (USPSTF). (2018b). Unhealthy alcohol use in adolescents and adults: Screening and behavioral counseling interventions. Retrieved October 23, 2020, from https://www.uspreventiveservicestaskforce.org/uspstf/document/RecommendationStatementFinal/unhealthy-alcohol-use-in-adolescents-and-adults-screening-and-behavioral-counseling-interventions#bootstrap-panel–6

U.S. Preventive Services Task Force (USPSTF). (2019). Abdominal aortic aneurysm: Screening. Retrieved October 31, 2020, from https://www.uspreventiveservicestaskforce.org/uspstf/recommendation/abdominal-aortic-aneurysm-screening

U.S. Preventive Services Task Force (USPSTF). (2020). Screening for cognitive impairment in older adults: US Preventive Services Task Force Recommendation Statement. *The Journal of the American Medical Association*, *323*(8), 757–763. https://doi.org/10.1001/jama.2020.0435

Vajaranant, T. S., Wu, S., Torres, M., & Varma, R. (2012). The changing face of primary open-angle glaucoma in the United States: Demographic and geographic changes from 2011 to 2050. *American Journal of Ophthalmology*, *154*(2), 303–314.e3.

Vogelsang, E. M. (2014). Self-rated health changes and oldest-old mortality. *Journals of Gerontology. Series B, Psychological Sciences and Social Sciences*, *69*(4), 612–621.

Walter, L. C., & Covinsky, K. E. (2001). Cancer screening in elderly patients: A framework for individualized decision making. *The Journal of the American Medical Association*, *285*, 2750–2756.

Wang, J. J., Baker, M. L., Hand, P. J., Hankey, G. J., Lindley, R. I., Rochtchina, E., Wong, T. Y., Liew, G., & Mitchell, P. (2011). Transient ischemic attack and acute ischemic stroke: associations with retinal microvascular signs. *Stroke*, *42*(2), 404–408.

Wang, X. M., Brisbin, S., Loo, T., & Straus, S. (2015). Elder abuse: An approach to identification, assessment and intervention. *Canadian Medical Association Journal*, *187*(8), 575–581.

Wang, Y. P., & Andrade, L. H. (2013). Epidemiology of alcohol and drug use in the elderly. *Current Opinion in Psychiatry*, *26*, 343–348.

Weinreb, R. N., Aung, T., & Medeiros, F. A. (2014). The pathophysiology and treatment of glaucoma: A review. *The Journal of the American Medical Association*, *311*(18), 1901–1911.

Wilson, J. F. (2011). In the clinic. Herpes zoster. *Annals of Internal Medicine*, *154*, ITC31–15; quiz ITC316.

Wooten, J. M. (2015). Rules for improving pharmacotherapy in older adult patients: part 2 (rules 6–10). *Southern Medical Journal*, *108*, 145–150.

Wooten, J. M. (2015). Rules for improving pharmacotherapy in older adult patients: part 1 (rules 1–5). *Southern Medical Journal, 108*, 97–104.

Yellowitz, J. A., & Schneiderman, M. T. (2014). Elder's oral health crisis. *The Journal of Evidence-Based Dental Practice, 14*(Suppl), 191–200.

Yeo, G. (2009). How will the U.S. healthcare system meet the challenge of the ethnogeriatric imperative? *Journal of the American Geriatrics Society, 57*, 1278–1285.

Yeo, G., Bell, C. L., Okamoto, L., & Mehta, K. (2017). The future of ethnogeriatrics. In: L. Cummings-Vaughn & D. Cruz-Oliver (Eds.), *Ethnogeriatrics*. Springer, Cham. https://ebrary.net/111446/health/future_ethnogeriatrics

ADDITIONAL READINGS

Fuoto, T. (2019). Palliative care nursing communication: An evaluation of the COMFORT model. *Journal of Hospice and Palliative Nursing, 21*(2), 124–130. https://doi.org/10.1097/NJH.0000000000000493

Lessig, M., Scanlan, J., Nazemi, H., & Borson, S. (2008). Time that tells: Critical clock-drawing errors for dementia screening. *International Psychogeriatrics, 20*(3), 459–470.

McDicken, E. (2019). Accuracy of the short-form Montreal Cognitive Assessment: Systematic review and validation. *International Journal of Geriatric Psychiatry, 34*(10), 1515–1525. https://doi.org/10.1002/gps.5162

GLOSSARY

abduction movement of a limb away from the trunk.

accommodation changes in the shape of the lens to focus the eye to see objects at various distances.

acoustic related to sound or sense of hearing.

acral pertaining to extremities (e.g., limbs, fingers).

active range of motion amount of motion at a given joint when the joint is moved by the patient.

activities of daily living (ADLs) six routine activities people do every day without assistance: eating, bathing, getting dressed, toileting, mobility, and continence of bladder and bowel functions.

adduction movement of a limb toward the trunk.

adenopathy disease or inflammation that involves the glandular tissue or lymph nodes.

adipose tissue a connective tissue containing stored fat that serves as a source of energy and cushions and insulates vital organs.

adventitious sounds abnormal lung sounds heard when listening to the chest as the person breathes; may be wheezes, crackles (rales), or stridor.

affect appropriateness of emotional response in context.

amblyopia known as "lazy eye," contributing to a decrease in visual acuity.

amenorrhea absence or abnormal cessation of the menses.

amplitude the forcefulness of a pulse, apical impulse, or the height of an EKG deflection.

anisocoria unequal pupil size.

anorexia lack or loss of appetite for food.

aphasia the inability to understand or express speech.

aphthous mouth sore.

areola pigmented skin encircling the nipple.

arthralgia pain in a joint.

ascites accumulation of fluid in the peritoneal cavity causing abdominal swelling.

assessment evaluate a patient by taking a history and performing a physical examination.

ataxia loss of full control of bodily movements.

atheroma a fatty thickening in the walls of arteries.

atherosclerosis the formation of fibrofatty deposits in the intimal lining of large and medium arteries leading to hardening and narrowing of the arteries.

auscultatory gap period of diminished or absent Korotkoff sounds during the manual measurement of blood pressure.

Babinski response dorsiflexion of the big toe and fanning of the other toes with plantar stimulation.

biases the attitudes or feelings attached to perceived differences; may be conscious (explicit) or unconscious (implicit).

body mass index (BMI) a weight-to-height ratio calculated by dividing one's weight in kilograms by the square of one's height in meters; used as an indicator of optimal weight.

bradykinesia extreme slowness of movement.

BRCA genes genetic mutations that result in a higher risk for breast cancer in women and prostate cancer in men due to the lack of suppression of tumor development.

bronchiolitis inflammation and congestion of the bronchioles, usually caused by a viral infection; usually occurs in children younger than 2 years old.

bronchophony the sound of the voice heard through the stethoscope over a healthy bronchus.

bruit also called vascular murmur, the abnormal sound generated by turbulent flow of blood in an artery due to either an area of partial obstruction or a localized high rate of blood flow through an unobstructed artery.

canthus corner of the eye.

carcinoma in situ of the testicle a form of testicular cancer, where the cancer cells have not yet spread outside the walls of the seminiferous tubules.

cardiac cycle a complete round of cardiac systole and diastole.

cholecystitis inflammation of the gall bladder.

circumcision removal of the foreskin of the penis.

circumduction movement of a limb in a circular manner.

claudication cramping pain that limits movement of the legs or arms occurring during exercise.

clonus a series of involuntary muscle contractions.

comprehensive health history provides the nurse with a full picture of the patient's health status as well as health promotion and risk reduction needs.

concussion a type of traumatic brain injury.

condyle a rounded protuberance at the end of some bones, forming an articulation with another bone.

confidentiality the duty of a nurse to refrain from sharing confidential patient information with others except with the express consent of the patient.

confrontation assesses peripheral vision.

congenital relating to a condition present at birth.

consensual reaction a reaction on one side when the other side has been stimulated (e.g., with a penlight shining in the eye causing the opposite eye to constrict).

constipation bowel movements are decreased in number and difficult to pass.

convergence movement of the two eyes to turn inward to look at a close object.

cough sudden, forceful air expulsion to clear irritants in the throat or airway.

crepitus a crackling or rattling sound made by a part of the body either spontaneously or during physical examination, for example, the grating of a joint in osteoarthritis.

cryptorchidism failure of one or both testes to descend into the scrotum.

cultural competence a set of skills necessary to care for people of different cultures.

cultural humility a process that requires individuals to continually engage in self-reflection and self-critique as lifelong learners and reflective practitioners keeping culture always in mind.

culture the system of shared ideas, rules, and meanings that influences how people view the world, experience it emotionally, and behave in relation to other people.

culture-bound syndromes illnesses defined by a particular culture but that have no corresponding illness in Western medicine.

cystocele protrusion of the bladder into the vagina.

deep tendon reflex assessed in the neurologic examination, each reflex corresponds to a specific area.

deep vein thrombosis a blood clot that forms in a deep vein and is accompanied by an inflammatory response in the vein wall; usually occur in the lower leg, thigh, or pelvis.

delirium a sudden state of severe confusion and rapid changes in brain function, sometimes associated with hallucinations and hyperactivity.

dementia general term for a group of symptoms affecting memory, thinking, and social interactions.

dermatome area of the body innervated by the sensory root of a single spinal nerve.

dermis the lower or inner layer of the two main layers of the skin; contains blood vessels, lymph vessels, hair follicles, and glands that produce sweat and sebum, which reach the skin's surface through pores.

diarrhea frequent bowel movements of loose, watery consistency.

diastasis recti separation of the two rectus abdominis muscles, causing a midline ridge, most apparent when the infant contracts the abdominal muscles.

diastole period in the heart cycle when the ventricles fill with blood.

diplopia double vision.

direct reaction constriction of pupil size in the eye in which light is directed.

disease the cause of a patient's symptoms.

drusen small, yellow deposits of fatty proteins (lipids) clustered under the retina.

dysarthria difficulty with articulating words.

dysconjugate failure of the eyes to turn together in the same direction.

dysesthesias abnormal sensations.

dyshemoglobinemia disorders in which the hemoglobin molecule is functionally altered and prevented from carrying oxygen.

dysmenorrhea pain with menses.

dyspareunia abnormal pain during sexual intercourse.

dyspepsia chronic or recurrent discomfort or pain centered in the upper abdomen.

dysphagia difficulty or discomfort swallowing.

dyspnea labored or difficult breathing, shortness of breath.

ectropion eversion, usually of the eyelid.

edema abnormal accumulation of fluid in the intercellular spaces of the body.

edentulous without teeth.

effusion accumulation of fluid in various spaces of the body frequently as a byproduct of injury.

egophony occurs during lung auscultation when the patient says "ee" but it is heard as "ay."

electrocardiogram a recording of the electrical activity of the heart.

emergency history data collection focused on the patient's emergent problem with a systematic prioritization of need based on the patient's presentation.

enterocele protrusion of the small bowel into the vagina.

entropion turning inward, usually of the eyelid toward the eye.

epidermis the outermost layer of the skin that does not contain nerves, blood vessels, or hair follicles.

epistaxis acute hemorrhage from the nostril, nasal cavity, or nasopharynx.

ethnicity self-identity of belonging to a group with shared values, ancestry, and experiences.

euphoria a state of happiness.

extension movement that increases the angle between two body parts.

facies the appearance of the face.

fasciculation involuntary contraction or twitching of muscle fibers visible under the skin.

fibrosis development of fibrous connective tissue as a reparative response to injury or damage.

flexion refers to a movement that decreases the angle between two body parts.

focused or problem-oriented assessment used when a known patient has a new problem or symptom.

follow-up history a form of focused assessment; the nurse "follows up" on the status of a previously identified problem.

fremitus a vibration that can be felt by a hand placed on the chest during coughing or speaking.

functional dyspepsia (nonulcer) signs and symptoms of indigestion without an obvious cause that recur.

functional incontinence urinary incontinence as a result of a disability (e.g., inability to recognize the need to use the toilet).

furuncle a bacterial or fungal infection of the hair follicle.

galactorrhea milky discharge unrelated to prior pregnancy or lactation.

gastroesophageal reflux disease (GERD) occurs when acidic stomach contents back up from the stomach into the esophagus.

general survey an overall review.

geriatric syndromes conditions typically seen with aging.

gingivitis inflammation of the gums.

Glasgow Coma Scale scoring system used to describe the level of consciousness.

gynecomastia enlargement of male breasts caused by an imbalance of estrogen and testosterone.

headache pain in the head.

health state of complete physical, mental, and social well-being.

health history holistic assessment of all factors affecting a patient's health status, including current and past medical issues, family history, and lifestyle.

Health Insurance Portability and Accountability Act (HIPAA) a 1996 law that sets strict standards for disclosure of patient information by both institutions and health care providers when sharing patient information.

heartburn irritation of the esophagus caused by stomach acid.

helix outer rim of the ear.

hematemesis vomiting of blood.

hematuria blood in the urine.

hemianopsia inability to see half of the visual field, generally on one side.

hemiparesis weakness of one half of the body.

hemiplegia paralysis of one side of the body.

hernia a condition in which part of an organ is displaced and protrudes through the wall of the cavity containing it (e.g., part of the intestine through the abdominal musculature).

hidradenitis skin lesions resulting from inflammation and infection of sweat glands.

hydrocele accumulation of serous fluid in a saclike cavity in the scrotum.

hydrocephalus enlargement of the ventricles of the brain, usually due to a blockage in the drainage system of the cerebral fluid.

hyperkinesia muscle spasm.

hypertension high blood pressure.

hyperventilation deep, rapid breathing resulting in decreased carbon dioxide levels and increased oxygen levels that produce faintness and tingling of the fingers and toes.

hypospadias a birth defect in which the opening of the urethra is on the underside of the penis instead of at the tip.

illness how the patient experiences disease, including its effects on relationships, functioning, and sense of well-being.

incisional hernia weak area in the abdomen from a previous surgical incision where intra-abdominal content can come through the site.

insight ability to see into or explain a situation.

instrumental activities of daily living (IADLs) activities and tasks beyond basic self-care that are necessary for living independently like mobility, cooking, using the telephone, cleaning the house, doing laundry, shopping, going to the bank, and managing medications.

integumentary system the skin, hair, and nails.

jaundice yellow discoloration of the skin, mucous membranes, and the whites of the eyes caused by increased amounts of bilirubin in the blood.

judgment ability to consider facts and come to a conclusion.

kinesthesia (proprioception) awareness of body position and movement.

Korotkoff sounds changes in the sounds of the blood flowing through the artery.

kyphosis exaggerated outward or convex curvature of the thoracic spine.

labyrinth inner ear.

lactation secretion of milk by the mammary glands.

lactiferous forming milk or a milky fluid.

lesion circumscribed pathologic alteration of the skin.

level of consciousness measurement of arousability and responsiveness.

lymphadenopathy enlargement of the lymph nodes with or without tenderness.

lymphedema swelling of a body part due to pooling of interstitial fluid caused by the blockage of a lymph node or vessel.

malodor unpleasant smell.

mastitis infection of the breast resulting in pain, redness, swelling, and warmth.

menarche beginning of menstruation.

menopause cessation of menses for 12 months.

menstruation cyclic endometrial shedding and discharge of bloody fluid from the uterus during the menstrual cycle.

mental status assessment of behavioral and cognitive functioning.

metatarsus adductus (pigeon-toed) the metatarsal bones are turned toward the midline.

mixed incontinence symptoms of both stress and urge incontinence.

motivational interviewing technique that helps patients identify, create, and implement changes in behaviors to improve or maintain health.

murmur a whooshing or swishing sound during the cardiac cycle made by blood moving through the heart and its valves; may be innocent due to increased blood flow through a valve or abnormal (e.g., when blood leaks backward through an incompetent heart valve).

muscle stretch reflex involuntary contractions of muscle brought on by a brisk stretch of the muscle.

muscle tone slight residual tension that remains in a relaxed muscle.

myalgia tenderness or pain in the muscles.

myelinated enclosed in a myelin sheath.

nocturia urinary frequency at night.

nonpitting edema (brawny edema) serum proteins accumulated in the interstitial space with water and coagulate; cannot be moved by finger pressure and frequently seen with local infection or trauma.

nursing health assessment set of questions to determine the best plan of care.

nutritional status balance between the intake of nutrients and the expenditure of nutrients in the processes of growth, reproduction, and health maintenance.

nystagmus involuntary, rapid, and repetitive movement of the eyes.

objective data obtained from direct observation and measurable information.

odynophagia pain with swallowing.

open-ended question a question that calls for a response using the patient's own knowledge and/or feelings in contrast to a close-ended question, which can be answered with "yes," "no," or a specific piece of information like date of birth.

ophthalmoscope instrument to inspect the eye.

orientation understanding of person, place, time, and event.

orthostatic hypotension a drop in blood pressure with change in position.

otalgia an earache.

otorrhea ear drainage.

overflow incontinence involuntary release of urine.

pain uncomfortable sensation.

palpebral fissure opening between the upper and lower eyelids.

palpitations a sensation of rapid or irregular beating of the heart; may be described as a sensation of thudding, fluttering, or throbbing under the sternum.

papilledema swelling of the optic nerve due to increased intracranial pressure.

paradoxical breathing seesaw breathing; the chest moves inward during inhalation instead of outward.

paralanguage the qualities of speech, such as pacing, tone, and volume.

paraplegia paralysis of the legs.

paresis impaired muscle strength.

paresthesia sensation of numbness, prickling, or tingling.

passive range of motion amount of motion at a given joint when the joint is moved by an examiner.

pectus excavatum "funnel chest," the sternum points inward.

peripheral arterial disease (PAD) narrowing or blockage of the vessels that carry blood from the heart to the extremities.

peripheral neuropathy damage to the nerves outside the brain and spinal cord.

peritonitis inflammation of the peritoneum.

photoreceptors cells in the retina that respond to light.

physical examination part of the physical assessment to check body systems.

pitting edema mobile interstitial water that can be translocated with the pressure exerted by a finger.

plagiocephaly positional, a flattening of the occipital or parieto-occipital region of an infant's head; synostotic, one or more fused cranial sutures.

plegia absence of muscle strength; also called paralysis.

pneumothorax a collection of air in the pleural cavity, "collapsed lung."

point of maximal impulse (PMI) area of the chest where the apical pulse can be felt, usually the fifth intercostal space at the left midclavicular line.

polyuria significant increase in 24-hour urine.

precordium the area on the anterior chest that overlies the heart and great vessels.

presbycusis age-related hearing loss.

presbyopia farsightedness due to decreased elasticity in the lens occurring with age.

pressure injury localized damage to the skin and/or underlying soft tissue, usually over a bony prominence or related to a medical or other device; results from intense and/or prolonged pressure or pressure in combination with shear force.

prodrome early symptom(s) before the onset of a disease.

proprioception (kinesthesia) awareness of body position and movement.

pulmonary embolism blockage in one of the pulmonary arteries caused by a blood clot, usually from the legs, that breaks loose and travels through the bloodstream to the lungs.

pulse contour the shape of the arterial pulse, an indicator of left ventricular stroke volume.

pulse oximetry a device that measures arterial oxygen saturation, or SpO_2.

pyelonephritis kidney infection.

quadriplegia paralysis of all four limbs.

race a socially constructed concept of dividing people into populations or groups on the basis of various sets of physical characteristics, usually stemming from genetic ancestry.

range of motion full movement potential of a joint, usually its range of flexion and extension.

regurgitation a backward flowing, as in the return of solids or fluids to the mouth from the stomach or the backflow of blood through a defective heart valve.

religion a system of beliefs or a practice of worship.

retractions inward movement of the skin between the ribs during inspiration.

retrocele protrusion of the posterior vaginal wall into the rectum.

rotation movement of the limbs around the long axis.

sarcopenia loss of muscle tissue as a natural part of the aging process.

scoliosis lateral curvature of the spine.

sebaceous glands produce sebum, a fatty substance secreted onto the skin surface through the hair follicles.

shoulder girdle a complex interconnected structure of four joints, three large bones, and three principal muscle groups.

social determinants of health (SDOH) social and economic conditions that impact health status.

source of history can be the patient (primary source) or a family member, friend, health care provider, or the medical record (secondary sources).

spina bifida occulta malformation of one or more vertebrae, sometimes called "closed" spina bifida.

spirituality all behaviors that give meaning to life and provide strength to the individual.

splenomegaly enlargement of the spleen.

stadiometer device for measuring height that typically consists of a vertical ruler with a sliding horizontal rod or paddle which is adjusted to rest on the top of the head.

standard precautions basic infection control practices to be used in the care of all patients every time.

stereognosis ability to identify an object using tactile information such as size, texture, and spatial properties.

strabismus eyes not directed at the same point; crossed eyes.

stroke blood supply to part of the brain is interrupted or reduced, depriving brain tissue of oxygen and nutrients; may be caused by bleeding from a cerebral artery or a blood clot in a cerebral artery.

stroke volume the amount of blood ejected by the left ventricle with each contraction.

subcutaneous tissue the lowermost layer of the integumentary system.

subjective data symptoms, information from the patient or family.

supernumerary one or more extra nipples of the breast located along the "milk line."

sweat glands include the eccrine glands, which open directly onto the skin surface, and help control body temperature, and the apocrine glands found chiefly in the axillary and genital regions.

syncope transient and usually sudden loss of consciousness accompanied by an inability to remain standing; fainting.

synovium membrane in the knee, hip, and other joints that produces fluid to lubricate the joint and supply nutrients to the cartilage.

systole period in the heart cycle when the ventricles contract and expel blood into the aorta and pulmonary arteries.

talipes equinovarus talipes calcaneovalgus, or clubfoot.

tamponade obstruction of the blood flow to or through an organ by external pressure.

tangential lighting lighting from the side to facilitate observation of small movements or pulsations of the body.

Tanner sexual maturity ratings (SMRs) used to assess the five stages of adolescent physical development during puberty.

thelarche the beginning of breast development.

thought content part of the mental status examination; describes what the patient is thinking and includes the presence or absence of delusional or obsessional thinking and suicidal ideations.

thought processes the actual thoughts described.

thrill a palpable vibration felt over the precordium or an artery due to blood turbulence, associated with grade 4 to 6 heart murmurs.

tibial torsion inward twisting of the shin bones causing the feet to turn inward, "pigeon-toed."

tinnitus a ringing or buzzing sound heard by the patient.

tonic–clonic type of seizure that involves violent muscle contractions and a loss of consciousness.

traumatic brain injury (TBI) occurs when an outside force traumatically injures the brain.

tripod position the patient sits or stands leaning forward and supporting the upper body with hands on the knees or on another surface. Often used by people experiencing respiratory distress.

turbinate bony structure inside the nose.

turgor the degree of skin elasticity.

tympanic clear, hollow, drum-like quality of the note heard during percussion over gas-filled organs, such as the stomach and bowels.

umbilical hernia portion of the intestine pushes through an opening in the abdominal muscles near the umbilicus.

urge incontinence sudden need to urinate when the bladder contracts, causing some urine to leak through the sphincter muscles holding the bladder closed.

urinary frequency urination many times day or night in normal or smaller amounts.

urinary incontinence involuntary leakage of urine.

values standards used to measure our own and others' beliefs and behaviors.

vasovagal syncope caused by a sudden drop in blood pressure, usually triggered by a reaction to an event.

venous insufficiency inadequate flow of blood back to the heart caused by inadequate valves in the veins, resulting in edema in the affected extremities.

venous thromboembolism (VTE) a clotting disorder that includes deep vein thrombosis (DVT) and pulmonary embolism (PE).

ventral hernia occurs along the vertical center of the abdominal wall, area of weakness where a loop of intestine or abdominal tissue pushes through.

vertigo the feeling of being in a state of constant movement, usually due to a problem with the inner ear but can also be caused by visual problems.

visual acuity vision is measured by assessing the ability to discern letters or numbers at a given distance.

visual fields area that can be seen when an eye is fixed straight at a set point.

vital signs used to determine how the body is functioning; blood pressure, heart rate, respiratory rate, and temperature.

vitreous humor clear gel that fills the space between the lens and the retina of the eye.

wheeze a musical respiratory sound that may be audible to the patient and others.

whispered pectoriloquy increased loudness of whispering heard during auscultation of the lung fields on a patient's chest.

INDEX

Note: Page numbers followed by b indicate boxed material, those followed by t indicate tables, and those followed by f indicate figures.